AF179611

ORTHOPAEDIC
KEY REVIEW CONCEPTS

Kingsley R. Chin, MD
Samir Mehta, MD
Resident Editor

ORTHOPAEDIC KEY REVIEW CONCEPTS

Kingsley R. Chin, MD

Department of Orthopaedics
Hospital of the University of Pennsylvania
Philadelphia, Pennsylvania

Samir Mehta, MD

Resident Editor
Fellow, Orthopaedic Traumatology
Department of Orthopaedics and Sports Medicine
Harborview Medical Center
University of Washington
Seattle, Washington

Wolters Kluwer | Lippincott Williams & Wilkins
Health

Philadelphia • Baltimore • New York • London
Buenos Aires • Hong Kong • Sydney • Tokyo

Acquisitions Editor: Robert Hurley
Managing Editor: David Murphy
Project Manager: Nicole Walz
Senior Manufacturing Manager: Benjamin Rivera
Marketing Director: Sharon Zinner
Art Director: Risa Clow
Cover Designer: Joseph DePinho
Production Services: Pine Tree Composition, Inc./Laserwords Private Limited
Printer: RR Donnelley-China

530 Walnut Street
Philadelphia, PA 19106 USA
LWW.com

Library of Congress Cataloging-in-Publication Data

Orthopaedic key review concepts / [edited by] Kingsley R. Chin, Samir Mehta.
p. ; cm.
Includes bibliographical references.
ISBN-13: 978-0-7817-7438-3
ISBN-10: 0-7817-7438-1
1. Orthopedics—Handbooks, manuals, etc. I. Mehta, Samir. II. Chin, Kingsley R.
[DNLM: 1. Musculoskeletal Diseases—Handbooks. 2. Orthopedic Procedures—Handbooks. 3. Orthopedics—Handbooks. WE 39 O772 2007]
RD732.5.O83 2007
617.4′7—dc22

2007007179

To purchase additional copies of this book, call our customer service department at (800) 638-3030 or fax orders to (301) 223-2320. International customers should call (301) 223-2300.

Visit Lippincott Williams & Wilkins on the Internet: at LWW.com. Lippincott Williams & Wilkins customer service representatives are available from 8:30 am to 6 pm, EST.

10 9 8 7 6 5 4 3 2 1

To all the residents who poured their hearts into this book and to those who will carry on their legacy in future editions.

To my family, friends, colleagues, teachers, mentors, and the many people who have helped me along the way: your unselfish support drives me to pursue excellence.

To my mother Loleta Blythe, who ensured that I focused on education and from whom I learned the value of persistence and resourcefulness.

—Kingsley R. Chin, MD

To my family who allowed me the time and provided me with the fortitude to pursue this endeavor.

To my co-residents and faculty who were an inspiration as well as a tremendous resource.

—Samir Mehta, MD

"If I have seen further, it is by standing on the shoulder of giants."

—Sir Isaac Newton

Preface

"Change is inevitable. In a progressive country change is constant."

(Benjamin Disraeli, 1867).

Many changes have occurred in recent years to produce an increase in the amount of orthopaedic information—information which residents will ultimately see in their conferences, on their in-training examination, and during their boards. Today's residents can access this information from a myriad of sources: the AAOS, the Internet, orthopaedic journals, review books, and texts. These resources can include summary statements, questions, annotated references, surgical techniques, or web links, but it is rare to find all of these in one source. Residents and practicing surgeons have less time to read through pages of text and even less time to review multiple sources to ascertain the important concepts for study. The increase in orthopaedic information has led residents to supplement current review texts with their own notes. This text was created from this need to efficiently and effectively gather, review, and retain this mass of information. In an effort to access the key orthopaedic concepts and to better prepare today's busy residents to score well on the Orthopaedic In-Training Examination (OITE) and the Orthopaedic Boards and for the busy practicing orthopaedic surgeon to pass the Re-certification Examination, the Orthopaedic Key Review Concept (OKRC) was founded.

In order to tailor the OKRC to today's residents and practicing physicians, residents training within the University of Pennsylvania Orthopaedic Residency Program were the primary authors on each chapter. Multiple references were used in an effort to create a timely, well-rounded, and thorough text including AAOS resources, previous in-training examinations, leading textbooks, and landmark journal publications. Each chapter presents the review material in a format that the residents felt focuses on the important concepts. Thus, the concepts were summarized and presented in a glossary-like format to explain only the important facts of each review concept. We avoided trying to present all possible information in orthopaedics in the text, but rather select only the important and testable concepts. Extraneous facts that were unlikely to be tested on a formal examination or asked of a resident during routine clinical practice were omitted or succinctly summarized. The material in this text provides answers to previous in-training examinations and review questions. The resident can therefore be assured that the text is up-to-date with the material from which the in-training and Board examinations are being developed.

The material in each chapter has been integrated into reasonable thought-lines thus making it intuitive in terms of finding certain topics. For example, we do not have a separate anatomy chapter but rather have placed the relevant anatomy at the beginning of each subspecialty chapter. We also separated statistics into its own chapter so we could cover this important topic in depth. The business chapter was also separated for the same reasons and we placed more pertinent information for the resident who is about to go into practice. The chapter on how to prepare for the OITE, boards, and re-certification examination contains valuable insights and statistics on success rates for the different examinations. To engender further confidence in this text, we received the approval of many of the leading orthopaedic surgeons in their respective subspecialties. Finally, we felt it was important to have the support of a major and respected publisher. We were fortunate to have Lippincott Williams & Wilkins overwhelmingly support the premise and format of this review and to lend their expertise and resources to ensure the highest quality of the final text.

In the end, the residents have written their own review book with the support of experts in their respective fields. This first edition is a testament to their need for a fresh review textbook and will form the foundation from which future editions will be written by subsequent groups of residents.

Kingsley R. Chin, MD

ACKNOWLEDGMENTS

We would like to thank Robert Hurley, Eileen Wolfberg, David Murphy, Sharon Zinner, Mark Moyer, Nicole Walz, Risa Clow, and the entire Lippincott Williams & Wilkins family for their recognition and support of this endeavor. Furthermore, we would like to thank Molly Connors at Dovetail Content Solutions, and Patty Donovan and Katie Boilard from Pine Tree Composition for creating a tangible textbook from our vision and our manuscript.

Foreword

I am extremely delighted and honored to be asked to write a foreword for this unique Orthopaedic text. It has become quite evident that the foundation of knowledge developed during one's Orthopaedic training will be critical, not only in application for credentialing and examinations, but also for the search for excellence in Orthopaedic patient care. Ever increasing scrutiny is being placed on our profession to maintain high levels of standards and this certainly begins in residency training. The continuous desire for knowledge, updating oneself with current developments, and recertifying as Orthopaedic surgeons has become the hallmark of our profession. What better way to present information that is fundamental to the foundation of Orthopaedic knowledge during residency by having it organized and consolidated by individuals who are on the same level. This is a unique concept but one that should prove to be exceptionally well accepted by all Orthopaedic residents.

This text is extremely organized, very well illustrated, and presents information in a concise yet very readable format. References are complete with key references highlighted and annotated. Furthermore at the end of each chapter a series of refresher questions will forward the reader a chance to self-assess their comprehension of the topic.

The text will provide the reader exposure to all of the basic specialty subjects in orthopaedics but also extends to biostatistics and even business and practice principles. I am certain that this will become the kind of reference that is utilized throughout all residency-training programs and served as well as an excellent source of review when preparing for future examinations.

I am personally delighted and honored as well to write this foreword because of the lead editor, Dr. Kingsley R. Chin. Dr. Chin was a resident in our program and from the first time I met him I became keenly aware that this was an outstanding individual who is destined to become a major contributor to our Orthopaedic knowledge and also to the educational efforts of our future Orthopaedic surgeons. Dr. Chin has, in a short time, developed an outstanding reputation and has become a well-respected educator and surgeon in his own institution. I can say with certainty that this text will be one of many stellar academic accomplishments from Dr. Chin and his colleagues and I am very pleased to have the opportunity to have been his teacher and mentor during his formative years in training.

Jesse B. Jupiter, MD
Director, Orthopaedic Hand Service
Massachusetts General Hospital
Hansjörg Wyss/AO Professor
Harvard Medical School

Contents

Contents Expanded

Contributors

Joshua D. Auerbach, MD
Resident, Orthopaedic Surgery
University of Pennsylvania School of Medicine
Philadelphia, Pennsylvania

Sepideh Baghian, MD
Hand Fellow, Orthopaedic Surgery
University of Massachusetts
Worcester, Massachusetts

Gregory Carolan, MD
Resident, Orthopaedic Surgery
University of Pennsylvania School of Medicine
Philadelphia, Pennsylvania

Kingsley R. Chin, MD
Assistant Professor of Orthopaedic Surgery
Department of Orthopaedic Surgery
University of Pennsylvania School of Medicine
Philadelphia, Pennsylvania

Denis S. Drummond, MD
Professor Emeritus, Orthopaedic Surgery
University of Pennsylvania School of Medicine
Philadelphia, Pennsylvania

Price Chipley French, RFC, CLU
Registered Financial Consultant
The French Financial Firm, LLC
Durham, North Carolina

Jonathan P. Garino, MD
Associate Professor, Orthopaedic Surgery
Chief, Adult Reconstruction Surgery
University of Pennsylvania School of Medicine
Philadelphia, Pennsylvania

Purushottom A. Gholve, MD, MBMS, MRCS
Clinical Instructor, Orthopaedics
Fellow, Pediatric Orthopaedics
Weill Medical College of Cornell University
Hospital for Special Surgery
New York, New York

Harish S. Hosalkar, MD, MBMS, FCPS, DNB
Pediatric Orthopaedic Surgeon, India & U.K.
Resident, Orthopaedic Surgery
University of Pennsylvania School of Medicine
Philadelphia, Pennsylvania

G. Russell Huffman, MD, MPH
Assistant Professor, Orthopaedic Surgery
Penn Sports Medicine Center
University of Pennsylvania School of Medicine
Philadelphia, Pennsylvania

Mary Ann Keenan, MD
Professor/Vice Chair for Graduate Medical Education
Department of Orthopaedic Surgery
University of Pennsylvania
Chief, Neuro-Orthopaedics Service
University of Pennsylvania School of Medicine
Philadelphia, Pennsylvania

Sharat Kumar Kusuma, MD, MBA
Resident, Orthopaedic Surgery
University of Pennsylvania School of Medicine
Philadelphia, Pennsylvania

Richard D. Lackman, MD
Paul B. Magnoson Professor of Bone
and Joint Surgery A&D
Chair, Department of Orthopaedic Surgery
University of Pennsylvania School of Medicine
Philadelphia, Pennsylvania

Samir Mehta, MD
Resident Editor Fellow, Orthopaedic Traumatology
Department of Orthopaedics and Sports Medicine
Harborview Medical Center
University of Washington
Seattle, Washington

Todd A. Michener, MD
Fellow, Orthopaedic Surgery/Sports Medicine
Steadman-Hawkins Clinic of the Carolinas
Spartanburg, South Carolina

Sameer Nagda, MD
Orthopaedic Surgeon
ProSport Orthopaedics
Las Vegas, Nevada

Luke S. Oh, MD, MS
Chief Resident
Department of Orthopaedic Surgery
Hospital for Special Surgery
New York, New York

Enyi Okereke, MD
Associate Professor, Orthopaedic Surgery
University of Pennsylvania School of Medicine
Chief, Division of Foot and Ankle Surgery
Hospital of the University of Pennsylvania
Philadelphia, Pennsylvania

Selene G. Parekh, MD, MBA
Assistant Professor, Orthopaedic Surgery
Adjunct Faculty, Kenan-Flagler School of Business
University of North Carolina
Chapel Hill, North Carolina

Sudheer C. Reddy, MD
Resident, Orthopaedic Surgery
University of Pennsylvania School of Medicine
Philadelphia, Pennsylvania

Richard Scarlett, MD
Resident, Orthopaedic Surgery
University of Pennsylvania School of Medicine
Philadelphia, Pennsylvania

Jeffery F. Sodl,
Faculty Fellow, Sports Medicine/Shoulder
and Elbow Reconstruction
USC Department of Orthopaedics
Keck School of Medicine
Los Angeles, California

David A. Spiegel, MD
Assistant Professor, Orthopaedic Surgery
University of Pennsylvania School of Medicine
Attending Orthopaedic Surgeon
Children's Hospital of Philadelphia
Philadelphia, Pennsylvania

Jesse T. Torbert, MD, MS
Resident, Orthopaedic Surgery
University of Pennsylvania School of Medicine
Hospital of the University of Pennsylvania
Philadelphia, Pennsylvania

Russell F. Warren, MD
Professor, Orthopaedic Surgery
Weill Medical College of Cornell University
Hospital for Special Surgery
New York, New York

Gautam Yagnik, MD
Resident, Orthopaedic Surgery
University of Pennsylvania School of Medicine
Philadelphia, Pennsylvania

Warren D. Yu, MD
Chief, Spine Section
George Washington University Hospital
Assistant Professor, Orthopaedic Surgery
George Washington University
Washington, D.C.

Miltiadis H. Zgonis, MD
Resident, Orthopaedic Surgery
University of Pennsylvania School of Medicine
Philadelphia, Pennsylvania

Chapter 1

Basic Science

SUDHEER C. REDDY, MILTIADIS H. ZGONIS, and JOSHUA D. AUERBACH

I. CELLULAR AND MOLECULAR BIOLOGY OF ORTHOPAEDICS

Deoxyribonucleic Acid (DNA). DNA has a double-helix-double-stranded shape with each strand representing a sugar molecule. Each strand has repetitive sequences of four nitrogenous bases (adenine, guanine, cytosine, and thymine). The strands are connected by these nitrogenous bases via hydrogen bonds. In the sequences, adenine links to thymine and guanine to cytosine. One strand plus a nitrogenous base makes up a nucleotide. The nucleotide sequence of one strand determines the sequence of the other strand because of the set pairing of the base pairs. The genetic sequence is then grouped into *codons*, three-letter words that specify one of the 20 possible amino acids (amino acids are the building blocks for proteins). The DNA of each cell resides in the nucleus within the chromosomes and is responsible for regulating all cellular function via protein synthesis. In humans, every cell has 46 chromosomes (23 pairs) that are made of both DNA and ribonucleic acid (RNA). Cellular function is controlled via gene transcription from DNA into RNA (initial production of a messenger RNA (mRNA) transcript that is then exported into the cytoplasm) and the subsequent translation of mRNA into protein by a process termed translation (Fig. 1.1). Each chromosome contains at least 150,000 genes, which are the portion of the DNA that codes for a specific enzyme (one gene equals one enzyme). Although every cell has the same genes, only selective genes are expressed in

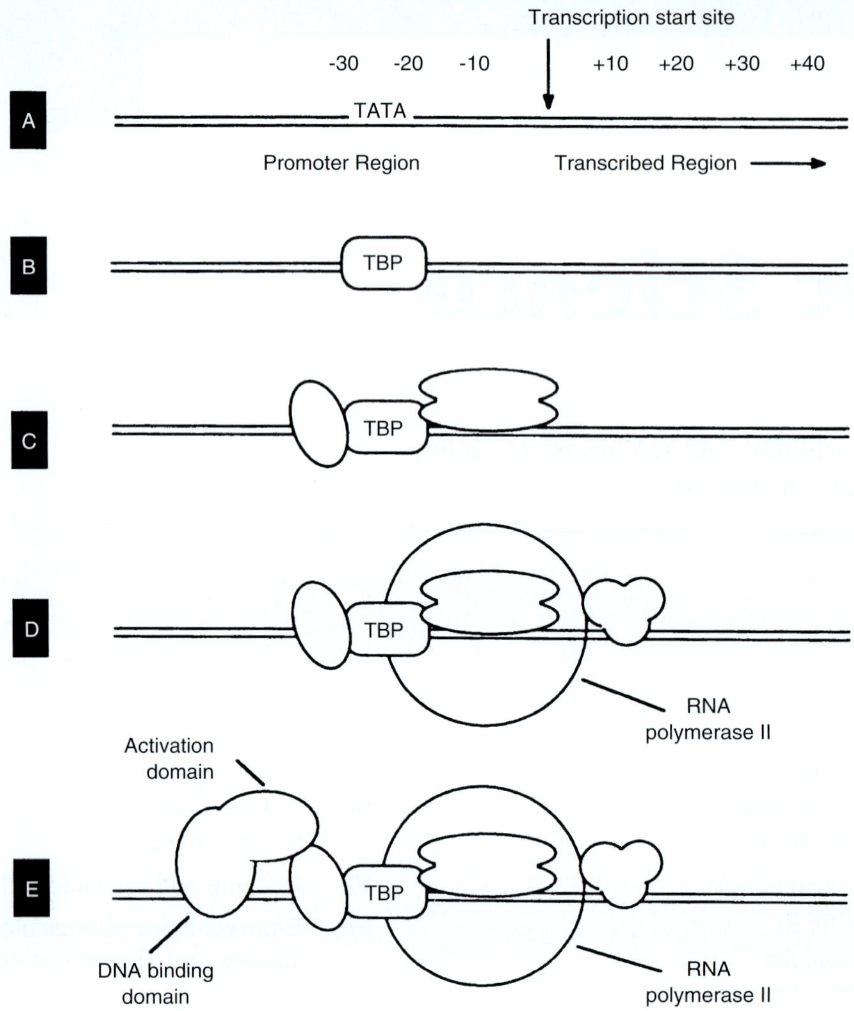

FIGURE 1.1 **The transcriptional complex is assembled sequentially (A), with the initial event being binding of the TATA-binding protein (TBP; also called transcription factor IID [TFIID]) to the TATA box (B). Subsequently, TFIIA and TFIIB associate with TBP (C), followed by binding of RNA polymerase II (D). Finally, regulatory transcriptional factors that control the rate of transcription associate with consensus sequences in the promoter region and the transcriptional complex of proteins (E). (*Source*: Shore EM, Kaplan FS. Tutorial: Molecular biology for the clinician: Part I. General principles. *Clin Orthop* 1994;306:264–283.)**

a given cell, thereby maintaining uniqueness of that cell. DNA controls DNA replication, transcription of mRNA, and regulates cell division and the production of mRNA.

Regulation of Transcription. Transcription is controlled via proteins termed *transcription factors* that are responsible for controlling the production of the mRNA. mRNA itself is composed of a series of sequences of three nucleotides, with each sequence termed a codon. These codons carry the genetic code information for the 20 amino acids that serve as the building blocks for all proteins. Specific noncoding sequences, termed regulating DNA, control transcription. Included within these noncoding sequences are gene promoters to which transcription factors attach and control the transcription of genes. Eukaryotic mRNA is termed *monocistronic* because one gene codes for one protein with a single start codon for the start of translation and a single stop codon for the end of translation. Each mRNA has a 5′-end and a 3′-end, with the 5′-end indicating the presence of a 5′-phosphate and the 3′-end indicating the presence of a 3′-hydroxyl at the end of the RNA being synthesized. Bacterial mRNA, on the other hand, is polycistronic with a single transcript possessing multiple start and stop codons with intervening untranslated sequences.

The mRNA transcript then undergoes splicing in which the actual coding sequences of the genes, exons, are spliced together to form the functional mRNA transcript. Prior to its export to the cytoplasm, the mRNA transcript undergoes several posttranslational modifications including (1) the placement of a guanine cap on the 5′-end and (2) adenylation, with the placement of the poly(A) tail on the 3′-end of the transcript. Once processed, the mRNA transcript is exported to the cytoplasm to undergo translation via ribosomes to produce the amino acid sequence of the protein.

Tools and Techniques of Molecular Biology. A number of molecular tools are available, collectively termed recombinant technology, that allow investigators to create limitless combinations of DNA sequences. This technology has enabled tremendous advances in the diagnosis of molecular diseases and inherited disorders. Restriction endonucleases (restriction enzymes) cut DNA into specific fragments called restriction sequences. These enzymes allow investigators to cut DNA into fragments that can be spliced together to create recombinant DNA. The restriction enzymes used by investigators cut at palindromic sequences. Hundreds of restriction enzymes have been identified, and approximately 50 to 70 have practical use. The ends of the restriction fragments are cohesive, meaning that they can anneal, or join, other restriction fragments. These ends are termed "*sticky ends.*" To further understand the tools and techniques of molecular biology, a few concepts and definitions need to be explained.

- *DNA ligation*—The joining of sticky ends, or joining of two DNA fragments, is termed *DNA ligation*, which is accomplished by enzymes termed *DNA ligases.*
- *Restriction mapping*—Once genetic material has been sectioned with restriction enzymes into restriction fragments, the fragments can be separated on the basis of size and charge via gel electrophoresis. Briefly, the gel is synthesized by creating a gel mold, which is then mixed with an electrophoresis buffer. The restriction fragments are then placed into the individual slots at the top of the gel and then migrate through the gel according to relative size and charge. The fragments, which are negatively charged (owing to the negatively charged phosphate groups), migrate to the positive pole. Digestion of the same DNA sample by different restriction enzymes and then subjection of the fragments to gel electrophoresis in parallel lanes allows one to create a restriction map (Fig. 1.2).
- *Gel electrophoresis*—Because DNA is negatively charged, when fragments of DNA are exposed to an electromagnetic field, they will preferentially migrate toward the positive pole of the field. The medium used in gel electrophoresis is typically agarose and will selectively restrict the migration of DNA fragments according to the molecular size

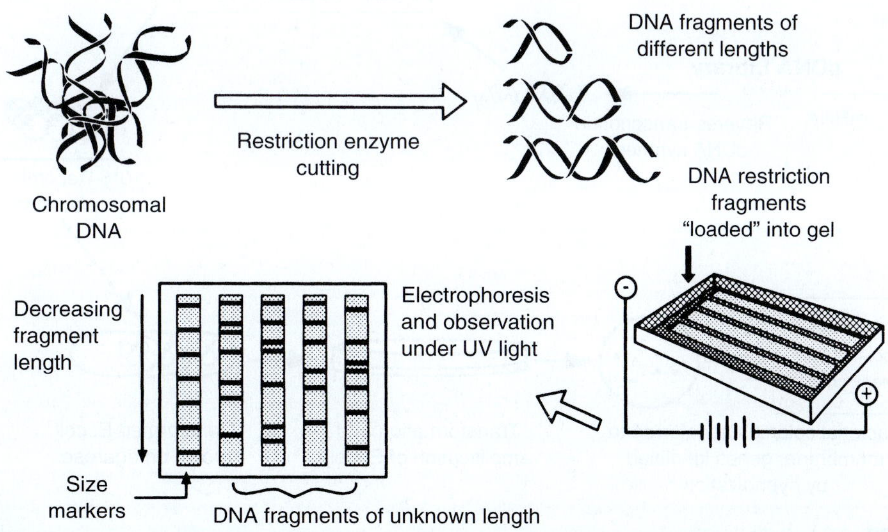

FIGURE 1.2 **Agarose gel electrophoresis of DNA involves placing DNA fragment in wells at the top of an agarose gel suspended in a buffer; an electric voltage is applied. The highly negatively charged DNA migrates toward the positive electrode, and the rate of migration is determined by the size of the fragment. Ethidium bromide binding to DNA can be visualized under ultraviolet light. (*Source*: Buckwalter JA, Einhorn TA, Simon SR. *Orthopaedic Basic Science: Biology and Biomechanics of the Musculoskeletal System*, 2nd ed. Rosemont, IL: American Academy of Orthopaedic Surgeons, 2000; 36, Fig. 15.)**

and thus is able to separate fragments of varying sizes, which can then be deduced by comparing to molecular markers of known size.

- *Plasmids*—Once the restriction sequences are formed and isolated, they can be inserted into plasmid, forming a recombinant plasmid. These plasmids are then introduced into bacteria (bacterial transformation). With bacterial replication, the plasmids and recombinant DNA are replicated as well, allowing for an exponential increase in the number of copies of the recombinant DNA.
- *Genomic libraries*—Genomic libraries consist of numerous cloned DNA fragments. Formation of a library allows investigators to isolate and clone a gene or fragment of a gene (Fig. 1.3).
- *Southern blotting*—Probes are DNA or RNA sequences with a label (usually a radioactive tracer such as ^{32}P-labeled radionucleotides). Southern blotting is the use of a probe or probes to identify a specific DNA fragment. Once a DNA specimen is digested with restriction enzymes, the fragments are isolated via gel electrophoresis and denatured. The gel is then placed against nitrocellulose with the single-stranded DNA fragments transferred to the nitrocellulose. The nitrocellulose is then incubated with the probe, allowing the probe to attach to the target sequence.
- *Northern blotting*—This technique utilizes the same concept as Southern blotting but is used to identify and quantify presence of RNA, usually mRNA.
- *Western blotting*—This technique also utilizes the same concept as Northern and Southern blotting but is used to identify protein sequences.
- *Polymerase chain reaction (PCR)*—PCR is method of amplifying a specific DNA sequence to levels that allow further investigative use. The process depends on the temperature-dependent hybridization (annealing) of primers to a DNA template, polymerization then subsequent denaturation, and then a new round of polymerization. A thermostabile DNA polymerase must be used to withstand the repeated cycles of annealing and denaturation.
- *Enzyme-linked immunosorbent assay (ELISA)*—This assay is a common method of detecting and quantifying specific proteins in solution. It relies on an antibody binding to the protein of interest followed

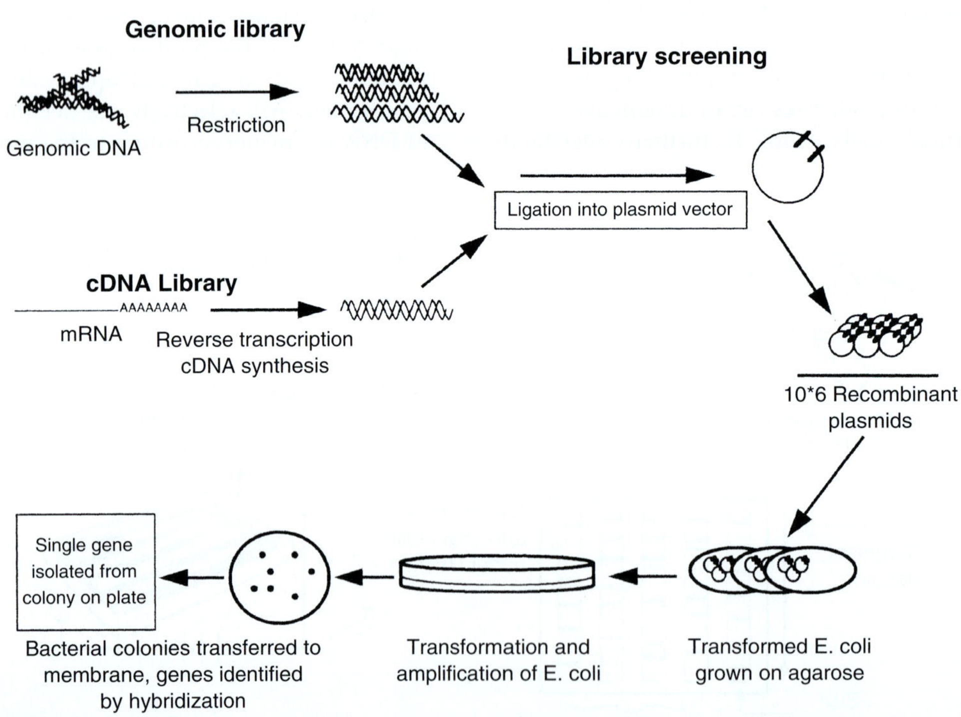

FIGURE 1.3 Library screening involves restriction digestion of genomic DNA or cDNA, followed by ligation of the restriction I fragments into plasmids. The plasmids are used to transform bacteria. Dilutions of the bacterial suspension are plated, and single colonies transferred to nitrocellulose membranes and hybridized with appropriate probe for gene of interest. Positive clones are then selected and grown in culture to produce the DNA fragment of interest. (*Source*: Buckwalter JA, Einhorn TA, Simon SR. *Orthopaedic Basic Science: Biology and Biomechanics of the Musculoskeletal System*, 2nd ed. Rosemont, IL: American Academy of Orthopaedic Surgeons, 2000; 41, Fig. 18.)

by the use of a secondary antibody linked to an enzyme. The enzyme is then incubated with its substrate with the resultant reaction producing a soluble, colored product that can be detected by measuring the absorbance of the solution at the appropriate wavelength. It is an excellent technique for the rapid and simple evaluation of large numbers of samples with a high level of sensitivity.

- *Transgenic animals*—These animals serve as libraries of selected transgenes that carry the gene of interest. The genome of these animals has the foreign gene of interest, which was inserted into the single-cell embryo and is transmitted to every cell in the organism via cellular replication.

Gene Therapy. The tools available to research investigators provide the technical avenues by which they can introduce normal genes to correct defects. Table 1.1 shows certain musculoskeletal disorders and their genetic defects. Different methods of gene therapy have been developed, including the use of viral vectors such as adenovirus or adeno-associated virus (AAV) to deliver specific genes to directed target sites as well as to introduce recombinant plasmids containing the gene of interest.

Regulation of the Cell Cycle. The cell cycle is divided into 4 active phases and 1 inactive phase (Fig. 1.4). The G_0 phase is a resting phase and represents the time spent by a cell before preparation for active division. The length of this phase depends on the cell type. Some cells, such as neurons, remain in this state for the life span of the cell. The entry phase of the cell cycle, G_1, lasts approximately 6 to 12 hours and is the time during which the cell is actively synthesizing RNA and protein. The cell then enters the S phase, during which the cell actively replicates its DNA content in preparation for cell division. The G_2 phase represents the stage during which the cell is preparing for mitosis; it lasts approximately 3 to 4 hours and is characterized by an increase in RNA and protein synthesis without further DNA synthesis. The M (mitotic) phase concludes the G_2 phase and signifies the period during which the replicated chromosomes segregate into the daughter cells.

Cell Signaling. Cells of the musculoskeletal system are differentiated in that certain genes are selectively expressed. The selective expression of genes is dependent on transcription factors that are coupled to signaling cascades in response to an external cellular signal (a process termed *signal transduction*). Numerous transcription factors have been identified

TABLE 1.1 Musculoskeletal disorders and their genetic defects

Musculoskeletal Genetic Disorder	*Genetic Mutation*
Achondroplasia	FGF receptor 3
Osteogenesis imperfecta	Type I collagen
Pseudoachondroplasia	Cartilage oligomeric matrix protein (COMP)
Marfan syndrome	Fibrillin
Spondyloepiphyseal dysplasia	Type II collagen
Multiple epiphyseal dysplasia	COMP or type IX collagen (COL9A2)
Thanatophoric dysplasia	FGF receptor 3
Diatrophic dysplasia	Sulfate transporter
Duchenne muscular dystrophy	Dystrophin
X-linked hypophosphatemic rickets	PEX (cellular endopeptidase)
Osteopetrosis	Carbonic anhydrase type II
Fibrous dysplasia	$G_{s\alpha}$ (receptor-coupled signaling protein)
Schmid metaphyseal dysplasia	Type X collagen
Jansen metaphyseal chondrodysplasia	PTH/PTHrP receptor
Multiple hereditary exostoses	EXT1, EXT2 genes
Hypochondroplasia	FGF receptor 3

FGF = fibroblast growth factor; COMP = cartilage oligomeric matrix protein; MCSF = macrophage-colony stimulating factor; PTH = parathyroid hormone; PTHrP = parathyroid hormone related protein.

Source: Buckwalter JA, Einhorn TA, Simon Sr. *Orthopaedic Basic Science: Biology and Biomechanics of the Musculoskeletal System.* Rosemont, IL: American Academy of Orthopaedic Surgeons, 2000.

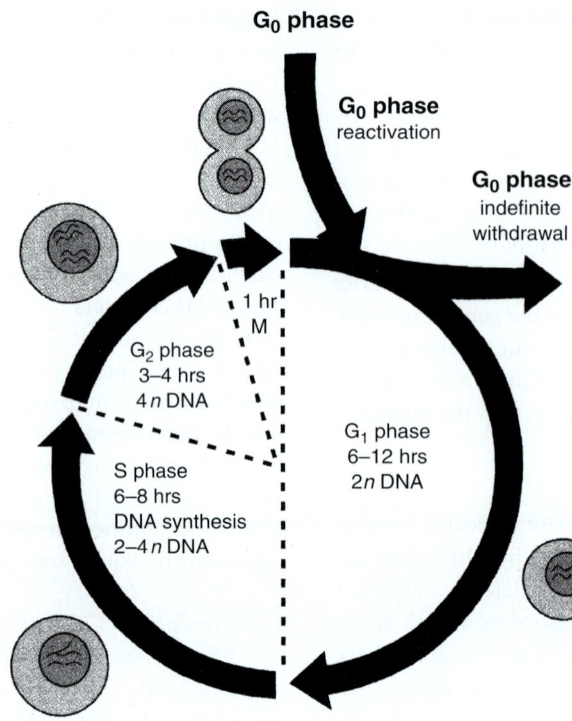

FIGURE 1.4 **The phases and approximate durations of the cell cycle. (*Reproduced with permission from* Lewin B. *Genes VI.* New York: Oxford University Press, 1997; 1089.)**

for mammalian cells. They help transcription enzymes (RNA polymerase) initiate transcription. They can often be classified according to their structural motifs (Table 1.2).

Apoptosis. Apoptosis is the phenomenon of programmed cell death. Contrary to cellular necrosis, it does not induce an inflammatory response. It is identified by several methods, including fragmentation of DNA and disassembly of the cell's organelles and nucleus via gelsolin activation. Ligand-mediated activation of the process can occur through receptors such as tumor necrosis factor receptor 1 (TNFR1) or CD95. Upon ligand binding, the "death domains" of the receptors and kinases called FADD interact, resulting in activation of caspase 8. Caspase 8 results in activation of other effector caspases, such as caspase 3, and dissociation of the CAD (caspase-activated DNAse) from its inhibitor, resulting in internucleosomal cleavage of DNA. The effector caspases also activate gelsolin, disrupting the cytoskeleton. The TNF receptor can also exhibit antiapoptotic effects in some cells through activation of a kinase called RIP, which activates a signaling protein (Traf2) resulting in both release of NF_B from its binding protein I_B and phosphorylation of c-jun by its kinase (JNK). These

TABLE 1.2 **Transcription factors classified by structure**

Type	*Structure*	*Examples*
Helix-Turn-Helix	Three DNA helices separated by short loop segments	Bacterial regulatory proteins, homeotic proteins
Zinc Fingers	Cysteine- and histidine-rich region complexing zinc	Steroid receptor proteins
Leucine zipper	DNA-binding domain contains lycine and arginine residues to facilitate dimmer formation required for DNA binding	Protooncogenes (c-fos,c-jun)

Source: Griffiths AJF., Miller, JH, Suzuki, DT, Lewontin, RC, Gelbart, WM. *An Introduction to Genetic Analysis*, 6th ed. New York: W.H. Freeman, 1996.

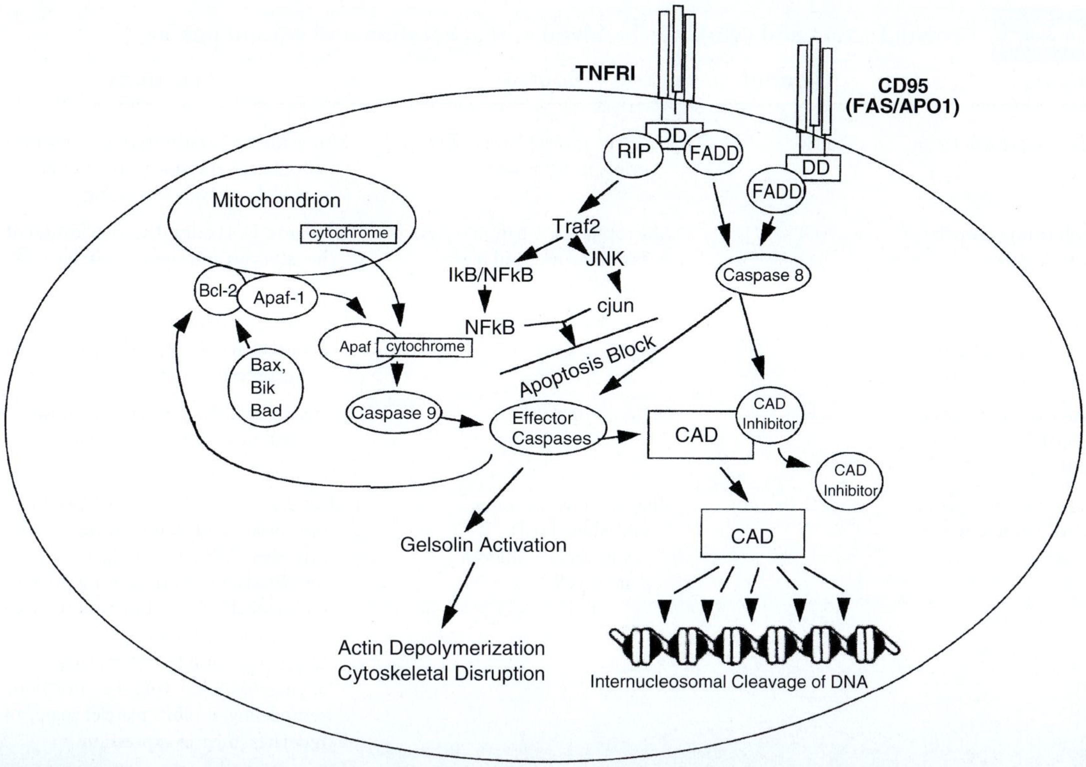

FIGURE 1.5 **Regulation of apoptosis occurs through complex intersecting pathways. (*Source*: Buckwalter JA, Einhorn TA, Simon SR. *Orthopaedic Basic Science: Biology and Biomechanics of the Musculoskeletal System*, 2nd ed. Rosemont, IL: American Academy of Orthopaedic Surgeons, 2000; 60, Fig. 33.)**

transcription factors can then block apoptosis. Other signals, including toxins, can cause apoptosis through activation of the caspase 9 pathway. In this pathway, Bcl-2 functions as an apoptotic inhibitor by binding of Apaf-l. Dimerization with proapoptotic proteins such as Bax, Bik, Bid, or Bad results in release of Apaf-l and a permeability transition in the mitochondrial outer membrane, which releases cytochrome c. Cytochrome c binds Apaf-l and activates caspase 9, which in turn activates effector caspases such as caspase 3, thus triggering apoptosis. The relative levels and states of phosphorylation of Bcl-2 and Bax family members control the levels of Apaf-l/caspase 9 activity. The expression of the Bcl-2/Bax families of anti- and proapoptotic control genes and their phosphorylation is in turn regulated by numerous signaling pathways (Fig 1.5).

Cancer occurs when this phenomenon of programmed cell death is not followed, leading to uncontrolled growth. It is dependent on several classes of genes, including oncogenes and tumor suppressor genes. Oncogenes encode for growth factor receptors, growth factors, or other proteins involved in regulating cellular proliferation. Mutations within these genes can lead to excess production of growth factors and/or their receptors, leading to uncontrolled growth. Tumor suppressor genes, in turn, control proteins that are responsible for regulation of growth. Mutations within these genes leads to the loss of regulation of cellular growth.

Growth Factors. Growth factors are central to a cell's homeostasis and communication with the external environment (see Table 1.3 for general list of growth factors and cytokines). A number of growth factors influence the musculoskeletal system, including PDGF (platelet-derived growth factor), TGF-β (transforming growth factor-β), and BMP (bone morphogenetic protein). BMPs are a subclass of the TGF-β superfamily of growth factors. Involved in regulation of growth and development, they possess the ability to induce differentiation of cartilage and bone. See Table 1.4 for functions of certain types of the BMP subclass.

Cytokines. Cytokines have a role similar to that of growth factors, and the distinction remains primarily historical in nature. They are produced in response to antigens, either self (which are perceived as foreign) or nonself. They play a critical role in inflammation and can be either proinflammatory or antiinflammatory

TABLE 1.3 Growth factors and cytokines involved in regeneration and wound healing

Cytokine	Symbol	Source	Functions
Epidermal growth factor	EGF	Platelets, macrophages, saliva, urine, milk, plasma	Mitogenic for keratinocytes and fibroblasts; stimulates keratinocyte migration and granulation tissue formation
Transforming growth factor alpha	TGF-α	Macrophages, T lymphocytes, keratinocytes, and many tissues	Similar to EGF; stimulates replication of hepatocytes and certain epithelial cells
Hepatocyte growth factor/scatter factor	HGF	Mesenchymal cells	Enhances proliferation of epithelial and endothelial cells, and of hepatocytes; increases cell motility
Vascular endothelial cell growth factor (isoforms A, B, C, D)	VEGF	Mesenchymal cells	Increases vascular permeability; mitogenic for endothelial cells (see Table 3-3)
Platelet-derived growth factor (isoforms A, B, C, D)	PDGF	Platelets, macrophages, endothelial cells, keratinocytes, smooth muscle cells	Chemotactic for PMNs, macrophages, fibroblasts, and smooth muscle cells; activates PMNs, macrophages, and fibroblasts; mitogenic for fibroblasts, endothelial cells, and smooth muscle cells; stimulates production of MMPs, fibronectin, and HA; stimulates angiogenesis and wound contraction; remodeling; inhibits platelet aggregation; regulates integrin expression
Fibroblast growth factor-1 (acidic),—2 (basic) and family	FGF	Macrophages, mast cells, T lymphocytes, endothelial cells, fibroblasts, and many tissues	Chemotactic for fibroblasts; mitogenic for fibroblasts and keratinocytes; stimulates keratinocyte migration, angiogenesis, fam wound contraction and matrix deposition
Transforming growth factor beta (isoforms 1, 2, 3); other members of the family are BMP and activin	TGF-β	Platelets, T lymphocytes, macrophages, endothelial cells, keratinocytes, smooth muscle cells, fibroblasts	Chemotactic for PMNs, macrophages, lymphocytes, fibroblasts, and smooth muscle cells; stimulates TIMP synthesis, keratinocyte migration, angiogenesis, and fibroplasia; inhibits production of MMPs and keratinocyte proliferation; regulates integrin expression and other cytokines; induces TGF-β production
Keratinocyte growth factor (also called FGF-7)	KGF	Fibroblasts	Stimulates keratinocyte migration, proliferation, and differentiation
Insulin-like growth factor-1	IGF-1	Macrophages, fibroblasts and other cells	Stimulates synthesis of sulfated proteoglycans, collagen, keratinocyte migration, and fibroblast proliferation; endocrine effects similar to growth hormone
Tumor necrosis factor	TNF	Macrophages, mast cells, T lymphocytes	Activates macrophages; regulates other cytokines; multiple functions
Interleukins	IL-1, etc.	Macrophages, mast cells, keratinocytes, lymphocytes, and many tissues	Many functions. Some examples: chemotactic for PMNs (IL-1) and fibroblasts (IL-4), stimulation of MMP-1 synthesis (IL-1), angiogenesis (IL-8), TIMP synthesis (IL-6); regulation of other cytokines
Interferons	IFN-α, etc.	Lymphocytes and fibroblasts	Activates macrophages; inhibits fibroblast proliferation and synthesis of MMPs; regulates other cytokines

BMP, bone morphogenetic proteins; PMNs, polymorphonuclear leukocytes; MMPs, matrix metalloproteinases; HA, hyaluronic acid; TIMP, tissue inhibitor of matrix metalloproteinase.

Modified from Schwartz SI: *Principles of Surgery*, McGraw Hill, New York, 1999.

Source: Kumar V, Abbas AK, Fausto N. *Robbins & Cotran Pathologic Basis of Disease*, 7th ed. Elsevier Science, 2004, as modified from Schwartz SI. *Principles of Surgery*. New York: McGraw Hill, 1999.

TABLE 1.4 BMP subclasses and their functions

BMP 1	Metalloproteinase that functions as a C-propeptidase for collagen types I, II, and III.
BMP 2	Osteoinductive factor that can induce chondrogenic differentiation of mesenchymal cells. Recombinant human BMP2 is also being used to induce bone regeneration in animal nonunion models and to enhance spinal fusion.
BMP 4	Overexpressed in the cells of patients with fibrodysplasia ossificans progressiva. Noggin is underexpressed in the cells of patients with FOP and is a secreted polypeptide that acts as an antagonist to BMP2, BMP4, and other BMPs by binding BMPs and preventing interaction with their transmembrane receptors.
BMP 5	Plays a role in osteoinduction.
BMP 6	Located in hypertrophic cartilage and promotes cartilage maturation and eventual endochondral calcification
BMP 7 (osteogenic protein 1)	Has a similar role to BMP6 but also is being used clinically to induce bone regeneration.

in nature. They are important in maintaining the health of the musculoskeletal system. As an example, transgenic mice deficient in interleukin-10 (IL-10) develop inflammatory bowel disease and have a reduced life span. See Table 1.5 for a list of cytokines that have proinflammatory properties.

Cytokines play an important role in the inflammatory arthritides such as rheumatoid arthritis and psoriatic arthritis. Anti-TNF-α biological therapies have resulted in clinical improvement of patients with rheumatoid arthritis owing to the destructive role that the proinflammatory cytokine TNF-α has in the pathogenesis of rheumatoid arthritis.

The pathogenesis of osteolysis can be attributed to the elaboration of interleukin-1 (IL-1) by macrophages in response to polyethylene particulate debris.

Prostaglandins. Prostaglandins are lipid-derived signaling molecules that mediate the inflammatory response (Fig. 1.6). They are the products of the cyclooxygenase pathway of arachidonic acid metabolism. Two forms of the cyclooxygenase enzyme exist and are termed COX-1 and COX-2. COX-1 is expressed constitutively and is important to the normal physiology of the gastrointestinal and renal systems. COX-2 is predominantly seen in inflammation. Nonsteroidal antiinflammatory drugs (NSAIDs) are responsible for nonselectively inhibiting the cyclooxygenase enzyme and are used to reduce the pain of inflammation. Selective COX-2 inhibitors have been developed to target the COX-2 enzyme to reduce inflammation yet also minimize gastrointestinal and renal side effects. However, several COX-2 inhibitors have come under scrutiny recently, and their use has been discontinued because of a possible increase in the risk of serious cardiovascular events.

Immunobiology. The immune system is critical to the development of an inflammatory response. Responses can be nonspecific, humoral (with the elaboration of antibodies), or cell-mediated. An example of the nonspecific inflammatory response is the elaboration of IL-1, interleukin-6 (IL-6), and TNF-α consequent to the phagocytosis of particulate material (polyethylene debris) that results in the activation of osteoclasts and the resorption of bone. The humoral response involves

TABLE 1.5 Cytokines with proinflammatory properties

Cytokine	*Cellular Source*	*Major Targets and Biological Effects*
TNF-α	Monocytes, Macrophages, T lymphocytes	Monocytes, macrophages, fibroblasts, chondrocytes, increased MHC class II expression, secretion of MMPs
IL-1	Monocytes, macrophages	Monocytes, macrophages, fibroblast proliferation, T cell proliferation, inhibition of matrix synthesis by chondrocytes, secretion of MMPs (leads to matrix degradation)
IL-6	Activated T cells	Stimulation of acute phase protein synthesis in liver, B and T cell proliferation, differentiation of hematopoietic precursor cells
TGF-β	Many cell types	Immune suppression, monocyte chemotaxis, anabolic for cartilage, differentiation of mesenchymal and epithelial cells

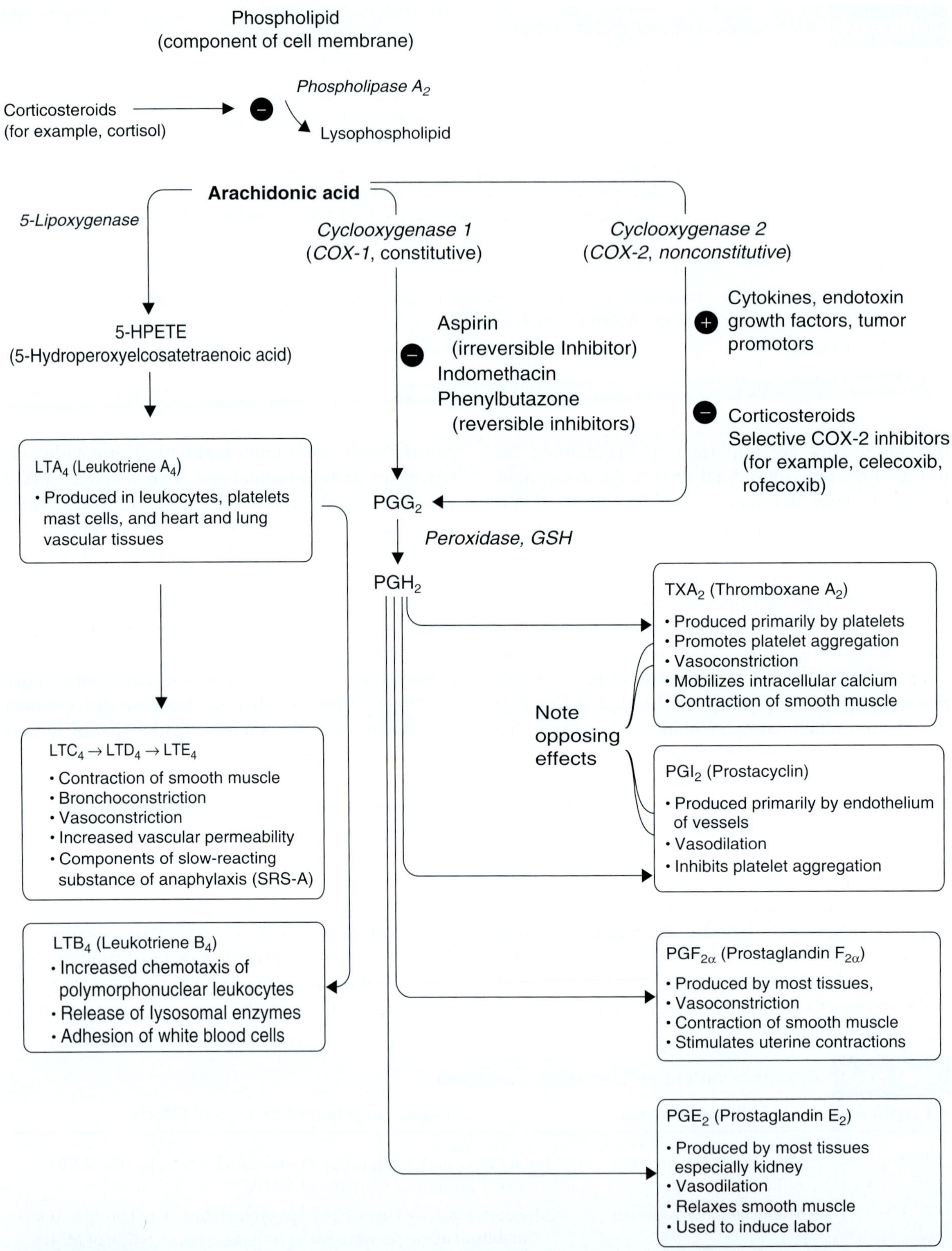

FIGURE 1.6 **Overview of the biosynthesis and function of some important prostaglandins, leukotrienes, and a thromboxane from arachidonic acid. (*Source*: Champe PC, Harvey RA, Ferrier DR. *Biochemistry*, 3rd ed. Philadelphia: Lippincott Williams & Wilkins, 2005; 213.)**

the T-helper lymphocytes (CD4 cells) interacting with B lymphocytes, which differentiate into plasma cells that produce immunoglobulins raised against certain antigens. The cytotoxic response involves the stimulation of cytotoxic T-cells (CD8 cells) that are activated through antigen-type I MHC (major histocompatibility complex) molecules. When activated, these cells elicit a cytotoxic response that contributes to the immune response (Fig. 1.7). Immunoglobulin types and functions are listed here.

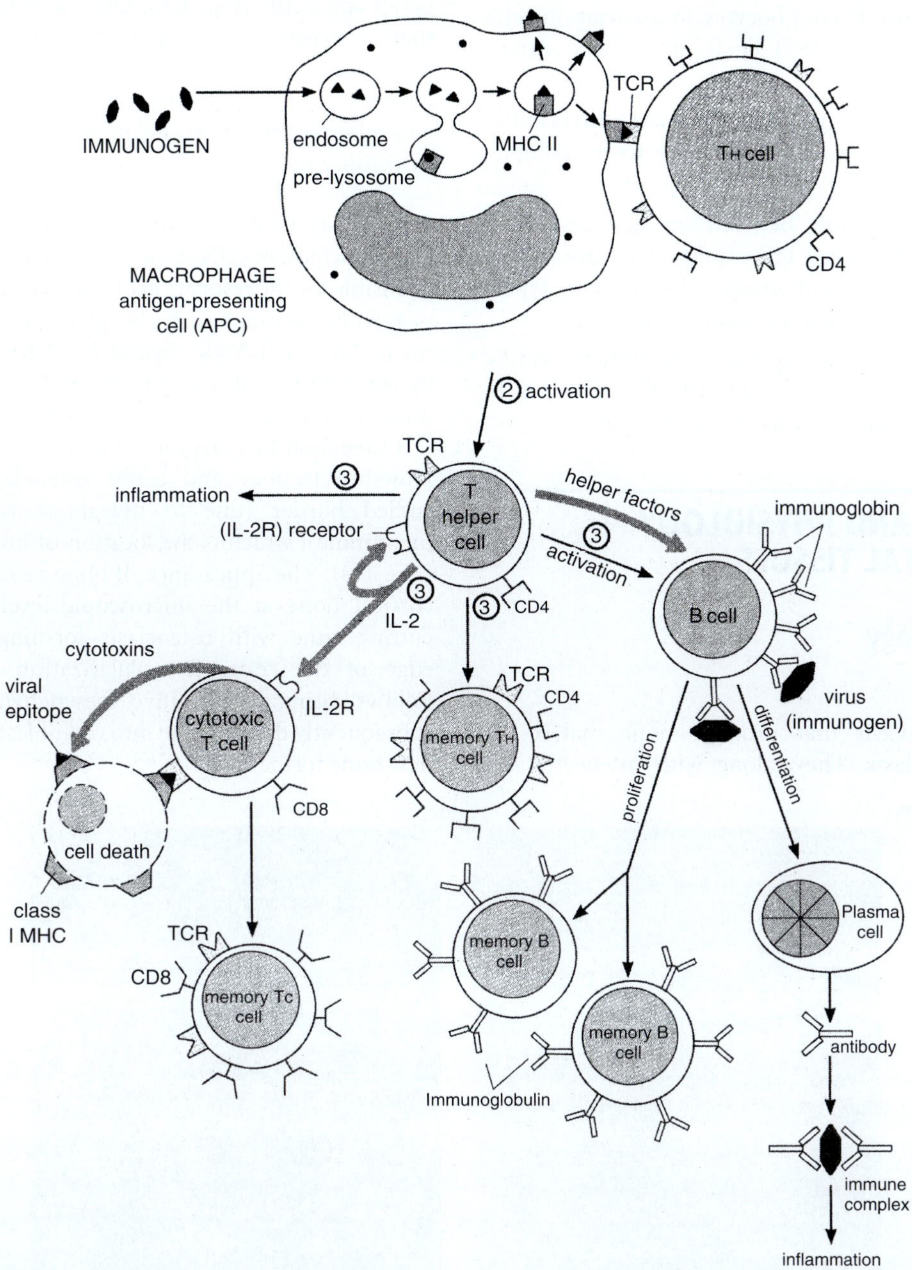

FIGURE 1.7 **Immune response stimulation involves internalization of an antigen by macrophages, which is then bound to a receptor, MHC II, and expressed on the cell surface. The CD4-expressing helper T cells are activated by receptor interaction with the antigen (2) if it is recognized as foreign. The activated CD4 cell elaborates factors that stimulate B cells to express antibody and inflammatory cytokines. B cells can differentiate into antibody-producing plasma cells or remain as memory cells. Similarly, the sensitized T cells can expand by proliferation and mediate cytotoxicity or be retained as memory cells. (*Source*: Stites DP, Terr AI, Parslow TG. *Medical Immunology*, 8th ed. Norwalk, CT: Appleton & Lange, 1994; 43–44.)**

TYPE	FUNCTION
IgA	Plays an important role in defense against viral and bacterial infections. Blocks transport of microbes across mucosal surfaces.
IgD	Present in low levels in serum. Found on most B lymphocytes in association with IgM, where it likely acts as an antigen receptor.
IgG	Only Ig that crosses placenta. Involved in complement pathway by fixing complement.
IgE	Interaction between antigen and mast cell–bound IgE results in release of histamine, leukotrienes. Involved in type I (IgE)–mediated hypersensitivity.
IgM	Seen in early, primary immune responses. Antibodies to the Rh factor (seen in erythroblastosis fetalis) are IgM.

II. FORM AND PHYSIOLOGY OF SKELETAL TISSUES

Bone Histology

Bone Cells

Osteoblasts. Cells that produce bone matrix are called osteoblasts. They, along with osteocytes, are the predominant bone-forming cells. They synthesize type I collagen, alkaline phosphatase, osteocalcin, and bone sialoprotein and are responsive to parathyroid hormone (PTH). The cytoplasm of the cell is geared toward protein synthesis and is composed primarily of the nucleus, rough endoplasmic reticulum, and the Golgi apparatus (Fig. 1.8). Once a mineralized bone matrix surrounds osteoblasts, the osteoblast becomes an osteocyte. The cellular composition of the osteocyte changes with a reduction in the amount of rough endoplasmic reticulum and an increase in the nucleus-to-cytoplasm ratio.

Osteoclasts. Large, multinucleate cells that are derived from pluripotent cells of the bone marrow. They are responsible for the resorption of bone via the production of tartrate-resistant acid phosphate. Receptor activator of NF-kB (RANK) ligand (RANKL) is produced by osteoblasts and is a critical regulator of osteoclast differentiation and resorptive activity.

Osteoclasts lie in regions of bone resorption termed Howship lacunae and active osteoclasts possess a ruffled border (due to invaginations of the cell membrane), which is the location of bone resorption (Fig. 1.9). The appearance of bone resorption within cortical bone at the microscopic level is that of a cutting cone with osteoclasts forming the leading edge of the cone. Revascularization of the bone follows, bringing primitive mesenchymal cells that subsequently differentiate into osteoblasts to stimulate new bone formation.

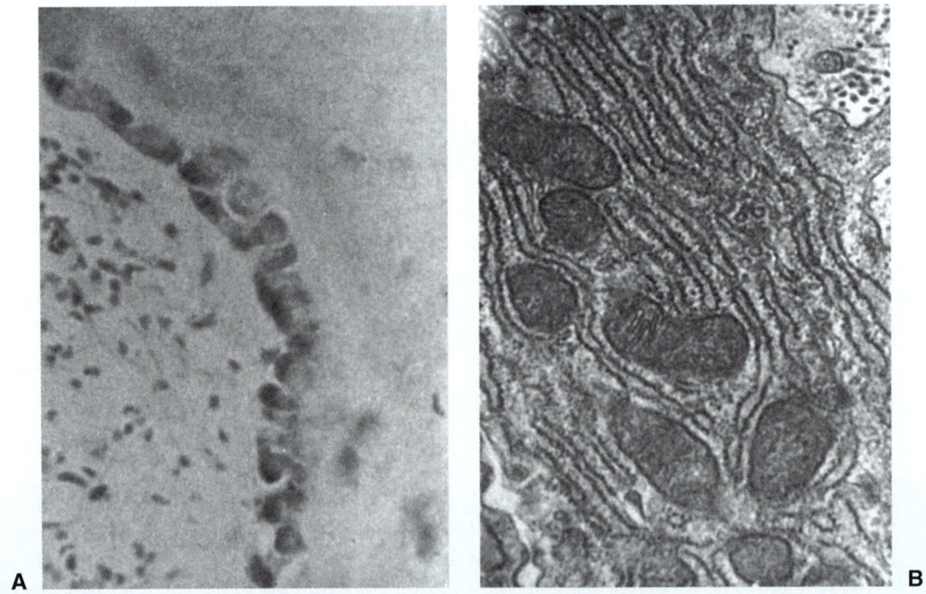

FIGURE 1.8 Light (A) and electron (B) photomicrographs of osteoblasts. (*Source*: Buckwalter JA, Einhorn TA, Simon SR. *Orthopaedic Basic Science: Biology and Biomechanics of the Musculoskeletal System*, 2nd ed. Rosemont, IL: American Academy of Orthopaedic Surgeons, 2000; 323, Fig. 7.)

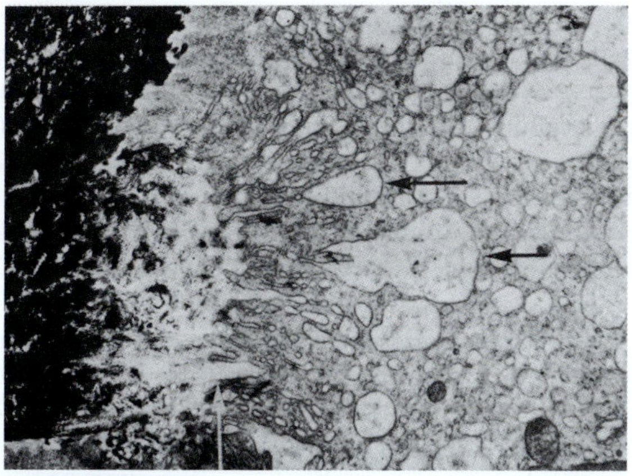

FIGURE 1.9 Electron micrograph of a section of a bone surface undergoing resorption. Calcified bone appears black at the left. The main part of the picture is occupied by the cytoplasm of an osteoclast; it consists of complex folds and projections that abut on the bone at the left. Between the ruffled border of the osteoclast and the heavily calcified bone is an area where the calcium content is much less, which suggests that the osteoclast is dissolving or otherwise removing mineral from this area. Black granules of mineral can be seen in some of the large vesicles, indicated by horizontal arrows, that probably form because of the bottom of crypts being pinched off. In the original print, a collagenic microfibril showing typical periodicity could be seen at this site, indicated by the vertical arrow (original magnification × 20,000). (*Source*: Boothroyd B, Hancox NM. In: Ham AW, Cormack DH (eds.), *Histology*, 8th ed. Philadelphia: JB Lippincott, 1979.)

Bone Matrix

Inorganic Phase. The inorganic phase of bone is composed of calcium hydroxyapatite that is present as a crystal and may contain impurities such as carbonate, chloride, or fluoride (Fig. 1.10). The crystals are approximately 2 × 9 × 25 nm in size. The impurities present can reflect the dietary, age, and health status of the individual. The inorganic phase comprises approximately 70% of the bone matrix; water, 5%; and the organic phase, the remainder. The inorganic phase

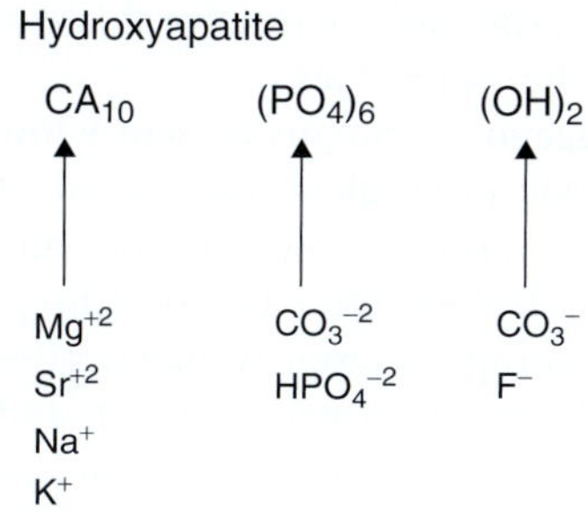

FIGURE 1.10 Bone mineral is an analog of the naturally occurring calcium phosphate, hydroxyapatite, the chemical formula of which is shown here. In bone, as illustrated here, there may be substitutions for calcium, phosphate, and hydroxide groups, the extent of such substitutions varying with age, dietary history, tissue site, and health status. (*Source*: Buckwalter JA, Einhorn TA, Simon SR. *Orthopaedic Basic Science: Biology and Biomechanics of the Musculoskeletal System*, 2nd ed. Rosemont, IL: American Academy of Orthopaedic Surgeons, 2000; 328, Fig. 10.)

is also composed of ostecalcium phosphate (brushite). Of note, crystals in woven bone are smaller in size than those in lamellar bone.

Organic Phase. Type I collagen is the predominant organic component of bone. Type I collagen contains three polypeptide chains that are each composed primarily of approximately 1,000 amino acids. Each polypeptide chain is organized into an α-helical structure (two $\alpha 1$ and one $\alpha 2$ chains). These three chains are then intertwined and held together via hydrogen bonding to form the α-helix. Collagen fibrils are formed by the parallel arrangement of the collagen molecules in a quarter-staggered array. The fibrils are then bundled together to form a collagen fiber. Because of the repetitive nature of the arrangement of the collagen molecules within the fibril, certain characteristic features can be seen under electron microscopy. Hole zones represent the individual spaces found between the ends of the molecules; pores represent spaces on the sides of the parallel molecules. It is in these spaces that mineral deposition requisite for ossification occurs. Once arranged, the individual collagen molecules are stabilized by cross-linking reactive aldehydes on lysine and hydroxylysine residues.

Noncollagenous proteins present within the bone matrix include osteocalcin, osteonectin, bone sialoprotein, and various growth factors and cytokines (TGF-β, interleukins, etc.). Osteocalcin, produced by osteoblasts, comprises approximately 10% to 20% of the noncollagenous protein content and is associated with mineralization of the bone matrix. It is thought to play a role in regulating bone mineralization. The synthesis of osteocalcin is increased by 1,25-dihydroxyvitamin D and is inhibited by parathyroid hormone (PTH) and corticosteroids. Osteonectin is produced by osteoblasts and platelets and is thought to regulate the calcium concentration within the bone matrix and potentiate mineralization. The presence of growth factors and cytokines are crucial to the process of bone remodeling and cellular turnover.

Bone Mineralization. As stated previously, the inorganic portion of bone is comprised predominantly of calcium hydroxyapatite. Mineralization occurs in two stages: initiation of mineralization (nucleation) and proliferation (addition of mineral deposits on the initial deposits). The combination of both processes is termed *multiplication*. Mineral aggregation occurs within the pores and holes between the collagen molecules (Fig. 1.11).

Heterotopic ossification is the formation of normal bone in an abnormal location (soft tissue). Causes of heterotopic ossification include trauma, CNS injury, and inherited disorders of ossification, such as fibrodysplasia ossificans progressive (FOP). FOP is an autosomal dominant disorder characterized by congenital malformation of the great toes and painful postnatal heterotopic ossification that immobilizes the joints of the axial and appendicular skeleton. Attempts to remove heterotopic bone in FOP patients lead to rampant new bone formation. Additionally, tumors such as synovial sarcoma can demonstrate intralesional calcifications. Classically, heterotopic ossification can be divided clinically into early, intermediate, and late findings, as seen in Table 1.6.

NSAIDs and radiation have been found to inhibit heterotopic bone formation and have been used as prophylactic agents for this purpose. Additionally, postoperative radiation in the dose of 6 Gy given within 3 days following total hip arthroplasty has also been shown to be effective in preventing heterotopic ossification.

Types of Bone (Structural vs. Microscopic). Structurally, bone is composed of trabecular (cancellous) and cortical bone. The former has approximately 4 times the mass of cancellous bone while the metabolic turnover of cancellous bone is 8 times that of cortical bone. Their structural differences allow them to withstand the different stress placed upon them. Cortical bone is best suited to resisting bending, torsional, and compressive forces. Cancellous bone is located primarily at the metaphysis and epiphyses of long bones and allows it to withstand a number of different stress patterns (primarily compression) (Fig. 1.12).

The microscopic composition of bone is divided into woven and lamellar bone. Woven bone primarily is present during fracture healing and in certain pathologic states, such as osteogenesis imperfecta and osteosarcoma. It is also seen normally in the fetus and newborn and in the metaphysis of growing bones. It is coarse, and there is no uniform orientation of the collagen fibers. Lamellar bone, on the other hand, is more organized in structure and results from the remodeling of woven bone. It is contained within trabecular and cortical bone that allows it to resist

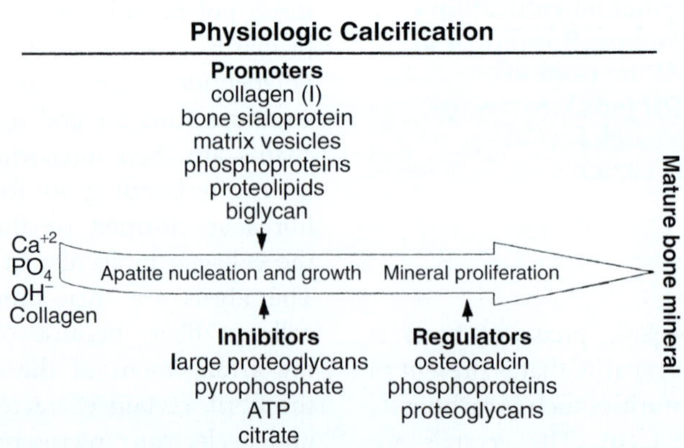

FIGURE 1.11 **Bone mineral deposition consists of several stages, which are dependent on a variety of matrix proteins as illustrated here. (*Source*: Buckwalter JA, Einhorn TA, Simon SR. *Orthopaedic Basic Science: Biology and Biomechanics of the Musculoskeletal System*, 2nd ed. Rosemont, IL: American Academy of Orthopaedic Surgeons, 2000; 330, Fig. 12.)**

TABLE 1.6 Clinical and laboratory findings in heterotopic ossification

Finding	Early (0–4 wks)	Intermediate (5–8 wks)	Late (9–12 wks)
Symptoms	Increased pain, swelling, stiffness	Pain, swelling, stiffness	Decreased pain, swelling, stiffness
Signs	Erythema, warmth, tenderness, induration, decreased ROM	Further decreasing ROM	Decreased ROM, possible ankylosis
Serum alkaline phosphatase	Elevated	Elevated, then plateaus	Returns to normal
Histopathologic Findings	Mesenchymal metaplasia	Osseous or chondroosseous differentiation	Bone
Radionuclide bone scan	Positive phases I–III	Positive phase III	Decreasing phase III
Radiographic findings	None or soft-tissue swelling	Early osteogenesis	Late osteogenesis with remodeling

Source: Kaplan FS, et al. Heterotopic ossification. *JAAOS* 12(2):116–125,2004.

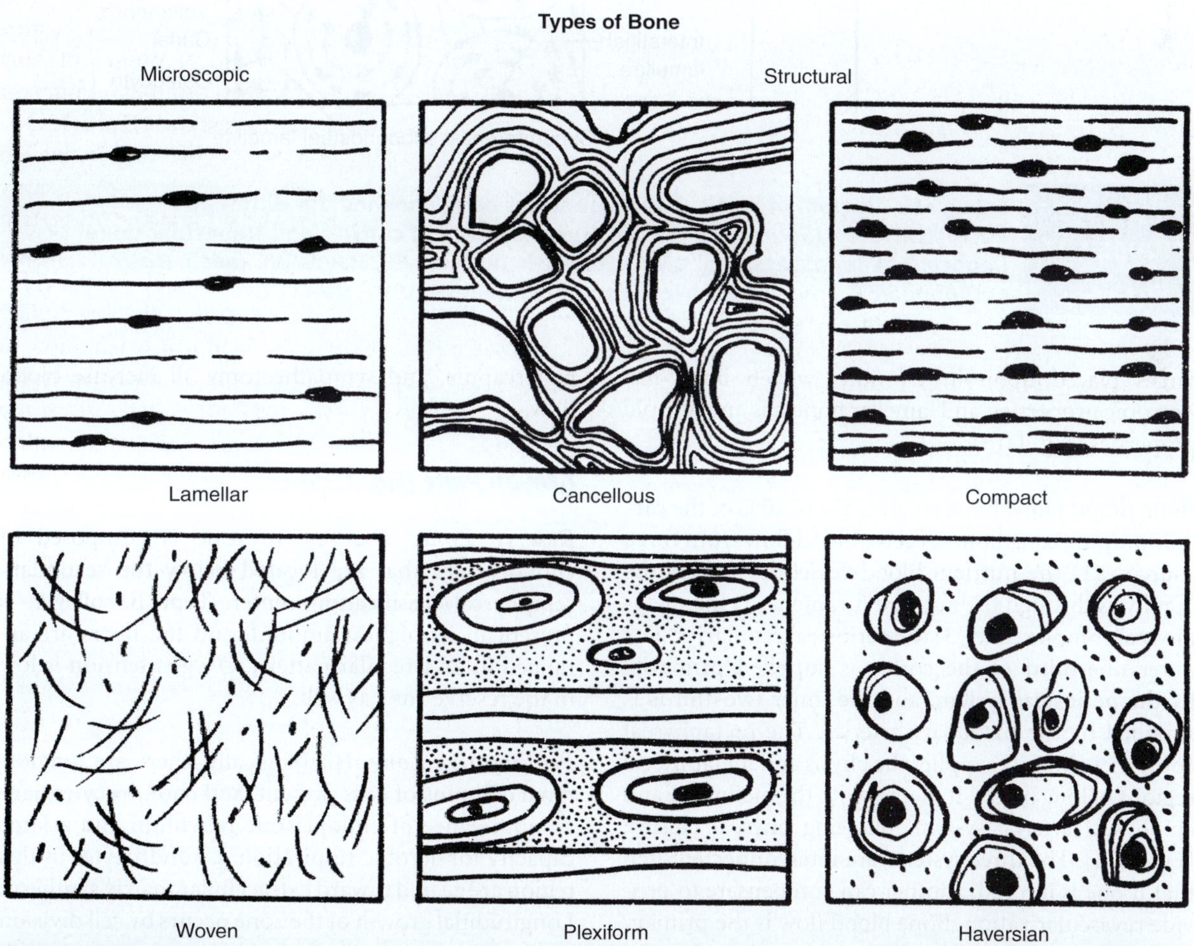

FIGURE 1.12 **Diagrams of types of bone. (*Source*: Buckwalter JA, Einhorn TA, Simon SR. *Orthopaedic Basic Science: Biology and Biomechanics of the Musculoskeletal System*, 2nd ed. Rosemont, IL: American Academy of Orthopaedic Surgeons, 2000; 320, Fig. 1.)**

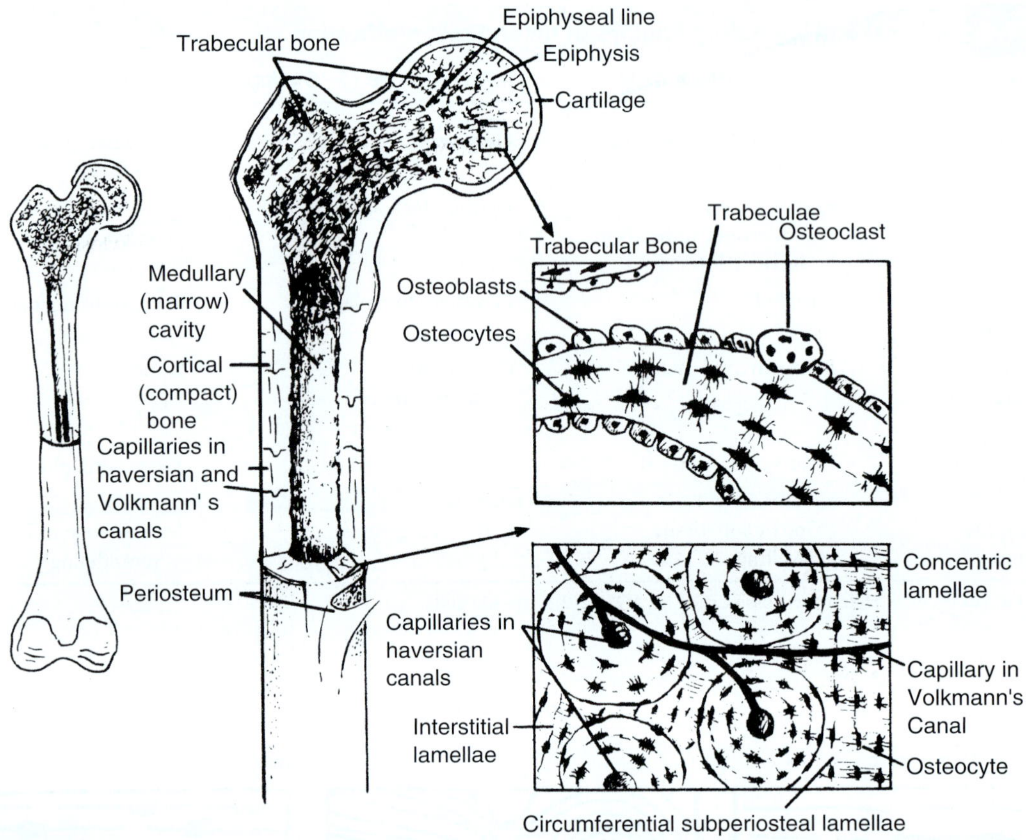

FIGURE 1.13 **Schematic diagram of cortical and trabecular bone showing the different microstructures. (*Source*: Hayes WC. Biomechanics of cortical and trabecular bone: Implications for assessment of fracture risk. In: Mow VC, Hayes WC (eds.), *Basic Orthopaedic Biomechanics*. New York: Raven Press, 1991; 93–142.)**

forces placed upon it. Of note, woven bone has isotropic properties, and lamellar bone has anisotropic properties (Fig. 1.13).

Bone Blood Flow. Bone receives 5% to 10% of the cardiac output. Long bones receive blood flow from three sources: (1) the nutrient blood vessel that enters the diaphysis through the nutrient foramen, (2) the metaphyseal complex, and (3) the periosteal capillaries. The outer one-third of the cortex is supplied primarily by the periosteal system, and the inner two-thirds is supplied by the medullary arteries. The metaphyseal complex primarily supplies the physis and metaphyseal regions of long bones. It merges with the medullary and epiphyseal arterial system following physeal closure (Fig. 1.14). The three systems are interconnected such that if one is injured, another can compensate to provide revascularization. Bone blood flow is the primary determinant of fracture healing, and it peaks at 2 weeks following fracture. After a fracture, blood flow initially decreases because of disruption of vessels, but within hours to days it increases, peaks at 2 weeks, and then normalizes again between 3 and 5 months. Hypoxia, hypercapnia, and sympathectomy all increase blood flow.

Growth Plate (Fig. 1.15)

Reserve Zone. The reserve zone is composed of chondrocytes that are located below the secondary (epiphyseal) ossification center. Type II collagen is present in its highest amount, and the fibers are arranged in an irregular pattern. Oxygen tension is low in the reserve zone as well.

Proliferative Zone. Histologically, there are longitudinal columns of cells present, and chondrocytes have an abundance of endoplasmic reticulum and a large capacity for aerobic respiration. Chondrocytes in this region are geared toward extracellular matrix synthesis. Longitudinal growth of the zone occurs by cell division of the chondrocytes in the proliferative zone. As with the reserve zone, the distribution of the collagen fibers is irregular. However, oxygen tension is high within this region owing to its rich vascular supply to support the aerobic metabolism that characterizes these

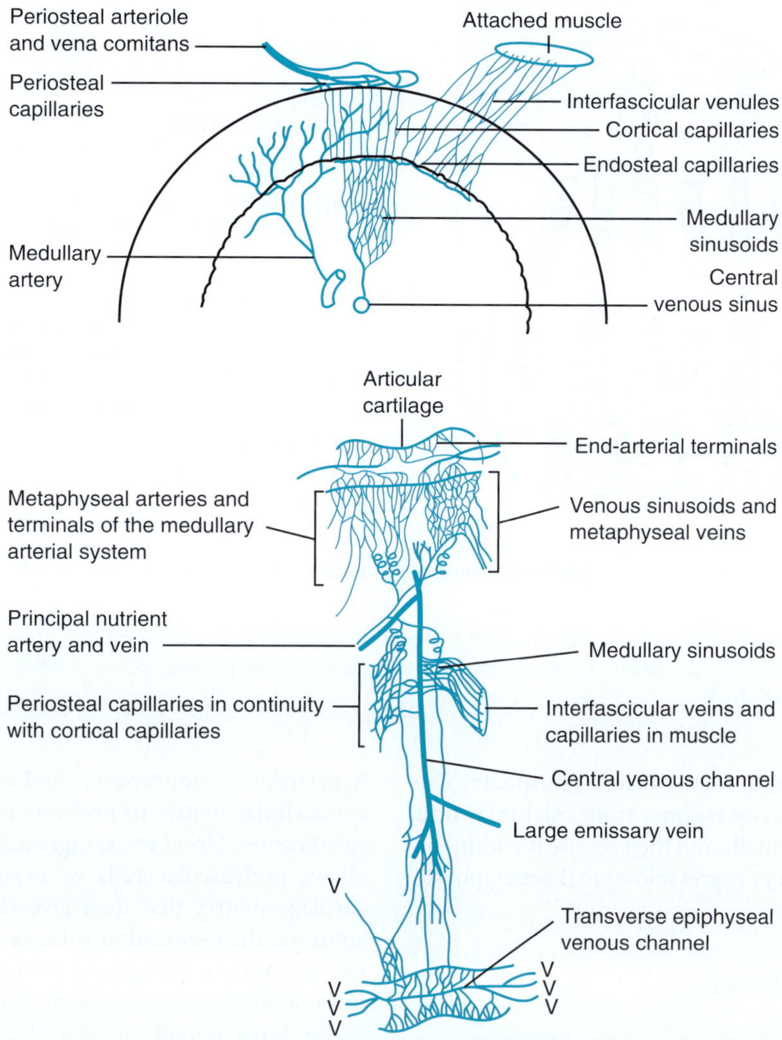

FIGURE 1.14 **Blood supply of a long bone. Three basic blood supplies are shown: (1) nutrient; (2) metaphyseal, which anastomoses with epiphyseal after epiphyseal closure; and (3) periosteal. The numerous metaphyseal arteries arise from periarticular networks and anastomose with terminal branches of ascending and descending medullary arteries. Periosteal capillaries emerge from the cortex (efferent blood flow). (4) A periosteal arteriole feeds capillaries that provide afferent blood flow to a limited outer layer of cortex. (*Adapted from* Rhinelander FW. Circulation of bone. In: Bourne GH (ed.), *The Biochemistry and Physiology of Bone*, 2nd ed. New York: Academic Press, 1972; 2.)**

chondrocytes. The majority of the longitudinal growth of the growth plate occurs in this zone.

Hypertrophic Zone. Cells in the hypertrophic zone are considerably larger than those in the proliferative zone. The zone is avascular, resulting in a low oxygen tension (similar to the reserve zone). The extracellular matrix undergoes progressive mineralization as the chondrocytes in this region prepare the matrix for mineralization and eventual calcification. Within the hypertrophic zone, there are three individual zones termed the *zone of maturation*, *zone of degeneration*, and *zone of provisional calcification*. It is within the zone of provisional calcification that true matrix calcification occurs.

Growth Plate Mineralization. Mineralization is dependent on matrix vesicles. They are produced by the chondrocyte plasma membrane and are rich in calcium ions and alkaline phosphatase. They are responsible for promoting calcification because they contain proteases that degrade aggregated proteoglycans and promote the hydrolysis of pyrophosphate, both of which hinder mineralization. In regards to the pyrophosphate, hydrolysis leads to the formation of phosphate ions that couple with the concentrated

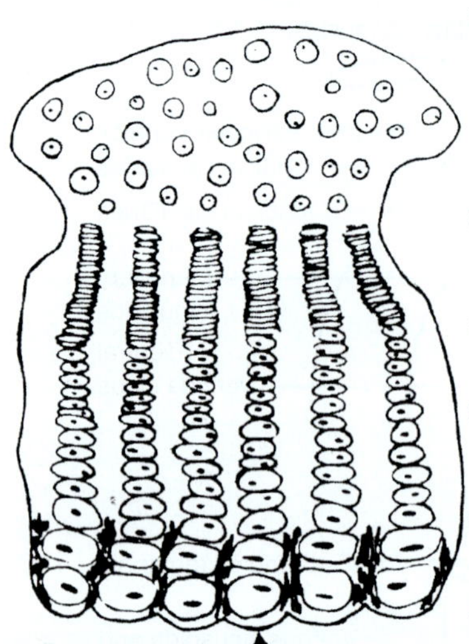

FIGURE 1.15 **Zonal structure, function, and intracellular calcium transfer in the growth plate. (*Source*: Brighton T. Structure and function of the growth plate. *Clin Orthop* 1978; 136:24.)**

calcium ions present to form calcium phosphate. The hypertrophic chondrocytes concentrate calcium within the mitochondria initially and then release it within the matrix vesicles as they progress closer to the metaphysic (Fig. 1.16).

Bone Injury and Repair

Fracture Healing. Fracture healing occurs via six stages.

1. Hematoma formation and inflammation
2. Angiogenesis and cartilage formation
3. Cartilage calcification
4. Cartilage removal
5. Bone formation
6. Bone remodeling

Hematoma formation serves as a repository for cytokines and growth factors required to initiate the fracture healing process. Over the first 10 days of fracture healing, both intramembranous and endochondral ossification are initiated to form the fracture callus. If the two ends of a fractured bone are not in continuity, a soft (bridging) callus is formed where endochondral ossification occurs that is then replaced by woven bone where intramembranous ossification occurs. Fracture callus calcification occurs approximately at 2 weeks following the initial fracture as hypertrophic chondrocytes become the predominant cell type. Calcification occurs in a fashion similar to that of the growth plate as matrix vesicles are produced by the hypertrophic chondrocytes and are released into the extracellular matrix to promote mineralization. With calcification, blood vessel ingrowth then occurs, which allows perivascular cells to invade the mineralized cartilage matrix that then give rise to osteoblasts to continue the ossification process. Osteoclasts also arrive and aid in cartilage removal to allow for continued intramembranous ossification. During the remodeling phase, bone initially produced by intramembranous ossification is replaced with lamellar bone to provide further strength.

It is important to note that with rigidly fixed fractures that are stabilized in compression with a plate, fracture healing occurs by the process of Haversian remodeling, without callus formation.

Fracture healing in cases in which the fracture fragments are not rigidly anatomically aligned (such as in a closed treatment) occurs with soft and hard callus formation. Fractures stabilized with locked plating that can prevent compression or that allow a certain degree of motion at the fracture site (such as with intramedullary nailing) also allow for callus formation. Table 1.7 displays the indications for both compression and locked plating (bridging internal fixator).

Disorders of Bone Mineralization and Bone Density

Osteomalacia. This is a condition of impaired bone mineralization. Osteomalacia manifested in children is rickets and leads to an inability to form primary spongiosa. Failure to maintain a proper serum calcium

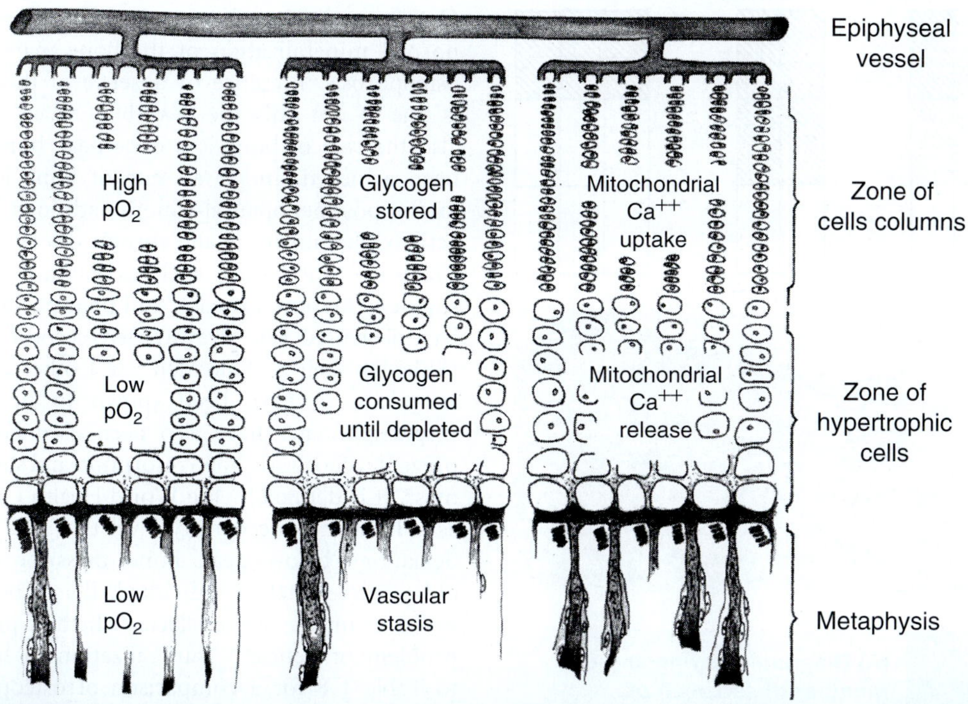

FIGURE 1.16 **Metabolic events in the growth plate. The growth plate showing the relative oxygen tensions in the various zones in the left-hand column, the change in glycogen storage and utilization in the center column, and the role of mitochondria in the right-hand column. (*Source*: Brighton CT, Hunt RM. The role of mitochondria in growth plate calcification as demonstrated in a rachitic model. *J Bone Joint Surg* 1978;60A:630–639.)**

and phosphate concentration leads to poor mineralization. Treatment is dependent on restoring normal serum levels of calcium and phosphorus (Fig. 1.17). Conditions resulting from vitamin D deficiency can be treated by administering vitamin D or 1,25-(OH_2) vitamin D. Diseases involving vitamin D resistance are treated by giving inorganic phosphate and 1,25-(OH_2) vitamin D.

Renal Osteodystrophy. The spectrum of pathologic bone changes seen in renal osteodystrophy is due to glomerular disease leading to phosphate retention and

TABLE 1.7 **Indications for compression or bridging internal fixator techniques**

Fracture Pattern	*Compression*	*Bridging*	*Combination*
Simple diaphyseal fractures	Yes	No	No
Simple metaphyseal fractures	Yes	No	No
Multifragmentary diaphyseal fractures	No	Yes	No
Multifragmentary metaphyseal fractures	No	Yes	No
Osteotomies	Yes	Yes	No
Articular fractures	Yes	No	No
Articular fractures with multiligamentary meta- or diaphyseal fractures			Yes
Segmental fractures with two different fracture patterns			Yes

Source: Gardner MJ, et al. Has locked plating completely replaced conventional plating? *Am J Orthopaedics* 9:440–446,2004.

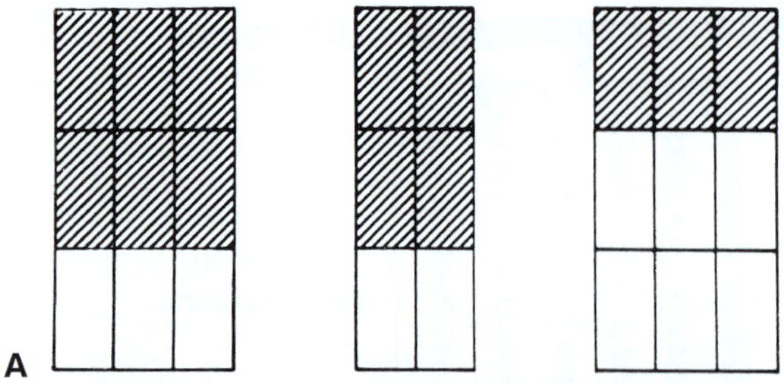

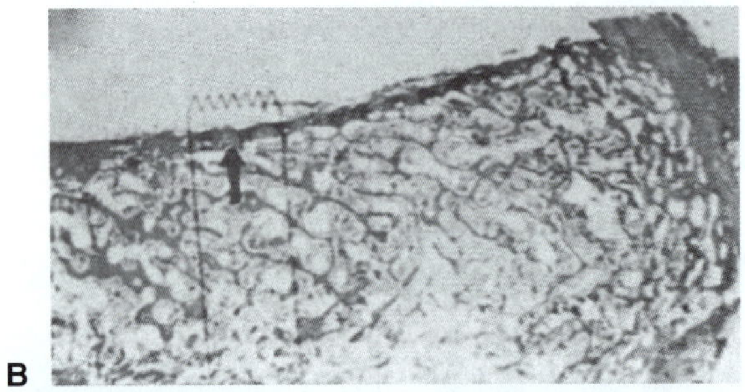

FIGURE 1.17 **(A) Diagram showing amount (number of sections) of normally mineralized (cross-hatched sections) and insufficiently mineralized (blank sections) bone matrix. (B) Photomicrograph of transcortical bone biopsy specimen, demonstrating sparse trabeculae with cortical resorption. (*Source*: Buckwalter JA, Einhorn TA, Simon SR. *Orthopaedic Basic Science: Biology and Biomechanics of the Musculoskeletal System*, 2nd ed. Rosemont, IL: American Academy of Orthopaedic Surgeons, 2000; Fig. 50.)**

low production of 1,25-(OH_2) vitamin D. Histologically, bone changes are manifested as osteitis fibrosa reflecting the excess PTH activity and extensive bone resorption. Acidosis seen in the chronic renal failure state exacerbates this condition. Osteomalacia seen in this condition is commonly due to aluminum toxicity as a result of aluminum-containing phosphate binders used to treat the hyperphosphatemia. Patients will often have chronic bone pain and can present with pathologic fractures. Serum studies reveal decreased calcium, increased phosphate, increased PTH, and increased alkaline phosphatase levels reflecting the increased bone turnover. Treatments include (1) phosphate binders, (2) suppressing the endogenous hyperparathyroidism, (3) aluminum chelation, and (4) renal transplant (Fig. 1.18).

Osteoporosis. A reduction in bone mass but with normal mineralization of the bone matrix is called osteoporosis. Presence or absence of this condition is due to not only the peak bone mass present but also the rate of bone loss once peak bone mass has been achieved. Increased rate of bone loss is seen in the postmenopausal state, conditions of reduced activity, malnutrition, and chronic disease conditions. Treatment modalities such as vitamin D, calcium supplementation, exercise, and pharmacologic agents have been used. Selective estrogen receptor modulators (SERMs) such as Raloxifene and other agents such as calcitonin have been shown to be successful. Bisphosphonates have also been used because they prevent osteoclastic bone resorption and stabilize bone mass. It is defined by the World Health Organization as a lumbar bone density level that is 2.5 standard deviations below peak bone mass of a 25-year-old gender-matched individual. It is a bone density problem unlike osteomalacia, which is principally a problem of deficient mineralization of bone. Refer to Table 1.8 for a comparison of osteoporosis and osteomalacia. Osteoporosis is classically categorized into two types: (1) type I (postmenopausal) affects trabecular bone (vertebrae, distal radius) primarily in postmenopausal women, and (2) type II osteoporosis (age-related) affects both genders equally and affects both trabecular and cortical bone. The DEXA (dual x-ray absorptiometry) is the most accurate test to diagnose osteoporosis and is commonly used as a screening test for osteoporosis. Patients are assigned a z-score that indicates the quantitative bone mass present in an individual and allows comparison to age- and gender-matched controls.

Paget Disease. Paget disease is a condition of abnormal bone turnover, as indicated by an increased level of alkaline phosphatase. It is a common disorder of the geriatric population, and signs and symptoms can be subtle. Common clinical scenarios of the patient with Paget disease relate to bone deformity and enlargement. Patients may complain of hearing loss owing to enlargement of the temporal bone, bony tenderness, hyperthermia (hyperemia of Pagetoid bone), asymmetric bone enlargement (such as leg-length discrepancy), and fractures. The high degree of bone turnover results in a dense, sclerotic bone with visible trabeculae (osteosclerosis). While mineralization is normal, the remodeling process is not. Fractures also heal at a slower rate than in normal bone, and although the bone is more dense, it is more prone to fracture because of the abnormal remodeling that occurs. Treatment modalities are directed at controlling bone resorption (such as with calcitonin or bisphosphonates).

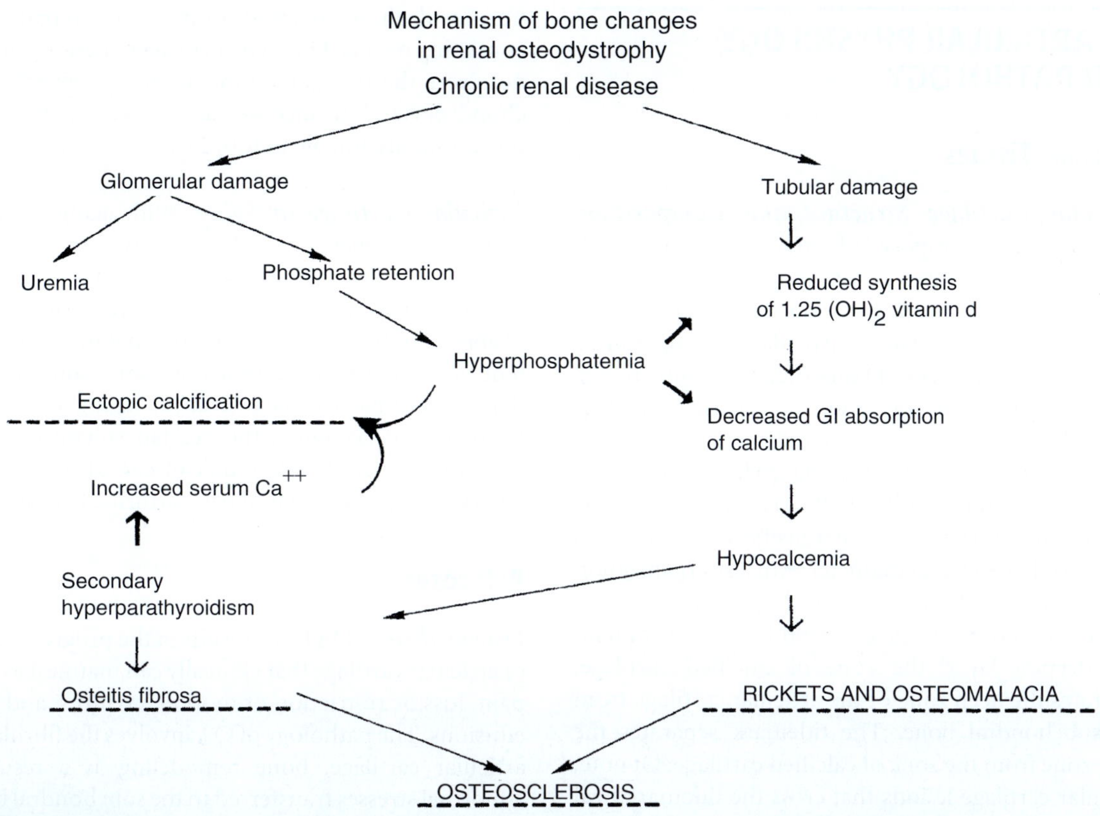

FIGURE 1.18 **Pathogenesis of bone changes in renal osteodystrophy. (*Source*: Buckwalter JA, Einhorn TA, Simon SR. *Orthopaedic Basic Science: Biology and Biomechanics of the Musculoskeletal System*, 2nd ed. Rosemont, IL: American Academy of Orthopaedic Surgeons, 2000; Fig. 52.)**

TABLE 1.8 **Comparison of osteoporosis and osteomalacia**

	Osteoporosis	*Osteomalacia*
Definition	Bone mass decreased	Bone mass variable
	Mineralization normal	Mineralization decreased
Age of Onset	Generally elderly, postmenopausal	Any age
Etiology	Endocrine abnormality	Vitamin D deficiency
	Age	Abnormality of vitamin D metabolic pathway
	Idiopathic	Hypophosphatemic syndromes
		Renal tubular acidosis
Symptoms	Pain referable to fracture site	Generalized bone pain
Signs	Tenderness at fracture site	Tenderness at fracture site and generalized tenderness
Lab Findings	Serum Ca, PO_4, alkaline phosphatase normal	Serum Ca, PO_4 low/normal Alkaline phosphatase elevated

Source: Buckwalter JA, Einhorn TA, Simon SR. *Orthopaedic Basic Science: Biology and Biomechanics of the Musculoskeletal System*, 2nd ed. Rosemont, IL: American Academy of Orthopaedic Surgeons, 2000.

III. ARTICULAR PHYSIOLOGY AND PATHOLOGY

Articular Tissues

Articular Cartilage Structure and Composition. Cartilage itself is composed of extracellular matrix with chondrocytes that are sparsely populated within the matrix. Chondrocytes are responsible for the overall maintenance of the matrix. Articular cartilage can be divided into four layers: (1) superficial, (2) transitional, (3) deep zone, and (4) zone of calcified cartilage (Fig. 1.19).

In the superficial zone, the collagen fibers are parallel to the surface and are suited to the elastohydrodynamic form of joint lubrication. The transition zone contains fibers that have a larger diameter with less organization than in the superficial zone. The deep zone contains a high content of proteoglycans and low water content. The deepest layer, the zone of calcified cartilage, separates the deep zone of the articular cartilage from the subchondral bone. The tidemark separates the deep zone from the zone of calcified cartilage. Of note, articular cartilage lesions that cross the tidemark heal with fibrocartilage (type I collagen). This is important because it pertains to abrasion chondroplasty, which results in the migration of undifferentiated precursor cells from the bone marrow into the articular surface defect. These precursor cells then differentiate along a fibrocartilaginous pathway to produce a repair tissue consisting primarily of type I collagen. Lesions that do not cross the tidemark stimulate the proliferation of chondrocytes, but since articular cartilage is avascular, the lesions are unable to fully heal.

Articular Cartilage in Aging. With aging, articular cartilage becomes less cellular relative to immature cartilage. As an organism ages, the water content of articular cartilage decreases and reaches a steady state (Table 1.9). It is important to note that the water content of osteoarthritic cartilage is significantly greater than in normal cartilage from an aging individual. Furthermore, in aging, the keratan sulfate increases until the age of 30, while that of chondroitin sulfate decreases (opposite that of osteoarthritic cartilage).

Arthroses

Osteoarthritis (OA). OA results in the progressive loss of articular cartilage that clinically can manifest as joint pain, loss or restriction of motion, crepitus, and joint effusions. The pathology of OA involves the fibrillation articular cartilage, bone remodeling as a result of abnormal stresses transferred to the subchondral bone, and osteophyte and bone cyst formation.

Articular cartilage fibrillation involves the erosion of articular cartilage surface with resulting ulceration and cleft formation within the articular cartilage (Fig. 1.20). Initially cleft formation is confined

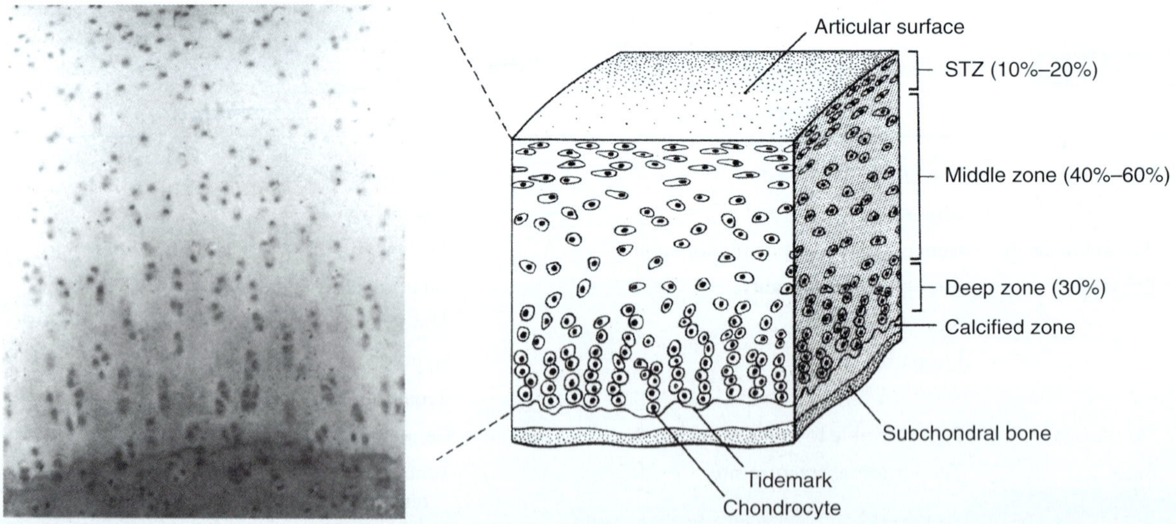

FIGURE 1.19 **(A) Histologic section of normal adult articular cartilage showing even Safranin O staining and distribution of chondrocytes. (B) Schematic diagram of chondrocyte organization in the 3 major zones of the uncalcified cartilage, the tidemark, and the subchondral bone. STZ = superficial tangential zone. (*Source*: Mow VC, Proctor CS, Kelly MA. Biomechanics of articular cartilage. In: Nordin M, Frankel VH (eds.), *Basic Biomechanics of the Musculoskeletal System*, 2nd ed. Philadelphia: Lea & Febiger, 1989; 31–57.)**

TABLE 1.9 Biochemical changes of articular cartilage

	Aging	*Osteoarthritis*
Water content (hydration, permeability)	Decreased	Increased
Collagen	Unchanged	Disordered structure (matrix degradation), content decreases in severe OA
Proteoglycan content	Decreased (length of protein core and glycosaminoglycan chains decrease)	Decreases
Proteoglycan synthesis	Decreased (maintenance of extracellular matrix)	Increased
Proteoglycan degradation	Decreased	Significantly increased
Chondroitin sulfate concentration	Decreased	Increased
Keratin sulfate	Increased	Decreased
Chondrocyte size	Increased	Increased
Chondrocyte number	Decreased	Increased*
Modulus of elasticity	Increased	Decreased

*Varies directly with severity of osteoarthritis to a point of failure, after which mitotic activity decreases.

to the superficial layers but can extend into the deeper layers as the disease progresses. Clefts can extend past the gliding (superficial) layer and into the transitional zone. Fragmentation of the articular surface develops and eventually results in remnants of articular cartilage attached to the exposed, eburnated subchondral bone. Synovial thickening is also seen with OA and can contribute to joint effusions that are frequently observed with this condition. Focal areas of inflammation as well as neovascularization can be seen within the synovium histologically. The surface of the synovium is hypervascular and friable. The synovium becomes markedly thickened with advanced disease. Bone remodeling occurs because of altered stress patterns transmitted to the subchondral bone owing to the loss of the compressive effect of the articular cartilage that progressively becomes more fragmented. Osteosclerosis (Fig. 1.21) develops along with fibrocartilage formation. Osteophyte formation that accompanies bone remodeling is thought to be a result of bone formation at the bony margins of the joint surface and is covered with hyalinelike cartilage.

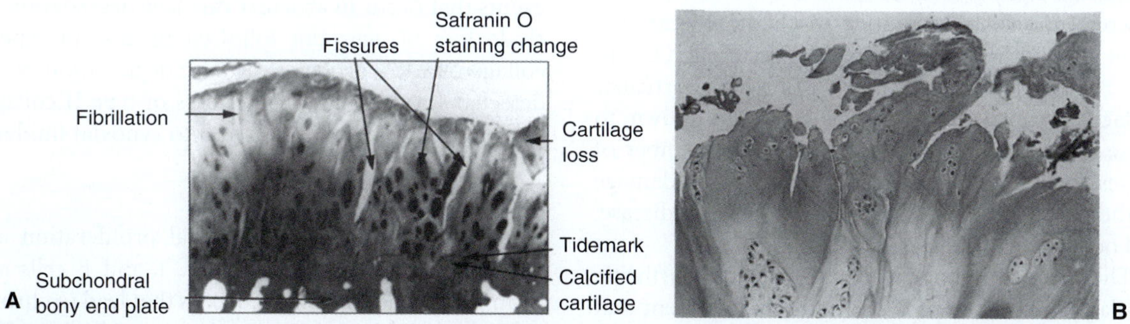

FIGURE 1.20 **(A) Low-power magnification of a section of a glenohumeral head of osteoarthritic cartilage removed at surgery for total shoulder replacement. Note the significant fibrillation, vertical cleft formation, the tidemark, and the subchondral bony endplate. (B) A higher power magnification of surface fibrillation showing vertical cleft formation and widespread large, necrotic regions of the tissue devoid of cells. Clusters of cells, common in osteoarthritic tissues, are also seen. (*Source*: Buckwalter JA, Einhorn TA, Simon SR. *Orthopaedic Basic Science: Biology and Biomechanics of the Musculoskeletal System*, 2nd ed. Rosemont, IL: American Academy of Orthopaedic Surgeons, 2000; Fig. 3.)**

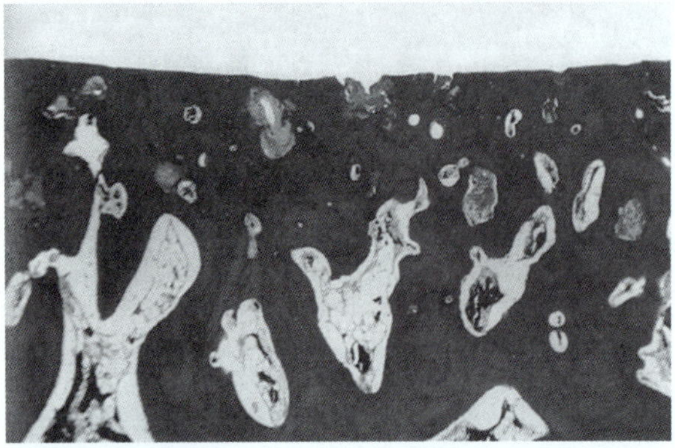

FIGURE 1.21 A histologic section of an eburnated section of bone with a dense sclerotic appearance. (*Source*: Buckwalter JA, Einhorn TA, Simon SR. *Orthopaedic Basic Science: Biology and Biomechanics of the Musculoskeletal System*, 2nd ed. Rosemont, IL: American Academy of Orthopaedic Surgeons, 2000; Fig. 5.)

It is thought to be a response of the bone to repair the articular cartilage surface. Subchondral osteoarthritic cysts are also a hallmark feature of the osteoarthritic joint and are located close to the joint surface. They often contain clear or gelatinous fluid.

Etiology of Osteoarthritis. The etiology of OA can be divided into primary and secondary. Primary OA (idiopathic) has no known cause, though it is thought that aging, increased metabolism, and changes in matrix composition all play a role. A common misconception is that routine mechanical wear as a result of long-term daily use can result in OA. In fact, routine submaximal loading of normal articular surfaces during a lifespan has not been shown to cause degeneration. Secondary OA has a number of causes, including posttraumatic? that result in damage to the articular surface, infection, metabolic disease, and neuropathy (Table 1.10)

The biochemical alterations seen in osteoarthritic cartilage include an increase in the water content that is often seen early in the disease process. Furthermore, there is a change in the matrix composition because of an increase in chondroitin-4-sulfate and a decrease in keratin sulfate production, resulting in an increase in the chondroitin-to-keratin sulfate ratio. It is thought that this composition more closely resembles immature articular cartilage. Collagen within osteoarthritic cartilage also becomes less orderly, allowing for increased water deposition within the matrix and resulting in a reduction in the tensile strength of the cartilage. This reduction in tensile strength is also what leads to fissuring and ulceration, as it is no longer competent to withstand the normal compressive forces seen in joint loading. Proteoglycans also have shorter chains than normal. Of note, osteoarthritic cartilage is also more permeable, allowing more synovial fluid and water to impregnate the articular cartilage that exacerbates the incompetence of articular cartilage. Additionally, chondrocytes from osteoarthritic cartilage are more metabolically active than in normal, intact cartilage with increased collagen synthesis and increased proteoglycan synthesis in response to the increased proteoglycan breakdown. The increased proteoglycan and matrix degradation is due to the increased activity of metalloproteinases, collagenases, and stromelysin. Furthermore, activity of these enzymatic degradation systems is a result of interleukin-1 (IL-1)–mediated activity. IL-1 is only a normal byproduct of inflammation but has also been shown to be produced by chondrocytes within the osteoarthritic cartilage.

Inflammatory Arthritides

Pathophysiology of Articular Cartilage Degradation. Articular cartilage degradation occurs as a result of cartilage erosion. Areas susceptible to cartilage erosion include the lateral aspects of the joint where the synovium is in contact with the articular cartilage. Central to this degradation are collagenases (matrix metalloproteinases), specifically MMP-1, MMP-8, and MMP-13. In particular, MMP-1 and MMP-13 have been shown to lead to collagen degradation in rheumatoid arthritis (RA). IL-1 and TNF-α are perhaps the best known stimulators of the metalloproteinases. Early events that occur in articular cartilage degradation include loss of aggrecan followed by loss of type II collagen. In RA, articular cartilage degradation can be detected via degradation products of type II collagen and aggrecan that are released into synovial fluid and serum.

Synovial Inflammation. Synovial proliferation and hyperplasia are hallmarks of RA. T and B cells also form part of the contingent of cells that lead to chronic inflammation that occurs in rheumatoid joints. This proliferative synovium can develop invasive characteristics and lead to degeneration of surrounding cartilage, bone, and ligaments, with the offending section of synovium termed *pannus*. The metalloproteinases family responsible for articular cartilage degradation is also part of the pathogenesis of destruction caused by rheumatoid pannus. It is thought that T cells play an integral role in mediating the inflammation seen with pannus-mediated destruction.

TABLE 1.10 Causes of joint degeneration (secondary osteoarthritis)

Cause	*Presumed Mechanism*
Intra-articular fractures	Damage to articular cartilage and/or joint incongruity
High-intensity impact joint loading	Damage to articular cartilage and/or subchondral bone
Ligament injuries	Joint instability
Joint dysplasias (developmental and hereditary joint and cartilage dysplasias)	Abnormal joint shape and/or abnormal articular cartilage
Aseptic necrosis	Bone necrosis leads to collapse of the articular surface and joint incongruity
Acromegaly	Overgrowth of articular cartilage produces joint incongruity and/or abnormal cartilage
Paget's disease	Distortion or incongruity of joints caused by bone remodeling
Ehlers-Danlos syndrome	Joint instability
Gaucher's disease (hereditary deficiency of the enzyme glucocerebrosidase, leading to accumulation of glucocerebroside)	Bone necrosis or pathologic bone fracture leading to joint incongruity
Stickler's syndrome (progressive hereditary arthro-ophthalmopathy)	Abnormal joint and/or articular cartilage development
Joint infection (inflammation)	Destruction of articular cartilage
Hemophilia	Multiple joint hemorrhages
Hemochromatosis (excess iron deposition in multiple tissues)	Mechanism unknown
Ochronosis (hereditary deficiency of enzyme, homogentisic acid oxidase)	Deposition of homogentisic acid polymers in articular cartilage leading to accumulation of homogentisic acid
Calcium pyrophosphate deposition disease	Accumulation of calcium pyrophosphate crystals in articular cartilage
Neuropathic arthropathy (Charcot joints, syphilis, diabetes mellitus, syringomyelia, meningomyelocele, leprosy, congenital insensitivity to pain, amyloidosis)	Loss of proprioception and joint sensation results in increased impact loading and torsion, joint instability and intra-articular fractures

(Reproduced with permission from Buckwalter JA, Mankin HJ: Articular cartilage: Degeneration and osteoarthritis, repair, regeneration and transplantation, in Cannon WD Jr (ed): *Instructional Course Lectures 47*. Rosemont, IL, American Academy of Orthopaedic Surgeons, 1998, pp 487–504.)

Osseous Inflammation. Rheumatism is accompanied by an increased osteoclastic activity that leads to periarticular osteopenia, which is characteristic of this disease. The osteoclasts are stimulated inflammatory mediators released as a result of the ongoing inflammation. There is also endosteal resorption and cortical thinning. Subchondral erosions have also been observed in this process.

Meniscus

Meniscal Anatomy. The medial meniscus is roughly semicircular in form and attaches anteriorly in the region of the anterior intercondylar fossa in front of the ACL. The anterior horns of the medial and lateral menisci are usually attached via a transverse ligament. The posterior horn is attached in the posterior intercondylar fossa between the attachments of the PCL and lateral meniscus. It is adherent to the tibial articular surface via the coronary ligament and is also attached to the deep part of the MCL. The lateral meniscus is more circular in shape and covers more of the tibial articular surface relative to the medial meniscus. It attaches behind the ACL and in front of the intercondylar eminence. The posterior horn of the lateral meniscus attaches behind the intercondylar eminence in front of the posterior horn of the medial meniscus and PCL. The posterior horn of the lateral meniscus is the site of attachment of the two meniscofemoral ligaments. The anterior meniscofemoral ligament (ligament of Humphrey) runs anterior to the PCL and attaches to the medial femoral condyle, while the lateral meniscofemoral ligament (ligament of Wrisberg) runs behind the PCL.

Histologically, the meniscus is composed predominantly of type I collagen (fibrocartilage). Two types of cells have been found within the substance of the meniscus: a fusiform cell in the superficial zone and fibrochondrocytes that are distributed throughout the remainder of the meniscus. The fibrochondrocytes is responsible for synthesizing the fibrous matrix of the meniscus. The meniscus also is roughly 75% water.

Meniscal Motion. The lateral meniscus is more mobile than the medial, with the lateral meniscus undergoing an excursion of approximately 11 mm (in an anterior–posterior direction) from terminal extension into 120 degrees of knee flexion. The medial meniscus undergoes approximately 5 mm of anterior–posterior excursion. The menisci are also able to undergo elastic deformation to maintain its congruity with the tibial and femoral articulating surfaces.

Meniscal Healing. The peripheral 25% of the meniscus, by width, is vascularized. Radial lesions of the meniscus within this peripheral rim have the capability of healing and can be repaired. Lesions in this region can form scar tissue by 10 weeks but take several months to form fibrocartilage. This peripheral rim is often termed the red-red zone. Medial to this zone is the red-white zone, in which the peripheral part is vascularized but the inner part is avascular. Lesions in this region can heal but depend solely on the peripheral blood supply on the outer region of this zone (red-white tears). Lesions in the inner zone of the meniscus are avascular and cannot heal by meniscal repair. Tears in this region must be resected via partial meniscectomy (white-white tears).

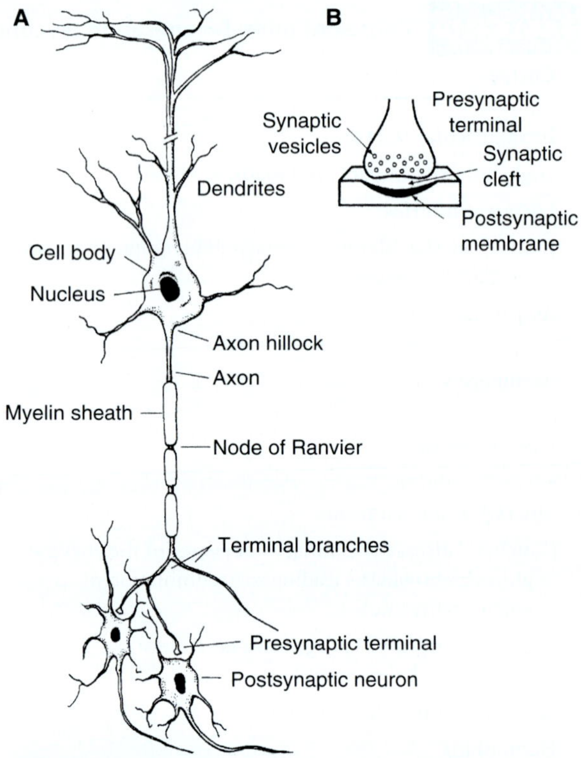

FIGURE 1.22 **(A) Main features of a typical vertebrae neuron. (B) Presynaptic terminal postsynaptic receptor. (*Source*: Buckwalter JA, Einhorn TA, Simon SR. *Orthopaedic Basic Science: Biology and Biomechanics of the Musculoskeletal System*, 2nd ed. Rosemont, IL: American Academy of Orthopaedic Surgeons, 2000; 618, Fig. 1.)**

IV. NEUROMUSCULAR AND CONNECTIVE TISSUE

Nervous System

Neurons and Signal Generation

Nerve Cells. A typical neuron is composed of four regions (Fig. 1.22).

- *Cell body*—Accounts for less than 10% of neuron size; contains the nucleus and is the metabolic center of the cell; gives rise to 1 axon
- *Dendrites*—Thin processes extending from the cell body that receive synaptic input from neighboring nerve cells
- *Axon*—Arises from the axon hillock; is the main conducting unit of the nerve; acts by propagating electrical signals in the form of action potentials over long distances
- *Presynaptic terminal*—Part of the axon near its target organ that is responsible for transmitting information to dendrites of other neurons

Giant Cells and Myelin Formation. Three types of cells are involved in myelin formation.

- *Schwann cells*—Myelinate peripheral nerve axons. Myelin is composed of 70% lipid and 30% protein. Myelinated axons conduct faster than nonmyelinated axons. A single peripheral axon can be myelinated by up to 500 Schwann cells, but each Schwann cell can myelinate only 1 axon.
- *Oligodendrocytes*—Located only within the central nervous system (CNS).

- *Astrocytes*—The most common glial cell but located only within the CNS. They have a supportive role within the CNS (Fig. 1.23).

Axoplasmic Transport. Molecules synthesized in the cell body are rapidly transported to the presynaptic terminals via axoplasmic transport. It is dependent on ATP, calcium, and microtubules. Transport can take place slowly or quickly and can be antegrade (delivery) or retrograde (returning of degradation materials). Reductions in transport capacity have been described in diseases such as diabetes, amyotrophic lateral sclerosis, Guillain-Barré syndrome, and peripheral neuropathies, which may contribute to clinical manifestations of neurologic disease.

Resting Potential. In a resting state, there is negative electrical potential within the cell (between −50 and −80 mV) compared with the external environment. This electrical difference results from an unequal distribution of charged ions, most notably Na^+, Cl^-, K^+, and organic ions, which are separated by the lipid bilayer of the cell membrane.

Action Potential. This electrical potential (Fig. 1.24) transmits signals rapidly and over long distances to

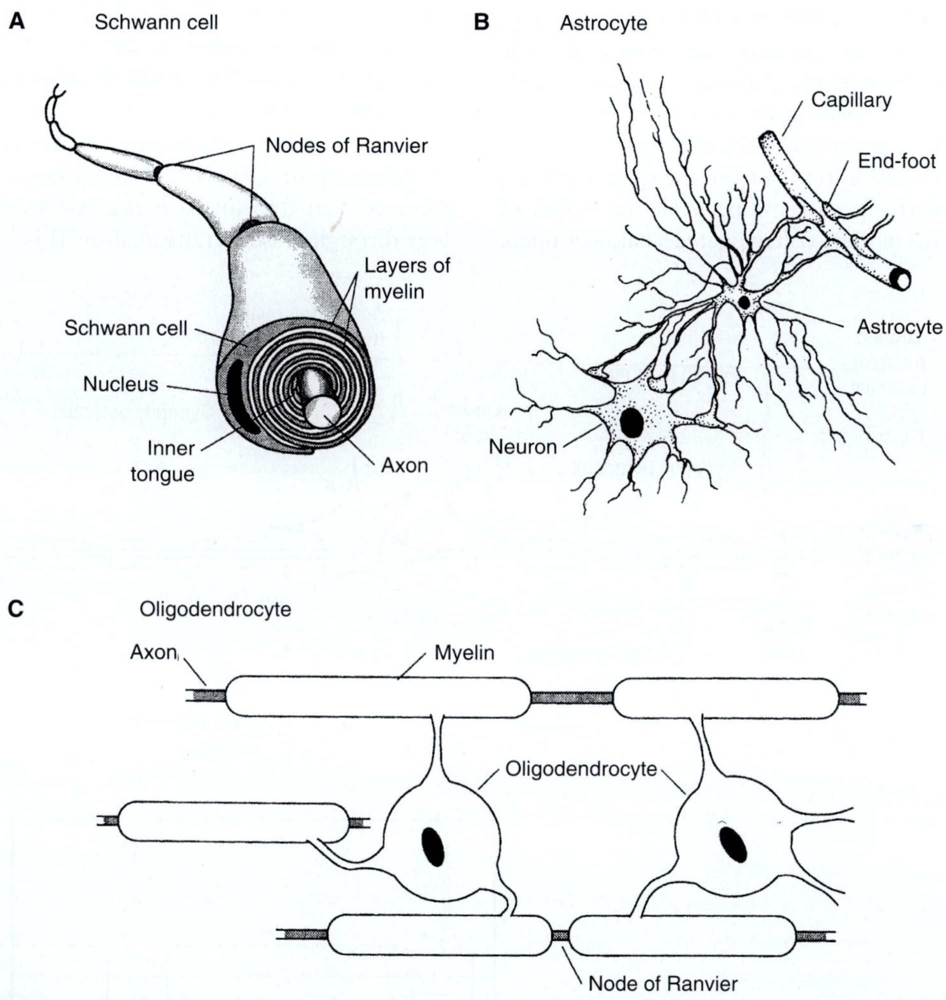

FIGURE 1.23 **The principal types of glial cells. (A) Schwann cells line up along the length of peripheral nervous system axons at regular intervals, each forming a segment of myelin sheath about 1 mm long. (B) Astrocytes are star-shaped and have end feet that contact both capillaries and neurons. (C) In white matter, oligodendrocytes participate in myelination of axons; a single oligodendrocyte can form myelin around several different axons. In gray matter, they surround the cell bodies of neurons. (*Source*: Buckwalter JA, Einhorn TA, Simon SR. *Orthopaedic Basic Science: Biology and Biomechanics of the Musculoskeletal System*, 2nd ed. Rosemont, IL: American Academy of Orthopaedic Surgeons, 2000; 619, Fig. 3.)**

other neurons or receptor organs, such as muscle. Graded potentials that do not achieve the threshold are able to communicate over short distances. Depolarization that reaches threshold potential changes cell membrane permeability and allows Na^+ to rush in via one of three types of gated ion channels: voltage-gated, mechanical-gated, and chemical transmitter–gated channels. Graded stretching of a muscle produces graded potentials in the terminal fibers of the sensory neuron. This potential spreads passively to the trigger zone, and if the potential is large enough, it will trigger an action potential, which is actively propagated without change along the axon to the terminal region. At the terminal of the afferent fiber, the action potential triggers the release of transmitter that diffuses across the synaptic cleft and interacts with the membrane of the motoneuron to initiate a synaptic potential in the motoneuron. The synaptic potential passively spreads to the axon hillock where an action potential is initiated if the membrane potential is above threshold. Action potential propagation results from the spread of local passive depolarizing currents between the nodes of Ranvier. At the nodes, voltage-gated channels open, producing an action potential (Fig. 1.25). Nongated channels are responsible for the resting membrane potential. The action potential propagates along the axon by both passive and active membrane changes. Larger diameter axons will conduct faster than smaller axons. Nodes of Ranvier represent specific foci along the axon without myelin but rich in voltage-gated Na^+ channels. Action potentials are evoked at the nodes and can "jump" from node to node via saltatory propagation.

Classification of Nerve Fibers

Sensory System. The sensory system receives information from the environment via different receptors, then transmits the data to the CNS where it is processed. Four attributes of a stimulus are recorded by the sensory system: modality (quality), intensity, duration, and location. The external stimulus activates a special sensor, such as a photoreceptor, mechanoreceptor, thermoreceptor, chemoreceptor, or nociceptor, which receives then transforms it into electrochemical energy through sensory transduction. This energy is then

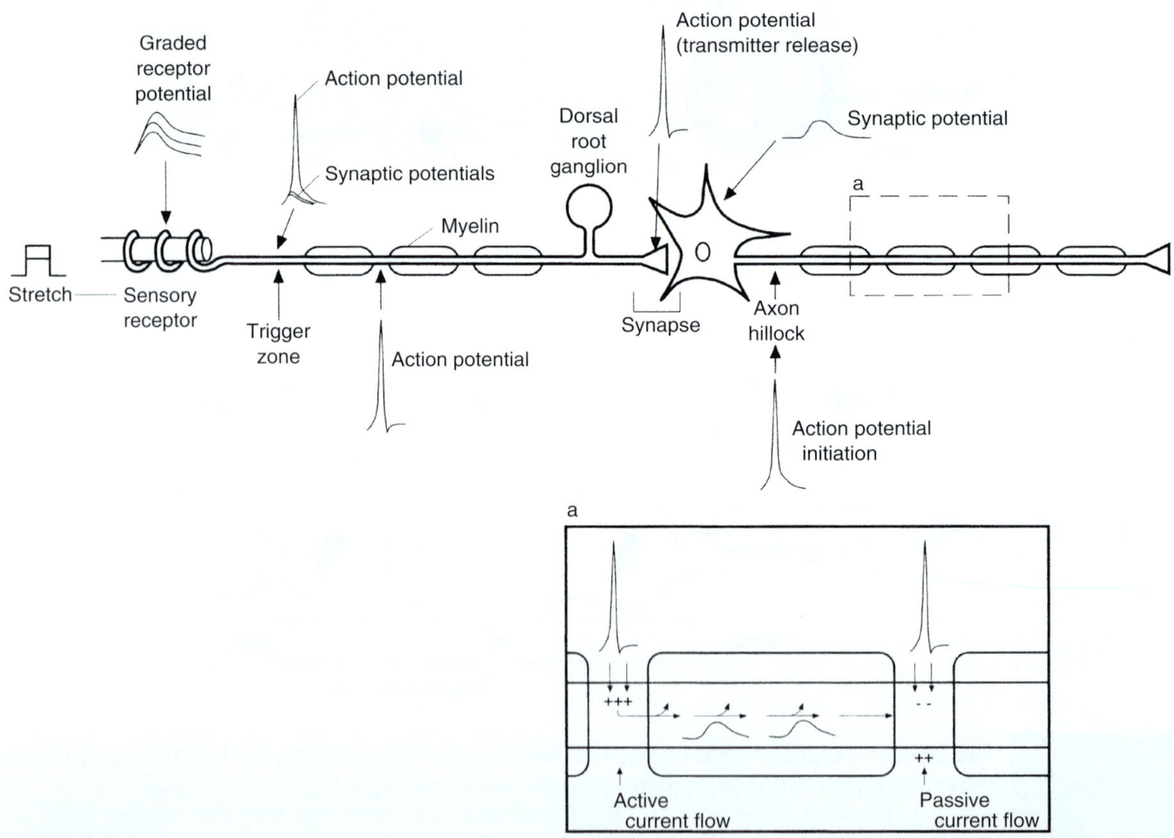

FIGURE 1.24 **Propagation of action potential and passive current flow. (*Source*: Nerve and muscle. In: Gamble JG (ed.), *The Musculoskeletal System–Physiologic Basics*. New York: Raven Press, 1988; 123, Fig 7.3.)**

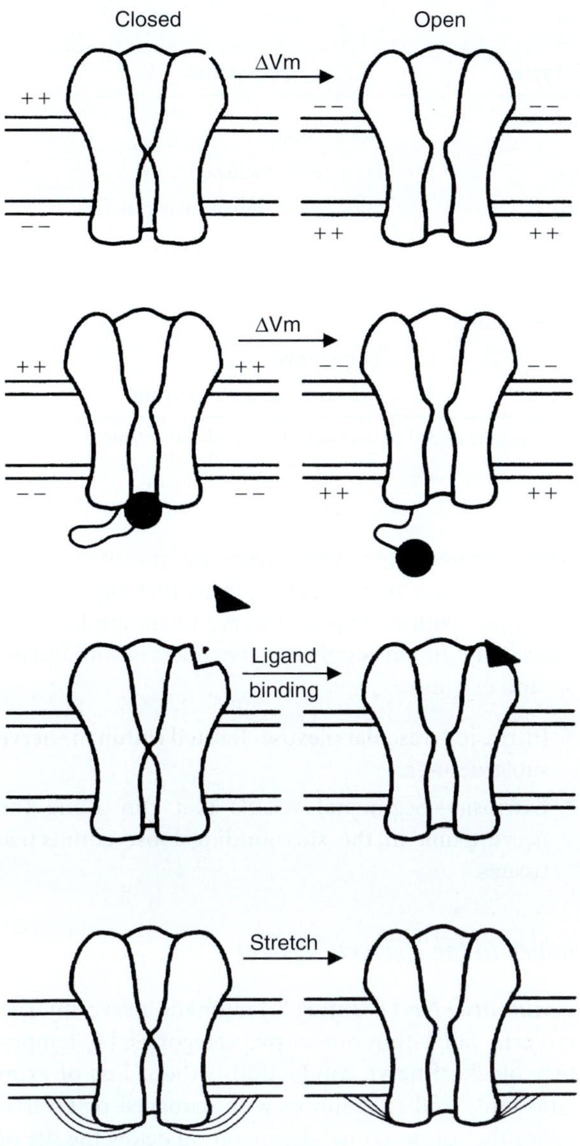

FIGURE 1.25 Channel gating is controlled by several types of stimuli. Changes in voltage can regulate a channel by causing a blocking particle to swing into or out of the channel mouth (often referred to as ball-and-chain model). Binding of a ligand to a receptor located on the channel or stretch or pressure can activate the channel by causing conformational changes in the channel. (*Adapted with permission from* Kandel ER, Schwartz JH, Jessell TM. *Principles of Neural Science*, 3rd ed. Norwalk, CT: Appleton & Lange, 1991; 75–76.)

transported to the CNS via action potentials for further processing.

Sensory information is conveyed to the brain via the dorsal column–medial lemniscal tract (touch and limb proprioception) and the anterolateral tract (pain and temperature). Specific sensory receptors are listed in Table 1.11. All somatosensory information (mechanical, pain, and temperature) is conveyed (via *afferent* fibers from the sensory system to the CNS) to the brain stem or spinal cord via dorsal root ganglion (DRG) neurons. The DRG facilitates sensory transduction and transmission of encoded stimuli (Fig. 1.26). Specific receptor types are listed in Table 1.12.

Motor System. Four major components comprise the motor system: spinal cord, brain stem and reticular formation, motor cortex, and premotor cortical areas (basal ganglia and cerebellum).

The spinal cord (Fig. 1.27) extends from the foramen magnum to the lower border of L1. Each spinal nerve contains a ventral (efferent) limb to transmit output to striated muscles and a dorsal (afferent) limb to carry sensory information from the somatic sensory receptors. The cell bodies of the afferent fibers are located within the DRG. The components of the motor system are as follows:

- *White matter*—Contains ascending and descending fiber tracts (both myelinated and unmyelinated nerve axons)
- *Gray matter*—Divided into the dorsal horn, intermediate zone, and ventral horn. Contains 3 types of neurons: (1) projections out of CNS via ventral roots (α- and γ-*motoneurons*), (2) *interneurons* (axonal projections that remain within the spinal cord), and (3) *tract cells*, which send ascending axonal projections to the supraspinal centers.
- *Lower motoneurons*—Movement is initiated by skeletal muscle contraction, which is innervated by lower motoneurons located within the ventral gray matter of the spinal cord.
- *Upper motoneurons*—Disruption of these motoneurons (by stroke, brain trauma, or spinal cord injury), which are located within the descending motor pathways, leads to common injury patterns (Table 1.13). Comparisons of upper and lower motoneuron lesions are listed in Table 1.14.
- *Motor unit*—Consists of an α-motoneuron and the fibers it innervates. Motor units are separated into 4 major types: (1) slow fatigue resistant (type S); (2) fast fatigue resistant (type FR); (3) fast fatigue intermediate (type FI); (4) fast fatiguable (type FF). See Table 1.15 for a summary.

TABLE 1.11 Sensory systems

Modality	Stimulus	Receptor Type	Receptors
Vision	Light	Photoreceptors	Rods, cones
Hearing	Sound	Mechanoreceptors	Hair cells (cochlear)
Balance	Head motion	Mechanoreceptors	Hair cells (semicircular canal)
Somatic	Mechanical	Mechanoreceptors	Dorsal root ganglion cells
	Thermal	Thermoreceptors	
	Noxious	Nociceptors, chemoreceptors	
Taste	Chemical	Chemoreceptors	Taste buds
Smell	Chemical	Chemoreceptors	Olfactory sensory neurons

Source: Kandel ER, Schwartz JH, Jessel TM (eds.). *Principles of Neural Science*, 3rd ed. Norwalk, CT: Appleton & Lange, 1991; 334.

Spinal Cord Reflexes. A reflex is a "stereotyped response" to a specific sensory stimulus that involves the receptor (sensory organ), the effector (motoneuron), and the bridging interconnecting neural elements, called interneurons (Table 1.16; Fig. 1.28).

- *Monosynaptic*—A reflex that involves only one synapse between the receptor and the effector organ.
- *Polysynaptic*—A reflex that involves more than one interneuron between the receptor and the effector organ.

Peripheral Nerve Anatomy. A peripheral nerve is a complex structure consisting of individual nerve fibers, vascular supply, and connective tissue. Figure 1.29 demonstrates the microarchitecture of a peripheral nerve. Individual nerve fibers, separated by *endoneurium* (loose collagenous matrix), are bundled into *fascicles*, which are surrounded by a dense connective tissue sheath, the *perineurium*. Fascicles are bound together by the protective *epineurium* layer, which protects the nerve from compressive forces and contains a rich vascular plexus that supplies the structures within. Types of nerve fibers are listed in Table 1.17. Blood supply to nerve fibers is both intrinsic and extrinsic.

- Intrinsic—vascular plexuses located within the nerve substructures.
- Extrinsic—Segmental vessels that run along the nerve trunk in the surrounding loose connective tissues.

Injury to the Nervous System

Traumatic Nerve Injury. Traumatic nerve injuries typically fall within one of two categories: (1) temporary block of nerve conduction without loss of axon continuity and (2) injuries with damaged or severed axons that cause axonal degeneration below the site of injury. Wallerian degeneration occurs, which is characterized by axon and myelin sheath disintegration

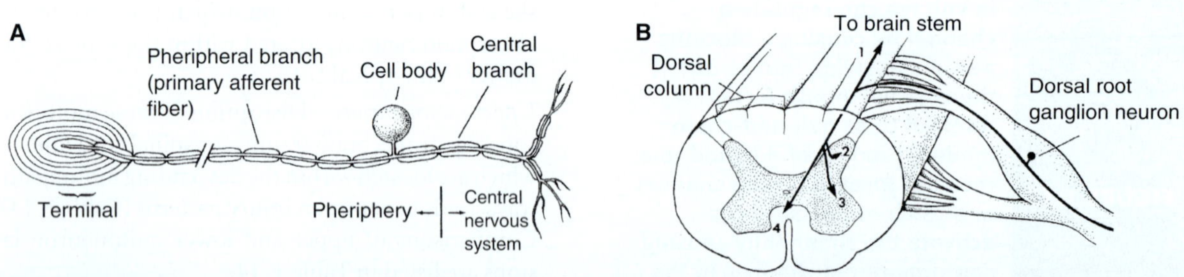

FIGURE 1.26 Projections of the central branch. The dorsal root ganglion cells that mediate pressure, touch, and proprioception have several central branches. The principal branch ascends in the dorsal column to the brain stem (1). The other branches terminate locally in the dorsal and ventral horns of the spinal cord (2, 3) or descend a few segments and terminate in the spinal cord (4). Branches 2, 3, and 4 participate in local spinal reflexes. (*Source*: Kandel ER, Schwartz JH, Jessell TM. *Principles of Neural Science*, 3rd ed. Norwalk, CT: Appleton & Lange, 1991; 287–342.)

TABLE 1.12 Receptor types

Receptor type	Fiber type	Quality
Nociceptors		
Mechanical	Aδ	Sharp, pricking pain
Thermal and mechanothermal	Aγ	Sharp, pricking pain
Thermal and mechanothermal	C	Slow, burning pain
Polymodal	C	Slow, burning pain
Cutaneous and subcutaneous mechanoreceptors		
Meissner's corpuscle	Aβ	Touch
Pacinian corpuscle	Aβ	Flutter
Ruffini corpuscle	Aβ	Vibration
Merkel's receptor	Aβ	Steady skin indentation
Hair-guard, hair-tylotrich	Aβ	Steady skin indentation
Hair-down	Aβ	Flutter
Muscle and skeletal mechanoreceptors		
Muscle spindle primary	Aα	Limb proprioception
Muscle spindle secondary	Aβ	Limb proprioception
Golgi tendon organ	Aα	Limb proprioception
Joint capsule mechanoreceptor	Aβ	Limb proprioception

Source: Kandel ER, Schwartz JH, Jessel TM (eds.). *Principles of Neural Science*, 3rd ed. Norwalk, CT: Appleton & Lange, 1991; 342.

along the myelin sheath distal to the site of injury. As a result, there is separation of the neuron cell body from the target organ (denervation). The response of the cell body is either regeneration or degeneration (cell death). Regeneration via axonal budding occurs after approximately a 1-month delay and occurs at the rate of 1 mm/day. Nerve injuries are typically classified into 3 types.

Neuropraxia	Reversible conduction block; local ischemia and selective demyelination of axon sheath; good prognosis
Axonotmesis	More severe injury characterized by disruption of the axon and myelin sheath, but the epineurium remains intact; prognosis fair
Neurotmesis	Complete nerve transection and connective tissue elements; prognosis poor

There are three primary causes of nerve injury.

Compression injury	Can be either acute or chronic. Nerve deficit results from both mechanical and ischemic factors (Fig. 1.30).
Double crush phenomenon	Injury characterized by nerve entrapment at one level with concomitant entrapment at another level within same extremity. Partial nerve entrapment may make the nerve more susceptible to compression at another site.
Nerve stretch injury	Can also be acute or chronic. Commonly occurs as a result of joint dislocations and fractures.

Neural Degeneration. Healing of nerve tissue is unique because it involves cellular repair, not tissue repair seen commonly in other areas following injury. The cell body of the neuron generates new axonal processes, which locate the target organ and reestablish synaptic capabilities. This process is demonstrated in Figure 1.31.

Axonal Regeneration. Regenerating axons from the proximal stump must cross the zone of injury to reach the distal stump. The reparative tissue in the gap between the stump ends resembles nerve tissue, but it is more extensive, denser, and more disorganized than the tissue between surgically reunited nerve ends.

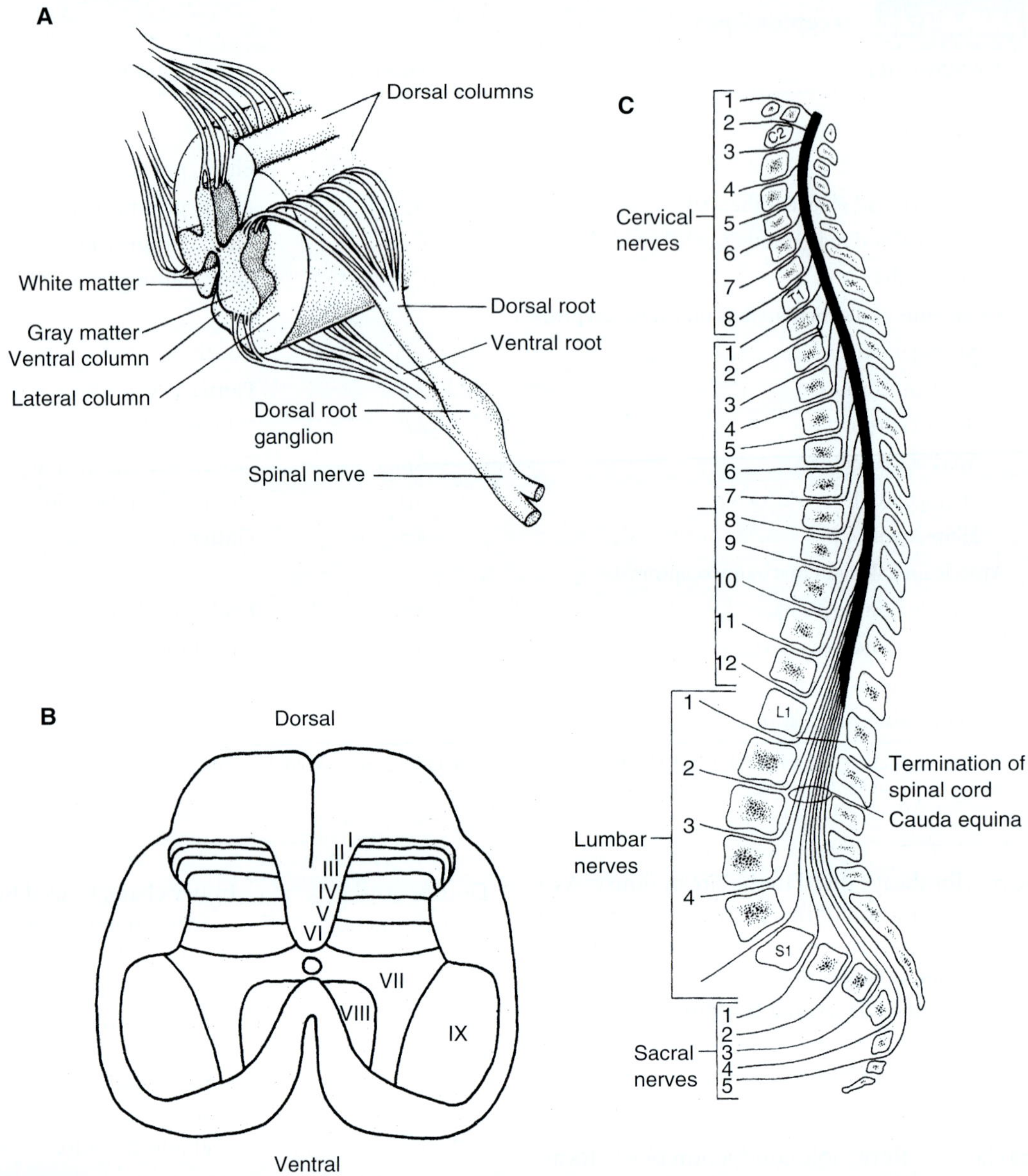

FIGURE 1.27 **Spinal cord anatomy. (A) Each spinal nerve has a dorsal and ventral root. The dorsal (sensory) root comprises the central branches of the dorsal root ganglion cells; the ventral (motor) root comprises the motor axons emerging from motoneurons in the ventral horn. (B) Location of Rexed's lamina within the dorsal and ventral horns of the spinal cord. (C) The individual spinal nerves are related to the 4 levels of the spinal cord. The adult spinal cord terminates at the border of L-1. The dorsal and ventral roots of the lumbar and sacral nerves within the vertebral column are collectively termed the cauda equina. (*Source*: A and C from Kandel ER, Schwartz JH, Jessell TM. *Principles of Neural Science*, 3rd ed. Norwalk, CT: Appleton & Lange, 1991; 285–286; B from Buckwalter JA, Einhorn TA, Simon SR. *Orthopaedic Basic Science: Biology and Biomechanics of the Musculoskeletal System*, 2nd ed. Rosemont, IL: American Academy of Orthopaedic Surgeons, 2000; 633, Fig 19.)**

TABLE 1.13 Findings in upper and lower motoneuron lesions

Findings	*Upper Motoneuron Lesion*	*Lower Motoneuron Lesion*
Stretch	Decreased	Decreased
Tone	Increased	Decreased
Deep tendon reflexes	Increased	Decreased
Superficial tendon reflexes	Decreased	Decreased
Babinski's sign	Present	Absent
Clonus	Present	Absent
Fasciculations	Absent	Present
Atrophy	Absent	Present

Source: Buckwalter JA, Einhorn TA, Simon SR. *Orthopaedic Basic Science: Biology and Biomechanics of the Musculoskeletal System*, 2nd ed. Rosemont, IL: American Academy of Orthopaedic Surgeons, 2000; 643.

The healing process that takes place is similar to that seen in other tissues, as previously described. Scar tissue in the gap acts to obstruct, delay, and slow down the development of advancing and regenerating axons. In the distal stump, the regenerating axon (from a myelinated nerve) stimulates the Schwann cells to form myelin. The rate of regeneration varies depending on the site and type of injury. Regeneration is typically slower following a transection compared with a crush injury. Human peripheral nerves typically regenerate at an average of 1 to 2 mm/day (Table 1.18).

Functional Recovery After Nerve Injury. Functional recovery is usually complete following a crush injury because the basement membrane and the endoneurium are intact, permitting the damaged axons a conduit for regeneration within their original endoneurial tubes. Following complete transection, recovery is poor because of misdirected regeneration of axons (scar) and inappropriate innervation of denervated muscles. Nerve regeneration is influenced by *contact guidance* (axon selects appropriate path according to molecular environment), *neurotrophism* (axons developing in correct path continue to be guided by nutritive or trophic factors), and *neurotropism* (axons guided by diffusible factors released from distal targets). Limited muscle recovery following denervation is related to (1) loss of muscle fibers, (2) loss of motor units, and (3) decreased capacity to increase muscle fiber size and reverse denervation-induced atrophy.

Surgical Nerve Repair. The main objectives of surgical repair are to maximize the number of axons that regenerate across the site of injury and to increase the accuracy of regenerating axons in reaching target

TABLE 1.14 Positive and negative symptoms observed in upper motoneuron lesions at various levels

	Level of Damage		
Damaged Pathway	*Spinal*	*Brain Stem/Caudal to the Red Nucleus*	*Brain Stem/Rostral to the Red Nucleus*
Pyramidal tract (corticospinal tract)	Weakness, loss of abdominal reflex, Babinski's sign	Weakness, loss of abdominal reflex, Babinski's sign, hyporeflexia, and hypotonia	Weakness, loss of abdominal abdominal reflex, Babinski's sign, seizure, apraxia, hyporeflexia, and hypotonia
Extrapyramidal tract (rubrospinal, reticulospinal, and vestibulospinal tracts)	Hyperreflexia, clonus spasticity, and clasp-knife reflex	Hyperreflexia, clonus spasticity, clasp-knife reflex, and decerebrate posture	Hyperreflexia, clonus spasticity, clasp-knife reflex, apraxia, and decorticate posture

Source: Buckwalter JA, Einhorn TA, Simon SR. *Orthopaedic Basic Science: Biology and Biomechanics of the Musculoskeletal System*, 2nd ed. Rosemont, IL: American Academy of Orthopaedic Surgeons, 2000; 643.

TABLE 1.15 General characteristics of motor unit types

Parameter	Motor Unit Types* FF	FR	S
Muscle unit physiology **			
Contraction time	Fastest	Slightly slower	Slowest
Sag	Present	Present	Absent
Maximum tension	Largest	Smaller	Smallest
Fatigue index	< 0.25	< 0.75–1.0	0.7–1.0
Muscle unit anatomy +			
Innervation ratio	2.9	2.1	1.0
Fiber cross-sectional area	1.3	0.98	1.0
Specific tension	1.4	1.2	1.0
Muscle unit metabolism			
Fiber type++	FG	FOG	SO
Myosin heavy chain	IIB	IIA	I
Glycogen	High	High	Low
Hexokinase	Low	Intermediate	High
Glycolytic enzymes	High	High	Low
Oxidative enzymes	Low	High	High
Cytochrome c	Low	High	High
Capillary supply	Sparse	Rich	Very rich
Motoneuron			
Cell body size	Largest	Slightly smaller	Smallest
Conduction velocity	Fastest	Slightly slower	Slowest
After-hyperpolarization duration	Shortest	Slightly shorter	Longest
Input resistance	Lowest	Slightly higher	Highest

* FF = fast fatigable; FR = fast fatigue resistant; S = fatigue resistant
** Data relative to the FF unit
+ Data relative to the slow unit
++ FG = fast glycolytic; FOG = fast oxidative glycolytic; SO = slow oxidative
Source: Buckwalter JA, Einhorn TA, Simon SR. *Orthopaedic Basic Science: Biology and Biomechanics of the Musculoskeletal System*, 2nd ed. Rosemont, IL: American Academy of Orthopaedic Surgeons, 2000; 634.

TABLE 1.16 Summary of spinal reflexes

Segmental Reflex	Receptor Organ	Afferent Fiber
Phasic stretch reflex	Muscle spindle (primary endings)	Type Ia (large myelinated)
Tonic stretch reflex	Muscle spindle (secondary endings)	Type II (intermediate myelinated)
Clasp-knife response	Muscle spindle (secondary endings)	Type II (intermediate myelinated)
Flexion withdrawal reflex	Nociceptors (free nerve endings), touch and pressure receptors	Flexor-reflex afferents: small unmyelinated cutaneous afferents (A-delta, C and muscle afferents, group III)
Autogenic inhibition	Golgi tendon organ	Type Ib (large myelinated)

Source: Buckwalter JA, Einhorn TA, Simon SR. *Orthopaedic Basic Science: Biology and Biomechanics of the Musculoskeletal System*, 2nd ed. Rosemont, IL: American Academy of Orthopaedic Surgeons, 2000; 639.

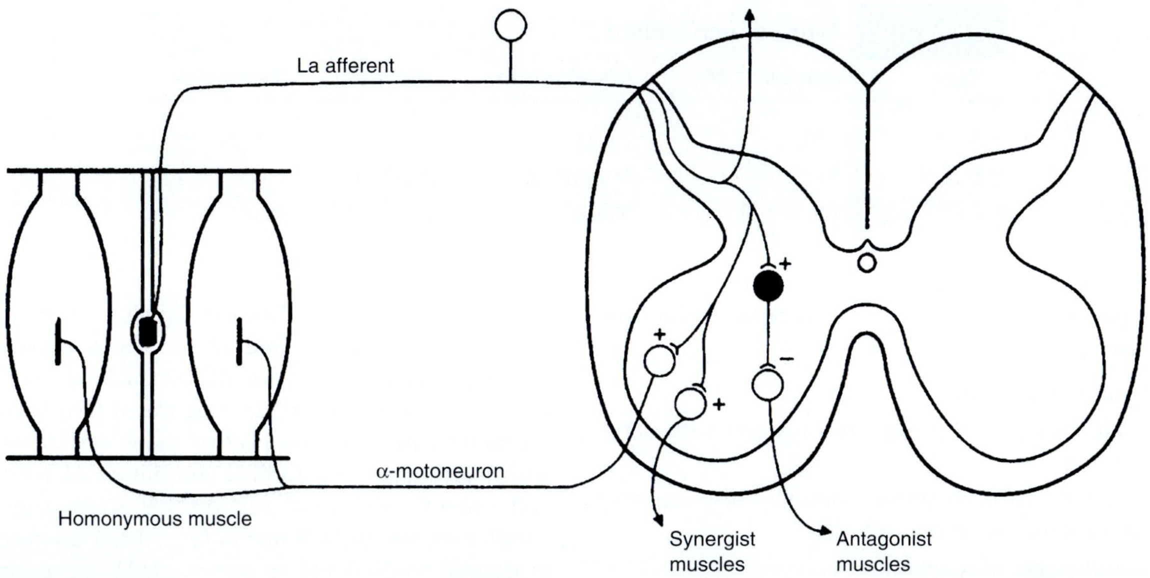

FIGURE 1.28 **The stretch reflex. Stretching the spindle activates the Ia afferent neuron, which synapses on the *a* motor neuron, producing efferent action potentials that cause the muscle to contract, relaxing the stretch on the spindle. *Adapted with permission from* Truex and Carpenter (1969). (*Source*: Costanzo LS. *Physiology*, 3rd ed. Philadelphia: Lippincott Williams & Wilkins, 2003; 56.)**

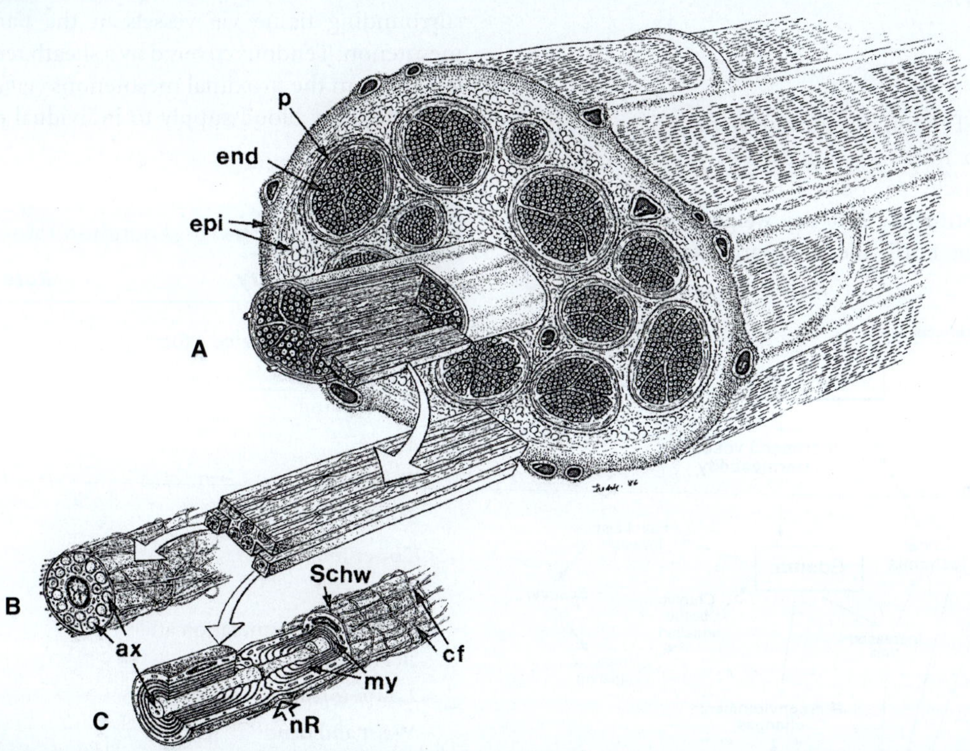

FIGURE 1.29 **Microanatomy of a peripheral nerve trunk and its components. (A) Fascicles surrounded by a multilaminated perineurium (p) are embedded in a loose connective tissue, the epineurium (epi). The outer layers of the epineurium are condensed into a sheath. (B) and (C) illustrate the appearance of unmyelinated and myelinated fibers, respectively. Schw = Schwann cell; my = myelin sheath; ax = axon; nR = node of Ranvier; cf = collagen fibrils. (*Reproduced with permission from* Lundborg G. *Nerve Injury and Repair.* New York: Churchill Livingstone, 1988; 33.)**

TABLE 1.17 Types of nerve fibers

Type	Diameter (μM)	Myelination	Speed	Examples
A	10–20	Heavy	Fast	Touch
B	< 3	Intermediate	Medium	ANS
C	< 1.3	None	Slow	Pain

organs. The basic principles in nerve repair include the following steps:

- Stump preparation
- Approximation of stump ends (careful with nerve tension)
- Coaptation of nerve stumps (optimal cross-sectional stump contact area apposition)
- Maintenance of coaptation

Several types of repairs have been described, including (1) direct muscular neurotization (insert proximal nerve stump directly into the muscle belly), (2) epineurial repair, and (3) grouped fascicular repair (reapproximation of individual fascicles under the microscope).

Tendon

Anatomy. Tendon is a composite material comprised of collagen fibrils in a matrix of proteoglycan that attach muscle to bone. Type I collagen is the major constituent (86% dry weight). Beginning with the collagen fibril, the microarchitecture of tendon increases in size by forming larger subunits of microfibrils, subfibrils, and fibrils. These units are closely packed in parallel orientation and held together to form fascicles (Fig. 1.32). Fascicles within tendon are bound by loose connective tissue (*endotenon*), which facilitates longitudinal movement of tendon and provides structural support for accompanying lymphatics, vessels, and nerves (e.g., flexor digitorum profundus tendon) and are surrounded by *epitenon.*

Tendon insertion into bone consists of four zones: tendon, fibrocartilage, mineralized fibrocartilage, and bone.

Blood Supply. Blood supply to the tendon comes from 3 sources: perimysium, periosteal insertion, and surrounding tissue via vessels in the paratenon or mesotenon. Tendons covered by a sheath receive blood supply from the proximal mesotenons (*vinculae*). The vinculae carry blood supply to individual portions of

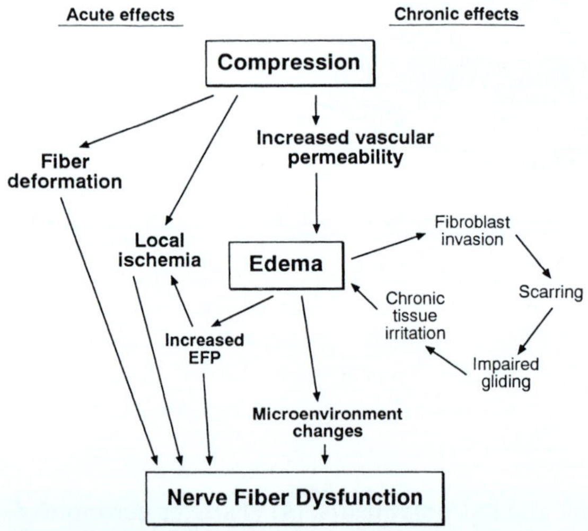

FIGURE 1.30 Effects of compression on intraneural tissues. (*Source:* Lundborg G. *Nerve Injury and Repair*. New York: NY, Churchill Livingstone, 1988; 64.)

TABLE 1.18 Axonal regeneration rate

Location of Injury	Rate (mm/day)
Rates of uncomplicated axon regeneration	
Root of limb	6
Elbow	4–5
Wrist	1–2
Hand	1–1.5
Lower limb	1–2
Ankle	1
Rates of axon regeneration after nerve suture	
Lower forearm	2
Wrist and hand	1
Upper leg	2
Lower leg	1.5
Ankle	1

Source: Buckwalter JA, Einhorn TA, Simon SR. *Orthopaedic Basic Science: Biology and Biomechanics of the Musculoskeletal System*, 2nd ed. Rosemont, IL: American Academy of Orthopaedic Surgeons, 2000; 674.

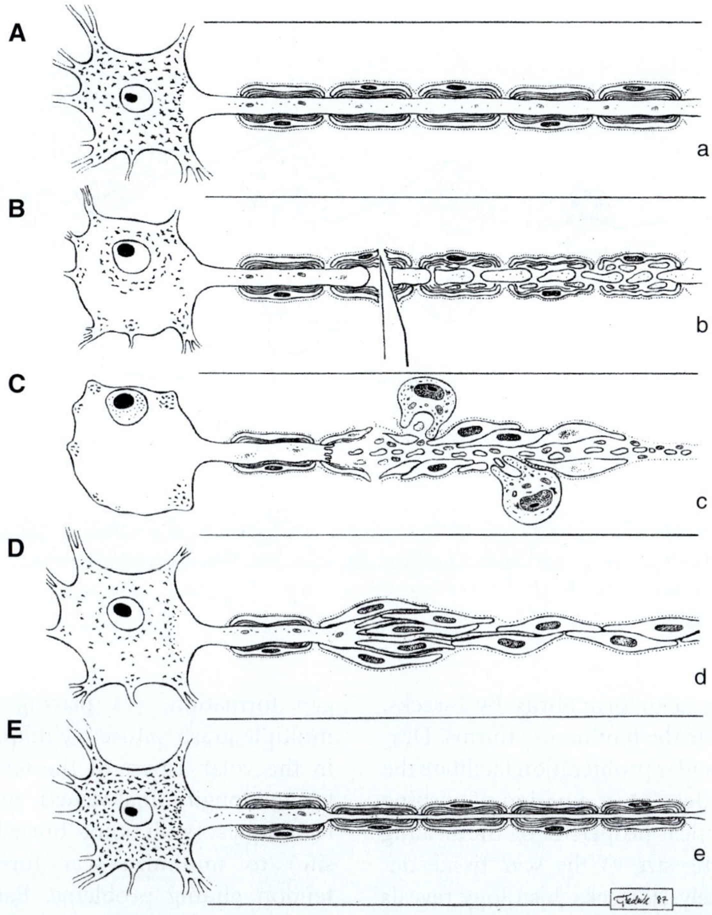

FIGURE 1.31 **Degeneration and regeneration of myelinated fiber. (A) Normal appearance. (B) Transection of the fiber results in distal fragmentation of axon and myelin. In the proximal segment, degeneration occurs at least to the nearest node of Ranvier. (C) In the distal segment, Schwann cells proliferate. Macrophages and Schwann cells phagocytose debris material. (D) The Schwann cells in the distal segment have lined up in bands of Büngner. Sprouting occurs from the cut axonal stump. Advancing sprouts are embedded in Schwann cell cytoplasm. (E) Axonal connection with periphery, maturation of nerve fiber. Sprouts that do not link up with the periphery may atrophy and disappear. The cell body response during these phases includes swelling, migration of the nucleus to the periphery, and condensation of basophilic material (chromatolysis). (*Source:* Lundborg G. *Nerve Injury and Repair.* New York: Churchill Livingstone, 1988; 151.)**

the tendon. Avascular areas that do not receive their own blood supply rely on diffusion from vascularized areas and from osseous insertions. Tendons covered by a *paratenon* (loose areolar connective tissue), however, are supplied by a rich source of peripheral vessels, which anastomose with a longitudinal system of capillary vessels and therefore heal better than sheathed tendons.

Sheathed Tendon Healing. Contrary to previous belief, recent studies have shown that tenocytes have intrinsic reparative capabilities. Specifically, a tissue cap forms on the lacerated tendon ends through proliferation and migration of cells originating from epitenon and endotenon. Following surgical tendon repair and controlled passive motion, the intrinsic healing response of the epitenon is dominant. With immobilization, however, the healing process is characterized by ingrowth of connective tissue from the digital sheath and cellular proliferation of the endotenon (Fig. 1.33).

Paratenon-Covered Healing. Animal studies have demonstrated that paratenon-covered tendon transection is immediately followed by an inflammatory process that initially provides no tensile strength. Disorganized fibroblasts infiltrate the gaps, and collagen synthesis begins as early as the third day. Collagen

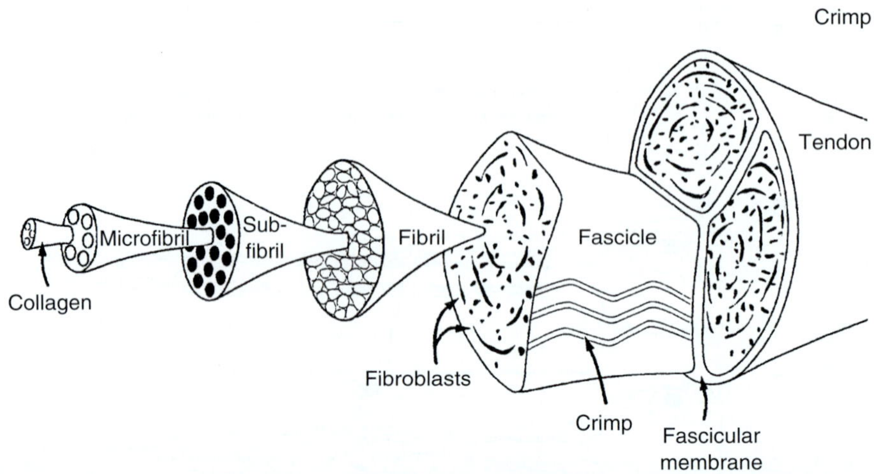

FIGURE 1.32 **Schematic representation of the microarchitecture of a tendon. (*Source*: Kastelic J, Baer E. Deformation in tendon collagen. In: Vincent JFV, Currey JD (eds.), *The Mechanical Properties of Biologic Materials.* Cambridge, England: Cambridge University Press, 1980; 397–435.)**

molecules begin to coalesce to form fibrils. By 2 weeks, a fibrous bridge connects the tendinous stumps. Dramatic fibroblast and vascular proliferation facilitate the uniting of the tendon edges. Over a period of ensuing months, the biomechanical properties of the healing tissue increase while the size of the scar tissue decreases. By approximately 20 weeks, histology reveals few differences between healed and native tendon. The ultimate biomechanical strength will depend on the loads applied to the healed tendon.

Tendon Repair. A variety of suture techniques have been described to optimize tendon healing potential (see Chapter 6). Key points include (1) minimizing gap formation, (2) placing multiple strands and multiple grasp suture techniques, (3) placing sutures in the volar aspect of the tendon to avoid dorsally located longitudinal vessels, and (4) using low-profile techniques (with knot buried within the lacerated site) to minimize scar formation and therefore tendon gliding problems. Early, controlled passive mobilization stimulates the repair and facilitates a strong repair. A careful balance must be achieved between stress and motion to promote healing without causing tendon damage. Tendon repairs are weakest at 7 to 10 days, regain most of their strength at 21 to 28 days, and achieve full strength at 6 months. Dynamic synergistic rehabilitation protocols provide the ideal amount of mobilization while protecting the repair, giving it time to heal.

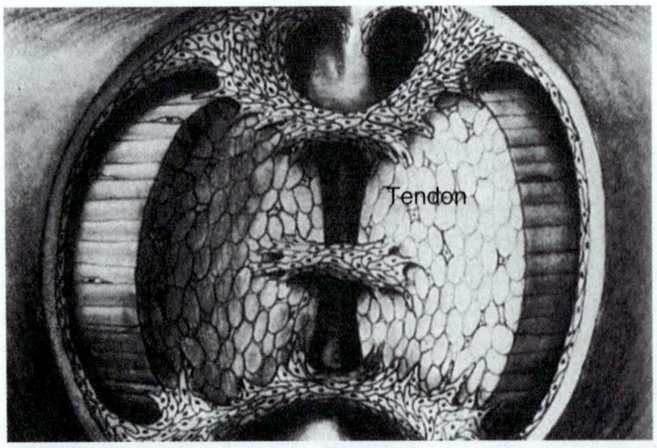

FIGURE 1.33 **Schematic drawing of an immobilized tendon illustrating extrinsic and intrinsic repair. (*Courtesy of* Dr. R. H. Gelberman, Boston.)**

Ligament

Anatomy. Ligaments are fibrous, flexible connections between bones. The structure and function of ligament is quite similar to tendons. Type I collagen predominates (70% dry weight). Compared with tendon, ligament has a higher content of *elastin*, which changes the mechanical properties of ligament. Direct ligamentous insertions into bone include 4 distinct zones of transition: ligament, fibrocartilage, mineralized fibrocartilage, and bone (Fig. 1.34).

Indirect ligamentous insertions (more common) are characterized by a superficial layer that connects directly with the periosteum and a deeper portion that connects to bone via *Sharpey's fibers* (Fig. 1.35).

Blood supply to ligaments has uniform microvascularity, which originates from the insertion sites and is

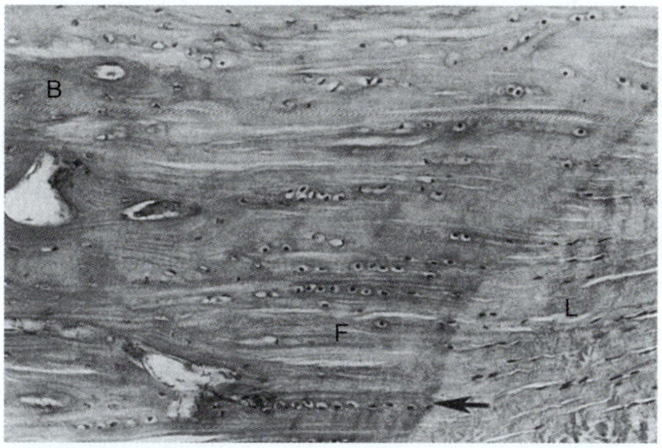

FIGURE 1.34 Femoral insertion of a rabbit MCL is typical direct insertion. The deep fibers of the ligament (L) pass into the bone (B) through a well-defined zone of uncalcified and calcified fibrocartilage (F). (*Source*: Woo SL-Y, Gomez MA, Sites TJ, et al. The biomechanical and morphological changes in the medial collateral ligament of the rabbit after immobilization and remobilization. *J Bone Joint Surg* 1987;69A:1200–1211.)

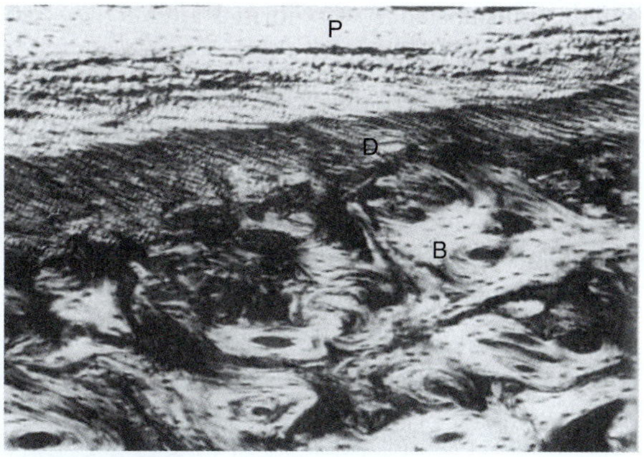

FIGURE 1.35 Indirect insertion of a rabbit MCL into the tibia showing superficial fibers (P) inserting into periosteum and the deep fibers (D) inserting obliquely into bone (B). (Hematoxylin and eosin, ×50.) (*Source*: Woo SL-Y, Gomez MA, Sites TJ, et al. The biomechanical and morphological changes in the medial collateral ligament of the rabbit after immobilization and remobilization. *J Bone Joint Surg* 1987;69A:1200–1211.)

responsible for the ongoing process of matrix synthesis and repair. Studies have shown that ligaments are innervated to some degree to provide pain sensation (spinal facet capsular ligaments) and proprioception (ACL, MCL).

Ligamentous Healing. There are three grades of ligamentous tears.

- *Grade I*—Mild sprains, which present with tenderness to palpation but no ligamentous laxity.
- *Grade II*—Reflect the incomplete disruption of some, but not all, ligamentous fibers. They are considered moderate sprains, which present with more pain and swelling and some detectable joint laxity.
- *Grade III*—These injuries are often less painful than grade II injuries but reflect complete disruption of all tendon fibers and therefore demonstrate significant joint laxity.

Healing of ligaments occurs in stages, as seen in the reparative process of other vascular tissues:

- *Phase I: Inflammation*—The torn ends of the ligaments are bathed in hematoma, which fills the gap and facilitates delivery of inflammatory mediators such as prostaglandins, vasodilators, histamine, and serotonin. Fibroblast proliferation occurs at the end of the inflammatory phase, which permits early scar formation. Most collagen produced in these early stages is type III, which is responsible for early stabilization of the collagen network.
- *Phase II: Matrix and cellular proliferation*—The ensuing 6 weeks is characterized by progressive organization of the fibrin clot, granulation tissue formation between torn ligament ends, and a transition to predominantly type I collagen. The improved mechanical properties of the scar reflect increasing type I collagen and proteoglycan concentrations.
- *Phases III and IV: Remodeling and maturation*—This phase is characterized by increase in collagen concentration, increased organization, and improved tensile strength. Complete remodeling is thought to occur by 12 months.

Immobilization and Remobilization. Although immobilization is often required in the early phases of healing, prolonged ligament immobilization may lead to altered mechanical properties, specifically a decrease in the elastic modulus. In a rabbit model, 9 weeks of immobilization decreased the load to failure by 66%. These detrimental effects on ligamentous properties reverse with remobilization. The ultimate load to failure at the ligament insertion reached 80% at 1 year, but the midsubstance was normal after 9 weeks of remobilization.

Skeletal Muscle

Structure and Function

Histology. The muscle fiber is a syncytium of many muscle cells fused together with multiple nuclei. Fiber arrangement can be either parallel or oblique (pennate, bipennate, multipennate) to the long axis of the muscle. Individual muscle fibers are surrounded by *endomysium*. Multiple fibers are arranged as *fascicles*, which are surrounded by *perimysium*. The entire muscle is encased in *epimysium*.

Muscle Membrane System. Electrical impulses from the *motor endplate* (point of contact between muscle fiber and nerve terminal) pass down a complex membrane system that facilitates communication between surface signals and the muscle fiber. *Transverse tubules*, located perpendicular to the axis of the cell, penetrate the fibers at the A-band and the I-band junctions and communicate with the *sarcoplasmic reticulum* (stores calcium). In response to the electrical impulse, calcium is released from the sarcoplasmic reticulum, which facilitates contractile proteins to interact and produce force (Fig. 1.36).

Structural Proteins of Muscle. Muscle fibers are composed of myofibrils, which itself is a collection of repeating units called *sarcomeres* (Fig. 1.37). Within each sarcomere, there are repeating light and dark bands. The dark band is the *A band*, which is composed of a parallel arrangement of thick filaments primarily composed of *myosin*. The myosin can bind to thin (*actin*) filaments and hydrolyzing ATP, which allows the fibers to slide past one another.

The *H band* contains only thick (myosin) filaments. The *I band* contains only thin (actin) filaments. These thin filaments are attached to the *Z line* (Fig. 1.38). Each sarcomere is bound by two adjoining Z lines.

Muscle Contraction. The chain of events that lead to muscle contraction is as follows: an electrical impulse generated in the cell body of a nerve traverses the length of the axon to reach the neuromuscular junction and the motor endplate. Presynaptic vesicles containing *acetylcholine* (Ach) are then released and traverse the synaptic cleft to bind a muscle membrane receptor. The binding of Ach triggers the release of calcium from the sarcoplasmic reticulum, which then binds to regulatory protein *troponin* on actin filaments. Binding of calcium to troponin induces a conformational change in *tropomyosin*, another regulatory protein, which can now no longer prevent the formation of cross-bridges on the actin filament. Contractile proteins actin and myosin are then free to interact, induce ATP hydrolysis, and slide past one another in the form of muscle contraction and the generation of force. Following muscle contraction, muscle relaxation occurs by driving calcium back into the sarcoplasmic reticulum, with subsequent restoration of troponin and tropomyosin on the actin filament to prevent cross-bridges and interaction with myosin.

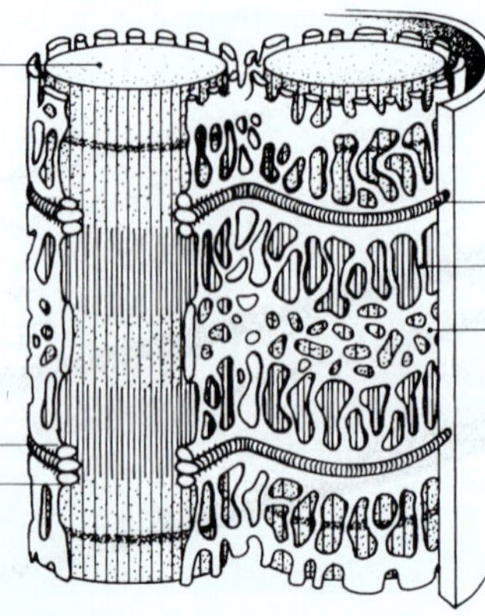

FIGURE 1.36 **Details of the sarcoplasmic reticulum (SR), the system of membranes responsible for transmission of the electrical signal from one muscle cell to the next. An action potential moving over the surface of the fiber passes down the transverse tubules and causes Ca^{2+} release from the outer vesicles of the SR. (*Source*: Buckwalter JA, Einhorn TA, Simon SR. *Orthopaedic Basic Science: Biology and Biomechanics of the Musculoskeletal System*, 2nd ed. Rosemont, IL: American Academy of Orthopaedic Surgeons, 2000; 687, Fig. 5.)**

Myotendinous Junction. The region of highly folded membranes at the muscle–tendon junction is called the myotendinous junction. It is responsible for transmission of forces from muscle fibers to limb for movement. It is a *common site of tears.*

Fiber Types and Adaptability of Muscle

Tonic muscles, located close to the skeleton, have a higher proportion of type I fibers. This is in contrast to phasic muscles, located more superficially, that contract faster and therefore have a higher proportion

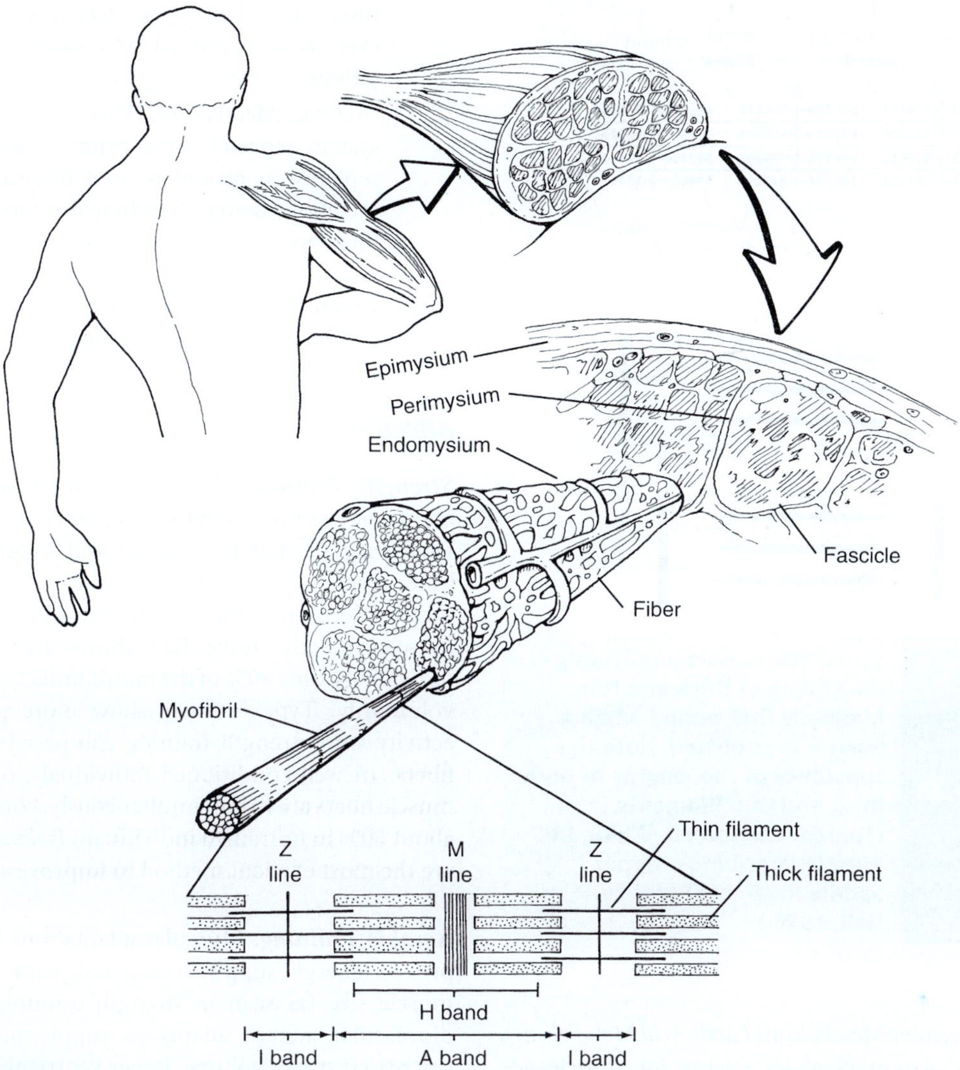

FIGURE 1.37 **Skeletal muscle architecture. (*Source*: Brinker MR, Miller MD. *Fundamentals of Orthopaedics.* Philadelphia: WB Saunders, 1999; 10.)**

of type II fibers. Similarly, endurance athletes will be more likely to have predominantly type I fibers, and sprinters type II fibers. Characteristics of muscle fiber types are listed in Table 1.19.

- Muscle fiber types (Table 1.20)
- Types of muscle contractions (Table 1.21)
- Energetics—Three systems supply energy stores for the generation of muscle activity. The predominant system is dependent on the intensity and length of time for which the muscular activity is required (Fig. 1.39).

1. *Phosphagen System (or Adenosine Triphosphate-Creatine Phosphate System)*. This energy storage system provides ATP (and high-energy phosphate compounds, or phosphagens) for muscle activities of short duration (~20 seconds), such as sprinting 100 to 200 meters. The production of energy from ATP hydrolysis and high-energy phosphate bonds is as follows:

$$\text{ATP} \diamond \text{ADP} + \text{P} + \text{Energy}$$

$$\text{ADP} \diamond \text{AMP} + \text{P} + \text{Energy}$$

This system does not require oxygen and does not produce lactate.

Another source of high-energy phosphate bonds is creatine phosphate (CP). In this system, however, energy is derived indirectly through the synthesis of ATP from ADP according to these equations:

$$\text{ADP} + \text{CP} \diamond \text{ATP} + \text{creatine}$$

$$\text{ADP} + \text{ADP} \diamond \text{ATP} + \text{AMP}$$

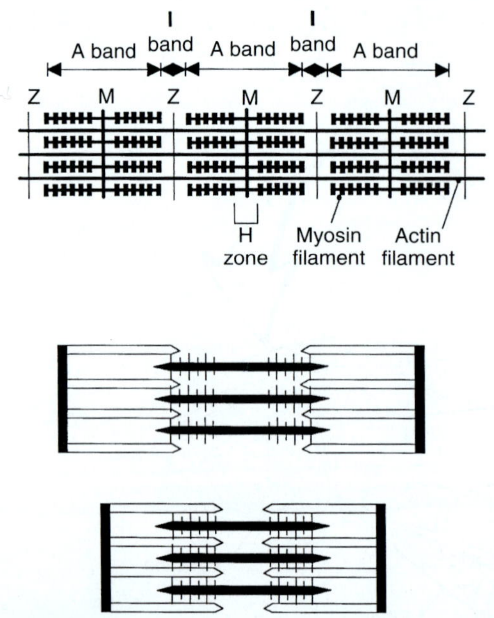

FIGURE 1.38 Schematic drawing indicating the sliding of thick and thin filaments that occurs when a muscle is stretched. Note the constancy of the lengths of both thick and thin filaments. (*Source*: Carlson FD, Wilkie DR. *Muscle Physiology.* Upper Saddle River, NJ: Prentice Hall, 1974.)

2. *Anaerobic Metabolism (Lactic Acid Metabolism).* This system provides energy for muscle activities of intermediate duration (~20 to 120 seconds), such as sprinting 400 meters. It involves the hydrolysis of glucose molecules to produce 2 molecules of lactic acid and 2 ATP molecules. The lactic acid produced, however, is toxic, which may cause acidosis and fatigue.
3. *Aerobic Metabolism.* This oxygen-dependent system represents the primary mode of ATP replenishment and is used in situations with metabolic demands of long duration and lower intensity muscular activities. Essentially, glucose or fatty acids are broken down to pyruvate, which then enters the Krebs cycle, and ATP is produced via oxidative phosphorylation.

Athletics

Strength Training. High-force (increased tension) and low-repetition activity increases muscle strength. Data suggests that hyperplasia and hypertrophy are both responsible for the increase in strength. An increase in motor-unit recruitment may also increase muscle strength. Studies have shown that in untrained individuals, only 80% of the motor units are stimulated voluntarily. Type II fibers show more pronounced activity with strength training compared with type I fibers. In well-conditioned individuals, over 90% of muscle fibers are firing simultaneously, compared with about 60% in untrained individuals. *Isokinetic exercises* are the most efficient method to improve strength.

Aerobic Training. Muscular adaptations involve improved energy supply, compared with changes in muscle size (as seen in strength training). The cardiovascular system adapts to supply more oxygen (increased stroke volume, larger ventricular size), and the circulatory system modifies arteriole control to improve blood flow to muscles. At the muscular-cellular level, increases in the numbers and density of mitochondria, capillary density, and oxidative capacity are

TABLE 1.19 Characteristics of human skeletal muscle fiber types

Other Names	*Type I* *Red, slow twitch (ST)* *Slow oxidative (SO)*	*Type IIA* *White, fast twitch (FT)* *Fast oxidative glycolytic (FOG)*	*Type IIB* *Fast glycolytic* *(FG)*
Speed of contraction	Slow	Fast	Fast
Strength of contraction	Low	High	High
Fatigability	Fatigue-resistant	Fatigable	Most fatigable
Aerobic capacity	High	Medium	Low
Anaerobic capacity	Low	Medium	High
Motor unit size	Small	Larger	Largest
Capillary density	High	High	Low

Source: Buckwalter JA, Einhorn TA, Simon SR. *Orthopaedic Basic Science: Biology and Biomechanics of the Musculoskeletal System*, 2nd ed. Rosemont, IL: American Academy of Orthopaedic Surgeons, 2000; 692, with permission.

TABLE 1.20 Muscle fiber types

Type	Metabolic Capacity	Function
I (red/slow twitch)	Aerobic (contain high numbers of mitochondria, enzymes, triglycerides; low amount of glycogen, glycolytic enzymes)	Endurance activities; first fibers lost without rehabilitation
II (white/fast twitch)	Anaerobic (contain high amount of glycogen, low triglyceride stores); high contraction speeds, quick relaxation times	High-intensity, short-duration activities

TABLE 1.21 Types of muscle contractions

Type of Muscle Contraction	Definition	Example	Phases
Isotonic	**Muscle tension is constant through the range of motion.** Muscle *length changes* through the range of motion. This is a measure of *dynamic strength.*	Biceps curls using free weights.	**Concentric contraction:** The muscle shortens during the contraction. Tension within the muscle is proportional to the externally applied load. An example of an isotonic concentric contraction is *the "curl"* (elbow moving toward increasing flexion) portion of a biceps curl. **Eccentric contraction:** The muscle "*lengthens*" during the contraction (internal force is less than external force). **Eccentric contractions have the greatest potential for high muscle tension and muscle injury.** An example of an isotonic eccentric contraction is "*the negative*" (elbow moving toward increasing extension) portion of a biceps curl.
Isometric	Muscle tension is generated, but the length of the muscle remains unchanged. This is a measure of *static strength.*	Pushing against an immovable object (such as a wall).	
Isokinetic	Muscle tension is generated as the muscle maximally contracts at a constant velocity over a full range of motion. Isokinetic exercises are *best for maximizing strength (specifically eccentric phase)* and are a measure of *dynamic strength.*	Isokinetic exercises require special equipment such as a Cybex machine.	Concentric; eccentric

Source: Miller MD. *Review of Orthopaedics*. Philadelphia: W.B. Saunders, 2004; 70.

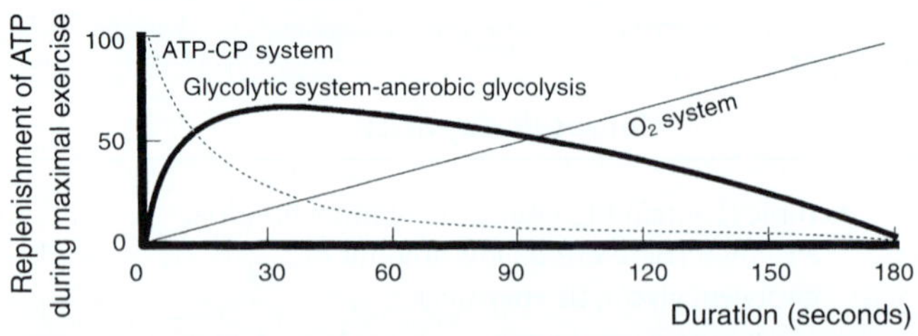

FIGURE 1.39 **Energy sources for anaerobic activity. (*Source*: Buckwalter JA, Einhorn TA, Simon SR. *Orthopaedic Basic Science: Biology and Biomechanics of the Musculoskeletal System*, 2nd ed. Rosemont, IL: American Academy of Orthopaedic Surgeons, 2000; 694, Fig. 12.)**

seen. There is also an increase in the percentage of oxidative IIA fibers.

Sprint or Power Training. One of the primary modifications in this type of activity is an increase in the level of stored phosphagens, in addition to elevated concentrations of enzymes responsible for glycolysis. *Plyometrics* ("bounding" exercises) are the most efficient method for improving power. They are characterized by a muscle stretch followed immediately by a rapid contraction. An example of a plyometric exercise is "jumping rope," in which the sequential stretch and contraction of the gastrocnemius/soleus complex allows one to repetitively perform this exercise.

Muscle Injury and Repair

Muscle Laceration. Following complete muscle laceration, full recovery is uncommon. In a rabbit model, muscle was shown to heal with a dense connective tissue scar. Mid-belly lacerations followed by suture repair recovered approximately 50% of their original tensile strength and shortened approximately 80% of normal.

Muscle Contusion. Mobilized muscles demonstrated improved recovery of tensile properties compared with immobilized muscle. Severe blunt injury may cause myositis ossificans (MO). In an animal model, the amount of bone formed was proportional to the number of episodes of injury and hematoma formation.

Muscle Strains. Most muscle strains occur at the myotendinous junction, commonly following a rapid *eccentric contraction*. Acutely, inflammatory changes and edema are seen at the site of the tear. Animal studies have shown significant scar formation at 1 week and a decreased ability to produce muscle tension, which approached normal level by 7 days postinjury.

Muscle Soreness. Muscular pain that develops 24 to 72 hours following intensive muscle activity. It is associated primarily with eccentric activities and reaches a maximum by about 1 to 3 days. Muscles may appear firm and swollen, suggesting an increase in intramuscular pressure. Soreness may be associated with changes in the I band of the sarcomere.

Muscle Cramps. The physiology of cramps is not completely understood. Cramps commonly occur following fatigue, prolonged muscle activity, dehydration, lowered levels of calcium and magnesium, or during sleep when the muscle remains in a shortened position.

Immobilization and Disuse. Muscle immobilized for a long period of time causes a reduction in muscle size, structure, and physiologic and metabolic properties. Disuse (bedrest, pain avoidance strategies) induces similar changes. Clinically, muscle atrophy, loss of muscle strength, and increased fatigability are seen. Such changes are more commonly seen in muscles immobilized under no tension. Insulin sensitivity of immobilized muscle is also dramatically reduced, thereby diminishing the ability of glucose to enter muscle.

Hormonal Effects on Skeletal Muscle

Insulin. Secreted by the pancreas, insulin increases the storage of glucose, fatty acids, and amino acids. Insulin demonstrates anabolic activity as it facilitates the entry of glucose into muscle, increased glycogen synthesis, and decreased protein catabolism.

Growth Hormone. Somatotropin, or growth hormone (GH), is synthesized in the anterior pituitary gland and is therefore under hypothalamic control. Its anabolic effects on muscle include the increasing amino acid transport and production of proteins in cells, which ultimately leads to increased synthesis of skeletal muscle. Other factors may more directly mediate muscle synthesis, including insulinlike growth factor-1 (IGF-1). Growth hormone is essential to proper development of bone, adipose tissue, and skeletal muscle. Excessive GH production before physeal closure leads to gigantism, and after physeal closure, to acromegaly. Deficiency before physeal closure leads to dwarfism.

Steroids. The precise mechanism by which anabolic steroids increases muscle protein synthesis, muscle size, and strength is currently unknown. Steroids have received much attention recently because of illegal steroid use by Olympic and professional athletes who participate in sports requiring large anaerobic energy (sprinting, weightlifting). The potentially serious and life-threatening side effects of anabolic steroids are well-documented. Side effects of anabolic steroids include virilization, increased aggression, sense of euphoria, decreased levels of high-density lipoprotein (HDL), stroke, myocardial infarction, liver dysfunction, oligospermia, azoospermia, voice changes, and premature physeal closure.

Testosterone. This hormone has a significant anabolic effect on skeletal muscle. Produced in the Leydig cells of the testicles and to a lesser extent in the adrenal cortex, its anabolic effects include increasing protein synthesis and decreasing catabolism in muscle cells. Like anabolic steroids, testosterone can also induce premature physeal closure in children and adolescents.

Creatine Supplements. Commonly used by athletes, creatine supplements rely on conversion of creatine to phosphocreatine, an additional energy store for ATP. Although creatine does not increase the peak force generated, it increases the amount of work in the first few maximum-effort anaerobic repetitions.

Intervertebral Disks

Anatomy

Disk Structure and Function. The intervertebral disk (IVD) is situated between two rigid bodies that together, with the IVD, comprise the *mobile spinal motion segment.* Thus, the disk must be soft enough to permit large, complex, three-dimensional motion and simultaneously stiff enough to provide stability to the motion segment and spinal column. This dichotomous behavior is achieved by the unique ability of the IVD to absorb and dissipate energy through the complex biomechanical interactions of the constituents of the IVD, described below.

Nucleus Pulposus. The nucleus pulposus is a gelatinous structure composed of a meshwork of loosely organized collagen fibrils located within the center of the IVD. Nondegenerate disks are well hydrated with a water concentration of approximately 70% to 80%, while collagens comprise about 20%. Proteoglycans account for about 50% of the dry weight of the nucleus. The major collagen constituent is type II, and the nucleus also receives contributions from collagen types V, VI, IX, and XII. The negatively charged glycosaminoglycans on proteoglycan molecules attract positively charged water molecules and provide large osmotic pressures, which resists *compressive* loads to which the spine is constantly subjected.

Annulus Fibrosus. The annulus is a fibrocartilaginous structure that surrounds the nucleus pulposus. It is composed of 15 to 40 concentric layers of collagen fibers oriented at approximately 30 degrees to the horizon. Water comprises about 65% of annulus tissue. Type I collagen is the main constituent of the stiffer outer annulus fibrosus, while the less-dense inner annulus reflects a shift toward a higher concentration of type II collagen, as in the nucleus. The annulus is primarily responsible for resisting the large *tensile* forces to which the disk is subjected during the activities of daily living.

Endplate. The cartilaginous endplate consists of type II collagen and is located at the superior and inferior margins of the vertebral bodies. This structure plays an important role in supporting and distributing the load from the disk to the vertebra

Disk Degeneration. Hallmark findings of disk degeneration include a loss of hydration; diminished proteoglycan concentration; changes in disk size; annular cracks, fissures, and tears; endplate calcification; and cell death. Related changes to surrounding structures include vertebral osteophytes, increased bone density or sclerosis, and facet joint arthrosis. Although disk degeneration is considered a major source of low back pain, the precise mechanisms by which disk degeneration causes back pain remain unclear.

V. ORTHOPAEDIC INFECTIONS AND MICROBIOLOGY

One the most common and devastating problems facing orthopaedics is infection of the musculoskeletal system. This topic is particularly of interest to orthopaedic surgeons in general not only because of its debilitating effects on patients but also because much infection is indeed the result of surgical intervention endeavoring to solve other orthopaedic problems. It is very important for the responsible orthopaedic surgeon to understand how musculoskeletal infections occur, how to effectively treat the resulting condition, and moreover, how to prevent such occurrences if possible.

This section provides a brief overview of the prominent orthopaedic infections and includes content on treatment and prophylaxis where appropriate.

Musculoskeletal Infections

Acute Hematogenous Osteomyelitis (AHO). Bone infection caused by blood-borne pathogens. AHO is most commonly seen in children; boys are affected more than girls. In children, AHO most commonly affects the metaphyseal or epiphyseal regions of the long bones but doesn't normally cross the physis. The reason AHO does not cross the physis is not completely understood, but is thought to be partly due to the orientation of the vasculature in the rapidly growing metaphysis in the area near the physis. Here the blood slows considerably and exhibits a decreased oxygen tension, which directly contributes to hematogenous bacterial seeding and to decreased immune function in that area (Fig. 1.40). Physical examination findings can include pain, fever, and the potential loss of function of the affected limb. Newborns with this condition, however, may not be febrile. In cases of AHO in the neonate, blood cultures can often be helpful in establishing a positive diagnosis. The basic laboratory work-up of patients with a suspected osteomyelitis includes a complete blood count (CBC) with differential, erythrocyte sedimentation rate (ESR), and C-reactive protein (C-RP). C-RP is the most sensitive indicator of infection in children with AHO. Generated by the liver, it is normally present in very small amounts in the plasma and can increase to significantly higher levels within a few hours of onset, eventually peaking around 2 days after onset. An elevated ESR and elevated WBC count may also be present.

Radiographic evidence includes soft-tissue swelling early on with loss of tissue planes. Bone lysis follows 1 to 2 weeks later. The infection can leave behind bacteria-laden devascularized necrotic bone, called a sequestrum, which can harbor bacteria and slow down (if not halt) antibiotic eradication. This condition is further complicated with the formation of new periosteal bone, called an involucrum, around the sequestrum some time later. If early radiographs are inconclusive but infection is still suspected, then another useful tool is technetium-99 m (Tc99m) triple-phase bone scan. The first two phases of this scintigraphic examination, which are completed within the first 5 minutes of the scan, are associated with determining blood flow and determining where the blood is pooling. The third phase, and the one most helpful in diagnosing osteomyelitis, is related to the incorporation of Tc99m diphosphonate into new lamellar bone by osteoblasts

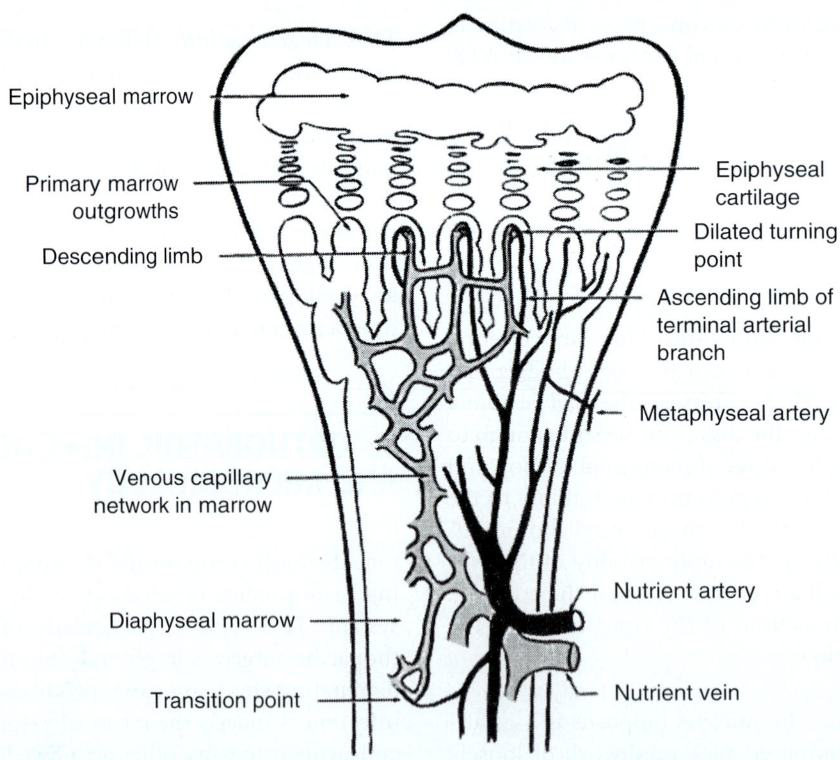

FIGURE 1.40 **Metaphyseal sinusoids where sluggish blood flow increases susceptibility to osteomyelitis. (*Source*: Tachdjian MO. *Pediatric Orthopaedics*, 2nd ed. Philadelphia: WB Saunders, 1990.)**

at the site of infection. Infection is strongly suggested if activity is detected in the bone within 3 hours. Tc99m triphasic bone scans are sensitive in detecting acute osteomyelitis, but false-positive results can occur in patients with underlying skeletal illness. False-negative results can occur frequently in neonates (under 6 months old). Other nuclear scans exist, such as gallium-67, indium-111, and newer Tc99m-hexamethylpropylene amine oxime complex (HMPAO) leukocyte labeling. All have their utility but can be difficult to do and time-consuming, and they are not necessarily better than Tc99m scintigraphy in all situations. In addition to these tests, positron-emission tomography (PET) scans have improved in their ability to detect bone infection, with some studies revealing very high accuracy rates. Unfortunately, they still suffer from a lack of volume in evidence and from expensive detection equipment. The newest methods, involving conjugation of isotopes to immunoglobulins (immunoscintigraphy), hold promise for detecting infection and inflammation, especially in evaluating infection in joints after total joint arthroplasties. A detailed discussion of the various scintigraphy investigations is beyond the scope of this chapter, but see Table 1.22 for a brief overview of the advantages and disadvantages of some in the evaluation of orthopaedic infection. Magnetic resonance imaging (MRI) is both highly sensitive and highly specific, and shows changes in bone and bone marrow before radiographs do. The shortcomings, however, are artifact in patients with prostheses and the expense of MRI testing. After obtaining cultures via aspiration or surgical drainage, empiric therapy should be started immediately (Table 1.23).

Indications for operative intervention include:

1. The need to drain an abscess
2. Débridement of infected tissues to prevent the spread of the infection and promote healthy tissue ingrowth
3. Refractory cases where nonoperative treatment has failed

Acute Osteomyelitis (Nonhematogenous). Acute osteomyelitis results from open fracture or open reduction with internal fixation (ORIF) procedures. The infection is most commonly populated by *Staphylococcus aureus* and *Pseudomonas aeruginosa*, although it can uncommonly be associated with coliforms. Empiric therapy includes a PRSP (i.e., nafcillin, methicillin) with a fluoroquinolone such as ciprofloxacin or vancomycin with a third-generation cephalosporin. Diabetics and others with peripheral vasculopathy can often manifest a mixed flora (polymicrobial) picture.

Subacute Osteomyelitis. As the name suggests, this manifestation of osteomyelitis has very few clinical cues aside from potentially painful local signs such as a painful gait or a limp. Subacute osteomyelitis includes an often normal WBC count and negative blood culture. It can arise from a nutrient-rich matrix such as a fracture hematoma but can also be the result of an incompletely treated acute osteomyelitis. It commonly affects the long bones of the leg (usually the femur and tibia) and can cross the physis. This can be evaluated radiographically with the presence of a Brodie abscess, a cortically confined radiolucency mostly seen in the metaphyseal region of the long bones. Elevated ESR and culture from the suspected bone can be beneficial in establishing a diagnosis. The radiographic appearance of a Brodie abscess in the metaphysis or in the epiphysis can be very much like the radiographic appearance of bony tumors such as Ewing sarcoma (metaphysis) or chondrosarcoma (epiphysis). Therefore, prudence must be exercised to rule out malignancy to ensure proper treatment. Interestingly, epiphyseal osteomyelitis is almost always caused by *S. aureus* and requires surgical intervention only if pus is present.

Chronic Osteomyelitis. Chronic osteomyelitis is a severe and often debilitating infection of the bone and marrow characterized by continued inflammation over time that leads to lysis, deformity, and sclerosis. The general radiographic picture of bone resorption and new periosteal bone formation may give the impression of dysplasia or malignancy. Therefore, as with a Brodie abscess, a biopsy may be necessary for a sure diagnosis. Chronic osteomyelitis may result from an incompletely treated acute condition, trauma, open fracture, direct spread from adjacent soft tissues, or iatrogenic causes like joint arthroplasties. Populations particularly at risk are the nutritionally deficient, the elderly, the immunosuppressed, IV drug abusers, and diabetics. Cierney and Mader, 1990 proposed an anatomic classification for chronic osteomyelitis (Fig. 1.41).

Type 1	Medullary or endosteal infection
Type 2	Superficial infection
Type 3	Localized, well-marked infection with sequestration and cavity formation
Type 4	Diffuse osteomyelitis

The most common organism causing chronic osteomyelitis is *S. aureus*, along with the less common *P. aeruginosa* and *Enterobacter*. Infection most commonly occurs in the metaphyses of the long bones. It is not reliable to determine specific microscopic organism causing chronic osteomyelitis based on stratification criteria such as age or history. Instead, one must obtain deep cultures to make a specific microbiologic diagnosis. Cultured sinus tract drainage, if a sinus tract exists, should not be used as a sole source

TABLE 1.22 Use of scintigraphic imaging in orthopaedic infections

Primary Imaging	Secondary Imaging	Advantages	Disadvantages
Acute Infection			
Bone scan		Readily available High sensitivity	2- to 3-hour delay between injection and imaging Low specificity
	Technetium (Tc99m) HMPAO* leucocyte scan	Infection/inflammation visualized more rapidly than indium	Time-consuming preparation Lower radiation dose Requires a specialized labeling facility
	Indium-111 (In111) leucocyte scan		Time-consuming preparation Requires specialized labeling facility
	Technetium-labeled (Tc99m) antigranulocyte antibody (immunoscintigraphy)	Kit product Readily available Rapid imaging Appears to have high sensitivity and specificity in prosthetic infection	Variable sensitivity
	Gallium-67 (Ga67)	No preparation needed	May need a delay to order the radiotracer High radiation dose High sensitivity but specificity is lower
	Fluorodeoxyglucose (FDG) PET	High accuracy reported in the literature	Cyclotron to produce radiotracer Expensive camera imaging Only small numbers of patients studied
Chronic Infection			
Bone scan		Readily available High sensitivity	2- to 3-hour delay between injection and imaging Low specificity
	Gallium-67 (Ga67)	No preparation needed	May need a delay to order the radiotracer High radiation dose High sensitivity but specificity is lower
	Indium-111 (In111) leucocyte scan	Specific for inflammation or infection	Time-consuming preparation Requires specialized labeling facility

TABLE 1.22 *(continued)*

Primary Imaging	Secondary Imaging	Advantages	Disadvantages
Infections of the Spine			
Bone scan		Readily available High sensitivity	2- to 3-hour delay between injection and imaging Low specificity
	? FDG PET	Imaging within 1 hour	Cyclotron to produce radiotracer
		Result available by the end of the day	Expensive camera imaging
			Only small numbers of patients studied
Prosthetic Joint Infections			
Bone scan		Readily available High sensitivity	2- to 3-hour delay between injection and imaging Low specificity
	Gallium-67 (Ga67)	No preparation needed	May need a delay to order the radiotracer High radiation dose High sensitivity but specificity is lower
	Indium-111 (In111) leucocyte scan		Time-consuming preparation Requires specialized labeling facility
	Technetium-labeled (Tc99m) antigranulocyte	Kit product	
	antibody (immunoscintigraphy)	Readily available Rapid imaging Appears to have high sensitivity and specificity in prosthetic infection	

* Hexamethylpropylene amine oxime
MRI is likely to be more useful and available than the secondary imaging technique.
Source: Adapted from Hain SF, et al. Functional imaging and the orthopaedic surgeon. *J Bone Joint Surg Br* 2002 Apr;84(3):315-21.

for culture because it may not reliably report the actual causative organism of the osteomyelitis.

Tc99m triple-phase bone scans have been found to be useful in evaluating disease activity, but other methods are available (Table 1.22). Pharmacological treatment of the infection should be based on the results of deep tissue culture; empiric therapy, unlike in the acute setting, is not indicated in chronic osteomyelitis. A thorough surgical débridement of infected, necrotic bone and tissue is the primary treatment for chronic osteomyelitis. Treatment should also include the complete removal of any associated orthopaedic hardware because the hardware acts as a nexus for continued bacterial adherence and growth. This situation often results in massive loss of bone and surrounding host tissue, and bone must subsequently be replaced by graft, placement of osteoinductive substances (e.g., BMP-2, rOP-1), or distraction osteogenesis to help regenerate a load-capable structure and avoid nonunion. The communicating sinus tracts commonly found in chronic osteomyelitis have the capability of developing into a Marjolin ulcer, a squamous cell carcinoma of inflamed tissue otherwise associated mostly with burns and other scars.

TABLE 1.23 Empiric pharmacological treatment of acute hematogenous osteomyelitis

Population/Age	Causative Agent	Antibiotic
Newborn (< 4 mos)	*S. aureus*, Gram-negative bacilli, Group B strep	Nafcillin or oxacillin and a 3rd-generation cephalosporin
Children > 4 mos and < 4 yrs	*S. aureus*, Gram-negative bacilli, group B strep, *H. influenzae* type B†	Nafcillin or oxacillin and a 3rd-generation cephalosporin
Children > 4 yrs	*S. aureus*, group A strep, coliforms	Nafcillin or oxacillin; vancomycin or clindamycin
Adults > 21 yrs	*S. aureus*	Nafcillin or oxacillin or cefazolin
Sickle Cell	*Salmonella* (characteristic)	Fluoroquinolones (adults only) or 3rd-generation cephalosporin
Hemodialysis/IVDA	*S. aureus, S. epidermidis, P. aeruginosa*	PRSP* (nafcillin) or vancomycin + ciprofloxacin

*PRSP = penicillinase-resistant semisynthetic penicillins, such as methicillin, nafcillin, or oxacillin, introduced in 1959.
†*H. influenzae* infection has been greatly mitigated by immunization programs since the early 1990s.

Chronic Sclerosing Osteomyelitis (of Garré). A rare, atypical type of osteomyelitis that is characterized by the circumferential proliferation of the periosteum in the diaphysis of the long bones. This produces the dense, sclerotic-looking bone from which this condition is named. It is primarily seen in adolescents and may be caused by many different organisms. As with all suspected infections in bone, neoplasia must be ruled out. This may also have a radiographic appearance similar to stress fracture, although stress fracture evolves much more rapidly on radiographic examination over several weeks and does not have as exuberant a periosteal response.

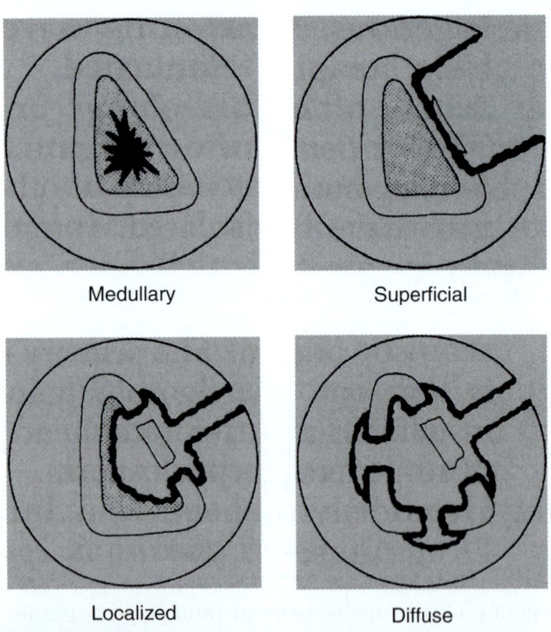

FIGURE 1.41 Cierney's anatomic classification of adult chronic osteomyelitis. (*Source*: Cierney, G., III. Chronic osteomyelitis: Results of treatment. *Instr. Course lect.* 39:495,1990.)

Chronic Recurrent Multifocal Osteomyelitis. Also rare, this condition occurs mostly in the long, tubular bones of children and adolescents, although it can affect other bones such as the clavicle, sternum, and scapula, among others. It is characterized by a prolonged, unpredictable course of recurring and remitting episodes of pain over many years. The radiographic and scintigraphic evidence usually indicates osteomyelitis, but multifocal lesions should suggest otherwise. Biopsy and histological evaluation are frequently inconclusive as to the causative agent. Historically, chronic recurrent multifocal osteomyelitis has been associated with an infectious agent, but this association has been the subject of some controversy over the past decade.

Soft-Tissue Infections (Table 1.24)

Infections of the Joint

Septic Arthritis. In children, the most commonly affected population, septic arthritis is often the result of metaphyseal osteomyelitis rupturing into the respective joint. This is particularly true in septic arthritis of the proximal femur, proximal humerus, radial neck, and distal fibula, whose metaphyses are actually enveloped by joint capsule. Patients with septic arthritis will usually complain of pain at or around a joint. Cardinal signs of redness, swelling, and warmth will further suggest an infectious cause. A history of fever, chills, or an inability to move a joint secondary

TABLE 1.24 Soft-tissue infections

Type	Most Common Organisms	Clinical Presentation	Diagnosis	Treatment (Antibiotics in Preferential Order)
Cellulitis/mastitis	Group A strep, *S. aureus*	Warm, painful, nonpruritic erythema w/o discharge	By clinical appearance; regional adenopathy favors strep, bullae favor *s. aureus*; lower extremity cellulitis tends to recur	Cefazolin 1gm IV q8h × 2 weeks; nafcillin 2gm IV q4h × 2 weeks; clindamycin 600 mg IV q8h × 2 weeks
Cellulitis, lower extremity	Group A strep, *S. aureus, E. coli, P. mirablis, K. pneumoniae*	Same as above	Same as above	Ceftizoxime 2 gm IV q8h × 2 weeks; cefotaxime 2 gm IV q6h × 2 weeks; 4th-generation quinolone
Erysipelas	Same as cellulitis	Resembles cellulitis, but raised and sharply demarcated	Same as cellulitis ± culture from skin lesion	Same as cellulitis
Mixed aerobic-anaerobic deep soft-tissue infection	*Enterobacteriae*, group A strep, *S. aureus*, anaerobes, fusobacterium	Acutely ill with gross gas deep in soft tissues and high fever	Gram stain and culture of aspirated fluid, discharge is foul-smelling; crepitance and prominent gas in soft tissue on x-ray suggests mixed aerobic/anaerobic infection, not gas gangrene	Meropenem 1 gm IV q8h × 2 weeks; imipenem 1 gm IV q6h × 2 weeks; piperacillin/tazobactam 4.5 gm IV q8h × 2 weeks; surgical débridement with antibiotics may be life-saving
Gas gangrene (clostridial myonecrosis)	*Clostridia* sp.	Fulminant infection of muscle with little or no fever; infected area is extremely painful, indurate, and discolored; rapid progression; death may occur within hours	Clinical; aspirate may show few PMNs with Gram-positive bacilli; not accompanied with high fever; diarrhea common; little visible gas on x-ray compared with mixed aerobic/anaerobic infection; rapidly progressive hemolytic anemia is characteristic	Penicillin G 10 million units IV q4h × 2 weeks; meropenem 1 gm IV q8h × 2 weeks; imipenem 1 gm IV q6h × 2 weeks; piperacillin/tazobactam 4.5 gm IV q8h × 2 weeks; surgical débridement is life-saving

(*continued overleaf*)

TABLE 1.24 *(continued overleaf)*

Type	Most Common Organisms	Clinical Presentation	Diagnosis	Treatment (Antibiotics in Preferential Order)
Necrotizing fasciitis	Group A strep, *enterobacteriae*, anaerobes, *S. aureus*	Acutely ill patient with high fever, extreme local pain w/o gas in tissue	Clinical with CT/MRI showing infection confined to one or more muscle compartments/fascial planes; no hemolytic anemia as with gas gangrene; foul-smelling aspirate suggests anaerobes	Meropenem 1 gm IV q8h × 2 weeks; imipenem 1 gm IV q6h × 2 weeks; piperacillin/tazobactam 4.5 gm IV q8h × 2 weeks; surgical débridement a must for control of infection/decompression of affected compartment(s)
Animal bite wound infection	Group A strep, *P. multocida*, Capnocytophaga (DF2), *S. aureus*	Cellulitis surrounding bite wound	By culture of bite wound exudates; deep bites may cause osteomyelitis	Piperacillin/tazobactam 4.5 gm IV q8h × 2 weeks; ampicillin/sulbactam 3 gm IV q6h × 2 weeks; meropenem 1 gm IV q8h × 2 weeks; imipenem 1 gm IV q6h × 2 weeks; amoxicillin/clavulanate 875 mg PO q12h × 2 weeks; tetanus prophylaxis as needed
Human bite wound infection (fight bite)	Oral anaerobes, *S. aureus*, group A strep, *E. corrodens*	Cellulitis surrounding bite wound	By culture of bite wound exudates; can also cause osteomyelitis; more likely than animal bites to contain anaerobes, *S. aureus*; fight bite has highest incidence of infection of any bite wound; must put MCP joints through entire ROM, with special attention to passive flexed position to assess tendon and joint involvement	Piperacillin/tazobactam 4.5 gm IV q8h × 2 weeks; ampicillin/sulbactam 3 gm IV q6h × 2 weeks; meropenem 1 gm IV q8h × 2 weeks; imipenem 1 gm IV q6h × 2 weeks; amoxicillin/clavulanate 875 mg PO q12h × 2 weeks; if any evidence of damaged tendon or penetrated joint capsule in noninfected case, must have operative I&D; tetanus prophylaxis as needed

Adapted from Cunha BA. *Antibiotic Essentials.* Royal Oak, MI: Physician's Press, 2002; 96–97.

TABLE 1.25 Etiology of and empiric therapy in septic arthritis based on population

Age	Most Common Pathogens	Empiric Therapy
Newborn (< 3 mos)	*S. aureus*, group B strep	PRSP* + 3rd-generation cephalosporin
Children (3 mos–14 yrs)	*S. aureus, S. pyogenes, H. influenzae,* Gram-negative bacilli	PRSP + 3rd-generation cephalosporin
Sexually active adults (monoarticular)	*N. gonorrhoeae, S. aureus*	Ceftriaxone (NG); nafcillin/oxacillin (*S. aureus*)
Adults not sexually active	*S. aureus*, strep, GNR	PRSP + 3rd-generation cephalosporin
Chronic monoarticular septic arthritis	Brucella	Tetracycline
Polyarticular septic arthritis	Borrelia, gonococci	Doxycycline

*PRSP = penicillinase-resistant semisynthetic penicillins

to pain should strongly suggest infection. Laboratory evaluation of these patients should mimic that of an acute osteomyelitis, with a CBC, ESR, and C-RP ordered. See Table 1.25 for a brief overview of causes and initial empiric antibiotic therapy of septic arthritis. Initial damage arising from septic joints appears in the articular cartilage, where the bacteria attack the GAG (glycosaminoglycans) units that form the core of the structure. Without GAGs, the cartilage loses its ability to retain water and thus loses its ability to withstand repeated compressive loads. Eventually, collagen type II, the predominant collagen in cartilage, begins to break down and the articular cartilage progresses to destruction. Untreated septic joints can also result in scar formation and severe contractures of the surrounding tissues. Treatment includes aspiration of joint space or actual surgical drainage of the joint capsule. The septic hip joint in particular calls for open or arthroscopic incision and drainage. The classic site of septic arthritis developing from osteomyelitis is the proximal femur.

Infections After Total Joint Arthroplasty (TJA). The most important historical cue suggesting infection after total joint arthroplasty is pain at rest. Interestingly, the patient might not exhibit other classic signs of infection, and concurrent inflammation such as fever, chills, redness, swelling, and warmth may not be present. Tests to evaluate the possibility of infection should include a CBC with differential, an ESR, and a C-RP level, as well as a possible joint aspiration with Gram staining. If these tests return negative, but clinical suspicion and patient progress are not favorable, a revision can be undertaken to investigate the area for aseptic loosening of the implant, and granulation tissue, if present, can be collected for frozen section and evaluation. The utility of this method of confirming the absence of infection has been supported in the literature.

Although its ability to confirm the presence of infection is still under debate, the definitive test for infection remains to be culture of inflamed joint tissue collected at time of surgery. Of note, prophylactic antibiotic therapy has been shown to reduce the prevalence of infection following total joint replacement. However, use should be judicious with a short duration of prophylaxis utilized to avoid fostering resistance.

Acute infections of less than 3 weeks' duration, although risky because of possible recurrence, can potentially be treated with a prosthesis salvage procedure involving a thorough surgical débridement and IV antibiotics if there is no evidence of loosening or lysis at the implant site. Infections of any greater length or severity should include removal of any implanted hardware or foreign bodies, followed by a rigorous débridement of infected or necrotic tissues. The decision of when to reimplant should be based on severity and chronicity of the infection and can be accomplished in multiple stages. While *S. epidermidis*, a common microbe found on the skin, remains the most common pathogen involved in total joint arthroplasty infections, hematogenous seeding of bacteria is also possible, especially after dental extractions or procedures involving dental surgery because of exposure of the circulation to virulent organisms living in the mouth. Certain populations of people are more apt to become infected after a dental procedure. These populations include the immunocompromised or otherwise immunosuppressed patient in addition to diabetics, hemophiliacs, and the malnourished. Previous TJA infection and recent TJA are also predisposing factors. Regimens for the prophylaxis of dental patients undergoing total joint arthroplasty are suggested in Table 1.26.

Foot Infections

Diabetic Foot Infections. Diabetic foot infections are commonly caused by multiple organisms. As in

TABLE 1.26 Suggested prophylactic regimens for TJA in patients after dental procedures

Patients Not Allergic to Penicillin	Cephalexin, Cephradine, or Amoxicillin: 2 g Orally 1 Hour Before Dental Procedure
Patients not allergic to penicillin but unable to take oral medications	Cefazolin 1 gram or ampicillin 2 grams IM/IV 1 hour before procedure
Patients allergic to penicillin	Clindamycin: 600 mg orally 1 hour before dental procedure
Patients allergic to penicillin and unable to take oral medications	Clindamycin: 600 mg IM/IV 1 hour before procedure

Adapted from the American Academy of Orthopaedic Surgeons Advisory Statement: Antibiotic Prophylaxis for Dental Patients with Total Joint Replacements.

most orthopaedic infections, surgical biopsy is much more accurate than superficial ulcer swabs in detecting the causative organism. Treatment depends on the extent of the infection. In more benign cases, such as superficial ulceration or mild cellulitis, antibiotic treatment may be sufficient, as there is adequate blood supply to carry to viable tissues. In more severe cases where there is necrotic tissue present, rigorous surgical débridement down to the level of viable tissue must be done. Once a culture has been acquired, broad-spectrum antibiotic treatment may be started until culture and sensitivity dictate otherwise. Table 1.27 reports incidences of the various microbes of the infected diabetic foot; Table 1.28 suggests first-line antibiotic choices based on culture results. Puncture wounds by a nail through a sneaker or tennis shoe most commonly show *P. aeruginosa*, and osteomyelitis can develop in 1% to 2% of children who sustain these puncture wounds. Treatment should include débridement of the nail tract, débridement of any involved bone, irrigation and drainage of affected joints, tissue biopsy for culture, removal of any foreign body such as a piece of shoe, packing of the wound, and administration of antibiotics to cover *P. aeruginosa.*

TABLE 1.27 Incidences of pathogenic bacteria in the diabetic foot

Organism	Incidence
Staphylococcus aureus	46%
Streptococcus species (nonenterococcal)	35%
Enterococcus species	29%
Proteus mirabilis	26%
Staphylococcus epidermidis	23%
Peptostreptococcus species	22%
Diphtheroids	19%
Pseudomonas aeruginosa	16%
Bacteroides species	16%

Source: Laughlin RT, Calhoun JH, Mader JT. The diabetic foot. *J Am Acad Orthop Surg* 1995;3:218–225.

TABLE 1.28 Antibiotic selection in the diabetic foot

Organism	Antibiotic
Staphylococcus (methicillin-sensitive)	First-generation cephalosporin, β-lactamase-resistant penicillins (oxacillin, nafcillin), vancomycin, rifampin
Staphylococcus (methicillin-resistant)	Vancomycin
Enterococcus (group D *Streptococcus*)	Ampicillin, β-lactamase inhibitor (sulbactam or ticarcillinclavu-lanate), vancomycin
Gram-negative (*Pseudomonas* species, *Proteus* species)	Ciprofloxacin, ofloxacin, ceftazidime
Anaerobes (*Bacteroides* species)	Clindamycin, metronidazole, ticarcillin-clavulanate

Source: Laughlin RT, Calhoun JH, Mader JT. The diabetic foot. *J Am Acad Orthop Surg* 1995;3:218–225.

Spinal Infections

Vertebral Osteomyelitis. The elderly, and men more than women, show a predilection for vertebral osteomyelitis. This manifestation of osteomyelitis is very similar to osteomyelitis elsewhere in the body in that it is most commonly caused by *S. aureus* and can arise via (1) a hematogenous route (likely a combination of arterial bacterial seeding near the vertebral endplate and retrograde venous flow from the pelvis, via (2) direct spread from surrounding infected tissue (e.g., retroperitoneal abscess), or via (3) direct inoculation (e.g., trauma, surgery).

Clinical manifestations of this condition almost always include neck or back pain in addition to paraspinal muscle pain that is not activity related. Neurologic symptoms are usually not present, although abscess formation can cause neural compression at its respective level. Laboratory studies should be the same as those ordered for a suspected osteomyelitis, namely the CBC with differential, ESR, and C-RP. These tests can be useful but are not any more specific for infection in this setting than they are in other forms of osteomyelitis. Closed biopsy of the affected region with a Craig biopsy needle or fine-needle aspiration under fluoroscopic or CT guidance should be undertaken to determine the causative organism. If this procedure fails to reveal the diagnosis, then open biopsy should be considered to establish it. Tissue should be sent for Gram stain, acid-fast stain, and culture, as well as histology to evaluate for possible neoplasia. Radiographs may show progressive osteolysis and vertebral endplate destruction with eventual collapse of adjacent disk spaces. Bone scan is very sensitive but can be nonspecific, especially in patients with existing degeneration. MRI is both highly sensitive and highly specific for vertebral osteomyelitis.

Treatment should include IV antibiotics based on culture and sensitivity results. Surgery should be done if medical management has not sufficiently decreased symptoms or if sufficient structural damage has taken place so that the vertebral column is unstable or that neurologic impairment is resulting.

Spinal Tuberculosis or Granulomatous Spinal Infection. Very uncommon in the United States, tuberculosis is endemic in some parts of the world. Most commonly caused by *Mycobacterium tuberculosis* (Pott disease), tuberculosis can also be more uncommonly caused by *M. africanum* or *M. avium*. Is most often a result of systemic disease with hematogenous seeding, with 10% of tuberculosis cases affecting the skeleton and 50% of those cases affecting the spine.

Clinical manifestations can include pain but are rather nonspecific. Populations at risk are the immunocompromised/immunosuppressed, the elderly, patients from South America or Southeast Asia, and patients with recent exposure to tuberculosis. Laboratory results are nonspecific; however, gene amplification techniques like PCR hold promise for future improvements in this area.

Radiographs of a patient with this condition will show osteolysis but will relatively spare the disk space, unlike vertebral osteomyelitis in which the disk space can be obliterated. A kyphotic deformity may also be present. Treatment is the same as with vertebral osteomyelitis, with a cocktail of antimycobacterial drugs like ethambutol, rifampin, and isoniazid for a period of 6 months. Surgical indications are also the same, with the goal of eradicating the organism if medical management has failed, stabilizing the vertebral column, and relieving neurologic compromise if present.

Pediatric Discitis. Anatomically, children are thought to be more prone to infections of the disk because their immature vertebra contain vascular channels that act as conduits for the bacteria, if present, to seed directly into the avascular nucleus pulposus. Clinical cues are inconsistent, but low-grade fever, pain on standing or sitting, refusal to weight-bear, and discomfort with spinal flexion are all symptoms. Children may also present with difficulty walking and back pain. C-RP is usually very elevated in pediatric discitis, and an elevated ESR can also occur.

All sources of infection should be cultured, and if the diagnosis cannot be established, biopsy of the affected region under fluoroscopic or CT guidance should be undertaken to determine the offending organism. Radiographs can show a spectrum from normal to disk space narrowing with endplate osteolysis and evidence of swelling in the surrounding tissue. Bone scan and MRI are much more useful in detecting early infection. Treatment involves immobilization in a brace. Since the infectious etiology of pediatric discitis is not universally accepted, some controversy exists as to whether or not to treat the condition with immobilization alone or in addition to a short course of parenteral antibiotics.

Epidural Abscess. In general, this condition is the result of direct extension from an established vertebral osteomyelitis or discitis. However, these abscesses can form insidiously in rare cases because of IV drug abuse or iatrogenic seeding of bacteria during a previous spinal procedure. Clinical presentation can include rapid onset of pain and difficulty with flexion/extension movements. Radiographs can be inconclusive, but MRI can visualize granulomatous lesions of the spine extremely well. Neoplastic processes should be ruled out, however, because they can sometimes mimic abscess in their appearance. Treatment almost always involves IV antibiotics and surgical incision and drainage of the abscess.

Viral Infections

Much focus is dedicated to the identification and eradication of bacterial infection in the orthopaedic setting. However, the importance of understanding viral illness in orthopaedics, especially HIV and hepatitis B and C, cannot be understated. These issues continue to affect the care of our patients and present a potential danger to health care professionals and the patients they serve, and deserve a mention in this section.

HIV. An estimated 850,000 to 950,000 persons in the United States are living with human immunodeficiency virus (HIV), including 180,000 to 280,000 who do not know they are infected. HIV is a retrovirus. All retroviruses are enveloped RNA viruses, meaning that the viral genome is made of RNA instead of DNA and is enveloped by a protein sheath. In order for the virus to replicate, it relies on a polymerase protein called reverse transcriptase to "reverse" engineer DNA from the RNA, which can then be incorporated into the host genome. The gene that codes for the protein envelope mutates quickly, which makes developing a vaccine for it extremely difficult. The gene that codes for the reverse transcriptase is relatively stable, though, and this makes the polymerase a target of therapy by reverse transcriptase inhibitor medications. There are two types: the first is nucleoside reverse transcriptase inhibitors (NRTIs), which are modified nucleosides that compete with normal nucleotides in the reverse transcription phase of infection. These modified nucleosides work because the viral transcription process is the most active process requiring nucleotides in the cell, and so they are preferentially incorporated by the reverse transcriptase. Once they are incorporated into the viral DNA, the process cannot continue, and the incomplete viral DNA cannot be incorporated into the host genome, thus halting the viral progression. The second is nonnucleoside reverse transcriptase inhibitors (NNRTIs), which are molecules that bind to reverse transcriptase and halt its activity. Certain strains of HIV have been shown to have mutated their reverse transcriptase so that current NNRTIs lose their ability to bind to the enzyme and stop it.

Another target of therapy is the protease enzyme essential in the assembly and packaging of the HIV virus once the host cell has replicated it. These protease inhibitors, while plagued with difficult treatment regimens and undesirable side effects, have improved significantly and have considerably reduced the morbidity and mortality among HIV patients over the past decade.

Diagnosis is made by ELISA, a highly sensitive and specific test for HIV. Positive results can be repeated and then confirmed by western blot (gold standard, but is more labor-intensive and takes longer). This combination produces an extremely low false-positive rate and is considered standard of care. AIDS (acquired immune deficiency syndrome) is defined by an HIV-positive status and either (1) a $CD4^+$ T-cell count of less than 200 cells/μL, or (2) an opportunistic infection as defined by CDC guidelines for AIDS-defining disease (Table 1.29). The risk of being infected with HIV after exposure to HIV-positive blood products depends on the circumstances of the exposure. The risk of infection after percutaneous inoculation is approximately 0.3%, and 0.1% with exposure to mucous membranes. Use of postexposure prophylaxis has been shown to significantly decrease the odds of infection. The risk of infection from transfusion of blood products is extremely low. It has steadily been declining over the years with more rigorous screening of donated blood, including screening for HIV-1 antibody. There is, however, a "window period" between infection and seroconversion in a recently infected individual of approximately 22 days, so that blood donated during this time can test negative for anti-HIV antibody. Therefore, the chance of infection from donated blood still exists, about 1 in 500,000 units. Newer tests, such as the p24 antigen test and a form of PCR called nucleic-acid amplification

TABLE 1.29 AIDS-defining opportunistic infections

Candidiasis of bronchi, trachea, or lungs
Candidiasis, esophageal
Cervical cancer, invasive
Coccidioidomycosis, disseminated or extrapulmonary
Cryptococcosis, extrapulmonary
Cryptosporidiosis, chronic intestinal (greater than 1 month's duration)
Cytomegalovirus disease (other than liver, spleen, or nodes)
Cytomegalovirus retinitis (with loss of vision)
Encephalopathy, HIV-related
Herpes simplex: chronic ulcer(s) (greater than 1 month's duration); or bronchitis, pneumonitis, or esophagitis
Histoplasmosis, disseminated or extrapulmonary
Isosporiasis, chronic intestinal (greater than 1 month's duration)
Kaposi sarcoma
Lymphoma, Burkitt (or equivalent term)
Lymphoma, immunoblastic (or equivalent term)
Lymphoma, primary, of brain
Mycobacterium avium complex or *M. kansasii*, disseminated or extrapulmonary
Mycobacterium tuberculosis, any site (pulmonary or extrapulmonary)
Mycobacterium, other species or unidentified species, disseminated or extrapulmonary
Pneumocystis carinii pneumonia
Pneumonia, recurrent
Progressive multifocal leukoencephalopathy
Salmonella septicemia, recurrent
Toxoplasmosis of brain
Wasting syndrome due to HIV

Source: Centers for Disease Control. 1993 Revised classification system for HIV infection and expanded surveillance case definition for AIDS among adolescents and adults. *MMWR* 1992;41 (no.RR-17).

testing (NAT), have decreased the "window period" by detecting HIV elements earlier and more accurately. Recent studies show a fourfold rate reduction in HIV transmission by transfusion of blood products, down to 1 in 2 million units transfused. Similar rates have been achieved in hepatitis C virus detection.

Hepatitis. Hepatitis is caused by a variety of viruses, ranging from Picornaviruses to Flaviviruses to delta viruses. The feature they share in common is inflammation of the liver, hence their common moniker. Types A through G have been identified, though types B and C are the types most clinically significant. Types A and E are generally not seen in developed countries but continue to be an issue in developing ones. They share clinical manifestations as self-limiting diseases that produce acute hepatitis without a chronic phase, and mortality is very low (−1%). Once infected by type A, the host will produce antibodies that confer immunity. A vaccine for type A is also available for prophylaxis.

Hepatitis B, a Hepadnavirus, is transmitted through exposure to bodily fluids containing the virus, including blood transfusions (now rare), unprotected sexual contact, from mother to child during childbirth, and reuse of contaminated needles and syringes from IV drug use. Roughly 95% of adults infected will clear the infection without treatment and produce antibodies conferring immunity. The other 5%, however, will not clear acute infection and will go on to become chronic carriers of the virus. These people have a greatly increased risk of developing cirrhosis of the liver and hepatic neoplasias such as hepatocellular carcinoma, especially if the individual is co-infected or superinfected with hepatitis D, an RNA virus that requires the replication machinery of hepatitis B virus to multiply. A vaccine is available for nonimmune patients and health care workers, which has significantly decreased infection rates. Hepatitis B immunoglobulin can be administered acutely to decrease the risk of infection in nonimmune patients after exposure and can serve as a first-line treatment along with various antiviral medications for chronic carriers in an attempt to clear the infection.

Hepatitis C is not considered a sexually transmitted disease and is mainly transmitted through exposure to contaminated blood. It leads to a chronic form of hepatitis, in many cases resulting in cirrhosis or hepatocellular carcinoma. It can remain asymptomatic for 10 to 40 years after infection. However, superinfection with other hepatitis types like A and B can result in a fulminant acute hepatitis. Therefore, it is recommended that seropositive hepatitis C carriers be vaccinated against type A and B if they are not already immune to those types. No vaccine is available for hepatitis C. It is commonly associated with IV drug abuse and is the most common form of hepatitis associated with blood transfusion, but this mode of transmission has decreased significantly with the advent of nucleic-acid amplification techniques (PCR).

Other Infections

Rabies. Rabies is caused by a Lyssavirus of the same name that is usually found in the saliva of infected animals, domesticated and otherwise. This virus preferentially infects neurons. After infection, the virus travels up the axon and in time infects the CNS, where encephalitis occurs. There is no known cure for symptomatic rabies in humans or animals, and if left untreated, it will lead to certain death by paralysis and asphyxiation. Treatment depends on the specific situation. The incubation period of the virus in dogs, cats, and ferrets is well known. If a patient is bitten by a healthy one of these animals, then the decision is to wait 10 days to see if symptoms arise in the animal. If not, then the patient requires no further treatment. If the animal shows signs of infection, or if the patient is bitten by a wild animal that is not available for inspection, infection is assumed and treatment is administered.

Treatment consists of two different shots:

1. A one-time dose of human rabies immunoglobulin based on the weight of the patient injected into the area of the bite.
2. A 28-day regimen of rabies vaccine (either human diploid cell vaccine [HDCV], rabies vaccine absorbed [RVA], or purified chick embryo cell culture vaccine [PCEC]) divided into 5 shots, beginning on day 0 at the emergency room.

Postexposure prophylaxis is efficacious in the case of rabies because there is some delay between the time of exposure and the time the virus infects the CNS.

Tetanus (Clostridium tetani). Tetanus is a condition of paralysis caused by the action of an exotoxin called tetanospasmin produced by the Gram-positive anaerobic bacillus Clostridium tetani. After an incubation period of 3 to 21 days, the result is either (rarely) local tetanus affecting only the muscles around the wound, (rarely) a cephalic type that affects mostly the muscles of the face, or (most common) a generalized tetanic contraction of skeletal muscles in the body beginning with the muscles of mastication (trismus or lockjaw), moving inferiorly to the neck and back, and affecting the accessory muscles of breathing. There is at least a 30% mortality rate associated with symptomatic tetanus. Treatment for symptomatic tetanus infection is supportive (diazepam to control muscle spasm) but should include penicillin and metronidazole to kill as many bacteria as possible, and human antitetanospasmin immunoglobulin should be administered to try to reduce the amount of active exotoxin. Treatment for a fresh wound is based on the suspicion that a wound is contaminated with *C. tetani* spores. Wounds that are older than 6 hours, wounds made by a projectile, wounds caused by burns or frostbite, and wounds that have necrotic tissue or are contaminated should be suspicious for tetanus. Patients who appear to have a tetanus-prone wound and have an uncertain immunization history require tetanus and diphtheria toxoid in addition to human antitetanospasmin immunoglobulin. Patients who appear to have a tetanus-prone wound and are fully immunized do not require any treatment unless the patient's last booster was more than 5 years ago. If so, then the patient should receive a new booster of tetanus toxoid. Patients who are not suspected of having tetanus do not require treatment unless they have an uncertain immunization history.

Cat Scratch Disease (Bartonella henselae). Cat scratch disease is a benign disorder, first described in 1889 by Henri Parinaud, most commonly found in children 1 to 2 weeks after being scratched by a cat. It is caused by the Gram-negative bacillus *Bartonella henselae*. The condition resolves spontaneously in all cases within 1 month with or without treatment, although painful swelling can occur in the lymph nodes, causing alarm and distress. Pain and swelling can be treated symptomatically with needle aspiration to relieve pain if need be, but full incision and drainage is contraindicated because the course is benign. More severe cases can present with fever, malaise, and anorexia.

Antibiotics

Antibiotics are among the orthopaedic surgeon's best weapons against infection occurring in the musculoskeletal system. Since the chance discovery of penicillin in 1928 by Alexander Fleming, many different types of bacteria have been discovered and developed to attack vital support processes in bacteria from as many angles as possible. The main ways that antibiotics carry out their role in stifling or killing bacteria are summarized in Table 1.30, but almost all routinely used antibiotics either (1) target bacterial cell wall synthesis, (2) inhibit protein synthesis, (3) inhibit DNA synthesis, or (4) interfere with cellular metabolism.

Bactericidal antibiotics cause lysis of bacterial cell wall viability either by activating enzymes that destroy the cell wall or by inhibiting cell wall synthesis. Penicillin and cephalosporins, vancomycin, and bacitracin are bactericidal. Clindamycin is an example of a bacteriostatic antibiotic and works by inhibiting protein synthesis.

Many bacteria, unfortunately, have developed genetic resistance mechanisms to protect themselves from the onslaught of antibiotics administered to kill them. By exhaustive usage of various antibiotics over the years, we have selectively grown a population of bacteria that have, through genetic mutation or by transmissible genetic elements, managed to (1) alter the vital target of the antibiotic so that it is no longer susceptible to its action; (2) produce proteins or structures that can inactivate the antibiotic, or (3) change their structure so that the antibiotic can no longer reach its intended target (Table 1.31). Penicillins, for example, enact their effect by virtue of a β-lactam ring that interferes with cross-linking of linear peptidoglycans and vital constituents of the bacterial cell wall. Many organisms have developed enzymes that can destroy the β-lactam ring (called β-lactamases or penicillinases), thus rendering the drug inactive. One way that researchers found to counteract this effect is to develop inhibitors to the β-lactamase enzymes found in these resistant organisms. Clavulanic acid, tazobactam, and sulbactam are commonly used β-lactamase inhibitors that, when coupled with penicillins (e.g., ampicillin/sulbactam or piperacillin/tazobactam), can counteract their defense mechanism and destroy the organism. *Staphylococcus aureus*, one of the most notorious offending organisms in orthopaedic infection, is but one of the myriad of bacteria that have exhibited this mutation phenomenon. Vancomycin, a glycopeptide antibiotic that inhibits cell wall synthesis, is the mainstay of treatment of methicillin-resistant *S. aureus* (MRSA), although strains of *S. aureus* have been found clinically that have developed at least a partial resistance to vancomycin (vancomycin-intermediate *S. aureus*, or VISA) or even a full resistance (vancomycin-resistant *S. aureus*, or VRSA). The fact that these two strains have seemingly developed their resistance mechanisms through two different mechanisms (mutation with VISA vs. gene transfer from enterococci in VRSA) underscores the tremendous challenge that scientists face today in developing novel antibiotics while keeping pace with current demand for effective treatment. Furthermore, it also should serve as a reminder that prudence should always be exercised when treating infections, with emphasis on properly identifying the causative organism through culture and sensitivities and using the lowest common denominator antibiotic that will eradicate the disease.

Orthopaedic infections can be difficult to eradicate and thus require high doses of antibiotics over an extended period. A typical patient with osteomyelitis, for example, may receive 1 to 2 weeks of IV antibiotics and 4 to 5 weeks of oral antibiotics. However, many antibiotics have toxicities associated with them when they are given systemically at high doses. Therefore, local antibiotic delivery methods have been developed to maximize antibiotic delivery to a target area in potentially higher doses than can be achieved by

TABLE 1.30 Mechanisms of action of common antibiotics

Antibiotic Class	*Mechanism of Action*	*Site of Action*
Beta-lactams (penicillins and cephalosporins)	Inhibition of cell wall production by prevention of peptidoglycan cross-linkage	Cell wall
Glycopeptides (vancomycin)	Inhibition of cell wall production by interference with addition of cell wall subunits	Cell wall
Bacitracin	Inhibition of cell wall production by interference with cell wall subunit carrier lipid	Cell wall
Aminoglycosides (gentamicin)	Inhibition of protein synthesis by binding with 30S ribosomal subunit	Protein synthesis
Macrolides (erythromycin)	Inhibition of protein synthesis by binding with 50S ribosomal subunit	Protein synthesis
Lincosamides (clindamycin)	Inhibition of protein synthesis by binding with 50S ribosomal subunit	Protein synthesis
Chloramphenicol	Inhibition of protein synthesis by binding with 50S ribosomal subunit	Protein synthesis
Tetracycline	Inhibition of protein synthesis by binding with 50S ribosomal subunit	Protein synthesis
Mupirocin	Inhibition of protein synthesis by interference with isoleucine t-RNA synthetase	Protein synthesis
Streptogrammin (synercid-investigational)	Inhibition of early and late stages of protein synthesis at ribosomal level	Protein synthesis
Oxazolidinones (linezolid-investigational)	Inhibition of protein synthesis by binding to 50S ribosomal subunit	Protein synthesis
Rifamycins (Rifampin)	Inhibition of DNA-dependent RNA polymerase	DNA synthesis
Fluoroquinolones (Ciprofloxacin)	Inhibition of DNA gyrase	DNA synthesis
Novobiocin	Inhibition of DNA gyrase	DNA synthesis
Metronidazole	Inhibition of DNA synthesis by generation of short-lived reactive intermediates by electron transfer system	DNA synthesis
Sulfonamides and trimethoprim	Inhibition of enzymes involved in folic acid biosynthesis	Cell metabolism

Source: Buckwalter JA, Einhorn TA, Simon SR. *Orthopaedic Basic Science: Biology and Biomechanics of the Musculoskeletal System*, 2nd ed. Rosemont, IL: American Academy of Orthopaedic Surgeons, 2000; 246.

systemic parenteral administration alone while keeping the systemic toxicities to a minimum. These include biodegradable polymers, implantable osmotic pumps, beads or cement of antibiotic impregnated PMMA, fatty acid dimers, and others. Care should be exercised when impregnating PMMA with antibiotic because (1) some antibiotics, such as chloramphenicol and tetracycline, can be deactivated by the polymerization of PMMA; and (2) the mechanical properties of the PMMA may be reduced with a high enough concentration of drug.

All antibiotics have contraindications for their usage. For example, fluoroquinolones cause arthropathy and tendon rupture in immature mammals and are therefore contraindicated in children. It is also useful to note the pharmacodynamics of the antibiotic of choice. Many antibiotics, such as amoxicillin/clavulanate, ciprofloxacin, or cefuroxime, have high oral bioavailability levels such that serum concentrations achieved with oral therapy can match that achieved with IV administration. Oral therapy also results in greater patient compliance and less morbidity from the IV site. An antibiotic's bioavailability, however, can be adversely affected by the microenvironment it is in after ingestion. An example of this is how ciprofloxacin has decreased absorption when taken orally with magnesium or aluminum-containing antacids. Conversely, serum levels are increased when taken with theophylline. Planning should also include foreknowledge of the distribution properties of the antibiotic. For example, clindamycin, a macrolide antibiotic exerting its effect on the bacterial 50S ribosomal subunit, achieves the highest concentration of all antibiotics in bone.

TABLE 1.31 Mechanisms of antibiotic resistance

Antibiotic Class and Type of Resistance	Specific Resistance Mechanism
Altered Target	
β-lactam antibiotics	Altered penicillin-binding proteins
Vancomycin	Altered peptidoglycan subunits
Aminoglycosides	Altered ribosomal proteins
Macrolides	Ribosomal RNA methylation
Quinolones	Altered DNA gyrase
Sulfonamides	Altered dihydropteroate
Trimethoprim	Altered dihydrofolate reductase
Rifampin	Altered RNA polymerase
Detoxifying Enzymes	
Aminoglycosides	Phosphotransferase, acetyltransferase, nucleotidyltransferase
β-lactam antibiotics	β-lactamase
Chloramphenicol	Acetyltransferase
Decreased Uptake	
Diminished permeability	
β-lactam antibiotics tetracycline, quinolones, trimethoprim	Alteration in outer membrane porins
Active efflux pumps	
Erythromycin	Membrane transport system
Tetracycline	Membrane transport system

(From Buckwalter JA, Einhorn TA, Simon Sr. *Orthopaedic Basic Science: Biology and Biomechanics of the Musculoskeletal System*, 2nd ed. Rosemont, IL: American Academy of Orthopaedic Surgeons, 2000; 247.

VI. PERIOPERATIVE ISSUES IN ORTHOPAEDICS

Embolism

Thromboembolic Disease

Understanding the incidence and pathophysiology of, and pharmacological methods of prophylaxis in, thromboembolic disease is extremely important to the orthopaedic surgeon because so much of it occurs as a consequence of orthopaedic surgery.

This is especially true in orthopaedic procedures involving the hip. Sources differ on the incidence of thromboembolism in total hip arthroplasties (THA) without thromboembolic prophylaxis, but the range is as high as 50% to 75% incidence of deep venous thrombosis (DVT) and up to 20% incidence of pulmonary embolism (PE), with 1% to 3% of those being fatal. Total knee arthroplasty (TKA) DVT rates without prophylaxis are even higher than THA, with DVT events occurring in up to 80% to 84% of surgeries.

Physiology of Coagulation

Intrinsic Pathway. Intrinsic pathway initiated by the contact of factor XII with exposed subendothelial collagen of damaged vessels. After a cascade of enzymatic activations involving factor XI and factor IX, this pathway leads to the activation of factor X. It is monitored by the activated partial thromboplastin time (aPTT).

Extrinsic Pathway. Extrinsic pathway is initiated by the release of thromboplastin by damaged cells. Thromboplastin then activates factor VII, which in turn leads to the activation of factor X. It is monitored by the prothrombin time (PT).

Common Pathway. Both the intrinsic and extrinsic pathways join a common pathway after the activation of factor X. The common pathway proceeds until factor II (prothrombin) is activated into thrombin, which in turn enzymatically induces soluble fibrinogen to precipitate as fibrin at the site of the injury (Fig. 1.42).

Predisposition to Venous Thrombosis. Patients are predisposed to developing venous thrombosis if they generally fulfill the *Virchow triad*:

1. Venous stasis
2. Hypercoagulable state
3. Vascular endothelial cell damage.

All of these conditions can be met in the postoperative setting: immobility can cause stasis, hypercoagulability can be a natural host response to anesthesia and surgical trauma, and endothelial cell damage can occur from relative venous dilation and distention from surgical manipulation of the extremities and from some anesthetic compounds used during surgery. The use of surgical instruments (e.g., Bovie electrocautery) near or on veins can cause intimal damage well. Other comorbidities and conditions after surgery or trauma can fulfill the Virchow triad in whole or in part and therefore predispose to formation of a thrombus (Table 1.32).

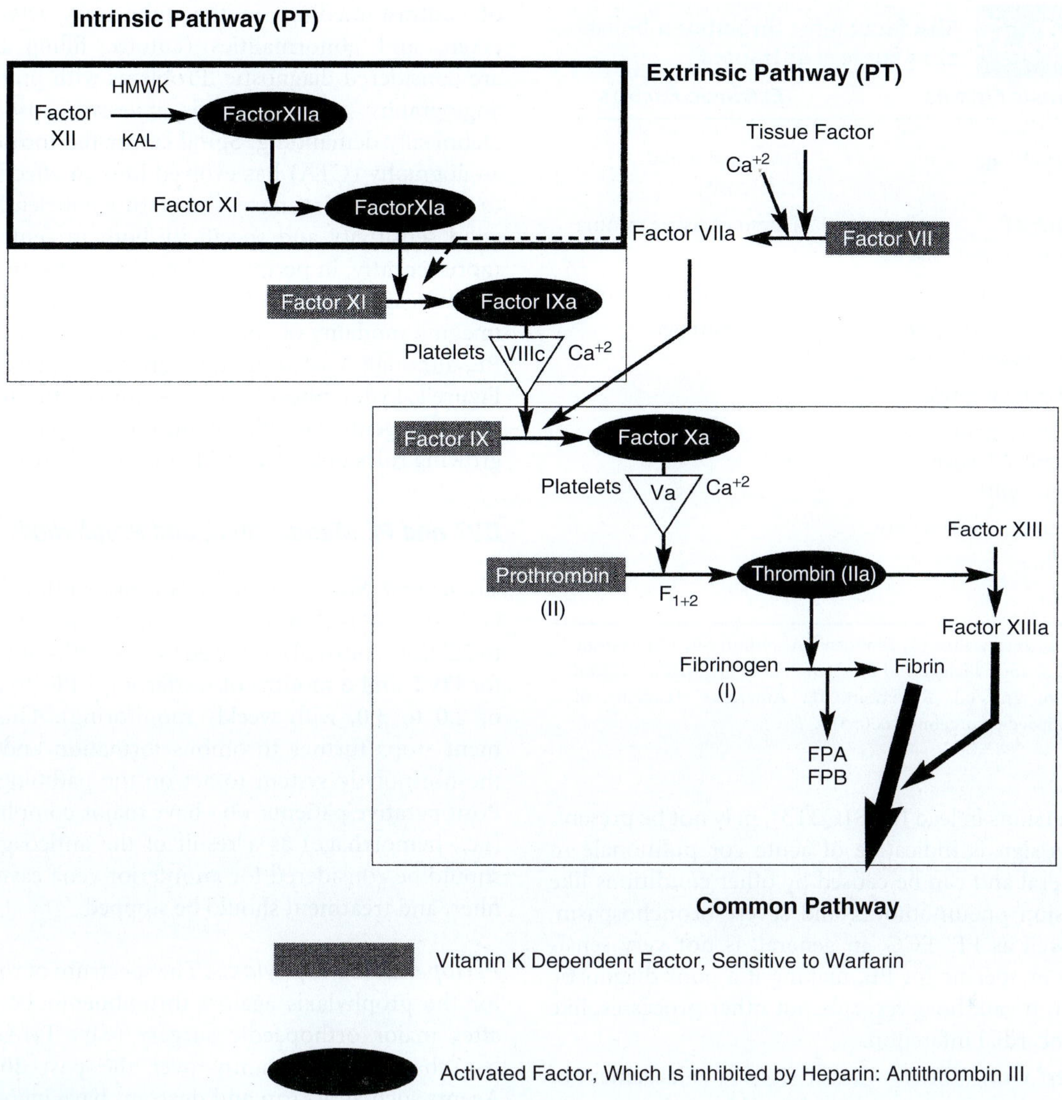

FIGURE 1.42 The coagulation pathway. Important features include the contact activation phase, vitamin K–dependent factors (affected by warfarin) and the activated serine proteases that are inhibited by heparin-antithrombin III. Prothrombin measures the function of the extrinsic and common pathways; the partial thromboplastin time measures the function of the intrinsic and common pathways. (*Source*: Stead RB. Regulation of hemostasis. In: Goldhaber SZ (ed.), *Pulmonary Embolism and Deep Venous Thromboembolism*. Philadelphia: WB Saunders, 1985; 32.)

Manifestations of Thromboembolic Disease in Orthopaedic Surgery

Deep Venous Thrombosis (DVT). Classic signs of DVT include calf tenderness, edema, venous distention, and calf pain on forced dorsiflexion (Homan sign). These signs are frequently absent, however. Clinical suspicion in a patient with a relative probability of thromboembolism should be tested using duplex ultrasound as a screening method, followed by a more definitive test such as venography if needed (Table 1.33).

Pulmonary Embolus (PE). Classic symptoms of PE (Fig 1.43) are dyspnea and pleuritic chest pain and can include signs like tachypnea (most common), tachycardia, and fever. Audible pleural friction rub can suggest pulmonary infarction. These signs are all nonspecific, however. Tests typically used for initial evaluation in the patient with suspected PE include:

- *Electrocardiography (ECG)*—Typically abnormal, with nonspecific signs of right-heart strain like T-wave inversion in the anterior leads. Classic S-waves in lead I, with Q-waves and T-wave

TABLE 1.32 Risk factors for thromboembolism after surgery or trauma

Intrinsic Factors	Extrinsic Factors
Advanced age	Increased blood viscosity
History of thromboembolism	Extent of tissue trauma
Varicose veins	Immobility or paralysis
Malignancy or other hypercoagulable state	Use of estrogen
Oral contraceptives	
Inherited factors (e.g., factor V Leiden mutation)	
Congestive heart failure	
Smoking	
Obesity	

Source: Buckwalter JA, Einhorn TA, Simon SR. *Orthopaedic Basic Science: Biology and Biomechanics of the Musculoskeletal System*, 2nd ed. Rosemont, IL: American Academy of Orthopaedic Surgeons, 2000; 313.

inversions in lead III (S1Q3T3), may not be present. This sign is indicative of acute cor pulmonale in general and can be caused by other conditions like tension pneumothorax and severe bronchospasm, as well as PE. ECG, in general, is not very sensitive or specific for PE, making it a poor diagnostic tool. It can, however, rule out other processes, like myocardial infarction.

- *Chest x-ray (CXR)*—Classic signs of enlargement of the pulmonary arteries and focal hyperlucency are seldom seen. The utility of CXR in evaluating the patient is, like the ECG, the ability to rule out other developments like pneumothorax, pneumonia, or congestive heart failure.
- *Arterial blood gas (ABG)*—PaO_2 less than 80 mmHg, $PaCO_2$ less than 35 mmHg, or O_2 gradient ($P_{(A-a)O2}$) greater than 20 mmHg can all indicate PE. ABG abnormalities can be absent, however. Pulse oximetry is not a viable substitute for an ABG.
- *Ventilation/perfusion scanning (V/Q scanning)*—Provides a noninvasive next step in diagnostic tests. Results are rated high, intermediate, or low probability of having PE. High probability results combined with high clinical suspicion have a positive predictive value of 96% of confirmed PE. It is considered diagnostic, and treatment is necessary. Low probability and low clinical suspicion for PE makes the diagnosis doubtful.

For other cases, PE can be verified, if possible, by pulmonary angiography (gold standard). Images of contrast medium in the pulmonary arteries are taken, and abnormalities (cutoffs, filling defects) are considered diagnostic. Problems with pulmonary angiography are that it is invasive, costly, and technically demanding. Spiral computed tomography angiography (CTA) has evolved into an effective way to visualize pulmonary vasculature efficiently with good sensitivity and specificity both in central and, more recently, in peripheral lung locations. In fact, in many hospitals, spiral CTA has become the first-line imaging modality of choice for evaluation of possible PE, although MRI techniques are developing as well. Figure 1.43 describes a basic algorithm for the diagnosis and management of PE, but one must keep in mind the growing roles of CTA and MRI in current diagnosis.

DVT and PE Management and Prophylaxis

Treatment. Standard care for diagnosed thromboembolic disease includes IV heparin (to an aPTT of 1.5 to 2.5 times normal) followed by 3 months of warfarin for DVT and 6 months of warfarin for PE (to an INR of 2.0 to 3.0, with weekly monitoring). This treatment stops further thrombus formation and allows the fibrinolytic system to act on the pathologic clot. Postoperative patients who have major complications (i.e., hemorrhage) as a result of the anticoagulation should be considered for an inferior vena cava (IVC) filter, and treatment should be stopped.

Perioperative Prophylaxis. The spectrum of regimens for the prophylaxis against thromboembolic disease after major orthopaedic surgery (e.g., THA, TKA) has changed significantly over the past 20 years. Agents such as aspirin and dextrans have increasingly been abandoned as more advanced therapies have been introduced. Current thinking supports the use of low-molecular weight heparin (LMWH) instead of unfractionated heparin and low-dose warfarin as an outpatient in prophylaxis. Some recent work has shown even newer agents (pentasaccharides, i.e., fondaparineux) to be superior to LMWH in terms of safety and efficacy. Other promising therapies on the horizon are oral direct thrombin inhibitors, which have the advantage of being PO like warfarin but show a much more favorable drug interaction profile, and can be as effective as LMWH. Table 1.34 shows a brief comparison among the most used prophylactic agents against venous thromboembolism.

Fat Embolism and Fat Embolism Syndrome (FES). Fat embolism refers to the presence of fat globules in the lung and peripheral vasculature, whereas fat embolism syndrome refers to a distinct condition generally consisting of a characteristic triad of respiratory distress, skin petechiae, and neurologic compromise 24 to

TABLE 1.33 Tools for diagnosing possible DVT

Test	*Advantages*	*Disadvantages*	*Notes*
Duplex Ultrasonography	Noninvasive, painless No radiation Inexpensive Can be done at bedside Can reveal other causes of pain (e.g., hematoma)	Highly user-dependent Technical proficiency is a must Less sensitive for DVT in calf than in thigh and can have difficulty with pelvic vessels	Excellent screening tool with high sensitivity and specificity, especially in the thigh
Venography	gold standard sensitivity and specificity approaching 100% in the thigh and calf	Expensive Procedure-related morbidity (e.g., discomfort, bleeding, complications from use of contrast) Limited by poor venous access	Indicated with ambiguous results from ultrasound; sensitivity can be less in pelvis because of dilution of contrast agent by blood from other converging veins
Magnetic Resonance Imaging (MRI)	Noninvasive, painless No contrast agent needed Simultaneous viewing of both lower extremities	Expensive Limited availability Contraindicated in patients with some implants (e.g., metallic heart valves, metal vascular clips)	Sensitivity can be greater than venography in the pelvis, but inferior in the calf; as good as venography in the thigh; test of choice when pelvic thrombi are suspected
Cuff-Impedance Plethysmography	Noninvasive, painless Inexpensive	Low sensitivity and specificity compared to other methods	Routine use not recommended with advent of better methods
^{125}I Fibrinogen	Can visualize thrombus in situ	Low sensitivity and specificity compared to other methods High rate of false-positives	Routine use not recommended with advent of better methods; injected agent no longer available in United States

48 hours after injury that are the fulminant, worst-case scenario result of fat embolus. It should be thought of as the most severe outcome on a spectrum of outcomes that can result from fat embolus. It is of particular importance to orthopaedic surgeons because of the high incidence of fat embolus after skeletal trauma. While fat embolism occurs in most (more than 90%) patients with traumatic injury, the fat embolism syndrome (FES) occurs in only 3% to 4% of patients with long-bone fractures. Why some patients remain subclinical with hypoxemia while others proceed onto FES is still a mystery. How fat enters the circulation and how it results in the devastating condition of FES is not entirely understood. Two contributing theories are (Fig. 1.44):

- *Mechanical theory*—Describes the mechanical extrusion of fat globules into the surrounding venous circulation due to a relative increase in intramedullary pressure after trauma (path of least resistance into torn venous vessels) or due to greatly increased intramedullary pressure in the long bones as seen in lower extremity arthroplasties (e.g., THA, TKA, femoral intramedullary nailing). Once the fat globules enter the venous circulation, they pass on to the lungs where they can either occlude the small capillaries or pass on to the arterial circulation, potentially lodging in capillary beds elsewhere in the body (e.g., brain, kidney). Once lodged in an end-organ capillary bed, they become a nidus for platelet adhesion and subsequent clot formation, which complicates the occlusion further and affects the end result of ischemia and/or infarction.
- *Biochemical theory*—Describes the process by which lung parenchymal lipases hydrolyze fat globules that

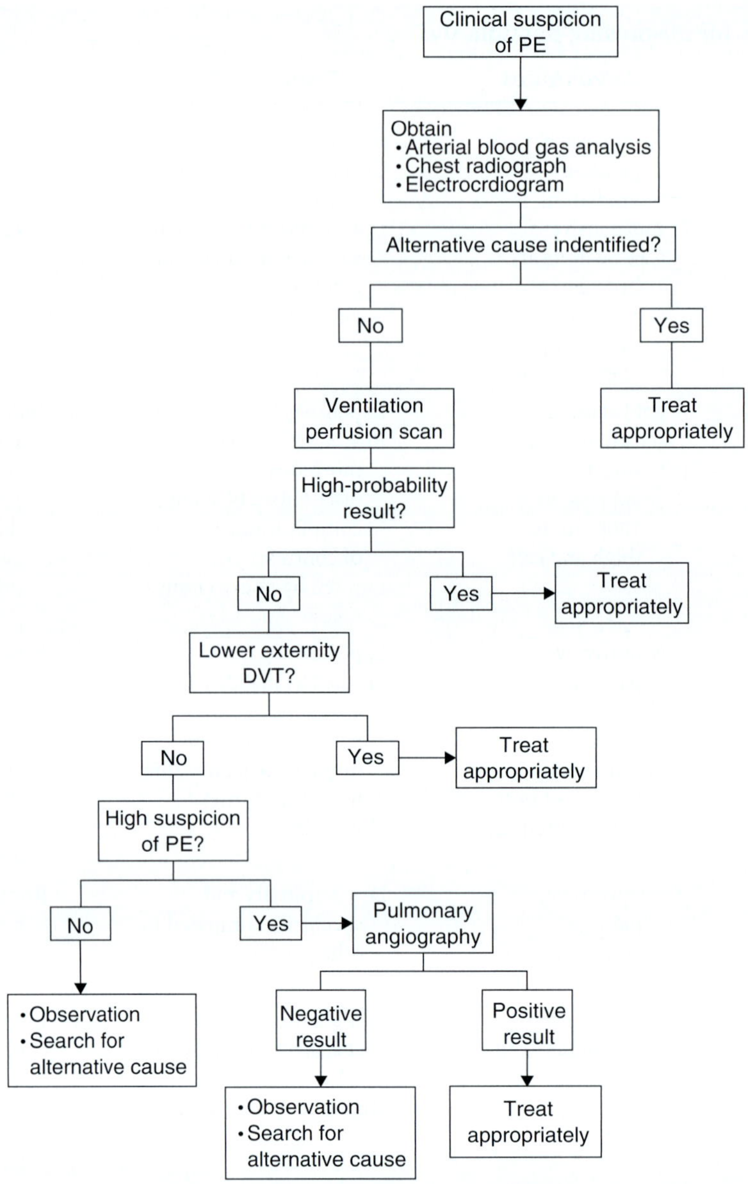

FIGURE 1.43 Algorithm for evaluation and treatment of suspected PE. (*Source*: Algorithm for evaluation and treatment of suspected PE. Thromboembolism after hip and knee arthroplasty: Diagnosis and treatment. *J Am Acad Orthop Surg* 1998;6:327–336, Fig. 2.)

have migrated to the area into biologically active fatty acids. These molecules then begin a cascade of inflammatory events that eventually lead to interstitial pulmonary edema. The final result resembles adult respiratory distress syndrome clinically and radiographically.

Diagnosis. There is no single laboratory test or radiographic examination that will definitively diagnose FES. FES should be suggested clinically by a number of signs and symptoms in the setting of sufficient trauma progressively worsening over the course of 24 to 48 hours after injury. Since introduced in 1974, Gurd and Wilson's criteria for the diagnosis of FES (Table 1.35) have been commonly used by physicians around the world to identify cases. Patients can manifest confusion and other mental status changes, petechiae, hypoxia, and tachycardia. EKG may or may not show changes. Laboratory studies, such as a CBC, serum lipase, fat globules in the urine or sputum, and ABG can be helpful in establishing the diagnosis. In the majority of patients with FES, the P_{O2} on an ABG will drop to less than 50 mmHg within 72 hours. Other causes of hypoxemia, such as pneumothorax or pulmonary embolus, should be ruled out with radiography and spiral CTA. Diffuse, bilateral infiltrates

TABLE 1.34 Perioperative DVT prophylaxis

Means	*Effect*	*Advantages*	*Disadvantages*
Unfractionated heparin (IV vs. SQ)	Binds to and potentiates antithrombin (AT) III inhibition of thrombin (IIa) and factor Xa, in addition to IXa, XIa, XIIa and kallikrein	Reversible via protamine sulfate	Bleeding; lower bioavailability than LMWH; heparin-induced thrombocytopenia (HIT) in 10% of patients
Enoxaparin (Lovenox)/low molecular weight heparin (LMWH)	Binds to and potentiates antithrombin (AT) III inhibition of thrombin (IIa); factor Xa, IXa, XIa, XIIa; and kallikrein	No monitoring; longer half-life than unfractionated heparin; improved bioavailability; less risk of HIT	Expensive; bleeding (less than unfractionated heparin)
Pentasaccharides (i.e., fondaparinux)	ATIII-mediated selective inhibition of factor Xa; does not affect thrombin already active	Stops further thrombin activation but allows thrombin present to continue activity, thus decreasing chance of bleeding; few side effects (no HIT); excellent performance	Expensive; bleeding (less than unfractionated heparin); not reversible as of yet
Coumadin	Inhibits vitamin K requiring clotting factors (II, VII, IX, X)	PO; reversible over a day with Vitamin K	3–5 days for full effect; requires monitoring (PT/INR); can be thrombogenic (prot. C&S); many drug interactions
Oral thrombin inhibitors (i.e., Melagatran)	Direct inhibition of thrombin	PO; wide therapeutic window; no monitoring; no known drug interactions	Expensive; bleeding; limited availability
ASA	Inhibits thromboxane A2, inhibiting platelet aggregation	PO; no monitoring	Weak efficacy
Pneumatic compression (foot pump)	Mechanical pump externally inducing blood flow, decreasing stasis	No drug interactions; reasonable efficacy; inexpensive	Bad compliance; unwieldy

(“snowstorm” pattern) on chest radiographs can be seen. There is a higher incidence of FES in patients with multiple fractures compared to single fractures.

Treatment. Treatment is largely supportive. Since there is no specific treatment for patients with FES, management should focus on supporting vital systemic processes such as mechanical ventilation for respiratory failure, nutrition, and optimizing blood parameters for maximized oxygen delivery to tissues.

Prevention. Much attention has been dedicated to the prevention of FES in high-risk patients. Many studies have shown the efficacy of low-dose steroids (e.g., methylprednisolone) in decreasing the severity of fat embolism sequelae, even with the potential chance that infection may occur as a result their use.

The mechanisms behind this protective phenomenon are not completely clear, but it is thought that (1) the steroids stabilize the pulmonary capillary membranes, thereby decreasing pulmonary infiltrates, and (2) the steroids counteract the inflammatory processes set off by the powerful fatty acid products of the fat embolism digestion. Studies show that the incidence of FES is significantly diminished with early fixation of fractures. The possibility that reamed intramedullary nailing of fractures increases incidence of FES versus unreamed nailing has not been definitively established.

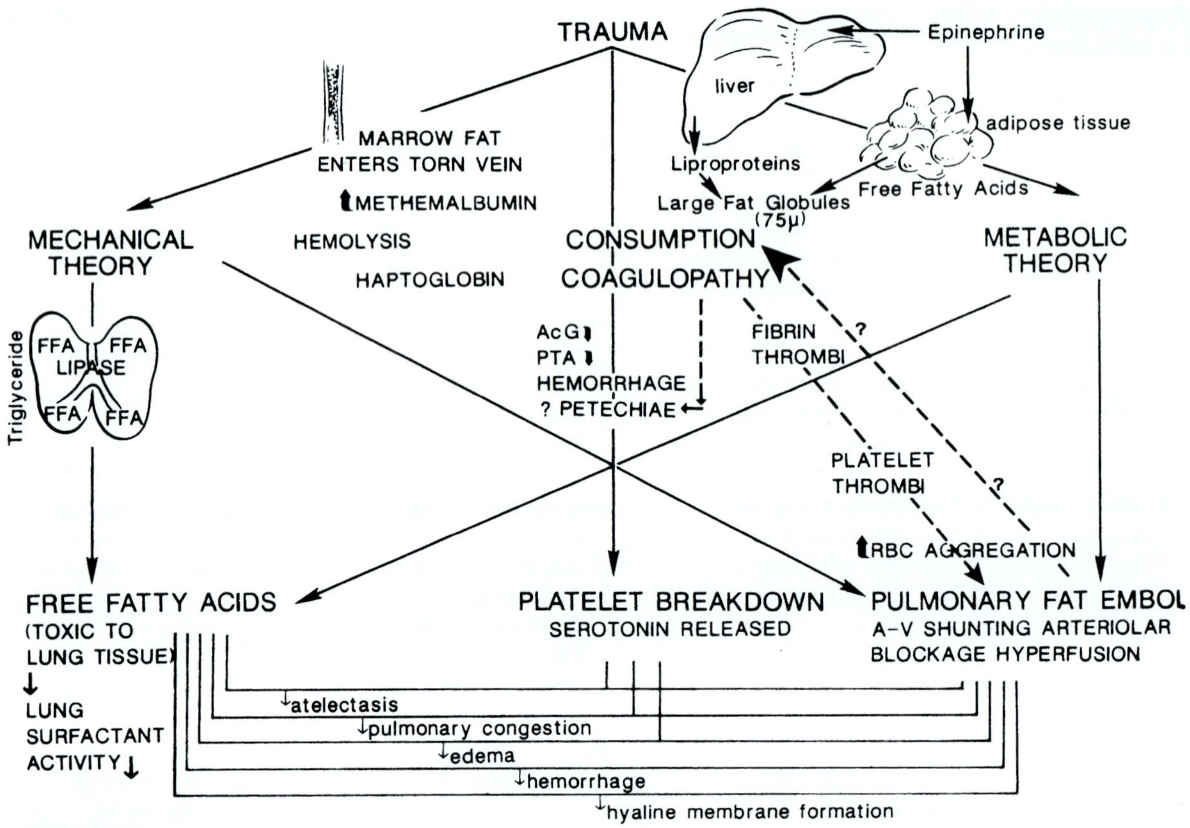

FIGURE 1.44 Pathological events of fat embolism syndrome. (*Source*: Simon SR (ed.). *Orthopaedic Basic Science*. Rosemont, IL: American Academy of Orthopaedic Surgeons, 1994; 502.)

Other Perioperative Issues

Shock. Acute failure of circulation leading to inadequate delivery of oxygen and nutrients to tissue due to a variety of causes, shock is most often broken down into the following groups (Table 1.36):

- *Hypovolemic*—Almost always associated with severe hemorrhage (Table 1.37) but can also be due to severe volume depletion (diarrhea, emesis, diuretic usage). It is also common in severe burns and in cases of severe third-space fluid loss, as in ascites.
- *Cardiogenic ("pump failure")*—Associated with a decline in cardiac output secondary to a serious heart condition such as myocardial infarction, pericardial tamponade, and progressive congestive heart failure, among others.
- *Septic*—Seen primarily in patients with bacteremia or severe abdominal or pelvic infections. Is the result of toxin-mediated vasodilation by primarily Gram-negative organisms. Toxic shock syndrome is a subset of septic shock caused by *Staphylococcus*. Incidence has decreased with the discontinuation of

TABLE 1.35 Gurd and Wilson's diagnostic criteria for fat embolus syndrome

Major Criteria	*Minor Criteria*
Axillary or subconjunctival petechia occurs transiently (4–6 hours) in 50%–60% of cases	Tachycardia (more than 110 beats per minute)
Hypoxemia (PaO_2, < 60 mmHg; $FiO_2 \leq 0.4$)	Pyrexia: temperature higher than 38.5°C (101.3°F)
CNS depression disproportionate to hypoxemia	Emboli present in retina on funduscopic examination
Pulmonary edema	Fat globules present in urine
	Sudden unexplainable drop in hematocrit or platelet values
	Elevated ESR
	Fat globules present in sputum

Must have at least 1 from major criteria and at least 4 from minor criteria.

TABLE 1.36 Types of shock and corresponding cardiovascular responses

Type	Preload	Afterload	Myocardial Contractility	Heart Rate (HR)	Stroke Volume (SV)	Cardiac Output (CO)	Systemic Vascular Resistance (SVR)
Hypovolemic (Hemorrhagic)	ʃ	)	Normal	)	No change or ʃ	No change or ʃ	)
Cardiogenic	)	)	ʃ	)	ʃ	ʃ	)
Septic	ʃ	ʃ	)	)	)	)	ʃ
Distributive (Neurogenic, Anaphylactic, etc.)	ʃ	ʃ	)	ʃ or normal	No change	ʃ	ʃ

extended-use tampons, which were a major cause of toxic shock syndrome due to staphylococcal growth within them while in the vagina.

- *Distributive*—This type of shock is typified by a severe loss of vascular tone, and includes neurogenic shock (spinal injury, etc.), anaphylactic shock (presence of IgE antibodies), and shock due to drug overdose with barbiturates and antihypertensives.

Pain Management After Major Orthopaedic Surgery

Pain management after major orthopaedic surgery is based on an individualized regimen depending on comorbidities, surgical procedure, and resources.

Opioids. Opioids (PO and IM) and IV patient-controlled analgesia (PCA) remain the modalities of choice for most patients recovering from orthopaedic surgery.

Epidural. Epidural analgesia (intermittent or continuous) uses local anesthetics alone or in combination with opioids to achieve a high level of targeted analgesia in patients who are experiencing severe pain.

Local. Local anesthetics interfere with local nerve conduction, resulting in the failure of nociceptive fibers to depolarize. Examples of local anesthetics include amides (lidocaine) and esters (metoxybutacaine, ethyl aminobenzoate). This method can also be coupled with a PCA device.

TABLE 1.37 Estimated fluid and blood losses based on patient's initial presentation in hemorrhagic shock†

	Class I	*Class II*	*Class III*	*Class IV*
Blood Loss (mL)	≤ 750	750–1500	1500–2000	> 2000
Blood Loss (% Blood Volume)	≤ 15%	15%–30%	30%–40%	> 40%
Pulse Rate	< 100	> 100	> 120	> 140
Blood Pressure	Normal	Normal	Decreased	Decreased
Pulse Pressure (mmHg)	Normal or increased	Decreased	Decreased	Decreased
Respiratory Rate	14–20	20–30	30–40	> 35
Urine Output (mL/hr)	> 30	20–30	5–15	Negligible
CNS/Mental Status	Slightly anxious	Mildly Anxious	Anxious, confused	Confused, lethargic
Fluid Replacement (3:1 rule)‡	Crystalloid	Crystalloid	Crystalloid and blood	Crystalloid and blood

†For 70-kg male
‡"3 for 1 rule": Empiric observation that patient in hemorrhagic shock requires approximately 300 mL of electrolyte solution for each 100 mL of blood loss
Source: Committee on Trauma. *Advanced Trauma Life Support Manual.* Chicago: American College of Surgeons 1997; 103–112.

Neuraxial. Any neuraxial analgesia holds risks, such as spinal hematoma, when associated with prophylactic anticoagulation. Other effective techniques include peripheral nerve blockade and continuous plexus block.

Nonsteroidal Antiinflammatory Drugs (NSAIDs). These drugs have an analgesic effect by blocking the production of prostaglandins via inhibition of the enzyme cyclooxygenase (COX). Both COX-1 and COX-2 inhibitors exist with COX-2 inhibitors selectively preserving the beneficial effects of the COX-1 enzyme: maintaining the gastric mucosa, renal blood flow, and endothelial protection. COX-2 inhibitors also limit the production of prostaglandins by inflamed synovium of arthritic joints more effectively than COX-1 inhibitors, making them effective arthritic medications.

VII. IMAGING AND SPECIAL STUDIES

Nuclear Medicine

Bone scans can be performed with a number of modalities. Tc99m, gallium citrate, and indium scans are all useful modalities, depending on the clinical situation present.

Technetium-99 m (Tc99m). Tc99m is a good compound for use in bone scans because it has a short half-life of 6 hours, and the energy it emits allows it to be imaged on a bone scan. Tc99m pyrophosphate complexes reflect an increase in blood flow and local metabolism. These complexes are absorbed onto the hydroxyapatite crystals of osseous tissue in infection, trauma, and neoplasia, allowing it to be useful to diagnose these clinical situations. A triple-phase bone scan is performed to localize a particular lesion and is performed with Tc99m-labeled phosphonate complex. There are 3 phases: the first phase (blood flow) displays blood flow through the arterial system; the second phase (blood pool—30 min) displays equilibrium of tracer throughout intravascular volume; the third is delayed (4 hrs) and displays sites in which tracer accumulates. A fourth scan can also be performed 24 hours after injection to better delineate tracer uptake by bone relative to soft tissue, but it is not typically needed to reach a diagnosis.

Gallium-67 Citrate. Gallium-67 citrate localizes in sites of inflammation and neoplasia because of the release of labeled serum proteins. The use of gallium citrate requires delayed imaging 1 to 2 days postinjection.

Indium-111. An indium-111 (In-111) WBC scan utilizes the tracer In-111 that accumulates in areas of inflammation and is useful in the diagnosis of acute infection.

MRI

T1 images are weighted toward fat, while T2 images are weighted toward water (H_2O).

T1 images best demonstrate anatomic structure (high signal-to-noise) ratio, while T2 images best for contrasting normal and abnormal tissues. This is particularly true in pathologic situations in which fluid (edema) accumulates. The magic angle phenomenon is seen when visualizing tendon or ligament. The tendon or ligament is oriented 55 degrees to the magnetic field, causing the specimen to appear bright on T1 imaging. Specific applications for MRI include (1) detection of osteonecrosis, (2) evaluation of occult hip fractures, such as those of the femoral neck, (3) detection of neoplasm, (4) identification of recurrent disk herniation (best diagnosed via MRI scan with gadolinium to differentiate between scar [absorb contrast] and disk [ring enhance]), and (5) diagnosis of PCL rupture, meniscal tears, and ACL rupture (95% sensitive).

Other Imaging Studies

Computed Tomography (CT). Useful for delineating the cross-sectional dural area of the cervical spine on axial imaging in order to diagnose cervical spinal stenosis (spinal stenosis present if area is less than 100 mm^2). It is the best study for demonstrating the bony anatomy and is important for evaluating the subtalar joint for tarsal coalitions. Plain radiographs using a Harris (axial) view can also identify talocalcaneal and tarsal coalitions. Dynamic CT scan is the best study for evaluating patients with atlantoaxial rotatory subluxation such as in Grisel syndrome occurring from inflammation of the soft tissues of the neck in patients with pharyngitis.

Discography. Discography is controversial but is one method used to identify a painful disk. Injection is done at low pressure (chemical reaction) and at high pressure (mechanical reaction).

Myelography. Procedure of choice to diagnose extramedullary intradural pathology.

Dual-Energy X-ray Absorptiometry (DEXA). DEXA is the most reliable method of quantifying bone mass and predicting fracture risk, especially in osteoporotic patients with a lower radiation dose than quantitative CT scan.

Electrodiagnostic Studies

Nerve Conduction Studies. Nerve conduction studies examine motor and sensory responses of peripheral nerves along their course. A nerve impulse is generated and recorded by surface electronic electrodes, and a conduction velocity is calculated. The time between the onset of the stimulus and response is the latency. Late response (F and H waves) provides information on proximal lesions, since the impulse travels to the spinal cord and returns.

Somatosensory Evoked Potentials (SSEP). SSEP can be used to study brachial plexus injuries and for spinal cord monitoring during surgery. Peripheral nerve entrapment syndromes have abnormal distal motor and sensory latencies of greater than 3.5 m/sec and velocities of less than 50 m/sec.

Electromyography (EMG). EMG uses intramuscular needle electrodes to assess for muscle denervation. The earliest signs are fibrillations at about 4 weeks after injury, sharp waves, and abnormal recruitment patterns.

VIII. BIOMECHANICS OF MUSCULOSKELETAL TISSUES AND TISSUE REPLACEMENTS

Basic Concepts

It is important to understand a few basic definitions regarding biomechanics. Biomechanics is the science of the action of forces, internal or external, on the living body. Statics is the study of the action of forces on bodies at rest (in equilibrium). Dynamics is the study of bodies in motion and the forces related to producing motion. The field of *kinetics* relates the effects of forces to the motion of bodies, while *kinematics* is the study of motion (displacement, velocity, and acceleration) without reference to the forces causing the motion.

Newton Laws. Central to understanding the principles of biomechanics and how they affect the skeletal system are three Newton laws governing forces. The first law, the law of inertia, is simply stated as follows: if the net external force acting on a body is zero, the body will remain at rest or move uniformly (zero acceleration). This allows for static analysis of the forces acting upon a body via the equation $\Sigma F = 0$. The second law, the law of acceleration, is the principle that the net force acting on an object is the product of the object's mass and its acceleration. Newton's third law, the law of reactions, states that there is an equal and opposite reaction. An understanding of these forces allows one to analyze the action of forces on bodies (free body analysis). Free body analyses are useful for understanding stresses in bone and bone remodeling in response to these stresses.

Biomechanics

Joint Biomechanics

Degrees of Freedom. Joint motion is described as rotations and translations occurring in the x, y, and z planes, requiring 6 parameters or degrees of motion (freedom to function). It is important to note that not all joints exhibit 6 degrees of freedom because of anatomic constraints to motion.

Hip. The hip is a joint that does exhibit 6 degrees of freedom and is termed a ball-and-socket joint. The stability of the joint is largely based upon the ball-and-socket design. The bone of the hip is also designed to withstand the significant stress that is placed upon it during daily activities. In fact, the reactive force of the hip can reach 3 to 6 times body weight, primarily due to the contraction of muscles that cross the hip joint. These muscles, primarily the abductor group (the gluteus medius and minimus), confer stability to the hip and are important in stabilizing the pelvis during gait. Table 1.38 shows the range of motion that the hip joint is capable of producing.

Knee. In contrast to the hip, the knee exhibits only 4 degrees of freedom: internal and external rotation, flexion and extension. The knee is a hinge joint, and stability is conferred upon it by the ligamentous structures that surround it. For example, the collateral and cruciate ligaments confer coronal plane stability with the knee in extension. While there is purely rotational movement about the hip, the knee does allow for translational motion during flexion and

TABLE 1.38 Range of motion of hip joint

	Average Range (Deg)	Functional Range (Deg)
Flexion	115	90 (120 to squat)
Extension	30	Not required
Abduction	50	20
Adduction	30	Not required
Internal rotation	45	0
External rotation	45	20

TABLE 1.39 Range of motion of knee joint

	Average Range (Deg)	Functional Range (Deg)
Extension	−10 (hyper-extension)	0
Flexion	130	90*
Internal rotation (at 90 deg of flexion)**	30	Not required#
External rotation (at 90 deg of flexion)**	45	Not required#

*117 deg required for squatting and lifting; 110 deg required to arise from a chair following a total knee arthroplasty.
**True rotation of the knee varies with degree of flexion.
#During the last 15 deg of extension, the femur internally rotates on the tibia, allowing full extension. This is called the "screw home" mechanism.

extension and is rather a complex series of rotations and translations about an instantaneous center of rotation. While understanding this complex series of motions of the knee is beyond the scope of this text, it is important to note that the knee does undergo additional motions besides flexion and extension and that the functional range of motion is different than the total range of motion that the knee is able to undergo. Table 1.39 shows the actual and functional range of motion of the knee.

Joint Reaction Force. Forces are generated within a joint in response to forces acting on the joint (both intrinsic and extrinsic). Muscle contractions about a joint are the major contributory factor to the joint reaction force. As an example, the gluteus medius and minimus attach to the greater trochanter of the proximal femur and create an abductor moment on the hip. When they contract, pulling the femur proximally, the force of contraction creates a joint reactive force against the acetabular wall by the femoral head.

Instant Center of Rotation. This is the point about which a joint rotates. For some joints, the instantaneous axis of rotation (IAR) is static, and for others it is dynamic (changes during the arc of motion, such as in the knee and unconstrained total disk replacement). It is helpful in understanding the types of motion that various joints undergo.

Rolling/Sliding Motion. Most joints, such as the knee, exhibit simultaneous rolling and sliding motion. Pure rolling occurs when the instant center of rotation is at the rolling surfaces and the contacting points have zero relative velocity. Pure sliding occurs with pure translation or rotation about a stationary axis; there is no angular change in position and no instant center of rotation.

Friction/Lubrication. The predominant mechanism of lubrication during dynamic joint function is *elastohydrodynamic.* With joint function and loading, there is deformation of the articular cartilage (hyaline cartilage), which leads to an efflux of fluid from the cartilage, contributing to the lubrication of the joint (which has a thin film of joint lubricant separating the surfaces) and reducing the coefficient of friction between the articular surfaces. The coefficient of friction in joints is a function of synovial fluid, an ultrafiltrate of blood plasma produced by the synovial membrane. Synovial fluid is produced by type B synovial cells (fibroblastlike). Of note, the type A synovial cells are important in phagocytosis.

Biomaterials

Critical to understanding the principles of tissue biomechanics is knowledge regarding the concepts of load, deformation, and stiffness. Load refers to the force(s) acting on a body and can be applied in compression, tension, shear or torsion, or some combination of these. Deformation is the change in shape produced in a body as a result of an applied load. This alteration can be temporary (elastic) or permanent (plastic). Stiffness describes the resistance of a body to deformation. Each of these properties is dependent on the geometry of a specimen and is therefore considered a *structural property.* Properties that are independent of geometry are termed *material properties* and include stress and strain, which are discussed in the next section. Stress is defined as force per unit area and can be normal (perpendicular) to a surface or can act in shear (parallel to the surface). It is typically reported in N/m^2 (pascals). Strain can also be normal or shear and is defined as the change in length/original length of a specimen. Because strain is a proportion, it is unitless. Modulus (Young's modulus of elasticity) is the measure of the ability of a material to resist deformation and is equal to stress and strain.

The Stress–Strain Curve. A stress–strain curve plots stress against strain for a specimen under uniaxial load. As illustrated in Figure 1.45 a specimen will typically exhibit linearly elastic behavior up to a limit, which is referred to as the proportional limit, or *yield point.* In this region, the material obeys *Hooke law,* which states that stress is proportional to strain or $F/A = E(Dl/l_0)$, where F is the force (or load)

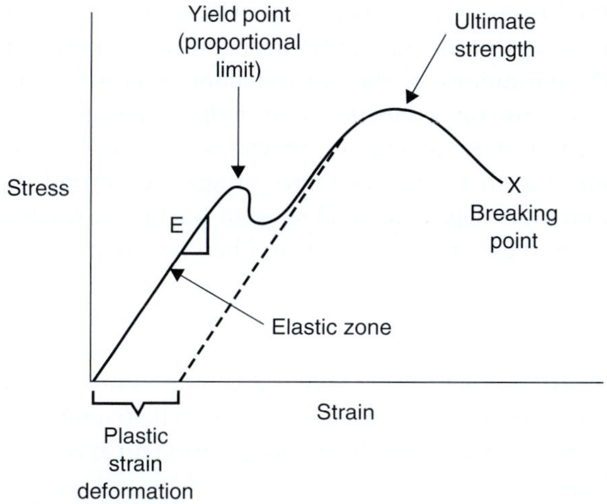

FIGURE 1.45 Stress-strain curve. (*Source:* Miller MD. *Review of Orthopaedics,* 2nd ed. Philadelphia: WB Saunders, 1996; 102.)

applied to the specimen, A is its cross-sectional area, and Dl/l_0 is the resultant strain. The proportionality constant, E, is referred to as *Young's modulus* and is an important property of the material because it measures its resistance to deformation. This property is independent of specimen geometry. Beyond the yield point, stress is no longer proportional to strain and deformation is no longer fully recoverable because of damage to the internal microstructure of the specimen. Other important features of the stress–strain curve are the *ultimate strength* (the maximum stress value attained by the specimen), the *breaking point* (the point at which the specimen fails), and the *plastic deformation* (the change in length after removing the load in the plastic range, before the breaking point). In addition to this information, the stress–strain curve can also be used to calculate *strain energy*, or *toughness*, which is the energy required to bring the specimen to failure and is represented by the area under the curve. Strain energy is a useful measure because injuries transfer energy to a body, which results in deformation and possibly fracture. By determining how much energy can be absorbed by a material before failure, it may be possible to enhance fracture prevention. Strain energy may also be useful in determining possible causes of existing fractures. Based on the concepts outlined in this section, several categories exist that describe material characteristics and behavior:

- *Brittle*—Brittle materials exhibit a linear stress–strain curve to failure and elastic deformation only. An example of a brittle material encountered in orthopaedics is polymethylmethacrylate (PMMA).
- *Ductile*—Ductile specimens, such as metals, undergo a large amount of plastic deformation before reaching failure.
- *Elastic*—Stress is directly proportional to strain for elastic materials, and deformation is fully recovered when a load is removed. The properties of elastic materials are insensitive to the rate of loading.
- *Viscoelastic*—The stress–strain behavior of viscoelastic materials depends on time and rate of loading. Viscoelasticity is a function of internal friction in the material. For such materials, a constant force will produce *creep*, that is, the deformation will increase with time as long as the force is maintained on the material, until equilibrium is reached. Conversely, a constantly held deformation will cause *stress relaxation* to occur, that is, the force required to maintain the deformation will diminish with time until equilibrium in reached. An example of this is bending a piece of copper wire: the copper wire will deform in response to the initial force applied. With time, the wire will remain in its deformed state (and require no force to maintain it in this state) or will require less force to attain this deformed state. Articular cartilage, intervertebral disk, ligament, tendon, and bone exhibit pronounced viscoelastic behavior.
- *Isotropic*—Isotropic materials have the same mechanical properties in all directions.
- *Anisotropic*—Mechanical properties vary with the direction of applied load in these materials. Biologic tissues are anisotropic in nature.

Mechanical Properties of Bone

Composition. Bone is a composite material consisting of minerals, proteins, water, cells, and other macromolecules (lipids, sugars, etc.), and its composition varies with anatomic site, age, diet, and the presence of disease. In general, however, approximately 90% of the organic matrix of bone is collagen, and the main constituent of its mineral phase is hydroxyapatite. Collagen has a low modulus, good tensile strength, and poor compressive strength. Hydroxyapatite is a stiff, brittle material with good compressive strength. This combination yields an anisotropic material that is strongest in compression, weakest in shear, and intermediate in tension.

Cortical and Trabecular Bone. The mineral content is the main determinant of the elastic modulus of cortical bone. Cortical bone is excellent in resisting torque, while trabecular bone is good in resisting compression and shear. Trabecular bone is 25% as dense, 10% as stiff, and 500% as ductile as cortical bone. Trabecular bone density varies significantly with anatomic location and age, and such variations directly impact the mechanical properties of the tissue. For example, trabecular bone properties within the proximal tibia can vary by up to 2 orders of magnitude because of changes in density alone. To further complicate matters, the mechanical properties of trabecular bone also depend on architecture, which, like density, depends on anatomic site and age. While cortical bone is essentially a low-porosity solid, trabecular bone is best described as an open-celled porous foam, composed of a series of thin and thick interconnecting trabeculae. Depending on the type and orientation of these basic cellular structures, the mechanical properties can vary by at least an order of magnitude.

Dynamic Properties. Bone is a dynamic material capable of self-repair and adaptation. Whereas prolonged immobilization induces bone weakness, exercise increases bone strength. With aging, the mechanical properties of cortical bone progressively deteriorate. This deterioration has been demonstrated in cortical bone samples taken from the femoral middiaphysis, which showed a decrease in elastic modulus and ultimate strength of approximately 2% per decade after 20 years of age. Probably the most significant change in terms of fracture risk, however, is the approximately 7% reduction in energy absorption that occurs with aging. Taken together, these data indicate that cortical bone becomes less stiff, weaker, and more brittle with aging. To offset age-related loss in mechanical properties, bone remodels its geometry to increase the inner and outer cortical diameters, thus minimizing bending stresses.

Wolff Law. Wolff law is the ability of bone to adapt structurally to changing loads. As an example, the trabecular patterns in the femoral head and neck are distributed in a pattern to allow the proximal femur to withstand the typical forces experienced by the hip in daily activities. Both the primary and secondary compression groups of trabecular lines are centered on the proximal, medial cortex (calcar), allowing it to withstand the compressive forces that are placed on it during gait. These stress patterns develop as a person first learns to walk. In pathologic situations, Wolff law may no longer hold true because bone loses its ability to remodel to stress, which increases the propensity of abnormal bone to fail under normal loading conditions, leading to a pathologic fracture.

Fractures

Type Based on Mechanism of Injury

Stress Fractures. Stress fractures can occur as a result of fatigue damage. In fatigue fractures, there are three characteristic stages: crack initiation, crack growth, and final fracture. In cortical bone, Haversian canals and lacunae serve as crack initiators because they represent discontinuities in the cortical bone microstructure. The most important factor in fatigue damage is the second stage of crack propagation, as microcracks join together once they have progressed beyond the initiation stage. The final stage of fracture is reached when these cracks coalesce and become large enough to overcome the absorptive properties of the Haversian system.

Tension Fractures. Tension fractures occur by muscle pull with the bone failing in tension. The fracture line is transverse, perpendicular to the load and axis of the bone.

Compression Fractures. Compression fractures occur by axial loading of bone, with cancellous-type bone failing typically. It results in a crush type of fracture, such as a buckle fracture in a child.

Shear Fractures. Shear fractures occur with a load that is parallel to the bone surface, with the resultant fracture parallel to the direction of loading. It is a component in spiral fracture patterns.

Butterfly Fragment. Fractures that are produced as a result of a bending force produce a characteristic called a *butterfly fragment* that is indicative of this fracture pattern. The fracture starts on the tension side of the bone and continues transversely (or obliquely) to the compression side of the bone. The bone bifurcates, producing a butterfly fragment.

Spiral Fractures. Spiral fractures result from tensile and shear forces. In a long bone that undergoes torsion, the greatest stress on the bone is experienced on the periosteal (outer) surface as opposed to the endosteal surface.

Comminuted Fractures. Comminuted fractures result from high-energy injuries without a specific force or force pattern creating the fracture. It is a function of the amount of energy transmitted to the bone, resulting in comminution. Furthermore, with high-energy injuries (such as those from a motorcycle), the energy can be dissipated to the surrounding soft tissues, resulting in soft-tissue damage (muscle, vascular, and skin damage).

Factors Affecting Fracture Risk

To estimate the degree of fracture risk of a particular bone in an individual, one must know three parameters about that particular bone: (1) the geometry of the bone, (2) the mechanical properties of the materials from which the bone is made, and (3) the location and direction of the loads to which the bone is subjected. In order to obtain this information, one must know not only the bone in question but also the activity of the individual in question. For example, critical clues in the patient's history, such as frequent stair ascent, falls, or repeated bending and/or lifting of objects, can lead a clinician to believe that an individual is at a higher risk of fracture. The geometry of the bone and the mechanical properties of the bone also play a critical role in allowing bones to resist the forces placed upon them during daily living. Osteoporosis is a classic example of how important these two concepts are to the structural integrity of the bone.

Aging. As the body ages, bone mass is lost, resulting in a decrease in overall bone density. The age-related reduction in bone mass is termed *senile osteoporosis*. It results in an increase in trabecular-bone fragility. Histomorphometric studies have shown that the number and thickness of the trabeculae decrease, while the intertrabecular spaces increase. This loss of trabeculae (termed *double jeopardy* because of the reduction in the number and thickness of the trabeculae) results in an increase in the porosity of the trabecular bone and a resultant reduction in its resistance to failure (Fig. 1.46). This age-related geometric change is reflected in the propensity for fracture of certain anatomic sites, such as the spine, proximal femur, and distal radius, which are largely trabecular bone structures. Fatigue fractures of these sites are most commonly seen in the elderly population. Elderly females are particularly at risk because peak bone mass in females is lower than it is in males. Furthermore, postmenopausal osteoporosis results in a disproportionate decrease in bone mineral density in women. In fact, in the lumbar spine in females, trabecular bone density has been shown to decrease approximately 50% from 20 to 80 years of age.

Mineral Content. The mineral content of bone is the most important determinant of the strength of bone, with hydroxyapatite being the most important mineral within bone. Various conditions of bone mineralization, such as those that relate to calcium and phosphate metabolism, can adversely affect bone mineralization and increase the propensity for fractures. As an example, familial hypophosphatemic rickets is an X-linked dominant disorder in which there is an impaired renal tubular reabsorption of phosphate, interfering with proper bone mineralization.

Mechanical Properties

Tendon and Ligament. Tendons and ligaments are anisotropic and viscoelastic and can sustain 5% to 10% tensile strain before failure (vs. 1% to 4% in bone). A typical stress–strain curve for these tissues (Fig. 1.45) can be divided into a low modulus (toe) region, followed by a linear region with higher modulus. The toe region has been attributed to the straightening of the crimped fibrils and to nonuniform recruitment of individual fibers. Tendon, which has one of highest tensile strengths of any soft tissue in the body, consists

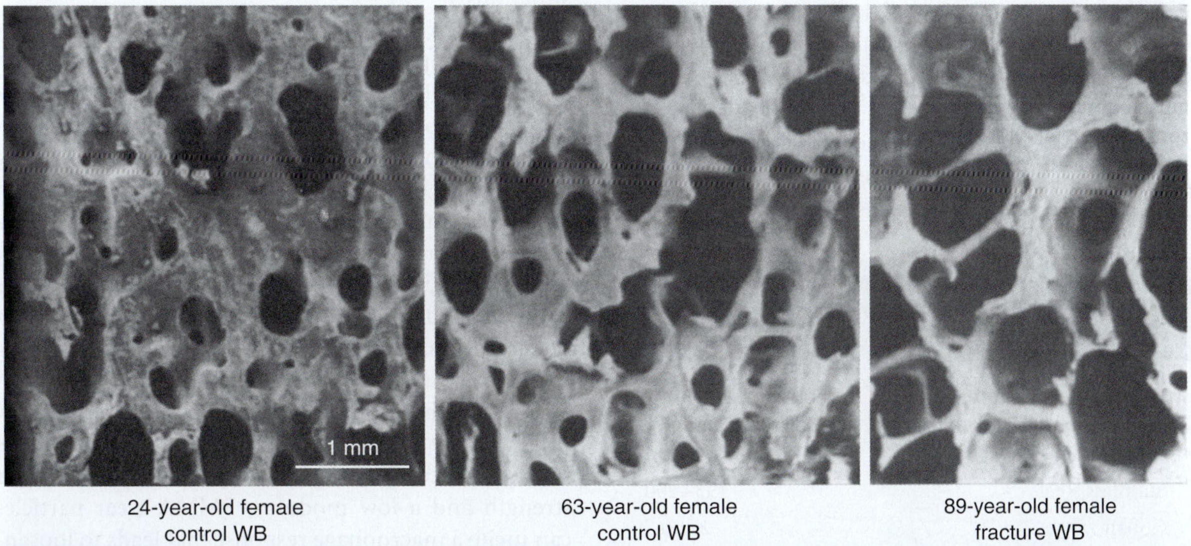

FIGURE 1.46 **Age-related changes in apparent density and architecture of human trabecular bone from the lumbar spine. (*Source*: Buckwalter JA, Einhorn TA, Simon SR. *Orthopaedic Basic Science: Biology and Biomechanics of the Musculoskeletal System*, 2nd ed. Rosemont, IL: American Academy of Orthopaedic Surgeons, 2000; 347, Fig. 38.)**

almost exclusively of fibers oriented along a single direction of force. Ligament, however, has a broader distribution of fiber directions because of more varied loading conditions in vivo.

Intervertebral Disk. Intervertebral disks are anisotropic and viscoelastic, and also exhibit toe and linear regions in tensile extension. The annulus fibrosus exhibits high values for Young's modulus, stiffness, and failure stress, all of which indicate that this tissue is well equipped to sustain the large tensile stresses that it endures in situ. In particular, the outer annulus is ideally suited for minimizing disk bulging. Because tensile properties depend on the pathologic state of tissue, however, annulus degeneration can lead to disk herniation. The nucleus pulposus acts predominantly as fluid under static load, generating large hydrostatic pressures that help to maintain disk height and support and transfer load.

Cartilage. Similar to the other orthopaedic soft tissues, cartilage is anisotropic and viscoelastic. It exhibits toe and linear regions in tensile extension. Its ultimate tensile strength is only 5% that of bone, but it is well suited for compressive loading because of its highly viscoelastic properties.

Tissue Replacement Mechanics

Materials. A comparison of Young's modulus for common artificial materials encountered in orthopaedics can be seen in Table 1.40, along with the values of this property associated with biologic tissues. Following is a description of the basic categories into which these replacement materials may fall and a description of their related uses and concerns.

Metals. Metals are used as structural elements in joint prostheses. They demonstrate relatively good corrosion resistance and reasonable fatigue life, and their moduli exceed that of bone. Orthopaedic implants are typically made of stainless steel (e.g., 316 L), cobalt-chromium (Co-Cr), or titanium alloys. The properties of each, such as modulus (Table 1.40), are varied and are important when choosing the optimal material for each application. Titanium, for instance, is extremely biocompatible with a high-yield strength and a modulus closer to that of bone than exhibited by stainless steel or Co-Cr. Titanium, however, has poor resistance to wear, raising some concerns regarding its use in implants because the release of corrosion products may incite a macrophage response. Co-Cr alloy generates less metal debris than titanium. Its increased modulus along with that of stainless steel, however, make these metals more likely to induce a condition known as stress shielding, in which normal stress is transferred from the bone to the implant, often with detrimental effects.

TABLE 1.40 Modulus of elasticity (Young's modulus) for various materials (GPa)

Polymethylmethacrylate (PMMA)	3–4
Cortical bone	17.0
Titanium alloys	104–116
Stainless steel	193–200
Cobalt	211.0
Chromium	248
Molybdenum	320
Aluminum oxide (alumina ceramic, Al_2O_3)	393

Polymers. There are two specific applications in orthopaedics in which polymers have proved useful, and in both cases, the appropriate mechanical properties of the polymer are of major importance. First, polymers are used as articulating surface components in joint prostheses. Thus, they must have a low coefficient of friction and low wear rate when they are in contact with the opposing surface, which is usually made of metal or ceramic. Second, polymers are used for fixation as a structural interface between the implant component and bone tissue. This usually requires that the polymers be able to minimize plastic deformation and resist creep under the stresses found in clinical situations.

Examples of polymers with orthopaedic applications include polyethylene, PMMA, and silicone. Ultrahigh molecular weight polyethylene (UHMWPE) is often used to fabricate weight-bearing implant components, such as acetabular cups and tibial trays, owing to its tough, ductile nature as well as its low friction properties and resistance to wear. Wear damage to a UHMWPE articulating surface is most often caused by foreign body inclusions, and the associated wear debris is the main factor affecting the longevity of these joint replacements. PMMA is frequently used as a grouting material for fixation of implants and distribution of load at the bone–implant interface. It functions by mechanically interlocking with bone, and while it is strongest in compression, it has poor tensile and shear strength and a low modulus. PMMA wear particles can incite a macrophage response that leads to loosening of the implant. Unlike polyethylene and PMMA, silicones are polymers that are most often found in nonweight-bearing joints. Their poor strength and inability to resist wear can lead to frequent synovitis with prolonged use.

Ceramics and Glass. Ceramics contain metallic and nonmetallic elements and include inert materials, such as alumina (Al_2O_3), as well as bioactive (degradable) substances such as bioglass. They are brittle (no elastic deformation), have a high modulus, high compressive strength, low tensile strength, low yield strain, and exhibit favorable wear characteristics but poor crack resistance. Ceramics and glass ceramics have played an increasingly important role in implants and have been used primarily in two different applications. The first is their use as articulating surfaces, for which ceramic properties such as resistance to oxidation (i.e., inertness in the body), high modulus, and low friction and wear rates are highly desirable. Al_2O_3, for instance, has proven quite successful for use in paired femoral head and acetabular components in total hip arthroplasty. The second application takes advantage of the osteophilic surface of certain ceramics and glass ceramics. These materials, termed *bioglasses*, provide an interface of such biological compatibility with osteoblasts that these cells lay down bone directly next to the material. Several of these compositions have seen wide use as implant materials. The use of bioglass on the metallic stems of hip prostheses provides an alternative approach to fixation instead of using PMMA.

Composites. From the previous description of bone properties and a comparison with the corresponding properties of the various metals, polymers, and ceramics, it is clear that there is considerable disparity among these materials. This mismatch fueled the idea that it might be possible to optimize implant properties by combining materials and thus sparked an interest in composite materials. An area where composites may provide an interesting and important application is in bone plates. The rigidity and stiffness of the metallic plates generally used are much greater than that of the adjacent bone. Even after healing is well underway, the plate continues to carry a major portion of the load, thereby stress shielding the underlying bone and delaying, if not preventing, full healing. Eventually, a second operation is required to remove the plate. This situation is one in which composites may offer a superior solution. For instance, totally bioresorbable composite plates have been made from polyglycolic acid (PGA) fibers embedded in a polylactic acid (PLA) matrix. Because the degradation rate of such composites can be controlled via the design process, it is conceivable to design a plate that would remain stiff and rigid enough to support the loads of physical activity until the bone has healed sufficiently to do so without assistance. Consequently, instead of continuing to divert part of the load away from the underlying bone, the plate would gradually degrade and increasing amounts of load would be transferred to the bone, thus providing the proper loading conditions for full healing to proceed. Another orthopaedic application of composites is in replacement of tendons and ligaments. In this capacity, biodegradable polymers such as PLA have acted as a scaffold, allowing ingrowth of collagenous tissue in an attempt to reform the damaged connective tissue.

Engineered (Living) Tissue. These constructs typically consist of a cell-seeded scaffold, with or without bioactive elements, and are capable of self-adaptation and repair. With new technologies evolving rapidly, the future of tissue engineering for musculoskeletal tissue repair looks bright. Growth factors, introduced during fabrication or delivery of the constructs, hold promise for improving repair quality. In addition, the quality of the engineered tissue might be further enhanced through mechanical stimulation of the constructs during the fabrication process. All of these factors, however, are likely to be tissue and site specific and must be delivered thoughtfully and appropriately if tissue engineers expect to stimulate early cell proliferation and subsequent matrix synthesis. This matrix must also be deposited and rapidly organized if the repair is to be capable of resisting the large in vivo forces of daily activities. Scaffolds must also be identified with enough compliance that the cells can organize the construct but with enough stiffness to resist the expected in vivo loading regimes. These materials should initially attract, anchor, and protect the cells, but then degrade at controlled rates that prevent mechanical disruption of the repair and ensure biocompatibility. Many of these treatments are now being investigated and offer exciting potential for the repair of hard and soft tissue injuries.

References

1. Aquaro S, et al. Limited development and progression of resistance of HIV-1 to the nucleoside analogue reverse transcriptase inhibitor lamivudine in human primary macrophages. *J Antimicrob Chemother* 2005 Apr 21.
2. Babalis GA. Prevention of posttraumatic hypoxemia in isolated lower limb long bone fractures with a minimal prophylactic dose of corticosteroids. *Injury* 2004 Mar;35(3):309–317.
3. Boachie-Adjei O, Squillante RG. Tuberculosis of the spine. *Orthop Clin North Am* 1996;27:95–103.
4. Boyle BA. Considerations in selecting protease inhibitor therapy. *AIDS Rev* 2004 Oct–Dec;6(4):218–225.
5. Buckwalter JA, Einhorn TA, Simon SR. *Orthopaedic Basic Science: Biology and Biomechanics of the Musculoskeletal System*, 2nd ed. Rosemont, IL: American Academy of Orthopaedic Surgeons, 2000.
6. Bullough PG. Normal bone structure and development. In: *Bullough and Vigorita's Orthopaedic Pathology*, 3rd ed. London: Mosby-Wolfe, 1997.

7. Centers for Disease Control and Prevention (CDC). Case-control study of HIV seroconversion in health-care workers after percutaneous exposure to HIV-infected blood—France, United Kingdom, and United States, January 1988–August 1994. *MMWR* 1995 Dec 22;44(50):929–933.
8. CDC. Exposure to blood: What health-care personnel need to know. Available at: www.cdc.gov/ncidod/hip/Blood/Exp_to_Blood.pdf.
9. CDC. *HIV/AIDS surveillance report: HIV infection and AIDS in the United States.* 2003.
10. Chao EYS, Aro HT. Biomechanics of fracture fixation. In: Mow VC, Hayes WC (eds.), *Basic Orthopaedic Biomechanics*, 2nd ed. Philadelphia: Lippincott-Raven, 1997;317–351.
11. Chen FS, Frenkel SR, DiCesare PE. Repair of articular cartilage defects: Part I. Basic science of cartilage healing. *Am J Orthop* 1999;28:31–33.
12. Chen FS, Frenkel SR, DiCesare PE. Repair of articular cartilage defects: Part II. Treatment options. *Am J Orthop* 1999;28:88–96.
13. Chun CSY. Chronic recurrent multifocal osteomyelitis of the spine and mandible: Case report and review of the literature. *Pediatrics* 2004 Apr;113(4):e380–e384.
14. Cierny G, III. Chronic osteomyelitis: Results of treatment. *Instr Course Lect.* 1990;39:495–508.
15. de Winter F, van de Wiele C, Vogelaers D, de Smet K, Verdonk R, Dierckx RA. Fluorine-18 fluorodeoxyglucose-positron emission tomography: A highly accurate imaging modality for the diagnosis of chronic musculoskeletal infections. *J Bone Joint Surg Am* 2001 May 1;83(5):651–660.
16. Della Valle CJ, Bogner E, Desai P, et al. Analysis of frozen sections of intraoperative specimens obtained at the time of reoperation after hip or knee resection arthroplasty for the treatment of infection. *J Bone Joint Surg* 1999;81:684–689.
17. Erikkson BI, Agnelli G, Cohen AT, et al. Direct thrombin inhibitor melagatran followed by oral ximelagatran in comparison with enoxaparin for prevention of venous thromboembolism after total hip or knee replacement. *Thromb Haem* 2003;89:288–296.
18. Ferrari E, et al. The ECG in pulmonary embolism. *Chest* 1997;111:537–543.
19. Fingeroth RJ. Single dose 6Gy prophylaxis for heterotopic ossification after total hip arthroplasty. *Clin Orthop* 1995;317:131–140.
20. Gamble JG, Rinsky LA. Chronic recurrent multifocal osteomyelitis: A distinct clinical entity. *J Pediatr Orthop* 1986;6:579–584.
21. Gardner MJ, et al. Has locked plating completely replaced conventional plating? *Am J Orthopaedics* 2004;9:440–446.
22. Goodman S. Wear particulate and osteolysis. *Orthop Clin North Am* 2005 Jan;36(1):41–48, vi.
23. Gurd AR, Wilson RI. The fat embolism syndrome. *J Bone Joint Surg Br* 1974;56:408.
24. Gurd AR. Fat embolism: An aid to diagnosis. *J Bone Joint Surg* 1970;52B:732–737.
25. Haake DA, Berkman SA. Venous thromboembolic disease after hip surgery: Risk factors, prophylaxis, and diagnosis. *Clin Orthop* 1989;242:212–231.
26. Hain SF, et al. Functional imaging and the orthopaedic surgeon. *J Bone Joint Surg Br* 2002 Apr;84(3):315–321.
27. Hayes WC, Bouxsein ML. Biomechanics of cortical and trabecular bone: Implications for assessment of fracture risk. In: Mow VC, Hayes WC (eds.), *Basic Orthopaedic Biomechanics*, 2nd ed. Philadelphia: Lippincott-Raven. 1997; 69–111.
28. Joseph TN. Use of antibiotic-impregnated cement in total joint arthroplasty. *J Am Acad Orthop Surg* 2003;11:38–47.
29. Kallenbach J, Lewis M, Zaltzman M, Feldman C, Orford A, Zwi S. 'Low-dose' corticosteroid prophylaxis against fat embolism. *J Trauma* 1987 Oct; 27(10):1173–1186.
30. Kaplan FS. Heterotopic Ossification. *JAAOS* 2004;12(2): 116–125.
31. Kishiyama JL, Adelman DC. Allergic and immunologic diseases. In: Tierney LM, McPhee SJ, Papadakis MA (eds.), *Current Medical Diagnosis and Treatment*, 40th ed. New York: McGraw Hill, 2001;19.
32. Koval KJ (ed.), *Orthopaedic Knowledge Update 7*. Rosemont, IL: AAOS, 2002;3–18.
33. Kropfl A, Berger U, Neureiter H, Hertz H, Schlag G. Intramedullary pressure and bone marrow fat intravasation in unreamed femoral nail. *J Trauma* 1997;42:946–954.
34. Levy D. Fat embolism syndrome: A review. *Clin Orthop* 1990 Dec;(261):281–296.
35. Mackowiak PA, et al. Diagnostic value of sinus-tract cultures in chronic osteomyelitis. *JAMA* 1978 Jun 30;239(26):2772–2775.
36. Manganelli D, Palla A, Donnamaria V, Giuntini C. Clinical features of pulmonary embolism: Doubts and certainties. *Chest* 1995;107(suppl 1):25S–32S.
37. Mauerhan DR, Nelson CL, Smith DL, et al. Prophylaxis against infection in total joint arthroplasty: One day of cefuroxime compared with three days of cefazolin. *J Bone Joint Surg* 1994;76A:39–45.
38. Modic MT, Feiglin DH, Piraino DW, et al. Vertebral osteomyelitis: Assessment using MR. *Radiology* 1985;157:157–166.
39. Musso AD, Mohanty K, Spencer-Jones R. Role of frozen section histology in diagnosis of infection during revision arthroplasty. *Postgrad Med J* 2003 Oct;79(936):590–593.
40. Neal BC, et al. A systematic survey of 13 randomized trials of non-steroidal anti-inflammatory drugs for the prevention of heterotopic bone formation after major hip surgery. *Acta Orthop Scand* 2000;71:122–128.
41. Ostermann PA, Seligson D, Henry SL. Local antibiotic therapy for severe open fractures: A review of 1085 consecutive cases. *J Bone Joint Surg* 1995;77B:93–97.
42. Pape HC, Auf'm'Kolk M, Paffrath T, Regel G, Sturm JA, Tscherne H. Primary intramedullary femur fixation in multiple trauma patients with associated lung

contusion: A cause of post-traumatic ARDS? *J Trauma* 1993;34:540–548.

43. Perron MD, Miller AD, Brady WJ. Orthopedic pitfalls in the ED: Fight bite. *Am J Emerg Med* 2002 Mar;20(2):114–117.
44. Pfeltz RF, Wilkinson BJ. The escalating challenge of vancomycin resistance in Staphylococcus aureus. *Curr Drug Targets Infect Disord* 2004 Dec;4(4):273–294.
45. Pruit BA, McManus WF, McManus AT, et al. Infections: Bacteriology, antibiotics and chemotherapy, In: Jupiter JB (ed.), *Flynn's Hand Surgery*, 4th ed. Baltimore: Williams & Wilkins, 1991;713.
46. Quiroz R, et al. Spiral CT for pulmonary embolism: The paradigm has shifted. *Am Heart Hosp J* 2003 Fall;1(4):281–288.
47. Ratner BD, Hoffman AS, Schoen FJ, Lemons JE (eds.), *Biomaterials Science: An Introduction to Materials in Medicine*. San Diego: Academic Press, 1996.
48. Regmi A, Fuson T, Yang X, et al. Suramin interacts with RANK and inhibits RANKL-induced osteoclast differentiation. *Bone* 2005 Feb;36(2):284–291.
49. Rugo, HS. Cancer. In: Tierney LM, McPhee SJ, Papadakis MA (eds.), *Current Medical Diagnosis & Treatment*, 40th ed. New York: McGraw Hill, 2001.
50. Sande MA, Kapusnik-Uner JE, Mandell GL. Antimicrobial agents, In: Gilman AG (ed.), *Goodman and Gilman's The Pharmacological Basis of Therapeutics*, 8th ed. New York: McGraw, 1990;1019.
51. Schonfeld SA, Ploysongsang Y, DiLisio R, et al. Fat embolism prophylaxis with corticosteroids. A prospective study in high-risk patients. *Ann Inter Med* 1983 Oct;99(4):438–443.
52. Scoles PV, Quinn TP. Intervertebral discitis in children and adolescents. *Clin Orthop* 1982;162:31–36.
53. Shuford, Jennifer A. Steckelberg, James M. Role of oral antimicrobial therapy in the management of osteomyelitis. *Curr Opin Infect Diseases* 2003 Dec;16(6):515–519.
54. Sivakumar B, Paleolog E. Immunotherapy of rheumatoid arthritis: Past, present and future. *Curr Opin Drug Discov Devel* 2005 Mar;8(2):169–176.
55. Solomon SD, McMurray JJ, Pfeffer MA. Adenoma prevention with celecoxib (APC) study investigators. Cardiovascular risk associated with celecoxib in a clinical trial for colorectal adenoma prevention. *N Engl J Med* 2005 Mar 17;352(11):1071–1080.
56. Stramer SL, et al. Detection of HIV-1 and HCV infections among antibody-negative blood donors by nucleic acid-amplification testing. *N Engl J Med* 2004 Aug 19;351(8):760–768.
57. Stulberg BN, Insall JN, Williams GW, Ghelman B. Deep-vein thrombosis following total knee replacement: An analysis of six hundred and thirty-eight arthroplasties. *J Bone Joint Surg Am* 1984;66:194–201.
58. Stumpe KD, Dazzi H, Schaffner A, Von Schulthess GK. Infection imaging using whole body FDG-PET. *Eur J Nucl Med* 2000;27:822–832.
59. Tay BKB, Deckey J, Hu SS. Spinal infections. *J Am Acad Orthop Surg* 2002;10:188–197.
60. Turpie AGG, Bauer KA, Eriksson BI, Lassen MR. Fondaparinux vs Enoxaparin for the prevention of venous thromboembolism in major orthopaedic surgery. *Arch Intern Med* 2002;162:1833–1840.
61. Value of the ventilation/perfusion scan in acute pulmonary embolism. Results of the prospective investigation of pulmonary embolism diagnosis (PIOPED). The PIOPED Investigators. *JAMA* 1990;263:2753–2759.
62. van Beek EJ. MRI for the diagnosis of pulmonary embolism. *J Magn Reson Imaging* 2003 Dec;18(6):627–640.
63. Wakitani S, Goto T, Pineda SJ, et al. Mesenchymal cell-based repair of large, full thickness defects of articular cartilage. *J Bone Joint Surg* 1994;76A:579–592.
64. Wenger DR, Bobechko WP, Gilday DL. The spectrum of intervertebral disc space infection in children. *J Bone Joint Surg Am* 1978;60:100–108.
65. Wiley AM, Trueta J. The vascular anatomy of the spine and its relationship to pyogenic vertebral osteomyelitis. *J Bone Joint Surg Br* 1959;41:796–809.
66. Woo SL-Y. Ligament, tendon, and joint capsule insertions into bone. In: Woo SL-Y, Buckwalter JA (eds.), *Injury and Repair of the Musculoskeletal Soft Tissues*. Park Ridge, IL: American Academy of Orthopaedic Surgeons, 1988;134–135.
67. Zimlich RH, et al. Current status of anticoagulation therapy after total hip and total knee arthroplasty. *J Am Acad Orthop Surg* 1996;4:54–62.

Key References

Baldwin KM, Winder WW, Holloszy JO. Adaptation of actomyosin ATPase in different types of muscle to endurance exercise. *Am J Physiol* 229:422–426,1975.

Higher concentrations of actomyosin were found in the red portion of the vastus lateralis and in the white portion of the vastus lateralis muscle than in the soleus or heart in rats. A strenuous program of treadmill running lasting 18 weeks or longer did not significantly affect the amount of actomyosin recovered from the different types of muscle. No changes in actomyosin ATPase occurred in fast-twitch white (white vastus) or heart muscles in response to the exercise training. In contrast, a decrease of approximately 20% occurred in the specific activity of actomyosin ATPase of fast-twitch red (red vastus) muscle (0.635 ± 0.029 mumol Pi/min per milligram for sedentary vs. 0.529 ± 0.021 mumol Pi/min per milligram for trained), while the actomyosin ATPase activity of slow-twitch red (soleus) muscle increased about 20% (0.209 ± 0.033 vs. 0.257 ± 0.031 mumol Pi/min per milligram). There was a close correlation (r = 0.99, P less than 0.001) between actomyosin ATPase activity and phosphofructokinase activity in the 3 types of skeletal muscles and in heart muscle of exercise-trained and untrained animals, providing further evidence in support of the concept that the glycogenolytic capacity of a muscle and its actomyosin ATPase activity are regulated in parallel.

Booth FW. Physiologic and biochemical effects of immobilization on muscle. *Clin Orthop* 219:25–27,1987.

Muscle strength rapidly declines during limb immobilization because of a decrease in muscle size and a decrease in tension per unit of muscle cross-sectional area. Muscle fatigability also increases rapidly after limb immobilization. Muscles within limbs fixed by plaster casts have lower levels of resting glycogen and adenosine triphosphate (ATP), a more rapid depletion of muscle glycogen and ATP during work, a greater increase in lactate during work, and a decreased capacity to oxidize fatty acids during work. The greatest loss of absolute muscle mass occurs at the beginning of muscle wasting with subsequent loss of muscle being exponential. A significant decrease in the rate of protein synthesis in muscles is observable at the sixth hour of limb immobilization, which most likely initiates the net loss of muscle protein. A change in the amount of either translational or elongational factor is most likely responsible for the early decrease in this rate of protein synthesis.

Buckwalter JA. Articular cartilage. *Instructional Course Lecture* 32:349–370,1983.

Cartilage is not simple, inert, homogeneous, bearing surface but rather a complex, living tissue. It has the capacity to provide a low friction surface, participate in joint lubrication, and distribute loads to subchondral bone, all with a very limited capacity for repair and without evidence of abrasive wear over a lifetime of use. The macromolecules of the cartilage matrix, collagen, proteoglycans, noncollagenous proteins, and glycoproteins give it its mechanical and biologic properties, and the cells produce and maintain the matrix. The interaction between the cells and matrix is critical for normal function of the tissue, as are the influences of mechanical loads and motion on the tissue, but study of these important areas is only beginning. Significant advances in the understanding and treatment of joint disease depends on further knowledge of cartilage structure and function as well as the factors that maintain and restore the cartilage matrix.

Burchardt H. The biology of bone graft repair. *Clin Orthop* 174:28–42,1983.

Cancellous and cortical autografts histologically have three differences: (1) cancellous grafts are revascularized more rapidly and completely than cortical grafts; (2) creeping substitution of cancellous bone initially involves an appositional bone formation phase, followed by a resorptive phase, whereas cortical grafts undergo a reverse creeping substitution process; (3) cancellous grafts tend to repair completely with time, whereas cortical grafts remain as admixtures of necrotic and viable bone. Physiologic skeletal metabolic factors influence the rate, amount, and completeness of bone repair and graft incorporation. The mechanical strengths of cancellous and cortical grafts are correlated with their respective repair processes: cancellous grafts tend to be strengthened first, whereas cortical grafts are weakened. Bone allografts are influenced by the same immunologic factors as other tissue grafts. Fresh bone allografts may be rejected by the host's immune system. The histoincompatibility antigens of bone allografts are presumably the proteins or glycoproteins on cell surfaces. The matrix proteins may or may not elicit graft rejection. The rejection of a bone allograft is considered to be a cellular rather than a humoral response, although the humoral component may play a part. The degree of the host response to an allograft may be related to the antigen concentration and total dose. The rejection of a bone allograft is histologically expressed by the disruption of vessels, an inflammatory process including lymphocytes, fibrous encapsulation, peripheral graft resorption, callus bridging, nonunions, and fatigue fractures.

Evans GA, Arulanantham K, Gage JR. Primary hypophosphatemic rickets: Effect of oral phosphate and vitamin D on growth and surgical treatment. *J Bone Joint Surg* 62(A):1130–1138,1980.

Failure to diagnose and treat hypophosphatemic rickets during childhood resulted in stunted growth and progressive deformities of the lower limb. When the deformities were treated surgically, recurrent deformity and nonunion of osteotomies developed, and further major operative procedures were required to remedy these complications. Treatment from early childhood with oral phosphate and vitamin D improved the rate of growth and controlled the progression of bowleg deformity. Residual varus deformity was corrected by osteotomy through the proximal tibial metaphysis at skeletal maturity, when the results were predictable. Genu valgum deformity was corrected by stapling the medial part of the distal femoral epiphysis prior to skeletal maturity. With early postoperative mobilization and adequate medication, the complications of delayed tibial union and failure to correct the femoral valgus deformity were avoided.

Jardon OM. Malignant hyperthermia: A Potentially fatal syndrome in orthopaedic patients. *J Bone Joint Surg* 61(A):1064–1070,1979.

Malignant hyperthermia is an inherited muscular disorder and a cause of sudden death in afflicted patients. Stress arising from trauma, surgery, and other causes can initiate the syndrome. We studied the types of orthopaedic problems commonly seen in patients with this condition as well as the clinical manifestations and pathophysiology of the syndrome. Recognition, management, and understanding of the pathophysiology of malignant hyperthermia can be aided by a study of its similarities to porcine stress syndrome. We performed experimental studies of muscle and prophylaxis in swine. We also demonstrated the extension of the prophylactic use of dantrolene sodium in a management protocol in 80 surgical procedures in humans.

Mankin HJ, Thrasher AZ. Water content and binding in normal and osteoarthritic human cartilage. *J Bone Joint Surg* 57(A):76–80,1975.

Water binding in normal and osteoarthritic cartilage slices from human femoral heads was studied using tritiated water to measure the water binding after short exposure, total water content, and avidity with which water is held. In osteoarthritic cartilage, compared with normal cartilage, there was no increase in water binding, but water content increased by 9% and the avidity with which the newly bound water was held also increased. These findings were almost exactly duplicated by partial extraction of the proteoglycan from normal tissues with 4 molar guanidinium hydrochloride.

Patzakis MJ, Wilkins J, Moore TM. Considerations in reducing the infection rate in open tibial fractures. *Clin Orthop* 178:36–41,1983.

During the period from 1979 to 1980, 109 patients with open tibial fractures were treated by a cephalosporin and an aminoglycoside, and by saline and topical antibiotic wound irrigation; partial closure was used for Types I and II open tibial wounds, and all Type III wounds were left open. Stabilization was accomplished by plaster alone, external pins in plaster, or an external fixator with full transfixion pins. The overall infection rate was 4.5% (5 of 109 wounds) in this study. This represents a significant reduction from the previous infection rate of 14% in 254 open tibial fractures treated by the authors in previous years by all methods.

Sumner DR, Turner TM, Purchio AF, Gombotz WR, Urban RM, Galante JO. Enhancement of bone ingrowth by transforming growth factor-β. *J Bone Joint Surg* 77(A):1135–1147,1995.

Enhancement of bone ingrowth with transforming growth factor-β was evaluated in a canine model. Ten dogs had bilateral implantation of a titanium-fiber-metal-coated rod in the proximal part of the humerus. A 3-millimeter gap between the outer surface of the porous coating and the surrounding cancellous bone was created to impair bone ingrowth. All of the implants were plasma-flame-sprayed with hydroxyapatite and tricalcium phosphate. In each animal, one implant was also treated with recombinant transforming growth factor-β 1 while the other implant, which was not so treated, served as a paired control. Two doses of transforming growth factor-β 1 were used: 335 micrograms in 5 animals and 120 micrograms in the other 5. At 4 weeks, the amount of bone ingrowth in the implants that had been treated with 120 micrograms of transforming growth factor-β 1 was threefold higher than that in the paired controls ($p = 0.009$), but with the numbers available there was no significant increase in bone ingrowth with the higher dose. The amount of new-bone formation in the 3-millimeter gaps adjacent to the treated implants was twice that in the gaps of the paired controls, regardless of the dose. The differences between the treated and control implants with regard to the architecture of the new bone in the gap indicate that the mechanism of action of transforming growth factor-β 1 may include both proliferation of osteoprogenitor cells and production of matrix by committed osteoblasts. Compared with the findings in a previous study in which this canine model was used, the data from the present investigation indicate that enhancement of bone ingrowth in implants that have been treated with a combination of a hydroxyapatite-tricalcium phosphate coating and transforming growth factor-β 1 may exceed that obtainable with grafting of the gap with autogenous cancellous bone.

Urist MR. Bone: Formation by autoinduction. *Science* 150:893–899,1965.

Wandering histiocytes, foreign body giant cells, and inflammatory connective-tissue cells are stimulated by degradation products of dead matrix to grow in and repopulate the area of an implant of decalcified bone. Histiocytes are more numerous than any other cell form and may transfer collagenolytic activity to the substrate to cause dissolution of the matrix. The process is followed immediately by new-bone formation by autoinduction in which both the inductor cells and the induced cells are derived from ingrowing cells of the host bed. The inductor cell is a descendant of a wandering histiocyte; the induced cell is a fixed histiocyte or perivascular young connective-tissue cell. Differentiation of the osteoprogenitor cell is elicited by the local alterations in cell metabolic cycles that are as yet uncharacterized.

Refresher Questions

1. The predominant method of lubrication of the native joint during dynamic joint function is:
   a) Elastohydrodynamic
   b) Boundary
   c) Hydrodynamic
   d) Mixed
   e) Weeping

2. Metabolic turnover of cancellous bone is approximately how many times greater than that of cortical bone?
   a) 4 times
   b) 8 times
   c) 10 times
   d) 12 times
   e) none of the above

3. What percentage of the meniscus, by width, is vascularized?
   a) 10%
   b) 20%
   c) 25%
   d) 40%
   e) 50%

4. What zone is most responsible for the longitudinal growth of the growth plate?
   a) Reserve zone
   b) Hypertrophic zone
   c) Proliferative zone
   d) Primary spongiosa
   e) Zone of provisional calcification

5. Tendon repairs are weakest at what time point postsurgery?
   a) 2 days
   b) 5 days
   c) 7 to 10 days
   d) 2 weeks
   e) 4 weeks

6. What is the first stage of bone healing?
   a) Hematoma formation/inflammation
   b) Angiogenesis
   c) Cartilage formation
   d) Bone formation
   e) Bone remodeling

7. Serum markers of renal osteodystrophy demonstrate the following pattern?
   a) Increased Ca, Increased phosphate, decreased PTH, increased alkaline phosphatase
   b) Decreased Ca, Increased phosphate, increased PTH, increased alkaline phosphatase
   c) Decreased Ca, Decreased phosphate, decreased PTH, decreased alkaline phosphatase
   d) Normal Ca, decreased phosphate, increased PTH, normal alkaline phosphatase
   e) Increased Ca, increased phosphate, increased PTH, increased alkaline phosphatase

8. The four layers of articular cartilage are as follows (starting from the articular surface):
   a) Superficial, transitional, deep zone, zone of calcified cartilage
   b) Transitional, superficial, deep zone, zone of calcified cartilage
   c) Superficial, zone of calcified cartilage, transitional, deep zone
   d) Deep zone, superficial, zone of calcified cartilage, transitional

9. Which of the following describes articular cartilage as it ages:
   a) Decreased water content, decreased chondroitin sulfate, increased keratan sulfate
   b) Normal water content, normal chondroitin sulfate, normal keratan sulfate
   c) Increased water content, increased chondroitin sulfate, increased keratan sulfate
   d) Decreased water content, increased chondroitin sulfate, increased keratan sulfate

10. Tendons covered by a sheath receive their blood supply by which of the following structures:
   a) Natatory ligaments
   b) Spiral cord
   c) Vincula
   d) Oblique retinacular ligament
   e) Perimysium

11. Tendon repairs reach full strength at what time point:
   a) 1 mo.
   b) 2 mos.
   c) 3 mos.
   d) 6 mos.
   e) 1 yr.

12. Type I fibers are differentiated from type II fibers by what characteristic:
   a) Increased mitochondria
   b) Low triglyceride content
   c) Ability to perform high-intensity activities
   d) Last to be lost without rehabilitation
   e) Less vascular

13. Which of the following nerve injuries has the best prognosis:
   a) Axonotmesis
   b) Neurotmesis
   c) Neuropraxia
   d) Wallerian degeneration

14. Human peripheral nerves regenerate at what rate:
   a) 0.5 mm/d
   b) 1 to 2 mm/d
   c) 3 to 4 mm/d
   d) 4 to 5 mm/d
   e) 7 to 8 mm/d

15. Which of the following exercises is the best method to improve power:
   a) Isotonic exercises
   b) Isometric exercises
   c) Plyometrics
   d) Isokinetic exercises

Chapter

2

Pediatric Orthopaedics

HARISH S. HOSALKAR, PURUSHOTTAM A. GHOLVE,
DAVID A. SPIEGEL, and DENIS S. DRUMMOND

I. SKELETAL DYSPLASIAS

Skeletal dysplasias are also known as osteochondrodysplasias and are a heterogeneous group of conditions characterized by generalized disorders of growth and development of bone and cartilage. The inheritance pattern and genetic defects of selected dysplasias are enumerated in Table 2.1. Disproportionate short stature is characteristic of the skeletal dysplasias, which differentiates these conditions from endocrine (e.g., absent growth hormone) and metabolic (e.g., rickets) disorders that cause proportionate short stature. Dwarfing conditions frequently are referred to as short-limb or short-trunk dysplasias, according to whether trunk or limbs are more extensively involved. Disproportionate involvement of the trunk is known as microsomia; disproportionate involvement of the limbs is known as micromelia. In short-limb dysplasias, the extremities are disproportionately short

TABLE 2.1 Inheritance pattern and genetic defects in skeletal dysplasias

Dysplasia	*Inheritance*	*Genetic defect*
Achondroplasia	AD	FGFR3
• Pseudoachondroplasia	AD	COMP
• Hypochondroplasia	AD	FGFR3
Chondrodysplasia of metaphysis	AD	PTHRP
• Jansen	AR	Unknown COMP and Type II collagen
• McKusick	AD	Type X collagen
• Schmid		
Cleidocranial dysplasia	AD	CBFA1
Diastrophic dysplasia	AR	Sulfate transport protein
Kniest syndrome	AD	Type II collagen
Mucopolysaccharidosis		
• Hunter	XR	
• Hurler	AR	
• Morquio	AR	
• Sanfilippo	AR	
Spondyloepiphyseal dysplasia	AD (Congenita) XR (Tarda)	Type II collagen

compared with the trunk. In contrast, short-trunk dysplasias produce greater shortening of the spine relative to the limbs.

- Short-limb dwarfism—micromelia
- Rhizomelia: proximal segment (arm, thigh)
- Mesomelia: middle segment (forearm, leg)
- Acromelia: distal segment (hand, foot)
- Short-trunk dwarfism—microsomia

Achondroplasia. Achondroplasia is the most frequent short-limb dwarfism with a prevalence of approximately 1 in 30,000 to 50,000. It is transmitted as an autosomal dominant trait with 80% spontaneous mutation presumably due to a point mutation for the gene encoding a fibroblast growth factor. Short stature is caused by rhizomelic shortening of the limbs, characteristic facies with frontal bossing and mid-face hypoplasia, limitation of elbow extension, genu varum, and trident hand (Fig. 2.1). The mutation has been mapped to chromosome 4. The primary defect is abnormal endochondral bone formation in the cartilaginous proliferative zone of the physis. Increased risk of having a child with achondroplasia is directly proportional to paternal age after 36 years. The typical facies includes frontal bossing and mid-face hypoplasia. Trunk height tends to be normal, but arm span and standing height are diminished. Radial heads may be subluxated. Developmental motor milestones are frequently delayed, although normal motor coordination is achieved in later childhood. Many children do not walk independently until 2 to 3 years. Hypotonic ligamentous laxity, relatively large head, and disproportionate trunk and limbs may contribute to the problem. Obesity is common. Patients have normal intelligence, but early speech may be difficult because of tongue thrust; this difficulty usually resolves by school age. Kyphosis at the thoracolumbar junction usually improves spontaneously. Ligamentous laxity is present in most patients, and the knees are most commonly in varus alignment but may be in excessive valgus. Facial bones, skull base, and foramen magnum are underdeveloped. Cranial bones are normal. Foramen magnum stenosis is common. Significant respiratory problems develop in 10% of affected individuals because of an abnormal thoracic cage configuration, midfacial hypoplasia, upper airway obstruction, or spinal cord compression at the foramen magnum. Three percent of affected individuals have hydrocephalus, and detection is difficult because head size may run above the 97th percentile. In the lumbar spine, central and foraminal stenosis is common. Interpedicular distance decreases from L1 to L5. The vertebral bodies have a scalloped appearance. The pelvis characteristically appears broad and flat, with squared iliac wings (champagne glass pelvis). The long bones are short and thick with metaphyseal flaring. Angulation is common at both

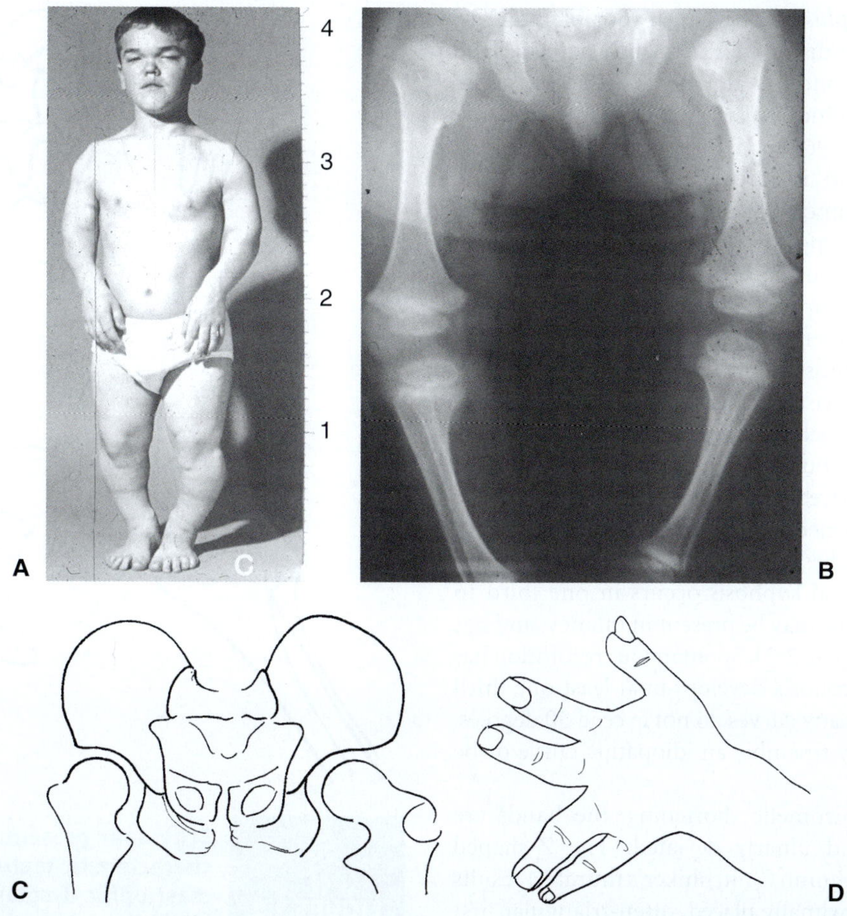

FIGURE 2.1 Achondroplasia. (A) Clinical picture. (B) Genu varum. (C) Champagne glass pelvis. (D) Trident hand.

the distal femoral and the proximal tibial metaphyses. Lumbar spinal stenosis is the most common and disabling problem. Onset of symptoms is typical in the third decade. Spinal decompression may be indicated in these circumstances. Because instability rarely develops, primary fusion is generally not indicated. Between 10% and 15% of patients retain kyphosis, which can increase the risk of symptomatic stenosis. Bracing is indicated if the deformity is accompanied by significant and progressive structural changes in the anterior vertebral bodies. Failed bracing needs posterior spinal fusion. The treatment of genu varum usually involves surgical correction by proximal tibiofibular realignment osteotomy.

Hypochondroplasia. Hypochondroplasia resembles achondroplasia but is less severe. This dysplasia is also transmitted as an autosomal dominant trait, and its gene defect also encodes for FGFR3. The mutation occurs in a different region of the gene from that occurring in achondroplasia (the tyrosine kinase domain in hypochondroplasia, in contrast to the transmembrane domain in achondroplasia.) Except for mild frontal bossing, the facial appearance is normal. Spinal deformities are rarely seen, although mild ligamentous laxity may persist. Mild spinal stenosis has been reported in one third of patients. Varus angulation of the knees is mild and may resolve with growth. Significant genu varum occurs in less than 10% of these patients.

Pseudoachondroplasia. Pseudoachondroplasia often has a similar presentation to achondroplasia with a prevalence of 4 per million. The dysplasia is characterized by normal facies and rhizomelic short-limb dwarfism, where both the epiphyses and metaphyses are involved. Other characteristics include cervical instability; short stature; scoliosis with increased lumbar lordosis; lower limb deformities; contractures at the hip, knee, and elbow; and a predisposition to premature osteoarthritis. Histologic studies of cartilage from patients with pseudoachondroplasia reveal noncollagenous protein accumulated in the rough endoplasmic reticulum of chondrocytes. The defect is on chromosome 19 within the cartilage oligomeric matrix protein (COMP).

Diastrophic Dysplasia. The Greek root of the term diastrophic means distorted, which aptly describes the ears, spine, joints, and feet of patients with diastrophic dysplasia. Diastrophic dysplasia was described by Lamy and Maroteaux in 1960 and is inherited as an autosomal recessive trait and is rare except in Finland. The defect is on chromosome 5 in the gene that codes for a sulfate transporter protein called diastrophic dysplasia sulfate transporter. Histopathology reveals that chondrocytes appear to degenerate prematurely and collagen is present in excess.

Facial characteristics include prominent cheeks (cherubic). The nasal bridge is flattened, and the cartilage of the trachea is abnormally soft. The ear is normal at birth but develops a peculiar swelling of the pinna at 3 to 6 weeks in most patients. The cartilage hardens in a deformed shape called a "cauliflower ear." The posterior arches of the lower cervical spine are often bifid. Cervical kyphosis occurs in one third to one half of patients, may be present in infancy, and has a variable course (Fig. 2.2). Spontaneous resolution has been reported. Scoliosis develops in at least one third of patients, but many curves do not exceed 50 degrees. The scoliosis may resemble an idiopathic curve or be sharply angular.

Because of rhizomelic shortening, the hands are short, broad, and ulnarly deviated. The Z-shaped deformity of the thumb ("hitchhiker's thumb") results from a short, proximally placed, often-triangular first metacarpal that may be hypermobile. The Z-shaped deformity of the thumb occurs in up to 95% of patients with diastrophic dysplasia. The proximal interphalangeal joints of the fingers are often fused.

The hips maintain a persistent flexion contracture. The proximal femoral epiphyses progressively deform and may subluxate. Epiphyseal flattening and hinge abduction develop in many patients. Arthritic changes develop by early to middle adulthood. The knees usually have flexion contractures. Excessive valgus is also common. One fourth of patients have a dislocated patella. Although patients with diastrophic dysplasia are described as having clubfoot, many foot complications exist in these patients. The big toe may be in additional varus, beyond the degree commonly occurring in idiopathic clubfoot. The big toe in varus is analogous to the Z-shaped deformity of the thumb. These foot complications cause stiffness, bony malformations, and contracture, and are as difficult to correct as clubfoot. Approximately 8% of patients die in infancy from respiratory causes or during childhood from cervical myelopathy.

Prenatal diagnosis can be made. Demonstration of long-bone measurements at least 3 standard deviations below normal, clubfoot, and adducted thumbs can be detected through the sonogram. The vertebrae are poorly ossified. The cervical spine may demonstrate kyphosis in infancy and early childhood, usually having an apex at C4. Spina bifida occulta occurs in over three fourths of patients with diastrophic dysplasia. The interpediculate distances narrow only slightly at descending levels of the lumbar spine, unlike in achondroplasia.

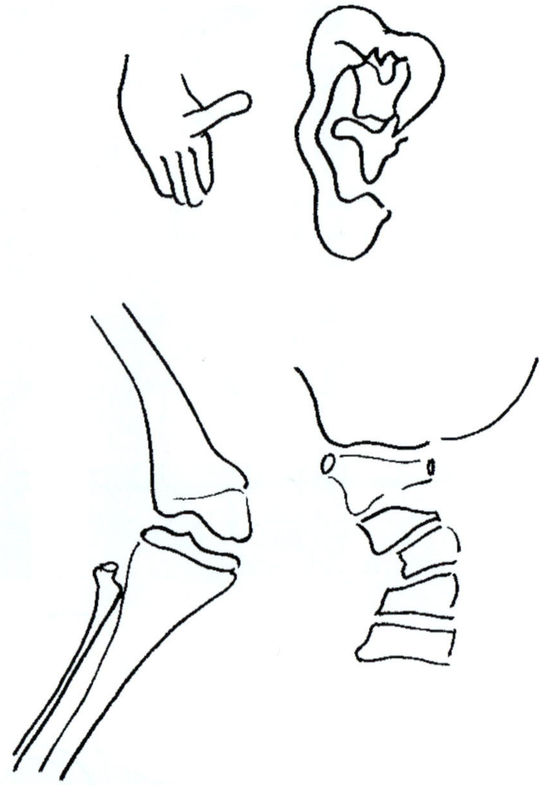

FIGURE 2.2 Schematic presentation of characteristic features of diastrophic dysplasia: hitchhiker's thumb, cauliflower ears, genu valgum, and cervical kyphosis.

The first metacarpal is small, oval, and proximally placed. Although the proximal interphalangeal joints of the digits are ankylosed, a radiolucent space is present early and later demonstrates bridging. The diaphyses of the long bones are short and broad. The epiphyses of both the proximal and the distal femur are delayed in appearance. The capital femoral epiphyses may show signs of osteonecrosis well into childhood. Arthrograms show flattening of both the proximal and the distal femur, accounting for the stiffness observed clinically. The proximal femur is usually in varus. Hip dysplasia or subluxation may develop progressively with time.

Patients with cervical kyphosis should be followed with clinical and radiographic examinations every 6 months. Progressive deformities with instability may need surgical fusion. Scoliosis often begins early in childhood. For curves smaller than 45 degrees, bracing is recommended. Sharply angular curves with kyphosis usually do not respond to brace treatment. Surgical intervention is required to prevent progression for curves over about 50 degrees. Posterior spinal fusion is the mainstay of the treatment. Femoral head deformity and joint contractures make reduction of dislocated hip challenging in patients with diastrophic dysplasia. The dislocations are teratologic in nature and therefore do not respond to closed forms of treatment.

Knee flexion contractures require soft tissue releases, which may be combined with simultaneous release of the hip flexion contractures. Genu valgum is common but does not require corrective osteotomy in most cases. Patellar subluxation/dislocation should be treated surgically in order to improve extensor power. Equinovarus foot deformity is common. The feet are usually rigid and resistant to conservative treatment by serial casting. Surgical treatment is required in most cases to achieve a plantigrade foot.

Kniest Dysplasia. Disproportionate short-trunk dwarfism, kyphoscoliosis, typical facial features, large stiff joints with contractures, and hearing and visual impairment characterize this dysplasia. Histopathologic findings include a disorganized physeal growth plate; soft, crumbly cartilage with a "Swiss-cheese" appearance; and diastase-resistant intracytoplasmic inclusions in the resting chondrocytes. Scanning electron microscopy demonstrates striking fragmentation and disintegration of collagen fibrils resulting in large, open, cyst-like spaces and deficiency and disorganization of the collagen fibrils.

Contractures and joint stiffness cause delayed motor development. Significant disproportionate short-trunk dwarfism and rhizomelic involvement of the limbs is characteristic. The face is often flat with widely spaced prominent eyes and a flat nasal bridge. Kyphoscoliosis and marked lumbar lordosis with hip flexion contractures further contribute to the short stature. Osteopenia is characteristic. Abnormalities of the odontoid with atlantoaxial instability and hypoplasia of the cervical vertebrae may occur. There is kyphosis, and often mild scoliosis, in the thoracolumbar spine. The pelvis is characteristic, with short and broad iliac crests and small insufficient acetabula. The epiphyses are irregular in shape and therefore lead to angular deformities of the lower extremities. The dumbbell-shaped long bones have very short, broad metaphyses leading to the appearance of joint enlargement.

Spondyloepiphyseal Dysplasia (SED) Congenita. This form of dysplasia is characterized by short-trunk dwarfism with primary involvement of the vertebrae and epiphyseal centers. It is the most common type, with an estimated prevalence of about 3 to 4 per million. Head circumference is normal with flattened facies and wide-set eyes. The neck is short and the chest is barrel-shaped in combination with pectus carinatum deformity. Scoliosis and kyphosis usually develop in adolescence. Angular deformities of the lower extremities, including coxa vara and, more commonly, genu valgum, may be seen. A waddling gate is produced by the coxa vara. The most common foot deformity is equinovarus. Patients should be screened for associated retinal detachment and myopia.

Various degrees of platyspondylia (delayed ossification) may exist. The odontoid may be hypoplastic or absent, leading to atlantoaxial instability that may cause neurologic compromise. Progressive kyphoscoliosis may develop in late childhood. The ossification centers of the proximal femur, distal femur, and proximal tibia are delayed, with flattening and irregularity of the articular surfaces. Genu valgum is more common than genu varum. Early osteoarthritis is likely in the hips, more so than in the knee. The carpals are delayed in ossification, but the tubular bones of the hands are near normal.

Spondyloepiphyseal Dysplasia Tarda. SED tarda is a disorder of endochondral bone formation characterized by disproportionate short stature with short neck and trunk. It can be distinguished from SED congenita by the later age at diagnosis and milder pattern of involvement.

The patient's stature is mildly shortened. It affects primarily the spine and the large joints, in which the changes become evident between 10 and 14 years of age. The initial diagnosis may be bilateral Perthes disease. Hip changes are very typical and include abnormal femoral heads (with coxa magna, flattening, and subluxation), acetabular insufficiency, and premature osteoarthritis (Fig. 2.3). Notably, in SED involvement is symmetric, while in bilateral Perthes disease involvement is discordant, with one hip more radiographically affected than the other. All patients should be evaluated for atlantoaxial instability, and cervical fusion should be considered if significant instability is detected.

Multiple Epiphyseal Dysplasia. Multiple epiphyseal dysplasia (MED) is one of the most common skeletal dysplasias characterized by delayed epiphyseal ossification, mild short stature, limb deformities, and early-onset osteoarthritis. It affects many epiphyses, produces symptoms mainly in those joints with significant load bearing, and has few changes in the physes or metaphyses. MED is broadly categorized into more severe Fairbank (type I) and milder Ribbing (type II)

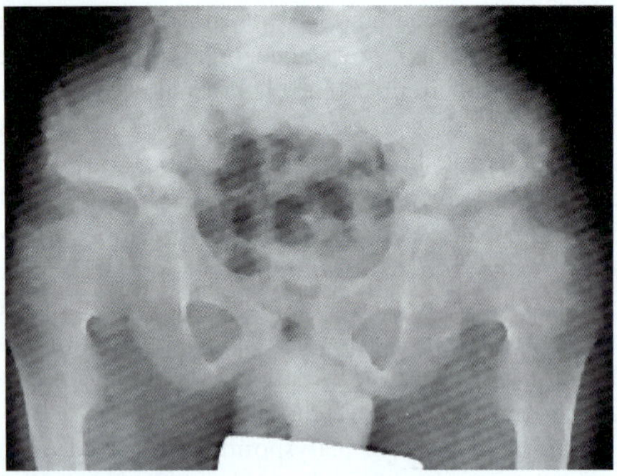

FIGURE 2.3 **Bilateral hip involvement in spondyloepiphyseal tarda.**

types. In the majority of patients, the dysplasia is inherited by autosomal dominant transmission. A rare autosomal recessive form also exists.

Often, the diagnosis is not made until early adolescence. The head and face are normal with minimal involvement of the spine that is usually asymptomatic. Angular deformities of the lower limbs, including coxa vara, genu varum, and genu valgum, are common. There may be flexion contractures of knees and elbows. Shortening of the digits of the hands and feet is the only typical clinical feature of patients with MED. There is no visceral involvement, and the intelligence is not affected. The principal finding is a delay in the appearance of the ossification centers. In the growing patient, the epiphyses are fragmented, mottled, and small in size. In adulthood, major joints develop premature osteoarthritis, which is most common and most severe in the hips. The radiographic changes are symmetric and fairly synchronous in MED, in contrast to asymmetric and metachronous involvement in Perthes disease.

Avascular necrosis occurs frequently in the hips of patients with MED. Angular deformities of the lower limbs may occur because of asymmetric physeal growth. Coxa vara may occur but is not necessarily bilateral. Radiographs of the knee may show valgus deformity, with flattened femoral condyles and shallow intercondylar notch. Valgus deformities at the ankles are common with changes occurring.

Mucopolysaccharidoses. Mucopolysaccharidoses (MPS) are a group of inherited metabolic disorders caused by deficiency of specific lysosomal enzymes, which results in intracellular accumulation of partially degraded glycosaminoglycans. Incidence of the MPS is 1 in 25,000 live births. The MPS are subdivided on the basis of their enzyme deficiency and the type of substance that accumulates (Table 2.2). Although there is phenotypic variability, these disorders share some common clinical features, such as facial dysmorphism, short stature, organomegaly, cardiac problems, and joint contractures.

Most of the MPS show similar changes in the cartilage; resting cartilage consists of uniformly stained matrix, with chondrocytes that are larger than normal and stain positively for glycosaminoglycans. Biochemical analysis of the urine can lead to the diagnosis of the specific MPS. Identification of the MPS is also possible through skin fibroblast culture. The fibroblasts are assayed for specific enzyme activity known to be abnormal in the different MPS. Molecular genetic research determines the specific mutations that result in MPS.

The clinical diagnosis of MPS is usually made between 6 months and 10 years of age, depending on the type. A flat nasal bridge, hypertelorism, and corneal clouding are typical facial features seen in children with MPS. Short stature, short neck, and joint contractures occur in most types. Cervical instability and thoracolumbar kyphoscoliosis are common spinal problems. Dysplasia of the pelvis and broadening and shortening of the long bones may be seen. Generalized joint laxity is a feature of Morquio syndrome (most common), making it distinctly different from the other MPS, in which joint stiffness is the rule. The patients with MPS I (Hurler syndrome) and MPS IV (Morquio syndrome) are usually more severely affected than the other types.

Radiographic changes are commonly seen in the skull; the skull is enlarged, with a thick calvarium. The clavicles are broad, especially medially. The ribs are oar-shaped and broader anteriorly than posteriorly. The vertebral bodies are ovoid when immature. Scoliosis and kyphosis are frequently present. The iliac wings are flared, and the acetabulae are dysplastic. Coxa valga is common, and the long bones often have thickened cortices. There is delay in ossification of the carpal bones. It is difficult to differentiate the various types of MPS on the basis of radiographic findings alone.

Genetic counseling is essential for all children diagnosed with MPS. Orthopaedic treatment usually consists of symptomatic corrective measures: fusion of cervical spine instability and conservative or surgical treatment of spinal curvatures and joint contractures.

Chondrodysplasia Punctata. Chondrodysplasia punctata is a rare skeletal dysplasia characterized by short-limb dwarfism and multiple punctate epiphyseal calcifications that are present at birth and resolve over the first year of life. Typical facial features, including hypertelorism, a depressed nasal bridge, and a bifid nasal tip, characterize patients with Conradi-Hünermann syndrome (autosomal dominant). A dysmorphic face

TABLE 2.2 Mucopolysaccharidoses and specific enzyme deficiencies

Mucopolysaccharidoses (MPS)	Enzyme deficiency	Gene locus	Urinary Excretion
MPS I (Hurler syndrome)	α-L-iduronidase	chromosome 4 (AR)	Dermatan/heparin sulfate
MPS II (Hunter disease)	Iduronate-2-sulfatase	X chromosome	Dermatan/heparin sulfate
MPS III (Sanfilippo syndrome)	Heparan sulfate sulfatase	chromosome 12 (AR)	Heparin sulfate
type A	α-N-acetylglucosaminidase		
type B	Acetyl CoA: α-glucosaminide-N-acetyltransferase		
type C	*N*-acetyl-glucosaminide-6-sulfatase		
type D			
MPS IV (Morquio syndrome)	Galactosamine-6-sulfate sulfatase	(AR)	Keratan sulfate
type A	β-galactosidase		
type B			
MPS V (polydystrophic dysplasia)	Arylsulfatase B	chromosome 5	

Adapted from Erol B, Moroz LA, Dormans JP. Skeletal dysplasia. In: Dormans JP (ed.), *Core Knowledge in Orthopaedics*. Philadelphia: Elsevier Mosby, 2005.

with a depressed nasal bridge is also a characteristic of rhizomelic type (more severe, autosomal recessive, usually fatal during the first year). These patients frequently have symmetrical shortening of the proximal limbs, contractures of the joints, subluxation/dislocation of the hips, limb-length inequality, and coxa vara. Spinal findings include atlantoaxial instability, congenital scoliosis, and kyphosis. Equinovarus or other foot deformities may be seen along with cataracts.

Metaphyseal Chondrodysplasias. Metaphyseal chondrodysplasias are a group of disorders characterized by metaphyseal deformity and irregularity adjacent to the physes, with little or no epiphyseal involvement. The real defect is in the growth plate itself (proliferative and hypertrophic zones) with the metaphyseal changes being the end results.

Schmid Metaphyseal Chondrodysplasia. The Schmid type is the most common form of metaphyseal chondrodysplasia. It is an autosomal dominant disorder with a mutation in the gene for the α-1 chain of type X collagen (COL10A1). On histologic examination, cartilage islands that extend into the metaphyses can be seen. Patients are normal at birth and are diagnosed at 2 to 3 years of age. Patients usually present with leg pain, a waddling gait, varus angulation of the knee, or short stature. Spinal changes occur infrequently. Radiographic changes characteristically occur at the metaphyseal regions of the long bones; the metaphyses are widened and scalloped, and may have cysts. The proximal femoral metaphysis is particularly irregular and splayed, and there is medial beaking. Some widening of the physis occurs, but not to the extent that is observed in rickets. Coxa vara is present to varying degrees. Shortening and bowing of the long bones and genu varum may be seen.

McKusick Metaphyseal Chondrodysplasia. McKusick metaphyseal chondrodysplasia, also known as cartilage-hair hypoplasia, is particularly prevalent in the Amish community, as well as in Finland. It is an autosomal recessive disorder, and the gene defect is located on chromosome 9.

McKusick metaphyseal chondrodysplasia is diagnosed at 2 to 3 years of age. Patients with this disorder have light-colored, sparse hair. Patients have markedly short adult stature. These patients have generalized ligamentous laxity, but the elbow extension may be limited. Scoliosis may be present in up to one fourth of patients. Pectus excavatum or carinatum may be observed. Mild genu varum is common. Atlantoaxial instability and some minimal changes in the thoracolumbar spine, which are not of much clinical importance, may be seen in McKusick metaphyseal chondrodysplasia. The metaphyseal involvement is more evenly distributed, and there is more shortening and less varus angulation of the long bones than seen in Schmid type. Radiographic changes in the thorax, including changes at the costochondral junctions, Harrison grooves, and a prominent sternum, occur in two thirds of the patients.

Jansen Metaphyseal Chondrodysplasia. Jansen metaphyseal chondrodysplasia is a rare autosomal dominant disorder characterized by abnormal growth plate maturation and laboratory findings that are indistinguishable from hyperparathyroidism. This dysplasia is usually apparent at birth because of severe short stature, excessive shortening of the limbs, frontal bossing, widely spaced eyes, and exophthalmos. The angular deformities of the lower limbs and flexion contractures of the major joints may develop. Radiographs show bulbous expansion of the metaphyses. Abnormal laboratory findings are typical and include hypercalcemia, hypophosphatemia, and increased renal excretion of phosphate, cAMP, and hydroxyproline, despite normal or undetectable levels of PTH and PTHrP. The genetic defect is in PTHrP.

Cleidocranial Dysplasia (Dysostosis). This autosomal dominant dysplasia involves multiple skeletal abnormalities, especially in bones of intramembranous origin. Classic features of cleidocranial dysplasia include a widening of the cranium, as well as dysplasia of the clavicle and pelvis. Cleidocranial dysplasia is inherited as an autosomal dominant trait. The defect is in CBFA1 (a transcription factor for osteocalcin).

Typically, the disease is identified within the first 2 years of life. The shoulders look droopy, and the upper thorax is narrow. Sternal abnormalities result from the abnormal intramembranous ossification, and pectus excavatum is common. The clavicles are partially or completely absent. The most common defect is loss of the lateral end of the clavicle, with failure of development of the middle third of the clavicle second in frequency. Hypermobility of the shoulders is very typical; many patients are able to completely appose the shoulders anteriorly. Coxa vara is a frequent problem and may result in limitation of abduction and a Trendelenburg gait. Clavicular defects found in patients with cleidocranial dysplasia do not require surgical intervention. The coxa vara is usually progressive and treated by proximal femoral valgus osteotomy if the neck shaft angle is less than 100 degrees. If there is acetabular dysplasia, a pelvic osteotomy may be recommended to improve the containment of the hip.

Larsen Syndrome. Multiple congenital dislocations of large joints, facial dysmorphism, ligamentous laxity, and foot deformities characterize Larsen syndrome. Autosomal dominant as well as recessive forms have been described. The disorder is similar to arthrogryposis. Larsen syndrome is recognizable at birth. A broad face with hypertelorism, depressed nasal bridge, and prominent forehead is typical. Congenital spinal deformities are frequently seen. Ligamentous laxity and congenital joint dislocations are very common. The knee deformity spans a spectrum from simple congenital hyperextension deformity to complete anterior dislocation. The hips are often teratologically dislocated. The elbows frequently demonstrate radiohumeral dislocation with lateral prominence of the radial heads even in the infant, and there may be more extensive dislocation with a total disruption of the radiocapitellar and the humeroulnar joints. Characteristic foot deformities include equinovarus and equinovalgus. One of the characteristic findings in Larsen syndrome is the presence of accessory calcaneal or carpal ossification centers. Shortened metacarpals and terminal phalanges are also noted.

Hereditary Multiple Exostoses. Hereditary multiple exostoses is one of the most common skeletal dysplasias seen by orthopaedic surgeons; it has an estimated prevalence of approximately 1 in 18,000. It is characterized by cartilage-capped prominences that develop from the epiphyses of the long bones. The disorder is of autosomal dominant inheritance, with penetrance approaching 96%. Numerous genetic studies have found anomalies on at least three different genes, termed exostosin (EXT) genes, making this a genetically heterogeneous disorder. The three described EXT loci have been recently mapped: EXT1 on chromosome 8, EXT2 on chromosome 11, and EXT3 on chromosome 19.

The exostoses usually appear after age 3 to 4 years. On presentation, 5 or 6 exostoses typically may be found, involving both the upper and lower limbs (Fig. 2.4). Over time, the upper and lower extremities may appear short in relation to the trunk. Shortening of the limbs is usually disproportionate. Distal femur, proximal tibia, proximal humerus, scapula and ribs, proximal fibula, and distal radius and ulna are the most commonly involved sites. Problems from this condition may be divided into four categories: (1) local prominence and impingement by the exostoses; (2) asymmetric growth of two-bone segments, such as the forearm and the leg; (3) limb-length inequality; and (4) late degeneration into chondrosarcoma. Malignant transformation in the pediatric age group is very rare and is difficult to monitor.

Like solitary osteochondromas, they may grow perpendicular to the bone in a sessile or pedunculated fashion. The cortex of the exostosis is contiguous with

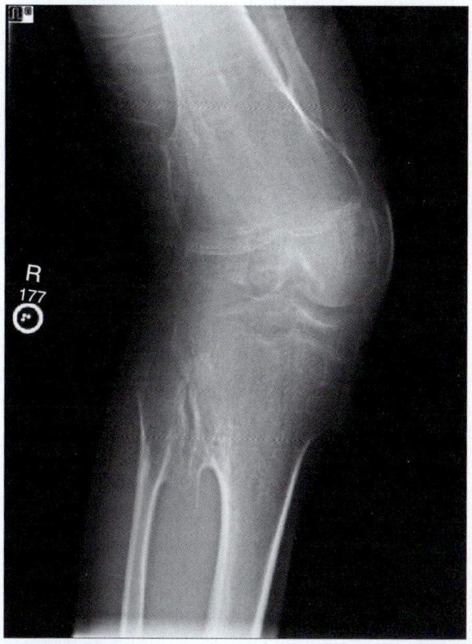

FIGURE 2.4 Knee x-ray in MHE showing multiple osteochondromas and genu valgum.

that of the bone itself. Subluxation/dislocation of the radial head occurs and is usually associated with a negative ulnar variance. The femoral necks are usually wide and in valgus Genu valgum and ankle valgus may be seen.

Any exostoses causing significant symptoms should be excised. Reasonable indications include pain, growth disturbance leading to angular deformity or limb-length discrepancy, joint motion compromised by juxtaarticular lesions, soft tissue impingement or tethering, false aneurysm produced by an osteochondroma, painful bursa formation, obvious cosmetic deformity, and a rapid increase in the size of a lesion. Significant valgus deformities of the knee and ankle are treated by osteotomy or hemiepiphyseodesis in young patients or corrective varus osteotomy in older (near maturity) patients.

II. CHROMOSOMAL AND TERATOLOGIC DISORDERS

Down Syndrome (Trisomy 21). A very common chromosomal abnormality associated with advanced maternal age is Down syndrome. Only 3% to 5% of cases are inherited; the remainder arise from nondisjunction of chromosome 21 during meiosis. These patients have typical facies with a wide forehead, flat nose, widely spaced eyes, flat occiput, and mental retardation. Other medical and surgical issues are celiac disease, Hirschsprung disease, gastroesophageal reflux, epilepsy, xerosis, blood disorders (AML), abnormal thyroid function, and cardiac anomalies (endocardial cushion defects). Orthopedic problems are scoliosis, hip instability, slipped capital femoral epiphysis, patellar instability, flat foot, metatarsus primus varus, and most importantly, atlantoaxial instability. The atlantodens interval (ADI) is measured on flexion-extension lateral radiographs of the cervical spine (Fig. 2.5). An ADI between 5 and 10 mm with no neurologic symptoms are observed with yearly radiographic and neurologic examinations. Surgical stabilization is indicated in asymptomatic ADI of more than 10 mm or symptomatic ADI between 5 and 10 mm. All children with Down syndrome should have cervical spine clearance before they participate in sports. Asymptomatic children with instability should avoid contact sports, diving, and gymnastics.

Turner Syndrome (45, XO). The two main clinical features of Turner syndrome are short stature and nonfunctioning ovaries. The diagnosis is usually made on the basis of a delay in puberty. Other physical features are webbed neck, flat chest with widely spaced nipples, low hairline, low-set ears, and a high-arched palate. It is associated with anomalies of the urinary tract system and coarctation of the aorta. No treatment is required for the increased cubitus valgus angle and short fourth and fifth metacarpals. Idiopathic scoliosis should be treated in the standard fashion. Malignant hyperthermia is common with anesthetic use.

Noonan Syndrome. Present only in boys, Noonan syndrome is characterized by short stature, droopy and wide-set eyes, low hairline, blue or gray eyes, and chest deformities. Cubitus valgus doesn't require any intervention. The incidence is reported to be 1 in 1,000 to 2,500 children. It is similar in presentation to Turner syndrome, except there is normal gonadal development, mental retardation, and more severe scoliosis.

Prader-Willi Syndrome. This syndrome is caused by abnormalities in genes located in 15q11q13 (partial chromosome 15 deletion from father) and has an incidence of 1 in 12,000 to 15,000 newborns. The major clinical criteria are neonatal and infantile hypotonia, dolichocephaly, narrow face, almond-shaped eyes, hypogonadism, and mild to moderate mental retardation or learning difficulties. Patients with Prader-Willi syndrome have hyperphagia, food foraging, and an obsession with food. Hip dysplasia and scoliosis is also observed.

Menkes Syndrome. Menkes syndrome is an X-linked recessive disorder affecting copper metabolism.

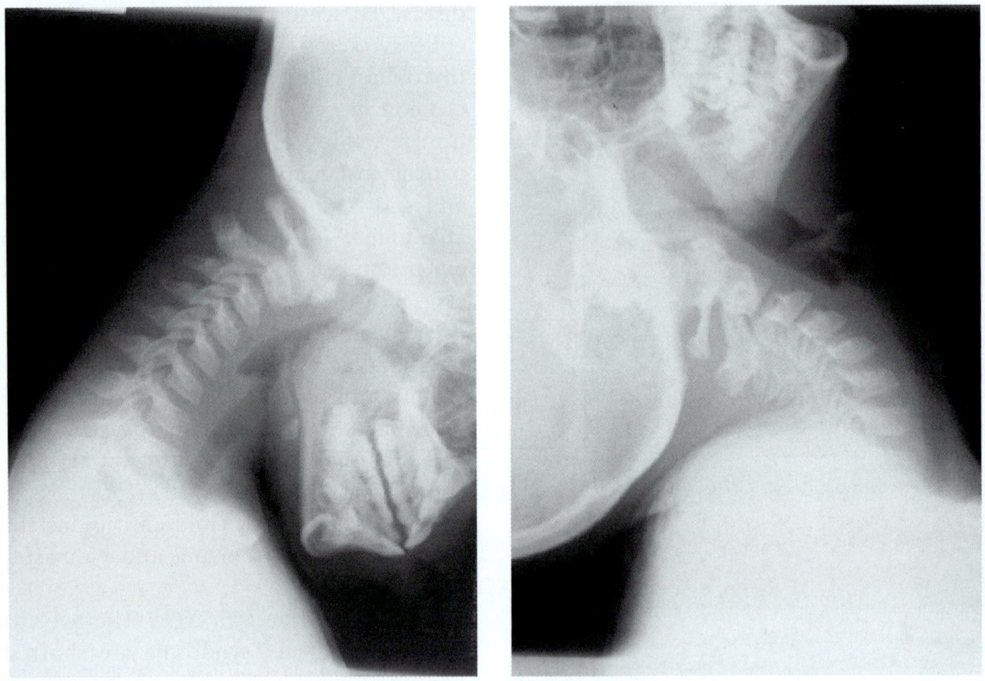

FIGURE 2.5 **Flexion–extension radiographs of cervical spine in a patient with Down syndrome.**

Abnormal copper transport causes a progressive, genetic, neurodegenerative disorder characterized by degeneration of the CNS gray matter with distinctive facies and hair and progressive neurological deficit. Clinical features are expressionless face and sparse, tangled, and fragile hair, which is lightly pigmented or white. Patients with Menkes syndrome also have hypotonia, seizures, and hypothermia.

Rett Syndrome. Two genes, MECP2 and CDKL5, are implicated in Rett syndrome. It is typically observed in females at 6 to 18 months of age when they fall off the growth curve. They lose achieved motor and speech skills and develop repetitive hand movement, irregular breathing pattern, extreme motor control problems (including spasticity), and seizures. Orthopedic problems are dislocation of the hips, talipes equines, joint contractures, and scoliosis, which is unresponsive to conservative treatment and requires surgery if severe. Spinal surgery for correction must include all of the kyphotic and C-shaped scoliotic deformity.

III. HEMATOPOIETIC DISORDERS

Gaucher Disease. Gaucher disease is a common lysosomal storage disorder caused by deficiency of enzyme β-glucocerebrosidase leading to accumulation of glucocerebroside in Gaucher cells. Autosomal recessive inheritance is associated with chromosome 1, and the disease is classically seen in Ashkenazi Jews. Type 1 Gaucher disease is more common and presents with involvement of liver, spleen, and bone marrow and sparing of the nervous system. Histologic analysis reveals lipid-laden histiocytes. Symptoms most frequently begin in adulthood with enlargement of the liver and spleen causing anemia, bruising, and abnormal clotting. Bone marrow involvement causes bone pain (Gaucher crisis), joint pain and avascular necrosis of hip. Arthritis due to avascular necrosis secondary to Gaucher has been treated with hip replacement, which requires special consideration for intraoperative bleeding, infection, and loosening. The radiographs of the femur demonstrate an Erlenmeyer flask deformity. Although enzyme replacement therapy is expensive, it has been successful in reducing all manifestations of Gaucher disease.

Niemann-Pick Disease. Niemann-Pick disease is an autosomal recessive disease frequently found in Jews of East European descent. Deficiency of sphingomyelinase leads to accumulation of sphingomyelin in the reticuloendothelial system and the CNS. Clinical features are enlargement of liver and spleen, jaundice following birth, cherry-red spot in the retina, sudden loss of muscle and tone, and progressive loss of motor skills. There is expansion of long bones with thinning of the cortices. The disease is often lethal in childhood.

Sickle Cell Anemia. Sickle cell disease (SCD) is a heterogeneous disorder, with clinical manifestations including chronic hemolysis, an increased susceptibility to infections, and vaso-occlusive complications. Early manifestations are splenic sequestration and dactylitis. Sickle cell crisis presents with severe pain in abdomen, chest, or bones. Treatment is analgesia, fluids, oxygen, and in severe cases, exchange transfusion. Bone infarcts cause osteonecrosis of the femoral and humeral heads. Biconcave "fish" vertebrae and septic arthritis are common. Although *Salmonella* osteomyelitis is associated with SCD (encapsulated bacteria due to asplenia), *Staphylococcus aureus* is the more common causative organism. Radiographs demonstrate osteoporosis, bone thinning, and infarcts. Hydroxyurea has been used to increase the fetal hemoglobin and decrease the incidence of painful crisis.

Thalassemia. The fundamental abnormality in thalassemia is impaired production of either the alpha or beta hemoglobin chain differentiating as alpha or beta thalassemia. Accelerated bone marrow activity to produce red blood cells leads to enlargement of the marrow cavity and thin cortices. Patients present with anemia, fatigue, flat facies, and bone pains. Treatment is blood transfusions and iron chelators.

Hemophilia. Hemophilia is the oldest known hereditary bleeding disorder with an X-linked recessive inheritance. Hemophilia A has abnormal factor VIII and hemophilia B (Christmas disease) has abnormal factor IX. Because of deficiency of the clotting factor, patients with hemophilia present with abnormal bleeding spontaneously or following trauma. Typically, bleeds occur deep within muscles and in joints. The iliacus is the most commonly involved muscle, presenting with abdominal or hip pain, flexion deformity, and swelling (pseudotumor) of the hip. Ultrasonography is very helpful in delineating the cause. Hemarthrosis presents with pain, swelling, and restricted motion (most commonly in the knee). Acute medical management of the disease often includes factor replacement and splinting of the affected joints. It is important to determine the factor inhibitor level so that factor levels can be raised to at least one fourth of the baseline in major bleeds. Some of the radiologic features include osteopenia, thinning of the bones, overgrowth of bones, and squaring of the patella.

Recurrent bleeds cause deposition of hemosiderin in the synovium and the articular cartilage, leading to early destruction of joints and causing chronic hemophilic arthropathy. Surgical interventions include arthroscopic or open synovectomy, arthrodesis, or joint replacement. Factor replacement is necessary before any surgical procedure, and the presence of antibody inhibitors is no longer a contraindication for elective surgery.

IV. METABOLIC DISORDERS OF BONE

Calcium and Phosphate Metabolism. If the concentrations of Ca^{2+} and HPO^{-}_{4} exceed the critical solubility product, ectopic calcification will occur. The irritability and conductivity of nervous tissue and muscle tissue (smooth and skeletal muscle) are inversely proportional, and the irritability and conductivity of cardiac muscle is directly proportional, to the concentrations of Ca^{2+}. With hypocalcemia, there is hypertonia, hyperreflexia, convulsions, and death in diastole. With hypercalcemia, there is hypotonicity, hyperreflexia, obtundation, and death in systole. Calcium cannot cross cell membranes without a transport system. The cell barrier–transport system for calcium includes 1,25-dihydroxyvitamin D (activated vitamin D), cytosolic phosphate, and to a lesser extent, parathyroid hormone (PTH). 1,25-dihydroxyvitamin D increases the synthesis of calcium-binding proteins such as calbindin and cholecalcin, while phosphate acts at the membrane transport level and PTH acts via adenyl cyclase–cAMP to increase calcium entry to the intracellular space as well as activate the release of calcium from the mitochondria. The role of PTH is primarily to balance the action of vitamin D through its differential effects on calcium and phosphorus metabolism.

Maintenance of Serum Calcium. The absorption of calcium from the gastrointestinal tract, reabsorption of calcium from the renal tubule, and bone–blood exchange are the three major components of the calcium control system (Fig. 2.6). All these components are under the control of the 1,25-dihydroxyvitamin D and PTH synergistic transport system. The lowered serum calcium level stimulates the production and release of PTH, which activates the synthesis of 1,25-dihydroxyvitamin D. Together, the two agents act to increase calcium absorption from the gut, tubular reabsorption of filtered calcium in the kidney, and resorption of bone. Bone resorption occurs by lysis of the crystalline apatite through osteoclastic resorption. Any excess phosphate that appears as a result of the breakdown of bone, under the influence of PTH, is rapidly excreted by the kidney by means of a marked decrease in the tubular reabsorption of phosphate.

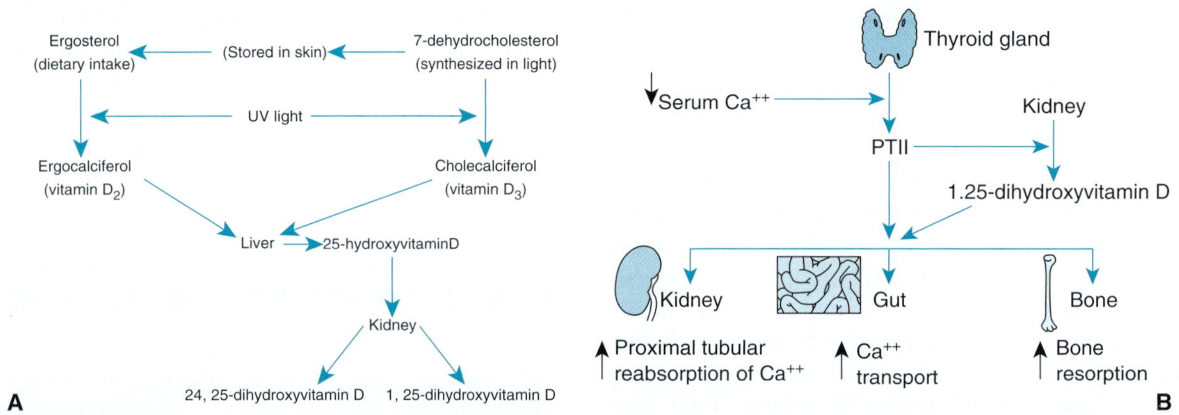

FIGURE 2.6 **(A) Biology of vitamin D. (*Adapted from* Erol B, Dormans JP, States L, Kaplan FS. Skeletal dysplasia and metabolic disorders of bone. Musculoskeletal tumors in children. In: Dormans JP [ed.], *Pediatric Orthopaedics and Sports Medicine*. Philadelphia: Mosby, 2000.) (B) Maintenance of serum calcium. (*Adapted from* Bulent E, Dormans JP. Metabolic disorders of Bone. In: Dormans JP [ed.], *Core Knowledge in Pediatric Orthopaedics*. Philadelphia: Elsevier Mosby, 2005.)**

Rickets. In rickets, the primary disturbance in bone is a failure of calcification of cartilage and osteoid tissue in the hypertrophic zone of the growth plate. There is failure of deposition of calcium along the mature cartilage cell columns, followed by disorderly invasion of cartilage by blood vessels, lack of reabsorption at the zone of provisional calcification, and increased thickness of the growth plate. The chondrocytes multiply normally, but the normal process of maturation of cartilage columns fails to take place. There is also failure of mineralization of newly formed bone. Osteoid formation proceeds normally; however, osteoclastic resorption of the uncalcified osteoid does not take place. Serum calcium levels are normal to mildly decreased, phosphate levels are low, and vitamin D levels are decreased, but PTH and alkaline phosphatase levels are high.

Generalized muscular weakness, lethargy, and irritability characterize rickets. Frontal bossing and enlargement of the suture lines (e.g., caput quadratum) are common. Enlargement of the costal cartilages (e.g., rachitic rosary), indentation of the lower ribs where the diaphragm inserts (i.e., Harrison groove), and occasionally pectus carinatum can be seen on physical examination. The spine is commonly affected, most characteristically with a long thoracic kyphosis. The long bones are deformed and shortened, usually with bowing abnormalities in the lower limbs. Apparent enlargement of the elbows, wrists, knees, and ankles, due to metaphyseal enlargement, may be detected on physical examination.

General radiographic findings include osteopenia, thin cortices, and small trabecula with overall decreased bone mass. The appearance of the growth plate, including irregular widening or cupping, is the most classical finding. Looser's lines are ribbonlike linear radiolucencies extending transversely from one cortex across the medullary canal and represent areas of weakening or incomplete fractures. They may become complete transverse fractures, sometimes with only minor trauma. Bowing of the femur and tibia and angular deformities of the lower extremities, including coxa vara, genu varum, and genu valgum, are common radiographic findings.

Renal Osteodystrophy. Glomerular damage leads to phosphate retention, and tubular injury causes decreased production of 1,25-dihydroxyvitamin D, the active form of vitamin D. These two factors severely inhibit the gut's ability to absorb calcium. The resultant hypocalcemia triggers severe secondary hyperparathyroidism, which remains ineffective in increasing intestinal absorption of calcium. Therefore, the body's only means of increasing serum calcium levels is by bone resorption. Patients with chronic renal disease are hyperphosphatemic, and even when there is reduced pH that shifts the solubility product, they depend on decreased serum calcium to avoid precipitation of the relatively insoluble $CaHPO_4$. If for any reason (e.g., dietary indiscretion, spontaneous improvement, or dialysis) calcium increases to near-normal levels, calcium salts may be precipitated to a variety of ectopic sites.

Features of rickets and renal osteodystrophy include increased fragility fractures with minor trauma. The periarticular calcification and ossification can cause severe limitation and pain in one or more joints. Ligamentous laxity and muscle weakness may be seen.

Genu valgum is the most commonly seen deformity in the lower extremities, but genu varum may occur in some patients. A "salt-and-pepper" skull, absence of a cortical outline on the outer centimeter of the clavicles, subperiosteal resorption of the ulnas, terminal tufts of the distal phalanges, and medial proximal tibias are radiographic findings. Slipped epiphyses and valgus alignment of the knees are also frequently seen in patients with renal osteodystrophy. Brown tumors appear as expanded destructive bone lesions and are usually round or ovoid with indistinct margins. These "tumors" may be present in the long bones or pelvis and, when associated with thinning of the cortex, may be the site of pathologic fractures.

Scurvy. Scurvy is caused by a nutritional deficiency of vitamin C (ascorbic acid). Vitamin C is necessary for the hydroxylation of lysine and proline to hydroxylysine and hydroxyproline, two amino acids crucial for proper cross-linking of the triple helix of collagen. The deficiency results in primitive collagen formation, seen throughout the body. Blood vessels become excessively permeable and rupture readily, normal bone formation is reduced, and bone that forms is lacking in tensile strength and is defective in structural arrangement. The greatest effect on bone formation is observed in the metaphysis. Deficiency of vitamin C produces a decrease in chondroitin sulfate synthesis, and a deficiency in collagen cross-linking is seen in the metaphysis. The microscopic appearance of the cartilaginous portion of the growth plate is normal, but the metaphysis is quite abnormal. It appears that the deficiency in metaphysis is related to the large amount of type I collagen normally found in this region.

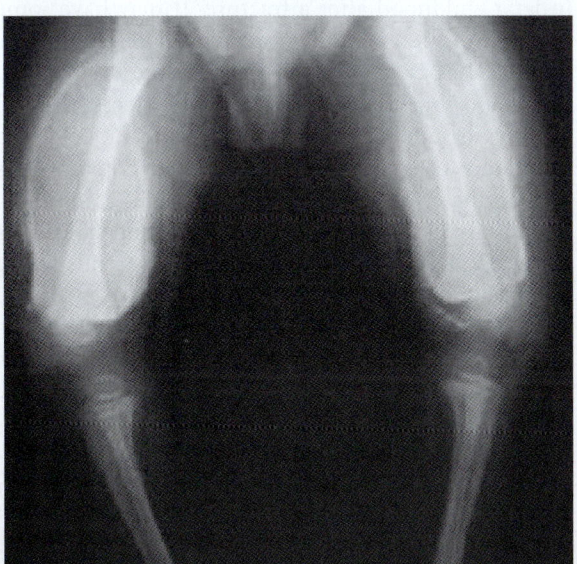

FIGURE 2.7 **Bilateral subperiosteal hemorrhage in scurvy.**

Subperiosteal hemorrhage is a distinctive sign, occurring most commonly in the distal femur and tibia and the proximal humerus (Fig. 2.7). Hemorrhages may also develop in the soft tissues, including the joints, the kidneys, and the gut, and petechiae may be seen. Hemorrhage of the gums is a common finding leading to swollen gums that are bluish in color. Anemia and impaired wound healing are common.

The zone of provisional calcification (i.e., white line of Fraenkel) increases in width and opacity because of failure of resorption of the calcified cartilaginous matrix and stands out compared to the severely osteopenic metaphyses. Brittleness of the zone of provisional calcification may lead to fractures and marginal spurs (i.e., Pelken sign). The epiphyseal nucleus is markedly radiolucent with relatively sclerotic margins, producing an appearance of ringed epiphyses (i.e., Wimberger sign).

Serum levels of vitamin C may be difficult to interpret in scurvy. A more reliable test is the absence of vitamin C in the buffy coat of centrifuged blood. Treatment is replacement of the deficient vitamin C. Rapid recovery is usual, with pain and tenderness resolving. Minimal daily requirements are 30 mg for infants and 50 mg for adults. Therapeutic dosages may be 200 mg or higher.

Osteogenesis Imperfecta (OI). Varying degrees of severity, from an infant with multiple fractures to a child who has only a few fractures before maturity, can encompass this disease. At least 90% have an identifiable genetically determined quantitative and/or qualitative defect in type I collagen formation. Type I collagen is the major structural protein found in bone, skin, tendon, ligament, cornea, sclera, and dentin. It is a triple helix, composed of two α-I chains and one α-II chain. The mutations in OI involve one of the two genes that encode the chains of type I collagen. The COL1A1 gene on chromosome 17 encodes the α-1 chain and COL1A2 gene on chromosome 7 encodes the α-2 chain. Mild forms result from a reduced amount of type I collagen of normal composition, while severe forms often result from structural abnormalities in type I collagen.

Sillence is the most commonly used classification system (Table 2.3). Treatment varies according to the variety of the disease. In the severe congenital form (Sillence type II), multiple fractures from minimal trauma during delivery or in utero cause the limbs to be deformed and short. The skull is soft and membranous. This type is usually fatal, with death secondary to intracranial hemorrhage or respiratory

TABLE 2.3 Sillence classification of osteogenesis imperfecta

Type	Severity	Features	Sclerae	Inheritance
IA, IB	Mild	Most common, mild to moderate bone fragility, little or no deformity	Blue	AD
II	Lethal, rarely survive infancy	Extremely fragile bones, severe deformity, perinatal	Blue	AR
III	Severe	Progressively deforming, moderate to severe deformity, progressive, neonatal fractures	Normal	AR
IVA, IVB	Moderately severe	Mild to moderate bone fragility, long bone/spine deformity, A with dental involvement	Normal	AD

insufficiency; the infant is stillborn or lives only a short time. In the nonlethal forms of the disease (Sillence type I, III, IV), fragility of the bones is the most prominent feature. Fractures heal at a normal rate, and frequency of fractures declines sharply after adolescence. Deformities of the long bones due to fractures or microfractures usually develop. Severe spinal deformities may develop.

Prenatal diagnosis can be made by ultrasound. The ultrasonographic features of type II OI include long-bone deformity (implying fracture), severely reduced femoral length, and decreased echogenicity of the skull. Some degree of generalized osteopenia is detected in almost all patients with OI. The osteopenic vertebrae may fracture easily, resulting in a flattened or biconcave shape. Thoracic or thoracolumbar scoliosis frequently is detected. The pelvis may show protrusion acetabuli. The long bones may be thin and bowed with thin cortices and a poorly developed trabecular pattern. Deformities may result from multiple fractures. The goal of orthopaedic treatment is to maximize the affected patient's function, prevent deformity and disability resulting from fractures, correct deformities that have developed, and monitor for potential complicating conditions associated with OI. Callus formed in response to the fracture is identical in structure with the rest of the skeleton; it is plastic and easily deformed by mechanical forces. Intramedullary rods (load-sharing devices) are preferable to plates and screws, which tend to dislodge from the weakened bone. Deformities of the long bones may require surgical treatment. Realignment of the deformed bone is provided by multiple osteotomies and intramedullary fixation with expansile rods. Pseudoarthrosis develops in up to 20% of the patients. Scoliosis is a difficult problem to treat in OI as in other disorders with osteopenia. Segmental instrumentation is performed because of the poor quality of bone.

Osteopetrosis. There is failure of bone resorption due to functional deficiency of the osteoclasts in osteopetrosis. There are 3 different forms of osteopetrosis: infantile-malignant form, intermediate form, and adult-tarda form. Infantile osteopetrosis is an autosomal recessive trait and maps to chromosome 11q13. The intermediate form is also transmitted as an autosomal recessive type. The adult form is inherited in an autosomal dominant pattern, and its gene locus is suspected to be on chromosome 1p21. In infantile osteopetrosis, pancytopenia can develop because of an inability of the bone marrow to participate in hematopoiesis. Bony overgrowth of the cranial foramina causes cranial nerve palsies, which result in blindness and deafness. Pathologic fractures occur frequently in the fragile, brittle bones. The intermediate form of osteopetrosis usually is diagnosed in later childhood after a fracture. It may have some features of the infantile form, but presentation is milder. The patients with adult form have a normal life expectancy but many orthopaedic problems. Clinical findings include mild anemia, pathologic fractures, and premature osteoarthritis. In rare cases, osteomyelitis may characterize the clinical picture. Radiographically, there is no distinction between cortical and cancellous bone, because the intramedullary canal is filled with bone (Fig. 2.8). Flaring of the metaphyses of the long bones (best seen in the distal femur), bone-within-a-bone appearance of the pelvis, and "rugger jersey" appearance of the spine are typical radiographic findings.

Treatment for infantile osteopetrosis is bone marrow transplantation at a young age with marrow from an appropriately HLA-matched donor. A successful transplant may resolve the hematologic abnormalities and can result in a gradual restoration of patent marrow cavities. High-dose 1,25-dihydroxyvitamin D therapy with a low-calcium diet has been employed because of its ability to stimulate osteoclasts and bone

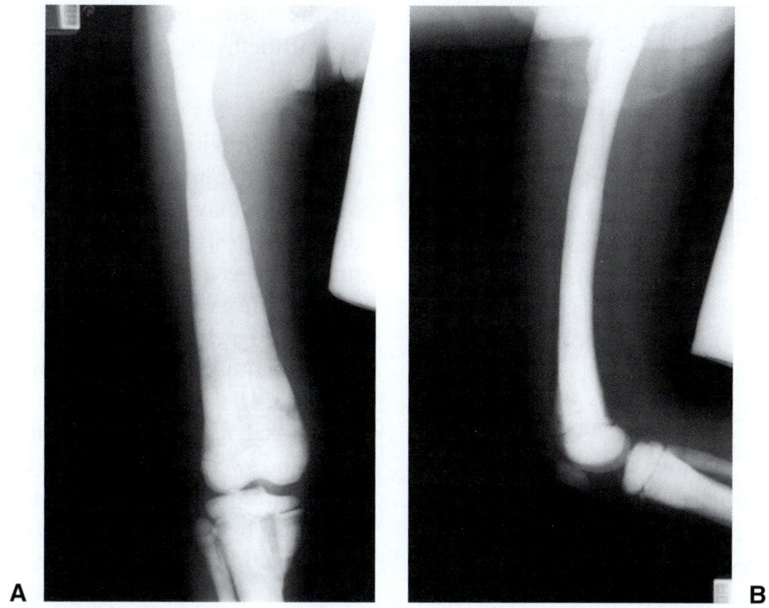

FIGURE 2.8 (A) Anterior-posterior and (B) lateral radiographs of femur in osteopetrosis. Absence of medullary canal.

resorption. Fractures in the intermediate and adult forms are common and require appropriate treatment. Healing does occur but may be delayed.

Infantile Cortical Hyperostosis. This is a self-limited disorder in infants presenting with soft tissue swelling, bone changes, and irritability. Two types have been noted: the familial and the sporadic. The familial form has an onset as early as 6 to 8 weeks, while the sporadic form presents around 9 to 11 weeks. Patients typically present with a triad of swelling, bone lesions, and irritability. Other features are a high fever, failure to grow, and sudden, deep, tender swelling. It involves multiple bones, the most common being the mandible, ulna, tibia, clavicle, and scapula. The etiology is unknown, and no treatment is required because it is self-limiting. It is to be differentiated from scurvy, hyperphosphatemia, hypervitaminosis A, child abuse, Ewing sarcoma, and metastatic neuroblastoma.

Hyperparathyroidism. Primary hyperparathyroidism results from hyperplasia of the parathyroid glands. The increased PTH stimulates osteoclastic resorption of bone, which produces hypercalcemia. The presenting symptoms are lethargy, bone pain, and abdominal complaints. The irritability and conductivity of nervous tissue are decreased by hypercalcemia. Prolonged hypercalcemia leads to ectopic calcification and renal calculi formation; the critical solubility product of calcium and phosphorus is exceeded. Hypertension is commonly present. Radiographic findings include generalized osteopenia, cortical thickening, and bony resorption at the terminal tufts of the distal phalanges and the distal clavicles. The classic laboratory findings in patients with hyperparathyroidism are elevated serum calcium, decreased serum phosphorus, and elevated alkaline phosphatase. Treatment is directed toward correcting the underlying cause of hyperparathyroidism. Fractures can occur and need to be managed by customary principles. Hypercalcemic crisis is treated by hydration and replacement of sodium losses.

Hypoparathyroidism. Hypoparathyroidism is caused by failure of the parathyroid glands to produce PTH. An autosomal dominant type is the result of mutations on chromosome 3q13 in the gene encoding for the G protein–coupled Ca^{2+}–sensing receptor, which regulates PTH secretion. Hypoparathyroidism is also associated with deletions in chromosome 22q11 (the gene responsible for DiGeorge syndrome) and cardiac defects. Other autosomal recessive types associated with growth retardation, seizures, and severe mental retardation, as well as an X-linked recessive type, have been described.

Irritability of nervous and muscle tissue, tetany, paresthesias, and alteration in mental status may be seen. The skin is dry, the hair brittle and scant. If hypocalcemia occurs early in development, mental retardation may result. Radiographic findings include increased density of the long bones and skull. Soft tissue calcifications can occur, including the basal ganglia. Laboratory findings reveal decreased total and serum ionized calcium and elevated serum phosphorus.

V. CONNECTIVE TISSUE SYNDROMES

Marfan Syndrome. AD with 30% of cases following a sporadic mutation. Mutation in gene fibrillin-1 causes a defect in the scaffolding for elastic tissues in the body. Clinical features include myopia, lens dislocation (superiorly), retinal detachment, aortic regurgitation, dissecting aortic aneurysm, and mitral valve prolapse. Prominent skeletal issues are joint laxity, protrusio acetabuli, and scoliosis. Bracing is recommended for progressive curves, many of which will require surgical fusion. Early echocardiogram and eye examination are part of routine care.

Ehlers-Danlos Syndrome (EDS). At least nine different types of EDS have been identified. Types I and II are most common and present with soft fragile skin, easy and severe bruising, eye problems, nearsightedness, joint laxity, double jointedness, and frequent dislocations in shoulder, knee, and hip. The other types have gum disease, weak blood vessels, easy rupture of the intestine and uterus, clotting problems, and scoliosis. Physical therapy and bracing are helpful in the majority of patients. Spinal arthrodesis is required for progressive scoliosis. Soft tissue procedures are avoided if possible due to the risk of complications, and recurrence of deformities.

Homocystinuria. AR trait with deficiency of cystathionine-β-synthase. The defect lies in the metabolism of the amino acid methionine leading to accumulation of homocysteine. Clinical features are failure to thrive, visual problems, mental retardation, and tendency to clot. It has several features resembling Marfan syndrome, such as dislocation of lens (inferiorly); long, spidery fingers (arachnodactyly); pes cavus; genu valgum; and scoliosis. The diagnosis is made on enzyme assay or detecting homocysteine in the urine. There is no specific cure for the disease, but vitamin B_6, low methionine diet, and trimethyglycine have been tried with variable success.

Juvenile Rheumatoid Arthritis (JRA). JRA is a chronic inflammatory disorder of the synovium, which over time, may result in contractures and ultimately destruction of the joint. While the etiology remains unknown, genetic predisposition, an environmental trigger, infection, and an autoimmune process have all been suggested. Schaller proposed different types of JRA depending on type and number of joints involved (Table 2.4).

Clinical features include morning stiffness, joint pain, and swelling. The joint is warm and has restricted range of motion. The diagnosis is made clinically and with the help of some tests. Clinical signs include onset before 16 years of age, arthritis or restricted range of motion, more than 6 weeks of duration, and exclusion of other forms of juvenile arthritis. Extraarticular manifestations are fever, rash, iridocyclitis, hepatosplenomegaly, pleuritis, and pericarditis. Twice yearly examination of the eye is essential to prevent complications from iridocyclitis or uveitis. Sedimentation rate and C-reactive protein are elevated during the acute phase. ANA is present in pauciarticular and polyarticular disease, while rheumatoid factor may or may not be positive. The aim of treatment is to preserve joint function and arrest progression of the disease. Nonsteroidal anti-inflammatory agents such as aspirin are the mainstay of therapy and methotrexate is used as a second-line drug. Physical therapy, splinting, and occasionally synovectomy, are all helpful in selected cases. Progressive inflammation with joint destruction may require arthrodesis or joint arthroplasty.

Ankylosing Spondylitis. Ankylosing spondylitis is an inflammatory disorder of unknown origin affecting primarily the axial and peripheral joints. Its prevalence

TABLE 2.4 Schaller classification of juvenile rheumatoid arthritis

Type	ANA	RF	Joints	Systemic Symptoms and Signs
Pauciarticular I (F)	+	–	Large	Iridocyclitis
Pauciarticular II (M)	–	–	Large	HLA-B 27 +, spondylitis
Polyarticular/RF –	1/3	–	Many	Mild fever
Polyarticular/RF +	1/3	+	Many	Mild
Systemic-Still's	–	–	Many	Fever, rash, organomegaly

Source: Schaller JG. Chronic arthritis in children: Juvenile rheumatoid arthritis. *Clin Orthop* 182:79–89,1984.

TABLE 2.5 Modified Jones criteria for the diagnosis of rheumatic fever

Major Manifestations	Minor Manifestations
Carditis	Prolonged P-R interval
Polyarthritis	Arthralgia
Sydenham chorea	Fever
Erythema marginatum	Elevated ESR or CRP
Subcutaneous nodules	

in men is 3 to 4 times that in women and normally starts by second to third decade. The initial complaint is low back pain and morning stiffness lasting at least 1 hour and improving with exercise. The examination demonstrates decreased motion in the spine (Schober test), decreased chest expansion, and obliteration of lumbar lordosis. Peripheral joint involvement is common with the hips and shoulder. Radiographs of the pelvis show early irregularities and erosions in the sacroiliac joint, which progresses to complete bony fusion. Spine radiographs show scalloping of the vertebrae and fusion of the spine with ossification in the interspinous ligaments (bamboo spine). The diagnosis is based on clinical and x-ray findings. HLA B27 is positive in 90% to 95% of patients with ankylosing spondylitis. Treatment is focused on NSAIDs, physical therapy, and an exercise program. Rarely, lumbar or cervical spine osteotomy is required to correct severe, fixed kyphotic deformities. Joint arthroplasty may be required to treat arthritis of the hips and/or shoulder.

Acute Rheumatic Fever. Acute rheumatic fever is caused by the immunologic response following infection with group A β-hemolytic streptococci. It presents 1 to 3 weeks following a throat infection in children 5 to 15 years old. The diagnosis is based on the Jones criteria (Table 2.5). The common findings are carditis, polyarthritis, erythema marginatum, chorea, and subcutaneous nodules. Management is with aspirin, antibiotics, and prompt cardiology referral.

VI. CEREBRAL PALSY

Overview. Cerebral palsy is a disorder of movement and posture resulting from damage to the immature brain. While the central nervous system lesion is nonprogressive, musculoskeletal abnormalities can progress throughout growth and development. Though the exact cause is unknown in most cases, and the etiology may be prenatal, may occur at the time of birth, or may be postnatal, common associations include prematurity, low birth weight, maternal infection such as chorioamnionitis and prenatal intrauterine infections (TORCH), birth anoxia, congenital brain malformations, and meningitis. The upper motor neuron lesion causes weakness, loss of voluntary movement, and spasticity leading to contractures and deformity. The manifestations change with growth and development. Other higher functions like speech, vision, and intellect may also be affected.

Classification. There are several common classification schemes. In the physiologic classification, patients are categorized based upon the type of movement disorder. In most cases, more than one physiologic type is present.

- *Spastic*—This is the most common type and occurs in about 60% to 75% of the cases. Spasticity is one form of hypertonicity, and is defined as a rate dependent change in muscle tone. Findings include increased muscle tone, hyperreflexia, and clonus. The simultaneous contractions of agonists and antagonists cause slow and restricted movement. Spasticity leads to contractures and deformities, which are amenable to surgery.
- *Athetoid/Dyskinetic*—Patients with this type of cerebral palsy present with abnormal, slow, writhing, involuntary movement due to involvement of basal ganglia. One common association, now mainly of historical interest, is erythroblastosis fetalis with kernicterus. Other features are dysarthria; abnormal, distal, jerky movement (chorea); and often normal intelligence. Patients are less likely to develop fixed deformities, and orthopaedic surgery is typically not indicated. This type is most difficult to correct with surgery.
- *Ataxia*—This type presents with deficits in balance and co-ordination, unsteadiness, a wide-based gait, and intentional tremor. These findings are secondary to involvement of the cerebellum.
- *Hemiballistic*—This type of cerebral palsy is characterized by sudden, continuous, violent, uncoordinated, involuntary muscular activity involving the axial and proximal appendicular musculature.
- *Hypotonic*—Hypotonic cerebral palsy is rare, however a subset of patients may initially be hypotonic, only to develop spasticity over the first 2 to 4 years of life.
- *Mixed*—Most patients will exhibit features of more than one physiologic subtype, and often one type predominates.

Geographic Classification:

- *Hemiplegia*—Both upper and lower limbs are involved on the same side. This type may occur following a cerebrovascular accident involving the middle cerebral artery. Spasticity is typically greater in the upper limb than the lower. All hemiplegics are expected to ambulate independently.

- *Diplegia*—Involvement of the lower limbs is greater than the upper limbs, in this type of cerebral palsy. Common associations are low birth weight (< 1500 grams) and prematurity associated with periventricular leukomalacia. Most diplegics will eventually walk. IQ may be normal, and strabismus is common.
- *Quadriplegia*—All four extremities are involved, and these patients usually have a variety of other manifestations including abnormalities in speech and swallowing, gastrointestinal problems (reflux, hypomotility), and seizures.

Orthopedic Assessment. The physical examination focuses on presence and degree of spasticity, range of motion at the joints of the upper and lower extremities, selectivity of muscular control, muscle strength testing (when possible), and in ambulators an observational gait analysis should be performed as well. The goals of treatment depend upon functional status. For children who walk, the goal is to improve the ease and efficiency of ambulation. In nonambulators, treatment is aimed at providing comfortable sitting, ideally maintaining a straight spine over a level pelvis. The most important priority for adults with cerebral palsy is communication, followed by activities of daily living, and only then mobility.

Nonoperative Management. Nonoperative management consists of physiotherapy, serial casting, the use of orthotics, and strategies to decrease spasticity (oral agents and intramuscular injections). Physical therapy helps with promoting the neurodevelopmental sequence, as well as with strengthening exercises and gaining or maintaining range of motion. Occupational therapists utilize a variety of interventions to improve upper extremity function. Oral agents, such as valium and baclofen, may reduce muscle tone, however dose dependent side effects (drowsiness) limit the ability to achieve the maximal benefit. Intramuscular injections of botulinum toxin A (BOTOX), or phenol, result in a reversible chemical denervation at the neuromuscular junction, lasting typically from 3 to 8 months. A decrease in muscle tone facilitates rehabilitation and the use of orthoses, and delays (or occasionally prevents) the need for orthopaedic surgical interventions. Serial casting may be employed to restore motion at the knee or ankle, or in the upper extremity. Orthotics (most commonly variants of an ankle-foot orthosis) may be employed to facilitate ambulation, or as a night splint to delay the progression of contractures.

Operative Management. Operative treatment may be directed towards spasticity (neurosurgical), or to the effects of spasticity on the growth of musculoskeletal tissues (orthopaedic).

Neurosurgical procedures to decrease spasticity include selective dorsal rhizotomy and implantation of an intrathecal baclofen pump. Selective posterior rhizotomy involves sectioning of a subset of dorsal rootlets, and requires a laminectomy or laminoplasty. The ideal patient is a community level ambulatory who is young (4 to 8 years), has adequate underlying muscle strength, has reasonable motor control, and who has no fixed deformities. The procedure offers permanent tone reduction in selected patients, which has a positive impact upon ambulation. Reduction of spasticity unmasks underlying muscle weakness, so an extensive period of rehabilitation is required. Intrathecal baclofen has been used most often in the nonambulatory patients with severe spastic quadriplegia to improve function and ease of care.

Orthopaedic surgical procedures typically involve lengthening of contracted muscle groups, transferring muscle groups that are contributing to the genesis of a deformity, osteotomies to correct rotational deformities or angular deformities, and rarely arthrodesis. While it may be difficult on bench examination to differentiate a dynamic deformity (spasticity) from a myostatic deformity (actual shortening of the muscle tendon unit), an exam under anesthesia may help to determine the true range of motion and to finalize the treatment plan.

Gait Disorders. Abnormal gait is a common problem in the hemiplegic and diplegic populations, as well as in the small number of quadriplegic patients who are able to ambulate. Observational gait analysis is a standard component of the physical examination, and instrumented motion analysis is being utilized with greater frequency to gain more detailed information with which to refine the problem list and decide upon the final treatment plan. Gait problems usually reflect abnormalities at multiple levels (hips, knees, ankles), and all levels must be addressed in the treatment plan. Surgical procedures to improve gait include osteotomies (femur, tibia, hindfoot), muscle lengthening procedures (iliopsoas, hamstrings, gastrosoleus), muscle transfers (rectus femoris, tibialis posterior or anterior), and rarely an arthrodesis (subtalar, triple). Surgery is typically delayed until children reach a plateau in their ambulation, usually around 6 to 8 years of age. The current trend is to perform multiple lower extremity procedures under the same anesthetic. Extensive postoperative physical therapy is required, and it takes up to one year to maximize function. Contractures are most common in diarthrodial muscles (rectus femoris, hamstrings, gastrosoleus), and care must be taken to address all levels of deformity (hips, knees, ankles).

Spinal Disorders. Scoliosis may be diagnosed in up to 70% of nonambulators by adulthood. Two types of curves have been identified; the type I curve is a single thoracic curve, or thoracic and lumbar curve, without any pelvic obliquity. The type II curve is a lumbar or thoracolumbar curve with marked pelvic obliquity. Progressive curves more than 20 to 30 degrees may be considered for bracing, and a soft spinal orthosis is tolerated best. While braces cannot be relied upon to arrest the progression of neuromuscular deformities, they improve function and may delay the need for surgical intervention. Wheelchair modifications may also provide sufficient trunk support to allow comfortable sitting. Progressive curves greater than 50 to 60 degrees, which are symptomatic or create functional impairment, are treated by an instrumented posterior spinal fusion with segmental fixation, typically from the upper thoracic spine (T2) to the pelvis (when there is pelvic obliquity.) Rigid curves, in which the trunk cannot be balanced relative to the pelvis on traction or bending radiographs, require an anterior release in addition to a posterior spinal fusion. Given the high risk of complications following these procedures, a detailed preoperative medical evaluation is mandatory. The perioperative issues to be considered are nutrition, blood loss, and ileus.

Hip Dysplasia. While neuromuscular dysplasia is rare in the ambulatory population, torsional abnormalities of the proximal femur (internal) commonly require surgical correction. Neuromuscular dysplasia is very common in nonambulators, and is due to the effects of spasticity and muscle imbalance (flexion/adduction > extension/abduction). Hip screening has been shown to decrease the incidence of neuromuscular dislocation, and the physical examination should be repeated at 6 month intervals in growing children with spastic quadriplegia to facilitate the early detection of neuromuscular dysplasia.

- *Hip at risk*—An increase risk of progressive dysplasia may be associated with both clinical factors (passive abduction in extension of less than 45 degrees) and radiographic factors (migration percentage greater than 30%). While clinical screening in high-risk patients should be performed every 6 months, radiographs are only obtained with such frequency when the clinical exam places that patient at high risk, or in the case of preexisting radiographic abnormalities. Surgical treatment for the hip felt to be at risk is early soft tissue release (adductors, iliopsoas), which may be effective in patients with a significant adduction contracture and a migration percentage below 40%. The procedure will fail when the migration percentage is greater than 60%. Most surgeons avoid performing a neurectomy of the anterior branch of the obturator nerve.
- *Subluxed hip*—In the presence of significant subluxation, which is typically associated with established bony deformity, bony procedures are required in addition to a soft tissue release. The most common procedure is a soft tissue release followed by a varus derotational proximal femoral osteotomy (often with shortening to decrease muscular forces), and usually a volume reducing pelvic osteotomy (DEGA or variants) if there is coexisting acetabular dysplasia (AI > 25 to 27 degrees).
- *Dislocated hip*—Ideally, dislocations can be prevented by screening, early diagnosis, and treatment. The treatment of dislocation depends upon the duration of dislocation and the presence of symptoms. For an established dislocation of short duration, consideration can be given to reconstruction. This requires, in addition to a soft tissue release, both a proximal femoral osteotomy and an acetabular osteotomy, and some suggest that an open reduction is required as well to limit the chances of resubluxation or dislocation. In cases where the dislocation is felt to be of intermediate duration, and the femoral head does not appear to be deformed on imaging studies (plain films or advanced imaging), consideration can be given to reconstruction, but an open reduction should be performed first to assess the shape of the femoral head and the status of the articular cartilage. If there is deformity or breakdown of cartilage, then a salvage treatment option should be selected. In chronic, symptomatic dislocations, the femoral head is often deformed, and the articular cartilage may be broken down; as such, salvage options are suggested, including resection of the femoral head and neck (perhaps the most common procedure, performed at the level of the lesser trochanter), a valgus osteotomy to redirect the damaged femoral head, resection/valgus osteotomy/interposition (McHale procedure), prosthetic reconstruction (total hip arthroplasty or with a humeral head prosthesis), or rarely an arthrodesis.

Knee Abnormalities. Two deformities that are most noticeable are knee flexion contracture and quadriceps contracture. The flexion contracture is caused by hamstring tightness. Treatment involves proximal or distal lengthening of the hamstrings. Attention must be paid to any psoas, equinus, and unnoticed quadriceps contracture, which may lead to other deformities. The quadriceps contracture causing stiff, extended knee is due to rectus femoris shortening. Treatment is lengthening of rectus femoris or out-of-phase transfer of rectus femoris to sartorius or intertrochanteric band.

Foot and Ankle Deformities.

- *Ankle equinus/equinovarus*—Progressive equinus contracture involves the gastrosoleus complex, and often just the gastrocnemius will be contracted. The contribution from each muscle is assessed by the Silverskiöld test, in which the foot is dorsiflexed with the knee both flexed (test soleus) and fully extended (test gastrocnemius and soleus). Several techniques are available for lengthening of the tendoachilles. The Strayer procedure is indicated when only the gastrocnemius is contracted. When there is also contracture of the soleus, lengthening can be achieved by a recession technique at the musculotendinous junction (Vulpius, Baker), or by lengthening the tendoachilles (percutaneous or open sliding lengthening, Z-lengthening). While the risk of overlengthening is greatest with a Z-lengthening technique, the recession techniques preserve better push-off power but have a higher risk of recurrence. Care should be taken to avoid over-lengthening of the Achilles tendon, especially in spastic diplegia, as a calcaneus gait is more difficult to treat than mild residual equinus.
- *Equinovalgus foot*— This condition is most common in spastic diplegia, and is associated with contracture of the tendoachilles, with or without peroneal spasticity/contracture. While the mild cases may respond to soft tissue lengthening of the tendoachilles and peroneus brevis, children with more significant deformities require additional measures for reconstruction. The most popular approach involves a hindfoot osteotomy coupled with soft tissue lengthening. The lateral column lengthening procedure involves an osteotomy of the anterior process of the calcaneus, and insertion of a trapezoidal wedge results in a three dimensional realignment of the hindfoot. Concomitant soft tissue procedures are required, and patients with residual forefoot deformity may require a plantar-based closing wedge osteotomy of the medial cuneiform as well. An alternative is an extraarticular subtalar arthrodesis, however osteotomy is currently favored because motion is preserved. For severe, rigid equinovalgus deformities in older patients, triple arthrodesis may be required to realign the hindfoot.
- *Equinovarus foot*—The dynamic equinovarus foot interferes with pre-positioning for stance phase, as well as stance phase stability (roll onto the lateral border of the foot). In addition to contracture of the tendoachilles, the equinovarus foot may be associated with dynamic overactivity of the tibialis posterior, the tibialis anterior, or both. It may be challenging to define the etiology based upon the physical examination, and a dynamic EMG study (one component of an instrumented motion analysis study) may help to distinguish which muscles are responsible for the deformity. Milder deformities may be treated by lengthening of the tendoachilles and the tibialis posterior (intramuscular). The deformities are classified as dynamic (flexible) and fixed. Tendon transfers are helpful to rebalance forces around the hindfoot, and split transfers are recommended, as the chance of over correction is high when the entire tendon is transferred. As a prerequisite for tendon transfer is a full range of motion, restoration of motion by soft tissue lengthening or release, and occasionally an osteotomy, may be required. If the tibialis posterior is responsible, then a split transfer of one half of the tibialis posterior to the peroneus brevis (or through the interosseous membrane to the dorsum of the foot) is recommended. When the tibialis anterior is causing the deformity, a split tibialis anterior transfer to the cuboid may be performed. Another option is a combined procedure involving a split tibialis anterior transfer and intramuscular lengthening of the tibialis posterior.

Upper Limb. Surgery is indicated to improve function, enhance hygiene, or improve appearance. Overall, a small, carefully selected group of patients stand to benefit from upper extremity surgery. In addition to spasticity, muscle imbalance, the development of fixed contractures, and loss of selective motor control, nearly 50% of patients will also have underlying deficits in sensation and proprioception. Common deformities of the upper extremity include flexion contracture at the elbow, forearm pronation, wrist/finger flexion, and the thumb in palm deformity. Shoulder position is usually not a limiting factor with regards to function. In severe cases, lengthening of the subscapularis and pectoralis major muscles can be performed to correct an internal rotation contracture.

Wrist flexion deformity directly impairs finger function and the ability to grasp and release. Transfer of the flexor carpi ulnaris to the extensor carpi radialis or extensor digitorum communis should be considered, and a concomitant transfer of the extensor carpi ulnaris to the midline can enhance wrist and finger extension. When the wrist is placed into extension and passive digital extension is not possible in this position, concomitant lengthening of the finger flexors (flexor digitorum profundus and/or superficialis) is necessary. If active finger extension is not present, additional tendon transfer to the finger extensor tendons may be necessary. The thumb-in-palm deformity is extremely difficult to correct. Examination of the thumb muscles often reveals spasticity of the intrinsic muscles (thenar and adductor pollicis muscles) and deficiencies within the extensor mechanism. Release of the thenar and adductor pollicis muscles from their origins allows these muscles to slide and diminishes their force. Augmentation of thumb extension and abduction is achieved by rerouting of the extensor pollicis longus tendon through the first dorsal compartment or other tendon transfers.

VII. NEUROMUSCULAR DISORDERS

Arthrogryposis Multiplex Congenita. Arthrogryposis is a nonprogressive disorder with multiple contractures. It is associated with decreased anterior horn cells. Intelligence is often normal. Evaluation should include neurologic studies, enzyme tests, and muscle biopsy (at 3 to 4 months). Affected patients typically have a normal facies, normal intelligence, multiple joint contractures, and no visceral abnormalities. The typical upper extremity deformity is shoulder adduction/internal rotation, elbow extension, and wrist flexion/ulnar deviation. Osteotomies can be considered after the age of 4. The typical lower extremity deformity consists of teratologic hip dislocations, knee contractures, resistant feet, and a vertical talus. Treatments for the lower extremity include early (6 to 9 months) soft tissue releases for knee contractures and medial open reduction with femoral shortening for hip dislocations.

Myelodysplasia (Spina Bifida). Spina bifida is a result of incomplete spinal cord closure or secondary rupture of the developing cord due to hydrocephalus. It can be classified into spina bifida occulta (vertebral arch defect with confined cord and meninges), meningocele (sac without neural elements protruding through the defect), myelomeningocele (sac protrusion with neural elements), and rachisis (neural elements exposed without coverage). Diagnosis can be made in utero with elevated α-fetoprotein levels and is related to folate deficiency in utero.

Function is primarily related to the level of the defect and associated congenital abnormalities, the most common of which is the Arnold-Chiari malformation. The myelodysplasia level is based on the lowest functional level with L4 being a key level because quadriceps function can allow for independent community ambulation.

Treatment utilizes a team approach with proper orthotic use, muscle balancing (through surgery), and deformity correction. Latex-free environments should be provided because these patients are noted to be extremely sensitive. Anterior hip release is often performed for patients with thoracic or high lumbar myelomeningoceles due to unopposed hip flexors or prolonged sitting. Hip dislocation is most common at the L3/L4 level, and treatment is controversial but often limited to those with a functioning quadriceps. Knee deformities can be treated with KAFO for quadriceps weakness or hamstring lengthening/posterior capsule releases for severe flexion deformities. The objective of treating the ankle and foot is to obtain a braceable, plantigrade foot with muscular balance. Fractures are common in myelodysplasia patients and may be associated with redness, warmth, and swelling; and are treated conservatively.

Spinal deformities are often severe and progressive, resulting from the spine disorder itself or other congenital malformation. Nearly all patients with thoracic-level paraplegia develop scoliosis. Bracing is unsuccessful, and curve progression can be rapid, often associated with a tethered cord.

Friedreich Ataxia. This autosomal recessive disorder with problems in the frataxin gene is a spinocerebellar degenerative disease with mean onset between 7 and 15 years of age. Patients present with a staggering gait, nystagmus, cardiomyopathy, cavus foot, and scoliosis. EMG reveals motor and sensory defects with an increase in polyphasic potential.

Charcot-Marie-Tooth Disease (CMT). CMT is part of a larger group of hereditary motor sensory neuropathies (HMSN). The two types of CMT have been classified as HMSN I and HMSN II. HMSN I is the autosomal dominant motor sensory demyelinating neuropathy, which is hypertrophic and has an onset during the second decade of life. The neuronal (HMSN II) type has a variable inheritance pattern, an onset during the third or fourth decade of life, and more extensive foot involvement. Diagnosis is made most reliably by DNA testing for duplication of chromosome 17. Physical manifestations include intrinsic wasting in the hands. The most severely affected muscles are the tibialis anterior, peroneus longus, and peroneus brevis. Motor defects are more pronounced than sensory defects. Treatment includes plantar release, posterior tibial tendon transfer (hindfoot must be flexible), and triple arthrodesis versus calcaneal osteotomies (fixed deformity).

VIII. MUSCULAR DYSTROPHIES

Genetics and Molecular Biology

Genetic research in molecular biology has tremendously enhanced the understanding of the genetic aspects of many muscular dystrophy disorders.

Dystrophin. The gene is located at the Xp21 region and spans 2.4 million base pairs. It includes 79 exons (coding regions) that encompass only about 2% of the gene and encodes the 427-kDa protein dystrophin. The large size of the gene correlates with the high rate of spontaneous mutation (approximately one third of cases). The distribution of dystrophin within skeletal, smooth, and cardiac muscle and within the brain correlates well with the clinical features in Duchenne and Becker muscular dystrophy.

When to Suspect a Disease of Muscle Hypotonia and Weakness. At birth, decreased fetal activity, sluggish newborn reflexes, poor head control on traction response (i.e., Moro reflex), slip-through at the shoulder girdle, poor weight-bearing, sluggish feeding, and increased respiratory effort are indicative of a neuromuscular disease. The timing of onset of symptoms and the rate of progression are key factors pointing toward a particular neuromuscular disorder. Unexplained cardiomyopathy should always prompt a search for an underlying muscular dystrophy or myopathy. Family history of a neuromuscular disorder is also a risk factor. Elevation of serum creatine kinase (CK) may be found incidentally and suggests an underlying muscle disease, though modest elevations can also be seen in some neuropathic conditions and in otherwise healthy teenage males.

The exam of the young infant focuses on functional indicators of weakness such as the extent of head lag on traction from supine to sitting, slip-through at the shoulder girdle when held vertically under the arms, and capacity to actively bear weight on extended legs. The scarf sign also demonstrates shoulder girdle weakness. For the older infant and young child, the evaluation should include sitting posture, ability to roll over, sitting, pulling into a standing position, rising from the supine to standing (Gowers maneuver) or from a chair to standing, and stair-climbing. Standard manual muscle testing on the 0 to 5 Medical Research Council scale and quantifiable measures of strength using a hand-held myometer can be used reliably in the school-aged child of normal intelligence. When used serially, quantified functional measures of endurance (e.g., time to walk/run 30 feet, climb 4 stairs, Gowers maneuver) can assess progression of disease and response to treatment.

Treatment. Treatment of the child with a muscular dystrophy is often best coordinated through a neuromuscular clinic with the combined help of the orthopedist, neurologist, rehabilitation specialist, cardiologist, pulmonologist, and physical, occupational, and speech therapists. Once a specific diagnosis has been established, a treatment algorithm can be formulated for that patient on the basis of the knowledge of the natural history of that condition.

Duchenne Muscular Dystrophy. Duchenne muscular dystrophy (DMD) is the most common form of muscular dystrophy, and is an X-linked recessive myopathy affecting only males. Its incidence ranges from 13 to 33 per 100,000 live births, of which one third arise from new mutations. This progressive disease results in the infiltration of muscle with fibrofatty tissue, resulting in progressive loss of muscle power and contractures. Typically, proximal muscles such as those around the shoulder and hip girdles are involved initially, followed by more distal muscle groups. Corticosteroids have been demonstrated to slow the rate of progression of weakness in Duchenne MD and may also transiently improve strength in some cases. Options include Deflazacort (not currently available in the United States) and prednisone is 0.75 mg/kg/day. The benefits must be weighed against the side effects for each individual patient. The administration of steroids has been shown to prolong ambulation, to delay the development of scoliosis, and to enhance longevity.

In DMD, joint contractures develop as weakness progresses, and are commonly observed at the ankle (equinus, equinovarus), the knee (flexion), and the hip (flexion/abduction). With progressive weakness around the hip girdle and lower extremity, coupled with equinus or equinovarus deformities, walking becomes difficult and could result in frequent falls. The muscles responsible for standing upright, particularly the extensors of the hips and knees become weak early, and compensatory mechanisms during gait include hyperlordosis of the lumbar spine to maintain upright balance. It remains unclear whether tendoachilles lengthening, with or without transfer of the tibialis posterior to the dorsum of the foot, will extend the time of ambulation in this group of patients.

More than 90% of patients will develop a progressive scoliosis, usually within a year or two after losing the ability to ambulate, and an instrumented posterior spinal fusion is offered for progressive curves greater than 20 degrees. Ideally, the procedure is performed early, before any significant decline in cardiopulmonary function.

IX. MUSCULOSKELETAL INFECTIONS

Epidemiology. Osteomyelitis can be defined as an infection of bone, whereas septic arthritis is a joint infection. Most cases occur from hematogenous seeding, although direct inoculation from penetrating trauma or surgical procedures can initiate the process. The most common site for bone infection is the metaphysis because of the characteristically rich blood supply in children (Fig. 2.9). The majority of these infections are bacterial, with *Staphylococcus aureus* currently isolated as the most common organism in

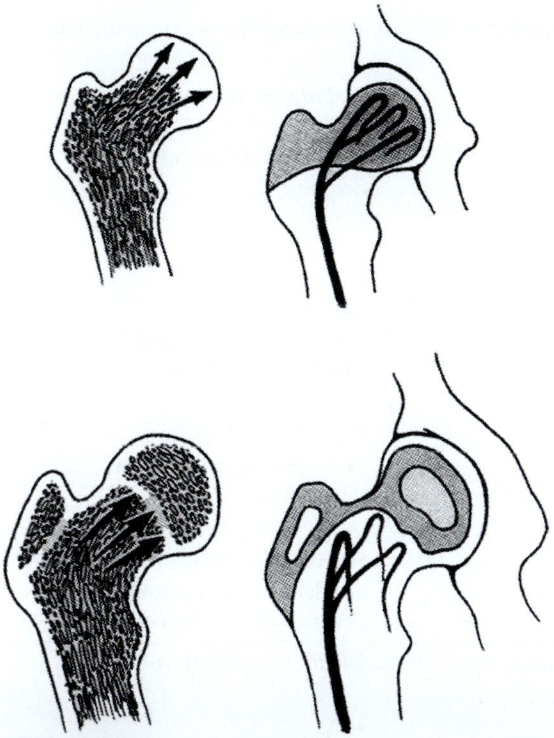

FIGURE 2.9 **Relation between metaphyseal and epiphyseal circulation in children younger than 18 months (top) versus children older than 18 months (bottom).** ***Source*: Dormans JP, Drummond DS. Pediatric hematogenous osteomyelitis: New trends in presentation, diagnosis and treatment. *J Am Acad Orthop Surg* 1994;2:333–341.**

all age categories. Other organisms frequently involved are listed in Table 2.6.

Evaluation. Relevant history includes time of onset, nature and location of symptoms, presence of constitutional symptoms, recent infection or treatment with antibiotics, refusal to walk or bear weight, and history of trauma. Relevant physical findings include focal tenderness, warmth, erythema, swelling, limited range of motion, pseudoparalysis, limp, and joint effusion.

Laboratory Studies. Initial studies include a complete blood count (CBC) with differential, erythrocyte sedimentation rate (ESR), C-reactive protein (CRP), and blood cultures.

Sequential determination of the CRP is perhaps the most important laboratory test used in evaluating and treating musculoskeletal infection. The serum value begins to rise within 6 hours of the stimulus and increases several hundredfold, reaching a peak within 36 to 50 hours of onset. Blood cultures yield positive results in only 30% to 50% of cases. However, they are indispensable because they may render the only isolate of an organism that may serve as a guide to treatment.

Aspiration. Aspiration has the greatest yield in cases of suspected septic arthritis. Generally, cell counts greater than 50,000/mL with greater than 75% polymorphonuclear (PMN) leukocytes suggest infection, while those less than 15,000/mL with less than 75% PMN leukocytes suggest inflammation. Bone aspiration in cases of suspected osteomyelitis should always be considered.

Plain Radiography. Soft tissue swelling is the first radiographic manifestation and changes in the bone may not occur for 10 to 14 days after the onset of infection.

Ultrasound. The advantages of ultrasound include low cost, absence of radiation exposure, noninvasive nature, and the ability to detect and localize joint effusions, and in some cases subperiosteal fluid collections.

Nuclear Medicine. A three-phase bone scan is comprised of an initial flow phase (essentially a radionuclide angiogram), a blood pool phase (performed after a brief period to evaluate soft tissue pooling), and delayed images (performed 2 to 3 hours later to evaluate the calcium phosphate deposition in bone). Gallium-67 citrate imaging may be a useful study when the technetium scan is normal.

Magnetic Resonance Imaging (MRI). MRI findings consistent with osteomyelitis include dark marrow on T1-weighted images and increased marrow signal intensity on T2-weighted images. The study should be completed with intravenous gadolinium whenever an infection is suspected. This facilitates the identification of any abscesses, which demonstrate rim enhancement.

Osteomyelitis

Acute Hematogenous Osteomyelitis (AHO). The acute, focal bone pain is often, but not always, accompanied by systemic findings of fever or malaise.The differential diagnosis includes trauma, leukemia, malignant tumors such as Ewing sarcoma or osteogenic sarcoma, and bone infarction from sickle cell crisis. The initial evaluation includes laboratory studies (blood cultures if febrile), and aspiration of any potential sites of infection is helpful. Imaging studies help to make the diagnosis.

Subacute Osteomyelitis. Subacute osteomyelitis may be pain without signs of systemic illness. The pain has usually been present for at least two weeks, but possibly

TABLE 2.6 Common causative organisms and empiric antibiotic selection for septic arthritis or osteomyelitis according to age

Age	*Organism*	*Empiric Antibiotic (IV)*
Neonate (up to 8 weeks)	*S. aureus* *Streptococcus* sp. *S. epidermidis* *Enterococcus, E. coli, Salmonella* sp. *N. gonorrhoeae*	Nafcillin and Gentamicin or Cefotaxime
Infant and Child (3 and younger)	*S. aureus* *K. kingae* *S. pneumoniae* Group A *Streptococcus*	Nafcillin, Oxacillin, Clindamycin, or Cefazolin Non-Hib-immunized: Cefuroxime
Children (4 and older)	*S. aureus* Group A *Streptococcus* *P. aeruginosa* (foot puncture) *Salmonella* sp. (SSD)	Nafcillin, Oxacillin, Clindamycin, or Cefazolin Ceftazidime Cefuroxime
Adolescents	*S. aureus* *N. gonorrhoeae* (sexually active)	Nafcillin, Oxacillin, Clindamycin, or Cefazolin Ceftriaxone or Cefotaxime

Source: Copley LB, Dormans JP. Musculoskeletal infection. In: Dormans JP (ed.), *Pediatric Orthopaedics and Sports Medicine: The Requisites in Pediatrics.* St Louis: Mosby, 2005.

for months. Laboratory studies are often unremarkable, although the ESR may be elevated. While it has been suggested that empiric antibiotics may suffice when the characteristic benign radiographic findings are present, some feel that biopsy is required in all cases. Biopsy is certainly required when aggressive features are present, such as a periosteal reaction, abscess, or bony destruction. A biopsy is required to establish the diagnosis, and a débridement can be performed at the same time. Antibiotics are the mainstay of treatment once the diagnosis is established.

Chronic Osteomyelitis. Classic features include the presence of devitalized bone (sequestrae) and soft tissue, and a host response involving periosteal new bone formation (involucrum). Sequestrae may be partially or completely resorbed. Sequestrae serve as a nidus for recurrent episodes of clinical infection, and chronic draining sinuses may be observed. Treatment involves establishing the diagnosis by biopsy and cultures (deep tissues or implants, not sinus tracts or drainage), followed by débridement of all necrotic tissue, and then reconstruction of any bony or soft tissue defects. Antibiotics serve as an adjunct, and are usually administered via an intravenous route for 6 weeks, often followed by oral agents for an additional period of time. With an aggressive treatment approach, the majority of cases of chronic osteomyelitis may be cured.

Chronic Recurrent Multifocal Osteomyelitis (CRMO). CRMO is an inflammatory disease of bone, and while the etiology remains unknown, it may involve an autoimmune process. It has been suggested that CRMO may fall within the spectrum of spondyloarthropathies, and also that it may be associated with the SAPHO syndrome (synovitis, acne, pustulosis, hyperostosis, and osteitis). Patients usually present with the gradual onset of pain, and laboratory findings include a normal WBC and a mild elevation in the ESR. The radiographic and histologic findings are suggestive of osteomyelitis. However, cultures of bone and blood are negative. Patients are usually treated initially by empiric antibiotics, since the diagnosis is difficult to make at the time of presentation. The treatment is by NSAIDs.

Septic Arthritis. Septic arthritis involves a bacterial infection of a joint, and organisms usually gain access via a hematogenous route. Other cases may follow direct inoculation of the joint following trauma, postoperative infections, and spread of a metaphyseal focus of osteomyelitis. The infection usually involves the synovium, and an effusion is present. The major concern is the potential destruction of joint cartilage from proteolytic enzymes, which are released from the white blood cells and synovium. The earliest changes occur during the first 24 hours, and irreversible damage may occur over several days in the absence of treatment. Septic arthritis secondary to metaphyseal osteomyelitis occurs in those joints in which the metaphysis lies within the capsule, namely the hip, the proximal humerus, the proximal radius, and the distal fibula. In infants, septic arthritis commonly involves more than one joint, and a comprehensive physical examination, supplemented with imaging studies, is required. Septic arthritis of the hip is a surgical emergency, and requires prompt diagnosis and surgical drainage. In the smaller joints, septic arthritis may also be managed by repeated aspirations.

Initially, all patients are started on empiric therapy after fluid is sent for culture (aspiration of surgical drainage), and recommendations are altered based upon the results of culture and sensitivities. The initial choice depends upon the age of the patient, as well as local variables. The prevalence of community acquired methicillin-resistant *Staphylococcus aureus* has risen, and in many centers clindamycin is used initially. The duration of antibiotic therapy for uncomplicated osteomyelitis is approximately 4 to 6 weeks and that for uncomplicated septic arthritis is approximately 2 to 4 weeks. Patients most commonly receive antibiotics at home through a PIC line. Patients are followed closely to assess both the clinical response, and the trend in laboratory values, to determine the duration of therapy.

X. LOWER EXTREMITY PROBLEMS

Rotational Deformities of Femur. Excessive femoral anteversion is the most common deformity presenting as an intoeing gait. Femoral rotation decreases from approximately 35 degrees at 1 year to 15 degrees by 16 years. It is commonly seen from 3 to 6 years of age. Children are in the habit of sitting in the W position or sleeping prone. While the diagnosis is made clinically, a CT scan will quantify the degree of rotation of the femoral head and neck relative to the shaft. Treatment consists of observation, as normally it corrects by 8 to 10 years of age. Indications for surgery include severe persistent deformity and/or unacceptable cosmesis, functional impairment, anteversion > 45 degrees and no external rotation beyond neutral are some of the indications for operative intervention. Surgical treatment involves a femoral derotational, and should not be considered until the patient is at least 10 to 12 years of age.

Medial Tibial Torsion. Medial tibial torsion presents with intoeing and may be associated with metatarsus adductus (or varus), or femoral anteversion. The diagnosis is made clinically, using the thigh-foot axis or the transmalleolar axis. Clinically there is a decreased thigh-foot and transmalleolar angle. The torsion generally improves over the first 6 to 8 years of life. Bracing has not been shown to alter the natural history, and is not recommended. Persistent deformity with functional impairment may be treated by supramalleolar osteotomy after the age of 6 to 8 years.

Lateral Tibial Torsion. Lateral tibial torsion is less common than medial tibial torsion, and may be associated with contracture of the iliotibial band. In contrast to medial torsion, lateral torsion does not improve with time, and may actually worsen. If symptomatic, a supramalleolar osteotomy can be performed. The triad of external tibial torsion, increased femoral anteversion, and genu valgum presents in adolescents with knee pain and is referred to as miserable malalignment syndrome. In such cases, consideration can be given to derotational osteotomy of both the femur and the tibia to correct the malalignment and improve patellofemoral alignment.

Hip and Femur Conditions

Developmental Dysplasia of the Hip (DDH). Developmental dysplasia of the hip represents a spectrum of abnormalities relating to the growth and development of the hip joint. Risk factors include family history, breech, oligohydramnios, female, and first-born.

Diagnosis. Tests for neonatal instability include the Ortolani and Barlow maneuvers. The Barlow maneuver is a stress test in which gentle posterior pressure is exerted with the hip in adduction. A positive test indicates that the hip is subluxatable or dislocatable, indicative of significant neonatal laxity. The Ortolani maneuver assesses whether a dislocated hip is reducible, and involves gentle abduction of the hip coupled with anterior translation of the head of the femur. Physical findings in older infants with a subluxated or dislocated hip may include limited passive abduction (adduction contracture), positive Galeazzi sign (difference in knee heights when both hips are flexed to 90 degrees and held together), and asymmetric thigh folds. The femoral capital epiphysis appears by 3 to 6 months and interpreting radiographs of hips becomes easier at this time. Prior to this, ultrasound is the best way to diagnose this condition. Graf classified the dislocation in four types on the basis of alpha angle obtained on static ultrasound (Fig. 2.10 A and B). The normal angle is greater than 60 degrees and anything less than 43 degrees is classified as dislocation. The dynamic ultrasound is performed in coronal plane while maneuvering the hip as in the Barlow test. Ultrasound not only assists diagnosis but also is useful to confirm reduction and assess the reduction in follow-up. Plain radiographs are useful once the ossific nucleus has appeared. The femoral head or metaphyseal beak should lie in the inner and lower quadrant formed by Perkins line and Hilgenreiner line (Fig. 2.10 C). An arthrogram is more useful for assessment of reduction of hip following examination under anesthesia. It also allows interpreting the structures obstructing the reduction of the hip.

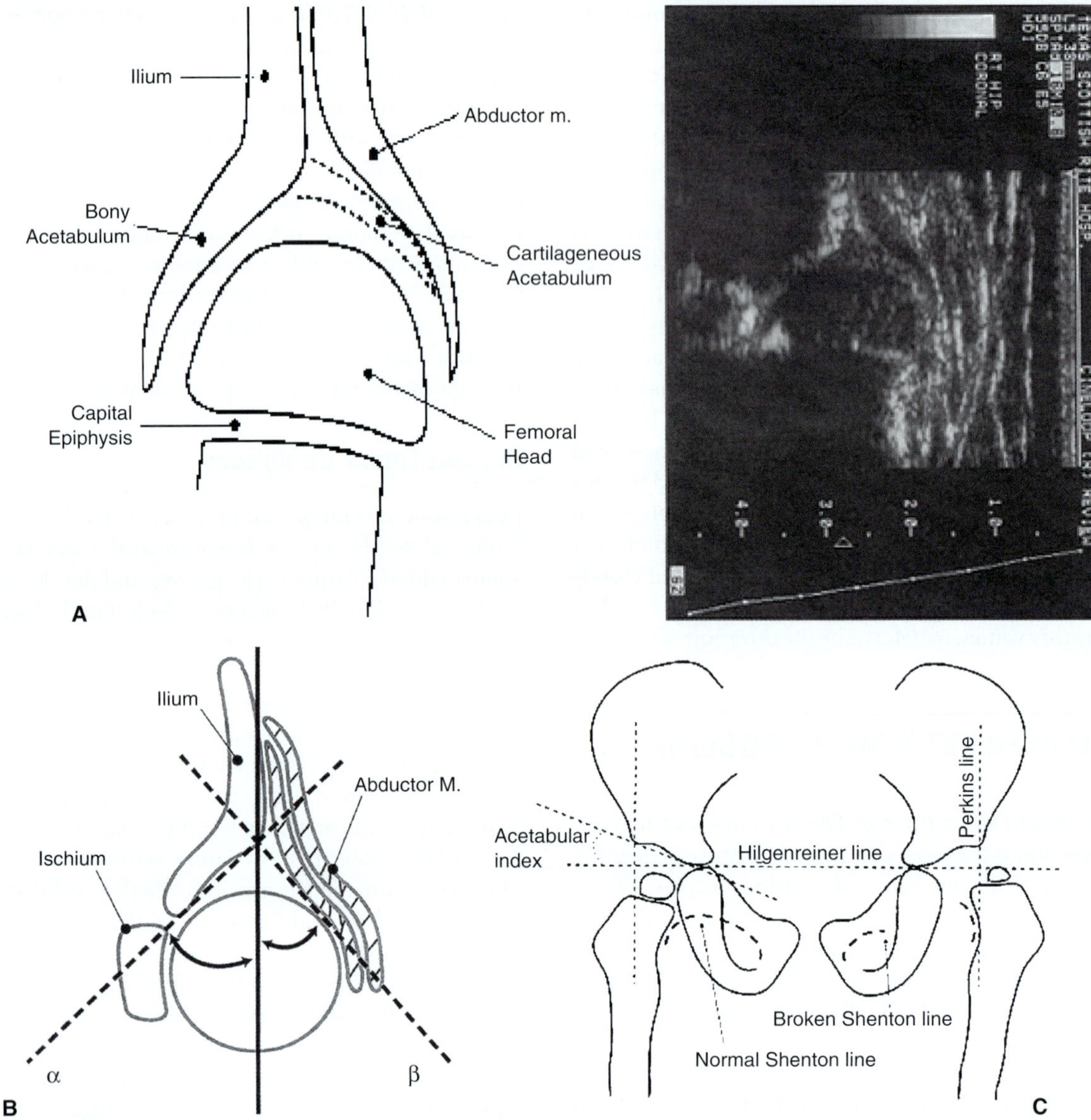

FIGURE 2.10 **(A) Images of normal ultrasound of an infant. (B) Schematic ultrasound image to demonstrate the alpha and beta angles in the hip. (A and B from Herring J. *Tachdjian's Pediatric Orthopedics.* Philadelphia: WB Saunders, 2001.) (C) Radiographic lines used in diagnosis of DDH. Acetabular index, Hilgenreiner, Perkins, and Shenton, lines.**

Treatment. The aim of treatment is a stable and concentrically reduced hip. The type of treatment depends on age and ease of achieving reduction. Most patients presenting during the first few months of life may be managed with a Pavlik harness. Ultrasound is useful in confirming and following up the reduction while in the harness. The treatment continues until the hip is stable and the radiographic appearance is satisfactory. The weaning period for the harness is double the time it was worn full time. The hip that fails to reduce concentrically in the acetabulum will be complicated with inferior dislocation as the hip is flexed beyond 90 degrees in a Pavlik harness. If reduction is not achieved by 2 to 3 weeks, then alternative methods of treatment should be considered. Those presenting after 6 months of age and irreducible hips are treated with closed reduction under general anesthesia. The use of traction prior to closed reduction remains controversial. In presence of tight adductors, an adductor tenotomy is recommended in order to improve the safe zone. While an exam under anesthesia is required to document the arc of stability, the typical position for immobilization in a hip spica cast is flexion (90 to 100 degrees) and abduction. Care should be taken to stay within the safe zone of abduction, and to avoid hyperabduction (beyond 60 degrees), which increases the risk of avascular necrosis. Intraoperative arthrogram is useful to assess the reduction and any obstructing structures. Postoperatively, the reduction should be assessed by computed tomography (limited study with cuts through the acetabulum) or by magnetic resonance imaging, as a posterior subluxation or dislocation may not be apparent on plain radiographs. The initial hip spica is replaced under anesthesia after 6 weeks, and often removed after an additional 6 weeks, depending upon the age of the patient. The total duration of casting is 3 to 4 months for most patients. Open reduction is performed when closed reduction fails, or in older patients, generally more than 18 months of age. Obstacles to closed reduction include an hourglass constriction of the capsule by the iliopsoas tendon, inverted labrum, hypertrophic ligamentum teres, and pulvinar (fibrofatty tissue). The most common surgical approach is anterolateral, however a medial approach may also be used in younger patients. The medial approach allows one to remove the obstacles to reduction, but does not provide access to perform a capsulorrhaphy.

Osteotomies. A subset of patients may require an osteotomy during treatment for DDH. In infants/toddlers who have a developmentally dislocated hip and are undergoing an open reduction, depending upon age and tension when the hip is reduced, a femoral shortening osteotomy is commonly performed to reduce the risks of avascular necrosis. In older patients with untreated dislocation, or in those with persistent dysplasia, a femoral and/or pelvic osteotomy may be recommended. Bony abnormalities in children with hip dysplasia commonly include increased femoral anteversion (variable) and acetabular dysplasia (deficiency is commonly anterior and lateral). A concentric reduction is a prerequisite for these osteotomies. Femoral osteotomies commonly involve shortening and derotation, and varus is infrequently required. A variety of pelvic osteotomies may be performed, depending upon the age of the child and the specific pathology being treated. While most osteotomies aim to cover the femoral head with healthy articular cartilage (reconstruction), several others are useful for salvage. For toddlers and children with acetabular dysplasia, a Salter innominate osteotomy (redirectional) or a Pemberton (volume reducing, hinges down the acetabular roof through the triradiate cartilage) may achieve the desired degree of coverage. In older children and adolescents, these procedures are more limited in their ability to provide the desired degree of realignment, and options for redirecting the acetabulum in this age group include the double innominate osteotomy (Sutherland), the triple innominate osteotomy (Steele), the Ganz osteotomy, and others. In many cases, a CT scan with three-dimensional reconstructions may help to better define the acetabular anatomy, and a CT scan can also be used to quantify the degree of femoral version. For patients with an incongruent joint, or in whom symptomatic degenerative changes are present, options to improve coverage of the femoral head include the Shelf procedure and the Chiari osteotomy. In the former, bone grafts are used to enlarge the size of the acetabulum and therefore improve coverage. In the latter, a medial displacement osteotomy is performed, which not only improves coverage of the femoral head, but also medializes the hip, which reduces the joint reactive force.

Congenital Coxa Vara. Coxa vara is defined as a decrease in the neck shaft angle to less than 120 degrees, and the developmental form is associated with abnormal ossification of the femoral neck. Acquired forms of coxa vara are secondary to metabolic, neoplastic, or traumatic conditions and include ricketic coxa vara, fibrous dysplasia, proximal physeal injury, and premature closure. Patients may present with a waddling gait (bilateral) or limp. On examination, an abductor lurch may be present owing to inefficiency of the abductors associated with proximal femoral varus alignment, and the Trendelenburg sign is usually positive. There is commonly asymmetric rotation at the hip as well. The anteroposterior radiographs of the hip demonstrate the decreased neck shaft angle, with an ossification defect in the inferomedial aspect of the neck. The Hilgenreiner epiphyseal angle (HEA) is the angle subtended by the horizontal Hilgenreiner line through the triradiate cartilages and an oblique line through the proximal femoral capital physes. An angle of less than 45 degrees is associated with a good prognosis. Surgical treatment is indicated for all with an HEA greater than 60 degrees and those with a limp and an HEA between 45 and 60. A proximal femoral valgus osteotomy (with derotation) is performed.

Legg-Calvé-Perthes Disease. Perthes disease describes idiopathic avascular necrosis of the femoral head in children, and the clinical course and imaging findings depend upon the extent of involvement (segmental versus the entire capital femoral epiphysis). Evidence to support a heritable coagulopathy is controversial, and while a family history is documented in 10% to 20%, there is insufficient evidence to classify this as a heritable disease. Perthes has been associated with secondhand smoke inhalation. It is estimated that 4% of patients with transient synovitis of the hip will ultimately be diagnosed with Perthes disease. The majority of patients exhibit short stature, and bone age is delayed in most patients. Attention deficit hyperactivity disorder is present in up to one third of patients. The disease is most commonly diagnosed in boys between 4 and 8 years of age, who present with a painless limp and/or pain in the groin, thigh, or knee. The discomfort is typically relieved by rest. While symptoms of the disease typically resolve by 18 to 24 months, radiographic healing may take several years. Perthes is bilateral in 10% to 12% of cases, and on radiographs the presentation is asymmetric and rarely simultaneous, in contrast to the epiphyseal dysplasias. The natural history of Perthes is characterized by an inciting event, which causes osteonecrosis of the capital femoral epiphysis. Reconstitution of the damaged area is by creeping substitution, and the process of healing occurs through various stages. Remodeling may also occur after healing is complete. This sequence of events has been classified by Waldenström into four radiographic stages, including subtle changes in density, fragmentation, reossification, and final healing (Table 2.7).

Several radiographic classification schemes have been proposed, including the Catterall, Salter and Thompson, and the lateral pillar (Herring). This classification is based on involvement of the lateral pillar of the capital femoral epiphysis in the fragmentation stage (Table 2.8, Fig. 2.11). In Group A there is no loss of the lateral pillar and a good outcome. In Group B, less than 50% of the lateral pillar is involved and prognosis for this is good for those with skeletal age less than 6 years, while not so good for older children. In Group C there is more than 50% involvement of lateral pillar and poor prognosis for all age groups. Some of the indicators associated uniformly with poor results are female sex, bone age less than 6 years, uncovering of the femoral head in excess of 3 mm in comparison to other hip, and Group C from Herring classification. Catterall's radiological head-at-risk signs are lateral subluxation of the head, calcification lateral to epiphysis, whole head involvement, metaphyseal cysts, Gage sign, and horizontal physis. Presence of any of these sign has poor prognosis.

While some patients present with a painless limp, discomfort in the groin, thigh, or knee is very common. Physical findings include a loss of abduction and rotation, and some patients will develop a flexion contracture. Examination demonstrates limitation and pain on motion, particularly internal rotation of the hip. The Perthes treatment has changed its course with increased understanding and long-term follow-up of the patients. The ultimate aim is to achieve a spherical, congruent, and well-covered head. Symptomatic treatment is indicated as and when the symptoms are bad. Acute episodes of hip irritability are treated

TABLE 2.8 Lateral pillar classification

Group A: No involvement of the lateral pillar; lateral pillar is radiographically normal; possible lucency and collapse in the central and medial pillars, but full height of the lateral pillar is maintained

Group B: Greater than 50% of the lateral pillar height is maintained; lateral pillar has some radiolucency, with maintenance of bone density at a height between 50% and 100% of the original height of the lateral head

Group C: Less than 50% of lateral pillar height is maintained; lateral pillar becomes more radiolucent than in type B, and any preserved bone is at a height of less than 50% of the original height of the lateral pillar

TABLE 2.7 Radiographic stages of Legg-Calvé-Perthes disease

Initial (osteonecrosis)

Early signs: Lateralization of the femoral head and smaller ossific nucleus

Later signs: Subchondral fracture, increased density of the femoral head, and metaphyseal lucencies

Fragmentation

Lucent areas appear in the femoral head

Segments of femoral head are demarcated

Increased density resolves

Acetabular contour is more irregular

Reossification (healing)

New bone formation occurs in the femoral head

Lucencies are replaced by new (woven) bone

Residual femoral head is fully reossified

Gradual remodeling of head shape occurs until skeletal maturity

The acetabulum also remodels

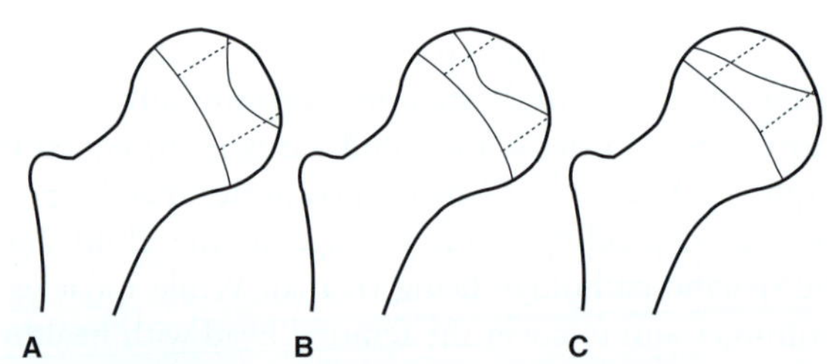

FIGURE 2.11 Lateral pillar classification for LCPD. Group A: No involvement of lateral pillar. Group B: More than 50% of the lateral pillar height is maintained. Group C: Less than 50% of the lateral pillar height is maintained. *Source:* Bulent E, Dormans JP. Hip disorders. In: Dormans JP (ed.), *Core Knowledge in Pediatric Orthopaedics.* Philadelphia: Elsevier Mosby, 2005.

with bed rest and skin traction, walking with crutches and non-steroidal anti-inflammatories (NSAIDs). The long-term abduction bracing or broomstick plasters have been ineffective for containment of the head. Surgical containment of the hip is considered in Herring Group B with skeletal age over 7 years and Herring Group C. Another criteria is presence of Catterall's radiological head-at-risk signs. The procedures are varus derotation osteotomy, Salter osteotomy, and Shelf osteotomy. In case of late presentation where the head is deformed and causes pain due to impingement on the acetabular margin, then salvage procedures are recommended. The Chiari osteotomy, cheilectomy, and valgus-flexion osteotomy are performed. The treatment of Perthes is still controversial and may improve with further long-term studies.

Slipped Capital Femoral Epiphysis (SCFE). Slipped capital femoral epiphysis is more common in African American males, and the average age at presentation is 12 to14 years, and earlier in females. The associated factors are obesity, hormonal imbalance (panhypopituitarism, hypothyroidism), and rapid growth. Various causative theories are proposed, including mechanical causes such as increased retroversion, increased weight, and slope of the growth plate. The slip occurs through the hypertrophic zone in a posterior and inferior direction. The slip following renal failure as a result of secondary hyperparathyroidism, occurs through the metaphyseal spongiosa. Patients present with pain in the hip, knee, or thigh. Examination demonstrates intoeing gait and obligatory external rotation on flexion of the hip. Acute slip is one with symptoms of less than 3 weeks while chronic slip has been symptomatic for more than 3 weeks. Acute-on-chronic slip presents with symptoms of more than 3 weeks with sudden exaggeration of pain. Weight bearing is observed in the stable group, while not in the unstable group. AVN is more likely to appear in the unstable group, leading to unsatisfactory outcome.

The diagnosis is based on anteroposterior and frogleg lateral view of the affected hip. Radiographs of both hips are necessary as the incidence of bilateral involvement is 25%. In mild displacement, the Klein's line does not pass through the epiphysis (Trethowan sign) and in pre-slip the physis is widened (Fig. 2.12 A). The bone scan may be of help in diagnosis of pre-slip stage. Depending on the angle of the epiphysis it is classified in three types; Type 1 is less than 30 degrees, Type 2 ranges from 30 to 60 degrees, and Type 3 is greater than 60 degrees. The important aspect in management of SCFE is not to attempt reduction as any attempts at reduction increases the risk of AVN. The capital femoral epiphysis is stabilized with a single in situ screw (Fig. 2.12 B). In a history of definite trauma, two screws and minimal reduction may be attempted, but this is still controversial. Reinhold Ganz has proposed safe surgical dislocation of the hip with anatomic reduction of slipped epiphysis. This should be attempted by surgeons trained in this procedure to avoid any complications. Post-operative patients are non-weight bearing for 6 weeks with gradual increase of weight bearing after that. Care should be taken when placing the screws in center of the epiphysis, as screw cut-out causes severe complications. Prophylactic pinning of the other hip is considered in pre-slip stage or in patients diagnosed with endocrinopathy.

Proximal Femoral Focal Deficiency (PFFD). This developmental defect of the proximal femur is recognizable at birth as a short, bulky thigh that is flexed, abducted, and externally rotated. PFFD is associated

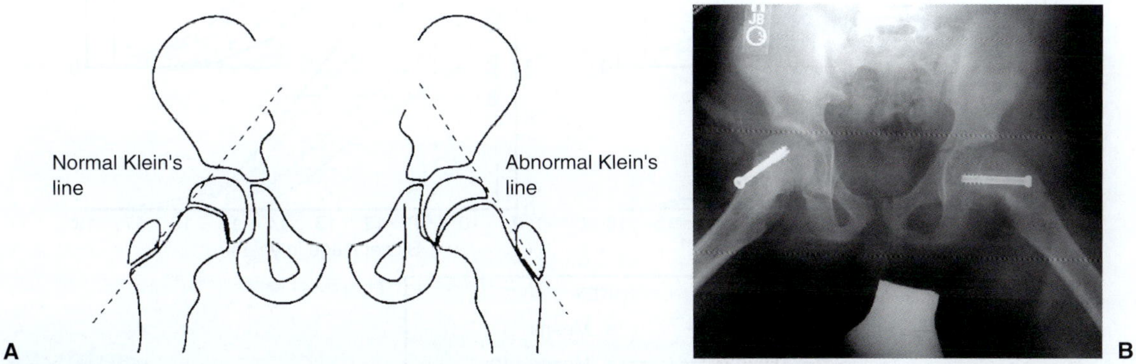

FIGURE 2.12 **(A) Klein's line, drawn along the superior cortex of the femoral neck on the anteroposterior view of the pelvis, normally intersects the lateral capital epiphysis. (*Source:* Bulent E, Dormans JP. Hip disorders. In: Dormans JP [ed.], *Core knowledge in Pediatric Orthopaedics*. Philadelphia: Elsevier Mosby, 2005.) (B) Anterior-posterior radiograph of pelvis demonstrating slipped capital femoral epiphysis fixed with in situ screw.**

with coxa vara, fibular hemimelia, and congenital knee ligamentous deficiency. Treatment is based on the individual leg-length discrepancy and associated foot deformities. The percentage of shortening remains constant during growth. The Aiken classification system divides PFFD into four groups. Types A and B have a femoral head, which allows for the potential of reconstructive procedures including limb lengthening. The acetabulum is dysplastic in patients with type B. Types C and D do not have a femoral head, and types D does not have an acetabulum either; therefore, treatment includes amputation, femoral–pelvic fusion (Brown procedure), Van Ness rotation plasty, and limb lengthening.

Leg Length Discrepancy. The leg length inequality leads to inefficient gait, postural scoliosis, back pain, and equinus contracture of ankle. The physical examination will help determine if it is a true or apparent shortening and also assess associated changes like scoliosis and pelvic obliquity. The CT orthoscanogram is the best test to determine the exact limb measurements and can be compared with bone age obtained from wrist radiographs. The treatment plan is based on prediction of ultimate height at completion of skeletal maturity. The Anderson and Green growth remaining chart, Moseley straight-line method, and Paley multiplier method are used to calculate final height and also the effects of epiphysiodesis (Fig. 2.13).

Final predicted inequality of less than 2 cm doesn't require any treatment, 2 to 5 cm can be dealt with epiphysiodesis of the longer leg, 5 to 7 cm could be treated with limb lengthening, and more than 7 cm with contralateral epiphysiodesis and ipsilateral lengthening. The actual epiphysis to be fused and the bone to be lengthened depends on the etiology and the bone that is shorter.

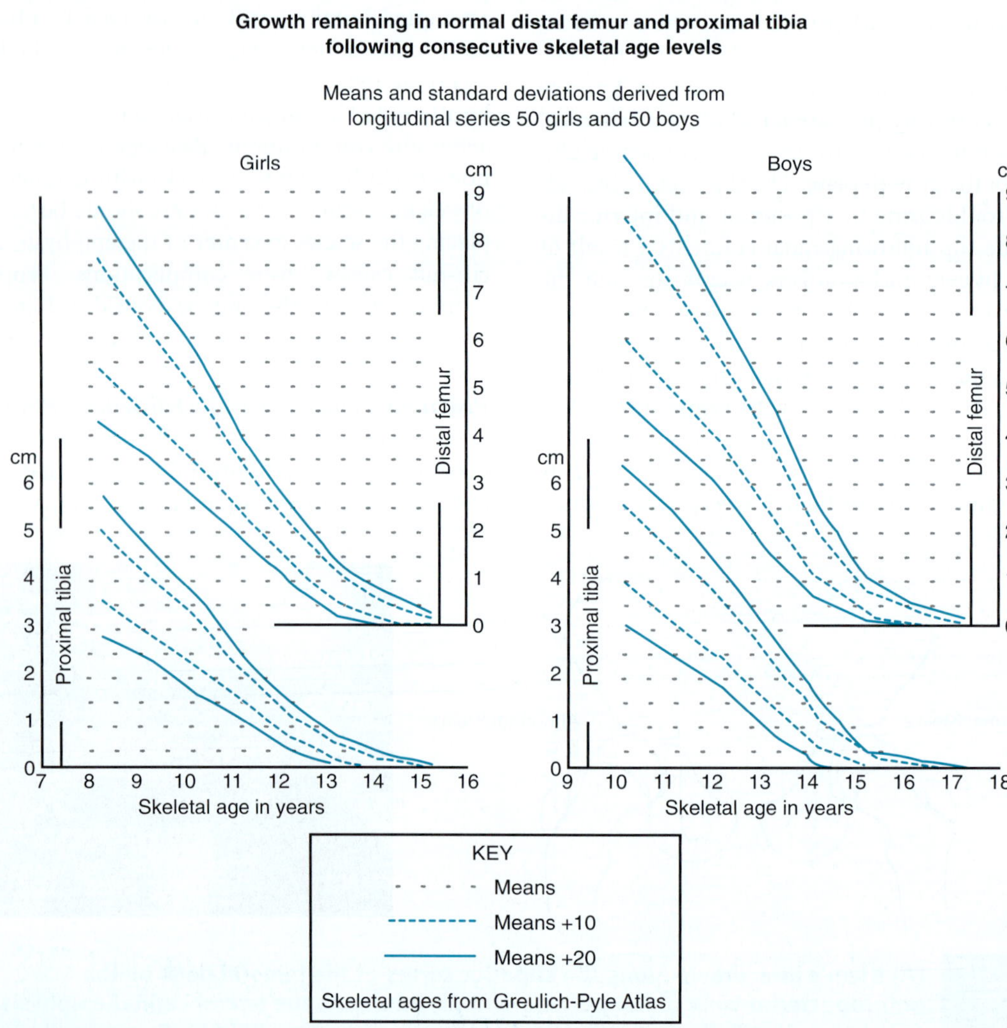

FIGURE 2.13 **Green-Anderson chart for prediction of leg-length discrepancy. *Adapted from* Anderson M, Green WT, Messner M. Growth and predictions of growth in the lower extremities. *J Bone Joint Surg Am* 1963;45A:1–14.**

Flexion contractures and angular deformities of a limb cause inaccurate limb-length measurement results with most clinical methods. A CT scanogram is more accurate than standard scanograms for determining limb length in patients with knee flexion contractures of 30 degrees or more.

Knee and Leg Problems

Genu Varum. The normal tibiofemoral angle at birth is 10 to 15 degrees of physiological varus. The alignment changes to zero degrees by 18 months and normal valgus of 7 degrees by 4 years of age. Persistence of varus beyond 2 years of age may be pathological. The differential diagnosis includes metabolic bone diseases (vitamin D–deficiency rickets, hypophosphatasia), assymmetric growth arrest (trauma, infection, tumor, Blount), bone dysplasia (dwarfism, metaphyseal dysplasia), and congenital and neuromuscular disorders. It is prudent to differentiate physiological bowing from Blount disease (Table 2.9).

Blount disease (tibia vara) is a growth disorder of the medial aspect of the proximal tibial epiphysis, leading to varus angulation and medial rotation of the tibia. It has a predilection for children of African American origin, obesity, female gender, walking at an early age, and family history. The disease progresses through 6 radiographic stages with increasing severity, as described by Langeskiöld (Fig. 2.14 B).

It has been divided into 2 types depending on the age of onset. Infantile Blount presents before 3 years of age and is usually bilateral. Radiographs may show a metaphyseal–diaphyseal angle abnormality and metaphyseal beaking. Drennan angle of greater than 16 degrees is considered abnormal and is formed between the metaphyseal beaks (Fig. 2.14 A).The treatment depends on the age and Langeskiold radiographic stage. In patients under 3 years and at Langeskiöld stage 1, 2, or 3, bracing is effective and can prevent progression of the disease. For those older than 3 years and above Langeskiöld stage 3, patients require surgical treatment. Early varus corrective osteotomy before 4 years of age prevents further progression of the deformity and Langeskiöld stage. After 4 years of age, corrective osteotomy is combined with additional procedure like proximal lateral epiphyseal hemiphysiodesis, excision of bony bar, and intraarticular osteotomy to elevate the depressed medial physis.

TABLE 2.9 Differences between physiological bowing and blount disease

Physiological Bowing	Blount Disease
Gentle and symmetric deformity	Asymmetric, abrupt, and sharp angulation
Metaphyseal–diaphyseal angle less than 11 degrees (Fig. 2.14 A)	Metaphyseal–diaphyseal angle greater than 11 degrees
Normal appearance of the proximal tibial growth plate	Medial sloping of the epiphysis
	Widening of the physis
	Fragmentation of the metaphysis
No significant lateral thrust	Significant lateral thrust

Adolescent Blount disease (older than 10 years) is usually unilateral and presents in obese children with less structural deformity; its incidence is on the rise. It may be associated with slipped capital femoral epiphysis. Deformity is multiplanar with varus, rotation, procurvatum, and compensatory deformity of the distal femur and distal tibia. A complete evaluation with long-leg anteroposterior and lateral radiographs is necessary. The goal is to achieve a leg with normal mechanical axis. Proximal varus corrective osteotomy with correction of rotation and procurvatum is normally done. This procedure is combined with upper tibial lateral hemiepiphysiodesis and correction of distal femur and tibia. Leg-length discrepancy (LLD) is to be considered, and treatment should incorporate its correction.

Genu Valgum. Variation up to 15 degrees of valgus is possible until 6 years of age, and hence physiological valgus has a good chance of correction on its own in this age group. Pathological conditions leading to valgus are metabolic bone disease (rickets, renal osteodystrophy), skeletal dysplasia, trauma, tumors, and infection. Increased valgus at the knee may be associated with increased femoral anteversion and external tibial torsion, sometimes referred to as miserable malalignment syndrome. All three increase the quadriceps Q angle and thus the chance of developing anterior knee pain. Deformities above 15 degrees and in patients over 7 years of age are unlikely to correct on their own and require surgical management. If the patient is skeletally immature, then medial tibial epiphyseal hemiepiphsiodesis could suffice for the correction. In the skeletally mature, an osteotomy is necessary at the center of rotation of angulation (CORA), which is usually situated in the distal femur.

Posteromedial Tibial Bowing. This type bowing, occurring between the middle and distal third of the tibia, is usually physiologic and therefore has a good potential to correct itself. It could be associated with secondary valgus of the distal tibia. Calcaneovalgus foot deformity should improve with stretching or modified

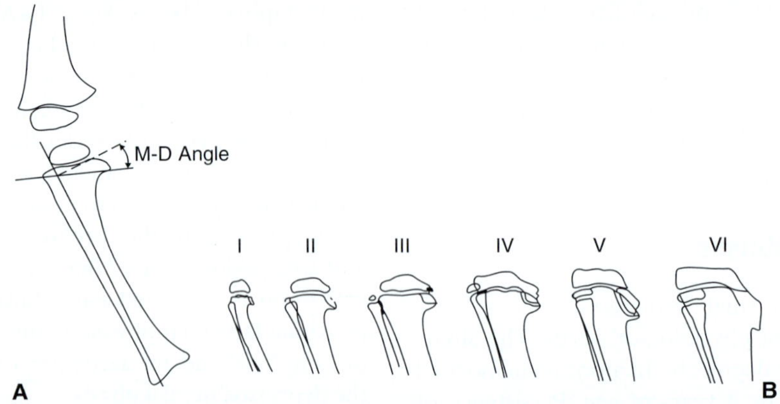

FIGURE 2.14 (A) Metaphyseal–diaphyseal angle (*Source:* Morrissy, RT, Weinstein (eds.). *Lovell and Winter Pediatric Orthopedics*, 3rd ed. Philadelphia: Lippincott Williams and Wilkins, 1990.) (B) Stages of infantile Blount disease. (*Source*: Langeskiold A. Tibia vara [osteochondrosis deformans tibiae]: A survey of 23 cases. *Acta Chir Scand* 1952;103:1.)

shoe wear but may require an ankle-foot orthosis. Although the bowing tends to correct on itself, growth lags behind the contralateral tibia, leading to LLD. Predicted LLD less than 4 cm is managed with age-appropriate epiphysiodesis of the normal leg. If the predicted LLD is greater than 4 cm, then management involves a combination of contralateral epiphysiodesis and ipsilateral lengthening. A corrective osteotomy for distal tibial valgus may be required and can be done in the same setting while correcting LLD.

Anteromedial Tibial Bowing. Fibular hemimelia is the most common cause of anteromedial bowing of the tibia. Along with anteromedial bowing, fibular hemimelia is associated with ankle instability, equinovarus foot (with absent lateral rays), tarsal coalition, and femoral shortening. The fibular deficiency can be complete or incomplete. The condition may be bilateral, and 15% of all cases have a femoral deficiency. The Achterman-Kalamchi classification places patients in two major types: type I consists of partial fibular presence. Type I is further divided into A and B: type IA consists of a short fibula with both a proximal and distal physis. Type IB consists of a severely shortened proximal fibula and no articulation with the tibia distally. Type II consists of an absent fibula.

Preservation of the foot and lengthening of the limb should be considered only when there is minimal or no ankle valgus and the projected shortening is less than 15 cm. For complete fibular hemimelia, ankle disarticulation may be necessary. A Syme or Boyd amputation can be performed when the child is beginning to stand. Indications include a projected shortening greater than 15 cm, bowing of the tibia, severe foot deformity, and an abnormal distal tibial growth plate. A tibial osteotomy may be necessary because of the bowing. Partial fibular hemimelia needs individualized treatment. Whereas a minor deformity with a relatively normal foot may be lengthened, a more severe deformity may eventually require amputation. Progressive knee valgus is a common problem and may require a lateral proximal tibial epiphyseodesis to improve the limb alignment.

Anterolateral Tibial Bowing. Anterolateral tibial bowing is associated with congenital pseudarthrosis of the tibia (Fig. 2.15). Fifty percent of the patients with anterolateral tibial bowing have neurofibromatosis, while only 10% of those with neurofibromatosis have this lesion. The pseudarthrosis or site of nonunion is typically situated between the middle and distal third of the tibia. Boyd has classified it in increasing severity depending on the presence of cystic and dysplastic changes. The treatment for this condition has been very frustrating with poor results. Bracing has been recommended to prevent fracture early in its course; however, bracing has not been successful. Numerous surgical interventions have been attempted to achieve union, including single and dual onlay grafting with rigid internal fixation, as well as vascularized fibular grafts. Intramedullary pinning with or without bone grafting and Ilizarov devices have also been attempted. Osteotomies to correct the anterolateral bowing are contraindicated. Amputation (Syme) and prosthetic fitting are indicated after 2 or 3 failed corrective procedures.

Tibial Longitudinal Deficiency. Tibial hemimelia (TH) is a deficiency of the tibia, the cause of which is unknown, but it has a known autosomal dominant inheritance pattern. Other skeletal anomalies are commonly seen, including foot deformities, hip dysplasia, and symphalangism of the hand.

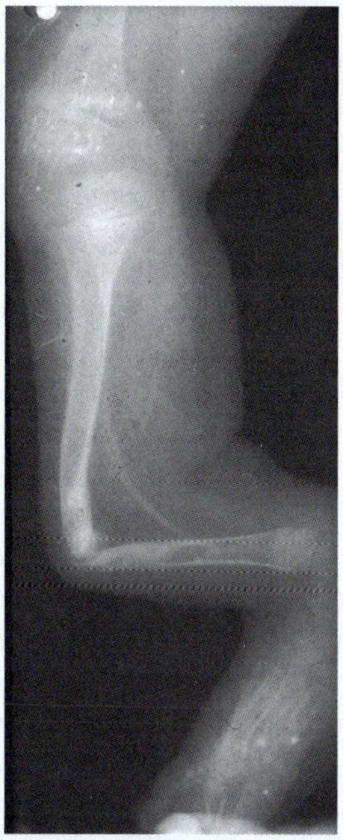

FIGURE 2.15 Lateral radiograph showing pseudarthrosis of the distal tibia with anterolateral bowing.

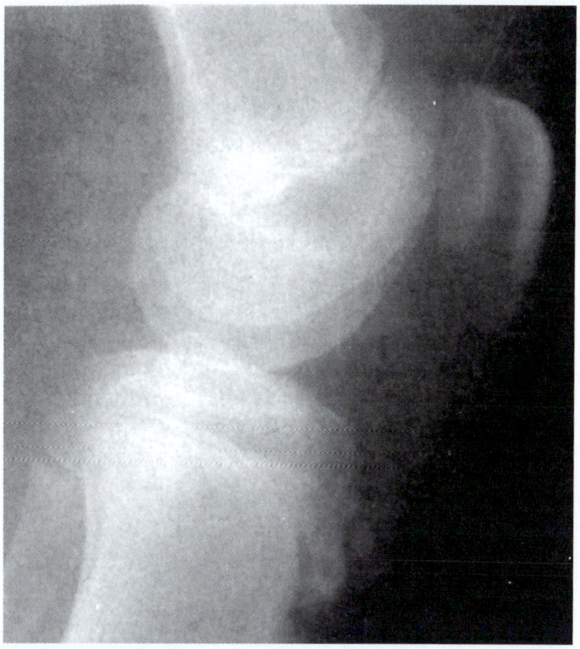

FIGURE 2.16 Osgood-Schlatter disease.

The Jones classification describes four types of TH. Type I has an absent tibia and further differentiates patients on the basis of whether the distal femoral epiphysis is hypoplastic or normal. The presence of a normal distal femoral epiphysis indicates that the proximal tibial epiphysis is present but late in ossifying. Type II is a partial deficiency in which the proximal tibia is ossified. Type III is also a partial (proximal) deficiency; however, the distal tibia is ossified. Type IV consists of a short tibia with diastasis of the tibia and fibula distally. There is a lack of distal articular surface.

Treatment revolves around presence of a proximal tibial anlage and functional quadriceps mechanism. In the absence of a proximal tibial anlage, knee disarticulation with prosthesis is recommended. In type II TH, the tibial anlage is present and the management comprises of early Syme amputation followed later by synostosis of fibula with the tibia and a below knee prosthesis. Type III is rare and management principle is Syme amputation with prosthesis. Type IV deformity is associated with ankle diastasis which requires stabilisation of ankle and correction of LLD at a later stage.

Miscellaneous Knee Disorders

Osgood-Schlatter Disease. Osgood-Schlatter disease is osteochondrosis of the upper tibial apophysis associated with a rapid growth spurt (Fig. 2.16). The presentation usually involves pain over the tibial tuberosity following athletic activities. Quadriceps stretch over the growing apophysis is one of the causes for pain over the tibial tuberosity. Radiographs show irregularities and fragmentation of the tibial tuberosity apophysis. MRI is associated with definite signal changes in the surrounding soft tissues. Treatment is nonsurgical because the disease is self-limiting, and complete recovery occurs in 95% of patients. Nonsurgical management involves activity modification, ice application, NSAIDs, and stretching exercises.

Discoid Meniscus. Discoid meniscus is a relatively infrequent cause of pain. The Watanabe classification divides it as type 1, which is complete discoid meniscus; type 2, which is incomplete discoid meniscus, and type 3 (the Wrisberg variant), which lacks a posterior capsular attachment. The lateral meniscus is more often discoid. It can be bilateral in 20% of cases. These children present with mechanical symptoms of clicking, snapping, catching, and locking. Radiographs can show a widened joint spacc on the affected side with flattening of the femoral coondy, but diagnosis is often based on the MRI scan. An MRI not only identifies the discoid nature of the meniscus but also accurately defines any intrasubstance tears. Treatment depends on the symptomatology and type of the discoid meniscus. In type 1 and 2 defects, partial meniscectomy is preferred, preserving the remaining meniscus. In type 3, the meniscus is stabilized by repairing it to the posterior capsule and then performing partial meniscectomy or contouring the meniscus centrally.

Popliteal Cyst. Popliteal cysts are commonly found in children and may be associated with JRA. The cysts are commonly located between the medial gastrocnemius and semimembranosus muscle. Relatively infrequent, they can be found in other bursas around the knee joint. The differential diagnosis of swelling in this region includes synovial sarcoma, popliteal artery aneurysm, and pigmented villonodular synovitis. The popliteal cyst is soft and fluctuant, transilluminates, and has no pulsations or bruits. In adults, the cyst is accompanied by meniscal pathologies, but not so in children. The majority of these cysts resolve spontaneously, and hence early surgical excision is not recommended.

Feet

Idiopathic Clubfoot. Idiopathic clubfoot is one of the most common foot deformities occurring in 1 in 1,000 live births with a 2:1 predominance in males. The true etiology is not yet known. Different theories of pathogenesis include arrested growth in cartilage, neuromuscular disorders, and retracting fibrosis. Associated disorders include hand anomalies (Streeter dysplasia), diastrophic dwarfism, arthrogryposis, prune belly, tibial hemimelia, and mylemoenincele. The deformity comprises the forefoot in adduction, cavus, and supination with the hindfoot in equines and varus. The heel is small and empty, with atrophy of the calf. The talar neck is medial and has plantar deviation with medial rotation of the calcaneus and medial displacement of the navicular and cuboid.

Early radiographs of the feet are not routinely performed unless a very resistant deformity is present or in the case of an atypical deformity. The talocalcaneal angle is assessed on both the anteroposterior (Kite) and dorsiflexed lateral (Turco) view of the foot. The talocalcaneal angle is decreased on both the AP (less than 20 degrees) and lateral (less than 35 degrees) views in comparison to the normal foot.

Casting is always the preferred initial method of treatment. Currently, the Ponseti technique is recommended because of its long-term results. This technique involves weekly plaster changes for 6 to 8 weeks. Initially, the cavus is corrected by supination of the forefoot followed by abduction of the supinated forefoot. This maneuver is done with the fulcrum over the lateral aspect of the talar head. Once the foot is abducted to 60 degrees, then the equinus is corrected with dorsiflexion of the foot. A percutaneous tenotomy of the tendoachilles is necessary in rigid equinus. After complete correction in 6 to 8 weeks, the foot is placed in a Denis-Browne bar shoe full time for 3 months. After that, an abduction shoe is required only during nighttime. With better experience in casting, the need for surgical posteromedial release has decreased. In resistant clubfeet, posteromedial release is considered at 6 to 9 months. In the case of recurrent deformity, an anterior tibial tendon transfer to the dorsum of the midfoot can be done. The affected foot has less growth potential and is smaller than the contralateral foot. The range of motion of the ankle and plantarflexion strength is also less in comparison to the normal foot. Untreated late presentation of clubfoot is rare in the United States, but bony procedures are essential in its correction. Medial opening or lateral column shortening is preferred from 3 to 10 years of age. After age 10, a triple arthrodesis is the appropriate procedure.

Teratologic clubfeet (those caused by a neuromuscular condition like spina bifida or arthrogryposis, or following diastrophic dwarfism) are more resistant to casting, and the majority require surgical correction. In spina bifida, the clubfoot is treated with a posteromedial release (tenotomy can be done) and lengthening of the tibialis anterior. Further, the talonavicular and subtalar joint can be pinned in a reduced position. In arthrogryposis, initial casting is done to make the foot more flexible and is followed by a posteromedial release. In many cases, this treatment may not suffice, and the patient may require primary talectomy or cuboidectomy. At skeletal maturity, any recurrent or residual deformity is treated with triple arthrodesis.

Metatarsus Adductus. Metatarsus adductus is a forefoot adduction deformity with an otherwise normal plantigrade hindfoot. Though the etiologic factor is not known, intrauterine fetal foot position is believed to be important. Beck has classified the deformity as mild, moderate, and severe according to the heel bisector line. The other assessment criteria are the flexibility and correction of the deformity. Mild deformity doesn't require any active treatment and can be observed. Moderate to severe deformities or noncorrectable adductus are initially treated with stretching and manipulation casting for 3 to 4 months. The rigid deformities require surgical intervention in the form of abductor hallucis longus lengthening and medial capsulotomy. Once the bony structural changes are set in, bony procedures are necessary (e.g., Evans calcaneal osteotomy, medial opening cuneiform, and lateral closing cuneiform, or metatarsal osteotomies). Long-term prognosis is good, and 90% of the deformities spontaneously correct by 5 years of age.

Pes Cavovarus. This deformity comprises an exaggeration of the longitudinal arch of the foot due to plantarflexion of the forefoot (mainly the first metatarsal) and a varus hindfoot. Although the majority of these are idiopathic in nature, a thorough search is necessary to rule out neuromuscular cause. Charcot-Marie-Tooth disease, postpolio residual paralysis, Friedreich ataxia, and cerebral palsy are all causes of cavovarus deformity. Intraspinal pathologies, like filum terminale syndrome, tethered cord, or tumors, may present with unilateral or bilateral deformities. The Coleman block test is done to check whether the hindfoot varus is fixed or correctible. The investigation work-up includes lateral weight-bearing radiographs of the feet, electromyography of the affected limb, MRI of the spine, creatinine phosphokinase levels, muscle and sural nerve biopsy, and a neurology referral.

Mild correctible deformities are managed with shoe modification or soft tissue procedures, including plantar fascia release, Achilles tendon lengthening, and extensor tendon recession. The claw toe deformities require flexor tenotomies with flexor-to-extensor transfer or extensor tendon recession. The bony procedures are done for rigid deformities.

Congenital Vertical Talus. Congenital vertical talus results in a rigid flat foot. The deformity consists of a rigid, rocker-bottom type of planovalgus foot, with the hindfoot in equinus and the forefoot abducted and dorsiflexed. The pathogenesis is excessive plantarflexion of the talus pointing toward the sole. The navicular is dislocated and lying over the anterosuperior aspect of the talar neck. The anteroposterior and plantarflexed radiographs demonstrate that the axis of talus passes below the first metatarsal–cuneiform axis, and the talocalcaneal angle is greater than 40 degrees. Initial treatment is manipulation and casting of the feet for 2 to 3 months. For failed conservative treatment, surgery is performed between 6 and 12 months of age. The surgery for a vertical talus is more radical than in clubfoot. It involves an extensile approach, with lengthening of the extensors, tibialis anterior, and Achilles tendon. Wide capsulotomies of the tibiotalar, subtalar, and calcaneocuboid joints are necessary. The navicular is reduced with the talar head and further stabilized by temporary pinning. The valgus hindfoot is corrected by peroneal lengthening, or in severe cases by extraarticular subtalar arthrodesis (Grice-Green procedure). For an irreducible talonavicular joint, the navicular is completely removed. The long-term prognosis is good in 60% to 80% of the patients, though some of them will have a stiff but functional foot.

Tarsal Coalition. Tarsal coalition occurs because of failure of the primary mesenchymal segmentation in the hind foot leading to fusion of the tarsal bones. Three types of coalitions are observed, and the most common is calcaneonavicular, which ossifies between 8 and 12 years of age. The second most common coalition is talocalcaneal, and it ossifies between 12 and 16 years of age. The third and relatively infrequent talonavicular coalition occurs between 3 and 5 years of age. The most common presentation is a painful flat foot with a rigid hindfoot. The examination is remarkable for a stiff hindfoot and restricted subtalar motion with uncorrectible valgus of the hindfoot. The oblique 45-degree radiographs of the hindfoot demonstrate the calcaneonavicular bar, while the Harris view shows the talocalcaneal bar. Since 20% of these patients have more than one bar and some of the bars are fibrous and cartilaginous, computed tomography (Fig. 2.17) or MRI is preferred for diagnosis.

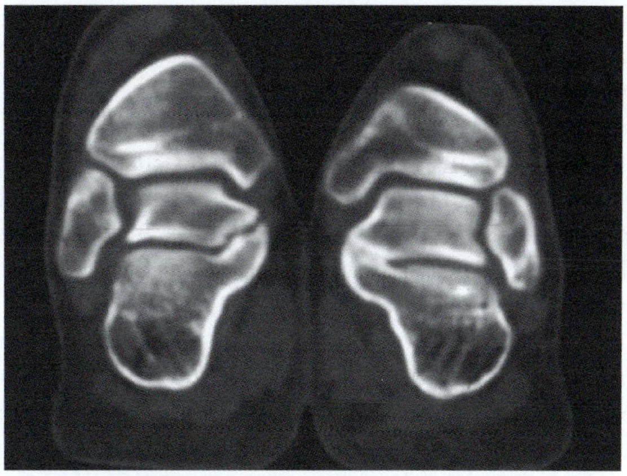

FIGURE 2.17 CT scan showing left talocalcaneal coalition.

A symptomatic coalition of any type is initially treated with immobilization for 4 to 6 weeks. Other nonoperative interventions are activity modification and NSAIDs. The nonresponders are treated with surgery. Those who have a talocalcaneal bar involving less than 50% of the middle facet are best treated with excision of the bar, while those who have greater than 50% involvement are treated with subtalar fusion. Patients with a recurrence of pain or advanced degenerative changes may require a triple arthrodesis.

Kohler Disease. Kohler disease is osteochondrosis of the tarsal navicular bone and presents with symptoms of pain. The age of presentation is usually between 5 and 8 years and is occasionally bilateral. Attachment of the tibialis posterior to the navicular leads to tendon dysfunction and mild flat-foot deformity. Radiographs of the feet demonstrate increased density and sclerosis of the navicular. Treatment consists of rest, NSAIDs, and immobilization of the ankle in equinus and slight varus. Because it is self-limiting, the pain disappears over a period of 10 months. No long-term sequelae are noted, and the navicular is completely reconstituted.

Pes Planus. Pes planus is characterized by the absence or a reduced medial longitudinal arch of the foot. The deformity is mild if the arch disappears on weight bearing, while a severe deformity lacks the arch even while nonweight bearing. Usually, the majority of the neonates have flat feet, and the arch becomes more apparent with age. It is commonly familial and bilateral and occasionally associated with generalized ligamentous laxity. Pes planus has a relatively benign natural history, but it is important to separate it from other causes of flat feet, such as tarsal coalition, congenital vertical talus, skew foot, and ankle valgus.

The examination of the foot should include evaluation for a tight Achilles tendon and flexibility of the hindfoot. Persistently painful flat foot or severe pain should alert the physician of the possibility of tarsal coalition, tight Achilles tendon, or tumor of the tarsal bone. Radiographs and computed tomography of the feet are necessary to diagnose these conditions and rule out any occult cause. Treatment of pes planus is nonsurgical in the form of shoe modification and inserts and stretching of a tight tendoachilles. Unabated pain in an adolescent may require bony surgery.

Accessory Navicular. It is characterized by the presence of an accessory ossicle that is medial and proximal to the navicular and in continuity with the tibialis posterior tendon. The incidence is 2% to 12%, and it ossifies around 9 years of age. The symptoms predominate with pain over the medial aspect of the foot, bony prominence, and flat foot. The external and internal oblique view is necessary to identify it on plain radiographs of the foot. The majority of patients will have spontaneous recovery. In rare circumstances, excision of the ossicle is done, followed with repair of the insertion of the tibialis posterior tendon to the navicular.

Congenital Toe Disorders

Syndactyly. This disorder presents with fusion of the soft tissues of the two neighboring toes, more often between the second and third toes. Simple syndactyly consists of fusion involving soft tissues, while complex syndactyly involves fused bones, nerves, blood vessels, and tendons. Generally, simple syndactyly does not require any treatment, and patients do well. Complex syndactyly is released between the ages of 6 months and 2 years. The new web space is created by using full-thickness skin grafts.

Congenital Hallux Varus. The metatarsophalangeal joint is usually medially subluxed and may be associated with polydactyly. The pathology consists of short and thick first metatarsal and contracted hypertrophied abductor hallucis longus. Severe deformities require surgery to correct them. The hypertrophied abductor is released, and the joint is reduced with a split lateral transfer of the extensor hallucis longus.

Overlapping Toe. Often, this deformity is familial and bilateral. The fifth toe overlaps the fourth toe. The deformity consists of dorsiflexion and adduction of the fifth toe. Nonoperative management in the form of stretching and spacers or neighbor strapping is the treatment of choice. The surgical management involves extensor tenotomy, medial collateral ligament release, and a dorsal capsulotomy. In rare circumstances, syndactylization of the fourth and fifth toes may be performed.

Curly Toe. This condition involves malrotation and flexion of the lateral three toes and is generally bilateral. Patients are usually asymptomatic and hence do not require any active treatment. If symptomatic, the toes can be surgically corrected by tenotomy of the contracted flexor digitorum longus and brevis. The surgery is ideally donc between 3 and 4 years of age.

Polydactyly. Polydactyly is more often seen in African Americans and women and is usually transmitted as an autosomal dominant trait, but occasional sporadic cases can occur following mutation. This deformity may be associated with polydactyly in the hand or hypoplasia of the tibia. Polydactyly of toes is most often postaxial or on the lateral side of the foot. The supernumary digits cause problems with shoe wear, and hence early surgical removal before walking age is recommended. Asymptomatic toes can be left alone.

XI. UPPER EXTREMITY PROBLEMS

Radial Deficiency. The degree of preaxial deficiency can range from mild thumb hypoplasia to complete absence of the radius. Regardless of the degree of expression, all forms warrant systemic evaluation for syndromes or associations. Holt-Oram syndrome, thrombocytopenia-absent-radius syndrome, VACTERL (vertebral abnormalities, anal atresia, cardiac abnormalities, tracheoesophageal fistula, esophageal atresia, renal defects, radial dysplasia, lower limb abnormalities) association, and Fanconi anemia are the primary concerns.

The basic goals of treatment are to (1) correct the radial deviation of the wrist; (2) balance the wrist on the forearm; (3) maintain wrist and finger motion; (4) promote growth of the forearm; (5) reconstruct thumb deficiency; and (6) improve the function of the extremity.

Ulnar Deficiency. Ulnar deficiency is 4 to 10 times less common than radial deficiency and affects the postaxial border of the limb. Ulnar deficiencies are not associated with systemic conditions but with other musculoskeletal abnormalities such as congenital scoliosis. Treatment is dependent on forearm stability, available elbow motion, and function. Unfortunately, surgery cannot restore motion for synostosis across the elbow and/or forearm.

Syndactyly. Syndactyly is defined as an abnormal interconnection between adjacent digits and is described according to the magnitude and extent of the linkage. The syndactyly may involve only skin and fibrous tissue (simple) or include bone (complex). Simple syndactyly of any considerable degree warrants surgical reconstruction of the web space for improved function and appearance. Border digits (thumb-index and ring-small web spaces) have marked differences in their respective lengths and should be separated within the first few months of life. Skin graft may be required during release of the syndactyly, which should never be placed within the commissure to avoid interdigital contracture and motion limiting scar. Complex syndactyly is associated with an increased incidence of neurovascular anomalies and is more challenging to treat, especially as the quantity of bony union intensifies. Similar surgical principles are used during separation of adjacent digits.

Polydactyly. Polydactyly can occur on the preaxial (radial) or postaxial (ulnar) side of the limb. In postaxial polydactyly, the digit is either well developed (type A) or rudimentary and pedunculated (type B). Usually, type B digits can be excised under local anesthesia. Type A requires operative ablation with preservation and transfer of important functional parts (e.g., ulnar collateral ligament and abductor digiti quinti) to the adjacent finger. The most common type of preaxial polydactyly involves duplicated proximal and distal phalanges that share a common articulation with a bifid metacarpal head. Treatment often requires using portions of each component (so-called spare parts) to construct a properly aligned and functional thumb.

Camptodactyly. Camptodactyly is a painless flexion contracture of the small finger proximal interphalangeal (PIP) joint that usually is gradually progressive. It is bilateral in approximately two thirds of the cases, although the degree of contracture is usually not symmetrical. Treatment is difficult and surgery is reserved for flexion deformities greater than 30 degrees that impair function. Surgical approach consists of a combination of release of tight and anomalous structures along with tendon transfer to augment proximal interphalangeal joint extension.

Clinodactyly. Clinodactyly typically affects the small finger middle phalanx and produces an angulation of the distal interphalangeal joint. The deviation is usually in a radial direction. On occasion, clinodactyly can involve several digits and is usually related to one or more delta-shaped middle phalanges. Many genetic syndromes and chromosomal abnormalities, however, have clinodactyly as a physical finding, most notably Down syndrome. Thumb clinodactyly is a prominent feature of Apert syndrome, Rubinstein-Taybi syndrome, diastrophic dwarfism, and triphalangeal thumbs.

Synostosis. Synostosis is a generic term that indicates an osseous union between bones that are normally separate. It most commonly involves the elbow. The synostosis can be isolated or associated with a radial head dislocation. A delay in diagnosis of radioulnar synostosis is common. Shoulder and wrist motion can compensate for lack of forearm rotation during many daily activities of childhood. The lack of forearm rotation becomes evident as the complexities of daily activities, such as catching a ball or eating soup, amplify. Mild degrees of fixed pronation or supination are well tolerated and require no treatment. Extremes of position create functional handicaps and may require rotational osteotomy through the fusion mass to a more functional position. Synostosis can also occur in other parts of the upper extremity. A radiohumeral joint synostosis can occur as part of ulnar deficiency. Metacarpal transverse synostosis occurs most commonly between the ring and small fingers and is frequently bilateral (60% to 80%).

Thumb Hypoplasia. Thumb hypoplasia occurs in varying grades and most commonly is part of radial deficiency. The main distinction between a thumb that can be reconstructed and thumb that requires ablation is the presence or absence of a stable carpometacarpal joint. A stable carpometacarpal joint provides a foundation for thumb reconstruction. Pollicization is the procedure of choice when the carpometacarpal joint is absent. Pollicization is a complex procedure that involves neurovascular transposition of the index digit to the thumb position with reconstruction of the intrinsic muscles of the thumb. Early good results have been shown to persist into adulthood.

Sprengel Deformity. Sprengel deformity is the most common abnormality of shoulder in children. The common associations are Klippel-Feil syndrome, congenital scoliosis, genitourinary anamolies, and cardiac defects. The defect is undescended medially rotated scapula with hypoplasia of the affected side. An abnormal bony omovertebral bar may be present in as many as 30% of the patients. It has been classified in 3 types depending on the severity and visibility of the deformity. The only functional impairment is restriction of the abduction. Surgery is indicated for unsightly deformity or functional impairment. The operation involves excision of all abnormal muscles/bands and the bony bar between the scapula and the vertebrae. The scapula is distally advanced and stabilized by tightening the lower muscles (Woodward procedure). The operation is recommended in patients between 3 and 6 years old.

Little League Elbow. Often observed in those who pitch in Little League baseball, this condition presents with increasing pain in the elbow of the throwing arm. The examination reveals tenderness over the lateral extensor origin and increase in pain on pronation of the forearm. The process of repeated throwing places tensile force on the medial side and compressile on the posterolateral side. The term Little League refers to a variety of symptoms in the elbow region of the growing athlete. The radiographs of the elbow show a pattern of irregular ossification in the capitellum and in advanced cases may appear as osteochondritis dissecans or osteochondrosis. The medial ligaments are normal and rarely show calcification or medial growth arrest. Treatment involves rest and activity modification, and most cases resolve with these nonoperative interventions.

XII. SPINE

Adolescent Scoliosis

Overview. Adolescent idiopathic scoliosis is the most common type of scoliosis and is a lateral deviation and rotational deformity of the spine without an identifiable cause. Most patients have a positive family history, but there is variable expressivity. The deformity is described as right or left according to the apical convexity. Right thoracic curves are the most common, followed by double major (right thoracic and left lumbar), left lumbar, and right lumbar curves. In adolescents, left thoracic curves are rare and should prompt further investigation of the spine with MRI to rule out cord abnormalities.

Risk Factors. Risk factors for curve progression include curve magnitudes (greater than 20 degrees), younger age (under 12 years old), and skeletal maturity (Risser stage 0 or 1) at presentation. Peak growth velocity is the best predictor of progression, which is based on age, menarchal status, and Risser stage. Risser stage can be determined by examining the ossification of the iliac crest apopohysis and grading it between 0 and 5. Severe curves (greater than 90 degrees) may be associated with cardiopulmonary dysfunction, early death, pain, and decreased self-image.

Physical Examination. School screenings are often a source of referrals with a threshold level of 7 degrees noted on forward flexion screenings. Physical examination findings include shoulder elevation, waistline symmetry, trunk shift, limb-length inequality, spinal deformity, and rib deformity. Neurologic evaluation is essential, especially in left thoracic curves, with particular attention to abnormal or asymmetric abdominal reflexes due to syringomyelia.

Imaging. The Cobb method is used to calculate curves on the standing PA and lateral radiographs. There is usually a hypokyphosis of the apical vertebra in the sagittal plane, since scoliosis is a lordoscoliotic deformity. An MRI is indicated in for patients with juvenile onset scoliosis (over the age of 11), structural abnormalities on radiographs, excessive kyphosis, rapid curve progression, neurologic involvement, and left thoracic curves.

Treatment. Treatment is based on the maturity of the patient, magnitude of the deformity, and rate of curve progression. Treatment options include observation, bracing, and surgery. Bracing can halt or slow curve progression but cannot reverse curve progression. Patients with thoracic lordosis or hypokyphosis are not good candidates for bracing. Outcomes of bracing are directly related to the amount of time the brace is worn per day.

Surgical options for scoliosis include anterior spinal fusion (ASF) with instrumentation, posterior spinal fusion (PSF) with instrumentation, or both. The indications for ASF and PSF in indiopathic scoliosis are severe deformities (greater than 75 degrees) and crankshaft phenomenon (Risser stage 0, girls under 10 years old or boys under 13 years old, prior to or during peak growth). The crankshaft phenomenon involves a rotational deformity around a fused posterior segment of the spine due to the presence of open anterior growth plates. ASF should be considered for patients with thoracolumbar and lumbar cases because better coronal, axial, and sagittal correction can be achieved while saving lumbar fusion levels. The advantage of ASF is saving levels and improved correction, while the disadvantages are lumbar kyphisism, thoracic hyperkyphosis, and pseudoarthrosis. PSF remains the gold standard for thoracic and double major curves.

Fusion Levels. The goal is to fuse the spine levels necessary to establish a well-balanced spine in the coronal and sagittal planes. Fusion levels include (1) the stable zone (1 level above and 2 levels below the end vertebra if they fall within vertical lines drawn up from the lumbosacral facet joints), (2) the neutral vertebra (the first level to show no rotation and symmetric pedicles), and (3) the stable vertebra (the most proximal vertebra that is most closely bisected by the center sacral line). Every attempt should be made to stop the fusion above

L3 because fusion to lower levels has been associated with increased low back pain.

Complications. Attempting excessive correction with sublaminar wires is associated with an increased risk of neurologic damage. This risk can be avoided with intraoperative SSEP/MEPs, wake-up tests, and clonus tests. Flat-back syndrome (early fatigability and pain due to a loss of lumbar lordosis) can be avoided with rod contouring in the sagittal plane and effective use of compression/distration tools. Treatment of flat-back syndrome requires revisions surgery consisting of a posterior closing-wedge osteotomy.

Other Forms of Scoliosis

Infantile Scoliosis. This condition presents in children under 3 years of age, with a left-sided thoracic scoliosis, predominantly in boys with plagiocephaly (skull flattening) and other congenital defects. The two factors most commonly affecting progression are curve magnitude and the apical rib–vertebral angle (RVA) difference of Mehta. Most curves of less than 25 degrees and an RVA of less than 20 degrees resolve spontaneously. Surgical options for severe curves include instrumentation (growing rods) without fusion or with ASF and PSF. All children with infantile scoliosis should obtain an MRI.

Juvenile Scoliosis. JID occurs in children between the ages of 3 and 10 and is similar to adolescent scoliosis in presentation and treatment. Seventy percent of children require treatment, with 50% requiring surgery. Fusion should be delayed until the onset of the growth spurt unless the curve is beyond 50 degrees. Consideration should be given to growing rods or ASF and PSF with instrumentation to prevent crankshafting.

Neuromuscular Scoliosis. Neuromuscular curves are larger, involve more vertebral levels, and are less likely to have compensatory curves. These curves tend to progress rapidly and may progress even after maturity. The curves are associated with pelvic obliquity, bony deformities, cervical involvement, and pulmonary complications, including decreased pulmonary function, pneumonia, and atelectasis. Curve progression may force wheelchair-bound individuals to be bedridden full time. Fusion is usually performed after age 12 (braced until then) to provide permanent correction. Surgical technique usually involves fusing more levels than in idiopathic scoliosis, with pelvic fixation often being included.

Progressive scoliosis develops in most patients with Duchenne muscular dystrophy. The onset of spinal deformity typically follows the cessation of walking, and curves can be expected to progress about 10 degree every year. Posterior spinal fusion should be performed as soon as a curve of 25 degree or greater is documented and before deterioration of pulmonary function (an FVC of less than 30 degree) precludes surgery.

Congenitial Disorders

Overview. This set of disorders within the spine results from developmental defect in formation of the mesenchymal anlage during the fourth to sixth week of development. Three basic types of defects are noted: failure of segmentations (vertebral bar), failure of formation (hemivertebra), and mixed. Spinal MRI scan should be obtained before any surgery to assess for intraspinal anomalies. Associated anomalies outside the spine include GU, cardiac, and dysraphism. Renal ultrasound is performed to rule out renal abnormalities.

Congenital Scoliosis. This is the most common congenital spinal disorder. Risk of progression is dependant on vertebral morphology. A fully segmented hemivertebra is free with normal disk spaces on both sides (higher risk of progression), whereas an unsegmented hemivertebra is fused above and below (lower risk). An incarcerated hemivertebra has a better prognosis than an unincarcerated hemivertebra. A unilateral unsegmented bar is a common disorder that is likely to progress. The best prognosis is with a block vertebra (bilateral failure of segmentation). The worst prognosis is seen with a unilateral unsegmented bar with a contralateral, fully segmented vertebra and is an indication for surgery at presentation. The treatment for this last entity is convex anterior and posterior hemiepiphysiodesis or ASF/PSF in situ. Other deformities should be observed and demonstrate progression before surgical intervention. Posterior spinal fusion in situ is the gold standard of treatment for most progressive curves, being aware of the crankshaft phenomenon.

Congenital Kyphosis. Congenital kyphosis may result from failure of formation (type I), failure of segmentation (type II), or mixed (type III). Failure of formation is the most common and has the worst prognosis for progression and neurologic involvement (paraplegia). The presence of a significant type I curve is an indication for surgery in children under 5 years and curves less than 50 degrees undergoing posterior fusion.

Neurofibromatosis. An autosomal dominant disorder of neural crest origin, neurofibromatosis is the second most likely cause of paraplegia (congenital kyphosis is the leading cause). It is associated with neoplasia and skeletal abnormalities and characterized by café-au-lait spots and neurofibromas. Radiographs will reveal vertebral scalloping; enlarged foramina; severe apical rotation; short, tight curves; or a paraspinal mass. The classic deformity is kyphoscoliosis in the thoracic region with dystrophic changes. Nonoperative treatment for dystrophic deformities with curves greater than 20 degrees is futile, and surgical intervention includes ASF/PSF. MRIs should be obtained on all patients prior to surgery. Cervical spine abnormalities include kyphosis and atlantoaxial instability.

Thoracic Spine

Low Back Pain. Complaints of low back pain can be related to mechanical, developmental, or infectious/tumor etiologies. Mechanical causes of low back pain include a muscle strain, herniated disk (often self-limiting), or spodylolysis (a stress fracture of the pars interarticularis). Single photon emission computed tomography (SPECT) is the most sensitive medical imaging technique for identifying and localizing small lesions of bone, particularly in the spine. It will identify abnormalities not detected by routine technetium 99m scans.

Activities with repetitive hyperextension of the lumbosacral spine (gymnastics, wrestling) are considered risk factors. A CT or bone scan can be used to aid in diagnosis. Spondylolisthesis is a forward slippage of the proximal vertebra on the distal vertebra and often occurs at the L5-S1 level. The larger the slip, the greater the chance of progression. Treatment should start with observation or activity modification with bracing. If conservative treatment fails, the fusion (if at L5) or repair of the pars (L4 or higher) is appropriate. Discitis is an infectious cause of low back pain, which presents as a refusal to sit or walk, increased ESR, and disk-space narrowing with endplate preservation.

Scheuermann Disease. The classic definition of Scheuermann disease is increased thoracic kyphosis with 5 degrees or more of anterior wedging at three sequential levels. Other radiographic findings include disk narrowing, endplate irregularities, scoliosis, and Schmorl nodes. This disease is more common in males, and it presents during adolescence with poor posture and pain, tight hamstrings, and irreversible hyperkyphosis. Treatment consists of bracing for patients with progression and more than 1 year of growth remaining. Bracing may improve the curve by 5 to 10 degrees but is less effective for curves greater than 75 degrees. For skeletally mature patients with curves greater than 75 degrees, anterior release, interbody fusion, and posterior spinal fusion are indicated.

Cervical Spine

Klippel-Feil Syndrome. The classic triad (occurring in less than 50% of patients) of Klippel-Feil syndrome includes low-posterior hairline, short "web" neck, and limited cervical range of motion. The disease is caused by failure of normal segmentation of cervical segments during 3 to 8 weeks of gestation. It is associated with congenital scoliosis, renal aplasia, Sprengel deformity, congenital heart disease, and brainstem abnormalities. Most therapy is conservative, but pain and instability may require surgery. Disk degeneration is universal, and contact sports should be avoided.

Atlantoaxial Instability. Anterior–posterior instability is associated with Down syndrome, JRA, and os odontoideum. In patients with Down, a normal neurologic examination and avoidance of contact sports is appropriate treatment, but progression requires posterior spinal fusion. An ADI of up to 4 mm in children is considered normal. Children with Down syndrome have increased ligamentous laxity, with atlantoaxial instability occurring in as many as 15% to 20% of patients. These patients are at risk for catastrophic injury following minor trauma and should be routinely screened for instability, generally beginning when the patient starts to walk. Patients with ADI of greater than 5 mm should avoid contact sports and high-risk activities such as gymnastics, diving, the high jump, and the butterfly stroke. The American Academy of Pediatrics Committee of Sports Medicine and Fitness guidelines recommend that lateral views of the cervical spine in neutral, flexion, and extension should be obtained in all children with Down syndrome who wish to participate in sports.

Rotatory atlantoaxial subluxation may be seen with torticollis and can be caused by retropharyngeal inflammation. It is likely due to secondary ligamentous laxity and is best treated early with traction and bracing. Diagnosis is performed by dynamic CT scanning through C1-C2. Late diagnosis may have to be treated by C1-C2 fusion.

Os Odontoideum. Previously thought to be caused by the failure of fusion of the base of odontoid, it appears like a type II odontoid fracture. More recent evidence suggests that it is likely due to a residual traumatic injury. Treatment is conservative unless there is instability (more than 10 mm of ADI or less than 13 mm SAC or neurologic symptoms) necessitating posterior C1-C2 fusion.

XIII. TRAUMA

Child Abuse. Approximately 1% of all children are victims of child abuse. Of these, 35% will be reinjured and 1% to 5% will die if they return to their original environment. Most children who are abused are under the age of 3. Risk factors include families with substance abuse, age under 3, premature infants, stepchildren, and disability. History and physical examination findings consistent with child abuse include multiple healing bruises, skin marks, burns, unreasonable histories, and signs of neglect. Fractures highly specific for nonaccidental injuries include corner or bucket-handle fractures, scapular fractures, posterior rib fractures, old fractures, multiple fractures of different ages, and spinous process fractures. Diaphyseal fractures are 4 times more likely to occur than metaphyseal fractures. Spinal fractures are not pathogonomic for abuse. A skeletal survey should be performed if suspicions arise indicating child abuse. A bone scan may be a more sensitive examination in children over 5 years of age. The physician must maintain a high index of suspicion, and all suspected cases of child abuse must be reported to the appropriate authorities. A multidisciplinary approach to the evaluation and treatment of these children must be applied.

Basic Principles. Fractures and dislocations are unique in the pediatric population because of open physeal plates, thick periosteum, increased remodeling, and increased bony ductility. Physeal or metaphyseal bone is the most likely site of failure rather than ligamentous rupture. Torus and greenstick fracture patterns are unique to children and imply a partial fracture with some part of the bone intact. Stiffness and contractures are less of a problem in children, allowing for prolonged immobilization (e.g., elbow). Remodeling can occur up to 10 degrees per year in the average metaphysis, is proportional to growth in a region, and is least in the torsional plane. Physeal fractures classically occur through the zone of provisional calcification within the zone of hypertrophy. The most common physeal injuries occur in the distal radius followed by the distal tibia. The Salter-Harris classification system is used to describe physeal injuries (Table 2.10). Physeal bars or bridges result from an injury to only a portion of the growth plate, thus leading to angular growth and deformity. The physeal bar or bridge can be resected and replaced with fat or interposition in patients who have more than 2 cm of growth remaining and less than 50% physeal involvement. MRI and CT scan can help determine the amount of physeal injury.

Upper Extremity

Distal Radius Fracture. Distal radial physeal fractures are the most common growth plate injury in children and often occur as Salter-Harris II fractures in children over age 10 (under this age, they are often buckle fractures). Because of the dorsal displacement of the fracture, the volar periosteum is often disrupted. The remodeling potential is one of the most important reasons that most distal radius fractures can be treated with cast immobilization (as opposed to surgical fixation in adults). Typically, angulation of about 10 degrees per year is corrected with remodeling. Radialward angulation of the distal radius, caused by pull of the brachioradialis, corrects more slowly. Bayonet apposition remodels reliably in young children; however, rotational malalignment will not remodel but can often be compensated for by shoulder rotation.

If the fracture is nondisplaced on anterior–posterior and lateral radiographs, a splint or short-arm cast can be applied in the emergency room. Displaced fractures should be reduced under sedation and a long arm cast used to hold the reduction. The cast should remain for 4 weeks. In children with 1 to 2 years of growth remaining, up to 50% displacement is acceptable. Repeat reductions more than 3 days after injury are thought to risk physeal arrest. Surgery, consisting of smooth wire fixation, is indicated for irreducible fractures. The long-term outcomes are usually excellent, with physeal arrest occurring less than 10% of the time.

Radius and Ulna Diaphyseal Fracture. The limits on acceptable reduction of the radial and ulnar shafts are more stringent, and therefore these injuries are

TABLE 2.10 Salter-Harris classification of physeal injuries

Type	Definition	Outcome
I	Through and parallel to physis	Excellent
II	Through the physis with a metaphyseal fragment	Excellent
III	Through the physis and epiphysis	Good, but may require ORIF because of potential intraarticular deformity
IV	Vertical fracture perpendicular to the physis (through epiphysis and metaphysis)	Good, but unstable fracture requires ORIF
V	Physeal crush	Poor (growth arrest)
VI	Perichondrial ring injury	Good (possible angular deformities)

more difficult to treat. Understanding the mechanism of injury—often a fall on an outstretched hand with a significant rotational component—is valuable in reducing these injuries because the rotational component plays a pivotal role in the management of the greenstick fracture. In fractures with dorsal angulation, the distal fragment is pronated; in fractures with volar angulation, the distal fragment is supinated. Malunion after a both-bones forearm fracture can lead to a permanent loss of pronation and supination. The most common cause of upper extremity compartment syndrome is this injury.

In all angulated or displaced fractures, a closed reduction should be performed. Acceptable reduction is 10 to 20 degrees of angulation in children under 10 years of age, but no more than 10 degrees of angulation in older children. Bayonet apposition is acceptable at union, but correction to near anatomic should be obtained at the time of injury. The injury should be placed in a well-molded long-arm cast for at least 6 weeks with frequent assessment for loss of reduction. If a loss of reduction is noted, surgical management can include intramedullary fixation, single-bone fixation with supplemental casting, and adult-style plating.

Monteggia Fractures. This constellation of injuries includes radial head subluxation or humeral dislocation and an ulnar fracture. Most of these injuries occur in children under 10. The Bado classification is used to describe these injuries. Type I injuries involve anterior dislocation of the radial head and are the most common. Type II injuries include posterior dislocation of the radial head. Type III fractures involve a lateral dislocation of the radial head. Type IV fractures are segmental radius fractures with dislocation of the radial head. In each case, the ulnar fracture angulates in the direction of the radial head dislocation.

Neurological evaluation may lead to discover of an associated 20% nerve injury rate, usually the PIN in Bado type III fractures. Closed reduction of the ulna often leads to relocation of the radial head, but close follow-up is necessary. If reduction cannot be maintained, surgical fixation of the ulna often provides stability to the radiocapitellar joint as well.

Radial Head Fractures. Radial head fractures are extremely common in the pediatric population, but many fractures are minimally displaced. The radial nerve should be examined in all suspected radial head fractures before an attempted closed reduction. While only minimal translation is acceptable, up to 30 degrees of angulation is acceptable.

Supracondylar Fractures. These fractures occur most frequently in children under 8 years of age. Because of ligamentous laxity, these injuries often result from elbow hyperextension, allowing the olecranon to act as a wedge in the olecranon fossa. These injuries can be quite severe and result in skin necrosis and nerve injury in 10% to 15% of cases. Usually, the AIN is injured; however, in posteriorly and medially displaced fractures, the radial nerve is at risk. The extension-type of supracondylar fractures are those that are most at risk for vascular injury.

The Gartland classification divides supracondylar fractures into three types. Type I fractures are nondisplaced, type II fractures are angulated with an intact posterior cortex, and type III fractures are completely displaced. In type III fractures, the humeral metaphysis will often tear through the brachialis muscle and can be palpated directly under the skin. If the anterior humeral line intersects the capitellum and there is no collapse of the medial column, the injury can be casted for 3 weeks. Otherwise, closed reduction and percutaneous pinning are indicated. Possible fixation strategies include 2 lateral pins, crossed medial and lateral pins, or 2 lateral pins and 1 medial pin. Postoperative complications include a transient neuropraxia, cubitus varus, and loss of motion. The "gunstock" deformity typically is only cosmetic and does not require further surgical intervention.

Lateral Condyle Fractures. Fractures of the lateral condyle are the second most common elbow fractures in children. The Milch classification is most commonly used to describe these injuries. Type I fractures are Salter-Harris IV fractures that pass from the metaphysis through the capitellar ossification center into the joint. The elbow is usually stable in these injuries. The Milch II fracture line passes medial to the capitellum into the trochlear groove of the distal humerus (and therefore is a Salter-Harris II fracture). The Milch II fracture is more common than Milch I. Treatment is usually operative. Nonoperative treatment is reserved for fractures with less than 2 mm of displacement. Complications can include nonunion and ultimately cubitus valgus with a tardy ulnar nerve palsy.

Medial Epicondyle Fractures. These injuries predominantly occur in adolescent males and are caused by a valgus force and contraction of the forearm flexor-supinator complex. This is the same mechanism of injury for elbow dislocations, and the examination should therefore include ruling out a dislocation. The physical examination should also pay particular attention to the ulnar nerve. Nondisplaced fractures or fractures displaced less than 5 mm can be treated nonoperatively, while fractures with more than 5 mm of displacement should be internally fixed. The treatment for medial condyle fractures remains controversial, though. The main complication with medial epicondyle fractures is a loss of terminal extension.

Humeral Shaft Fractures. The incidence of humeral shaft fractures is highest in children younger than 3 and older than 12 years. The radial nerve is especially vulnerable to a traction neuropraxia in this injury pattern. Children under 5 can tolerate 70 degrees of angulation and total displacement, children 5 to 12 can tolerate 40 to 70 degrees of angulation, and children older than 12 can tolerate 40 degrees of angulation and 50% apposition.

Clavicle Shaft Fractures. Neonatal fractures often occur as a result of direct trauma during birth. They can often be missed initially and present with pseudoparalysis or a bump over the fracture site after 7 to 10 days. In older children, this injury usually results from a fall on the shoulder or direct trauma. Radiographs can aid in the diagnosis and also rule out a congenitial pseudoarthrosis of the clavicle, which is usually on the right side. Most fractures can be treated simply in a sling, with or without a figure-8 splint.

Lower Extremity

Femur Fractures. Most femur fractures are low-energy events, primarily in the 6- to 10-year age group. Femur fractures in children under the age of 2 years should raise the concern for child abuse. Initial management should include ABCs and splinting of the involved extremity. Treatment varies by age group (Table 2.11).

Tibial Spine Fractures. These injuries are the pediatric equivalent of an anterior cruciate ligament injury and are thought to result because the incompletely ossified tibial spine of a child fails before the ACL. The mechanism of injury is hyperextension of the knee. Tibial spine fractures are classified by the Myers-McKeever system: type I have minimal or no displacement of the anterior margin, type II have an elevation of the anterior portion with an intact posterior hinge, and type III are completely displaced. Radiographs usually reveal the bony injury; however, MRI may aid in the diagnosis of lateral or medial meniscal tears or fracture interposition with soft tissue (e.g., the lateral meniscus). Type I and II injuries can be managed nonoperatively by placing the knee in extension (or hyperextension) or 10 to 20 degrees of flexion, but this treatment is controversial. Frequent postreduction radiographs should be performed to assess reduction. In type II injures that fail closed treatment, arthroscopic or open reduction should be performed. Type III injuries will require not only arthroscopic or open reduction but also fragment fixation via sutures, anchors, wires, or a screw.

Tibial Shaft Fractures. The tibia is the most commonly fractured bone in the lower limb. If the fibula is involved as well, then the likely mechanism of injury is direct injury. However, it is not uncommon for the fibula to be intact with a tibia fracture, often resulting from an indirect mechanism. Radiographs are often diagnostic. Closed reduction and cast immobilization is the first line of treatment because these fractures have a large remodeling potential. For children younger than 10 years, 15 degrees of varus angulation, 10 mm of shortening, 10 degrees of apex anterior angulation, and 15 degrees of external rotation have been well tolerated. Indications for internal or external fixation are open fractures, unstable closed fractures, neurovascular injuries, multiple trauma, and soft tissue abnormalities.

Triplane and Tillaux Fractures. Both triplane and Tillaux fractures occur in the adolescent age group with incompletely fused or closed distal tibial physis. Closure usually occurs over a 19-month period during skeletal maturity. It begins in the central portion of

TABLE 2.11 Femoral shaft fracture treatment by age

Treatment Modality	0–2 years	3–5 years	6–10 years	11 years	Closed Physis
Spica cast	X	X			
Traction and spica cast		X	X	X	
TEN		X	X		
Trochanteric antegrade nail				X	
Retrograde nail					X
Ex-fix		X	X	X	
Screw or plate		X	X	X	

the distal tibial physis, proceeds in a circular fashion medially, and ends at the anterolateral quadrant of the tibia. The mechanism of injury is external rotation stress on a planted foot. Radiographs are usually diagnostic. Closed reduction should be followed by repeat radiographs or a CT scan to assess the articular surface. If there is an articular incongruity or a diastasis greater than 2 mm, open reduction and internal fixation should be considered.

Stress Fracture. Bone scan or MRI can be diagnostic in patients with lower extremity pain with an appropriate repetitive loading mechanism (e.g., runners). The most essential component to treatment is rest for 6 to 8 weeks. Special attention should be paid to female athletes with stress fractures because these patients may suffer from the female athlete triad of amenorrhea, osteoporosis, and anorexia.

References

1. American Academy of Pediatrics Committee of Sports Medicine and Fitness. Atlantoaxial instability in Down syndrome. *Pediatrics* 1995;96:151–154.
2. An HS, Thometz GJ. Angular and torsional deformities of lower extremities in children. In: Chapman MW (ed.), *Operative Orthopedics*, 3rd ed. Philadelphia: JB Lippincott, 2001;4287–4335.
3. Anderson DJ, Schoenecker PL, Sheridan JJ, Rich MM. Use of an intramedullary rod for the treatment of congenital pseudarthrosis of the tibia. *J Bone Joint Surg Am* 1992;74:161–168.
4. Bassett GS. Orthopedic aspects of skeletal dysplasias. *Instr Course Lect* 1991;39:381–387.
5. Beaty JH (ed.), *Orthopaedic Knowledge Update 6*. Rosemont, IL: American Academy of Orthopaedic Surgeons, 1999;635–651.
6. Bellah RD, Summerville DA, Treves ST, et al. Low-back pain in adolescent athletes. Detection of stress injury to the pars interarticularis with SPECT. *Radiology* 1991;180:509–512.
7. Blanco JS, Taylor B, Johnston CE. Comparison of single pin vs. multiple pin fixation in treatment of slipped capital femoral epiphysis. *J Pediatr Orthop* 1992;12:384–389.
8. Bleck EE. Orthopaedic management in cerebral palsy. *Clin Dev Med* 1987;99:100.
9. Boden SD, Kaplan FS, Fallon MD, et al. Metatropic dwarfism. Uncoupling of endochondral and perichondral growth. *J Bone Joint Surg* 1987;69A:174.
10. Bowen JR, Ortega K, Ray S, et al. Spinal deformities in Larsen's syndrome. *Clin Orthop* 1985;197:159.
11. Bulman W, Dormans JP, Ecker M, Drummond DS. Posterior spinal fusion for scoliosis in patients with cerebral palsy: A comparison of Luque rod and unit rod instrumentation. *J Pediatr Orthop* 1996;16:314–323.
12. Carney BT, Weinstein SL. Natural history of untreated chronic slipped capital femoral epiphysis. *Clin Orthop* 1996;322:43–47.
13. Chin KR, Kharrazi FD, Miller BS, Mankin HJ, Gebhardt MC. Osteochondromas of the distal aspect of the tibia or fibula. Natural history and treatment. *J Bone Joint Surg Am* 2000 Sep;82(9):1269–1278.
14. Christensen F, Soballe K, Ejsted R, et al. The Catterall classification of Perthes disease: An assessment of reliability. *J Bone Joint Surg Br* 1986;68:614–615.
15. Cooperman DR, Bartucci E, Dietrick E, Millar EA. Hip dislocation in spastic cerebral palsy. Long-term consequences. *J Pediatr Orthop* 1987;7:268–276.
16. Darras BT. Neuromuscular disorders in the newborn. *Clin Perinatol* 1997;24(4):827–844.
17. Delgado ED, Schoenecker PL, Rich MM, Capelli AM. Treatment of severe torsional malalignment syndrome. *J Pediatr Orthop* 1996;16:484–488.
18. Dickhaut SC, DeLee JC. The discoid lateral–meniscus syndrome. *J Bone Joint Surg* 1982;64(7):1068–1073.
19. Dietz FR, Mathews KD. Update on the genetic bases of disorders with orthopaedic manifestations. *J Bone Joint Surg Am* 1996 Oct;78(10):1583–1598.
20. Diggs LW. Bone and joint lesions in sickle cell disease. *Clin. Orthop* 1967;52:119–143.
21. Dormans JP, Drummond DS. Pediatric hematogenous osteomyelitis: New trends in presentation, diagnosis, and treatment. *J Am Acad Orthop Surg* 1994;2(6):333–341.
22. Dormans JP, Pellegrino L. *Caring for Children With Cerebral Palsy: A Team-Based Approach*. Baltimore: Brookes, 1998.
23. Drennan JC. Congenital vertical talus. *Instr Course Lect* 1996;45:315–322.
24. Drummond DS, Hosalkar H. *Treatment of Cervical Spine Instability in the Cervical Spine*, 5th ed. Philadelphia: Lippincott Williams & Wilkins, 2005.
25. Dubowitz V. *Color Atlas of Muscle Disorders in Childhood*. Chicago: Year Book Medical Publishers.
26. Elliot S, Morton RE, Whitelaw RAJ. Atlantoaxial instability and abnormalities of the odontoid in Down syndrome. *Arch Dis Child* 1988;63:1484–1489.
27. Emery AE. The muscular dystrophies. *Lancet* 2002;359 (9307):687–695
28. Erdman WA, Tamburro F, Jayson HT, Weatherall PT, Ferry KB, Peshock RM. Osteomyelitis: Characteristics and pitfalls of diagnosis with MR imaging. *Radiology* 1991;180:533–539.
29. Erol B, Dormans JP, States L, et al. Skeletal dysplasias and metabolic disorders of bone. In: Dormans JP (ed.), *Pediatric Orthopaedics and Sports Medicine: The Requisites in Pediatrics*. Philadelphia: Mosby, 2004.
30. Fernandez-Palazzi F, Bendahan J, Rivas S. Congenital deficiency of the tibia: A report on 22 cases. Review. *J Pediatr Orthop B* 1998 Oct;7(4):298–302.
31. Finkel RS. Muscular dystrophy and myopathy. In: Maria BL (ed.), *Current Management in Child Neurology*. Hamilton, Ontario: BC Decker. 2001.

32. Gallagher KT, Roberts RL, MacFarlane JA, Stiehm ER. Treatment of chronic recurrent multifocal osteomyelitis with interferon gamma. *J Pediatr* 1997;131:470–472.
33. Ganz R. Safe surgical dislocation of hip for treatment of slipped capital femoral epiphysis. *Instr Course Lect* 2005.
34. Glorieux FH, Bishop NJ, Plotkin H, et al. Cyclic administration of pamidronate in children with severe osteogenesis imperfecta. *N Engl J Med* 1998;339:947.
35. Green NE, Griffin PP, Shiavi R. Split posterior tibial-tendon transfer in spastic cerebral palsy. *J Bone Joint Surg* 1983;65(A):748–754.
36. Greene WB, McMillan CW. Nonsurgical management of hemophilic arthropathy, In: Barr JS (ed.), *Instructional Course Lectures XXXVIII*. Park Ridge, IL: American Academy of Orthopaedic Surgeons, 1989;367–381.
37. Grogan DP, Gasser SI, Ogden JA. The painful accessory navicular: A clinical and histopathological study. *Foot Ankle* 1989;10(3):164–169.
38. Herring JA. *Tachdjian's Pediatric Orthopedics*. Philadelphia: WB Saunders, 2001.
39. Herring JA, Neustadt JB, Williams JJ, Early JS, Browne RH. The lateral pillar classification of Legg-Calve-Perthes disease. *J Pediatr Orthop* 1992;12:143–150.
40. Herring JA. *Tachdjian's Pediatric Orthopaedics*, 3rd ed. Philadelphia: WB Saunders, 2002.
41. Herring JA. Disorders of brain. In: Herring JA (ed.), *Tachdjian's Pediatric Orthopaedics*, 3rd ed. Philadelphia: WB Saunders, 2002;2:1121–1248.
42. Hosalkar HS, Johnston DR, Pill S, Flynn JM. Multiple epiphyseal separations in a child with scurvy and cerebral palsy. *Am J Orthop* 2005 Jun;34(6):295–298.
43. James MA, McCarroll HR, Manske PR. The spectrum of radial longitudinal deficiency: A modified classification. *J Hand Surg* 1999;24A:1145–1155.
44. Johnson DC, Damiano DL, Abel MF. The evolution of gait in childhood and adolescent cerebral palsy. *J Pediatr Orthop* 1997;17:392–396.
45. Jones DHA, Hosalkar HS, Jones S. The orthopaedic management of osteogenesis imperfecta. *Curr Orthop* 2002 Oct;16(5)374–388.
46. Jones KL (ed.), *Smith's Recognizable Patterns of Human Malformations*, 5th ed. Philadelphia: WB Saunders, 1997.
47. Kim HKW, Alman B, Cole WG. A shortened course of parenteral antibiotic therapy in the management of acute septic arthritis of the hip. *J Pediatr Orthop* 2000;20:44–47.
48. Kling TF Jr, Hensinger RN. Angular and torsional deformities of the lower limbs in children. *Clin Orthop Relat Res* 1983 Jun;(176):136–147.
49. Knudsen CJ, Hoffman EB. Neonatal osteomyelitis. *J Bone Joint Surg Br* 1990;72:846–851.
50. Kozin SH, Weiss AA, Webber JB, Betz RR, Clancy M, Steel HH. Index finger pollicization for congenital aplasia or hypoplasia of the thumb. *J Hand Surg* 1992;17A:880–884.
51. Kozin SH, Syndactyly. *J Am Soc Surg Hand* 2001;1:1–13.
52. Lateur LM, Van Hoe LR, et al. Subtalar coalition: Diagnosis with the C sign on lateral radiographs of the ankle. *Radiology* 1994;193(3):847–51.
53. Laville JM, Lakermore P, Limouzy F. Larsen's syndrome: A review of the literature and analysis of thirty-eight cases. *J Pediatr Orthop* 1994;14:63.
54. Lewin JS, Rosenfield NS, Hoffer PB, Downing D. Acute osteomyelitis in children: Combined Tc-99m and Ga-67 imaging. *Pediatr Radiol* 1986;158:795–804.
55. Loder RT, Aronsson DD, Greenfield ML. The epidemiology of bilateral slipped capital femoral epiphysis: A study of children in Michigan. *J Bone Joint Surg* 1993;75A:1141–1147.
56. Loder RT, Aronsson DD, Dobbs MB, Weinstein SL. Slipped capital femoral epiphysis. *Instr. Course Lect* 2001;50:555–570.
57. Loder R, Lee C, Richards B. Orthopedic aspects of Rett syndrome: A multicenter review. *J Pediatr Orthop* 1989;9:557–562.
58. Loder RT, Richards BS, Shapiro PS, et al. Acute slipped capital femoral epiphysis: The importance of physeal stability. *J Bone Joint Surg* 1993;75A:1134–1140.
59. Lourie GM, Lins RE. Radial longitudinal deficiency: A review and update. *Hand Clin* 1998;14:85–99.
60. MacKenzie WG, Gassett GS, Mandell GA, et al. Avascular necrosis of the hip in multiple epiphyseal dysplasia. *J Pediatr Orthop* 1989;9:666.
61. Makitie O, Kaitila I. Cartilage-hair hypoplasia: Clinical manifestations in 108 Finnish patients. *Eur J Pediatr* 1993;152:211.
62. Mankin HJ. Rickets, osteomalacia and renal osteodystrophy: An update. Review. *Orthop Clin North Am* 1990;21:81.
63. Mankin HJ, Rosenthal DI, Xavier R. Gaucher disease: New approaches to an ancient disease. *J Bone Joint Surg Am* 2001;83A(5):748–62.
64. Manske PR. Redirection of extensor pollicis longus in the treatment of spastic thumb-in-palm deformity. *J Hand Surg* 1985;10:553–569.
65. McCarthy JJ, Glancy GL, Chang FM, Eilert RE. Fibular hemimelia: Comparison of outcome measurements after amputation and lengthening. *J Bone Joint Surg Am* 2000 Dec;82A(12):1732–1735.
66. McKay DW. New concept of an approach to clubfoot treatment: Section II, correction of the clubfoot. *J Pediatr Orthop* 1983;3(1):10–21.
67. Norlin R, Hammerby S, Tkaczuk H. The natural history of Perthes disease. *Int Orthop* 1991;15:13–16.
68. Online Mendelian Inheritance in Man, OMIM. McKusick-Nathans Institute for Genetic Medicine, John Hopkins University (Baltimore, MD) and National Center for Biotechnology Information, National Library of Medicine (Bethesda, MD), 2000. Available at: http://www.ncbi.nlm.nih.gov/omim/.
69. Paulos L, Coleman S, et al. Pes cavovarus: Review of a surgical approach using selective soft-tissue procedures. *J Bone Joint Surg Am* 1980;2:942–953.

70. Perlman MH, Patzakis MJ, Kumar PJ, Holtom P. The incidence of joint involvement with adjacent osteomyelitis in pediatric patients. *J Pediatr Orthop* 2000;20:40–43.
71. Peterkofsky B. Ascorbate requirement for hydroxylation and secretion of procollagen: Relationship to inhibition of collagen synthesis in scurvy. *Am J Clin Nutr* 1991;54:1135.
72. Pimentel L. Scurvy. Historical review and current diagnostic approach. *Am J Emerg Med* 2003 Jul;21(4):328–332.
73. Ponseti IV, Becker JR. Congenital metatarsus adductus: The results of treatment. *J Bone Joint Surg Am* 1966;48:702–711.
74. Ponseti IV. *Congenital Clubfoot: Fundamentals of Treatment*. New York: Oxford University Press, 1996.
75. Rees D, Jones MW, Owen R. Scoliosis surgery in the Prader-Willi syndrome. *J. Bone Joint Surg* 1989;71:685–688.
76. Roberts JM, Drummond DS, Breed AL, Chesney J. Subacute hematogenous osteomyelitis in children: A retrospective study. *J Pediatr Orthop* 1982;2:249–254.
77. Salenius P, Vankka E. The development of the tibiofemoral angle in children. *J Bone Joint Surg Am* 1975;57A:259–261.
78. Salter RB, Hansson G, Thompson GH. Innominate osteotomy in the management of residual congenital subluxation of the hip in young adults. *Clin Orthop Relat Res* 1984 Jan-Feb;(182):53–68.
79. Schaller JG. Chronic arthritis in children: Juvenile rheumatoid arthritis. *Clin Orthop* 1984;182:79–89.
80. Shapiro F, Glimcher MJ, Holtrop ME, et al. Human osteopetrosis: A histological, ultrastructural, and biochemical study. *J Bone Joint Surg* 1980;62A:384.
81. Shapiro F. Consequences of an osteogenesis imperfecta diagnosis for survival and ambulation. *J Pediatr Orthop* 1985;5:456.
82. Shapiro F. Osteopetrosis: Current clinical considerations. *Clin Orthop* 1993;294:34.
83. Sheffield LJ, Halliday JL, Danks DM, et al. Clinical, radiologic, and biochemical classification of chondrodysplasia punctata. *Am J Med Gen* 1989;45(suppl A):A64.
84. Sillence DO. Osteogenesis imperfecta: An expanding panorama of variance. *Clin Orthop* 1981;159:11.
85. Simon SR (ed.), *Orthopaedic Basic Science*. Rosemont, IL: American Academy of Orthopaedic Surgeons, 1994;185–217.
86. Smith R. Idiopathic juvenile osteoporosis: Experience of twenty-one patients. *Br J Rheumatol* 1995;34:68.
87. Sponseller PD. The skeletal dysplasias. In: Morrissy RT, Weinstein SL (eds.), *Lovell and Winter's Pediatric Orthopaedics*, 5th ed. Philadelphia: Lippincott Williams & Wilkins, 2001.
88. Staheli LT, Chew DE. Slotted acetabular augmentation in childhood and adolescence. *J Pediatr Orthop* 1992 Sep-Oct;12(5):569–580.
89. Staheli LT, Coleman SS, Hensinger RN, et al. Congenital hip dysplasia. *Instr. Course Lect* 1984;33:350–363.
90. Staheli LT. Rotational problems in children. *Am Acad Orthop Surg Instr Course Lect* 1994;43:199–209.
91. Stanitski DF. Limb-length inequality: Assessment and treatment options. *J Am Acad Orthop Surg* 1999;7:143–153.
92. Steele HH. Triple osteotomy of the innominate bone. *J Bone Joint Surg Am* 1973;55:343–350.
93. Sutherland DH, Greenfield R. Double innominate osteotomy. *J Bone Joint Surg Am* 1977 Dec;59(8):1082–1091.
94. Suzuki S, Yamamuro T. Avascular necrosis in patients treated with the Pavlik harness for congenital dislocation of the hip. *J Bone Joint Surg Am* 1990 Aug;72(7):1048–1055.
95. Tachdjian MO. *Pediatric Orthopedics*. Philadelphia: WB Saunders, 1990;2867–2870.
96. Tamai J, Erol B, Dormans JP. Hip disorders. In: Dormans JP (ed.), *Pediatric Orthopaedics and Sports Medicine. The Requisites in Pediatrics*. St. Louis: Mosby, 2004;175–212.
97. The osteochondrodysplasias. In: Morrissy RT (ed.), *Lovell and Winter's Pediatric Orthopedics*. 3rd ed. Philadelphia: JB Lippincott, 1990;1:91–142.
98. Thompson GH, Price CT, Roy D, Meehan PL. Legg-Calve-Perthes disease: Current concepts. *Instr Course Lect* 2002;51:367–384.
99. Thompson GH. Gait disturbances. In: Kliegman RM (ed.), *Practical Strategies in Pediatric Diagnosis and Therapy*. 2nd ed. Philadelphia: WB Saunders, 2003.
100. Unkila-Kallio L, Kallio MJT, Peltola H. The usefulness of C-reactive protein levels in the identification of concurrent septic arthritis in children who have acute hematogenous osteomyelitis. *J Bone Joint Surg* 1994;76A(6):848–853.
101. Viere RG, Birch JG, Herring JA, Roach JW, Johnston CE. Use of the Pavlik harness in congenital dislocation of the hip. An analysis of failures of treatment. *J Bone Joint Surg Am* 1990 Feb;72(2):238–244.
102. Wallach DM, Davidson RS. Pediatric lower limb disorders. In: Dormans JP, (ed.) *Pediatric Orthopaedics: Core Knowledge in Orthopaedics.* 1st ed. Philadelphia: Elsevier Mosby, 2005;197–223.
103. Waters PM, Van Heest A. Spastic hemiplegia of the upper extremity in children. *Hand Clin* 1998;14:119–134.
104. Weinstein SL, Mubarak SJ, Wenger DR. Developmental hip dysplasia and dislocation: Part I. *J Bone Joint Surg* 2003;85A:1824–1832.
105. Wenger DR. Congenital hip dislocation. *Instr. Course Lect* 1989;38:343–354.
106. Winters TF, Gage JR, Hicks R. Gait patterns in spastic hemiplegia in children and young adults. *J Bone Joint Surg* 1987;69(A):437–441.
107. Zaleske DJ. Metabolic and endocrine abnormalities. In: Morrisy RT, Weinstein SL, (eds.), *Lovell and Winter's Pediatric Orthopaedics*, 5th ed. Philadelphia: Lippincott Williams & Wilkins, 2001.

Key References

Suk SI, Lee Ck, Kim WJ, et al. Segmental pedicle screw fixation in the treatment of thoracic idiopathic scoliosis. *Spine* 1995;20:1399–1405.

The authors retrospectively compared the results of correction of adolescent idiopathic scoliosis using pedicle screws and hooks. The major coronal curve corrected 55% with hooks and 72% with pedicle screws. Patients with hypokyphosis and rotational deformities had better correction with segmental pedicle screws.

Sussman MD. Advantage of early spinal stabilization and fusion in patients with Duchenne muscular dystrophy. *J Pediatr Orthop* 1984, Sept;4:532–537.

This study reported improved outcome with surgical stabilization and fusion of scoliosis. Surgical patients had a lower complication rate, shorter hospital stay, improved curve correction and overall balance, and more rapid return to daily life. The author recommends fusion in patients with progressive scoliosis between 30 and 40 degrees.

Comstock CP, Leach J, Wenger DR. Scoliosis in total body-involvement cerebral palsy: Analysis of surgical treatment and patient and caregiver satisfaction. *Spine* 1998, June 15;23:1412–1424.

The authors retrospectively reviewed patients followed for a minimum of 2 years. There was a 30% rate of late progression of the scoliosis, pelvic obliquity (more than 75%), and decompensation (more than 4 cm). Twenty-one percent of patients had revision surgery, but 85% of the parents and caregivers were satisfied with the results of surgery.

Fredrickson BE, Baker D, McHolick WJ, et al. The natural history of spondylolysis and spondylolisthesis. *J Bone Joint Surg* 1984;66A:699–707.

This study evaluated radiographs of 500 first-grade children and found a 4.4% incidence of spondylolisthesis among children, which increased to 6% in adulthood. Progression was unusual. Spina bifida occulta and a trapezoidal L5 vertebra were found to be significantly associated with spondylolisthesis. There was also a strong genetic factor contributing to the pars interarticularis defect. The authors recommended no limitation to the lifestyle of children with spondylolisthesis.

Hosalkar HS, Cain EL, Horn D, Chin KR, Dormans J, Drummond D. Traumatic atlanto-occipital dislocation in children. *J Bone Joint Surg Am* 2005 Nov;87(11):2480–2488.

The authors retrospectively reviewed 16 children with AOD. They concluded that prompt recognition and treatment of traumatic atlanto-occipital dislocation in children and adolescents can result in improved survival. They recommend surgical arthrodesis from the occiput to C2 (or the nearest adjacent intact and stable vertebra caudal to C2) for all children who survive a traumatic atlanto-occipital dislocation, particularly those with an incomplete spinal cord injury.

Jones D, Parkinson S, Hosalkar HS. Oblique pelvic osteotomy in the exstrophy/epispadias complex. *J Bone Joint Surg Br* 2006 Jun;88(6):799–806.

The authors reviewed retrospectively 45 patients (46 procedures; 92 osteotomies) with bladder exstrophy treated by bilateral oblique pelvic osteotomy in conjunction with genitourinary repair. The operative technique and postoperative management with or without external fixation are described. Authors conclude that bilateral oblique pelvic osteotomy with or without external fixation is useful in the management of difficult primary closure in bladder exstrophy, failed primary closure, and secondary reconstruction.

Ricchetti ET, States L, Hosalkar HS, et al. Radiographic study of the upper cervical spine in the 22q11.2 deletion syndrome. *J Bone Joint Surg Am* 2004 Aug;86-A(8):1751–1760.

Seventy-nine consecutive patients with the 22q11.2 deletion underwent clinical and radiographic evaluation of the occiput and cervical spine. The 22q11.2 deletion syndrome encompasses a wide spectrum of abnormalities including cardiac, palate, and immunological anomalies. At least one developmental variation of the occiput or cervical spine was observed in every patient. Authors present the various upper cervical spine anomalies in patients with this syndrome. The occipital variation most common was platybasia in 52 (91%) of the 57 patients.

Refresher Questions

1. A 12-year-old girl with bilateral knee pain reveals excessive femoral anteversion and excessive external tibial torsion. The patient has no patellofemoral instability. Nonsurgical management consisting of muscle strengthening and nonsteroidal medication has failed to relieve the patient's pain. Treatment should now consist of
   a) a patellar realignment procedure.
   b) internal rotation of the distal part of the femur.
   c) external rotation of the distal part of the tibia.
   d) arthroscopic retinacular release.
   e) corrective osteotomy with internal rotation of distal tibia and/or external rotation of the femur.

2. A 2-week-old infant has been referred for evaluation of nonmovement of the left hip. History reveals that the patient was delivered 6 weeks premature by cesarean section. Examination reveals no fever, and there is mild swelling of the thigh. Passive movement of the hip appears to elicit tenderness and very limited hip motion. A radiograph of the pelvis shows mild subluxation of the left hip. The next step in evaluation should consist of
   a) aspiration of the left hip.
   b) application of a Pavlik harness.
   c) A gallium scan.
   d) An MRI scan of the spine.
   e) Modified Bryant traction.

3. An asymptomatic patient with Down syndrome wants to participate in a Special Olympics running event. The flexion-extension lateral radiographs of the spine demonstrate atlanto-dens interval (ADI) of 6 mm. The neurologic examination is normal. Management should consist of
   a) MRI scan of cervical spine.
   b) fusion from the occiput to C2.
   c) fusion of C1-C2.
   d) application of a cervical collar and no participation in any sports.
   e) periodic follow-up examinations and no contact sports.

4. In a longitudinal study of children with spastic diplegia, analysis of long-term function will most likely reveal
   a) a deterioration of gait stability and an increase in double support time.
   b) a deterioration of gait stability and a decrease in double support time.
   c) improved excursion about the knee, ankle, and pelvis.
   d) improvement in the popliteal angle.
   e) increases in single support time.

5. Posterior spinal fusion for scoliosis should be performed on a patient with Duchenne muscular dystrophy when
   a) the patient is still ambulatory.
   b) lordotic posture is present.
   c) the forced vital capacity (FVC) is less than 30% of the predicted value.
   d) curve magnitude measures 25 degrees or greater.
   e) Orthotic management fails.

6. Which of the following is considered the most accurate test to determine the amount of limb-length discrepancy in a patient with a knee flexion contracture of 35 degrees?
   a) standing block test
   b) standing AP radiograph of the pelvis with blocks under the foot of the short leg
   c) CT scanogram
   d) scanogram
   e) measurement from the umbilicus to the medial malleolus.

7. The right thumb of a 9-year-old boy with spastic hemiparesis is adducted and flexed across the palm. He is unable to actively extend the metacarpophalangeal joint, but he can actively hyperextend the interphalangeal joint. Treatment should include
   a) lengthening of the flexor pollicis longus.
   b) redirection of the extensor pollicis longus.
   c) a bone block between the first and second metacarpal.
   d) fusion of the metacarpophalangeal joint of the thumb.
   e) transfer of the flexor carpi ulnaris to the extensor carpi radialis brevis.

8. In children, scurvy has the greatest effect on bone formation in the
   a) physis
   b) diaphysis
   c) epiphysis
   d) metaphysis
   e) articular surface

9. A 14-year-old female gymnast has severe low back pain as a result of a fall. Standard radiographs of the lumbar spine are within normal limits. What imaging modality is the most sensitive for detecting a stress fracture of the pars interarticularis?
   a) CT scan
   b) MRI scan
   c) SPECT scan
   d) lateral tomography scan
   e) technetium 99m scintigraphy

10. What is the diagnosis in a 3-year-old girl who has rhizomelic shortening of the limbs associated with cauliflower ears, hitchhiker's thumb, and flexion contractures of the hips, knees, and elbows?
    a) achondroplasia
    b) pseudoachondroplasia
    c) diastrophic dysplasia
    d) metaphyseal chondrodysplasia
    e) multiple epiphyseal dysplasia

Chapter 3

Sports Medicine

JEFFREY F. SODL, LUKE S. OH, GAUTAM YAGNIK, and RUSSELL F. WARREN

I. KNEE

Surgical Anatomy. Tables 3.1 and 3.2 review the muscles of the thigh and surgical approaches to the knee.

Nerves about the Knee. The sciatic nerve gives off the tibial and peroneal branches that supply the muscles of the lower extremities. The *tibial nerve* travels deep in the thigh to the long head of the biceps before entering the popliteal fossa, where it crosses over the popliteus muscle before splitting the two heads of the gastrocnemius muscle. From there it passes deep to the soleus, courses behind the medial malleolus and terminates as the medial and lateral plantar nerves. The muscles of the posterior leg are supplied by motor branches of the tibial nerve. The *common peroneal* nerve is smaller than the tibial nerve. It runs lateral to the popliteal fossa between the medial border of biceps and lateral head of the gastrocnemius. It then travels around the neck of the fibula deep to the peroneus longus, where it divides into superficial and deep branches. The superficial branch runs along the border between the lateral and anterior compartments, supplying branches to the peroneus longus and brevis before terminating as two cutaneous branches supplying the dorsal foot. The deep peroneal branch, also called the anterior tibial nerve, runs along the anterior surface of the interosseous membrane to supply the muscles of the anterior compartment. The *saphenous nerve* travels subcutaneously on the medial aspect of the knee between the sartorius and gracilis. It is at risk from meniscal repair. It is a branch of the femoral nerve and supplies sensation to the medial aspect of the foot. The *sural nerve* is another cutaneous nerve formed from branches of the tibial medial sural cutaneous and the common peroneal lateral sural

TABLE 3.1 Muscles of the thigh

Muscle	Origin	Insertion	Innervation
Anterior			
Vastus lateralis	Iliotibial line/greater trochanter/lateral linea aspera	Lateral patella	Femoral
Vastus medialis	Iliotibial line/medial linea aspera/supracondylar line	Medial patella	Femoral
Vastus intermedius	Proximal anterior femur	Patella	Femoral
Posterior			
Biceps (long head)	Medial ischial tuberosity	Fibula head/lateral tibia	Tibial
Biceps (short head)	Lateral linea aspera/lateral intermuscular septum	Lateral tibial condyle	Peroneal
Semitendinosus	Distal medial ischial tuberosity	Anterior tibial crest	Tibial
Semimembranosus	Proximal lateral ischial tuberosity	Oblique popliteal ligament Posterior capsule Posteriomedial tibia Popliteus Medial meniscus	Tibial

cutaneous nerves. It lies on the lateral aspect of the leg and foot. It is often used for nerve grafting.

Vessels around the Knee. The femoral artery becomes the popliteal artery in the fossa behind the knee. The *popliteal artery* enters the fossa between the biceps and semimembranosus then descends beneath the tibial nerve between the heads of the gastrocnemius to divide into the anterior and posterior tibial artery. The *anterior tibial artery* is the first branch of the popliteal artery and terminates as the dorsalis pedis artery in the foot after traveling on the anterior surface of the interosseous membrane between the tibialis anterior and EHL. The *posterior tibial artery* travels in the deep posterior compartment obliquely to pass behind the medial malleolus, where it terminates into medial and lateral plantar arteries. The posterior tibial artery gives off a main branch (*peroneal artery*) 2.5 cm distal to the popliteal fossa, which runs lateral to the posterior tibial artery between the tibialis posterior and FHL before terminating as the calcaneal branches. The knee receives several geniculate branches from the popliteal fossa, including the medial and lateral geniculates (supply the menisci) and the middle geniculate (supply

TABLE 3.2 Surgical approaches to the knee

Approach	Superficial Muscle (Innervation)	Deep Muscles (Innervation)	Structures at Risk
Medial parapatellar	Vastus medialis (femoral)	Rectus femoris (femoral)	Saphenous nerve (infrapatellar branch)
Medial	Vastus medialis (femoral)	Sartorius (femoral)	Saphenous nerve (infrapatellar branch)
Lateral	ITB (superior gluteal)	Biceps femoris (sciatic)	Peroneal nerve/lateral superior geniculate artery
Posterior	Semimembranosus/lateral gastrocnemius (tibial)	Biceps femoris/lateral gastroc (tibial)	Medial sural cutaneous nerve/tibial nerve/peroneal nerve
Lateral	Vastus lateralis (femoral)	Biceps femoris(sciatic)	Peroneal nerve/lateral superior geniculate artery

the cruciate ligaments). The *superolateral geniculate artery* is located between the femur and vastus lateralis and is commonly injured during lateral releases of the knee. The *descending geniculate artery* branches off the femoral artery proximal to Hunter canal and supplies the vastus medialis at the anterior border of the intermuscular septum. The *lateral inferior geniculate artery* runs posterior to the LCL between the lateral head of the gastrocnemius and the posterior capsule.

Anterior Cruciate Ligament (ACL). One of four ligaments that provide support to the knee joint, the ACL originates from a broad, oval-shaped area just anterior to and between the intercondylar spines of the tibia and inserts in a semicircular area on the posterior medial aspect of the lateral femoral condyle (Fig. 3.1). The average length is 33 mm and the average width is 11 mm in adults. It consists of the *anteromedial bundle*, which is tight in flexion, and the *posterolateral bundle*, which is tight in extension. The blood supply is via the middle geniculate artery and fat pad. A proprioceptive role is provided by mechanoreceptors. The ACL is composed of 90% type I collagen (10% type III). It is the primary restraint (85%) to anterior tibial translation. With the posterior cruciate ligament (PCL), it helps regulate the "screw home" mechanism (i.e., external tibial rotation with terminal knee extension). The average tensile strength is 2,160 N (younger patients, about 2,500 N). For reconstruction, the tensile strength of a 4-strand hamstring graft is about 4,500 N, while for a bone–patellar tendon–bone graft (10 mm), it is about 2,600 N.

ACL Injuries. A Segond fracture, seen on an AP x-ray (lateral capsular sign) is a capsular avulsion from the lateral tibial metaphysis that is highly associated with

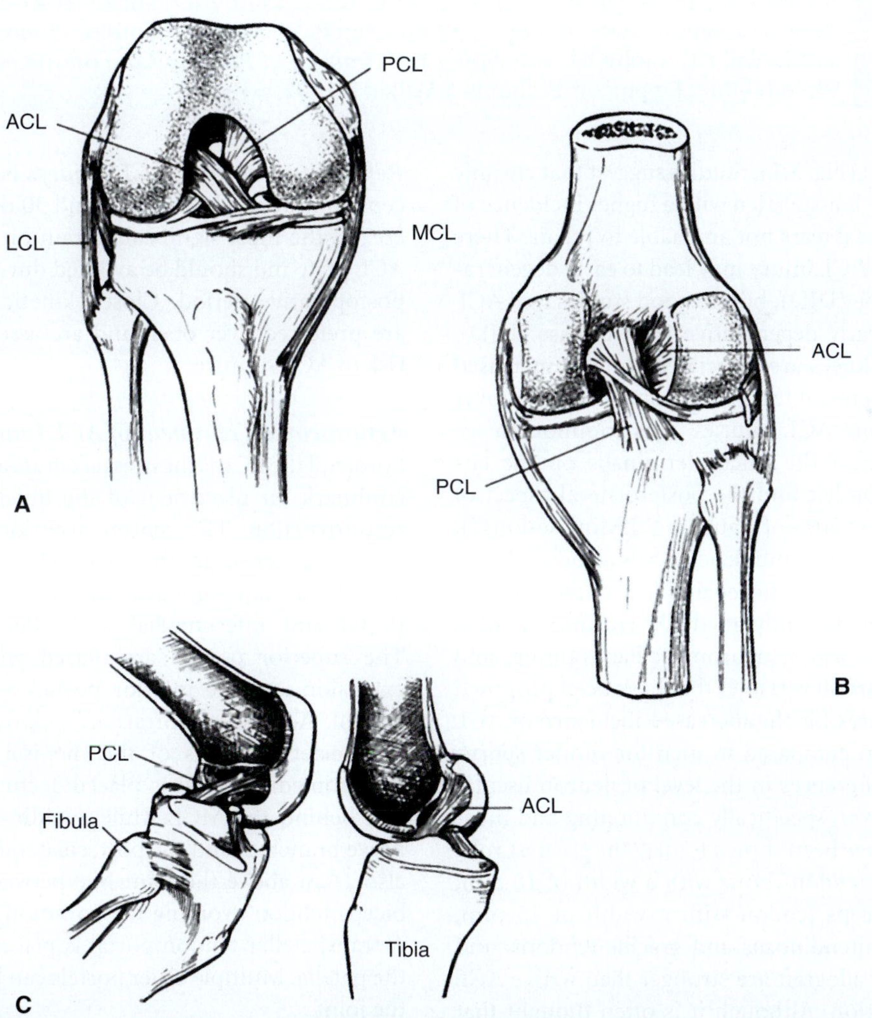

FIGURE 3.1 **(A) Anterior view of anterior and posterior cruciate ligaments. (B) Posterior view of anterior and posterior cruciate ligaments. (C) Lateral view of anterior and posterior cruciate ligaments. (*Source*: Fu FH, Stone DA. *Sports Injuries,* 2nd ed. Philadelphia: Lippincott Williams & Wilkins, 2001; 1105.)**

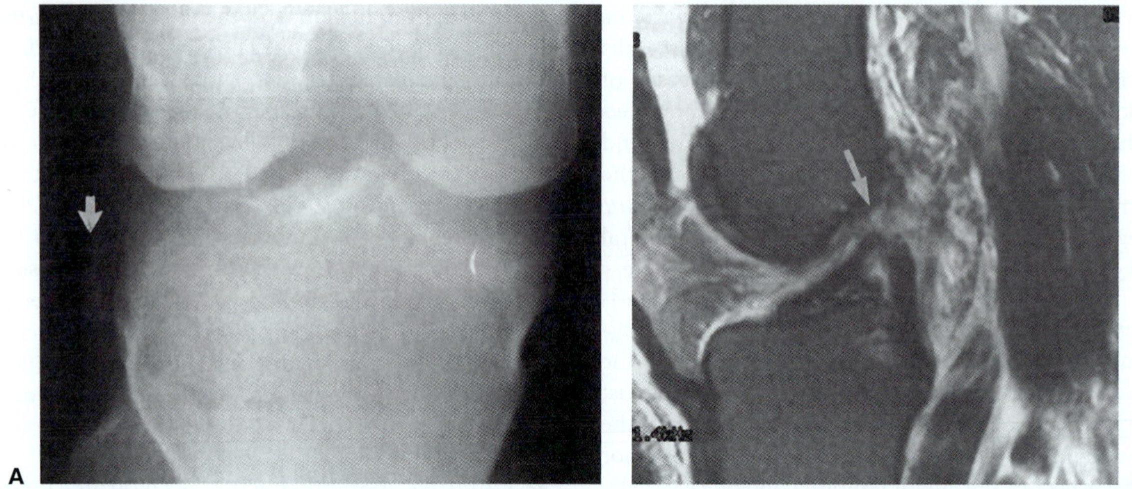

FIGURE 3.2 **This 22-year-old male fell while skiing and heard a *pop*. (A) Plain anterior–posterior (notch) reveals a flake fracture from the posterolateral tibial plateau *(arrow)*, a Segond fracture. (B) The sagittal FSE with fat saturation (3500/75Ef) shows avulsion of ACL from femoral origin *(arrow)*. A large joint effusion is also quite apparent. (*Source*: Garrett WE, Kirkendall DT, Squire DL. *Principles and Practice of Primary Care Sports Medicine*. Philadelphia: Lippincott Williams & Wilkins, 2001; 64.)**

ACL disruption (Fig. 3.2). Studies suggest that chronic ACL deficiency is associated with a higher incidence of complex meniscal tears not amenable to repair. There is concern that ACL injury may lead to early degenerative joint disease (DJD), but no good studies link ACL deficiency to early degenerative joint disease (DJD). ACL-deficient knees are associated with an increased incidence of meniscal tears and chondral injuries over time. After acute ACL injuries, it is common to see bone bruises near the sulcus terminalis on the lateral femoral condyle and the posterolateral aspect of the tibia in over 50% of patients ("kissing lesions"). Chronic ACL injuries and deficiency is associated with a higher incidence of unrepairable complex meniscal tears (predominantly medial). Hormones, ACL strength, notch width, neuromuscular training, and leg alignment are all variables that have been proposed as possible causes for the increased incidence of ACL tears in women compared to men for similar sports. The general differences in the level of neuromuscular training, however, specifically conditioning and muscle strength, have been shown to play the greatest role. Bone–patellar tendon–bone with a width of 10 mm, central quadriceps tendon with a width of 15 mm, quadruple semitendinosus and gracilis tendons, and tibialis tendon allograft are stronger than native ACL for reconstruction. Although it is often thought that the bone–tendon–bone graft is the strongest (maximum load to failure) when selecting a graft source for ACL reconstruction, biomechanical studies show that quadruple semitendinosus and gracilis tendons are the strongest of the tissues mentioned.

Rehabilitation after ACL Injury. Isometric quadriceps contraction between 15 and 30 degrees of flexion creates the most significant strain on a reconstructed ACL graft and should be avoided during rehabilitative postoperative period. Closed kinetic chain exercises are preferred over open and are associated with less risk of ACL rupture.

Arthroscopic Treatment of ACL Injury. The anterior border of the PCL is the most accurate and reproducible landmark for placement of the tibial tunnel in ACL reconstruction. The central insertion point is 10 to 11 mm anterior to the PCL. The standard portals include a superomedial or superolateral outflow portal and inferomedial and inferolateral portals. The superior portals are placed with the knee in extension and the inferior portals with the knee in flexion. Additional portals are helpful for visualizing the posterior horns of the menisci and PCL. The posteromedial portal is placed 1 cm above the joint line behind the MCL while avoiding the saphenous nerve branches, and the posterolateral portal is placed also 1 cm above the joint line between the LCL and biceps tendon avoiding the common peroneal nerve. A transpatellar tendon portal is placed 1 cm distal to the patella. Multiple other portals can be placed within the joint.

Posterior Cruciate Ligament (PCL). Originating from the broad crescent-shaped area on the anterolateral aspect of the medial femoral condyle, the PCL inserts on an extraarticular sulcus of the posterior tibia, which is

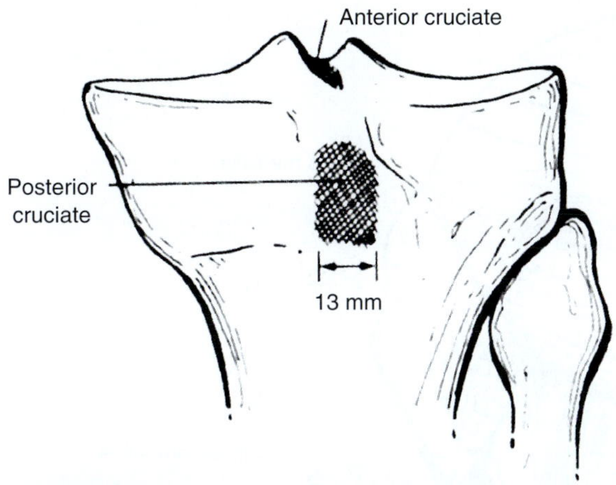

FIGURE 3.3 Dimensions of the tibial insertion of the posterior cruciate ligament. (*Source*: DeLee JC, Bergfeld JA, Drez D Jr (eds). *Orthopaedic Sports Medicine. Principles and Practice.* Philadelphia: WB Saunders, 1994.)

below the articular surface (Fig. 3.3). In adults it averages 38 mm in length and 13 mm in width. It is composed of 2 bundles: (1) the anterolateral bundle, which is tight in flexion and 2 times larger than the (2) posteromedial bundle, which is tight in extension. Intraoperative tensioning of a double-bundle PCL reconstruction should tension the anterolateral bundle in 90 degrees of flexion and the posteromedial bundle in 0 degrees of flexion to reproduce the most anatomic knee biomechanics. The blood supply is via the middle geniculate artery branches. Variable meniscofemoral ligament insertions onto the PCL include Humphrey ligament, which attaches from the lateral meniscus to the PCL (anterior), and the Wrisberg ligament, which attaches from the lateral meniscus to the PCL (posterior) (Fig. 3.4). The PCL is the primary restraint (95%) to posterior tibial translation and regulates the screw-home mechanism in conjunction with the ACL. The PCL acts synergistically with the posterolateral corner to resist posterior translation and posterolateral rotation and is the secondary restraint to varus–valgus and rotational stability.

Medial Collateral Ligament (MCL). A broad, flat ligament that originates from the medial femoral epicondyle and inserts onto proximal medial tibia, the superficial MCL (tibial collateral ligament) is the primary restraint to valgus force. The deep MCL (medial capsular ligament) is a thickening of the joint capsule that is intimately associated with medial meniscus via coronary ligaments. The posterior oblique component has twice the stiffness and tensile strength of the ACL. Injuries most commonly occur at the femoral insertion. The Pellegrini-Stieda lesion is seen on anterior–posterior plain radiographs and represents calcification of the MCL, usually near the femoral insertion, secondary to a chronic MCL injury (Fig. 3.5). Layers of medial structures are listed here:

LAYER	STRUCTURES
I	Fascia and sartorius muscle
II	Superficial MCL, posterior oblique ligament, semimembranosus muscle
III	Deep MCL, capsule

Lateral Collateral Ligament (LCL). A cordlike ligament that originates from the lateral femoral epicondyle and inserts on the lateral aspect of the

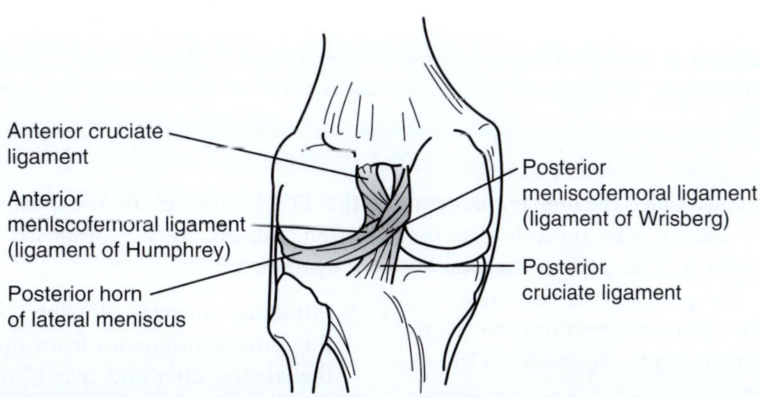

FIGURE 3.4 Relationship of the meniscofemoral ligaments to the posterior cruciate ligament. (*Adapted from* DeLee JC, Bergfeld JA, Drez D Jr, et al. The posterior cruciate ligament. In: DeLee JC, Drez D Jr (eds.), *Orthopaedic Sports Medicine: Principles and Practice.* Philadelphia: WB Saunders, 1994.)

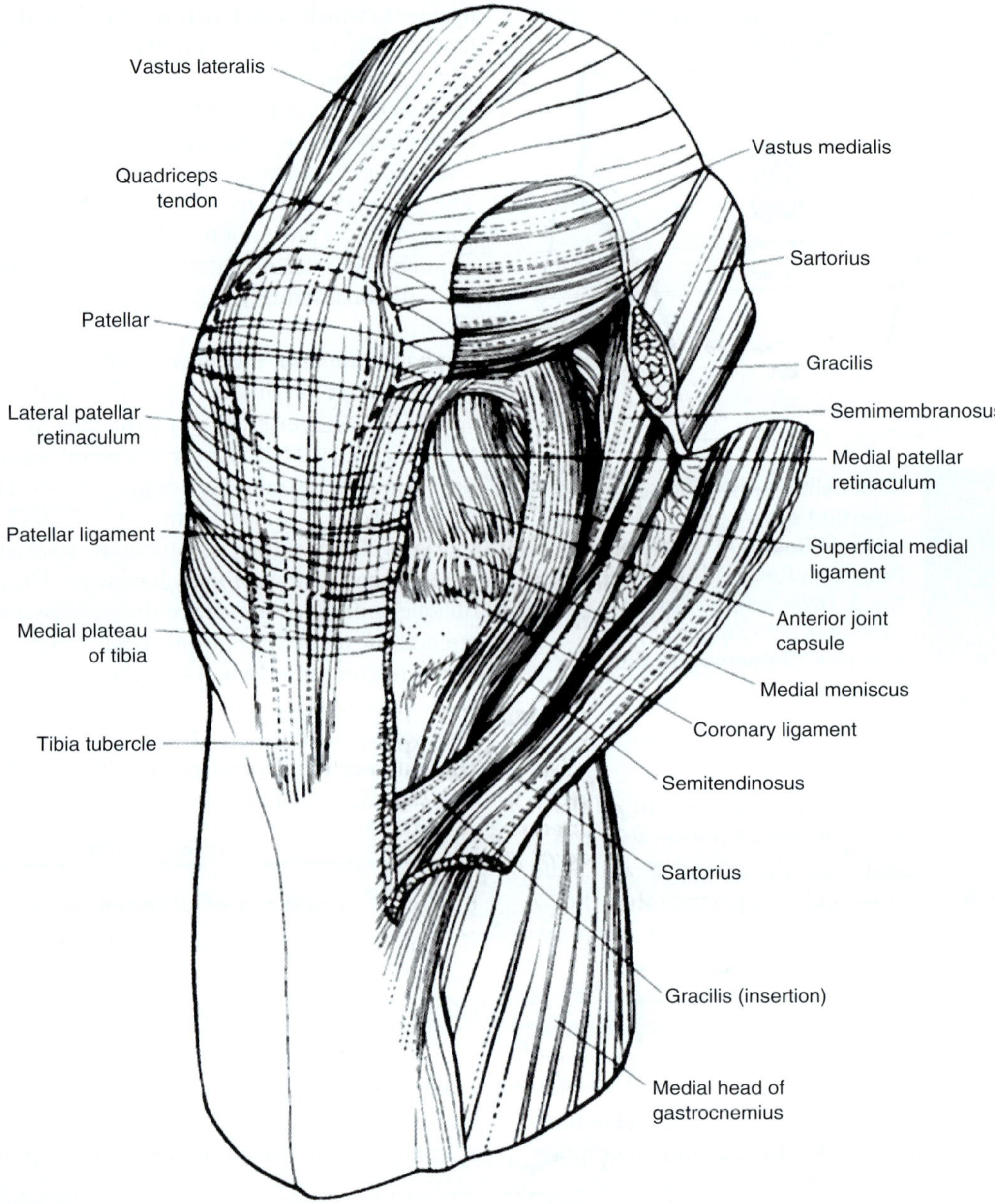

FIGURE 3.5 **Anatomy of the medial aspect of the knee. (*Source*: Hoppenfeld S, deBoer P. *Surgical Exposures in Orthopaedics: The Anatomic Approach.* Philadelphia, Lippincott 1984; 408.)**

fibular head, the LCL is also called the fibular collateral ligament. It inserts proximal and posterior to the popliteus tendon insertion. The LCL is tightest in extension because it lies posterior to the knee axis of rotation. It is the primary restraint to varus force and has an average tensile strength of 750 N (Fig. 3.6).

The Posterolateral Corner. The posterolateral corner functions with the PCL to resist posterior translation and posterolateral rotation (see Fig. 3.6). It is rarely injured in isolation (usually in conjunction with the PCL). Injuries to the posterolateral corner are often missed. It is composed of 2 muscles and 2 ligaments:

- **Popliteus muscle**—Possibly the most important, this muscle originates from the posterior aspect of the medial tibia and inserts medial, anterior, and distal to the LCL. The popliteus attaches to the head of the fibula as the popliteal fibular ligament.
- Lateral head of the gastrocnemius muscle
- Arcuate ligament complex
- LCL

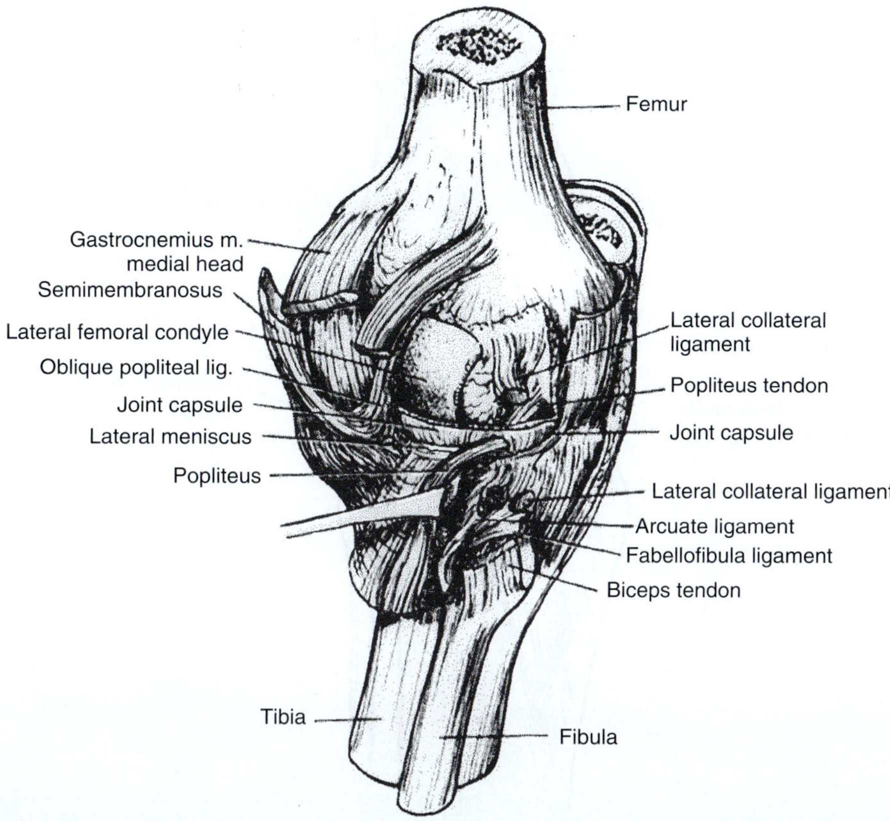

FIGURE 3.6 **The posterolateral corner of the knee. (*Source*: Seebacher JR, Inglis AE, Marshall JL, et al. The structure of the posterolateral aspect of the knee. *J Bone Joint Surg* 1982;64:536, with permission. Fu FH, Stone DA. *Sports Injuries,* 2nd ed. Philadelphia: Lippincott Williams & Wilkins, 2001, 1104.)**

Failure to diagnose and treat an injury of the posterolateral corner in a patient who has a tear of the ACL or PCL can result in failure of the reconstructed cruciate ligament. Chronic reconstruction of the posterolateral corner is associated with poor results, and thus acute anatomic repair is recommended. Techniques for repairing chronic injuries include posterolateral advancement, biceps tenodesis, popliteus bypass, and graft reconstruction of the LCL and popliteus/posterolateral corner. Layers of lateral structures are listed here:

LAYER	STRUCTURES
I	Fascia, iliotibial tract, biceps
II	LCL, patellar retinaculum, patellofemoral ligament
III	Arcuate ligament, fabellofibular

The Posteromedial Corner. An important contributor to rotatory stability, the posteromedial corner consists of the semimembranosus tendon, which fans out into 5 insertions, some of which contribute to capsular thickening posteriorly; the posterior oblique ligament (POL); and the oblique popliteal ligament, which is a thickening of the most posterior portion of the knee joint capsule (Fig. 3.7). An increased anterior drawer test with the tibia in external rotation indicates disruption of the posteromedial capsule and POL.

LIGAMENT	LIMIT
ACL	Anterior translation of the tibia
PCL	Posterior tibial displacement
MCL	Valgus angulation
LCL	Varus angulation

Patellofemoral Ligaments. Biomechanic studies have found the medial patellofemoral ligament is the major soft tissue restraint to lateral patellar displacement, providing a minimum of 50% of its stability.

Menisci. Crescent-shaped fibrocartilaginous structures called menisci deepen the articular surface of the tibial plateau and aid in load transmission, reduce stress on the articular surfaces, contribute to joint stability,

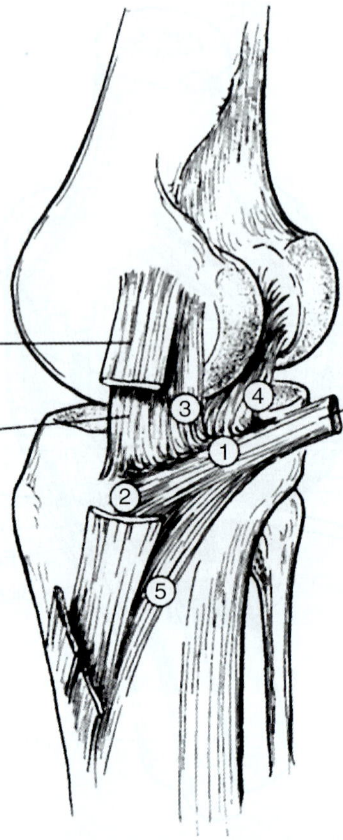

FIGURE 3.7 **The posteromedial corner of the knee. Numbers correspond to the insertions of the semimembranosus tendon and its sheath. (*Source*: From Warren LF, Marshall JL. The supportive structures and layers of the medial side of the knee. An anatomical analysis. *J Bone Joint Surg* 1979;61:56.)**

and aid in joint lubrication and chondral nutrition. Menisci are triangular in cross-section, tapering to a central free edge, and peripherally attach to the tibia via coronary ligaments. Blood supply in adults occurs via medial and lateral geniculate arteries that supply the peripheral 20% to 30% of the medial meniscus and the peripheral 10% to 25% of the lateral meniscus. The medial and lateral menisci are connected anteriorly by the transverse meniscal (intermeniscal) ligament. The medial meniscus is C-shaped, and abnormal strain is seen with ACL-deficient knee (posterior horn). The lateral meniscus is semicircular in shape and lacks peripheral attachment at the popliteal hiatus. It displaces 11 mm in the anterior–posterior direction during full knee flexion–extension (more than 2 times the displacement of medial meniscus). The lateral meniscus has twice the excursion of the medial meniscus during knee range of motion (ROM) and rotation. Collagen fibers in menisci are arranged radially and circumferentially/longitudinally. The circumferential fibers dissipate hoop stresses. The combined arrangement of fibers allows menisci to expand under compressive stresses and increase the contact area of joint (Fig. 3.8).

Fairbank Signs. Postmeniscectomy changes seen on plain anterior–posterior x-rays (Fig. 3.9), include

- Squaring of the femoral-condyle
- Narrowing of the joint space
- Lateral osteophyte formation (ridging)
- Peaking of intercondylar spines

Meniscal Tears. Meniscal tears represent 50% of knee injuries that require surgery. The medial meniscus is torn 3 times more commonly than the lateral meniscus. There are two main types of tears: traumatic and degenerative (Fig. 3.10). Traumatic tears occur in younger patients and are commonly sports related. These are usually more peripheral and amenable to repair. Degenerative tears occur in older patients and are usually of insidious onset. Complex tear patterns are near the free edge and are usually not amenable to repair.

Kinematics. The 4-bar cruciate linkage system explains flexion–extension kinematics of the knee joint and emphasizes the central role of the ACL in knee

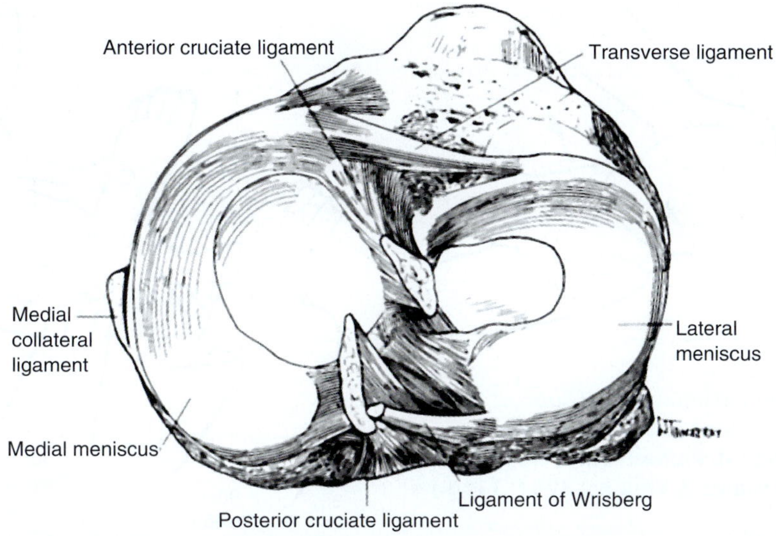

FIGURE 3.8 Tibial plateau showing the shape and attachments of the medial and lateral menisci. (*Source*: Warren RF, Arnoczky SP, Wickiewicz TL. Anatomy of the knee. In: Nicholas JA, Hershman EB (eds.), *The Lower Extremity and Spine in Sports Medicine.* St. Louis: Mosby, 1986; 657–694.)

kinematics. The 4 links include the ACL, the PCL, the femur, and the tibia. As the knee flexes, the instantaneous center of rotation moves posteriorly, forcing a combination of rolling and gliding between the articular surfaces. The ligaments anterior to the knee flexion axis become tight in flexion, and ligaments posterior to the axis become relaxed (the opposite occurs in knee extension).

Instability

Isolated instability is evidenced by laxity to stress in a *Single* plane.

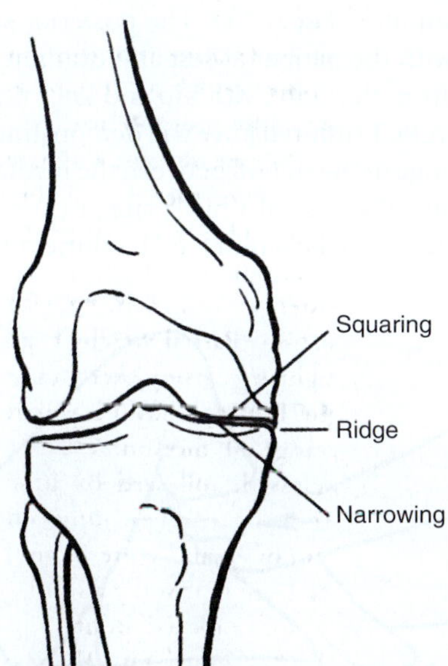

FIGURE 3.9 Fairbank radiographic changes of the knee joint after meniscectomy. (*Source*: Fu FH, Stone DA. *Sports Injuries*, 2nd ed. Philadelphia: Lippincott Williams & Wilkins, 2001; 1124.)

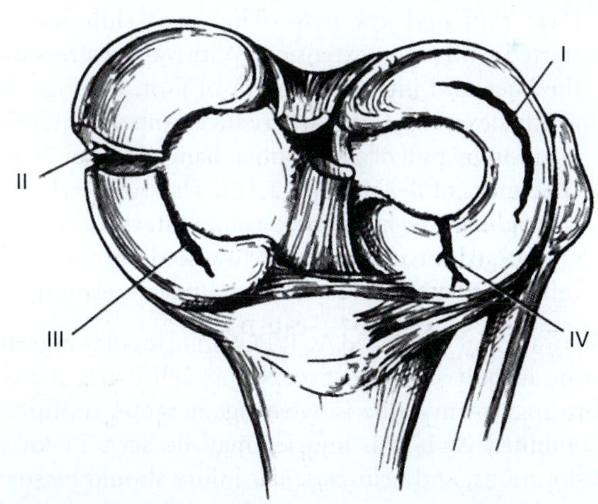

FIGURE 3.10 The four basic types of meniscal tear: I, longitudinal; II horizontal; III, oblique; IV, radial. (*Adapted from* Kalenak A, Hanks GA, et al. Arthroscopy of the knee. In: Evarts CM (ed.), *Surgery of the Musculoskeletal System.* New York: Churchill Livingstone, 1990; 3349, with permission.)

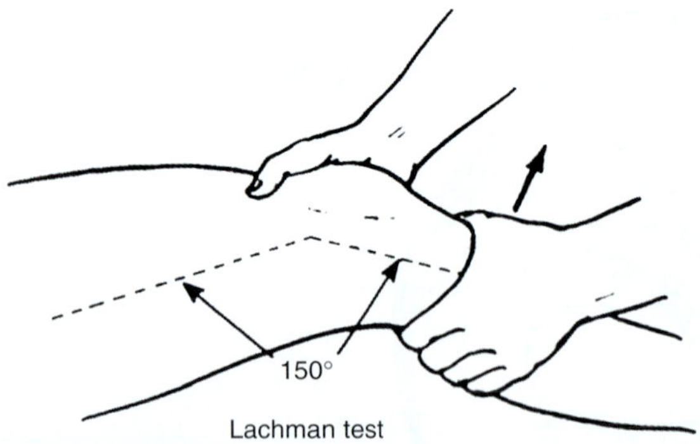

FIGURE 3.11 **The Lachman test. (*Source*: Fu FH, Stone DA. *Sports Injuries*, 2nd ed. Philadelphia: Lippincott Williams & Wilkins, 2001; 1116.)**

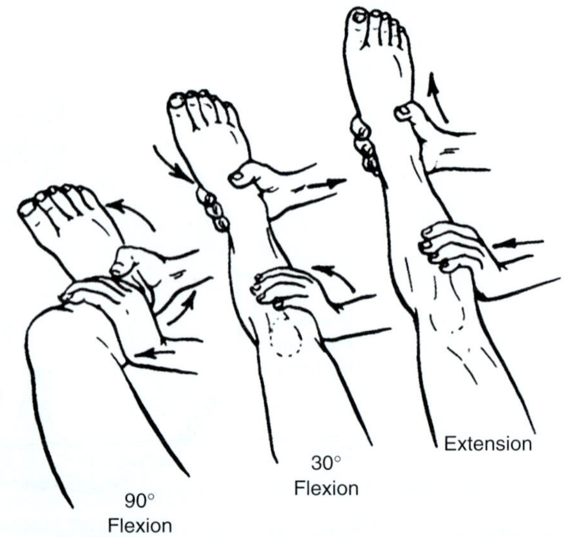

FIGURE 3.12 **The pivot shift test. As the knee is brought into flexion, the iliotibial band reduces the tibia from its anteriorly subluxated position. (*Adapted from* Insall JN. Examination of the knee. In: Insall JN (ed.), *Surgery of the Knee*. New York: Churchill Livingstone, 1984.)**

Anterior Instability. Anterior tibial translation can be tested with the knee partially flexed (Lachman test) or with the knee at 90 degrees of flexion (anterior drawer test) (Fig. 3.11).

- *Lachman test*—The most sensitive examination for assessing ACL laxity. It involves an anterior tibial translation with the knee flexed 20 to 30 degrees. Greater than 3 mm side-to-side difference is pathologic.
- *Finacetto test*—Lachman test with the tibia subluxing beyond the posterior horns of the menisci. It is suggestive of a severe ACL injury.
- *Pivot shift and jerk tests*—The pivot shift test is started with leg in extension. With valgus stress on the knee and internal rotation of foot, the knee is gently flexed. The tibia will reduce from an anterior position by pull of the iliotibial band (ITB) at 20 to 30 degrees of flexion (Fig. 3.12). The pivot jerk test is done with the knee in extension; internal rotation and valgus force are applied to also detect an ACL injury. These tests are best done under anesthesia.

Be aware that combined ACL/PCL injuries may appear to be in only one direction of instability and therefore may seem to be isolated ligamentous ruptures. Combined ACL/PCL injuries may be seen in knee dislocations, and neurovascular injury should be suspected in 30% to 50% of cases. Vascular studies should be done, and surgery may be delayed 5 to 12 days to ensure that there is no vascular injury unless there is popliteal artery injury, open dislocation, or irreducible dislocation. If an arthroscopy is to be performed, the use of an automated pump to maintain fluid pressure in the knee should be limited as this can lead to fluid extravasation and a potential compartment syndrome.

Posterior Instability. Posterior tibial translation. The posterior drawer test is the *most sensitive* examination for detecting isolated PCL injury. This occurs with posterior translation with the knee flexed 90 degrees (patient supine) (Fig. 3.13). The posterior sag sign is assessed with the patient at rest and examiner viewing the knee from the side (with hip and knee flexed to 90 degrees). A PCL-injured knee will demonstrate sag sign with a change in the stepoff between the medial femoral condyle and the medial tibial plateau (normally, the tibia is anterior to the femur). PCL injuries (Table 3.3)

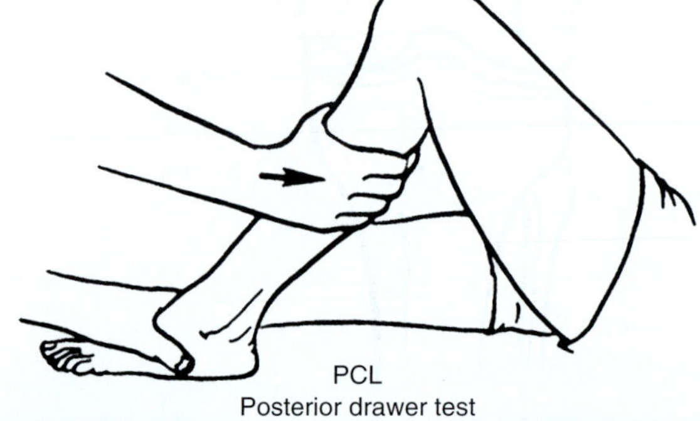

FIGURE 3.13 **The posterior drawer test. (*Source*: Fu FH, Stone DA. *Sports Injuries*, 2nd ed. Philadelphia: Lippincott Williams & Wilkins, 2001; 1122.)**

TABLE 3.3 Grading of PCL injuries

Grade of PCL Injury	Tibial Position
Normal	+10 mm
Grade I	+5 mm
Grade II	0 (tibia flush with femur)
Grade III	−5 mm or greater

usually result from a direct impact to the anterior tibia with the knee flexed, such as against the dashboard of a vehicle. Other mechanisms include a hyperflexed knee with a plantar-flexed foot without any impact to the knee or knee hyperextension. Nonoperative treatment is effective for isolated injuries, but bony avulsion fractures can be repaired primarily.

The quadriceps active test is positive when anterior translation of the tibia occurs from a sag position with a quadriceps contraction performed with the knee flexed 70 to 90 degrees. The majority of grade 1 and 2 PCL injuries can be treated with protected weight bearing and quadriceps rehabilitation with return to sports within 2 to 4 weeks. Grade 3 injuries require immobilization in full extension for 2 to 4 weeks followed by rehabilitation.

Varus–Valgus Instability. Varus stress and opening of the lateral joint at 30 degrees of knee flexion (with no laxity at 0 degrees) is indicative of an isolated collateral ligament injury (Table 3.4). Isolated LCL injury can be managed nonoperatively. Pain and instability with valgus stress at 30 degrees of knee flexion but not in full extension is indicative of MCL injury. These injuries most commonly occur at the femoral insertion. Isolated MCL injuries may be treated nonoperatively with a hinged knee brace. Opening at 0 degrees and 30 degrees of knee flexion is consistent with injury to the collateral ligament and other structures such as the PCL, ACL, posteromedial capsule, or posterolateral corner.

TABLE 3.4 Grading of collateral ligament injuries

Grade of Collateral Injury	Amount of Joint Space Opening
Normal	≤ 1 mm
Grade I	1–5 mm of opening (minimal tear/sprain)
Grade II	6–10 mm of opening (moderate tear)
Grade III	> 10 mm opening (complete tear)

Posterolateral Instability. The key element of examination is asymmetry of external rotation. The most reliable test for a relatively isolated posterolateral complex injury is asymmetric tibial external rotation, or dial test. Greater than 10 degrees of external rotation at 30 degrees when compared to the uninjured knee indicates damage to the posterolateral structures. The test is performed in both 30 and 90 degrees of knee flexion. If asymmetry occurs in 30 degrees of flexion only, then an isolated posterolateral corner injury is suspected. In contrast, if asymmetry occurs in 30 and 90 degrees, then a combined posterolateral corner and PCL injury is likely.

- *Posterolateral drawer test*—Increased posterior translation of the tibia occurs with the foot in external rotation. Also, with the foot in neutral, the lateral side of the tibia will move posteriorly on the femur but the medial side will not.
- *External rotation recurvatum test*—Raising both feet of a supine patient (by gripping the toes) will cause the injured side to fall into varus and recurvatum at the knee and the tibia to externally rotate. This test is not as reliable as the dial test in PLC injuries (Fig. 3.14).

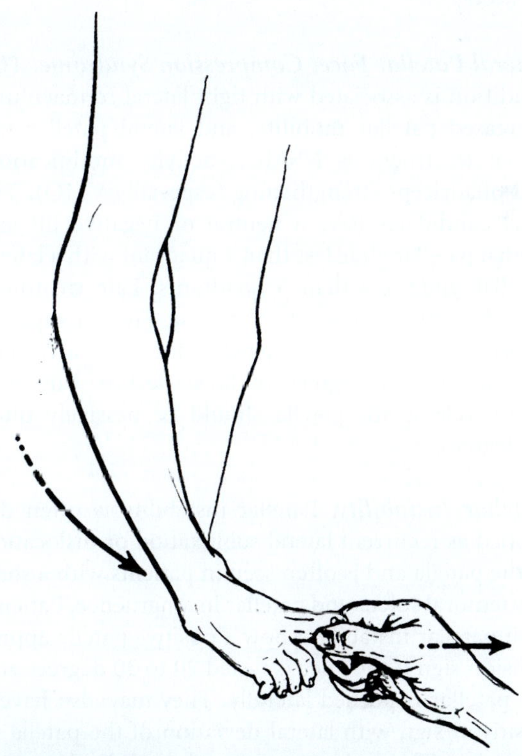

FIGURE 3.14 The external rotation recurvatum test. (*Source*: Fu FH, Stone DA. *Sports Injuries*, 2nd ed. Philadelphia: Lippincott Williams & Wilkins, 2001; 1122.)

- *Reverse pivot shift test*—Start with the knee flexed and leg held in external rotation, and gently extend knee. A posteriorly subluxated tibia will reduce at 20 to 30 degrees of flexion.

Combined Instability. Elicited in more than one direction using the examination findings described previously.

Patellofemoral Disorders

Patellar Tendinitis (Jumper's Knee). Patellar tendonitis causes pain and tenderness near the inferior pole of the patella, and the pain is usually *worse in extension*. This injury is common in jumping sports such as basketball and volleyball. Treatment is with NSAIDs, rest, and physical therapy with or without ultrasound treatment. Excision of degenerative tendon fibers is rarely necessary.

Prepatellar Bursitis (Housemaid's Knee). The most common knee bursitis is prepatellar bursitis. Typically, the patient has a history of prolonged kneeling, and the condition is also seen in athletes such as wrestlers. It is treated with knee pads, NSAIDs, and occasional cortisone injections. Bursal excision is rarely necessary.

Lateral Patellar Facet Compression Syndrome. This condition is associated with tight lateral retinaculum, decreased patellar mobility, and lateral patellar tilt. Initial treatment is NSAIDs, activity modification, and quadriceps strengthening (especially VMO). The ideal candidates have a neutral or negative tilt and medial patellar glide less than 1 quadrant with a lateral patellar glide less than 3 quadrants. Late treatment includes arthroscopic lateral release. From a superior arthroscopic portal, the patella does not articulate medially by 40 degrees of knee flexion, but after lateral release the patella should be passively tilted 80 degrees.

Patellar Instability. Patellar instability is often described as recurrent lateral subluxation or dislocation of the patella and is often seen in patients with a shallow femoral sulcus and patellar incongruence. Patients with patellar instability show a positive patella apprehension sign if the knee is flexed 20 to 30 degrees and the patellar is pushed laterally. They may also have a positive J sign with lateral deviation of the patella in extension. The main restraint to lateral displacement of the patella is the medial patellofemoral ligament. Femoral anteversion, genu valgum, and pronated feet may exacerbate symptoms, especially in adolescents. This condition is termed the miserable malalignment syndrome. Rehabilitation can be curative and is focused on quadriceps strengthening and stretching (especially VMO). Patients with malalignment often have an increased Q angle (ASIS-patella-tibial tubercle). Arthroscopic evaluation may be necessary in case of loose cartilaginous or osteochondral fragments. Acute repair of the medial patellofemoral ligament to the medial femoral epicondyle is often advocated, especially for first-time dislocations. Bracing and taping can also be effective.

Iliotibial Band Friction Syndrome. Abrasion between the ITB and the lateral femoral condyle causes ITB friction syndrome. Running uphill and cycling may predispose people to this syndrome. Examination reveals localized tenderness that is worse with the knee flexed 30 degrees. The Ober test shows tightness in the ITB with the patient in a lateral decubitus position and the hip abducted and hyperextended. Nonoperative rehabilitation is the mainstay of treatment, but for refractory cases, surgical excision of an ellipse of the ITB is sometimes successful.

Semimembranosus Tendinitis. This condition is often seen in male athletes in their early 30s. Nuclear imaging may be needed to make the diagnosis. Treatment involves stretching and strengthening.

Anterior Fat Pad Syndrome (Hoffa Disease). Knee trauma can lead to fibrotic changes in the fat pad, especially in patients with genu recurvatum. Treatment includes activity modification, ice, and knee padding. Arthroscopic excision may be beneficial.

Meniscal Examination. Joint-line tenderness to palpation, localized swelling, or a meniscal cyst are all suggestive of meniscal tears. Pain is often exacerbated by knee hyperflexion.

- *Squat test*—Involves asking the patient to squat or "duck walk" to reproduce knee pain or to see whether or not patient can perform the test secondary to pain.
- *McMurray test*—Involves starting with the patient supine with hip and knee flexed. Apply varus or valgus stress with tibial rotation while extending the knee. A positive test is a palpable or audible click or pop along the joint line, but pain may also be useful in diagnosis (Fig. 3.15).
- *Apley test*—The test is performed with the patient prone and knee flexed while applying compression. This can detect degenerative disk disease and meniscal pathology.

Discoid Lateral Meniscus. Discoid lateral meniscus is also called "popping knee syndrome" because patients may develop mechanical symptoms or "popping" with

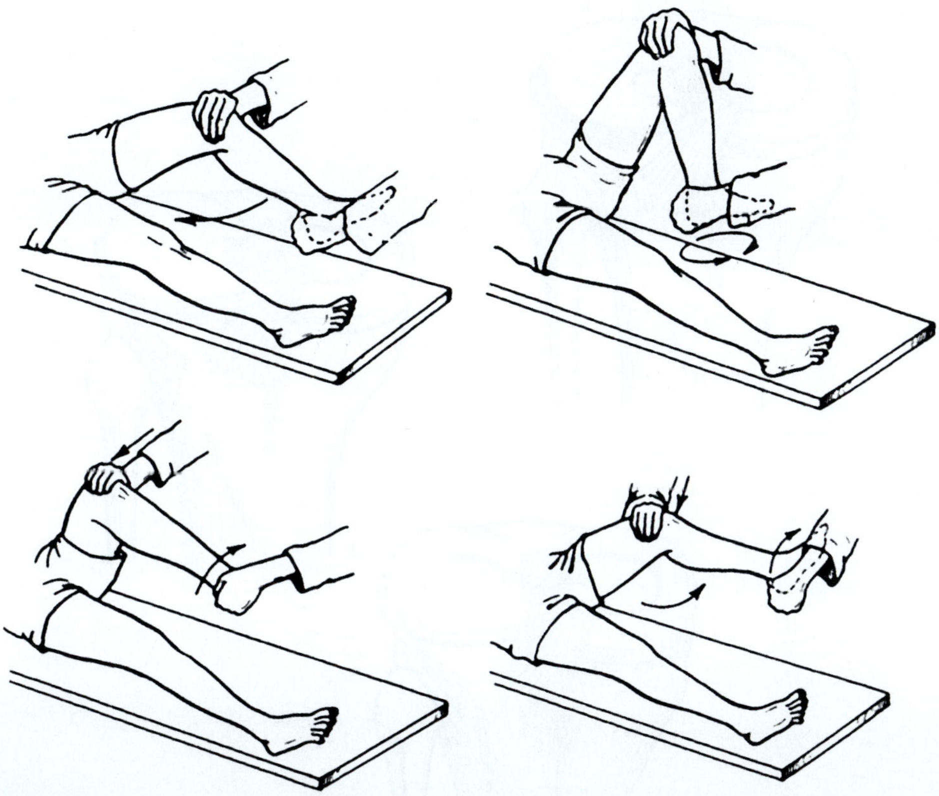

FIGURE 3.15 The McMurray test. (*Source:* Fu FH, Stone DA. *Sports Injuries,* 2nd ed. Philadelphia: Lippincott Williams & Wilkins, 2001; 1124.)

knee extension (Fig. 3.16). Loss of active extension may be seen on ROM testing. The cause is unknown but is not likely related to an arrest of embryologic meniscal development. Classic findings on AP x-ray include the following, but x-rays may be normal:

- Widened lateral joint space
- Squaring of the lateral femoral condyle
- Cupping of the lateral tibial plateau
- Hypoplastic lateral intercondylar spine

MRI is the diagnostic tool of choice, revealing a thick, flat meniscus generally seen on 3 consecutive MRI images. The Watanabe classification comprises the following categories.

- Incomplete
- Complete
- Wrisberg variant or lateral meniscal variant (absence of the posterior coronary ligament attachment to the tibia)

Complete or incomplete discoid menisci that are asymptomatic or found incidentally with no evidence of a tear should be treated with *observation*. Tears should be treated with saucerization of the meniscus, leaving a 6 to 8 mm rim of stable meniscus after the procedure. Some surgeons advocate complete meniscectomy for symptomatic Wrisberg discoid menisci; others recommend reattachment with meniscal repair techniques.

Meniscal Repair. The fibrochondrocyte is the cell responsible for healing tears. The clinician must take into account:

- Patient age and occupation
- Chronicity of injury
- Type, location, and length of tear
- Associated ligamentous injury (e.g., ACL)
- Relative urgency to return to sport or activity

For surgical consideration, the ideal candidate is a young patient with an acute, traumatic, longitudinal, peripheral meniscal tear that is 1 to 2 cm in length repaired in conjunction with an ACL reconstruction. Tear length, time from injury to repair, medial versus lateral meniscus, and the use of fibrin clot have not been shown to consistently affect meniscal healing.

Nonoperative healing is influenced mostly by the *rim width* (distance of the tear site from the peripheral meniscocapsular junction) (Fig. 3.17).

Meniscal cysts may occur commonly after horizontal cleavage tears of the lateral meniscus. They can be

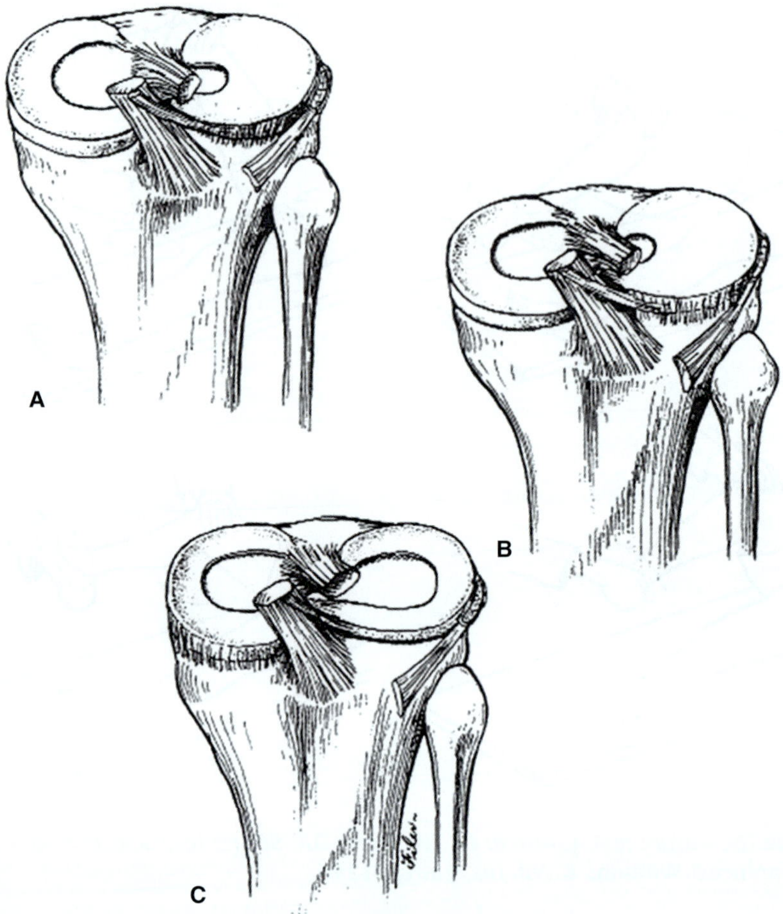

FIGURE 3.16 Three types of discoid menisci. (A) Partial (incomplete). (B) Complete. (C) Wrisberg variant. (*Source:* Neuschwander DC. Discoid meniscus. In: Fu FH, Harner CD, Vince KG (eds.), *Knee Surgery*. Baltimore: Williams & Wilkins, 1994: Fig. 1.60.)

treated with arthroscopic partial meniscectomy and decompression through the tear (Table 3.5). Popliteal cysts (Baker cysts) are associated with meniscus tears and usually resolve with treatment of the tear. Baker cysts are commonly located between the semimembranosus and medial head of the gastrocnemius muscles.

Osteochondral Pathology

Osteochondritis Dissecans (OCD). OCD is noted when a fragment of subchondral bone and its overlying cartilage are separated from the underlying bone. The etiology is uncertain but may be the result of trauma. The classic location is the lateral aspect of the medial femoral condyle (Fig. 3.18). There are many different classifications, but in general OCD can be classified as:

- In situ lesion
- Early separation lesion
- Incompletely detached lesion
- Completely detached lesion

Patients usually present with vague complaints of knee pain, with or without mechanical symptoms, swelling, effusion, and local tenderness. The Wilson sign is evidenced by pain with internal rotation and knee extension that is relieved with external rotation. Imaging studies should include a notch view and flexion weight-bearing AP view of the knee along with an MRI.

Treatment of children with open physes should include activity modification unless mechanical symptoms develop or fragment is loose on imaging. Ample evidence has shown that the prognosis of OCD in children is most influenced by the growth status of the physes. If physes are open, the chance of successful outcome is significantly greater than if closed.

Treatment in adults is guided by the general classification described previously.

- Type 1 lesions can be treated with retrograde drilling with or without bone graft.
- Type 2 lesions can be fixed with K-wires or absorbable pins to secure flap.

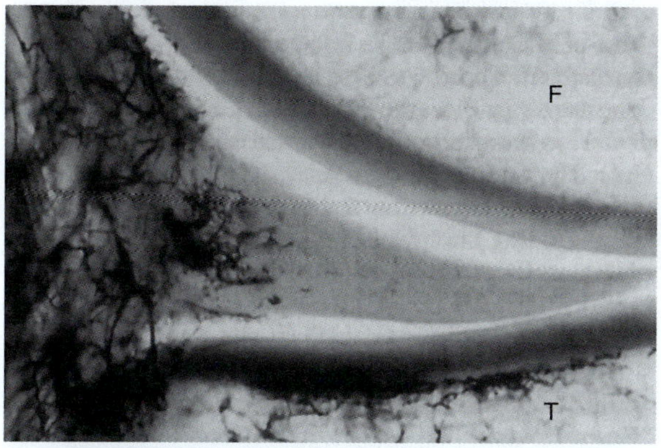

FIGURE 3.17 Five-millimeter-thick frontal section of the medial compartment of the knee after vascular perfusion with India ink and tissue clearing with a modified Spalteholz technique. Branching radial vessels from the perimeniscal capillary plexus (PCP) can be seen penetrating the peripheral border of the medial meniscus. *F*, femur; *T*, tibia. (*Source:* Arnoczky SP, Warren RF. Microvasculature of the human meniscus. *Am J Sports Med* 1982;10: 90–95.)

- Type 3 lesions involve removal of underlying fibrous tissue, abrasion chondroplasty or microfracture, possible bone grafting, then reduction and fixation of cartilage flap.
- Type 4 lesions involve removal of loose fragments, abrasion chondroplasty or microfracture, and consideration of osteochondral allograft transfer *(OATS procedure).*

Cartilage Injury. Pure isolated cartilage injury does not involve the subchondral bone. MRI is useful to distinguish between OCD and pure cartilage injury. Cartilage injuries are usually located on the weight-bearing surface of the medial compartment. Classification is based on the arthroscopic appearance because the x-rays are normal (unlike OCD lesions). MRI may be useful to distinguish from OCD (Fig. 3.19). Patients usually present with meniscal-like symptoms including effusion with or without mechanical symptoms. With a full-thickness cartilage lesion, a healing response is initiated with hematoma, stem cell migration, and vascular ingrowth. This response produces type I collagen and resultant fibrous cartilage rather than desired hyaline cartilage as produced by chondrocytes. This repair cartilage has diminished resiliency, stiffness, poor wear characteristics, and the predilection for arthritis. Type II collagen is found in normal articular cartilage.

Treatment is controversial and still evolving, but options include débridement and contouring for

TABLE 3.5 Meniscal repair techniques

Repair Technique	*Description*
Open meniscal repair	1. Capsular exposure through longitudinal incision 2. Preparation of meniscal rim and capsular bed 3. Placement of vertically oriented sutures at 5–10 mm intervals Note: *Vertically* oriented suture placement is strongest and yields most anatomic repair
Inside-out meniscal repair	1. Arthroscopic single- or double-barrel cannula is used to pass suture through meniscal tear after arthroscopic preparation of tear edges 2. Long Keith needle is retrieved by assistant through a small posterior incision taken down to capsule 3. Sutures are tied over capsule from outside
Outside-in meniscal repair	1. Uses separate 1–2 cm incisions for each suture pair 2. An 18-gauge spinal needle is placed across tear from outside the joint after arthroscopic preparation of meniscus 3. Suture is passed through needle into the joint and secured by a mulberry knot technique
All-inside technique	1. After arthroscopic preparation of the tear edges, a cannulated suture hook is used to pierce both sides of the tear, and suture is passed through the hook across the torn edges 2. Sutures are secured arthroscopically using a knot pusher

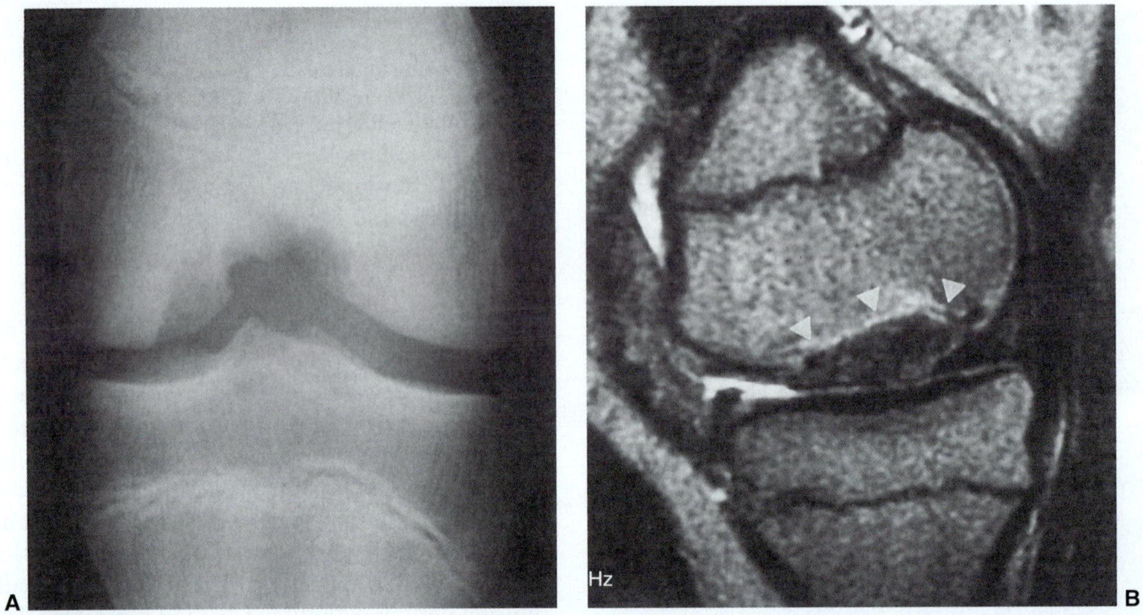

FIGURE 3.18 **Osteochondritis dissecans in an 18-year-old man. (A) Plain film shows a defect in lateral aspect of medial femoral condyle. (B) Sagittal T2-weighted spin-echo image showing slightly increased signal around the osteochondral fragment suggesting loosening (arrowheads). (*Source:* Garrett WE, Speer KP, Kirkendall DT. *Principles and Practice of Orthopaedic Sports Medicine*. Philadelphia: Lippincott Williams & Wilkins, 2000; 106.)**

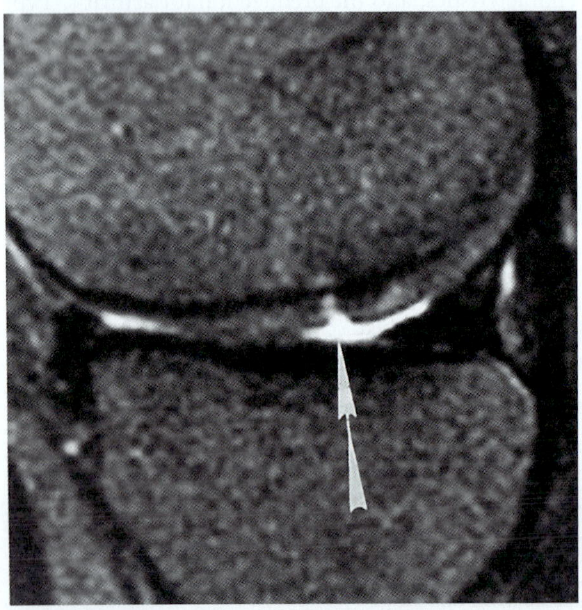

FIGURE 3.19 **Sagittal T2-weighted, fast spin-echo image that shows a focal full-thickness cartilage injury in a patient with medial pain with activity. (*Source:* Garrett WE, Speer KP, Kirkendall DT. *Principles and Practice of Orthopaedic Sports Medicine*. Philadelphia: Lippincott Williams & Wilkins, 2000; 105.)**

partial-thickness cartilage injuries. Chondroplasty or transfer/implantation can treat full-thickness injuries that extend down to bone. Additional options include:

- Microfracture for smaller lesions (less than 2 cm^2)
- Osteochondral plug transfer (OATS or mosaicplasty) for larger lesions
- Autologous chondrocyte implantation (ACI)
- Osteochondral allograft of large area of bone loss

Pigmented Villonodular Synovitis (PVNS). Emanates from the synovium. The knee joint is most commonly affected with arthroscopic appearance of brownish proliferative synovium. The etiology of PVNS is unknown and is categorized as diffuse or localized. The diffuse form is proliferative; the local form tends to be a nodular single lesion (Fig. 3.20). PVNS is histologically similar to giant cell tumor of tendon sheath and is characterized by histiocytes (foam cells), giant cells, hemosiderin deposition, and fibrous tissue. Patients tend to present with pain, swelling, and effusion (hemarthrosis). X-rays may demonstrate bony erosions, but MRI is the preferred imaging modality. Treatment is synovectomy, but there is a high recurrence rate with the diffuse type. Arthroscopic synovectomy is equal to open treatment, especially for the local nodular type. Significant disease extending to the popliteal fossa may be best reached with open technique. The popliteal fossa is bordered by the gastrocnemius muscles, semimembranosus, and

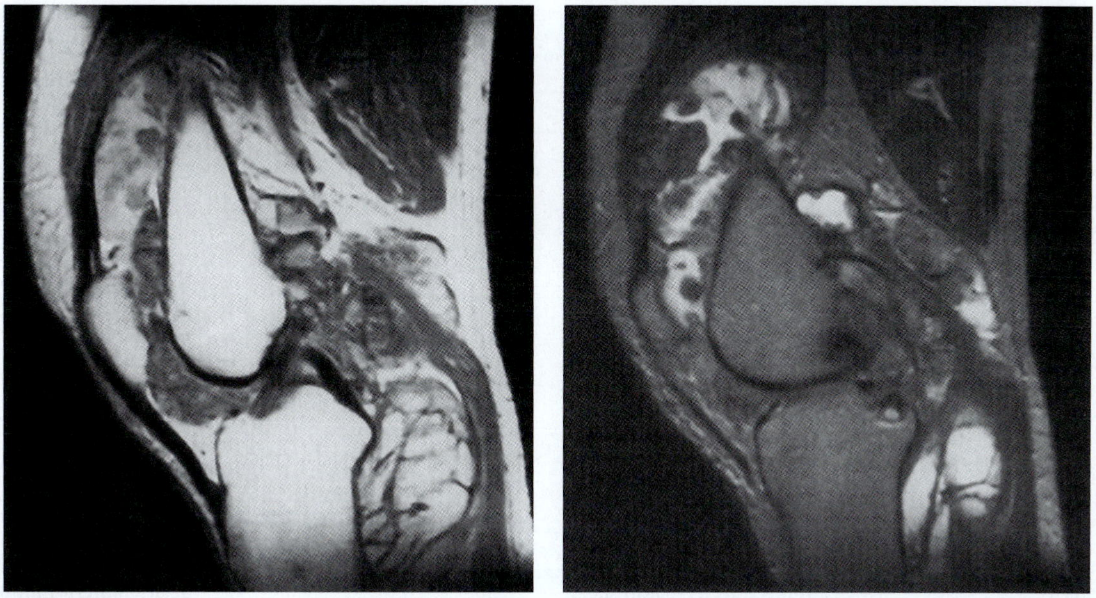

FIGURE 3.20 Sagittal SE 500/20 (A) and SE 2,000/60 (B) images of the knee in a patient with pigmented villonodular synovitis. Note the multiple large areas of decreased intensity in the distended joint on the T2-weighted sequence. (*Source:* Berquist TH. *MRI of the Musculoskeletal System*. Philadelphia: Lippincott Williams & Wilkins, 2001; 414.)

biceps. The plantaris muscle makes up the floor of the fossa.

Refractory cases may require local chemotherapy and radiation treatment.

Synovial Chondromatosis. This proliferative synovial disease leads to loose bodies in the joint. Treatment consists of loose body removal and synovectomy if indicated.

Synovial Plicae. Synovial plicae are synovial folds that represent embryologic remnants of partitions that originally separated the knee joint into three synovial compartments. Four plicae have been described on the basis of their location in relation to the patella (suprapatellar, infrapatellar, medial, and lateral). Medial patellar plica is the most common to be clinically significant because it passes over the medial femoral condyle. It may become irritated and thickened from trauma or inflammation. The diagnosis can be made clinically by eliciting tenderness and "snapping" over the medial femoral condyle at 30 to 40 degrees of knee flexion. Conservative treatment is recommended, but occasional arthroscopic resection is necessary. Plicae that are detected incidentally on arthroscopy should be observed.

II. HIP

Surgical Anatomy. Table 3.6 reviews surgical approaches to the hip.

Stress Fractures of the Femoral Neck. Femoral neck stress fractures may be seen in military personnel and athletes, especially cross-country skiers. Releasing the bindings may decrease the incidence. MRI and bone scan are the best studies for diagnosis. Treatment usually includes protected weight bearing, rest, cross-training, analgesia, and therapeutics. However, management depends on location of the lesion. Compression side fractures can be managed nonoperatively with rest and nonimpact cross-training until healed (generally 3 to 6 months). Tension (transverse) side fractures should be fixed operatively with multiple cannulated screws (Fig. 3.21).

Traumatic Hip Dislocations. Traumatic hip dislocations are rare sports injuries that may be encountered in high-impact sports like football. Subluxation of the hip may occur with a direct fall on a flexed knee. In dislocations without fracture, *osteonecrosis* is the most common complication, occurring in 15% of cases. Prompt, atraumatic reduction is the key to minimizing the risk of subsequent osteonecrosis. Nerve injuries are rare in this setting, and recurrent instability and dislocations are unusual in the absence of associated acetabular fracture. MRI should be performed 3 to 6 months after the injury to evaluate for osteonecrosis.

Muscle Contusion Injuries. Caused by a direct blow, muscle contusion injuries are treated with a 3-phase treatment program: (1) short period of immobilization with the muscle in a lengthened

TABLE 3.6 Surgical approaches to the hip

Approach	Superficial Muscle (Innervation)	Deep Muscles (Innervation)	Structures at Risk
Posterior iliac crest	Gluteus maximus (inferior gluteal)	Latissimus dorsi (thoracodorsal)	Clunial nerve, superior gluteal artery, sciatic
Anterior iliac crest	TFL/gluteus medius and minimus (superior gluteal)	External abdominal obliques (segmental)	ASIS/LFCN
Anterior (Smith-Peterson)	Sartorius/rectus femoris (femoral)	TFL/gluteus medius (superior gluteal)	LFCN, femoral nerve, ascending branch of LFCA
Anterolateral (Watson-Jones)	TFL (superior gluteal)	Gluteus medius (superior gluteal)	Femoral nerve, artery, vein/profunda artery
Lateral (Hardinge)	Splits gluteus medius (superior gluteal)	Splits vastus lateralis (femoral)	Femoral nerve, vein, artery/LFCA transverse branch
Posterior (Moore-Southern)	Splits gluteus maximus (inferior gluteal)		Sciatic, inferior gluteal artery
Medial (Ludloff)	Adductor longus/ adductor brevis (anterior division of the obturator)	Gracilis/adductor magnus (obt/tibial)	Anterior division obturator nerve/MFCA

position (flexion), (2) passive and active ROM exercises, and (3) strengthening. Hemorrhage and late myositis ossificans can result. Close monitoring for compartment syndrome is required.

Iliac Crest Contusions (Hip Pointers). The injuries result from a direct blow to the iliac crest and occur frequently in contact sports. In adolescents, avulsion of the iliac apophysis can accompany hip pointers. Treatment for both conditions is conservative and consists of rest, ice, and ROM exercises, followed by strengthening. Uneventful return to sports is the norm.

Quadriceps Contusions. Common in contact sports, quadriceps contusions are significant because of their potential to develop into myositis ossificans. Myositis ossificans is extraskeletal ossification that occurs in muscles and other soft tissues, generally as a result of trauma. Severe blunt trauma (e.g., football helmet

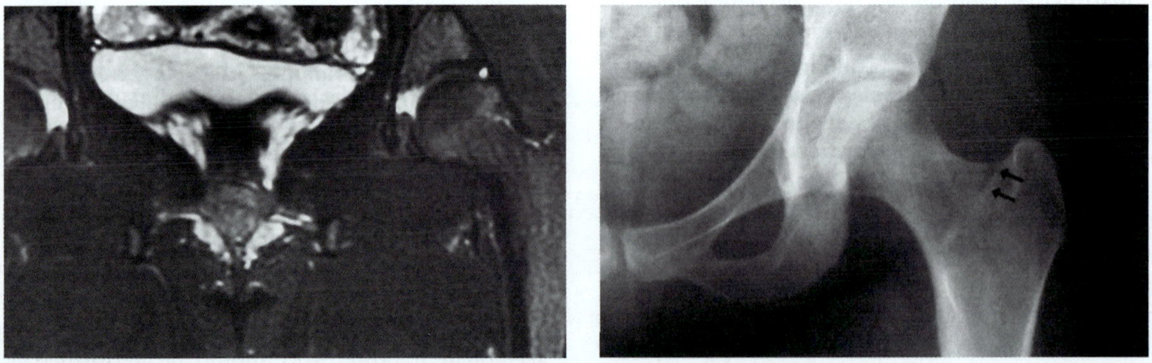

A B

FIGURE 3.21 (A) Magnetic resonance image demonstrating a stress fracture of the medial femoral neck. (B) The arrows indicate a stress fracture of the superior aspect of the femoral neck. (*Source:* Garrett WE, Speer KP, Kirkendall DT. *Principles and Practice of Orthopaedic Sports Medicine*. Philadelphia: Lippincott Williams & Wilkins, 2000; 573.)

to the thigh) causes an intramuscular hematoma that may result in delayed ossification. Myositis ossificans typically occurs in the quadriceps and presents as a painful, enlarging mass in the thigh. X-rays demonstrate soft tissue ossification not attached to bone with peripheral "egg shell" maturation, the reverse of that seen in a malignant tumor. Treatment consists of rest and brief immobilization followed by ROM exercise. Passive stretching is contraindicated during rehabilitation because it may potentiate the severity of myositis ossificans. Spontaneous resolution is the norm. In refractory cases, excision may be carried out but should not be performed prior to maturation of the lesion (minimum of 6 months).

Muscle Strains. Generally, muscle strains occur at the myotendinous junction of muscles that cross two joints and contain a high percentage of type II (fast-twitch) fibers. The hamstring is the most commonly injured muscle, although strains also occur in the adductors and rectus femoris. Initial treatment consists of rest, ice, elevation, NSAIDs, and compression for relief of pain and swelling. As pain and swelling decrease, physical therapy can be initiated to improve ROM and strength. Athletes may return to full activity once full ROM and strength are attained.

Bursitis. Thirteen bursae are present around the hip and thigh, and they all have the potential to develop inflammation and pain. Bursitis is difficult to diagnose and may often be confused with other pathology. Trochanteric bursitis is common in female athletes and is characterized by pain over the greater trochanter. Treatment includes NSAIDs, activity modification and stretching. Corticosteroid injections are reserved for refractory cases.

Piriformis Syndrome. Piriformis syndrome is best characterized by localized posterior buttock pain and radicular symptoms in the sciatic distribution. These symptoms are caused by compression of the sciatic nerve by the piriformis muscle. Treatment is conservative, although surgical decompression has been reported with some success.

Athletic Pubalgia (Sports Hernia). Athletic pubalgia is a distinct syndrome of lower abdominal and adductor pain that is most commonly seen in high performance male athletes, especially soccer. This syndrome can be caused by acute trauma or repetitive microtrauma. The diagnosis is one of exclusion and is primarily made clinically, although MRI can sometimes be helpful. This condition should be distinguished from osteitis pubis, which is painful inflammation of the symphysis pubis. Treatment is conservative, although surgical repair of the pelvic floor may be indicated in some high-performance athletes.

Snapping Hip (Coxa Saltans). This is characterized by an audible snapping of the hip that usually occurs during flexion and extension of the hip, coxa saltans is caused by either a thickened iliotibial band that snaps forward over the greater trochanter or by iliopsoas impingement over the hip capsule. Commonly seen in females with wide pelves and prominent trochanters, this condition may be exacerbated by running on banked surfaces. Diagnosis is made clinically, and most patients describe a snapping, painful sensation over the greater trochanter, which is readily reproducible with passive hip flexion from an adducted position. Note the difference from the less commonly diagnosed snapping iliopsoas tendon, which can be diagnosed with extension and internal rotation of the hip from a flexed and externally rotated position. Arthrography and/or bursography may aid diagnosis. Treatment is conservative and consists of stretching, avoidance of offending activities, and steroid injections. Bursectomies or surgical tendon lengthening are reserved for refractory cases with persistent pain and disability. Arthroscopic release can be performed but complete release may cause weakness.

Hip Arthroscopy. Hip arthroscopy is still infrequently performed in the United States largely because of the technically demanding nature of the procedure, the need for specialized equipment, and the risk of neurovascular injury from inaccurate portal placement. Many potential indications exist, but the clearest indications are for removal of loose bodies, débridement of labral tears, and irrigation and débridement of a septic joint. Impingement can be the result of a cam or pincer effect and may be treated arthroscopically with bony débridement. Most examination questions focus on portal placement and the neurovascular structures at risk during this placement. The three most common portals are the anterior portal, the anterior paratrochanteric portal, and the posterior paratrochanteric portal (Fig. 3.22). The structures at risk when placing the anterior portal include the lateral femoral cutaneous nerve superficially and the ascending branch of the deeper lateral femoral circumflex artery. The femoral artery and nerve are 3 to 4 cm away and should not be an issue unless portal misplacement occurs. The anterior and posterior paratrochanteric portals are placed laterally over the superior margin of the greater trochanter at its anterior and posterior borders. The anterior paratrochanteric portal is fairly safe, although the femoral neurovascular bundle can be damaged if the arthroscope is directed too anteriorly. The posterior paratrochanteric portal is potentially hazardous, and the hip should not be externally rotated because the sciatic nerve is brought into danger with this move.

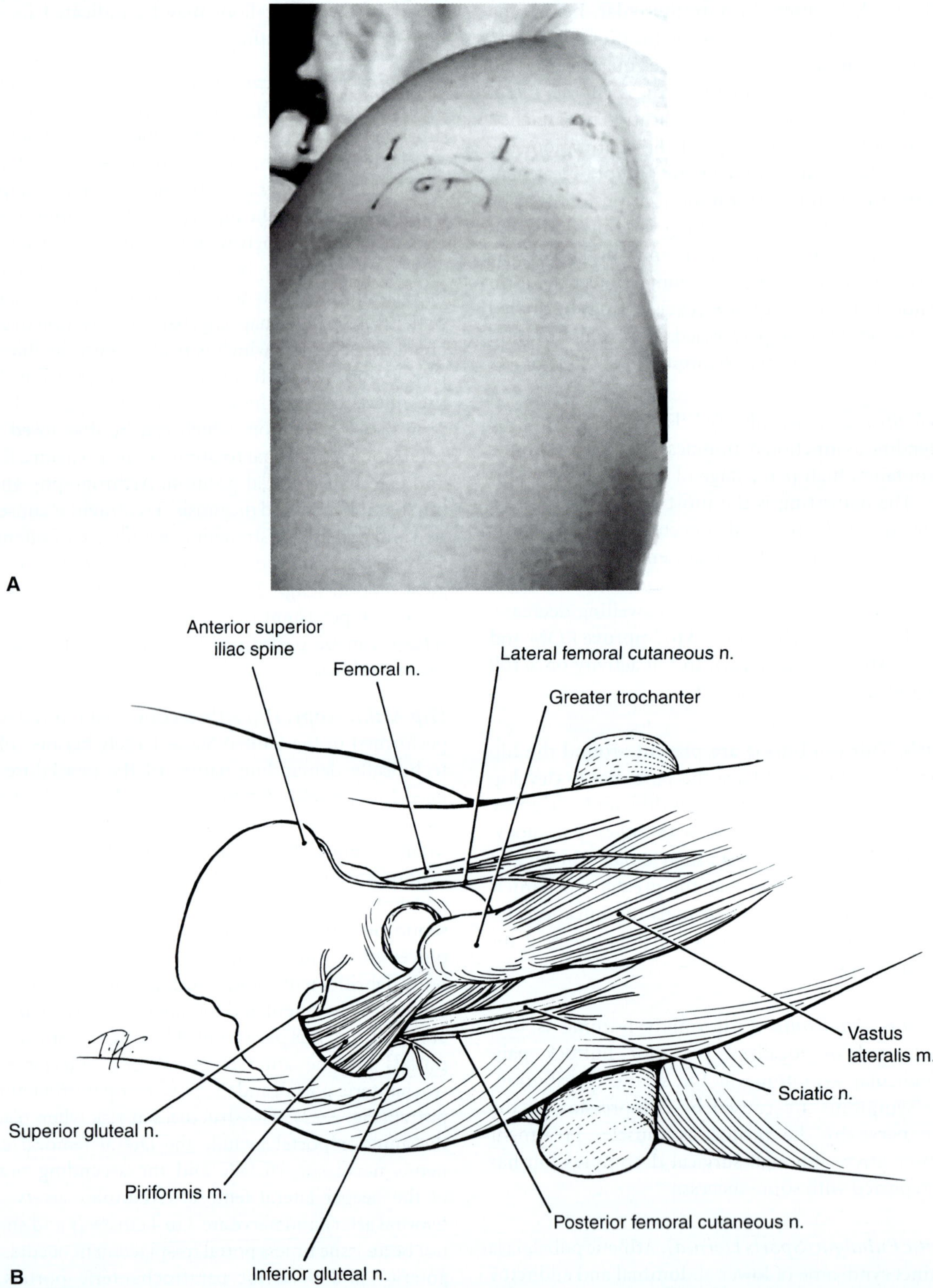

FIGURE 3.22 **(A) Main arthroscopic portals for hip arthroscopy. (B) Relevant hip anatomy in relation to portals. (*Source:* Buly RL, Maynard MJ. Arthroscopy of the hip. In: Craig EV (ed.). *Clinical Orthopaedics*. Philadelphia: Lippincott Williams & Wilkins, 1999.)**

III. FOOT AND ANKLE

Surgical Anatomy. Tables 3.7, 3.8, and 3.9 review the anatomic relationships and muscles of the leg and surgical approaches to the foot and ankle.

Peroneal Tendon Injuries

The peroneal tendons pass posterior to the fibula and are restrained by the superior peroneal retinaculum, the primary stabilizer of the tendons. (Fig. 3.23).

Subluxation/Dislocation. Subluxation or dislocation of the peroneal tendons is difficult to diagnose and often confused with lateral ankle sprains. Both injuries are common in skiers and associated with rapid dorsiflexion and inversion of the foot and ankle, which injure the fibro-osseous tendon sheath. Tenderness over the lateral retromalleolar region and apprehension or frank subluxation of the tendons with active dorsiflexion strongly suggests the diagnosis. An avulsion fracture of the distal tip of the fibula by the superior retinaculum is characteristic for peroneal tendon subluxation or dislocation. Treatment remains controversial, but most experts agree that initial management should consist of cast immobilization and protected weight bearing for 6 weeks. Surgery is reserved for recurrent or chronic conditions. Chronic reconstruction involves groove-deepening procedures, tissue transfer, or bone-block techniques.

Longitudinal Tears of the Peroneal Brevis. Tears of the peroneus brevis occur when the anterior portion of the tendon slips forward and is lacerated by the sharp posterior ridge of the fibula (Fig. 3.24). The increased use of diagnostic MRI has allowed this condition to be recognized as a distinct clinical entity. In general, conservative treatment is unsuccessful. Surgical options range from primary repair of the tendon to excision of the degenerated segment and tenodesis of the ends to the peroneus longus.

TABLE 3.7 Anatomic relationships of interest

Location	Structures
Knot of Henry	FDL–FHL intersection
Sustentaculum tali	Spring ligament (FHL inferior)
Base of fifth MT	Peroneus brevis/ plantar aponeurosis
Navicular tuberosity	Tibialis posterior
Cuboid groove	Peroneus longus
Sinus tarsi	Ligamentum cervis tali and EDB

Posterior Tibial Tendon. The high incidence of posterior tibial tendon inflammation is not surprising given the high functional strain placed on the tendon as it slingshots around the medial malleolus and inserts onto the navicular. Patients initially complain of pain and weak plantar flexion. Once complete rupture occurs, patients also demonstrate a hindfoot valgus and flatfoot deformity. Treatment depends on the level of involvement of the posterior tibial tendon. Swelling and inflammation of the tendon for only a few weeks warrants conservative treatment with 4 to 6 weeks of cast immobilization. Once complete rupture occurs, primary tendon repair or tendon reconstruction for chronic injuries using the flexor digitorum communis is indicated.

Achilles Tendon Injuries. Achilles tendon injuries encompass a continuum of disorders from tendonitis to complete rupture. Tendinitis and partial tendon ruptures are often the result of overuse and are commonly seen in runners. Treatment includes rest and physical therapy. Complete rupture of the Achilles tendon is caused by forceful plantar flexion while the foot is planted in a neutral position. Tendon rupture is often associated with a painful pop, and the patient may relate a feeling of being "shot" or "kicked" in the ankle. The diagnosis is made clinically by palpating a defect in the tendon and by eliciting a positive Thompson test (plantar flexion of the foot while squeezing the calf). In equivocal cases or in the presence of partial disruptions, MRI may aid in the diagnosis (Fig. 3.25). Treatment remains controversial, with surgical repair offering the advantage of a lower re-rupture rate and improved strength, but the disadvantage of wound complications and the potential for infection. Motion, pain, and recovery time are not specifically improved by surgical treatment. Chronic or neglected Achilles tendon ruptures can present a surgical problem, since end-to-end apposition of the tendon may not be accomplished without putting the foot in marked equinus. A tendon defect of greater than 5 cm requires the use of a tendon transfer (ideally the FHL) either alone or in combination with a V-Y advancement of the gastrocnemius. End-to-end tendon repair can reduce the recurrence rate.

Stress Fractures. Overuse injuries of the bone are commonly seen in athletes and military recruits. The etiology is multifactorial and believed to be caused by repetitive, submaximal loads on bones that cause an imbalance between bone resorption and formation. The classic presentation is the insidious onset of bony pain after an abrupt increase in the duration or

TABLE 3.8 Muscles of the leg

Muscle	Origin	Insertion	Action	Innervation
		Anterior Compartment		
Tibialis anterior	Lateral tibia	Medial cuneiform, first metatarsal	Dorsiflex, invert foot	Deep peroneal (L4)
Extensor hallucis longus	Middle fibula	Great toe distal phalanx	Dorsiflex, extend toe	Deep peroneal (L5)
Extensor digitorium longus	Tibial condyle/fibula	Middle and distal phalanges	Dorsiflex, extend toes	Deep peroneal (L5)
Peroneus tertius	Fibula and EDL tendon	Fifth metatarsal	Evert, plantar flex, abduct foot	Deep peroneal (S1)
		Lateral Compartment		
Peroneus longus	Proximal fibula	Medial cuneiform, first metatarsal	Evert, plantar flex, abduct foot	Superficial peroneal (S1)
Peroneus brevis	Distal fibula	Fifth metatarsal tuberosity	Evert foot	Superficial peroneal (S1)
		Superficial Posterior Compartment		
Gastrocnemius	Posterior medial and lateral femoral condyles	Calcaneus	Plantar flex foot	Tibial (S1)
Soleus	Fibula/tibia	Calcaneus	Plantar flex foot	Tibial (S1)
Plantaris	Lateral femoral condyle	Calcaneus	Plantar flex foot	Tibial (S1)
		Deep Posterior Compartent		
Popliteus	Lateral femoral condyle, fibular head	Proximal tibia	Flex, IR knee	Tibial (L5,S1)
Flexor hallucis longus	Fibula	Great toe distal phalanx	Plantar flex great toe	Tibial (S1)
Flexor digitorium longus	Tibia	Second to fifth toe distal phalanges	Plantar flex toes, foot	Tibial (S1-2)
Tibialis posterior	Tibia, fibula, interosseous membrane	Navicular, medial cuneiform	Invert/plantar flex foot	Tibial (L4-5)

intensity of exercise. Radiographs will pick up obvious fractures. However, bone scans and MRI are more sensitive and are often used to confirm the diagnosis.

Tibial Stress Fracture. The most common stress fractures seen in athletes are of the tibia. The transverse, anterior, tension-sided tibial stress fracture is particularly worrisome given its propensity to progress to complete fracture or nonunion. Initial treatment consists of rest with or without immobilization for a minimum of 4 to 6 months. Persistence of the fracture either clinically or radiographically after 4 to 6 months of rest mandates excision, bone grafting, and compression plating (Fig. 3.26). Tibial rodding has been performed for transverse tibial stress fractures, but incomplete, anterior, tension-sided tibial stress fractures at times require anterior compression plating.

Tarsal Navicular Stress Fracture. Typically seen in jumping athletes like basketball players, tarsal navicular stress fracture presents as the insidious onset of pain in the medial arch of the foot that is aggravated by activity. Most navicular stress fractures are oriented in the sagittal plane and involve the dorsal/central aspect

TABLE 3.9 Surgical approaches to the foot and ankle

Approach	*Superficial Muscle (Innervation)*	*Deep Muscles (Innervation)*	*Structures at Risk*
Anterior parapatellar	EHL (deep peroneal)	EDL (deep peroneal)	Saphenous nerve and vein
Posterior medial malleolus	Tibialis posterior	FDL	Saphenous nerve and vein
Posterolateral	Peroneus brevis (superficial peroneal)	FHL (tibial)	Sural nerve/small saphenous vein
Lateral fibula	Peroneus tertius (deep peroneal)	Peroneus brevis (superficial peroneal)	Sural nerve
Anterolateral	Peroneal muscles (superificial peroneal)	EDC and peroneus tertius (deep peroneal)	Deep peroneal nerve/ anterior tibial artery
Posteromedial	TP and FDL	FDL or FHL	Posterior tibial artery/ tibial nerve

of the navicular. These fractures are often difficult to recognize on plain radiographs because of the overlap of adjacent bones. Oblique x-rays offer the best view of navicular stress fractures. MRI can be helpful and usually shows a linear low-signal fracture line that usually extends to the talonavicular joint. Marrow edema and sclerosis usually surround the fracture line. Bone scanning may be useful to determine the chronicity of the fracture, and sequential CT scanning may be useful to evaluate healing after appropriate treatment has been provided. If diagnosed early, these fractures may be treated in a nonweight-bearing short-leg cast for 6 to 8 weeks. However, nonoperative treatment is associated with a high nonunion rate. In high caliber athletes or if symptoms have been present for several months, ORIF with bone grafting is generally recommended.

Fifth Metatarsal Stress Fracture. These fractures generally occur at the junction of the proximal metaphyseal–diaphyseal junction. Treatment depends on the stage of the lesion and the caliber of the athlete. If symptoms are present for more than 3 weeks and x-rays are positive for fracture, then treatment should include nonweight-bearing cast immobilization for 6 weeks. Internal fixation with a compression screw is indicated for high-demand athletes or in nonunions.

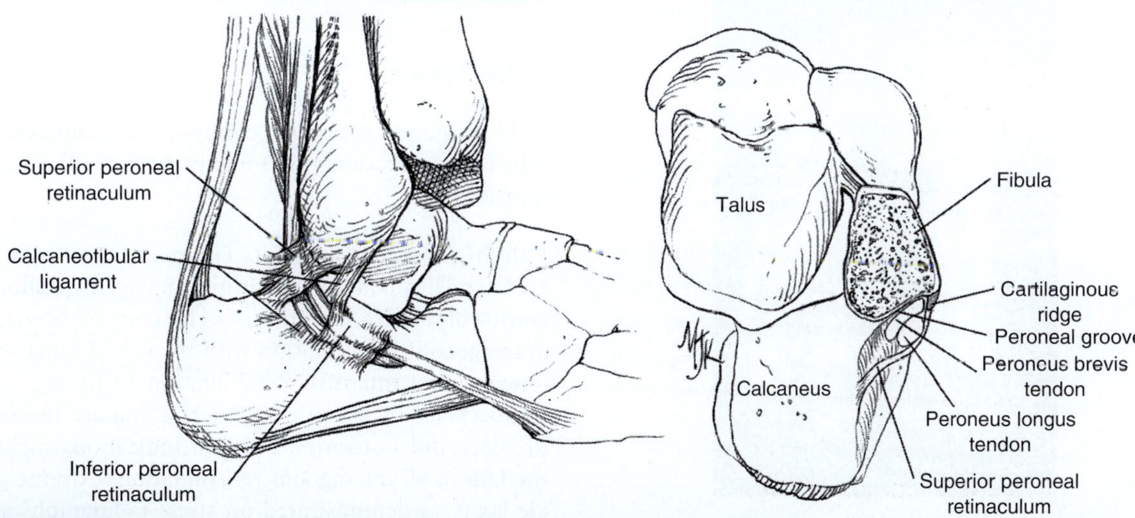

FIGURE 3.23 Anatomic relationships at the lateral aspect of the ankle. Note on the cross-section that the peroneal groove is supplemented by a fibrocartilaginous ridge. (*Source:* Garrett WE, Speer KP, Kirkendall DT. *Principles and Practice of Orthopaedic Sports Medicine.* Philadelphia: Lippincott Williams & Wilkins, 2000; 991.)

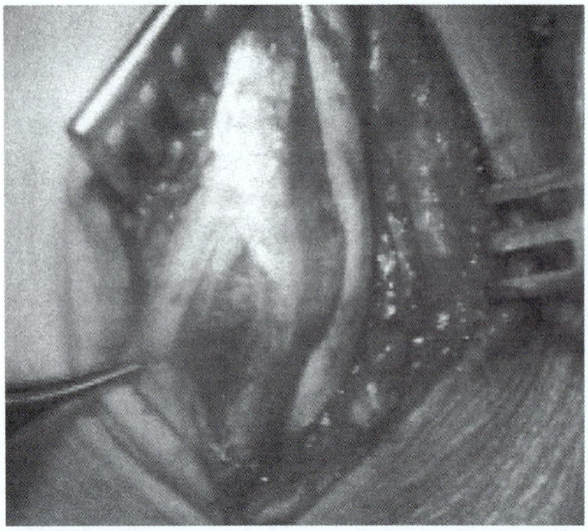

FIGURE 3.24 Complete longitudinal tear of the peroneus brevis, dislocated over the tip of the fibula. The peroneus longus remains reduced. (*Source:* Jones DC. Tendon disorders of the foot and ankle. *J Am Acad Orthop Surg* 1993;1: 90.)

Os Trigonum. An unhealed os trigonum fracture can cause impingement with plantar flexion, especially in ballet dancers. Nonoperative treatment includes local anesthetic injection and supportive footwear. Surgical excision is reserved for refractory cases.

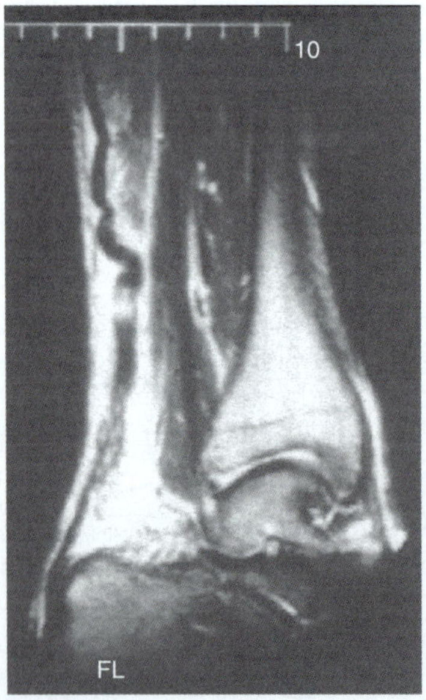

FIGURE 3.25 MRI of a partial longitudinal tear of the Achilles tendon. (*Source:* Jones DC. Tendon disorders of the foot and ankle. *J Am Acad Orthop Surg* 1993;1: 92.)

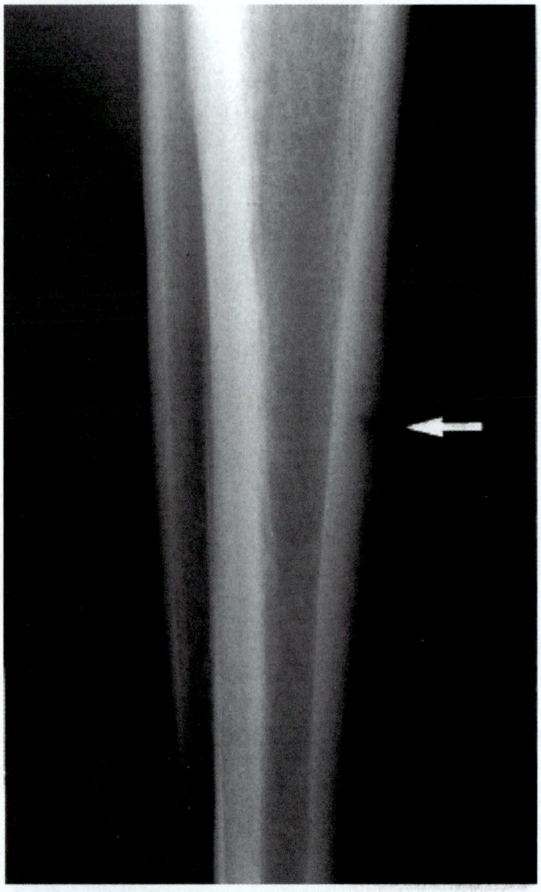

FIGURE 3.26 "Dreaded black line," anterior tibial stress fracture. (*Source:* Boden BP. High-risk stress fractures: Evaluation and treatment. *J Am Acad Orthop Surg* 2000;8: 346.)

Ankle Sprains

Ankle sprains are very common musculoskeletal injuries and account for roughly 40% of all athletic injuries.

Lateral Ligament Injuries. The majority of injuries are lateral ligament sprains. Initial management should consist of rest, ice, elevation, and bracing. Early weight bearing, controlled motion with the use of functional bracing, and intensive rehabilitation including neuromuscular and proprioceptive training are the keys to successful outcomes. Surgical indications include the failure of bracing and rehabilitation, extreme ankle laxity as demonstrated on stress radiographs and confirmed by clinical testing (anterior drawer and inversion/eversion stress testing), and recurrent ankle sprains with activities of daily living. The ATFL (anterior talofibular ligament) and the CFL (calcaneofibular ligament) are the primary stabilizers of the lateral ankle,

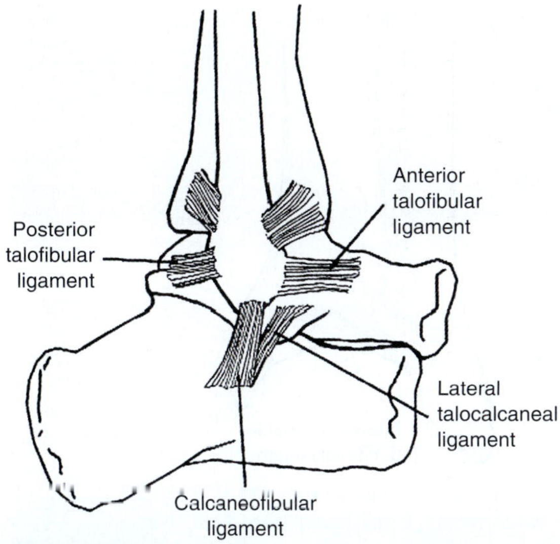

FIGURE 3.27 **Lateral ligaments of the ankle. (*Source:* Canale ST (ed.). *Campbell's Operative Orthopaedics*, 10th ed. St. Louis: Mosby-Year Book, 2003; 2132.)**

and surgical procedures should be aimed at restoring the normal function of these ligaments (Fig. 3.27). Direct repair of the ATFL and CFL with shortening and reattachment to the fibula has a high success rate. Augmented reconstructions using the peroneus brevis tendon should be reserved for patients with severe laxity or with insufficient tissue for direct repair.

Deltoid Ligament Injuries. Isolated injuries to the deltoid ligament are rare. Deltoid ligament injuries are usually associated with lateral malleolus fractures. Successful treatment of the lateral malleolus fracture, either by immobilization in a nonweight-bearing cast or by ORIF, concomitantly addresses the deltoid ligament injury (Fig. 3.28).

Syndesmotic Ankle Injuries. The distal lower extremity syndesmosis is made up of four ligaments and the interosseous membrane (Fig. 3.29). Disruption of the syndesmosis is most commonly associated with ankle fractures (Weber C) but also can occur without gross bone injury (high ankle sprain). Beware of a possible associated proximal fibula fracture. The mechanism of injury is commonly excessive external rotation of the pronated foot. The squeeze test and the external-rotation stress test are very sensitive clinical signs of a syndesmotic injury (Fig. 3.30). Tibiofibular clear space of greater than 6 mm on both anterior–posterior and Mortise is the most reliable predictor of early syndesmotic widening. If the diagnosis remains uncertain, stress radiographs, bone scan, or a CT scan of both ankles may be helpful. Gross instability indicated by clear space greater than 6 mm on standard radiographs or diastasis on stress radiographs generally requires closed reduction and stabilization with a transsyndesmotic screw. If gross instability is not present, treatment in a short-leg, nonweight-bearing cast for 4 weeks is adequate. High ankle sprains consistently require longer recovery times than typical lateral ankle sprains and can be associated with greater long-term disability. Removal of syndesmotic screws prior to weightbearing is controversial, but if performed, should be done so at about three months (prior to full-weightbearing on the ankle).

Exertional Compartment Syndrome. Athletes with exertional compartment syndrome have exercise-induced pain in the leg muscles that can linger

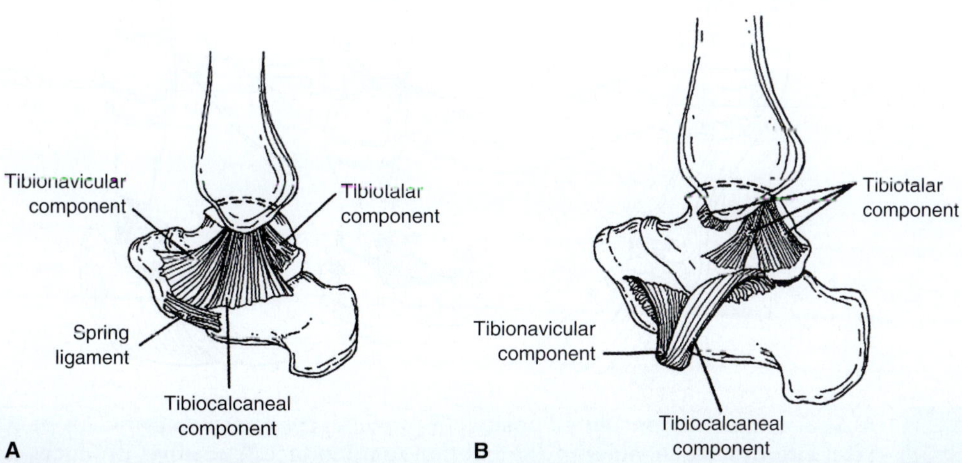

FIGURE 3.28 **Anatomy of the medial part of the ankle to show the (A) superficial and (B) deep deltoid ligament. (*Source:* Canale ST (ed.). *Campbell's Operative Orthopaedics*, 10th ed. St. Louis: Mosby-Year Book, 2003; 2132.)**

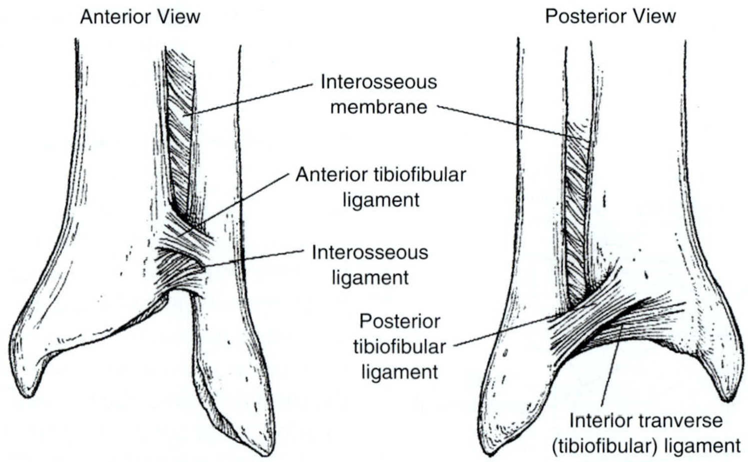

FIGURE 3.29 **Anatomy of the distal lower extremity syndesmosis. Four ligaments and the interosseous ligament combine to form the tibiofibular syndesmosis. (*Source:* Wuest TK. Injuries to the distal lower extremity syndesmosis. *J Am Acad Orthop Surg* 1997; 5:173.)**

for hours after cessation of activity. The condition is related to muscle ischemia caused by elevated compartment pressures, usually in the anterior and deep posterior compartments. Diagnosis is confirmed by intracompartmental pressure monitoring. Patients with the disorder have preexercise compartment pressure higher than 15 mm Hg and a 1-minute postexercise pressure higher than 30 mm Hg, or a 5-minute postexercise pressure higher than 20 mm Hg when compared to the other side. Treatment consists of subcutaneous fasciotomies using small incisions that may be assisted with a dry arthroscope to visualize fascial compartment release (Fig. 3.31).

Anterior Ankle Impingement. Anterior ankle impingement is characterized by chronic anterior ankle pain and swelling caused by the overuse of dorsiflexors in athletes. This condition is frequently observed in competitive soccer, rugby, track (jumpers), and football players. Other hallmarks include pain with forced dorsiflexion and anterior tibiotalar osteophytes on radiographs or MRI (Fig. 3.32). Treatment consists of

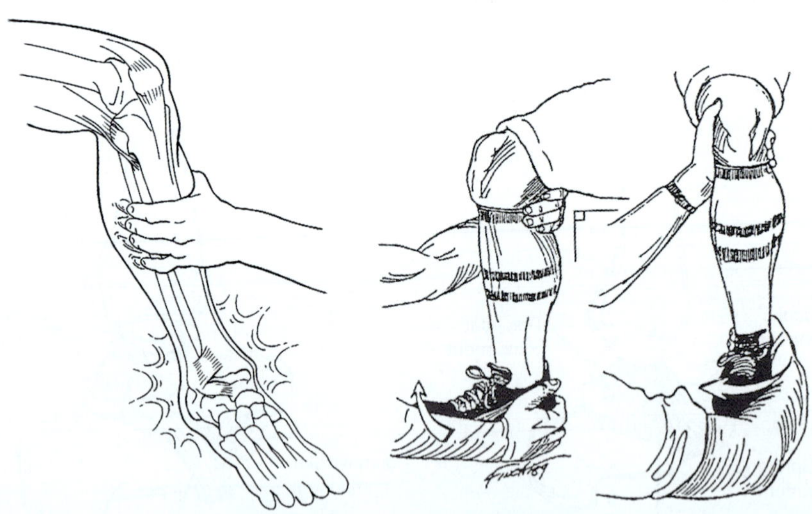

FIGURE 3.30 **(A) Squeeze test is considered positive if proximal compression produces pain in the distal interosseous ligaments. (B) External rotation test, if positive, produces pain over the anterior or posterior interosseous ligaments and over the interosseous membrane. (*Source:* Canale ST (ed.). *Campbell's Operative Orthopaedics*, 10th ed. St. Louis: Mosby-Year Book, 2003; 2137.)**

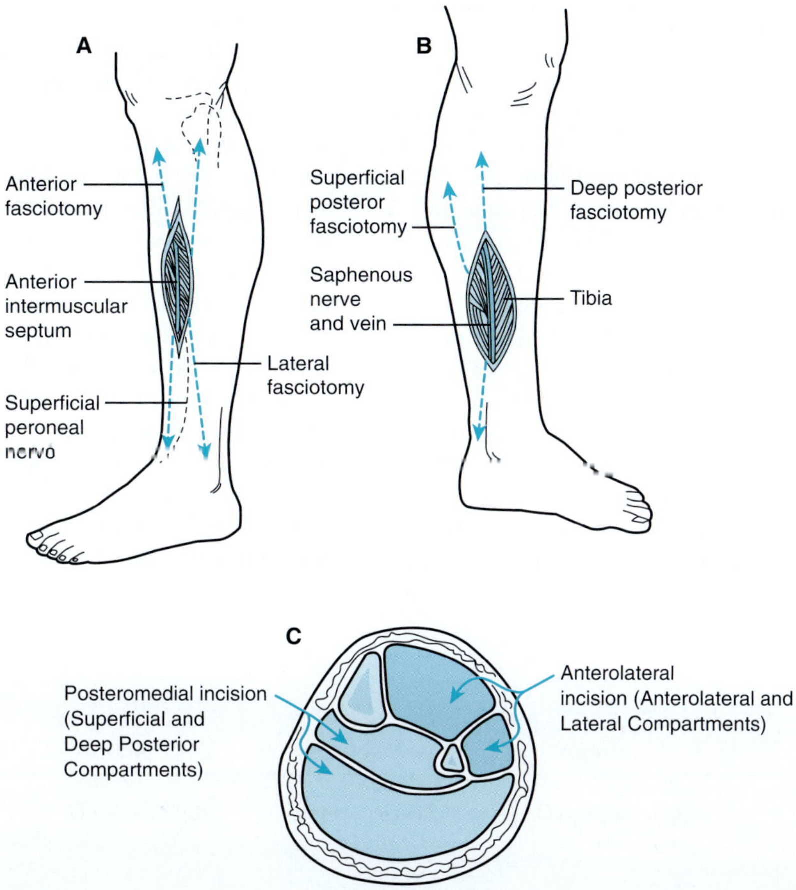

FIGURE 3.31 **Method for decompression of the compartments of the leg. (A) Anterolateral incision, (B) posteromedial incision, (C) decompression of all four compartments. (*Adapted from* Canale ST (ed.), *Campbell's Operative Orthopaedics*, 10th ed. St. Louis: Mosby-Year Book, 2003; 2454.)**

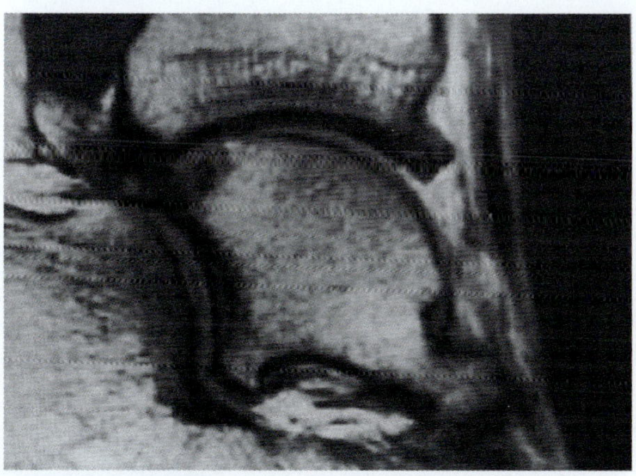

FIGURE 3.32 **T1-weighted sagittal MRI of the ankle demonstrating anterior impingement. (*Source:* Canale ST (ed.), *Campbell's Operative Orthopaedics*, 10th ed. St. Louis: Mosby-Year Book, 2003; 2151.)**

NSAIDs, immobilization, and cessation of offending activity. Arthroscopic débridement of anterior osteophytes is reserved for refractory cases.

Turf Toe A sprain of the first MTP joint caused by hyperextension is a turf toe. Hyperextension of the MTP joint results in subluxation followed by stretching of the plantar capsule and plantar plate. Patients present with pain, swelling, and stiffness of the joint. Treatment is conservative with rest, ice, elevation, and a stiff-soled shoe. Proximal migration of the medial sesamoid on stress lateral radiographs indicates severe traumatic disruption of the plantar plate. Complete disruption is unusual and should be treated surgically. Persistent symptoms may require a diagnostic bone scan for proximal phalanx fracture. Diastasis of bipartite sesamoid may occur. Dorsiflexion stress test can be performed to evaluate for widening of the syndesmosis. Treat with repair or excision of fragment.

IV. SHOULDER

Shoulder Anatomy. The shoulder consists of 3 bones and 4 articulations (see Tables 3.10, 3.11, and 3.12). The clavicle is an S-shaped bone articulating medially with the manubrium of the sternum at the sternoclavicular (SC) joint and laterally with the scapula at acromioclavicular (AC) joint (Fig. 3.33). It is the first bone in the body to ossify and the last to fuse (medial physis in early 20s). It has 2 primary and 1 secondary ossification center. The scapula has a complex osteology that allows 17 muscle origins and insertions. It articulates with the posterior chest wall and ribs 2 through 7, and it is angled 30 degrees anteriorly and 3 degrees cephalad. The coracoid is the origin for the conjoined tendon (short head of biceps and coracobrachialis) and insertion of pectoralis minor. The intrinsic ligaments of the scapula include the superior transverse scapular ligament (which separates the suprascapular nerve inferiorly and the vessels superiorly) and the coracoacromial ligament. The acromion is a broad, flat, lateral expansion of the scapular spine. It is the site of deltoid origin and trapezius insertion. The deltoid muscle should not be split more than 5 cm below the acromion during lateral shoulder approaches; otherwise, the axillary nerve is at risk. The arm should be abducted and externally rotated to move the nerve away from the surgical dissection. Surgical dissection should be avoided medial to the coracobrachialis for fear of injury to the musculocutaneus nerve, which penetrates the biceps/coracobrachialis 5 to 8 cm below the coracoid. This nerve enters these muscles closer than 5 cm about 30% of the time. The glenoid is the lateral projection of the scapula and provides the articulation with the humeral head. The average retroversion is 7 degrees with superior inclination of 5 degrees (Fig. 3.34).

TABLE 3.10 Muscles of the shoulder

Muscle	Origin	Insertion	Action	Innervation
Trapezius	Spinous process C7-T12	Clavicle, scapula (acromion, spine)	Rotate scapula	CN XI
Latissimus dorsi	Spinous process T6-S5, ilium	Intertubercular groove (ITG) of the humerus	Extend, adduct, IR humerus	Thoracodorsal
Rhomboid major	Spinous process T2-5	Scapula (medial border)	Adduct scapula	Dorsal scapular
Rhomboid minor	Spinous process C7-T1	Scapula (medial spine)	Adduct scapula	Dorsal Scapula
Levator scapulae	Transverse process C1-C4	Scapula (superior medial)	Elevate, rotate scapula	C3-C4
Pectoralis major	Sternum, ribs, clavicle	Humerus (L-ITG)	Adduct, IR arm	Medial and lateral pectoral
Pectoralis minor	Ribs 3–5	Scapula (coracoid)	Protract scapula	Medial pectoral
Subclavius	Rib 1	Inferior clavicle	Depress clavicle	Ulnar trunk
Serratus anterior	Ribs 1–9	Scapula (ventromedial)	Prevent winging	Long thoracic
Deltoid	Lateral clavicle, scapula	Humerus (deltoid tubercle)	Abduct arm	Axillary
Teres major	Inferior scapula	Humerus (M-ITG)	Adduct, IR, extend	Lower subscapular
Subscapularis	Ventral scapula	Humerus lesser tuberosity	IR arm, anterior stability	Upper and lower subscapular
Supraspinatus	Superior scapula	Humerus greater tuberosity	Abduct, ER arm, stability	Suprascapular
Infraspinatus	Dorsal scapula	Humerus greater tuberosity	Stability, ER arm	Suprascapular
Teres minor	Dorsolateral scapula	Humerus greater tuberosity	Stability, ER arm	Axillary

TABLE 3.11 Surgical approaches to the shoulder

Approach	Superficial Muscle (Innervation)	Deep Muscles (Innervation)	Structures at Risk
Anterior (Henry)	Deltoid (axillary)	Pectoralis major (medial/lateral pectoral)	MC nerve/cephalic vein
Lateral splitting	Deltoid (axillary)	Deltoid (axillary)	Axillary nerve
Posterior	Infraspinatus (suprascapular)	Teres minor (axillary)	Axillary nerve/posterior circumflex humeral artery
Anterolateral proximal humerus	Deltoid/pectoralis major (axillary/medial/lateral pectoral)		Radial and axillary nerve/anterior circumflex humeral artery

Humeral Head. The humeral head approximates a sphere with an average diameter of 43 mm. Normal retroversion is 30 degrees relative to transepicondylar axis. The articular surface inclines 130 degrees relative to the humeral shaft (Fig. 3.35). Greater and lesser tuberosities on opposite sides of the bicipital groove are sites of rotator cuff tendon insertions. The greater tuberosity is the insertion site for supraspinatus, infraspinatus, and teres minor, while the lesser tuberosity is the insertion site for the subscapularis. The SC joint is a gliding articulation with a complete intraarticular disk (Fig. 3.36). Elevation of the arm to 90 degrees abduction causes approximately 40 degrees of motion at the SC joint. Anterior dislocation is more common because the posterior SC ligament is stronger than the anterior SC ligament.

AC Joint. The AC joint has an incomplete intraarticular disk. AP (horizontal) stability is conferred through the AC ligaments/capsule. Superior/inferior (vertical) stability is conferred through the CC ligaments between the coracoid process and the lateral clavicle. The conoid ligament is medial, and the trapezoid ligament is lateral (Fig. 3.37).

TABLE 3.12 Four layers of the shoulder

Layer	Components
I	Deltoid
	Pectoralis major
II	Clavipectoral fascia
	Conjoined tendon, short head of biceps, coracobrachialis
III	Deep layer of subdeltoid bursa
	Rotator cuff muscles
IV	Glenohumeral joint capsule
	Coracohumeral ligament

Scapulothoracic Articulation. Scapulothoracic articulation occurs between scapula and posterior ribs 2 through 7. There are two major scapulothoracic bursae: the scapulotrapezial, between the trapezius and superomedial angle of scapula, and the infraserratus, between the chest wall and serratus anterior. The ratio of glenohumeral to scapulothoracic motion during shoulder abduction is 2:1.

Glenohumeral Joint. The glenohumeral joint is a congruent articulation with less than 2 mm of mismatch in the radius of curvature between the humeral head and glenoid. There is a lack of intrinsic stability to the joint. Only one third of the humeral head is covered by the glenoid in any given position of rotation. Stability is conferred through the capsule, labrum, and muscles.

Triangular Space. Bordered by the teres minor (superior), teres major (inferior), and long head of triceps (lateral), the triangular space contains the circumflex scapular artery.

Quadrangular Space. Bordered by the teres minor (superior), teres major (inferior), long head of triceps (medial), and lateral head of triceps (lateral), the quadrangular space contains the axillary nerve and the posterior humeral circumflex artery.

Triangular Interval. Bordered by the teres major (superior), long head of triceps (medial), and lateral head of triceps (lateral), the triangular interval contains the radial nerve and profunda brachii artery (Fig. 3.38).

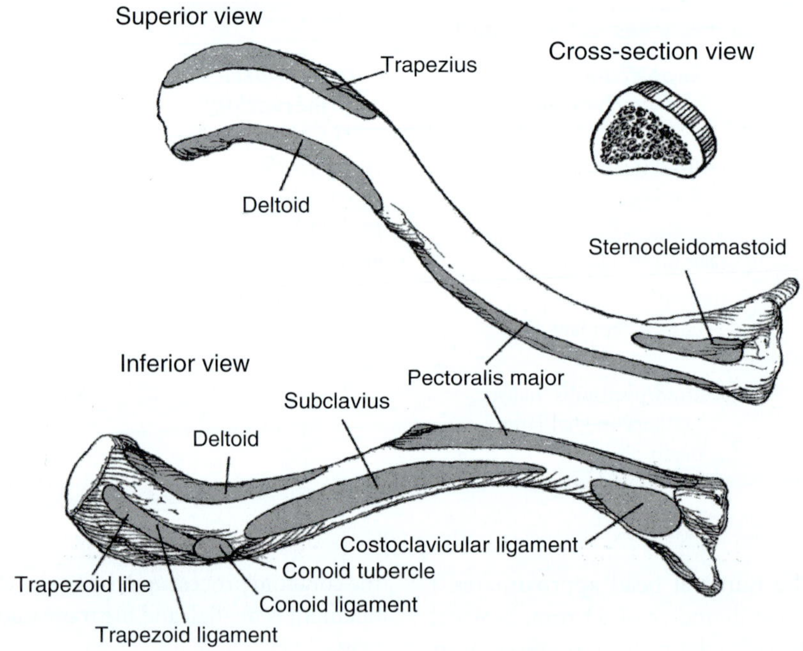

FIGURE 3.33 Anteroposterior, superoinferior, and cross-sectional views of clavicle. Note the triangular shape of the midclavicle on cross-section. The clavicle has a dual curvature with the medial portion convex anteriorly and the lateral portion concave anteriorly. (*Source:* Garrett WE, Speer KP, Kirkendall DT. *Principles and Practice of Orthopaedic Sports Medicine*. Philadelphia: Lippincott Williams & Wilkins, 2000; 330.)

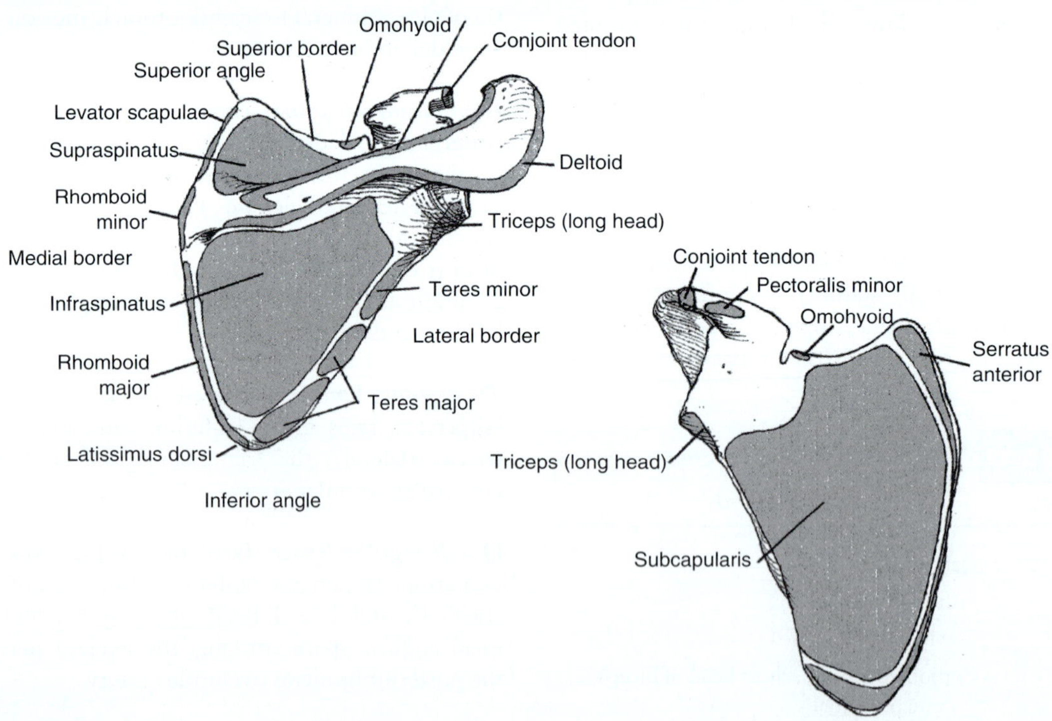

FIGURE 3.34 Dorsal and ventral views of the scapula. Note muscular origins and attachments. (*Source:* Garrett WE, Speer KP, Kirkendall DT. *Principles and Practice of Orthopaedic Sports Medicine*. Philadelphia: Lippincott Williams & Wilkins, 2000; 331.)

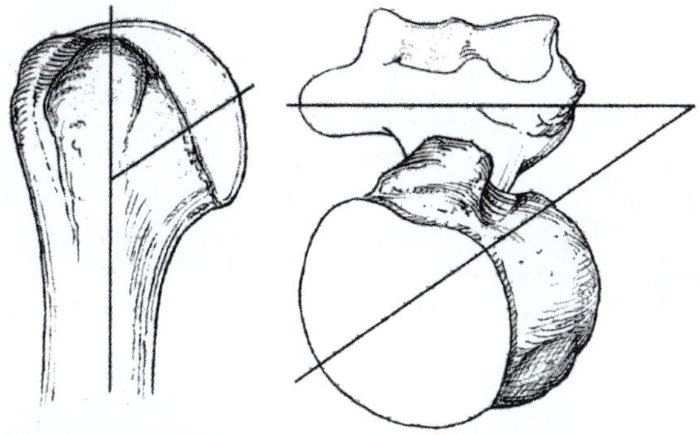

FIGURE 3.35 Version of the humeral head and neck in relation to the epicondylar axis. (*Source:* Garrett WE, Speer KP, Kirkendall DT. *Principles and Practice of Orthopaedic Sports Medicine.* Philadelphia: Lippincott Williams & Wilkins, 2000; 334.)

Rotator Cuff

Surgical Anatomy. The shoulder muscles are described in Table 3.13.

Biomechanics of the Shoulder. The shoulder is a minimally constrained articulation with soft tissue structures and bony architecture acting together to gain stability. Ligaments provide stability at the extremes of motion and muscles provide stability throughout the arc of motion.

Static Stabilizers

Articular Version of the Shoulder. The humeral head is retroverted 30 degrees. The glenoid is retroverted an average of 7 degrees. Increased anteversion or excessive retroversion is associated with instability.

Articular Conformity. Only one-third of the humeral head is in contact with the glenoid at any position of arm rotation. Conformity provides the basis for the *concavity-compression effect* of the rotator cuff musculature.

Glenohumeral Index (Described by Saha). The glenohumeral index is proportionate to the degree of stability and is calculated by dividing the diameter of the glenoid by the diameter of the humeral head. It is useful for determining glenoid dysplasia, glenoid fractures, and other injuries.

Glenoid Labrum. A fibrous ring attached to the glenoid articular surface, the glenoid labrum is firmly attached below the glenoid equator, but it is more mobile throughout the superior labrum. It increases the depth and surface area of the glenoid and also contributes to the concavity-compression effect through its deepening of the glenoid face. When intact, the superior labrum increases the ability of the shoulder to withstand excessive external rotational forces by an additional 32%. Detachment of the labrum leads to increased anterior translation of the humeral head.

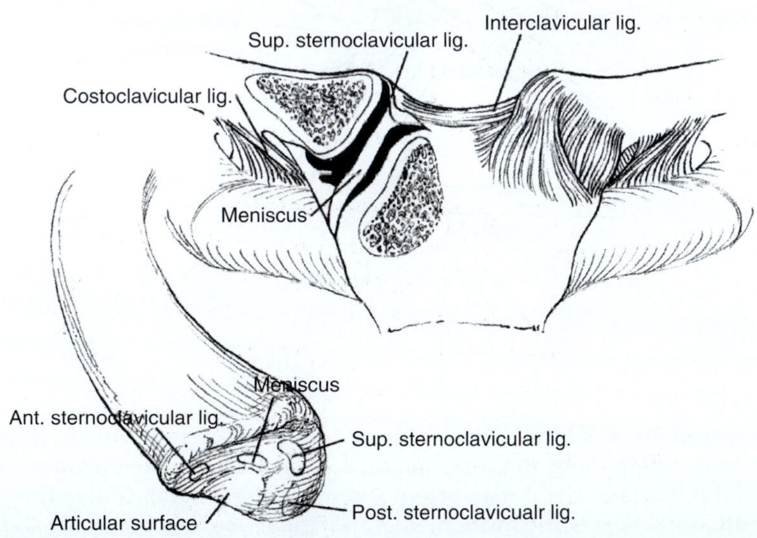

FIGURE 3.36 (A) Anteroposterior and (B) superoinferior views of the sternoclavicular joint. Note the relative incongruence of the joint and the ligamentous attachments, which provide stability in multiple planes. (*Source:* Garrett WE, Speer KP, Kirkendall DT. *Principles and Practice of Orthopaedic Sports Medicine*. Philadelphia: Lippincott Williams & Wilkins, 2000; 336.)

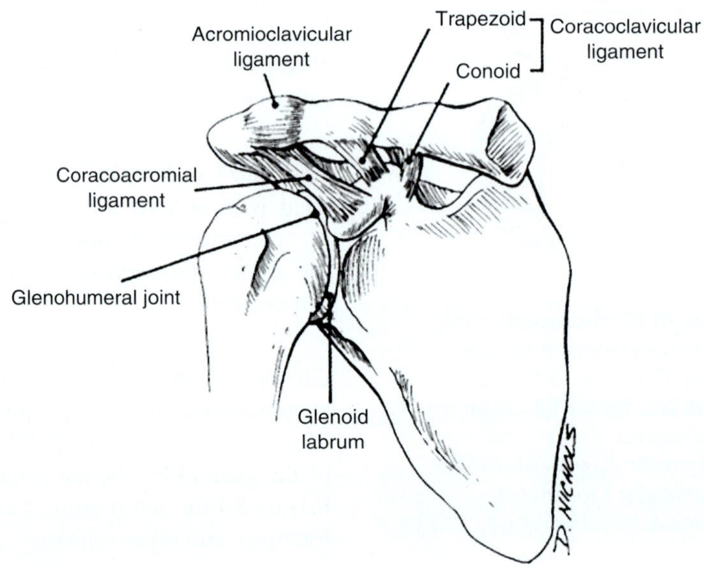

FIGURE 3.37 Ligamentous attachments of acromioclavicular, coracoclavicular, and coracoacromial ligaments. (*Source:* Andrews JR, Zarins B, Wilk KE. *Injuries in Baseball*. Philadelphia: Lippincott-Raven, 1998; 41.)

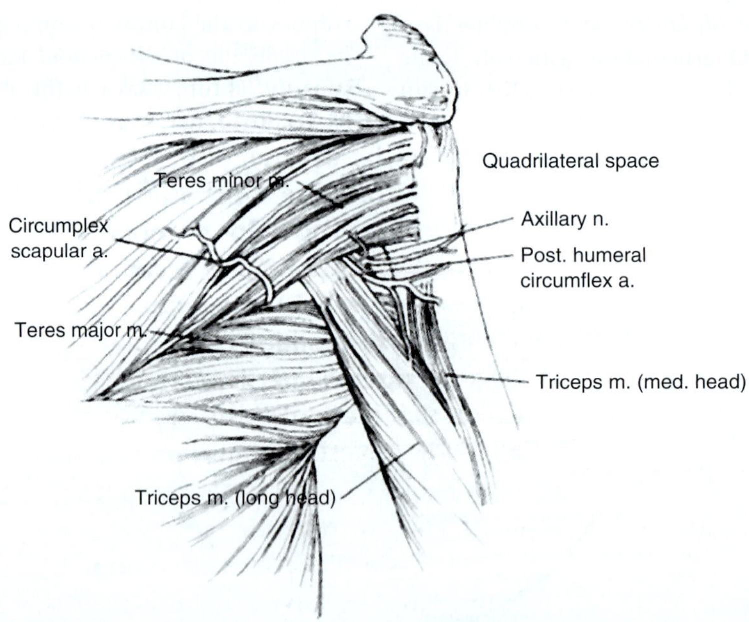

FIGURE 3.38 The quadrilateral space is bordered superiorly by the teres minor, laterally by the humerus, inferiorly by the teres major, and medially by the long head of the triceps. The posterior humeral circumflex artery and the axillary nerve course through the quadrilateral space. The more medial triangular space is bordered superiorly by the teres minor, laterally by the long head of the triceps, and inferiorly by the teres major. The circumflex scapular artery courses in this space. (*Source*: Garrett WE, Speer KP, Kirkendall DT. *Principles and Practice of Orthopaedic Sports Medicine*. Philadelphia: Lippincott Williams & Wilkins, 2000; 360.)

TABLE 3.13 Rotator cuff and other shoulder muscles

Muscle	Origin	Insertion	Innervation	Action
Supraspinatus	Supraspinatus fossa of scapula	Superior portion of greater tuberosity	Suprascapular nerve	Initiates abduction
Infraspinatus	Infraspinatus fossa of scapula	Middle portion of greater tuberosity	Suprascapular nerve	External rotation of humerus
Teres minor	Lateral scapula	Inferior portion of greater tuberosity	Axillary nerve	External rotation of humerus
Subscapularis	Subscapular fossa of scapula	Lesser tuberosity of humerus	Upper and lower subscapular nerve	Internal rotation and adduction
Trapezius	Spinous process C7-T12	Clavicle, scapula, acromion spinous processes	CN XI	Rotate scapula
Latissimus dorsi	Spinous process T6-S5, ilium	Humerus	Thoracodorsal	Extend, adduct, IR humerus
Rhomboid major	Spinous process T2-T5	Scapula medial border	Dorsal scapular	Adduct scapula

Negative Intraarticular Pressure. Clinically insignificant, negative intraarticular pressure creates a vacuum effect by the weight of the arm pulling the joint surfaces apart in a closed capsule.

Adhesion-Cohesion. Adhesion-cohesion is a clinically insignificant effect of the viscous joint fluid.

Capsuloligamentous Structures. Discrete capsular thickenings composed mostly of type I collagen, the capsuloligamentous structures are named according to their *glenoid* attachment. These structures function as static checkreins limiting excessive translation and rotation of the humeral head, principally at the extremes of motion and rotation (Fig. 3.39).

Superior Glenohumeral Ligament (SGHL). Superior glenoid tubercle to lesser tuberosity. It is present in more than 90% of individuals and limits inferior translation and external rotation when the arm is adducted.

Middle Glenohumeral Ligament (MGHL). Glenoid tubercle or anterosuperior labrum to lesser tuberosity. This ligament is present in 60% to 80% of individuals. The MGHL limits anterior and posterior translation of the partially abducted (45 degrees) and externally rotated humerus as well as external rotation of the adducted humerus. It also limits inferior translation of the adducted and externally rotated humerus.

Inferior Glenohumeral Ligament Complex (IGHLC). Inferior half of the glenoid neck or anterior inferior labrum to the lesser tuberosity below the MGHL insertion. The IGHLC is a discrete anterior and posterior band with axillary pouch interposed. It functions as a hammock-like structure. The complex moves posteriorly with internal rotation and anteriorly with external rotation. It limits anterior, posterior, and inferior translation between 45 and 90 degrees of arm abduction. The posterior band is the most important restraint to posterior translation with the shoulder in 90 degrees of flexion and internal rotation. Glenohumeral ligaments are described in Table 3.14 and Fig. 3.40.

Posterior Capsule. The posterior capsule is thinnest posteriorly proximal to the posterior band of the IGHLC. It may resist posterior translation in a flexed, adducted, and internally rotated arm.

Rotator Interval. The rotator interval is an area defined by the supraspinatus superiorly, the subscapularis inferiorly, the coracoid medially, and the biceps/humerus laterally (Fig. 3.41). It is reinforced by the SGHL and MGHL and may be devoid of tissue or have loosely arranged collagen representing a rotator interval capsular defect, which is normal in the stable shoulder. The rotator interval may contribute to inferior instability of the adducted arm. Tight rotator interval may be associated with adhesive capsulitis and limit external rotation.

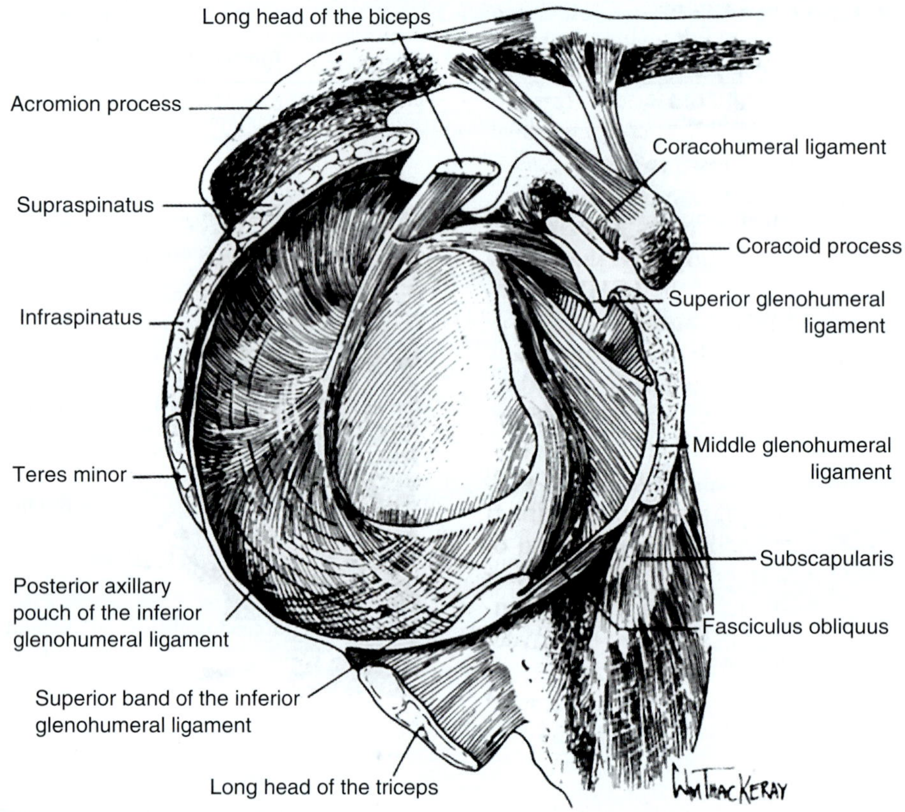

FIGURE 3.39 **Schematic of the glenohumeral ligaments and pericapsular tissues. (*Source*: Turkel SJ, Panio MW, Marshall JL, et al. Stabilizing mechanisms preventing anterior dislocation of the glenohumeral joint. *J Bone Joint Surg Am* 1981;63A:1208–1217.)**

Dynamic Restraints. Dynamic restraints function to maintain stability of the shoulder during midrange arm motion/rotation (capsuloligamentous restraints function at the extremes of motion). The posterior band of the inferior glenohumeral ligament is the most important restraint to posterior subluxation of the glenohumeral joint with the shoulder in 90 degrees of flexion and internal rotation. With the shoulder in external rotation, the subscapularis is an important stabilizer to posterior subluxation. When the shoulder

TABLE 3.14 Glenohumeral ligaments

GH Ligament	Origin	Insertion	Function
Superior (SGHL)	Supraglenoid tubercle	Lesser tuberosity	Restraint in adduction to inferior translation and external rotation
Middle (MGHL)	Glenoid tubercle or anterosuperior labrum	Lesser tuberosity	Limits anterior–posterior translation in partially abducted (45) externally rotated humerus
Inferior (IGHLC) anterior and posterior bands	Inferior glenoid neck or anteroinferior labrum	Lesser tuberosity below (MGHL)	Limits anterior–posterior and inferior translation in abducted arm; limits posttranslation in flexed, adducted, internally rotated arm

is in neutral rotation, the coracohumeral ligament is the primary stabilizer. The middle glenohumeral ligament functions primarily to resist anterior translation of the humeral head in the midrange of abduction. The supraspinatus muscle and tendon have relatively little contribution to anterior and posterior translation of the glenohumeral joint.

Joint Compression (Concavity-Compression Effect). The rotator cuff and biceps tendon center the humeral head on the glenoid during arm rotation (steering effect). Contraction of the rotator cuff tendons centers the humeral head and creates capsular tension through direct capsular attachments. During contraction, the rigid muscles and tendons of the rotator cuff restrain humeral head.

Scapular Rotators. The trapezius, rhomboids, latissimus dorsi, serratus anterior, and levator scapulae make up the scapular rotators. They function to maintain a stable glenoid platform during arm motion/rotation. Normally, the ratio of humeral-to-scapular elevation is 2:1.

Proprioception. Position sense receptors within the capsule are able to sense capsular stretch and humeral rotation, which activates a reflex mechanism that coordinates muscular contraction to counteract translation and instability.

Shoulder Instability. This pathologic condition presents as pain and dysfunction due to excessive translation of the humeral head on the glenoid during active shoulder motion. The shoulder is the most common

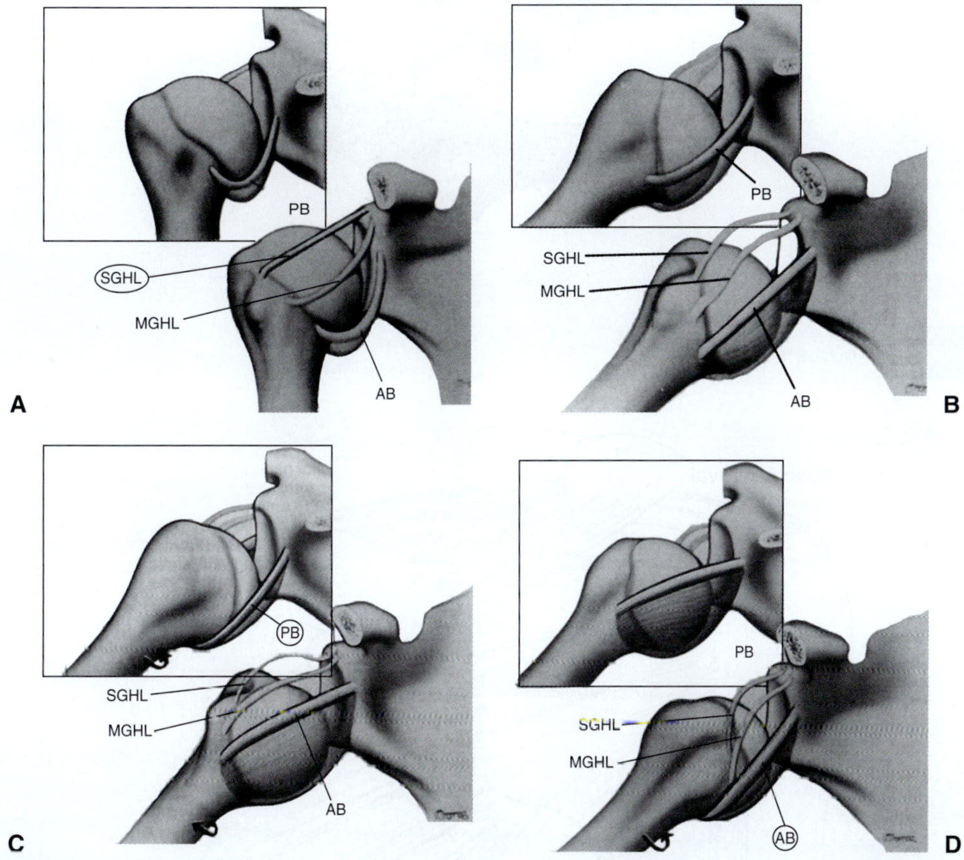

FIGURE 3.40 Diagrams of the function of the glenohumeral ligaments in various positions of humeral rotation and abduction. *SGHL*, superior glenohumeral ligament; *MGHL*, middle glenohumeral ligament; *AB*, anterior band; *PB*, posterior band. The posterior glenohumeral ligament is a prime restraint to inferior shoulder translation in the adducted shoulder (A). In 45 degrees of humeral abduction and external rotation, the anterior band moves superiorly (B), and the posterior band inferiorly. The opposite occurs with internal rotation (C). A similar mechanism takes place with 90 degrees of humeral abduction and rotation (E, F, G). (*Source*: Bowen MK, Warren RF. Ligamentous control of shoulder stability based on selective cutting and static translation experiment. *Clin Sports Med* 1991;10:757–782.)

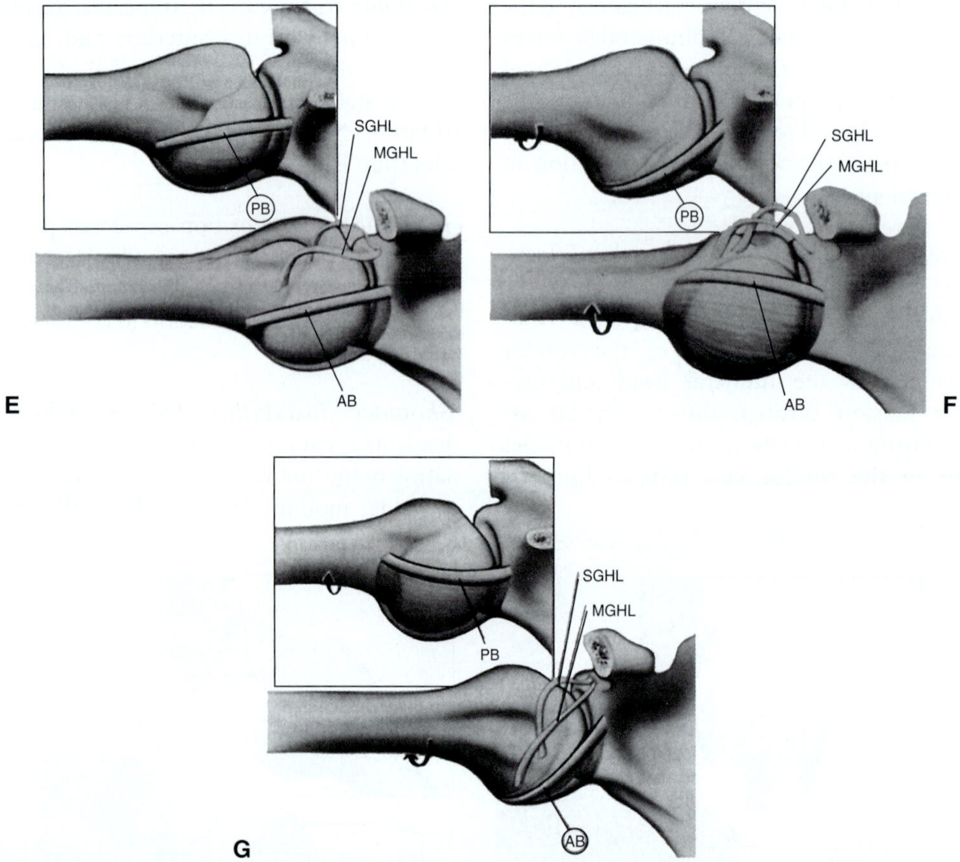

FIGURE 3.40 ***(continued)***

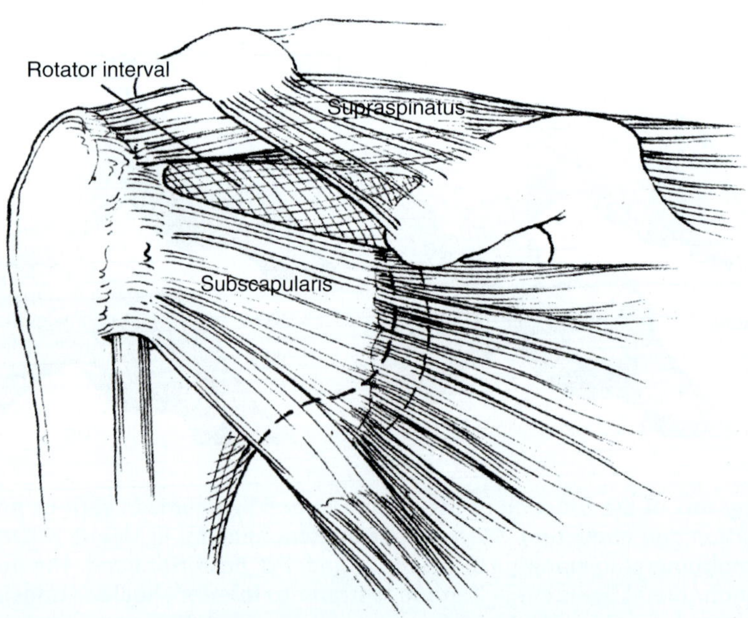

FIGURE 3.41 **Rotator interval. Note the triangular shape of the tissue with the base of the triangle medially at the coracoid. (*Source*: Garrett WE, Speer KP, Kirkendall DT. *Principles and Practice of Orthopaedic Sports Medicine*. Philadelphia: Lippincott Williams & Wilkins, 2000; 353.)**

joint to dislocate. Anterior dislocations are much more common than posterior. Anterior dislocations may be associated with greater tuberosity fractures, while posterior dislocations are associated with lesser tuberosity fractures. Axillary nerve injuries and rotator cuff tears may also occur with anterior dislocations, especially in older patients. There are two broad classifications of instability:

1. *TUBS*—Traumatic, unidirectional with a Bankart lesion. Often requires surgery. Often seen in young patients with 80% to 90% recurrence rate with nonoperative treatment.
2. *AMBRI(I)*—Atraumatic, multidirectional, bilateral dislocations often respond to rehabilitation and sometimes an inferior capsular shift interval (rotator interval) closure.

These two classifications represent the opposite ends of a continuum of instability associated with mixed pathology. The essential lesion of traumatic instability is thought to be the Bankart lesion.

Detachment of the anchor point of the IGHLC and MGHL from the glenoid is present in 80% to 95% of traumatic anterior glenohumeral dislocations. Recent cadaveric studies revealed only minimal increases of anterior translation in isolated Bankart lesions. Associated capsular pathology (such as ruptures, avulsions, intrasubstance tears, and plastic deformation) may contribute to instability. Hill-Sachs lesions are present in approximately 80% of traumatic anterior glenohumeral dislocations and up to 25% of subluxations. Bony architecture disruption such as bony Bankart lesions, glenoid fractures involving 30% or more of the glenoid surface, and dysplasia of the glenoid (including version abnormalities) may also contribute to instability (Fig. 3.42.)

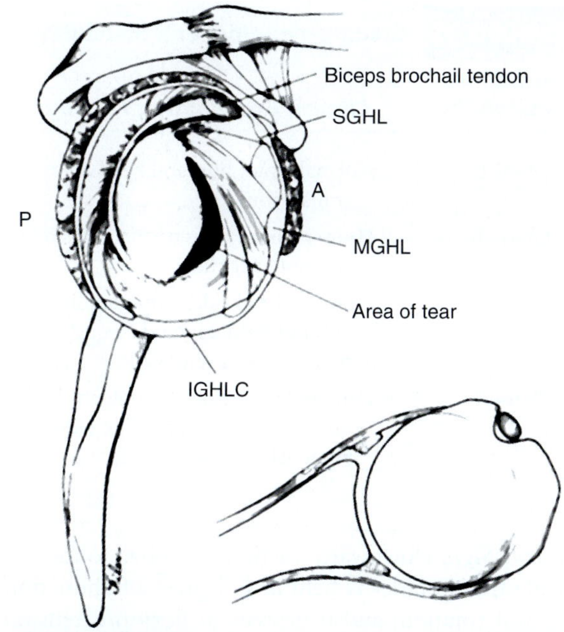

FIGURE 3.42 **Diagram of the Bankart lesion. *A*, anterior; *IGHL*, inferior glenohumeral ligament; *MGHL*, middle glenohumeral ligament; *P*, posterior; *SGHL*, superior glenohumeral ligament. (*Source*: Fu FH, Stone DA. *Sports Injuries, 2nd ed.*, Philadelphia: Lippincott Williams & Wilkins, 2001; 1016.)**

Traumatic Anterior Instability. Traumatic anterior instability is the most common form of shoulder instability and usually occurs with the arm in abduction and external rotation.

Posterior Dislocation. Posterior dislocation of the shoulder is much less common than anterior instability and may be missed in up to 50% of cases at first presentation. Common clinical scenarios that may lead to posterior instability include a history of alcohol abuse, seizure disorder, or electrocution. Nonoperative treatment focuses on strengthening of the external rotators and posterior deltoid. Posterior capsular shift may be helpful in refractory cases but is difficult because of the thin posterior capsule.

Multidirectional Instability. Inherent ligamentous laxity may be present in patients with multidirectional instability (MDI). MDI is not caused by an injury or repetitive overhead activities.

Load-and-Shift Test. The load-and-shift test is done by stabilizing the scapula with the patient in an upright position. Anterior and posterior stress is applied to the humeral head by grasping the proximal humerus.

A modified load-and-shift test is performed with the patient positioned supine with the affected shoulder in a scapular plane at the edge of the examining table. Force is applied to the elbow to concentrically reduce the humeral head into the glenoid fossa. Anterior and posterior forces are applied to the proximal humerus. Glenohumeral instability grades are provided in Table 3.15.

Apprehension-Relocation Test. The patient is positioned supine with the affected shoulder at the edge of the examining table. The arm is slowly abducted and externally rotated: A positive test reproduces the sensation of impending dislocation. Relocation sign is positive if a posterior force directed on the proximal humerus relieves the feeling of impending dislocation and a greater degree of external rotation is achievable.

TABLE 3.15 Grading glenohumeral instability

Grade of Instability	*Clinical Examination Findings*
Grade 0	Normal (trace humeral head translation)
Grade 1	Humeral head rides up glenoid slope but not over rim
Grade 2	Humeral head rides over glenoid rim but reduces *spontaneously* when stress is removed
Grade 3	Humeral head rides over glenoid rim and *remains* dislocated after removal of stress

Sulcus Sign. Downward traction is applied to the arm while the shoulder is held in 0 degrees of abduction, neutral rotation, and 0 degrees of flexion/extension. The acromiohumeral interval is measured to assess inferior glenohumeral laxity (Table 3.16).

Rotator Interval Test. While performing the sulcus test, externally rotate the arm. Healthy patients will have a reduction of inferior translation. No reduction in acromiohumeral interval is suspicious for rotator interval capsular deficiency.

Jerk Test. Start with the arm forward-flexed and adducted. Posterior-directed force will cause posterior translation in posterior instability. Moving the arm into the coronal plane may reduce the humeral head.

Treatment of Shoulder Dislocation

Nonoperative Treatment

- Prior to initiation of any nonoperative or operative therapy, a thorough neurovascular examination of both upper extremities as well as an evaluation of the integrity of the rotator cuff should be performed. Evaluation of the rotator cuff is particularly important in patients over 40 years old as these patients have a high rate of rotator cuff tear with dislocations.
- Immobilization for 2 to 4 weeks after the initial episode. Recent data suggests that immobilization in external rotation and slight abduction may yield better results and obviate surgical intervention by preventing medial healing of the anterior-inferior labrum to glenoid neck.
- Aggressive physical therapy focused on strengthening the dynamic shoulder stabilizers (see earlier discussion)
- Proprioceptive feedback and neuromuscular training may provide symptomatic relief
- Rehabilitation carries a success rate of 80% with nontraumatic causes of instability
- Success rate of 20% with traumatic instability; success rate is inversely proportional to age (younger people are more likely to redislocate)

TABLE 3.16 Inferior glenohumeral laxity grade

Grade of Laxity	*Acromial-Humeral Distance*
Grade 1	Interval < 1 cm
Grade 2	Interval 1–2 cm
Grade 3	Interval > 2 cm

Surgical Treatment

- There is data to suggest early stabilization of young patients who continue to engage in high-risk activities/athletics
- Examination under anesthesia
- Translation of humeral head graded (Table 3.15)
- Inferior laxity graded (Table 3.16)
- The shoulder should be tested in adduction, in 45 and 90 degrees of abduction, and in internal and external rotation to test capsuloligamentous structures and guide surgical treatment

Arthroscopic Stabilization Versus Open Stabilization. As there are no current randomized prospective published studies comparing arthroscopic versus open stabilization, the decision to proceed with one type of surgical stabilization over the other is based on surgeon preference, patient anatomy, and the advantages and disadvantages of each option. Advantages of arthroscopy include evaluation and treatment of concomitant intraarticular pathology, lower morbidity, better cosmesis, and less pain. However, disadvantages of arthroscopy include difficulty of procedures (learning curve), inability to address certain bony and capsular pathology, and complications of thermal capsulorrhaphy including capsule ablation and axillary nerve injury. Loss of external rotation after an anterior stabilization procedure for a Bankart lesion can lead to degenerative joint disease and posterior glenohumeral wear. Subscapularis tendon rupture is also a recognized complication of open anterior instability repairs when the subscapularis tendon is incised as part of the exposure.

Internal Impingement. Internal impingement occurs between the posterior labrum and rotator cuff, especially in throwing athletes, with external rotation and anterior translation (secondary impingement). Arthroscopic débridement and repair has good results.

Subcoracoid Impingement. This type of impingement is uncommon but can be associated with a laterally placed coracoid that impinges on the proximal humerus with forward flexion and internal rotation. Diagnosis can be made with CT with the arm in the provocative position and relief with local anesthetic injection. Resection of the lateral aspect of the coracoid process can be curative.

Subacromial Impingement. Subacromial impingement is a pathologic process that occurs when the rotator cuff is impinged upon by the anterior acromion, the coracoacromial ligament, or the AC joint. Always consider subtle glenohumeral instability as a cause of secondary impingement syndrome in younger patients.

Neer Stages of Impingement. The stages of impingement are provided in Table 3.17.

Outlet Versus Nonoutlet Impingement. Outlet impingement occurs when the coracoacromial arch encroaches on the supraspinatus outlet (Fig. 3.43). Nonoutlet impingement occurs secondary to thickening of the subacromial bursa or rotator cuff tendons.

Neer Impingement Sign. Passive forward elevation of the affected arm, in the scapular plane, beyond 90 degrees causes pain by impinging the supraspinatus tendon under the coracoacromial arch.

Hawkins Sign. Internal rotation of the forward flexed and adducted arm causes pain by impinging the rotator cuff between the anterior acromion and the greater tuberosity. Hawkins sign has greater sensitivity than Neer impingement sign but less specificity because the internal rotation of Hawkins sign tightens the posterior shoulder capsule (Fig. 3.44).

TABLE 3.17 Neer stages of impingement

Stage	*Age*	*Findings*
Stage 1	Under 25 years	Edema and hemorrhage of subacromial bursa and rotator cuff
Stage 2	Age 25–40 years	Irreversible changes of the rotator cuff: fibrosis and tendonitis
Stage 3	Age > 40 years	Chronic changes such as partial or complete tears of rotator cuff

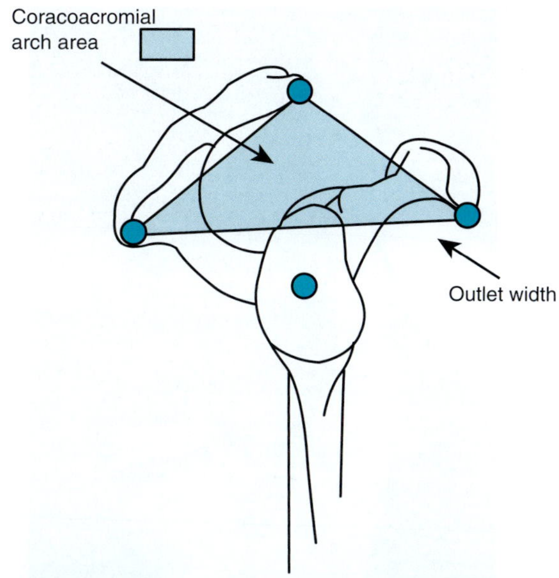

FIGURE 3.43 A reduction in the coracoacromial arch area has been correlated with an increased incidence of full-thickness rotator cuff tears providing further support for an extrinsic etiology in some cases of rotator cuff disease. (*Adapted from* Zuckerman JD, Kummer FJ, Cuomo F, et al. The influence of coracoacromial arch anatomy on rotator cuff tears. *J Shoulder Elbow Surg* 1992;1:8.)

Impingement Test. Injection of 10 mL of 1% lidocaine into the subacromial space relieves pain caused by the Neer or Hawkins tests. The impingement test is the most sensitive and specific test for impingement syndrome.

Treatment of Impingement Syndrome

Nonoperative Intervention. Most patients suffering from isolated impingement syndrome will improve with nonoperative treatment. Modalities include activity modification, NSAIDs, subacromial injections of steroids, and physical therapy. The recommended duration of nonoperative intervention varies by author, but a 6-month minimum is generally accepted.

Operative Intervention. If nonoperative intervention fails, anterior acromioplasty and resection of the coracoacromial ligament is recommended. It can be performed open or arthroscopically.

Open treatment carries risk of deltoid origin avulsion, longer recovery, and worse cosmesis.

Arthroscopic procedure risks incomplete acromioplasty and reoperation.

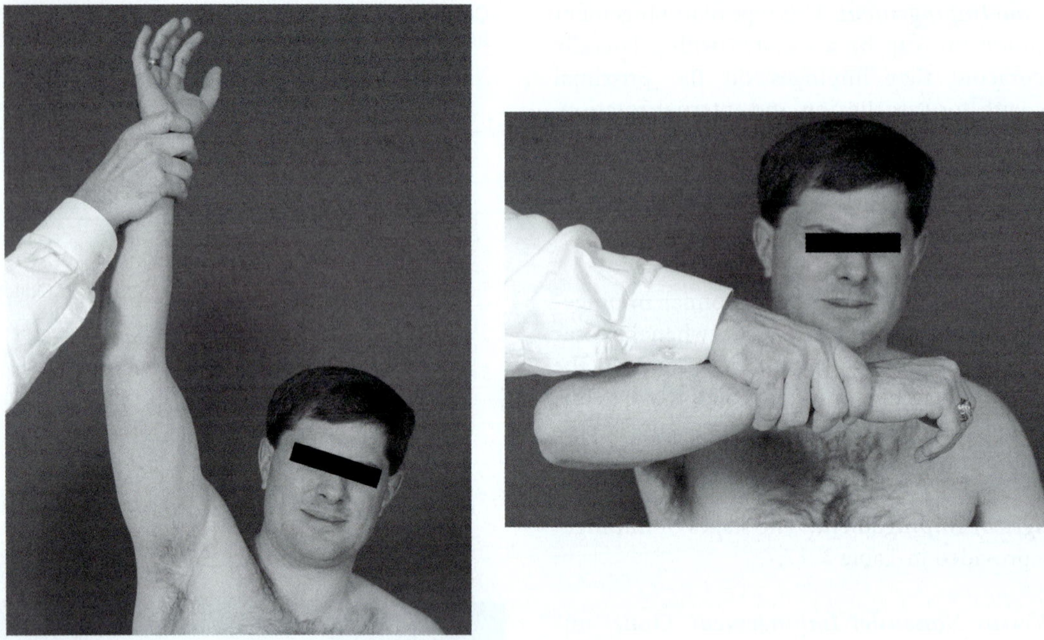

A B

FIGURE 3.44 Hawkins test (A) and Neer test (B) for impingement. The arm is raised in forward elevation. Pain near terminal elevation indicates impingement. (*Source*: Krishnan SG, Hawkins RJ, Warren RF. *The Shoulder and the Overhead Athlete*. Philadelphia: Lippincott Williams & Wilkins, 2004; 147.)

Rotator Cuff Pathology. Rotator cuff tears associated with chronic impingement syndrome typically begin on the bursal surface of the cuff or within the tendon substance (older patients). Rotator cuff tears associated with tension failure in overhead athletes usually occur on the articular side of the cuff (younger patients). Shoulder dislocations in older patients (over age 40) should always raise the suspicion of rotator cuff tears. Function and integrity of rotator cuff muscles can be tested.

Jobe Test. The Jobe test detects a supraspinatus tendon lesion. Resistance to examiner's force with arm in a pronated, forward-flexed position (60 degrees) in the plane of the scapula. Pain and weakness are sensitive for a supraspinatus tendon lesion. The Jobe test is not specific because of its similarity to the impingement position (it can be repeated with the arm in supination to remove the greater tuberosity from the undersurface of the acromion).

Adduction External Rotation Lag Sign. Failure of the patient to actively maintain the maximum passively externally rotated arm suggests tears involving the infraspinatus tendon.

Abduction External Rotation Lag Sign (Hornblower Sign). Failure of the patient to actively maintain the maximum passively externally rotated arm in the 90-degree abducted position suggests infraspinatus or teres minor tendon lesions.

Lift-Off Test. Inability of the patient to maintain the maximally internally rotated arm away from the lower back suggests subscapularis tendon pathology (more specific for lower subscapularis muscle injury) (Fig. 3.45).

Abdominal Compression Test. The abdominal compression test is an alternative to lift-off test (more specific for upper subscapularis muscle injury). It is useful in patients who experience pain with the lift-off test. The patient presses the hand against the abdomen while simultaneously maintaining the elbow anterior to the midaxillary line. This test is useful for detecting subscapularis pathology.

Drop Arm Test. Inability of the patient to maintain the passively positioned arm in fully forward-flexed position in the scapular plane suggests high-grade impingement syndrome or full-thickness rotator cuff tear.

Treatment of Rotator Cuff Tears

Nonoperative Intervention. Activity modification, rotator cuff and scapular stabilizer strengthening program, NSAIDs, ultrasound, and iontophoresis are nonoperative treatments for rotator cuff tears. Chronic

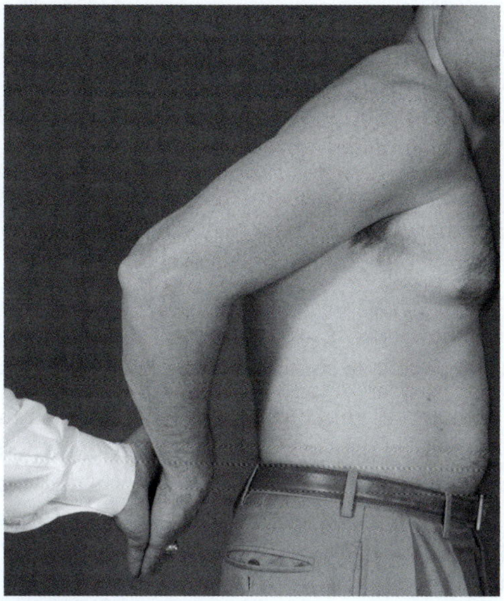

FIGURE 3.45 The lift-off test for subscapularis strength. With the hand behind the back, the patient attempts to push the hand off the back against resistance. (*Source*: Krishnan SG, Hawkins RJ, Warren RF. *The Shoulder and the Overhead Athlete.* Philadelphia: Lippincott Williams & Wilkins, 2004; 148.)

rotator cuff tears should be nonsurgically managed initially with a strengthening program; surgery is reserved for patients who continue to have pain and lose sleep despite physical therapy. Corticosteroid injections may provide temporary relief of symptoms but may cause biologic tendon weakening.

Operative Intervention. It is recommended that partial thickness tears of less than 50% of the tendon substance be treated with tendon débridement and subacromial decompression. Partial thickness tears of more than 50% are treated with rotator cuff repair. Rotator cuff tendon repair can be treated open, miniopen, or arthroscopically. Margin convergence (side-to-side closure of large U-shaped RTC tears) decreases the strain on the free margin of the repaired cuff and the sutures. Surgery reliably decreases pain (70% to 100%) and improves function and motion (70% to 80%) regardless of method chosen for repair.

Acromioclavicular Joint. The diarthrodial joint is vulnerable to degenerative disease as a consequence of its high load transmission to small surface area ratio. Intraarticular disk (incomplete disk) degeneration may begin as early as the second decade.

Diagnosis Triad for AC Joint Pathology

- Pain over the AC joint elicited by direct palpation
- Pain with forced cross-body adduction
- Relief of pain with injection of local anesthetic into AC joint

Symptomatic Primary Osteoarthritis of the AC Joint. This condition is uncommon despite radiographic changes in up to 50% of elderly. Posttraumatic arthritis may occur in up to 40% of patients with grades I and II AC joint sprains. Distal clavicle osteolysis is increasingly recognized in young weightlifters (osteopenia, osteolysis, tapering of clavicle, cystic changes). Conservative treatment involves NSAIDs, corticosteroid injection, and activity modification.

Primary osteoarthritis responds favorably to AC joint excision if nonoperative interventions fail.

AC Separations. AC joint separation typically results from a fall directly onto the shoulder. AC ligaments and capsule prevent AP translation. The coracoclavicular ligaments are responsible for preventing superior translation. The Rockwood classification system and treatment of AC joint injuries are shown in Tables 3.18 and 3.19 (Fig. 3.46).

Treatment of AC Separation. Dunn procedure is usually employed to treat AC separation. Treatments have

TABLE 3.18 Rockwood classification of AC joint injuries

Type of Injury	*Radiographic Findings*
Type I	AC sprain; intact ligaments
Type II	AC ligament rupture and CC ligament sprain
Type III	AC and CC ligament rupture; lateral clavicle superiorly displaced (25%–100%)
Type IV	AC and CC ligament rupture; posterior displacement of clavicle (poss through trap)
Type V	AC and CC ligament rupture; superior displacement of clavicle (100%–300%)
Type VI	AC and CC ligament rupture; inferior displacement of clavicle under conjoined tendon

Adapted from Williams GR, Nguyen VD, Rockwood CR. Classification and radiographic analysis of acromioclavicular dislocations. *Appl Radiol* 1989;Feb:29–34.

TABLE 3.19 Treatment of AC joint injuries

Rockwood Classification	Recommended Treatment
Type I	Symptomatic; sling and early ROM
Type II	Symptomatic; sling and early ROM; full painless ROM before sports
Type III	Controversial (most recommend nonoperative as in types I and II)
Type IV	Operative (Weaver-Dunn or pin)
Type V	Operative (Weaver-Dunn or pin)
Type VI	Operative (Weaver-Dunn or pin)

also included pins, plates, screws, and a combination of such devices, but these options pose risk of hardware breakage or *migration*.

Treatment of AC Joint DJD

Nonoperative Intervention. Activity modification, NSAIDs, corticosteroid injections into the AC joint, and physical therapy are used to treat DJD.

Operative Intervention. Open or arthroscopic distal clavicle resection should be considered if symptoms persist despite nonoperative treatments. Coplaning of the distal clavicle for spur formation may lead to painful AC joints in up to 35% of patients secondary to destabilization of the distal clavicle. Arthroscopic resection has the advantage of accurate resection (8 to 10 mm), preservation of superior AC ligaments/capsule, avoiding detachment of trapezius and deltoid, and quicker recovery (85% to 100% good to excellent results).

Sternoclavicular Joint. SC subluxation and dislocation are uncommon but potentially serious injuries caused by high-energy trauma or direct athletic injuries. Hoarseness, shortness of breath, or dysphagia are worrisome. CT scan should be obtained if suspected dislocation.

The medial epiphysis can be mistaken for traumatic injury because it is the last to ossify (18 to 20 years) and close (23 to 25 years). Anterior dislocation is much more common than posterior with a ratio of 20:1.

Treatment. Closed reduction is usually successful. Nonoperative neglect if closed reduction fails is generally acceptable. Open reduction of a *posterior* dislocation is recommended. Vascular surgery consult is recommended for risk of vessel injury. The use of hardware should be limited in this location. Spontaneous SC joint subluxation in patients is treated nonoperatively because it is a self-limiting condition.

Biceps Tendonitis. Biceps tendonitis presents with tenderness elicited over the bicipital groove of the proximal humerus.

It is often clinically associated with rotator cuff tears and impingement syndrome.

- *Yergason test*—Resisted supination of the forearm with the elbow slightly flexed elicits pain in the proximal biceps tendon.
- *Speed test*—Resisted forward elevation of the arm with the elbow in extension and the forearm fully supinated elicits pain in the long head of the biceps.

Treatment is initially nonoperative with strengthening (physical therapy) and local injection. Operative intervention usually includes subacromial decompression for associated impingement as well as arthroscopic biceps tendon release and tenodesis to the proximal humerus.

Biceps Tendon Subluxation. Medial displacement of the biceps tendon may be caused by tear in the medial portion of the coracohumeral ligament, the transverse humeral ligament, or the subscapularis tendon insertion. Best functional results requires repair of subscapularis tendon and biceps tenodesis. Tendon subluxation/dislocation can be palpated by bringing the arm into abduction and external rotation with a finger on the bicipital groove. High suspicion for rotator cuff or subscapularis tears is indicated if biceps subluxation exists on physical exam.

Treatment. Nonoperative treatment is similar to that for tendonitis. Operative intervention includes repair or reconstruction of the bicipital groove, biceps release, or tenodesis.

Superior Labrum Anterior and Posterior (SLAP) Tears. Tears of the superior labral complex and biceps anchor are associated with glenohumeral instability and rotator cuff disease. Superior labral tears from anterior to posterior were first described by Snyder and Wuh in the early 1990s. Patients complain of deep pain in the shoulder with or without a locking and catching sensation with overhead activities as a result of the torn labrum interposing between the glenoid and the humeral head. Tests suggestive of SLAP tears include those that place the biceps anchor or tendon on stretch.

O'Brien Sign. The O'Brien sign is deep anterior shoulder pain elicited with resisted downward force on the arm in an adducted (10 degrees) and 90-degree forward-flexed, maximally internally rotated shoulder. This pain may be relieved if the arm is brought into external rotation and supination. The Speeds test may also be positive in SLAP tears. Presence

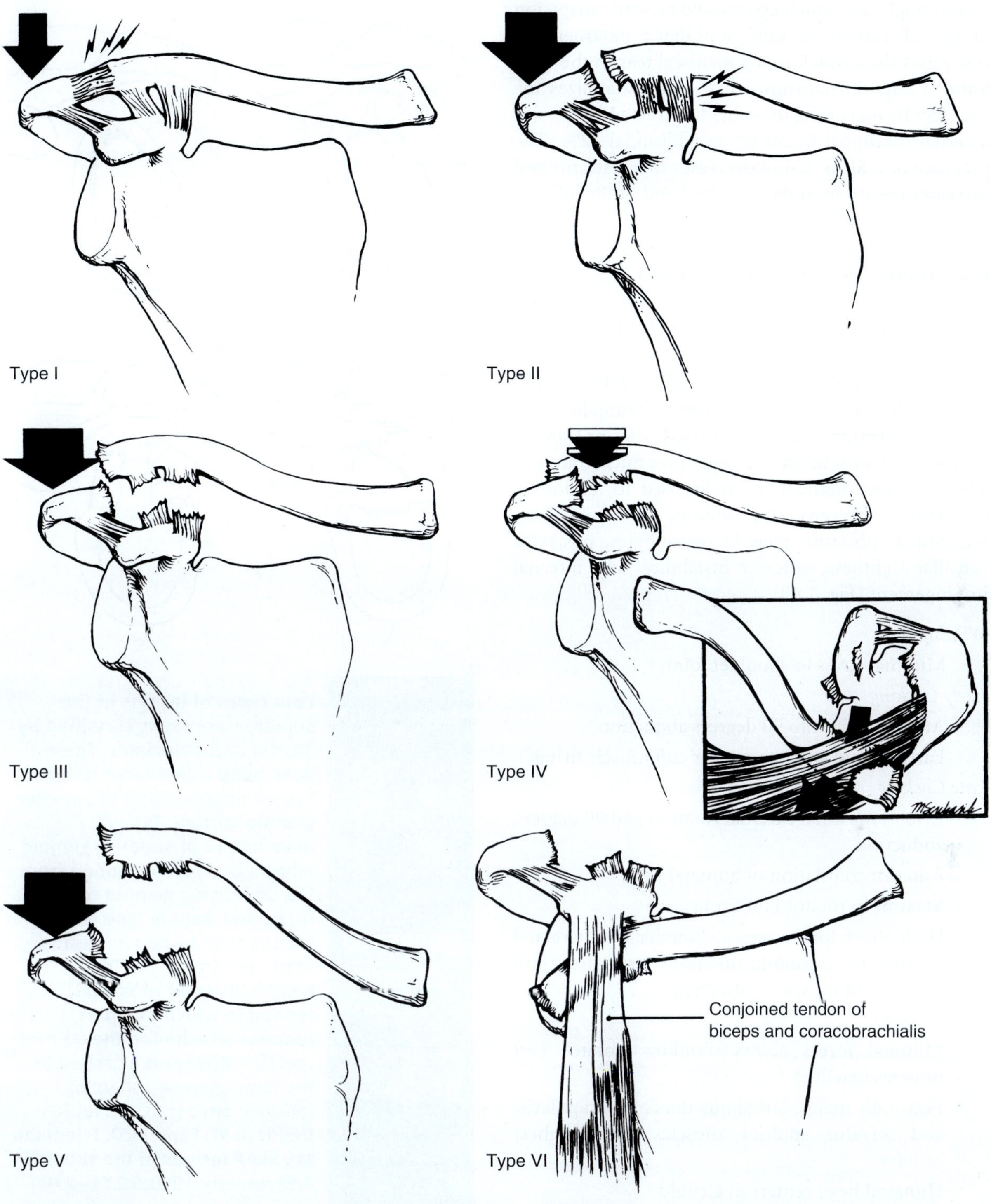

FIGURE 3.46 **Rockwood classification of injury to the acromioclavicular joint. (*Source*: Galatz LM, Williams GR. Acromioclavicular joint injuries. In: Bucholz RW, Heckman JD (eds.), *Rockwood and Green's Fractures in Adults*, 5th ed. Philadelphia: Lippincott Williams & Wilkins, 2001.)**

of a spinoglenoid notch cyst should raise the suspicion of a SLAP tear in the same way that a parameniscal cyst raises the suspicion of a meniscal tear in the knee joint. A superior labrum, when intact, stabilizes the shoulder by increasing its ability to withstand excessive external rotational forces by an additional 32%. The presence of a SLAP lesion decreases this restraint and increases the strain in the anterior band of the inferior glenohumeral ligament by over 100%.

Classification of SLAP Tears. See Fig. 3.47.

Treatment of SLAP Tears. See Table 3.20.

Throwing Shoulder. Forces exceeding 2 to 3 times body weight can be generated in the throwing shoulder, leading to overuse injuries. Increased anterior translation is noted on examination (repetitive microtrauma). The throwing shoulder is predisposed to tendonitis of rotator cuff/biceps, SLAP lesions, subacromial impingement, posterior glenoid osteophytes, posterior capsular tightness, anterior instability, and internal impingement (Fig. 3.48).

Windup

- Minimal stress to shoulder joint

Early Cocking

- Arm brought into 90 degrees abduction
- Early deltoid and late rotator cuff muscle firing

Late Cocking

- Arm in maximal external rotation and 90 degrees abduction
- Anterior translation of humeral head
- Maximum rotator cuff firing
- High shear forces across shoulder counteracted by labrum, capsuloligamentous structures, and rotator cuff muscle contraction

Acceleration

- Minimal forces across shoulder (rotator cuff muscles inactive)
- Pectoralis major, latissimus dorsi, subscapularis, and serratus anterior muscles show highest activity
- Humeral head centers in glenoid

Deceleration

- Most violent phase of throwing
- Highest torque measured across glenohumeral joint
- Muscle eccentric contraction to slow arm rotation (rotator cuff muscles show high activity)

Follow-through

- Remaining high compressive forces may lead to posterior capsule strain

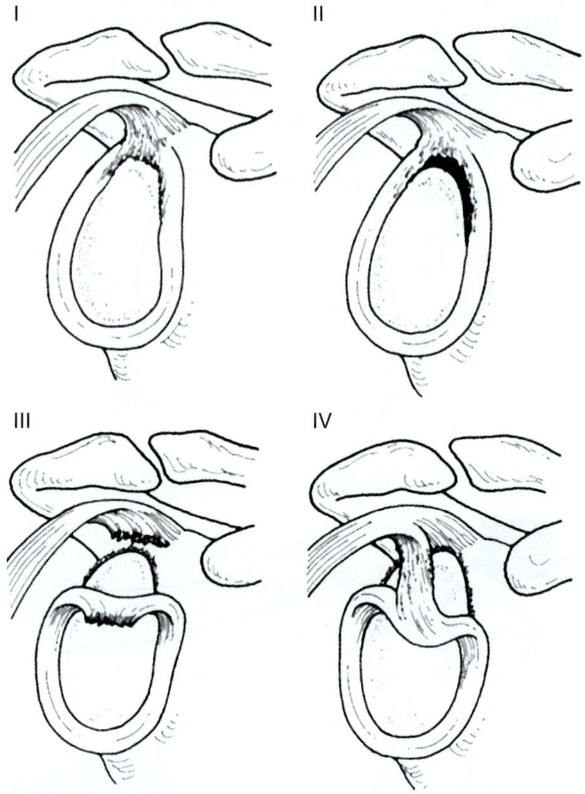

FIGURE 3.47 **Four types of lesions of the superior labrum as classified by Snyder and associates. These have been called SLAP lesions. Type I: degeneration of superior glenoid labrum. Type II: detachment of superior glenoid labrum and biceps tendon from the underlying glenoid rim. Type III: bucket-handle type tear of labrum with biceps tendon origin not torn. Type IV: Lengthwise tear of biceps tendon in which one part remains attached to the labrum and the other part attached to the supraglenoid tubercle. (*Source*: Snyder SJ, Karzel RP, DelPizzo W, Ferkel RD, Friedman MJ. SLAP lesions of the shoulder. *Arthroscopy* 1990;6:274–279.)**

- Loss of internal rotation occurs with an increase in external rotation commonly in overhead throwers and tennis players
- Posterior capsular stretching can improve symptoms (usually diffuse posterior deltoid pain) when accompanied by rest and gradual return to throwing; cortisone injection is not recommended because of possible false impression of

TABLE 3.20 Type-dependent treatment of SLAP tears

Type of SLAP Tear	Treatment
Type 1	Débride frayed labrum (anchor intact)
Type 2	Repair slap to stabilize anchor
Type 3	Débride labrum (biceps anchor attached)
Type 4	Repair labrum and biceps tear
Type 5	Repair
Type 6	Débride flap
Type 7	Repair labrum

improvement; pitching through the pain can cause further damage to the labrum and capsule; a sling and external rotator strengthening will not improve internal rotation

Brachial Plexus Injuries. Brachial plexus injuries result from compression of the brachial plexus, an injury commonly seen in football players as a result of tackling or falling on the shoulder and neck (Fig. 3.49). Burners or stingers, as they are commonly known, are the most frequent cervical spine injury in football players. The athlete usually complains of a transient, unilateral muscle paresis of the upper extremity with or without an accompanying burning or tingling sensation. Sometimes an athlete may present with a transient flail upper extremity. This injury is the result of traction to the upper trunk of the brachial

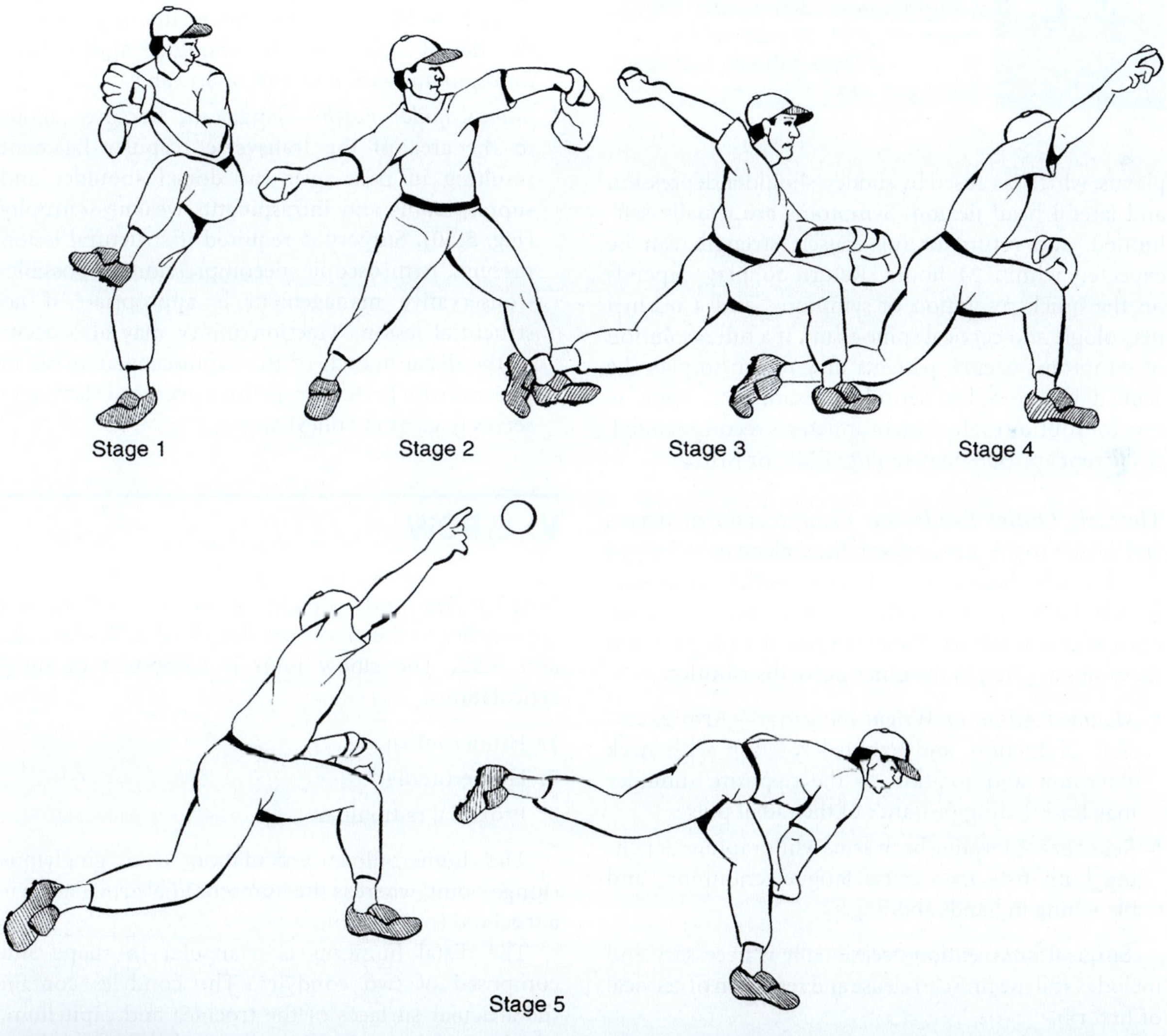

FIGURE 3.48 The five phases of the baseball pitch. (*Source*: Tibone JE, McMahon PJ. Biomechanics and pathologic lesions in the overhead athlete. In: Iannotti JP, Williams GR Jr (eds.), *Disorders of the Shoulder: Diagnosis and Management*. Philadelphia, Lippincott Williams & Wilkins, 1999.)

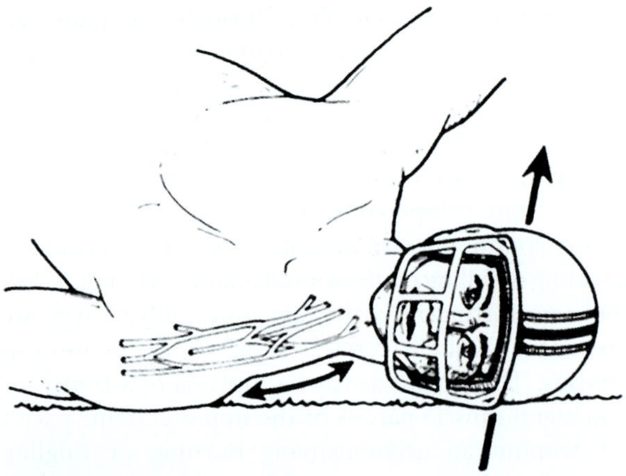

FIGURE 3.49 Mechanism of injury to the brachial plexus (burners). (*Source*: Zarins B, Prodromos LC. Shoulder injuries in sports. In: Rowe CR (ed.), *The Shoulder*. New York: Churchill Livingstone, 1988:411–433.)

plexus, which is caused by sudden shoulder depression and lateral head flexion. Symptoms are usually self-limited, and return of full muscle strength can be expected within 24 hours. Return to play depends on the quick resolution of symptoms and a normal neurologic and cervical spine exam. If a full resolution of symptoms occurs, patients may return to play the same day. A complete neurologic exam and c-spine x-rays for routine evaluation of athletes is recommended. Recurrent episodes may require EMG or MRI.

Thoracic Outlet Syndrome. Compression of nerves and vessels to the arm between the scalene muscles and the first rib characterizes thoracic outlet syndrome. It may be associated with a cervical rib or scalene muscle abnormalities. Patients present with pain and paresthesias often in the ulnar nerve distribution.

- *Modified Adson or Wright maneuver*—Arm extension, abduction, and external rotation with neck extension and rotation to the opposite shoulder may lead to disappearance of the radial pulse.
- *Roos test*—Elevating both arms while rapidly clenching both fists may cause fatigue, cramping, and blanching in hands and fingers.

Surgical intervention occasionally is necessary and includes scalene muscle release and resection of cervical or first rib.

Lateral Scapular Winging. Long, thoracic nerve palsy will result in scapular winging due to serratus anterior muscle dysfunction. The scapula assumes a position of elevation and medial translation with the inferior angle rotated medially. This condition is common in competitive swimmers and may have a viral etiology. Observation is recommended because scapular winging often resolves spontaneously by 18 months. Bracing may be effective because it avoids recurrent traction and helps nerve regeneration. Pectoralis transfer has been used for chronic cases.

Medial Scapular Winging. Cranial nerve XI (Spinal Accessory Nerve) palsy results in scapular winging due to trapezius muscle dysfunction. CN XI is vulnerable during cervical biopsy (lymph nodes). The shoulder will appear depressed and laterally translated because of unopposed serratus function.

Suprascapular Nerve. Compression may occur at various points along its path.

- *Spinoglenoid notch*—Cysts in this location may be caused by SLAP lesions and result in pain over the dorsal aspect of the shoulder and *isolated infraspinatus* weakness and/or atrophy.
- *Suprascapular notch*—Ganglia or fracture callous in the area of the transverse scapular ligament resulting in pain over the dorsal shoulder and supraspinatus and infraspinatus weakness/atrophy (Fig. 3.50). Surgery is required if structural lesion present. Arthroscopic decompression is possible. Conservative management is appropriate if no structural lesion. Traction injury may also occur to the distal branch of the suprascapular nerve in patients who perform repetitive overhead slams and serves (e.g., as in volleyball).

V. ELBOW

Surgical Anatomy. Muscles of the arm and surgical approaches to the elbow are described in Tables 3.21 and 3.22. The elbow joint is composed of three articulations:

1. Humeroulnar
2. Humeroradial
3. Proximal radioulnar.

The humeroulnar articulation is a ginglymus (hinge) joint, whereas the humeroradial articulation is a trochoid (pivot) joint.

The distal humerus is triangular in shape and composed of two condyles. The condyles contain the articular surfaces of the trochlea and capitellum, which articulate with the ulna and radial head respectively. The medial epicondyle serves as the attachment of the medial collateral ligament (MCL) and the flexor-pronator muscles of the forearm (FCR, FCU, FDS, pronator teres, and palmaris longus). The lateral

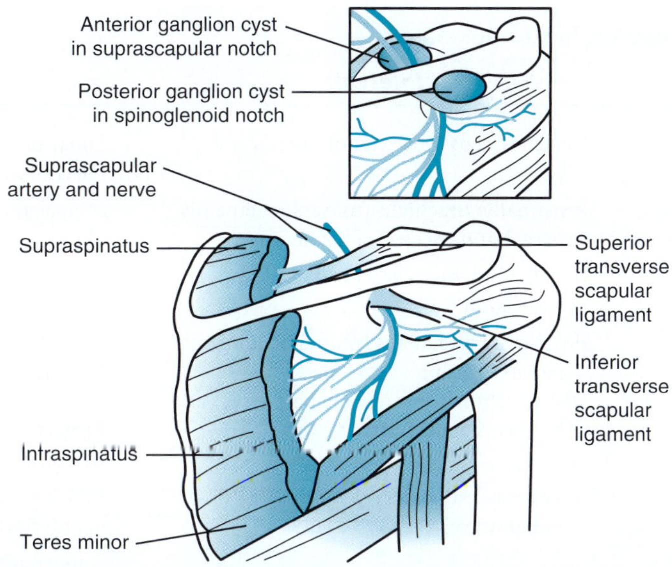

FIGURE 3.50 **The suprascapular nerve: potential sites of entrapment at the suprascapular and spinoglenoid notches; *lig.*, ligament. (*Adapted from* Fritz RC, Helms CA, Steinbach LS, Genant HK. Suprascapular nerve entrapment: Evaluation with MR imaging. *Radiology* 1992;132:438.)**

epicondyle serves as the attachment for the lateral collateral ligament (LCL) and the extensor muscles of the forearm (ECRL, ECRB, ECU, EDM, anconeus, and supinator).

The proximal ulna is composed of two curved processes: the olecranon and coronoid. The coronoid process is essential for the prevention of posterior subluxation.

The proximal radius is composed of the radial head, neck, and radial tuberosity. The radial head is an important secondary stabilizer against posterior displacement, and its integrity should be maintained in the setting of coronoid fractures.

Joint Articulations. The ulnohumeral joint is a congruous joint. In extension, the olecranon articulates with the olecranon fossa. In flexion, the radial head and coronoid articulate with their respective fossae. The ulnohumeral joint transmits 40% of an axial load, while the radiohumeral joint transmits 60%.

Nerves and Vessels of the Elbow. Numerous vessels and nerves of clinical significance surround the elbow. The location of these structures is a major determinant of surgical incisions and arthroscopic portal placement. The brachial artery lies medial to the biceps tendon, between the bicipital aponeurosis and brachialis

TABLE 3.21 **Muscles of the arm**

Muscle	*Origin*	*Insertion*	*Action*	*Innervation*
Coracobrachialis	Coracoid	Medial humerus	Flexion, adduction	Musculocutaneous
Biceps	Coracoid (SH)		Supination, flexion	Musculocutaneous
	supraglenoid (LH)	Radial tuberosity		
Brachialis	Anterior humerus	Ulnar tuberosity	Forearm flexion	Musculocutaneous radial
Triceps	Infraglenoid (LH)		Forearm extension	Radial
	Posterior humerus (Lat H)	Olecranon		
	Posterior humerus (Med H)			

SH, Short Head; LH, long head; Lat H, lateral head; Med H, medial head
Adapted from Miller MD. *Review of Orthopaedics, Anatomy*, 4th ed. Philadelphia: WB Saunders; 2004: 606, Table 11-6.

TABLE 3.22 Surgical approaches to the elbow

Approach	Interval	Risks
Posterior	Detach triceps or olecranon osteotomy	Ulnar nerve Olecranon nonunion
Medial	Proximally: Brachialis (musculocutaneous nerve) and triceps (radial nerve) Distally: Brachialis and pronator teres (median nerve)	Medial antebrachial cutaneous nerve
Anterolateral (Henry)	Proximally: Brachialis (musculocutaneous nerve) splitting Distally: Pronator teres (median nerve) and brachioradialis (radial nerve)	Lateral antebrachial cutaneous nerve Radial nerve Ligation of radial recurrent artery Protect brachial artery Important: Supinate forearm
Posterolateral (Kocher)	Anconeus (radial nerve) and ECU (PIN of radial nerve)	PIN (pronation moves PIN anteriorly and radially) Important: Pronate forearm

Adapted from Miller MD. *Review of Orthopaedics, Anatomy*, 4th ed. Philadelphia: WB Saunders; 2004: 606, Table 11.6.

muscle. It bifurcates at the cubital fossa to form the radial and ulnar arteries. The profunda brachii also contributes to the collateral circulation of the elbow.

The median, radial, and ulnar nerves traverse the elbow joint where they innervate the muscles of the forearm. The median nerve lies deep to the bicipital aponeurosis, anterior to the medial epicondyle and medial to the brachial artery. The radial nerve passes anterior to the lateral epicondyle and between the brachialis and brachioradialis. The ulnar nerve traverses the ulnar groove posterior to the medial epicondyle.

Biomechanics of the Elbow. The elbow is a hinge joint that allows slight varus and valgus motion as well as 3 to 5 degrees of rotational motion throughout flexion and extension. Normal ROM of the elbow includes extension to 0 degrees, flexion to 145 degrees, and pronation and supination to 90 degrees. However, activities of daily living require only a 100-degree arc of motion in flexion and extension (30 to 130 degrees) as well as in pronation and supination (50 to 50 degrees).

Both bony architecture and soft tissues contribute to the stability of the elbow joint. The bony articulation resists valgus and varus forces and has increased stability in extension. Soft tissue stability conferred to the elbow joint includes static and dynamic stabilization. Static stabilization is provided by the MCL, LCL, and joint capsule, especially in flexion. Dynamic stabilization is provided by the various muscles that cross the elbow joint. Since the flexor-pronator group is responsible for dynamic stabilization against valgus stress, this group of muscles must be incorporated in the rehabilitation program following MCL injury or reconstruction. Similarly, the supinator-extensor group must be strengthened after LCL injury or reconstruction because this group of muscles dynamically stabilizes the LCL. Of note, care must be taken not to disrupt the LCL during surgery for tennis elbow because that would result in iatrogenic instability.

MCL Injuries. During overhead motion, tensile forces are applied across the medial aspect of the elbow. Particularly during the late cocking and acceleration phases of throwing, excessive and repetitive stresses can injure the MCL. The anterior bundle of the MCL is the primary constraint to valgus instability of the elbow (Fig. 3.51). The MCL differs from the LCL in that it does not demonstrate isometry. The MCL undergoes a cam effect between the anterior and posterior bundles, which maintains ligamentous tension throughout the flexion-extension arc (Fig. 3.52). Clinically, MCL injuries may present as chronic or acute. Therefore, the chronology of past elbow symptoms and injuries should be reviewed. Most patients report an insidious onset of symptoms consistent with repetitive microtrauma associated with throwing sports. Acute MCL ruptures are rare but can occur. Acute ruptures are characterized by a "pop" and immediate pain at the medial aspect of the elbow. In either acute or chronic cases, tenderness is noted along the course of the ligament, which extends from the medial epicondyle to the sublime tubercle of the ulna. Valgus instability is present in approximately 25% of patients. Associated ulnar nerve involvement is common. Plain radiographs should be reviewed for avulsion fractures, posteromedial osteophytes, loose bodies, and osteochondritic lesions of the capitellum. Stress radiographs may demonstrate excessive medial joint opening. MRI is recommended to confirm the diagnosis. The use of

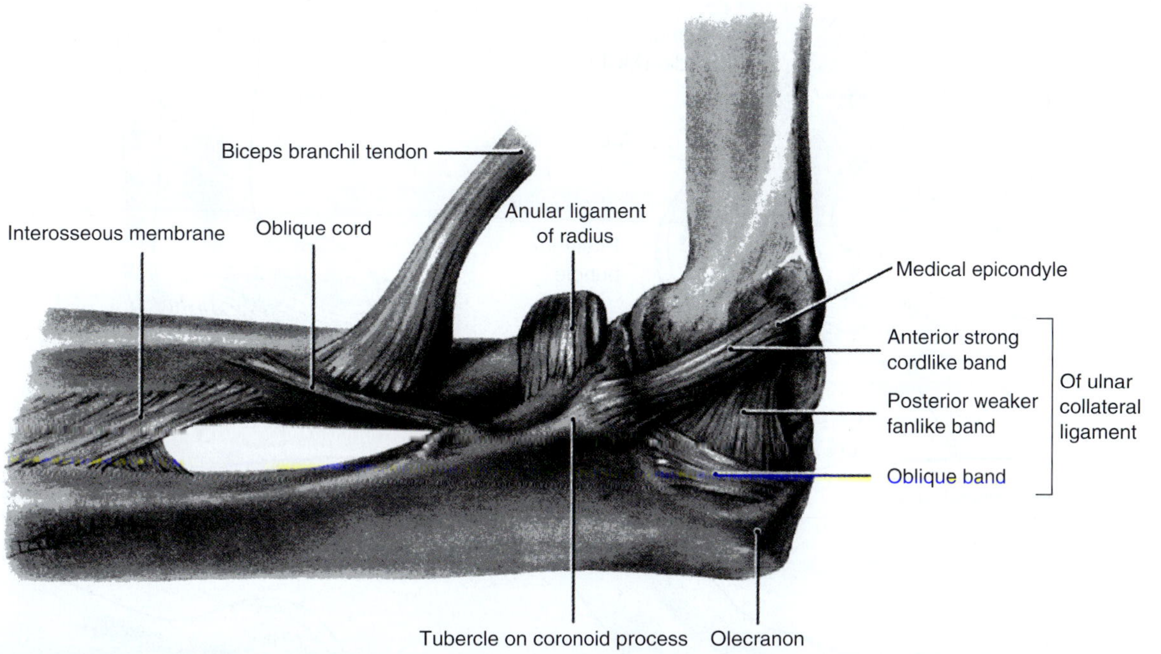

FIGURE 3.51 **Medial collateral ligament (MCL) anatomy. (*Source*: Agur AMR, Lee MK. *Grant's Atlas of Anatomy*, 10th ed. Philadelphia: Lippincott Williams & Wilkins, 1999: Fig. 6.51A.)**

contrast MRI may further delineate partial-thickness or undersurface tears.

Treatment of MCL Injuries. Initial treatment includes rest, physical therapy, and restoration of elbow motion. Surgery is indicated for competitive athletes who desire to return to overhead sports. Reconstruction is favored over repair. Approximately 80% of athletes with MCL reconstruction return to a previous or better level of performance. Palmaris longus tendon is the most commonly used graft and is passed through drill holes in a figure-of-8 manner. The ulnar nerve should be transposed in a subcutaneous fashion if symptomatic preoperatively. The patient can be expected to return to sports in approximately 1 year.

LCL Complex Injuries. The LCL complex is composed of the lateral collateral, lateral ulnar collateral, and annular ligaments (Fig. 3.53). The main function of the LCL complex is to provide stability to external rotation and varus stresses to the elbow joint as the elbow flexes. The LCL complex also plays a role in the stability of the radial head. Among the three components of the LCL complex, the lateral ulnar collateral ligament (LUCL) is referred to as the *essential lesion* and is the primary constraint against posterolateral rotatory instability (PLRI). It is the homologue of the anterior bundle of the MCL. Disruption of the LCL is usually caused by elbow dislocation or subluxation, and less commonly by varus stress. With elbow subluxation or dislocation, the LUCL is one of the first structures to be disrupted (Fig. 3.54). On physical examination, varus stress testing may not reveal any abnormality. However, PLRI can be demonstrated with the lateral pivot-shift test of the elbow. This test is performed by applying a valgus and external rotation force to the forearm (Fig. 3.55). In PLRI, the radial head subluxates posteriorly and reproduces symptoms. Surgery is indicated for patients with recurrent pain, instability, and mechanical symptoms. The *docking procedure* involves reconstruction with a palmaris longus tendon through a modified Kocher incision (Fig. 3.56).

Lateral Epicondylitis. Lateral epicondylitis, or tennis elbow, is thought to be caused by repetitive microtraumatic eccentric overload injury to the wrist and finger extensors, although the exact etiology is poorly understood. The primary pathologic lesion involves the origin of the ECRB. However, the origin of the ECRL and EDC can also be involved. Histopathology of the pathologic lesions demonstrates angiofibroblastic hyperplasia, suggesting that this condition is degenerative in nature rather than inflammatory. Therefore, lateral epicondylitis is more correctly described as a tendinosis rather then tendinitis. Diagnosis is made by history and physical examination, which include tenderness over the common extensor origin that is worsened with resisted wrist extension and supination. Plain radiographs may show soft tissue calcification around the epicondyle in some cases. MRI may be useful in confirming a tear and tendinosis of the ECRB.

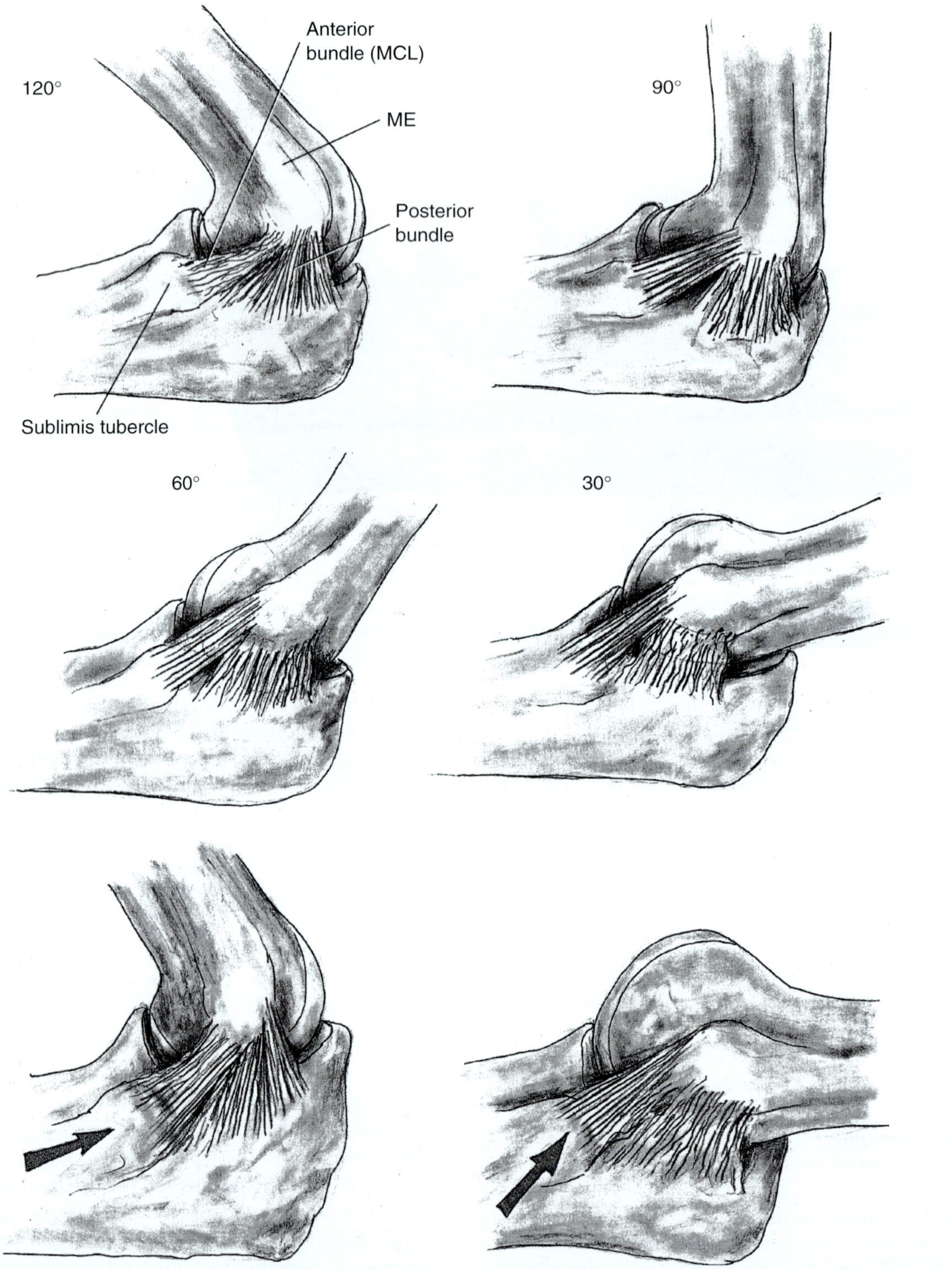

FIGURE 3.52 MCL cam effect. (*Adapted from* Callaway GH, Field LD, Deng XH, et al. Biomechanical evaluation of the medial collateral ligament of the elbow. *J Bone Joint Surg Am* 1997;79A:1223–1231.)

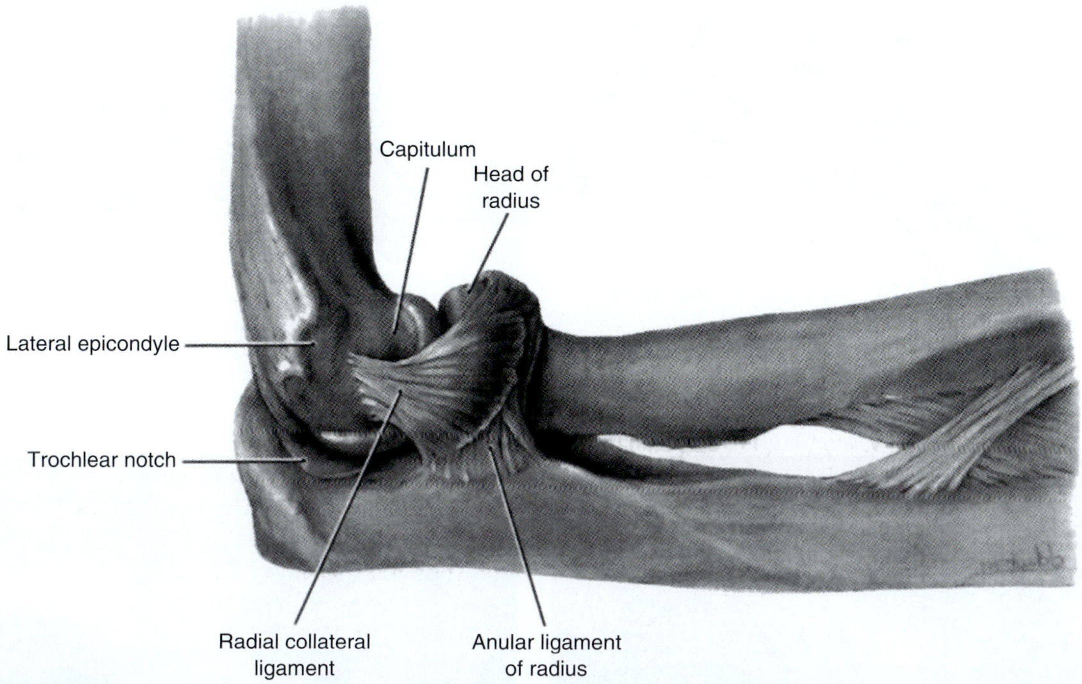

FIGURE 3.53 **LCL complex. (*Source*: Agur AMR, Lee MK. *Grant's Atlas of Anatomy,* 10th ed. Philadelphia: Lippincott Williams & Wilkins, 1999: Fig. 6.51B.)**

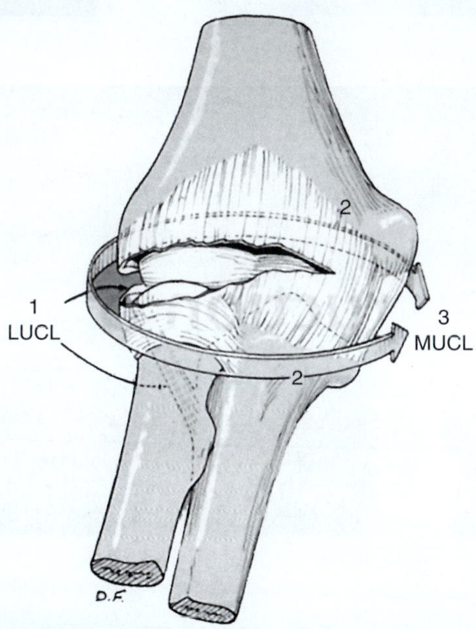

FIGURE 3.54 **Elbow dislocation disrupts LUCL. (*Adapted from* O'Driscoll SW, Morrey BF. Surgical reconstruction of the lateral collateral ligament. In: Morrey BF (ed.), *Master Techniques in Orthopaedic Surgery: The Elbow*, 2nd ed. Philadelphia: Lippincott Williams & Wilkins, 2002; 250: Fig. 15.1.)**

Treatment of Lateral Epicondylitis. Initial treatment is nonoperative and includes avoidance of offending activities and NSAID therapy. A tennis elbow counterforce brace and/or local injection may also be used. Nonoperative treatment is successful in approximately 90% of cases. Surgery is indicated in patients who fail conservative therapy. Surgical treatment of tennis elbow has evolved with increasing understanding of the true pathoanatomy. The current preferred procedure is an open release and débridement of the ECRB with closure of the extensor-supinator mass (Fig. 3.57).

Medial Epicondylitis. Medial epicondylitis, or golfer's elbow, is an overuse syndrome that results in tendinosis of the flexor pronator mass. Injury to the myotendinous junction at the medial epicondyle occurs in response to repetitive microtrauma resulting in tendon degeneration. Medial epicondylitis is much less common than lateral epicondylitis. Initial treatment is similar to that of tennis elbow. If surgery is indicated, the ulnar nerve on the affected upper extremity should be thoroughly evaluated because there is a high correlation between medial epicondylitis and ulnar nerve dysfunction. If the patient has any ulnar nerve deficit, the patient should undergo an ulnar nerve transposition in addition to removal of degenerated tendon tissue (Fig. 3.58).

Distal Biceps Avulsion. Distal biceps avulsion is a relatively uncommon injury that accounts for less

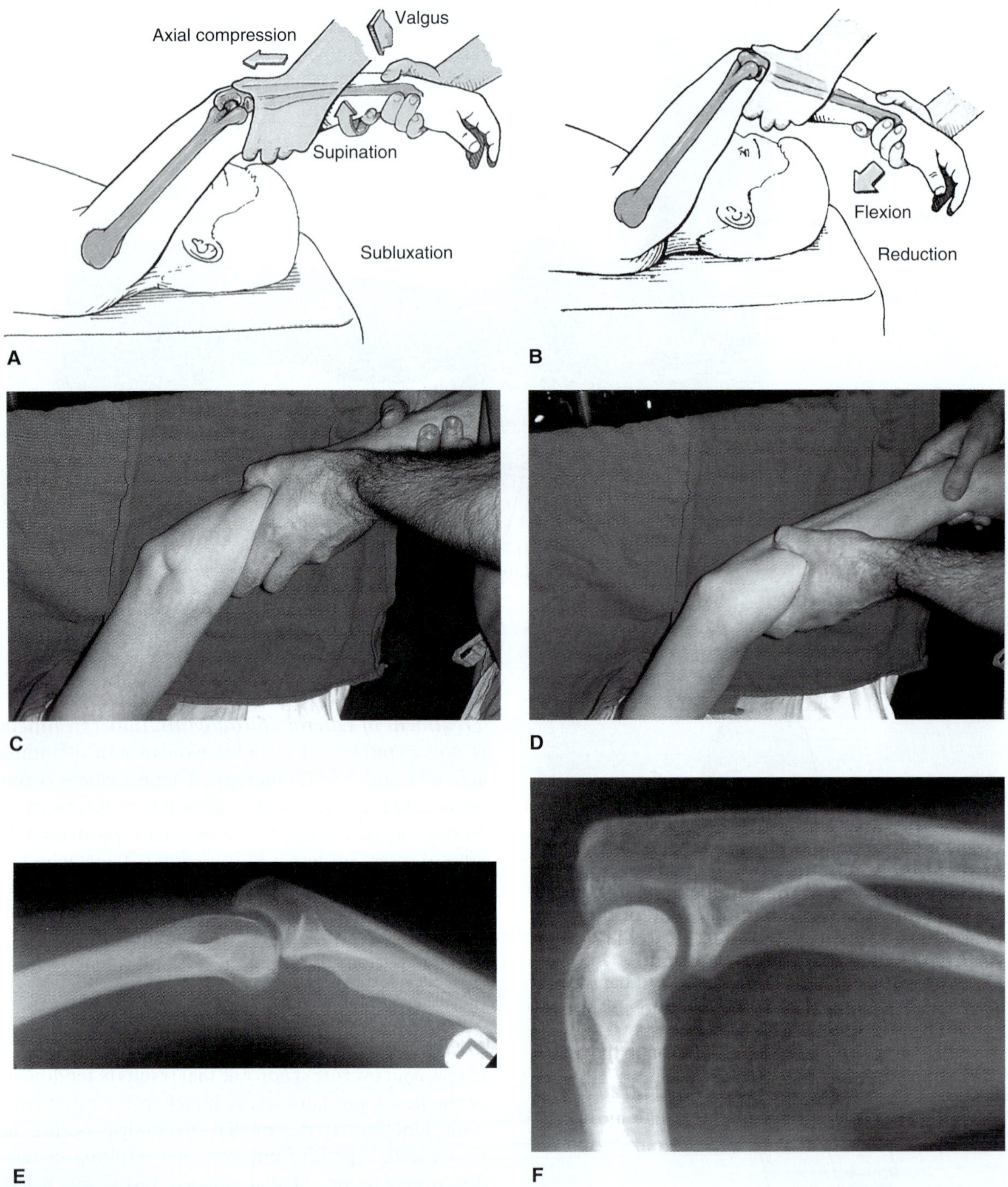

FIGURE 3.55 **Lateral pivot shift test of elbow. (*Adapted from* O'Driscoll SW, Morrey BF. Surgical reconstruction of the lateral collateral ligament. In: Morrey BF (ed.), *Master Techniques in Orthopaedic Surgery: The Elbow*, 2nd ed. Philadelphia: Lippincott Williams & Wilkins, 2002; 252: Fig. 15.3.)**

than 5% of all biceps ruptures. However, more cases have been reported in recent years with increasing frequency. The mechanism of injury involves the application of an eccentric load to the elbow with a sudden extension force while the elbow is in midflexion. This injury occurs predominantly in middle-aged men (30 to 50 years old) and usually affects the dominant extremity. Patients report hearing a "pop" with immediate pain, swelling, and ecchymosis in the antecubital fossa. Clinically, elbow flexion and forearm supination are weak. MRI may be used to confirm the diagnosis. Complete avulsion

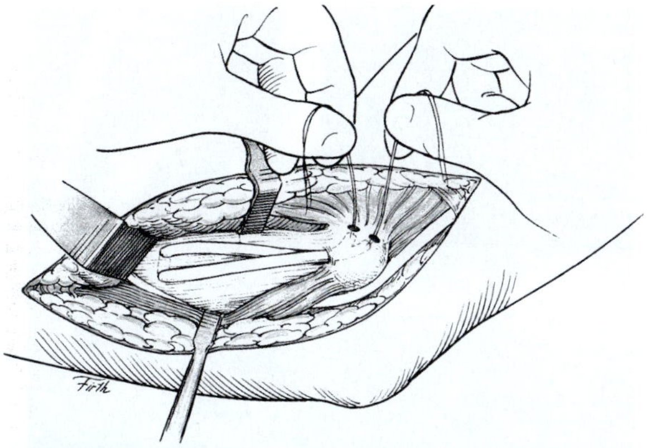

FIGURE 3.56 Docking procedure. (*Adapted from* O'Driscoll SW, Morrey BF. Surgical reconstruction of the lateral collateral ligament. In: Morrey BF (ed.), *Master Techniques in Orthopaedic Surgery: The Elbow*, 2nd ed. Philadelphia: Lippincott Williams & Wilkins, 2002; 241: Fig. 14.7.)

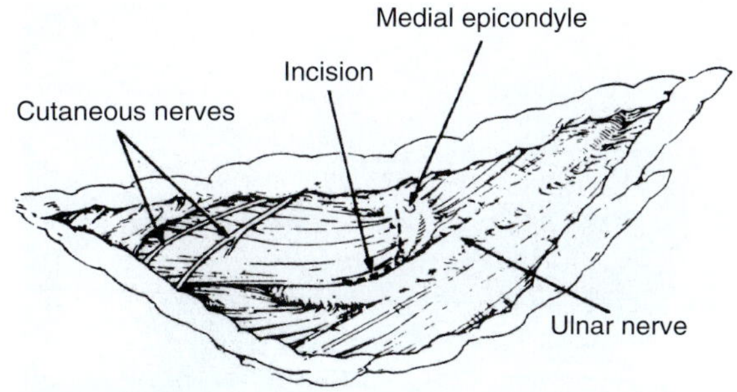

FIGURE 3.58 Indications for ulnar nerve transposition. (*Source*: David TS, Bast SC, Gambardella RA. Medial tendon injury: Open and arthroscopic treatment. In: Altchek DW, Andrews JR (eds.), *The Athlete's Elbow*. Philadelphia: Lippincott Williams & Wilkins, 2001; 86: Fig. 5.2.)

of the tendon from its insertion on the radial tuberosity is more common than partial ruptures of the tendon distally. Acute ruptures of the distal biceps tendon should be surgically reattached. Although acceptable to good results were reported in the past with nonanatomic reattachment of the distal biceps to the brachioradialis, recent studies support an anatomic repair to the radial tuberosity. Successful anatomic repairs may be achieved either by 1-incision or 2-incision techniques. The lateral antebrachial cutaneous nerve is vulnerable during the surgical dissection and approach to reattach the distal biceps tendon (Fig. 3.59). Other complications include heterotopic ossification and loss of elbow motion (particularly extension).

Distal Triceps Avulsion. Distal triceps avulsion is a rare injury. In the past 2 decades, only sporadic case reports of this injury were published. Different from distal biceps ruptures, distal triceps ruptures occur in both men and women. The mechanism of injury involves the application of a decelerating force to the arm during extension as the triceps muscle is

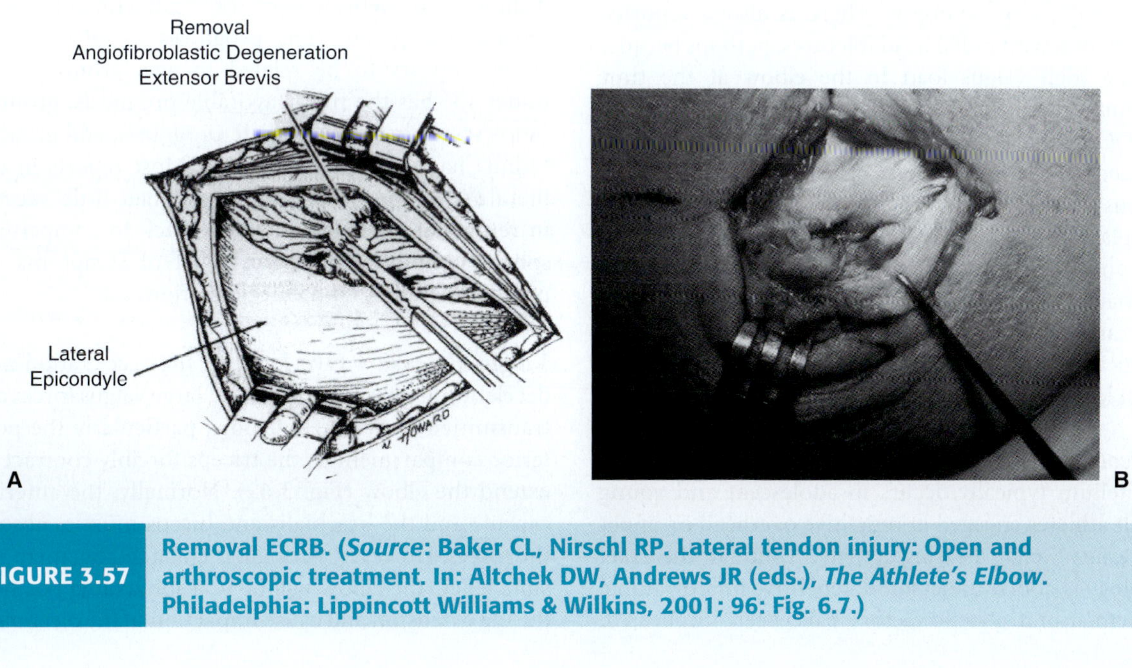

FIGURE 3.57 Removal ECRB. (*Source*: Baker CL, Nirschl RP. Lateral tendon injury: Open and arthroscopic treatment. In: Altchek DW, Andrews JR (eds.), *The Athlete's Elbow*. Philadelphia: Lippincott Williams & Wilkins, 2001; 96: Fig. 6.7.)

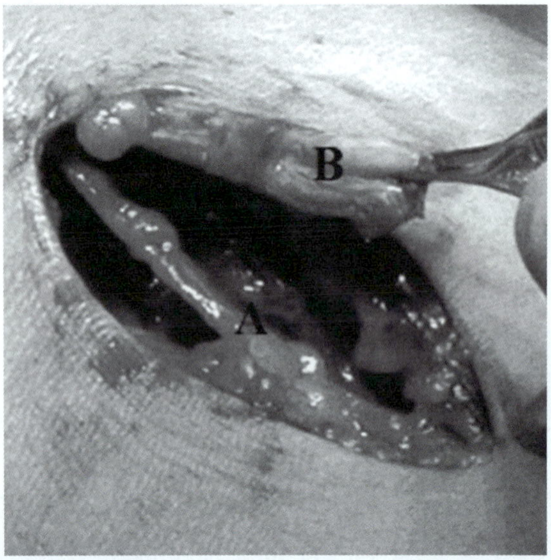

FIGURE 3.59 LABCN. (*Source*: Johnson DC, Allen Answorth A. Biceps and triceps tendon injury. In: Altchek DW, Andrews JR (eds.), *The Athlete's Elbow*. Philadelphia: Lippincott Williams & Wilkins, 2001; 106: Fig. 7.1.)

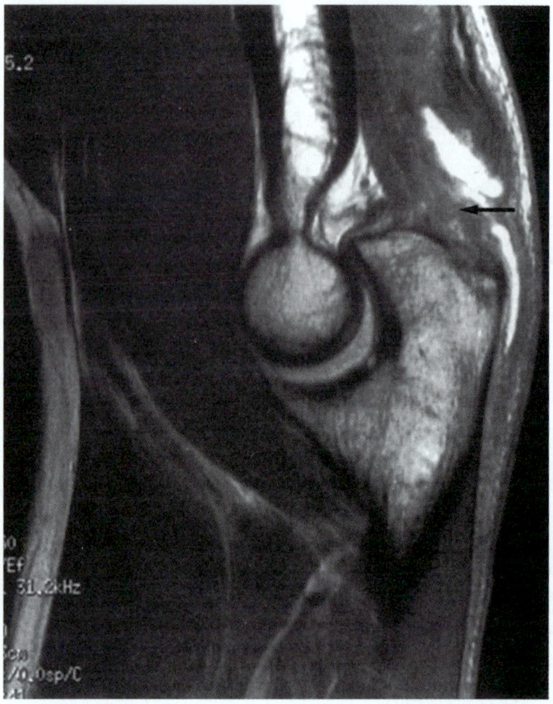

FIGURE 3.60 Distal triceps rupture. (*Source*: Johnson DC, Allen Answorth A. Biceps and triceps tendon injury. In: Altchek DW, Andrews JR (eds.), *The Athlete's Elbow*. Philadelphia: Lippincott Williams & Wilkins, 2001; 116: Fig. 7.15.)

contracting, such as after a fall on to an outstretched hand. This injury may be associated with steroid injections and chronic olecranon bursitis. Metabolic conditions such as Marfan syndrome, osteogenesis imperfecta, hypothyroidism, or renal osteodystrophy may also be a contributing factor. For example, elevated parathyroid hormone in patients with renal osteodystrophy can stimulate increased osteoclastic bone resorption, which may be a predisposing factor for distal triceps avulsion. There is also a reported association with radial head fractures, perhaps because of the high valgus load to the elbow at the time of injury. Clinically, patients sustain this injury after a FOOSH (fell onto outstretched hand) injury with immediate pain, palpable defect, and weak elbow extension. An avulsion fragment of bone may be seen on plain radiographs. Otherwise, MRI may be used to confirm the diagnosis (Fig. 3.60). Treatment is by primary reattachment of the avulsed tendon to the olecranon via transosseous tunnels (Fig. 3.61). After surgical treatment, the most common complication is a flexion contracture of the elbow.

Osteochondritis Dissecans (OCD). OCD of the capitellum typically occurs in adolescent and young adult athletes engaged in repetitive overhead or upper extremity weight-bearing activity. Although the exact etiology is poorly understood, repetitive microtrauma, ischemia, and genetic factors have been implicated. Plain radiographs and MRI are recommended to confirm the diagnosis. Treatment ranges from activity modification for an intact fragment to arthroscopic drilling and débridement or reattachment for a separated fragment. The prognosis of OCD of the elbow appears to be related to age: group 1 (age under 13) has the most favorable prognosis, group 2 (adolescent) has intermediate prognosis, and group 3 (adult) has the worst prognosis. Most reports in the literature suggest that surgery has had little success in returning patients with OCD back to competitive sports, obtaining long-term relief of symptoms, or preventing radiographic degeneration.

Valgus Extension Overload. In the acceleration and deceleration phases of throwing, large valgus forces are transmitted through the elbow, particularly the posterior compartment as the triceps forcibly contract to extend the elbow (Fig. 3.62). Normally, the anterior capsule and the brachialis and biceps muscles absorb the forces. However, with ulnar collateral ligament insufficiency, the elbow will be in a subluxated position during extension and cause impaction of the olecranon

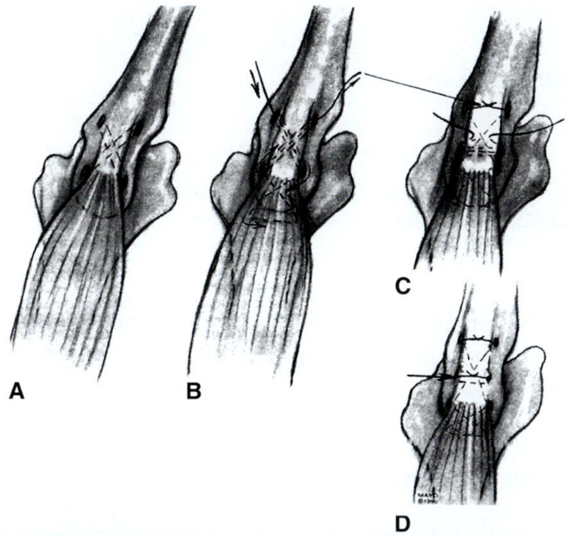

FIGURE 3.61 Distal triceps repair. (*Source*: Johnson DC, Allen Answorth A. Biceps and triceps tendon injury. In: Altchek DW, Andrews JR (eds.), *The Athlete's Elbow*. Philadelphia: Lippincott Williams & Wilkins, 2001; 117: Fig. 7.16.)

and the olecranon fossa posteromedially. As a result, posterior osteophytes develop and may lead to posterior impingement, loose bodies, and chondral defects. Clinically, patients report loss of extension and posterior elbow joint line tenderness. Elbow arthroscopy may be indicated to perform excision of osteophytes if conservative treatment has been ineffective.

Olecranon Stress Fractures. Stress fractures of the olecranon in baseball pitchers have been reported in the literature. High triceps forces coupled with isometric elbow extension during the acceleration phase of throwing can cause olecranon stress fractures. A throwing athlete with chronic posterolateral elbow pain that is recalcitrant to conservative therapy should undergo evaluation for a stress fracture. Imaging studies such as plain radiographs, bone scan, CT, or MRI should be part of the evaluation. Patients are initially treated by rest and activity restriction and may return to sports after documentation of healing and successful completion of an interval throwing program. Nonoperative management is usually effective for the treatment of olecranon stress fractures. However, refractory cases may need internal fixation with a cannulated screw.

Medial Epicondyle Fractures. In skeletally immature individuals, medial epicondylar physeal injuries may be the result of either acute trauma or repetitive stress. Adolescent throwers may present with either a widened

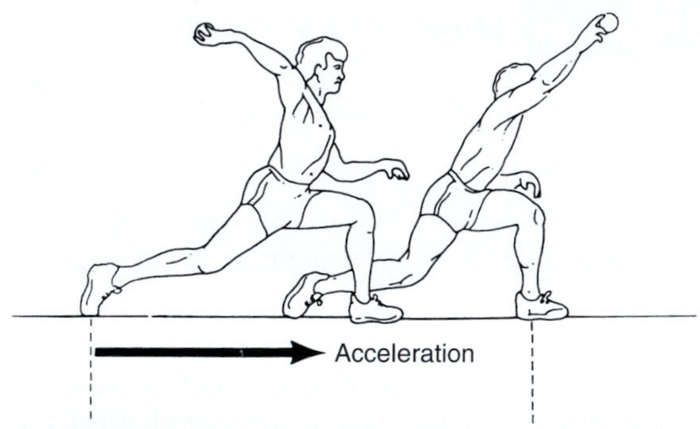

FIGURE 3.62 Acceleration phase. (*Source*: ElAttrache NS, Jobe FW. Treatment of ulnar collateral ligament injuries in athletes. In: Morrey BF (ed.). *Master Techniques in Orthopaedic Surgery: The Elbow*, 2nd ed. Philadelphia: Lippincott Williams & Wilkins, 2002; 230: Fig. 14.2.)

physis or stress fracture of the medial epicondylar physis as a result of repetitive valgus stress. Also known as Little Leaguer elbow, initial treatment with activity modification and immobilization is usually successful. Surgery is indicated if there is ulnar nerve involvement, displacement of medial epicondyle greater than 1 cm, or joint entrapment.

VI. HEAD AND SPINE INJURIES

Head Injuries

Concussions. Concussions are traumatically induced alterations in mental status that may or may not involve a loss of consciousness. Concussions can be subdivided by severity depending on whether loss of consciousness, amnesia, or associated neurologic sequelae has occurred. The major classification system is highlighted in Table 3.23. Athletes who experience loss of consciousness (LOC) for any period of time, even a few seconds, should not return to play that day. The official recommendation from the American Academy of Neurology is that the patient who experiences transient LOC may return to play in 1 week if completely asymptomatic. In cases of prolonged LOC, it is recommended that the patient be held out of play for 2 weeks. Management and return to play is dictated not only by the severity of the concussion but also by the number of concussions sustained by the athlete (Tables 3.23 and 3.24). Patients who suffer more than 2 grade 1 concussions in a season should not return to contact

TABLE 3.23 Concussion grading schemes

	Concussion grade and definition		
Guideline	**1**	**2**	**3**
American Academy of Neurology	No loss of consciousness Symptomatic < 15 minutes	No loss of consciousness Symptomatic 15 minutes	Any loss of consciousness

sports until next season. In some cases, concussions are followed by persistent complaints of physical, cognitive, affective, and behavioral symptoms, sometimes referred to as postconcussion syndrome. Controversy persists regarding the cause of persistent postconcussive symptoms and whether they arise from primarily physiological or psychological causes.

Second-Impact Syndrome. Second-impact syndrome is characterized by the rapid onset of catastrophic cerebral edema and brain swelling that can be life threatening and requires emergency medical treatment. It occurs in athletes who sustain minor head injuries shortly after a previous head injury from which they have not recovered.

Severe Head Injuries. More serious acute head injuries involve expanding mass lesions. High clinical suspicion and CT scans are often the key to diagnosis. Epidural hematomas are most commonly caused by skull fractures, leading to disruption of the middle meningeal artery and bleeding into the epidural space. The classic presentation is temporary LOC, followed by a "lucid interval" and then with rapid deterioration and brainstem compression. Surgical evacuation of the hematoma in a timely fashion is curative generally without any long-term sequelae. Subdural hematomas, intracerebral hematomas, and intraventricular hemorrhages also can occur in some badly injured athletes. These injuries require prompt hospitalization, neurosurgical consultation, and possible surgical intervention.

Spine Injuries

Cervical Spine Injuries. A wide variety of injuries can occur to the cervical spine during competitive athletics. The majority of these injuries are self-limited, and a full recovery and quick return to play is the norm. Because of the devastating complications that may result from mismanagement of cervical spine injuries, all suspected injuries should be treated with caution and vigilance.

Root and Brachial Plexus Neurapraxia. Burners or stingers are the most frequent cervical spine injury in football players. The athlete usually complains of a transient, unilateral muscle paresis with or without an accompanying burning sensation. This injury is the result of traction to the upper trunk of the brachial plexus, which is caused by sudden shoulder depression and lateral head flexion (see Fig. 3.49). Symptoms are usually self-limited, and return of full muscle strength can be expected within 24 hours. Return to play depends on the quick resolution of symptoms and a normal neurologic and cervical spine examination and plain radiograph. A player should be removed from competition until a cervical spine radiograph is

TABLE 3.24 Guidelines for management of first concussion

	Concussion grade and recommendations		
Guideline	**1**	**2**	**3**
American Academy of Neurology	May return to play if asymptomatic for at least 15 minutes	May return to play if asymptomatic at rest and after exertion for 1 week	May transport athlete to hospital emergency department; for momentary LOC, may return to play if asymptomatic for 1 week after momentary LOC and if asymptomatic for 2 weeks after prolonged LOC

Note. Recommendations for management differ for athletes with more than one concussion. LOC, loss of consciousness

TABLE 3.25 Nerve injury grade

Grade	*Classification*	*Physiology*
1	Neuropraxia	Demyelination of the axon sheath
2	Axonotmesis	Disruption of the axon and myelin sheath
3	Neurotmesis	Disruption of the epineureum and endoneureum

obtained if burners occur more than once. There are several grades of nerve injury (Table 3.25).

Acute Cervical Sprain. An acute cervical sprain, also known as whiplash, is a ligamentous injury resulting from a direct collision. These patients have no neurologic deficits but demonstrate reproducible focal tenderness and limited neck ROM. Because of the potential for instability, these patients should be protected in a hard collar and radiographs should be obtained. Once the acute symptoms have resolved, usually in 10 to 14 days, flexion-extension radiographs or an MRI should be obtained to assess for instability. Treatment is tailored to the severity of injury, and a hard collar should be worn until the patient demonstrates a pain-free neck ROM.

Acute Cervical Intravertebral Disk Herniation. Acute traumatic disk herniation can result in cord compression causing permanent or transient quadriplegia or quadriparesis. Injured players experiencing acute radiculopathy or motor weakness or paralysis of one or more extremities and decreased sensation should be suspected of an acute disk herniation. MRI confirms the diagnosis. Most common treatment consists of anterior diskectomy and fusion.

Cervical Stenosis. Cervical stenosis is the narrowing of the spinal canal in the anterior-to-posterior direction. Stenosis can be either congenital or acquired and is defined on the basis of a canal diameter of less than 13 mm. In order to minimize the inaccuracies of spinal canal measurements, the Pavlov ratio is often calculated from lateral radiographs. The Pavlov-Torg ratio is the ratio of the segmental sagittal diameter of the canal to the width of the vertebral body (Fig. 3.63). A ratio of less than 0.8 defines stenosis but may be artificially abnormal in patients with a larger vertebral body, especially male athletes, and therefore the spinal canal diameter is more reliable. Patients with congenital cervical stenosis may be at increased risk for neurapraxias of the cervical cord with transient quadriplegia or quadriparesis. Return to play for stenosis patients who suffer a cervical spine injury remains controversial. Spear tackler's spine refers to a dangerous constellation of cervical spine findings, which occurs in a subset of football players who employ improper tackling techniques. These findings include developmental stenosis, loss of the normal lordotic curve of the cervical spine, and various other posttraumatic abnormalities. Development of spear tackler's spine is an absolute contraindication for contact sports.

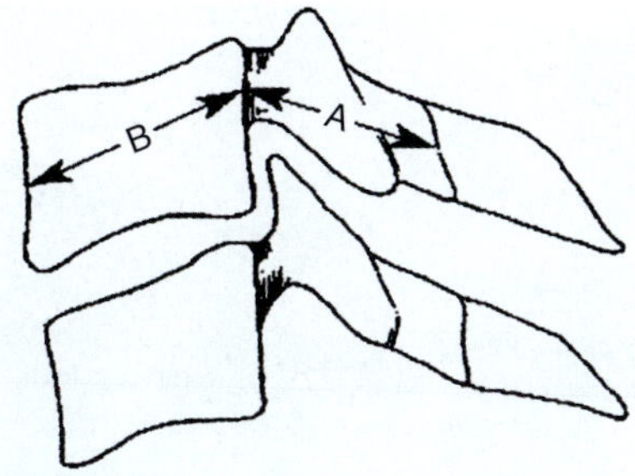

FIGURE 3.63 Pavlov ratio is calculated with the use of measurements on the lateral radiograph. The distance (A) is divided by the vertebral body (B). (*Source:* Thomas BE. Cervical spine injuries in football players. *J Am Acad Orthop Surg* 1999;7:338–347.)

Congenital Anomalies. The presence of congenital anomalies of the cervical spine alters the mechanical stability and greatly increases the risk for severe injury. Klippel-Feil syndrome is a failure of segmentation of the cervical spine resulting in the fusion of one or more motion segments (Fig. 3.64). This congenital fusion greatly alters the spine's ability to absorb and dissipate loads, thereby increasing the chance for injury. Congenital anomalies leading to a failure of formation of segments include odontoid agenesis or hypoplasia and developmental os odontoideum. These anomalies may cause significant atlantoaxial instability. While these conditions are frequently asymptomatic, if detected they are an absolute contraindication to contact sports.

Fractures and Dislocations. Most cervical spine fractures and dislocations that occur in sports are the result of axial loading of the cervical spine. Careful on-field management of serious cervical spine injuries is paramount. Proper acute management of the seriously injured athlete is important not only for appropriately treating life-threatening situations but also for preventing further morbidity. All unconscious athletes should be managed as if they have a cervical spine injury. The initial step consists of stabilizing the head and neck by manually holding them in

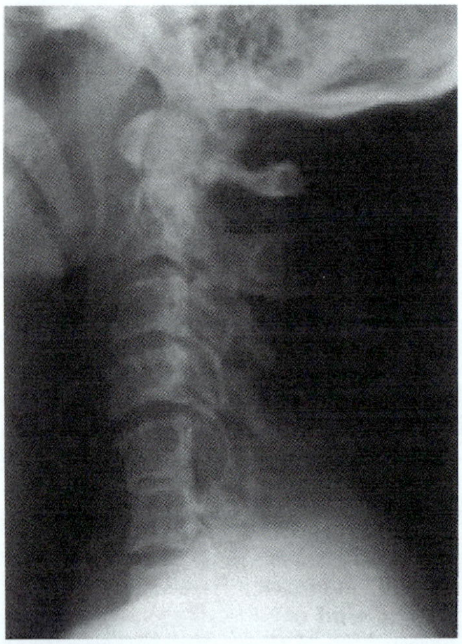

FIGURE 3.64 Lateral radiograph of a patient with Klippel-Feil syndrome demonstrating congenital failure of segmentation at C5-6. This patient should be restricted from contact sports. (*Source*: Thomas BE. Cervical spine injuries in football players. *J Am Acad Orthop Surg* 1999;7:338–347.)

a neutral position and logrolling the patient into a supine position. Next, ABCs and LOC are assessed. If the athlete is breathing, management should consist of mouth-guard removal and airway maintenance. If the athlete is not breathing, the face mask should be removed, with the helmet left in place. The airway must be established, followed by initiation of assisted breathing. CPR is instituted only when breathing and circulation are compromised. In the unconscious athlete or if cervical spine injury is suspected, the helmet should not be removed until the athlete has been transported to an appropriate facility and the cervical spine has been completely evaluated to avoid hyperextension of the cervical spine. Removal of the helmet and shoulder pads should be done simultaneously in the controlled setting of a hospital by 3 to 4 trained individuals.

Thoracic and Lumbar Spine Injuries. Most athletic thoracic and lumbar spine injuries involve the soft tissues surrounding the spine, including the paravertebral muscles and ligaments. Most of the strains and sprains are treated conservatively with rest, ice, analgesia, and physical therapy. Uneventful return to play is the norm. Disk herniation, primarily in the lumbar spine, is also commonly seen in athletes. Again, supportive therapy is generally successful, and surgery is reserved for patients with refractory sciatica. Spondylolysis is characterized by stress fractures of the pars interarticularis of the lumbar spine. This disorder presents as the insidious onset of lower back pain and is often seen in offensive linemen or gymnasts. Spondylolysis is thought to be caused by repetitive hyperextension of the spine, resulting in stresses on the pars interarticularis. Treatment is primarily supportive with rest and bracing. Surgery remains controversial but may be attempted to bridge the fracture with bone graft.

VII. MEDICAL MANAGEMENT OF THE ATHLETE

Medically Related Issues. The number one cause of sudden death in young athletes is myocardial pathology, with hypertrophic cardiomyopathy being the most common, while coronary artery disease is the most common in older athletes. Because of the muscle hypertrophy, the ventricular capacity is diminished and results in decreased cardiac output. During strenuous activity, the cardiac output cannot keep up with the demand, which leads to sudden death. A II/IV systolic ejection murmur is occasionally found in healthy athletes; however, when the murmur increases in intensity with maneuvers that decrease ventricular filling, such as standing or the Valsalva maneuver, dynamic obstruction that is the result of hypertrophic cardiomyopathy should be suspected. Commotio cordis can be caused by cardiac contusion from a direct blow to the chest (common in Little League baseball) and has a poor prognosis, even with immediate recognition and treatment. Normal EKG variants often seen in highly trained athletes include left ventricular hypertrophy, primary AV block, nonspecific STT wave changes in the lateral leads, and resting sinus bradycardia.

Traumatic Mydriasis. Traumatic mydriasis is a transient phenomenon during which the iris fails to constrict properly, resulting in a dilated pupil. The condition is caused by a contusion to the iris sphincter, usually from a direct blow to an athlete's eye. Physical examination reveals anisocoria (inequality in pupil size) but normal globe, normal extraocular movements, and grossly intact visual fields. More severe trauma can result in tear of the iris sphincter and permanent pupillary deformity.

Hyphema. Hyphema is blood in the eye associated with a vitreous or retinal injury in over 50% of cases.

Auricular Hematoma. Auricular hematoma is an acute, mildly tender, nonerythematous mass that occurs in the auricle (body) of the ear, generally in wrestlers who do not use protective headgear. The injury is related to blunt trauma and is not infectious in nature. Treatment consists of aspiration and application of a compressive dressing in order to reapproximate the perichondrium and limit reaccumulation of the fluid.

Amenorrhea. Amenorrhea may be due to low body-fat percentage and/or stress in female athletes. There is approximately a 50% incidence in elite runners and may be an underlying cause for stress fractures (osteopenia) and eating disorders. This condition is part of the female athlete triad and may be treated with birth control pills and dietary management.

Rib Stress Fractures. Rib stress fractures are the most common injury to the thorax in the rowing athlete. They generally occur during periods of intense training with a low stroke rate and heavy loads and are characterized by sudden onset of sharp, localized chest pain while rowing. One or more of the fifth through ninth ribs is generally affected. Diagnosis is best established with a bone scan.

On-Field Evaluation and Management of Seriously Injured Athlete. The initial step consists of stabilizing the head and neck by manually holding them in a neutral position. An athlete with suspected cervical spine injury may or may not be unconscious. All unconscious athletes should be managed as if they have a cervical spine injury. Next, ABCs and LOC are assessed. If the athlete is breathing, management should consist of mouth-guard removal and airway maintenance. If the athlete is not breathing, the face mask should be removed, with the helmet left in place. The airway must be established, followed by initiation of assisted breathing. CPR is instituted only when breathing and circulation are compromised. In the unconscious athlete or if cervical spine injury is suspected, the helmet should not be removed until the athlete has been transported to an appropriate facility and the cervical spine has been completely evaluated (Fig. 3.65).

Blunt Trauma. Blunt trauma to the torso can cause serious injury. Decreased breath sounds and hypotension can signify a tension pneumothorax and require immediate placement of a 14-gauge needle in the second intercostal space at the midclavicular line followed by a chest tube. The kidney is the most common organ injured, especially in boxing, followed by the spleen in football players.

Guidelines for Fluid and Electrolyte Replacement in Athletes. The goal of fluid replenishment should be to replace the sweat that has been lost. Sweat is mostly water, with a small concentration of salts and other electrolytes. Therefore, athletes should be encouraged to drink low osmolality (less than 10%) solutions before, during, and after athletic participation. Adding carbohydrates (glucose and maltodextrins) to the drink improves athletic performance by stimulating fluid absorption by the intestines. However, drinks that are high in fructose (orange juice) should be avoided because they slow intestinal absorption and may lead to GI distress and osmotic diarrhea. The water debt at the onset of exercise is most proportional to the magnitude of core temperature and heart rate increase in the high-demand athlete.

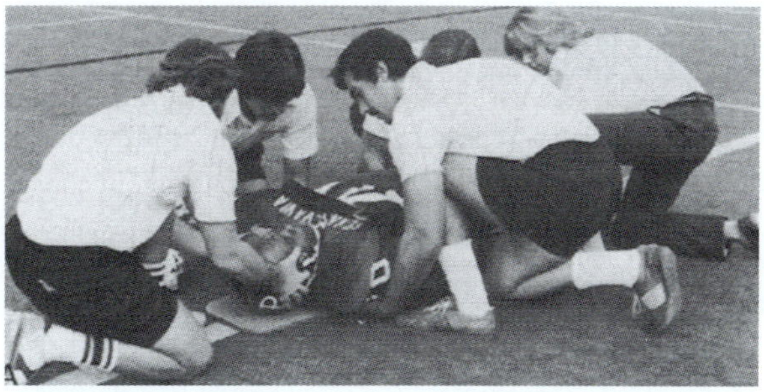

FIGURE 3.65 **In the severely injured athlete, assessment of ABCs and careful immobilization of the head and neck with the helmet still in place. (*Source*: Torg JS, Gennarelli TA. Head and cervical spine injuries. In: DeLee JC, Drez D (eds.), *Orthopaedic Sports Medicine*. Philadelphia: WB Saunders 1994; 421.)**

Doping. Anabolic steroids are a major problem in sports. These are derivatives of testosterone that act to build muscle mass, strength, and erythropoiesis. Associated adverse effects include liver dysfunction, hypercholesterolemia, cardiomyopathy, testicular atrophy, gynecomastia, and irreversible alopecia. Urine tests are commonly used to detect steroids. Human growth hormone is made from recombinant human DNA and has side effects similar to those of steroids, including hypertension and gigantism. Other drugs include amphetamines, diuretics, and laxatives.

Physical Therapy and Exercise. Physical therapy and exercise can have beneficial effects as treatment modalities and/or for prevention of injuries (Table 3.26). Stretching in conjunction with exercise is also beneficial.

TABLE 3.26 Exercise techniques

Exercise	Activity	Results
Isometric	Increased muscle tension but constant length	Muscle hypertrophy but not endurance
Isotonic	Weight lifting against a constant resistance through arc of motion	Improved motor function
Isokinetic	Weight lifting with constant velocity but variable resistance	Increased strength with less time
Plyometric	Rapid muscle shortening	Power generation
Functional	Aerobic fitness	

References

1. Abrams JS. Thermal capsulorrhaphy for instability of the shoulder: Concerns and applications of the heat probe. *Instr Course Lect* 2001;50:29–36.
2. Allen WC. Coxa saltans: The snapping hip revisited. *J Am Acad Orthop Surg* 1995;3:303–308.
3. Andrews JR, Timmerman LA. Outcome of elbow surgery in professional baseball players. *Am J Sports Med* 1995;23:407–413.
4. Arendt EA (ed.), *Orthopaedic Knowledge Update: Sports Medicine*. Rosemont, IL: American Academy of Orthopaedic Surgeons, 1999.
5. Baker CL, Uribe JW, Whitman C. Arthroscopic evaluation of acute initial anterior shoulder dislocations. *Am J Sports Med* 1990;18:25–28.
6. Barber FA. Coplaning of the acromioclavicular joint. *Arthroscopy* 2001;17:913–917.
7. Beiner JM, Jokl P. Muscle contusion injuries: Current treatment options. *J Am Acad Orthop Surg* 2001;9:227–237.
8. Bellier G, Dupont JY, Larrain M, et al. Lateral discoid menisci in children. *Arthroscopy* 1989;5:52–56.
9. Beynnon BD, Johnson RJ, Fleming BC, et al. The strain behavior of the anterior cruciate ligament during squatting and active flexion-extension: A comparison of an open and a closed kinetic chain exercise. *Am J Sports Med* 1997;25:823–829.
10. Blasier RB, Soslowsky LJ, Malicky DM, Palmer ML. Posterior glenohumeral subluxation: Active and passive stabilization in a biomechanical model. *J Bone Joint Surg Am* 1997;79:433–440.
11. Boden BP. High risk stress fractures: Evaluation and treatment. *J Am Acad Orthop Surg* 2000;8:344–353.
12. Bokor DJ, Hawkins RJ, Huckell GH, et al. Results of nonoperative management of full-thickness tears of the rotator cuff. *Clin Orthop* 1993;294:103–110.
13. Brinker M. *Basic Science in Review of Orthopaedics*, 3rd ed. Philadelphia: WB Saunders, 2000.
14. Brucker AJ. Diagnosis and management of injuries to the eye and orbit. In: Torg JS (ed.), *Athletic Injuries to the Head Neck and Face*, 2nd ed. St. Louis: Mosby Year Book, 1991;650–670.
15. Burkhart SS, Athanasiou KA, Wirth MA. Margin convergence: A method of reducing strain in massive rotator cuff tears. *Arthroscopy* 1996;12:335–338.
16. Burkhart SS. A stepwise approach to arthroscopic rotator cuff repair based on biomechanical principles. *Arthroscopy* 2000;16:82–90.
17. Callaway GH, Field LD, Deng X-H, et al. Biomechanical evaluation of the medial collateral ligament of the elbow. *J Bone Joint Surg* 1997;79A:1223–1231.
18. Canale ST (eds.). *Ankle injuries. Campbell's Operative Orthopaedics*, 10th ed. Philadelphia: Mosby, 1998;3:2131–2165.
19. Cannon LB, Hackney RG. Anterior tibiotalar impingement associated with chronic ankle instability. *J Foot Ankle Surg* 2000;39:383–386.
20. Chin KR, Barr SJ, Winalski C, Brick GW, MD. Treatment of advanced primary and recurrent diffuse pigmented villonodular synovitis of the knee: Comparison of open anterior and posterior synovectomy with and without adjuvant radiotherapy. *J Bone Joint Surg* 2002 Dec;84-A(12):2192–2202.
21. Chin KR, Brick GW, MD. Extraarticular pigmented villonodular synovitis of the knee: A cause for failed knee arthroscopy. *Clin Orthop* 2002 Nov;(404):330–338.
22. Colville MR. Surgical treatment of the unstable ankle. *J Am Acad Orthop Surg* 1998;6:368–77.
23. Conway JE, Jobe FW, Glousman RE, Pink M. Medial instability of the elbow in throwing athletes: Treatment by repair or reconstruction of the ulnar collateral ligament. *J Bone Joint Surg Am* 1992;74:67–83.
24. D'Alessandro DF, Shields CL Jr, Tibone JE, Chandler RW. Repair of distal biceps tendon ruptures in athletes. *Am J Sports Med* 1993;21:114–119.
25. Davison PA, Pink M, Perry J, Jobe FW. Functional anatomy of the flexor pronator muscle group in relation to the medial collateral ligament of the elbow. *Am J Sports Med* 1995;23:245–250.
26. DeHaven KE, Arnoczky SP. Meniscus repair: Basic science, indications for repair, and open repair. *Instr Course Lect* 1994;43:65–76.
27. Desio SM, Burks RT, Bachus KN. Soft tissue restraints to lateral patellar translation in the human knee. *Am J Sports Med* 1998;26:59–65.

28. Deutsch A, Altchek DW, Veltri DM, et al. Traumatic tears of the subscapularis tendon: Clinical diagnosis, MRI findings and operative treatment. *Am J Sports Med* 1997;25:13–22.
29. Durand P. On-field management of athletic head injuries. *J Am Acad Orthop Surg* 2004;12:191–95.
30. Federico DJ, Lynch JK, Jokl P. Osteochondritis dissecans of the knee: A historical review of etiology and treatment. *Arthroscopy* 1990;6:190–197.
31. Ferretti A, Cerullo G, Russo G. Suprascapular neuropathy in volleyball players. *J Bone Joint Surg Am* 1987; 69:260–263.
32. Fleisig GS, Escamilla RF. Biomechanics of the elbow in the throwing athlete. *Op Tech Sports Med* 1996;4:62–68.
33. Gisolfi CV. Guidelines for optimal replacement beverages for different athletic events. *Med Sci Sports Exerc* 1992;24:679–687.
34. Harmon KJ, Ireland ML. Gender differences in noncontact anterior cruciate ligament injuries. *Clin Sports Med* 2000;19:287–302.
35. Harner CD, Janaushek MA, Kanamori A, Yagi M, Vogrin T, Woo SL. Biomechanical analysis of a double-bundle posterior cruciate ligament reconstruction. *Am J Sports Med* 2000;28:144–151.
36. Haupt HA. Anabolic steroids and growth hormones: Current concepts. *Am. J. Sports Med* 1993;21:468–474.
37. Hawkins RJ, Bell RH, Hawkins RH, Koppert GJ. Anterior dislocation of the shoulder in the older patient. *Clin Orthop* 1986;206:192–195.
38. Hutchinson MR, Bae TS. Reproducibility of anatomic tibial landmarks for ACL reconstructions. *Am J Sports Med* 2001;29:777–780.
39. Iannotti JP, Williams GR. *Disorders of the Shoulder: Diagnosis and Management*, 1st ed. Philadelphia: Lippincott Williams & Wilkins, 1999;31–56.
40. Janarv PM, Hesser U, Hirsch G. Osteochondral lesions in the radiocapitellar joint in the skeletally immature: Radiographic, MRI, and arthroscopic findings in 13 consecutive cases. *J Pediatr Orthop* 1997;17:311–314.
41. Jobe FW, Moynes DR, Tibone JE, Perry J. An EMG analysis of the shoulder in pitching: A second report. *Am J Sports Med* 1984;12:218–220.
42. Jobe FW, Tibone JE, Jobe CM, Kvitne RS. The shoulder in sports, In: Rockwood CA, Matzen FA (eds.), *The Shoulder*. Philadelphia: WB Saunders, 1990;961–990.
43. Jones DC. Tendon disorders of the foot and ankle. *J Am Acad Orthop Surg* 1993;1:87–94.
44. Karlson KA. Rib stress fractures in elite rowers. *Am J Sports Med* 1998;26:516–520.
45. Kaufman BR. Sports related facial injuries. *Clin Sports Med* 1997;16:543–562.
46. Koffler KM, Kelly JD IV. Neurovascular trauma in athletes. *Orthop Clin North Am* 2002;33:523–534.
47. Koval KJ (ed.), *Orthopaedic knowledge update 7*. Rosemont, IL: American Academy of Orthopaedic Surgeons, 2002;407–416.
48. Koval KJ (ed.), *Orthopaedic Knowledge Update 7*. Rosemont, IL: American Academy of Orthopaedic Surgeons, 2002;99–110.
49. Kuhn JE, Plancher KD, Hawkins RJ. Scapular winging. *J Am Acad Orthop Surg* 1995;3:319–325.
50. Lintner S, Fischer T. Repair of the distal biceps tendon using suture anchors and an anterior approach. *Clin Orthop* 1996;322:116–119.
51. Lyons FR, Rockwood CA. Osteolysis of the clavicle. In: DeLee JC, Drez D (eds.), *Orthopaedic Sports Medicine*. Philadelphia: WB Saunders, 1994;541–546.
52. McSwain NE. Helmet removal from injured patients. *Bull of Am Coll Surg* 1997;82:42–44.
53. Meyer SA. Stress fractures of the foot and ankle. *Clin Sports Med* 1993;12:395–413.
54. Miller MD, Bergfeld JA, Fowler PJ, Harner CD, Noyes FR. The posterior cruciate ligament injured knee: Principles of evaluation and treatment. *Instr Course Lect* 1999;48:199–207.
55. Noonan TJ. Muscle strain: Diagnosis and treatment. *J Am Acad Orthop Surg* 1999;7:262–269.
56. Norns TR. Complications following anterior instability repairs. In: Bigliani LU (ed.), *Complications of Shoulder Surgery*. Baltimore: Williams & Wilkins, 1993;98–116.
57. Noyes FR, Butler DL, Grood ES, et al. Biomechanical analysis of human Ligament grafts Used in knee-ligament repairs and reconstructions. *J Bone Joint Surg Am* 1984;66:344–352.
58. Ollivierre CO, Nirschl RP, Pettrone FA. Resection and repair for medical tennis elbow: A prospective analysis. *Am J Sports Med* 1995;23:214–221.
59. Olsen BS, Sojbjerg JO, Dalstra M, Sneppen O. Kinematics of the lateral ligamentous constraints of the elbow joint. *J Shoulder Elbow Surg* 1996;5:333–341.
60. Petersson CJ. Spontaneous medial dislocation of the tendon of the long biceps brachii. *Clin Orthop* 1986;211:224–227.
61. Rodosky MW, Harner CD, Fu FH. The role of the long head of the biceps muscle and superior glenoid labrum in anterior stability of the shoulder. *Am J Sports Med* 1994;22:121–130.
62. Rozzi SL, Lephart SM, Gear WS, Fu FH. Knee joint laxity and neuromuscular characteristics of male and female soccer and basketball players. *Am J Sports Med* 1999;27:312–319.
63. Schenck RC, Heckman JD. Fractures and dislocations of the forefoot: Operative and non-operative treatment. *J Am Acad Orthop Surg* 1995;3:70–78.
64. Schepsis AA. Achilles tendon disorders in athletes. *Am J Sports Med* 2002;30:287–305.
65. Seiler JG III, Parker LM, Chamberland PD, Sherbourne GM, Carpenter WA. The distal biceps tendon: Two potential mechanisms involved in its rupture. Arterial supply and mechanical impingement. *J Shoulder Elbow Surg* 1995;4:149–156.
66. Stannard JP, Bucknell AL. Rupture of the triceps tendon associated with steroid injections. *Am J Sports Med* 1993;21:482–485.

67. Thomas BE. Cervical spine injuries in football players. *J Am Acad Orthop Surg* 1999;7:338–347.
68. Ticker JB, Bigliani LU, Soslowsky LJ, et al. Inferior glenohumeral ligament: Geometric and strain-rate dependent properties. *J Shoulder Elbow Surg* 1996;5:269–279.
69. Van Camp SP. Non-traumatic sports deaths in high school and college athletes. *Med Sci Sports Exerc* 1995;27:641–647.
70. Vegso JJ. Field evaluation and management of head and neck injuries. *Post Grad Adv Sport Med* 1987;10:2–10.
71. Veltri DM, Warren RF. Isolated and combined posterior cruciate injuries. *J Am Acad Orthop Surg* 1993;1:67–75.
72. Veltri DM, Warren RF. Posterolateral instability of the knee. *J Bone Joint Surg Am* 1994;76:460–472.
73. Warren LA, Marshall JL, Girgis F. The prime static stabilizer of the medial side of the knee. *J Bone Joint Surg Am* 1974;56:665–674.
74. Williams RJ III, Urquhart ER, Altchek DW. Medial collateral ligament tears in the throwing athlete. *Instr Course Lect* 2004;53:579–586.
75. Wilson TW, Zafuta MP, Zobitz M. A biomechanical analysis of matched bone-patellar tendon-bone and double looped semitendinosus and gracilis tendon grafts. *Am J Sports Med* 1999;27:202–207.
76. Wuest TK. Injuries to the distal lower extremity syndesmosis. *J Am Acad Orthop Surg* 1997;5:172–181.
77. Zvijac JE, Lau AC, Hechtman KS, Uribe JW, Tjin-A-Tsoi EW. Arthroscopic treatment of pigmented villonodular synovitis of the knee. *Arthroscopy* 1999;15:613–617.

Key References

Desio SM, Burks RT, Bachus KN. Soft tissue restraints to lateral patellar translation in the human knee. *Am J Sports Med* 1998;26:59–65.

This article examined soft tissue restraints to lateral patellar displacement. Biomechanic studies have found the medial patellofemoral ligament to be the major soft tissue restraint to lateral patellar displacement, providing a minimum of 50% of its stability.

Hawkins RJ, Bell RH, Hawkins RH, Koppert GJ. Anterior dislocation of the shoulder in the older patient. *Clin Orthop Relat Res* 1986 May;(206):192–195.

This paper was one of the first to identify a significant number of rotator cuff defects following a first-time dislocation in older patients (older than 40 years). Recurrence of instability in this group of patients is low; however, standard anterior repairs may be employed effectively in such situations. Knowledge of these facts will allow a better appreciation of the pathology associated with the anterior dislocation in the older patient.

Hutchinson MR, Bae TS. Reproducibility of anatomic tibial landmarks for ACL reconstructions. *Am J Sports Med* 2001;29:777–780.

This article examined anatomic landmarks that can be used for the placement of tibial tunnels in ACL reconstruction and found that the anterior border of the PCL is the most accurate and reproducible arthroscopic location for placement of this tunnel. Recommended placement is from 7 to 10 mm anterior to the border of the PCL.

Kraushaar BS, Nirschl RP. Tendinosis of the elbow (tennis elbow): Clinical features and findings of histological, immunohistochemical, and electron microscopy studies. *J Bone Joint Surg Am* 1999;81:259–278.

Treatment of lateral epicondylitis has evolved over the years as pathoanatomy of this condition became better understood. In 1979, Nirschl and Pettrone identified the primary pathoanatomic area of tennis elbow as the ECRB tendon. Twenty years later, Kraushaar and Nirschl defined the histopathology of this entity in precise detail using electron microscopy and histoimmunochemistry. These authors elucidated that tennis elbow is a condition characterized by angiofibroblastic tendinosis rather than an inflammatory process.

Mair SD, Viola RW, Gill TJ, Briggs KK, Hawkins RJ. Can the impingement test predict outcome after arthroscopic subacromial decompression? *J Shoulder Elbow Surg* 2004 Mar-Apr;13(2):150–153.

This paper showed that the satisfaction of patients after arthroscopic subacromial decompression was higher postoperatively if they had a positive preoperative impingement test (88%) compared to a negative preoperative impingement test (satisfaction 60%) at 12 months. Establishes the validity of the preoperative impingement test for postoperative outcomes after arthroscopic subacromial decompression.

Millett PJ, Willis AA, Warren RF. Associated injuries in pediatric and adolescent anterior cruciate ligament tears: Does a delay in treatment increase the risk of meniscal tear? *Arthroscopy*. 2002 Nov-Dec;18(9):955–959.

Evidence from this study supports the contention that associated injuries are common in young individuals with ACL tears. Furthermore, the data also show that a delay in surgical treatment is associated with a higher incidence of medial meniscal tears. Lateral meniscus tears were evenly distributed between patients treated acutely and chronically, while medial tears were found with much greater frequency (statistically significant) in the chronically treated group than in the acutely treated group.

Rohrbough JT, Altchek DW, Hyman J, Williams RJ III, Botts JD. Medial collateral ligament reconstruction of the elbow using the docking technique. *Am J Sports Med* 2002;30(4):541–548.

Surgical treatment of MCL insufficiency has continued to evolve from the original technique developed by Jobe and associates. This article describes a modification of MCL reconstruction using a single ulnar tunnel and single humeral tunnel that is performed through a muscle-splitting approach that usually does not require the need for ulnar nerve transposition. This modification is referred to as the docking technique.

Zvijac JE, Lau AC, Hechtman KS, Uribe JW, Tjin-A-Tsoi EW. Arthroscopic treatment of pigmented villonodular synovitis of the knee. *Arthroscopy* 1999;15:613–617.

The authors' experience showed that in the treatment of PVNS of the knee, arthroscopic synovectomy was equal to open treatment (synovectomy), especially for the local nodular type.

Refresher Questions

1. Which of the following variables has been shown to have the greatest influence on the higher rate of ACL tears in women when compared to men for similar sports?
   a) hormones
   b) ACL strength
   c) notch width
   d) neuromuscular training
   e) leg alignment

2. Which of the following tissues has the highest maximum load to failure?
   a) native ACL
   b) bone–patellar tendon–bone with a width of 10 mm
   c) central quadriceps tendon with a width of 15 mm
   d) quadruple semitendinosus and gracilis tendons
   e) tibialis tendon allograft

3. With a full-thickness articular cartilage, the body's healing response produces cartilage mainly composed of what type of collagen?
   a) I
   b) II
   c) III
   d) IV
   e) X

4. A 23-year-old baseball pitcher who has diffuse pain along the posterior deltoid reports pain during late acceleration and follow-through. Examination of his arc of motion from external rotation to internal rotation at 90 degrees of shoulder abduction reveals a significant deficit in internal rotation when compared to the nonthrowing shoulder. Initial management should consist of
   a) subscapularis muscle.
   b) supraspinatus muscle.
   c) middle glenohumeral ligament.
   d) inferior glenohumeral ligament.
   e) coracohumeral ligament.

5. Which of the following structures is the most important restraint to posterior subluxation of the glenohumeral joint when positioned in 90 degrees of flexion and internal rotation?
   a) subscapularis muscle
   b) supraspinatus muscle
   c) middle glenohumeral ligament
   d) inferior glenohumeral ligament
   e) coracohumeral ligament

6. A superior labrum anterior and posterior (SLAP) lesion doubles the strain in which of the following stabilizing structures?
   a) superior glenohumeral ligament
   b) middle glenohumeral ligament
   c) inferior glenohumeral ligament
   d) posterior inferior glenohumeral ligament
   e) subscapularis

7. An 18-year-old soccer player is struck in the head by an opposing player's knee during the opening moments of a game, resulting in a brief episode where the patient fell to the ground and experienced a loss of consciousness that lasted less than 1 minute. The athlete may return to play in the second half if
   a) the neurologic deficits are only motor.
   b) the neurologic deficits are only sensory.
   c) the patient reports only a headache without motor or sensory loss.
   d) the patient reports no persistent signs or symptoms.
   e) The patient should not return to play that day.

8. Which of the following is typical in an acute burner (stinger)?
   a) isolated motor weakness
   b) lower extremity symptoms
   c) bilateral upper extremity symptoms
   d) unilateral arm symptoms
   e) unilateral arm and leg symptoms

9. In throwing athletes, osteophytes around the posteromedial olecranon and olecranon articulation are most often formed by
   a) biceps or brachialis muscle weakness.
   b) forearm pronator and flexor muscle weakness.
   c) ulnar collateral ligament insufficency.
   d) radial Collateral ligament insufficiency.
   e) anterior capsular tears.

10. Which structure is the most common site of involvement in lateral epicondylitis?
    a) extensor carpi radialis longus
    b) extensor carpi radialis brevis
    c) extensor digitorum communis
    d) extensor carpi ulnaris
    e) anconeus

11. A 26-year-old professional downhill skier is found unconscious and face down after hitting a retaining fence during a race. The patient's helmet and face shield are intact. What initial management should be followed?

a) Remove the helmet to access the airway.
b) Logroll the patient and remove the helmet to access the patient.
c) Logroll the patient, immobilize the cervical spine, remove the face shield, and leave the helmet in place while accessing the airway.
d) Stabilize the cervical spine, logroll the patient, remove the face shield, and leave the helmet in place while accessing the airway.
e) Stabilize the cervical spine, logroll the patient, and remove both the face shield and the helmet to access the airway.

12. A division IA collegiate basketball player was diagnosed with a tarsal navicular stress fracture and was treated with short-leg-cast immobilization and no weight bearing for 6 weeks. The patient returns to the office today, still complaining of medial-sided pain and has an x-ray that demonstrates a sagittally-oriented fracture line with some callous formation. Management of this patient should consist of

a) application of a short-leg cast and full weight bearing for an additional 6 weeks.
b) application of a short-leg cast and no weight bearing for an additional 6 weeks.
c) a stiff-soled shoe and weight bearing as tolerated.
d) percutaneous pin fixation and application of a short-leg cast.
e) ORIF and bone grafting.

Chapter 4

Adult Reconstruction

SHARAT KUMAR KUSUMA and JONATHAN P. GARINO

I. HIP RECONSTRUCTIVE SURGERY

Surgical Anatomy

Tables 4.1 and 4.2 review the muscles around and surgical approaches to the hip.

Disorders Requiring Hip Replacement

Total hip arthroplasty (THA) is one of the most successful and efficacious procedures performed by orthopaedic surgeons. Annually, hundreds of thousands of patients gain functional improvements and pain relief after undergoing THA. Currently, the most common methods of performing total hip arthroplasty utilize combinations of cemented or noncemented acetabular and femoral components. Many historical studies demonstrate excellent long-term longevity of THA. This chapter reviews basic concepts of degenerative hip disease and THA.

Avascular Necrosis (AVN). Traumatic causes of AVN include hip dislocation and femoral neck fracture. Nontraumatic causes of AVN include high doses of steroids, which are often used to treat underlying diseases such as systemic lupus erythematosus (SLE) and rheumatoid arthritis (RA). AVN is also associated with high levels of alcohol intake. Other disorders associated with AVN include sickle cell disease, Gaucher disease, Caisson disease, HIV, pancreatitis, and liver and kidney disease. It is important to

TABLE 4.1 Muscles around the hip

Muscle	Origin	Insertion	Innervation
Flexors			
Iliacus	Iliac fossa	Lesser trochanter	(L2-4) femoral
Psoas	Transverse processes L1-L5	Lesser trochanter	(L2-4) femoral
Pectineus	Pectineal line of pubis	Femoral pectineal line	(L2-4) femoral
Rectus femoris	AIIS, acetabular rim	Patella to tibial tubercle	(L2-4) femoral
Sartorius	ASIS	Proximal medial tibia	(L2-4) femoral
Adductors			
Posterior adductor magnus	Inferior pubic ramus/ischial tuberosity	Linea aspera/adductor tubercle	(L2-4) obturator ad tibia
Adductor brevis	Inferior pubic ramus	Linea aspera/pectineal line	(L2-4) obturator
Adductor longus	Anterior pubic ramus	Linea aspera	(L2-4) obturator
Gracilis	Inferior symphysis/pubic arch	Proximal medial tibia	(L2-4) obturator
External Rotators			
Gluteus maximus	Ilium posterior to posterior gluteal line	Iliotibial band/gluteal sling(femur)	(L5-S2) inferior gluteal
Piriformis	Anterior sacrum/sciatic notch	Proximal greater trochanter	(S1-2) piriformis
Obturator externus	Ischiopubic rami/obturator membrane	Trochlear fossa	(L2-4) obturator
Obturator internus	Ischiopubic rami/obturator membrane	Medial greater trochanter (MGT)	(L5-S2) obturator internus
Superior gamellus	Outer ischial spine	MGT	(L5-S2) obturator internus
Inferior gamellus	Ischial tuberosity	MGT	Quadratus femoris
Quadratus femoris	Ischial tuberosity	Quadrate line of femur	Quadratus femoris
Abductors			
Gluteus medius	Ilium between posterior and anterior gluteal line	Greater trochanter	(L4-S1) superior gluteal
Gluteus minimus	Ilium between posterior and inferior gluteal line	Anterior border of greater trochanter	(L4-S1) superior gluteal
Tensor fascia latae	Anterior iliac crest	Iliotibial band	(L4-S1) superior gluteal

Source: Adapted from Miller MD. *Review of Orthopaedics*, 3rd ed. Philadelphia: WB Saunders, 2000; 560 (Anatomy, Table 11-8).

differentiate AVN from a similarly presenting disorder known as transient osteoporosis of the hip. Transient osteoporosis is most commonly seen in middle-aged men and pregnant women in the third trimester of pregnancy and is differentiated on MRI scan by increased signal throughout the femoral head and neck. This is in contrast to AVN, which appears as a discrete lesion in the femoral head on MRI scan. Transient osteoporosis is self-limiting and is treated conservatively, while AVN often requires surgical treatment. This important distinction also highlights the fact that MRI is the most sensitive and specific study for the diagnosis of AVN.

Rheumatoid arthritis (RA). Another condition that often requires THA is RA. Patients with RA demonstrate symmetric joint-space narrowing, osteopenia, periacetabular and femoral head erosions, and acetabular protrusio. Protrusio is often seen with rheumatoid arthritis but is also demonstrated in patients

TABLE 4.2 Surgical approaches to the hip

Approach	Superficial Muscle (Innervation)	Deep Muscles (Innervation)	Structures at Risk
Anterior (Smith-Peterson)	Sartorius/rectus femoris (femoral)	TFL/gluteus medius (superior gluteal)	LFCN, femoral, LFCA
Anterolateral (Watson-Jones)	Tensor fasciae latae (TFL) (superior gluteal)	Gluteus medius (superior gluteal)	Femoral NAV/profunda A
Lateral (Harding)	Splits gluteus medius (superior gluteal)	Splits vastus lateralis (femoral)	Femoral NAV/LFCA (transverse branch)
Posterior (Moore-Southern)	Splits gluteus maximus (inferior gluteal)		Sciatic, inferior gluteal artery
Medial (Ludloff)	Adductor longus/brevis (anterior div obturator)	Gracilis/adductor magnus (obturator/tibial)	Anterior div. obturator nerve/MFCA

LFCA, lateral femoral circumflex artery; MFCA, medial femoral circumflex artery; LFCN, lateral femoral cutaneous nerve
Source: Adapted from Miller MD. *Review of Orthopaedics*, Philadelphia: WB Saunders, 2000; 560 (Anatomy, Table 11-3).

with renal osteodystrophy, ankylosing spondylitis, and other metabolic bone diseases. In this condition, the center of hip rotation is moved posteriorly and medially. The ideal method of reconstructing these patients is to return the hip to an anterior and inferior position.

THA after Acetabular Fracture. Fractures of the acetabulum that meet criteria for operative intervention are most often best treated acutely with open reduction and internal fixation. Only in rare, isolated situations would THA be considered appropriate initial treatment for such fractures. However, despite anatomic reduction of such fractures, patients can often develop posttraumatic arthritis in the hip joint. Additionally, patients who are treated nonoperatively may have residual joint incongruities and possible malunion that will render subsequent THA more technically challenging. Overall, the results of THA after initial acetabular fracture are inferior to those of routine primary THA. The most often reported mode of THA failure after acetabular fracture is aseptic loosening of the acetabular component. Several reasons are proposed for this association, including diminished acetabular bone quality and blood supply. Additionally, the presence of increased scar tissue, possible prior nerve palsy, prior hardware, and heterotopic bone can compromise the results of THA following acetabular fracture.

DDH and THA. Patients with developmental dysplasia of the hip also pose treatment challenges. In general, patients with developmental hip dysplasia have acetabular malorientation with bony deficits in the anterolateral aspect of acetabulum. A useful radiographic parameter that can be used to determine the degree of acetabular insufficiency is the center-edge angle of Wiberg, which is determined on an anterior–posterior radiograph of the pelvis. Current published data indicates that for patient with a center-edge angle of 15 degrees or less, a periacetabular osteotomy can be performed. The false profile or faux provil x-ray is also an important component of the preoperative evaluation of a DDH patient and will demonstrate sagittal plane acetabular deficits. For performing a THA in a DDH patient, the acetabulum is best positioned anatomically in a medialized position. This position makes the best use of host bone coverage of the component.

THA in Chronically Dislocated Hips. Total hip replacement in the patient with congenital dislocation is technically more difficult than the same procedure in an unaffected individual. The classification systems that are most commonly used include those of Hartofilakidis and colleagues and the Crowe classification system. Hips with low and high dislocations present the surgeon with the most technically demanding problems, particularly with the issue of limb-length discrepancy. In general, a limb cannot be lengthened more than 4 cm without putting the sciatic nerve at great risk. With Crowe type IV hips, which are high dislocated hips that correspond with Hartofilakidis type III hips, the best results have been achieved with femoral shortening osteotomy combined with cementless, modular implants, which provide great flexibility in component size during the reconstruction. Despite these modifications, however, patients with dislocated hips demonstrate a much higher rate of revision surgery than patients with preoperatively unaffected or even subluxed hips. Additionally, the incidence of postoperative nerve injury is increased in dislocated hips because of the femoral lengthening discussed earlier.

THA in Ankylosing Spondylitis. These patients demonstrate good pain relief but a lower level of functional return than unaffected patients. This decrease in outcome is related to associated systemic diseases and spinal deformity. They also have a slightly higher incidence of postoperative infection and heterotopic ossification.

Nonarthroplasty Treatment of Hip Disease

Contraindications such as medical illness, young age, and infection may preclude patients from undergoing THA. In such patients, the physician must consider nonarthroplasty methods of treating hip arthrosis.

Conservative Management. Treatments that would be generally classified as "conservative" include such modalities as nonsteroidal antiinflammatory medications, weight loss, activity modification, and the use of an assistive device such as a cane or walker. Particularly when using a cane, patients should be instructed to place the device in the hand that is contralateral to the affected hip. In terms of activity modifications, patients should be instructed that if they are required to carry objects in their hands, they can reduce the forces across the diseased hip if they carry such objects using the upper extremity on the ipsilateral side of their affected hip. Although this may seem counterintuitive, studies have demonstrated that hip joint forces are smaller when patients carry loads using the upper extremity that is on the same side as the affected hip.

Osteotomies About the Hip

Relatively young patients with a history of developmental hip dysplasia who have mild to moderate joint arthrosis and severe hip pain can benefit from pelvic osteotomies. Ideally, pelvic osteotomies are done before the occurrence of severe joint degenerative changes. Outcomes are much improved when patients have well-maintained hyaline cartilage and no advanced degenerative joint disease (DJD). The best predictor of success of such procedures is still a simple functional radiograph, such as an abduction hip x-ray or a fluoroscopic study, which demonstrates an improved cartilage space interval with hip abduction maneuvers. The most common redirectional osteotomies include the Ganz periacetabular (PAO), Salter (single innominate), Sutherland (double innominate), and Steel (triple innominate). DDH patients with a painful but concentric, reduced hip joint are good candidates for a Ganz osteotomy. This procedure has several advantages, including the requirement of only one incision and its allowance for large amounts of rotational correction of the acetabulum. The Ganz procedure allows for early patient mobilization because of the limited need for internal fixation. Finally, this procedure maintains the vascular supply of the acetabulum through the inferior gluteal artery. Potential drawbacks include its technical difficulty and the possibility of anterior displacement of the hip joint, which may ultimately result in limited hip flexion. Although a Salter (single innominate) osteotomy may also be a reasonable option, this procedure offers only a limited amount of correction and lateralizes the hip joint, which increases the joint reactive force. Other osteotomies that may be performed in younger patients include the Dial (spherical) osteotomy, which is an intraarticular redirectional osteotomy that does not alter the position of the teardrop. The Chiari osteotomy is a salvage procedure that does not redirect the acetabulum and does not alter the position of the teardrop. It is best utilized in incongruent, subluxed hips. Figure 4.1 illustrates examples of acetabular osteotomies.

Intertrochanteric Osteotomies in Younger Patients. Another group of patients who are suboptimal candidates for THA include younger individuals with a history of femoral developmental anomalies such as coxa valga, coxa vara, Perthes disease, or slipped capital femoral epiphysis. Patients may also have traumatic proximal femoral deformities such as malunited intertrochanteric fractures or malunited femoral neck fractures with an intact femoral head. In such patients, the primary hip joint abnormality occurs in the proximal femur rather than the acetabulum; therefore, this group of patients can benefit from proximal femoral osteotomies that redirect the femoral head. However, it is important to note that in such patients, the major abnormality must be present in the proximal femur; if significant acetabular changes are present, then a femoral osteotomy alone is unlikely to fully address the hip pathology. Additionally, similar to pelvic osteotomy, the procedure should be performed prior to the development of advanced degenerative changes in the hip joint. Varus intertrochanteric osteotomy can be used in patients with coxa valga; however patients must have at least 15 degrees of passive hip abduction preoperatively to be considered for the procedure. The procedure is effective because it gives the hip more femoral offset, which increases the tension of the abductor muscles and thereby reduces hip joint reactive forces. This osteotomy does not affect the center-edge angle. Complications of the procedure include abductor lag, abductor lurch, and leg-length discrepancy, which results from shortening of the osteotomized extremity. Valgus intertrochanteric osteotomy is most commonly performed for nonunion of a Pauwel class

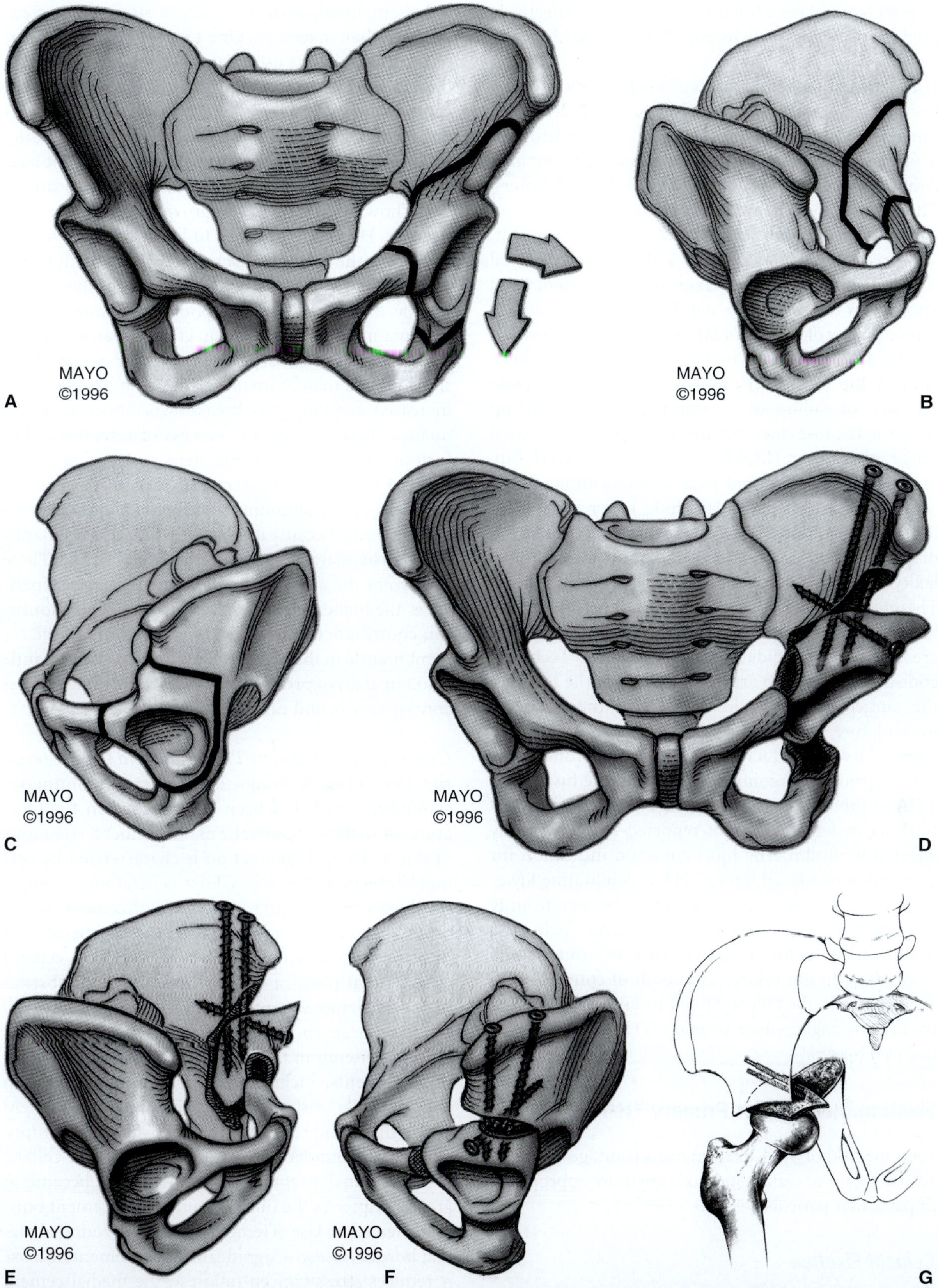

FIGURE 4.1 (A–F) Examples of acetabular osteotomies. (*Source:* Trousdale RT, Ganz R. Periacetabular osteotomy. In: Callaghan JJ, Rosenberg AG, Rubash HE [eds.], *The Adult Hip*. Philadelphia: Lippincott-Raven, 1998:793.) (G) Chiari osteotomy. (*Source:* Bailey TE, Hall JE. Chiari medial displacement osteotomy. *J Pediatr Orthop* 1985;5[6]:635–641.)

II or III femoral neck fracture. It can also be effectively used to treat early-stage osteoarthritis of the hip.

Hip Arthrodesis. The most common indication for hip fusion is severe but unilateral hip pain and decreased range of motion in a young patient. Hip arthrodesis is often thought to be a better option than proximal femoral osteotomy in patients who are heavy laborers. The optimal position for fusion is 30 degrees of flexion, which allows the hip to swing efficiently during gait, 5 degrees of adduction, and 5 degrees of external rotation; this positioning maximizes gait efficiency and also allows the patient to stand appropriately during stance phases of gait. Avoidance of abduction position during fusion reduces incidence of back and knee pain. A hip fusion on one side is likely to increase the rate of failure of a contralateral THA by up to 40% because the hip fusion requires increased range of motion (ROM) of the contralateral hip, thus increasing stress and wear. Complications of hip arthrodesis are many and include lower back pain, lumbar degenerative disease, accelerated degenerative disease of the contralateral hip, and ligamentous laxity with joint degeneration of the ipsilateral knee. Therefore, patients who have lumbar, ipsilateral knee, or contralateral hip degeneration preoperatively are not good candidates for arthrodesis. Technical considerations in hip arthrodesis include the fact that the surgeon must avoid damage to the abductor musculature during the procedure, and extensive damage to the abductor complex may prohibit the patient from undergoing conversion of the fusion to a THA in the future. Sexual function in both sexes and birthing in females are not reported to be adversely affected by fusion. The most common indication for conversion of a fused hip to THA is debilitating lower back pain. The back pain can often be significantly alleviated through conversion. However, pain and degeneration in the ipsilateral knee or contralateral knee often do not resolve as a result of conversion to THA. Overall, the failure rate of fused hips converted to THA is higher than primary THA in previously unfused hips.

Fixation Methods for Primary THA

Each method of THA fixation has advantages and disadvantages, and certain methods are more appropriate in particular patients.

Cement Fixation

Cement fixation of femoral and acetabular implants is based on the concept that the cement does not function as an adhesive but rather interdigitates within the bone. The cement itself is composed of polymethylmethacrylate, which is stronger in compression than in tension. One conceptual disadvantage of cement is that its use creates two separate interfaces that may fail: the cement–host bone interface and the cement–implant interface. The cement–bone interface is a static one, with no remodeling potential; thus, any areas of failure of the cement mantle do not have the ability to remodel. Nonetheless, numerous studies have shown that cement can provide stable, long-term fixation. However, in order to be successful over the long term, the cement must be prepared and implanted carefully at the time of surgery. The size of the cement mantle of the femoral component is thought to be best maintained at 2 mm or greater, particularly in the proximal medial aspect of the femur. Studies have shown that a mantle smaller than 2 mm demonstrates increased cracking and breakdown. Other technical nuances that increase the success of cemented THA include avoidance of varus stem positioning of the femoral stem and avoidance of gaps in the cement mantle. Varus positioning of cemented femoral stems is detrimental because it results in a thin cement mantle in the proximal medial and distal lateral femur. These are two of the areas where the cement mantle experiences the highest stress levels. Thus, varus positioning can contribute to early cracking and failure of the cement mantle in these areas. Gaps in the cement mantle result in areas of prosthesis–bone direct contact, stress concentration, and early failure.

Generations of Cement Technique and Characteristics. Cementing technique has undergone continuous evolution, which has been consolidated in the literature into three "generations" of cement technique (Table 4.3). Each generation is characterized by certain key technical practices. First-generation technique involved very elementary methods of cement preparation, including manual finger packing of cement into the femoral canal without the use of a cement gun, cement plug, or cement pressurization; absence of formal femoral canal preparation, and cast metal stems with sharp borders and thin medial borders. Second-generation technique introduced some major improvements, including femoral canal preparation with pulsatile washing and brushing, use of a cement gun with cement restricters, and alloy femoral components with rounded, broad medial edges and collars. Femoral canal preparation is important because it greatly improves the initial quality of the cement bone interdigitation. Use of femoral stems with rounded medial borders is also a significant improvement because it reduces stress concentration at the medial cement mantle, where failure can occur. Third-generation technique, which best represents present-day practices, includes such advances as vacuum preparation of cement to reduce porosity, pressurization of cement,

TABLE 4.3 Generations of cement technique

	Key Characteristics
First Generation	1. Finger packing 2. Unplugged femoral canal 3. Femoral components: sharp corners, narrow medial borders, stainless steel
Second Generation	1. Plugging of medullary canal 2. Pulse lavage cleaning of canal 3. Cement gun 4. "Super alloy" components 5. Removal of sharp corners 6. Broad medial border
Third Generation	1. Vacuum preparation of cement (porosity reduction) 2. Surface modifications of implants 3. PMMA application 4. Stem centralization proximally and distally

and use of stem centralizer. Porosity reduction and vacuum preparation of cement are important practices because they increase the ultimate strength of the cement.

Cemented Femoral Components. Overall, cemented femoral components have demonstrated excellent long-term survivorship, and several series have shown revision rates of 0% to 5% at 10-year follow-up. The Dorr classification of the femur can be helpful in determining which technique of femoral fixation to use (Fig. 4.2). This system radiographically characterizes the morphology of the proximal femur on the basis of the size and shape of the femoral canal and the thickness of the cortices. Dorr type A femora, which have small medullary canals, may be better suited for uncemented implants because of the difficulty in establishing a sufficient cement mantle. Dorr type B femora are equally treated with cemented or uncemented components. Alternatively, Dorr C femora may be better suited for cemented femoral components. Additionally, patients with poor bone quality that will not support uncemented implants may be better treated with cemented femoral components. Factors associated with early failure of cemented femoral components include varus stem positioning, obesity, and cement mantle defects. With regards to precoating of femoral stems, studies demonstrate that implants precoated with PMMA improve the interface between the stem and cement mantle. However, this mechanical improvement has not resulted clinically in lower rates of loosening, infection, or wear in precoated stems compared with nonprecoated stems.

Cemented Acetabular Components. On the acetabular side, cemented components have become less popular than cementless components. Studies have shown higher rates of loosening for cemented components in younger patients, patients with rheumatoid arthritis, acetabular protrusio, hip dysplasia, and bleeding diathesis. However, in patients without such comorbidities, several series demonstrate failure rates of such components at 17 to 20 years of 10% to 23%. Overall, cemented acetabulae perform better in older, lower demand patients. However, regardless of patient age or comorbidity, loosening is dependent on the quality of the bone–cement interface achieved intraoperatively.

Uncemented Components

Uncemented implants can have either a porous-coated or grit-blasted surface. Uncemented fixation, unlike cemented fixation, is a truly biologic method of implantation in that the coated surface of the metal implant is conducive to ingrowth or ongrowth of bone. The cortical bone actually grows into the porous channels within the metal implant to create a rigid interface. Of course, this implies that in order for uncemented technique to be successful, the implants must be seated against cortical bone and not cancellous bone. Unlike the cement–bone interface, the metal–bone interface has remodeling potential; if there is disruption of the bony intercalation into the implant, the bone can remodel and reestablish the rigid interface. Therefore, it is theoretically conceivable that uncemented implants may maintain rigid fixation longer than is possible with cemented implants. In recent years, as more THAs have been performed

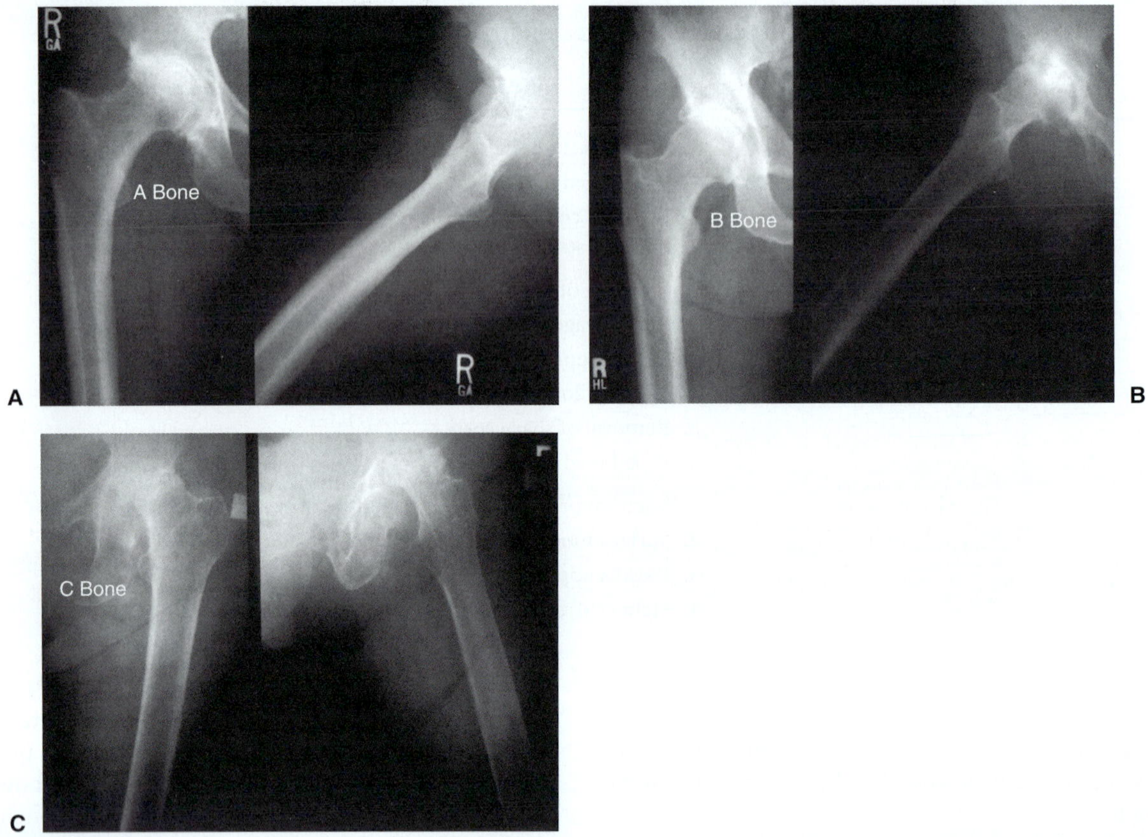

FIGURE 4.2 Dorr classification of femoral morphology. (A) Type A bone. (B) Type B bone. (C) Type C bone. (*Source:* Dorr LD, Said M. Proximal fixation of the noncemented stem. In: Callaghan JJ, Rosenberg AG, Rubash HE (eds), *The Adult Hip*. Philadelphia: Lippincott-Raven, 1998;1064.)

in younger patients who place higher demands on their prostheses, there has been an increase in the use of noncemented hips because of the potential life-long bond between the implant and the host bone. Many studies have demonstrated that cemented components have increased failure rates in younger patients, while complementary studies have shown in the short to medium term that uncemented components demonstrate improved performance and decreased loosening in young patients. Additionally, cementless implants may be ideal when patients have thick cortices, narrow femoral canals, and good bone quality.

Surfaces of Uncemented Implants. Uncemented implants can have a surface that is porous coated or grit-blasted. *Porous coated* describes a metallic surface that has been treated to have many microscopic pores of varying depths into which bone may grow. *Grit blasted* describes a slightly different uncemented metal surface; these implants have been bombarded with microscopic particles that create innumerable indentations on the metal surface onto which bone can grow. These indentations are analogous to jagged peaks and valleys on the metal surface. Technically speaking, porous-coated implants allow for bony ingrowth into the pores, while grit-blasted implants allow for bony ongrowth on the peaks and valleys.

With porous-coated implants, there are particular size distributions of the pores that optimize bony ingrowth. Studies have demonstrated that the optimum pore size is from 100 to 400 μm. The optimum porosity or pore density on the metal surface is on the order of 40% to 50%. When the surface porosity exceeds 50%, the porous coating can actually be sheared off of the metal surface of the implant (Table 4.4).

TABLE 4.4 Optimal characteristics of cementless implants

Optimum pore size	100–400 microns
Optimum porosity	40%–50%
Limits of micromotion	150 microns
Bone–implant distance	50 microns

Other conditions required for optimal porous ingrowth include a rigid, motion-free interface between the implant and the host bone.

Optimal Micromotion Between Implant and Bone. Micromotion between implant and bone should be reduced to a maximum of 150 μm. If motion between the bone and implant exceeds this value, weak fibrous tissue will grow into the pores. If micromotion is maintained below this amount, a rigid bony interface will develop. Another equally important parameter is the actual physical distance between the metal surface and the cortical bone. This distance should be kept at a maximum of 50 μm, because osteogenic cells and factors are unable to bridge a distance greater than this to create a rigid bony interface.

Rigid Fixation. With cementless implants, there are two techniques of achieving rigid fixation: line-to-line and press-fit.

- *Line-to-line technique*—Line-to-line technique is performed by reaming the acetabulum or femur to the same size as the component that is to be placed. With line-to-line acetabular technique, the use of supplemental fixation such as bone screws may be required to maintain a rigid, motionless interface between the host cortical bone and the component. The literature demonstrates that there are disadvantages to the use of acetabular screws. Studies have shown up to 99.1% 12-year survivorship of acetabular shells without screw fixation. Additionally, data demonstrates that the bone tracts created for the screws result in decreased acetabular surface area for bony ingrowth; these tracts also provide a conduit for wear debris, which can increase the extent of osteolysis. The screws are subject to backing out, placing them in direct contact with the nonarticular surface of the polyethylene, which can contribute to abrasive backside wear.
- *Press-fit technique*—The femur or acetabulum are reamed to a size that is 1 to 2 mm smaller than the component to be implanted. Press-fit technique does not often require supplemental fixation and relies on hoop stresses to maintain rigid fixation.

Grit-Blasted Implants. Grit-blasted implants also have certain physical characteristics that increase the rigidity of the bone–implant interface. The key characteristic of grit-blasted implants is the surface roughness; the roughness describes the average of the distance between all the peaks and valleys on the metal implant surface. Bone grows onto the peaks and valleys. Implants with a higher surface roughness concurrently exhibit a more rigid bone–metal interface. One theoretical disadvantage of grit-blasted components is that they require a larger proportion of their surface to be covered with a blasted surface; additionally, such components with large surface roughness values could abrade the cortical bone surface and produce metal debris.

The manner by which uncemented components have most frequently malfunctioned is through polyethylene failure and osteolysis. The mechanisms by which the polyethylene fails have included cracking or breaking of the polyethylene, excessive wear, and disengagement of the polyethylene from the metal shell due to inadequate locking mechanisms. However, many recent technological advances in implant design have largely curtailed the occurrence of such failures. Improvements in shell-liner engagement mechanisms have reduced the occurrence of dissociation between these two components. However, osteolysis continues to be one of the more elusive problems in joint replacement surgery; this topic is covered in a subsequent section.

Uncemented Acetabular Components. Uncemented acetabular components have an excellent track record. As mentioned earlier, medium-term data demonstrates that cementless acetabular components perform as well as or even better than cemented components, particularly in patients who place high mechanical demands on their prostheses. Survival rates as high as 98.8% at 10-year follow-up have been reported. Overall, among uncemented acetabular metal shells, the best-performing designs have been of the porous-coated variety. Shells with smooth metal backs have not performed as well. In patients under age 60, cementless, porous-coated, metal-backed acetabular components have shown the greatest survivorship at 10-year follow-up.

Uncemented Femoral Components. Despite initial difficulties with thigh pain and loosening, cementless femoral implants now enjoy a success rate very similar to that of the best cemented implants. Annual loosening rates of less than 0.5% have been demonstrated repeatedly in the literature. As discussed earlier, with cementless femoral implants, the surgeon must achieve rigid, motionless fixation between the host bone and the implant. The micromotion between the bone and implant should be maintained at a maximum of 150 μm to reduce the probability of fibrous ingrowth into the porous-coated femoral component. Various types of surface-coating materials have been used on porous-coated femoral components with the goal of improving the quality of the bony ingrowth interface. Among these various coating materials, hydroxyapatite may have a theoretical advantage in achieving bony ingrowth because it is an osteoconductive substance.

Porous Coating. Another design characteristic that has been heavily analyzed in recent years is the effect of the longitudinal extent of porous coating of the femoral implant on the femoral bone stock. Femoral implants can have a porous coating that covers only the proximal portion or the entire length of the prosthesis. The critical conceptual issue that relates to fully versus partially coated implants is that of stress shielding and osteolysis. Fully coated implants generally achieve rigid fixation throughout the length of the implant, with a large component of the fixation occurring in the more distal aspects of the femur. This distal fixation is evidenced radiographically as spot welds in the femoral diaphysis. Spot welds are areas of dense bony ingrowth between the cortex and femur, as seen on plain radiographs, that indicate distal fixation. When such distal fixation occurs, the force loads are transmitted to the more distal aspects of the femur, resulting in stress shielding in the proximal aspect of the femur, which leads to bone loss and osteopenia in this area. However, fully coated stems do have the advantage of providing a very large surface area for rigid fixation to occur. Femoral stems that are porous coated only proximally achieve rigid fixation only in these proximal regions of the femur. Therefore, force loads are transmitted in a more physiologic fashion, through the proximal femur, resulting in less stress shielding and proximal bone loss.

The *circumferential extent of porous coating around the implant* is also important in the clinical outcome of cementless femoral implants. Various designs of cementless femoral implants have utilized partial versus full proximal circumferential coating of the stem. These two design principles are important because they relate to the effective joint space and osteolysis. Implants that have only partially circumferentially coated designs have demonstrated failure to establish bony ingrowth around the entire perimeter of the proximal femur. Thus, such designs have left a conduit in the proximal femur where polyethylene wear debris can access the femoral diaphysis, thereby increasing the effective joint space. This wear debris has clinically resulted in greater osteolysis in the femoral diaphysis when such noncircumferentially coated designs have been used. By contrast, femoral stems that are fully coated proximally allow for full bony ingrowth around the entire perimeter of the proximal femur, thus effectively "sealing off" the femoral diaphyseal cavity from the effective joint space. Such circumferentially proximally porous-coated stems have performed better than noncircumferentially coated stems with regard to loosening, thigh pain, and osteolysis.

Stress Shielding. Stress shielding is also highly influenced by the stiffness of the femoral stem. Generally, stems that have increased mechanical stiffness can absorb more of the loads transmitted during weight bearing. Therefore, stiffer stems result in more stress shielding. Factors that influence the stiffness of stems include the radius of the stem, the geometry of the stem, and the intrinsic stiffness of the metal used for the stem. The radius of the stem is of critical importance because the stiffness is proportional to the fourth power of the radius. Therefore, small increases in stem radius lead to large increases in stiffness. The geometry of the stem also determines stiffness: stems that have flutes or that have been hollowed out have decreased stiffness. Finally, certain metals are intrinsically stiffer than others; concurrently, stems fashioned from cobalt-chrome are stiffer than those fashioned from titanium because cobalt-chrome itself is stiffer than titanium.

Design Considerations and Biomechanics

Offset of the Femoral Stem. An important intraoperative consideration is the offset of the femoral stem. Increasing the offset of the femoral stem can reduce the joint reactive force and improve the stability of the hip by increasing the tension of the abductor muscle complex. However, increased offset also leads to increased torsional loads on the stem and can cause trochanteric bursitis.

Elevated Rim Acetabular Liners. Liners can improve the anteversion of the acetabular component, which can ultimately decrease the probability of dislocation, particularly when a posterior approach is used. However, elevated posterior liners can also cause impingement of the femoral neck on the acetabulum and lead to dislocation.

Types of Liners. Other component design factors that influence ROM and stability include the use of elevated liners. Surgeons may choose to use posteriorly elevated acetabular liners in order to increase posterior stability of the hip. While such liners are effective in improving posterior stability, they also result in increased impingement and decreased primary arc range when the hip is extended. Therefore, the increased posterior stability afforded by posteriorly elevated liners comes at a cost. Finally, hip components that utilize constrained liners, in which the acetabular component nearly completely envelopes the femoral head, provide excellent stability but at the expense of a severely reduced primary arc range. Additionally, such constrained components result in a large amount of force being transmitted to the interface between the acetabular shell and the acetabular bone, which can result in accelerated mechanical loosening of the acetabular component.

Hip Stability

The topic of hip stability is critical in the discussion of primary THA because dislocation is a relatively common, preventable, and distressing complication, the incidence of which is most likely underreported in the literature. Dislocation rates of primary THAs are reported anywhere from 1% to 9% in the literature, with the true incidence most likely falling in the 2% to 3% range. The highest dislocation rate and risk occurs within the first 3 months after surgery. Early hip dislocations are considered as those that occur roughly within 1 year after the index procedure, while late dislocations are categorized as those that occur many years after the primary THA. Particular groups of patients that are at increased risk for postoperative dislocation include women, who have twice the risk of men; older patients; and as discussed earlier, patients who have had posterolateral approaches to the hip. Additionally, patients who have THA after acute femoral neck fracture also have increased dislocation rate. Finally, the literature has shown association between psychiatric problems such as dementia, depression, alcohol abuse, and increased dislocation. The most common direction of dislocation is posteriorly, with approximately three fourths of dislocations occurring in this direction. Studies have demonstrated that enhanced soft tissue repair of the hip external rotators and the capsule can decrease the rate of dislocation after primary THA with a posterior approach.

Assessment of Hip Stability. There are several key aspects of the primary THA that greatly influence its subsequent stability. These factors include the component configuration, the positioning of the components, and the abductor musculature.

Component Configuration. Several aspects of the component configuration affect the ultimate stability of the prosthetic hip. The parameters of the ball head and acetabular articulation are one of the most critical factors. Maximizing the femoral head–neck ratio through the use of larger ball heads and smaller diameter femoral necks can improve this ratio by improving the primary arc range and the excursion distance of the hip. The primary arc range is defined as the full ROM that the prosthetic articulation can tolerate before the femoral neck contacts the acetabular implant at the extremes of motion. At the limits of the primary arc range, the femoral neck will impinge upon the acetabulum. Therefore, it is clear that a larger head coupled with a thin femoral neck will allow for the largest primary arc range. Once the primary arc range has been reached, the implant still tolerates further motion before dislocation. The distance of this limit of motion after the primary arc range has been reached is defined as the excursion distance. This distance is normally one-half the diameter of the ball head. In relation to the head–neck ratio, studies have shown that the use of a larger femoral head while preserving the same head–neck ratio can result in improved stability without compromising the ROM. However, larger femoral heads do have the downside of increased volumetric wear of the polyethylene liner.

Other component design factors that influence ROM and stability include the use of elevated liners. Surgeons may choose to use posteriorly elevated acetabular liners in order to increase posterior stability of the hip. While such liners are effective in improving posterior stability, they also result in increased impingement and decreased primary arc range when the hip is extended. Therefore, the increased posterior stability afforded by posteriorly elevated liners comes at a cost. Finally, hip components that utilize constrained liners, in which the acetabular component nearly completely envelopes the femoral head, provide excellent stability but at the expense of a severely reduced primary arc range. Additionally, such constrained components result in a large amount of force being transmitted to the interface between the acetabular shell and the acetabular bone, which can result in accelerated mechanical loosening of the acetabular component.

Component Alignment. The orientation of the hip components within the patient's femur and acetabulum also critically influence hip stability. On the acetabular side, generally, implants placed in inadequate anteversion have increased risk of posterior dislocations, while those placed in excessive anteversion increase the risk of anterior dislocation. However, the surgical approach also impacts the degree of desired version. When posterior approaches are used, acetabulae are better placed in slightly higher ranges of anteversion to reduce the probability of posterior dislocation. Studies have demonstrated that for posteriorly implanted hips, between 15 and 20 degrees of anteversion result in excellent stability. This concept also extends to hips implanted through anterior approaches, which do not require the same increased anteversion that benefits the stability of posteriorly approached hips. The vertical orientation of the acetabular component also impacts the stability because implants that are inserted with an extreme vertical orientation or that have a large theta angle have higher risk of superior dislocation. The theta angle describes the degree of abduction or vertical alignment of the acetabular component.

In summary, although the optimal position of the acetabular component is a controversial issue, studies have demonstrated that the abduction should be between 30 and 50 degrees, while the anteversion should fall between 0 and 30 degrees depending on the surgical approach used. On the femoral side, studies have shown that the stem should be positioned between 0 and 15 degrees of anteversion. One final important concept is that the position of the hip components does not affect the absolute value of the primary arc range of the prosthesis; as discussed earlier, this primary arc range is a mechanical phenomenon that is a function of the primary femoral head–acetabular articulation. Changing component position results in a change in the position of this primary arc range within space. The goal of primary THA is to position the primary arc range of the prosthetic hip in the center of the functional ROM required by the patient. Such alignment will result in overall decreased dislocation and maximal ROM.

Tightness of the Abductor Complex. Another key factor impacting the stability of the implant is the tension conferred to the patient's hip abductor muscles by the prosthesis; this tension plays a critical role in generating sufficient force to maintain the prosthetic head within the acetabulum. The hip abductor muscles, consisting primarily of the gluteus medius and minimus, must be appropriately tensioned by the placement of the hip prosthesis. The maintenance of correct postoperative tension in these muscles requires that the femoral component have sufficient length and lateral offset to produce sufficient resting tension within these muscles to maintain a reduced prosthetic hip. An implant with a femoral neck that is too short in the cranial–caudal dimension will result in lax abductor muscles and compromised stability. The lateral offset of the implant is defined as the horizontal distance between the center of the femoral head and the center of the femoral shaft. An insufficient lateral offset will also result in lax abductor muscles and compromised stability. Therefore, placement of femoral components that maintain tension in abductors both in the cranial–caudal direction and medial–lateral direction is critical to achieving a stable THA. In general, increasing the femoral offset has the advantage of improving abductor tension and decreasing joint reactive force but has the disadvantage of increasing torsional loads on the femoral component, which could lead to earlier loosening. Finally, increased femoral offset is associated with trochanteric bursitis (Fig. 4.3).

Soft Tissue Function. The final critical component of THA stability relates to the actual preoperative status and functioning of the patient's abductor muscle complex. If the patient has very weak or damaged abductor muscles, even the perfect combination of lateral offset and neck length in the prosthesis will not result in a stable hip. Patients with deficient abductor function include those with central nervous system damage from cerebrovascular accidents, cerebral palsy, multiple sclerosis, Parkinson's disease, and cervical myelopathy. Peripheral nervous system dysfunction that results in weakened abductor muscles includes damage to the superior gluteal nerve, lumbar stenosis, and myelopathy. In such patients with abductor dysfunction, restoration of maximal abductor tension is even more critical than in unaffected patients. In extreme situations where the abductor complex is completely nonfunctional, the use of a constrained acetabular liner at the time of primary THA may be warranted.

Complications Following Hip Replacement Surgery

Although THA has been an extremely successful procedure, it is not without complications. Complications of THA can be divided into several categories based on the timing of their occurrence.

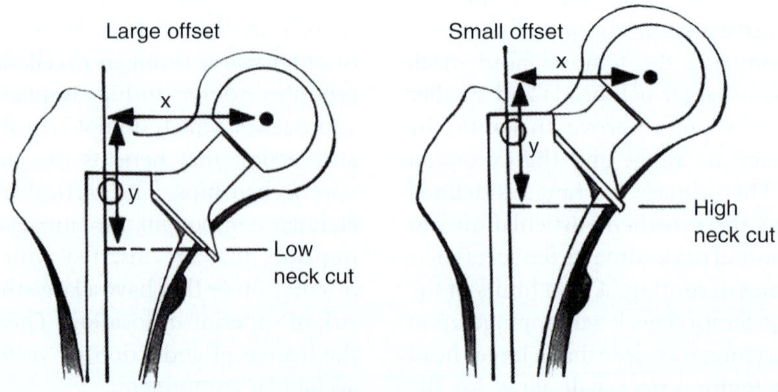

FIGURE 4.3 **Variations in femoral component offset depend on the patient's anatomy. (*Source:* Barrack RL. Preoperative planning. In: Callaghan JJ, Rosenberg AG, Rubash HE (eds.), *The Adult Hip*. Philadelphia: Lippincott-Raven, 1998;947.)**

Intraoperative Complications

The first group of complications occurs perioperatively. The major intraoperative complications include fracture of the femur or acetabulum, nerve injury, and vascular injury. Intraoperative fractures are more common in the femur than in the acetabulum and are more common during the implantation of uncemented components. The insertion of such components requires large amounts of force with the use of impacting devices in order to achieve the initial rigid fixation required for bony ingrowth. In the acetabulum, fractures occur when there is a large difference between the size of the last reamer used and the actual implant that is impacted. Fortunately, the majority of intraoperative acetabular fractures involve only partial cortical disruption of the posterior wall and therefore can be treated conservatively. Studies have suggested that the intraoperative detection of such a fracture is a good indication for the use of acetabular screws. The combination of the metal acetabular shell with the screw fixation actually allows the shell to function as an internal fixation device for the acetabular fracture. More extensive acetabular fractures may require formal open reduction and internal fixation with plating.

Fracture of the Femur or Acetabulum. On the femoral side, intraoperative fractures occur during broaching and implantation of the final component. As with the acetabulum, femur fractures happen when inappropriately large broaches or final implants or both are impacted with great force. Additionally, fractures may also occur in patients who have exceptionally poor bone quality or who have irregularly shaped metaphyseal and diaphyseal regions of the femur. Preoperative templating of femoral components with careful attention to the morphology of the femur can prevent intraoperative femoral fracture. The literature suggests that fractures of the metaphyseal region of the femur occur when proximally porous-coated implants are used, while fully porous-coated implants are more often associated with diaphyseal fractures. Most intraoperative femur fractures are partial cortical disruptions that can be treated with cerclage wiring. More extensive fractures that are full cortical disruptions with distal propagation may require the use of longer stem femoral implants with supplemental cerclage wiring.

Another observed intraoperative complication is nerve injury. Perioperative nerve injury can be caused by compression, traction, or ischemia. Nerve injury can be caused by errant retractor placement or by excessively forceful retraction for prolonged periods of time. Nerve injury can also be observed in the postoperative period when a large hematoma forms and compresses an adjacent peripheral nerve. In this situation, where hematoma compression is thought to be the cause of the injury, surgical exploration and hematoma evacuation is indicated. Nerve injury has been observed and documented in the literature in the sciatic, femoral, obturator, superior gluteal, and lateral femoral cutaneous nerves. The most commonly observed injury is to the peroneal branch of the sciatic nerve followed by the femoral nerve.

Nerve Injury. The obturator nerve can be injured during cemented THAs when cement escapes the confines of the pelvis. The lateral femoral cutaneous nerve (LFCN) can be injured secondary to positioning or pressure from pelvic positioners.

Risk Factors for Intraoperative Nerve injury

1. Female sex
2. DDH
3. Small stature
4. Associated lumbar disease
5. Peripheral neuropathy
6. Leg lengthening during THA

In general, leg lengthening–associated neuropraxia can be avoided if a nerve is not stretched by more than 6% of its preoperative length. Studies have also shown that lengthening of greater than 4 cm is associated with much greater risk of postoperative neuropraxia.

Vascular Injury. Although rare, vascular injury also represents an observed and reported intraoperative complication of THA. The most commonly damaged structures are the common femoral artery and the external iliac artery. Injury can be caused by careless placement of sharp retractors, by direct insult to a vascular structure with a knife or electrocautery, and by careless placement of acetabular screws that perforate a pelvic vessel. Errant placement of acetabular screws can be avoided by the surgeon's recognition of the acetabular quadrant system. This system divides the acetabulum into four equal quadrants, the anterior inferior and superior quadrants and the posterior superior and inferior quadrants. The compartments are delineated by two lines, the first of which starts at the anterior superior iliac spine and bisects the acetabulum, and the second of which is perpendicular to the first and also bisects the acetabulum. The safest area for screw placement is the posterior superior compartment, followed by the posterior inferior quadrant. The anterior inferior and anterior superior quadrants are both generally unsafe for screw placement (Fig. 4.4).

Early Postoperative Complications

The second category of THA complications can be considered as those that occur in the early postoperative

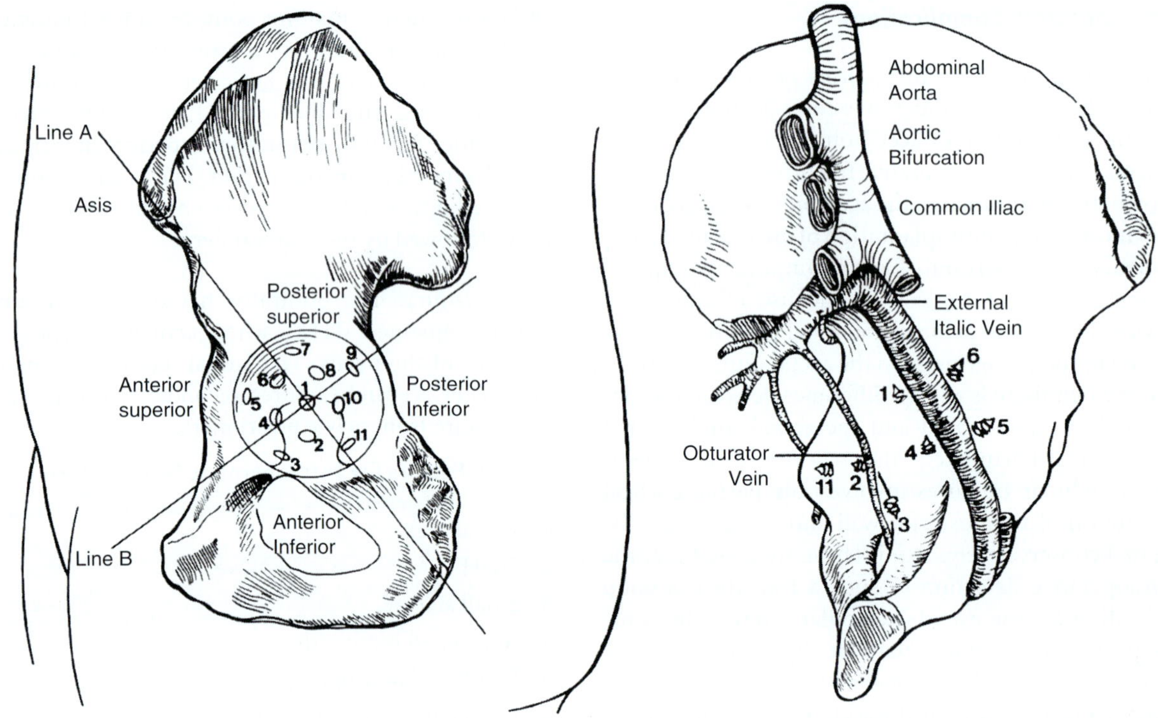

FIGURE 4.4 **Acetabular quadrant system for screw placement. (*Source:* Wasieleski RC, Cooperstein LA, Kruger MP, Rubash HE. Acetabular anatomy and the transacetabular fixation of screws in total hip arthroplasty. *J Bone Joint Surg* 1990;72A:501–508.)**

period and include infection, thromboembolic disease, and dislocation. The topics of infection and thromboembolic disease are covered here, but the subject of dislocation, because of its complexity, is covered in its own subsequent section.

Infection. Although it is quite uncommon, infection after THA represents a potentially devastating complication that can necessitate numerous repeat surgeries and long-term antibiotic treatments. The literature is clear that the most important factor for the prevention of infection is the administration of antibiotics approximately 1 hour before surgical incision is made. Other perioperative measures that have been shown to reduce infection include laminar flow operating rooms and full-body operative suits. Patients who have hip pain in the first 3 months after surgery with no radiographic evidence of dislocation or periprosthetic fracture must be evaluated for infection. For such patients, aspiration of the hip joint is the most specific and sensitive method by which to diagnose such early infection. Other useful tests for the diagnosis of infection include c-reactive protein (C-RP) and erythrocyte sedimentation rate (ESR). The sensitivity of these tests has been reported from 61% to 96%, while their specificity has ranged between 85% and 100%. Studies such as technetium Tc 99 bone scans are not helpful in early postoperative stages for diagnosis of infection; such studies will universally show increased uptake in the setting of recent THA. Additionally, it is important to note that patients with infected THA may not demonstrate systemic symptoms such as fever and chills and often do not exhibit elevated white blood cell count. Plain radiographs of recent THAs that demonstrate periosteal reaction suggest infection. Overall, the expeditious diagnosis of infection in recent THA may be critical because it may allow for early, aggressive surgical irrigation and débridement with avoidance of the removal of the components.

Thromboembolic Disease. Another issue related to early postoperative infection is that of antibiotic prophylaxis for surgical procedures that may result in the temporary seeding of the bloodstream with bacteria. Such procedures include dental, urological, and gastrointestinal procedures. Current American Academy of Orthopaedic Surgeons (AAOS) guidelines recommend antibiotic prophylaxis for 2 years following THA for such transient bacteremia-inducing procedures. Oral amoxicillin, 2.0 grams, is the most commonly recommended agent for penicillin-tolerant patients; alternative agents include cephalexin, clindamycin, and ciprofloxacin. Patients with special immunodeficiencies usually are advised to employ lifetime antibiotic prophylaxis for dental, urological, and gastrointestinal procedures after THA. Thromboembolic disease includes the occurrence of such complications as intra- and perioperative fat/marrow emboli and postoperative deep venous thrombosis that can result in pulmonary embolus. Thromboembolic disease is the most common complication following THA; however, most of these occurrences are of subclinical significance and do not adversely affect outcome. It is currently thought that most thromboembolic phenomena originate during the actual surgical procedures, particularly during reaming and broaching of the femoral canal, during insertion of the femoral stem, and during relocation of the dislocated hip. During insertion of femoral components, studies demonstrate that thrombogenic factors such as tissue thromboplastin are extruded into the femoral veins. Increased intramedullary pressure during insertion of the femoral component has been demonstrated as a critical event in the deposition of fat, marrow, and other thrombotic factors into the circulation. The occurrence of intraoperative thrombotic events is much more common with cemented femoral implants than with uncemented implants. The twisting of the femoral vessels that occurs during dislocation and relocation of the hip causes temporary venous stasis with subsequent release of thrombogenic substances into the circulation.

Gastrointestinal Complications. Postoperative ileus is observed after THA. Preoperative hypokalemia and extensive postoperative bedrest have been identified as risk factors for ileus after THA.

Delayed Complications

The final category of complications following THA includes those that occur in a delayed fashion, usually more than 3 months after performance of the procedure. Delayed or chronic infection can occur many months or years after THA and is included in this category. Periprosthetic fracture and heterotopic ossification are also seen many months after the index procedure.

Hip Loosening. Aseptic loosening of either the femoral or acetabular implant continues to be the most common indication for reoperation on a primary THA. Generally, with cemented THAs, the acetabulum is the first component to fail from loosening, while with cementless hips, the femoral component loosens more often as a result of osteolysis. Patients with loose implants generally complain of pain in three stages. The first stage occurs at startup, when weight bearing is initially commenced. In the second stage, after a short ambulation distance, the pain subsides somewhat, only to increase again after the patient ambulates further. Loose acetabular components generally cause buttock and groin pain, while loose femoral implants cause thigh pain. The diagnosis of loosening is best made by serial plain radiographs, which will demonstrate progressive radiolucencies around the components in consecutive images. Radiolucencies that involve the entire perimeter of a given component and that develop during a very brief time interval are more suggestive of a septic process. Authors have systematically described the radiographic patterns of loosening. Femoral component loosening is characterized by the Gruen system, which divides the femur as visualized on an anterior–posterior radiograph into 7 zones. Radiolucent lines documented in all 7 zones is highly indicative of a loose component. However, it is important to note that radiolucencies on the femoral side can also be the result of bone remodeling. The Gruen system also incorporates a description of 4 modes of cemented femoral component failure (Fig. 4.5).

The four mechanisms are as follows:

- *Pistoning behavior*—The stem and cement subside into the femur.
- *Medial stem pivoting*—A varus-positioned stem fails at the proximal medial and distal lateral areas.
- *Calcar pivoting*—Distal aspect of the stem can shift within the distal cement mantle.
- *Cantilever bending*—Actual stem may fracture because of loss of the cement mantle proximally, resulting in proximal stem bending and eventual breakage. With cantilever bending, the femur undergoes fatigue failure proximally because of repetitive loading at the compromised proximal cement implant interface.

Late Infection. Infection after THA can occur at any point, several months or years after the index primary THA, and therefore this complication can be considered as both an early and a late complication. The main difference between early and late infection is that early postoperative infection is more often the result of direct inoculation of the operative site during the primary THA, while late infection usually occurs through hematogenous seeding of the prosthetic joint. The infection originates at a distant body site and is hematogenously spread to the prosthetic joint. Late infections can be characterized as late acute or late chronic infections. Late acute infections are those that are discovered within approximately 3 weeks of the origination of infection in the prosthetic joint. Such infections can usually be treated with aggressive irrigation and débridement of the prosthesis with component retention and extended intravenous antibiotic treatment. Late chronic infections are those that have been present for more than 4 weeks. On the microscopic level, chronic infections are differentiated

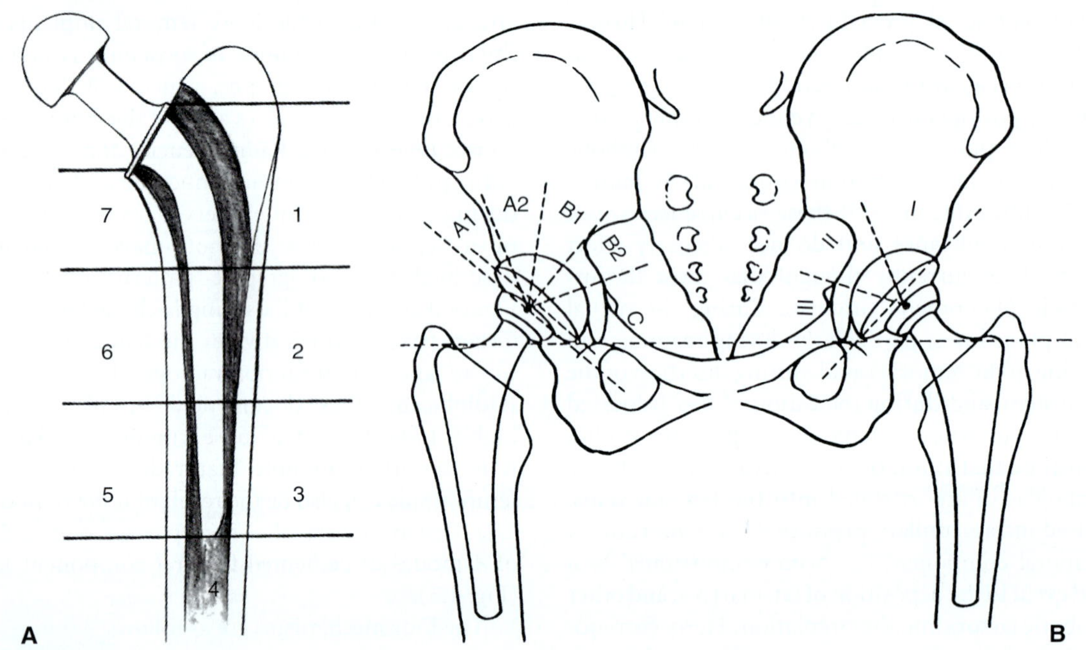

FIGURE 4.5 **(A) Gruen zones 1 through 7 as they would appear on anterior–posterior radiograph. (*Source:* Maloney WJ, Hartfor JM. The cemented femoral component. In: Callaghan JJ, Rosenberg AG, Rubash HE [eds.], *The Adult Hip*. Philadelphia: Lippincott-Raven, 1998;960.) (B) Acetabular zone systems. DeLee and Carnley are shown on the right, and that of Martell is shown on the left. (*Source:* Peters CL, Dunn HK. The cementless acetabular component. In: Callaghan JJ, Rosenberg AG, Rubash HE [eds.], *The Adult Hip*. Philadelphia: Lippincott-Raven, 1998;1006.)**

from acute infections by the presence of biofilm, which is a biologic polysaccharide that is deposited by infecting bacteria onto the prosthetic implants. The formation of such a layer necessitates the removal of all the components because irrigation and débridement of such chronic infections will not likely eradicate the bacteria. As with early postoperative infections, the diagnostic tests that are most helpful include hip aspiration, C-RP, and ESR. The one disadvantage of hip aspiration is the false-positive rate of 15%, but in combination with the ESR and C-RP, aspiration is still extremely valuable. The combination of a positive ESR and C-RP can be up to 96% sensitive in detecting infection. Bone scans are useful tests in differentiating septic and aseptic loosening if they are performed after a hip aspiration has been negative for infection.

Periprosthetic Hip Fracture. Periprosthetic hip fracture is most often a delayed complication that occurs several months or years after the index procedure. In general, cementless femoral stems fracture earlier than cemented stems because the aggressive broaching and reaming required for the placement of uncemented stems can create minute stress risers and cortical cracks that can propagate. This is in contrast to cemented femoral components, which are more often associated with fractures distal to the stem tip. Periprosthetic fractures are considered most simply by analyzing 3 main factors:

- The level of the fracture about the femur
- The quality of the fixation of the femoral stem at the time of the fracture
- The stability of the fracture

If both the fracture and prosthesis are stable, then nonoperative treatment can be utilized. A careful assessment of these 3 factors can often guide management of periprosthetic fractures. With a well-fixed prosthesis, the mechanism of fracture is usually such that the proximal femur, which is a bone—implant composite, is much stiffer than the distal femur. Therefore, there is a modulus mismatch between the proximal and distal femur, and fracture can result. The Vancouver classification is one of the more widely used systems to grade periprosthetic fractures. Vancouver type A fractures are peritrochanteric fractures, while type B includes those around the stem or distal to the stem tip; type C fractures are those well distal to the stem tip. Type B fractures are subclassified into B1, or those surrounding a rigidly fixed stem; B2, or those surrounding a loose stem; and B3, or those surrounding a stem with extensive osteolysis and bony destruction. Generally, type A fractures can be treated nonoperatively unless there is extensive osteolysis in the peritrochanteric region, in which case the debris-generating polyethylene component should be replaced along with débridement of sites of osteolysis. Type B1 fractures are treated with open reduction and internal fixation with the prosthesis left intact, with a combination of plating, cerclage wires, and screws. Generally, a well-fixed stem should not be revised, and ORIF is preferred. The preferred treatment for B2 fractures is revision of the femoral stem with a longer stem femoral component with supplemental cerclage wires or strut grafts. Type B3 fracture exhibit extensive proximal femoral bone loss and generally require reconstruction of the proximal femur with an allograft or tumor type prosthesis. Type C fractures, which are well distal to the femoral component, are best treated with open reduction and internal fixation.

Evaluation of Painful THA. Any patient with a painful THA that has no radiographic signs of fracture should initiate a work up for infection. Hip aspiration is a useful tool to help diagnose or rule out infection. Although the false-positive rate of aspiration is not insignificant, a negative hip aspiration makes infection highly unlikely. Other causes of pain in older patients with prior THA includes sacral insufficiency fractures.

Heterotopic Ossification (HO). The formation of heterotopic bone after THA is quite common, but fortunately it is not that often painful or clinically significant. The incidence in the literature is reported anywhere from 0.6% to 84%. HO is more common in males and also in patients with hypertrophic arthritis, ankylosing spondylitis, diffuse idiopathic skeletal hyperostosis (DISH); patients who have posttraumatic arthritis; patients with hip fusion that is converted to THA; and patients with Parkinson's disease, excessive osteophytosis, or enthesopathic radiographic changes on AP of pelvis, head injury, and/or spinal cord injury. HO is more commonly associated with anterior and lateral approaches to the hip and is related to the length of the surgical procedure and the extent of soft tissue disruption inflicted during surgery. HO is usually seen on hip x-rays 3 to 8 weeks postoperatively. HO is often classified using the Brooker system.

Grade I.	Islands of bone within the soft tissues
Grade II.	Bone off the pelvis or proximal end of femur with at least 1-cm gap
Grade III.	Bone off the pelvis or the proximal end of femur with less than 1-cm gap
Grade IV.	Bone connecting the pelvis and femur (ankylosis of the hip)

With the exception of grades III and IV, the presence of HO does not reliably correlate with clinical symptoms. Patients with grade III or IV disease that restricts motion are generally good candidates for surgical removal. Generally, HO need not be excised unless it causes significant restriction of motion or impingement of the hip. Surgical excision of HO is normally performed approximately 1 year after index THA. Additionally, postexcision prophylaxis in the form of radiation or pharmacotherapy should be utilized.

Prophylactic Measures for Prevention of HO. Prophylactic measures include radiation and pharmacotherapies; such treatments must generally be initiated within the first 72 hours after surgery to achieve maximal efficacy. The usual radiation protocol for prevention is to deliver 700 rads in one single dose within 24 hours after surgery. It is important to note that if radiation therapy is to be used, then cementless components should be protected because excessive radiation to such components can retard rigid bony ingrowth into the prostheses. Efficacious pharmacotherapies include indomethacin 75 mg/day for 6 to 8 weeks postoperatively, ibuprofen, and high-dose aspirin.

Miscellaneous Complications. Hypersensitivity to the metals used in THA has also been reported in the literature. Although rare, it is thought that nickel in cobalt-chromium components is the substance that most often induces hypersensitivity reactions.

Management of Dislocated THA. Most first and even second dislocations can be treated with closed reduction, abduction bracing, and patient education. The duration of bracing is usually on the order of 3 months to allow adequate scar tissue to form around the hip joint to augment stability. Approximately 66% of patients with dislocations will successfully maintain long-term stability with this protocol. The occurrence of a third dislocation is associated with an unfavorable prognosis, with a slim likelihood that nonoperative management will result in long-term stability. In such situations with repeated dislocations, the causes are many and include component malposition, component impingement, and abductor complex dysfunction. Surgical techniques that can be used to correct such issues include repositioning of malaligned components and increasing the femoral head–neck ratio; surgical techniques that may improve the tensioning of the abductor complex and thereby stability include increasing the femoral offset or neck length, and possible advancement of the greater trochanter. As described earlier, in situations where the abductors are severely dysfunctional, a constrained liner, in which the femoral head locks into the acetabular liner, may be utilized. Constrained liners increase stability but

TABLE 4.5 Classification of bony defects in revision THA

Acetabular Defects	Femoral Defects
1. Segmental: lysis of acetabular rim or medial wall	1. Segmental: loss of length of cortical bone
2. Cavitary: volumetric defects within acetabulum	2. Cavitary: loss of endosteal bone with preserved cortical bone

severely decrease primary arc range; they also transmit larger mechanical forces to the acetabulum, which can result in accelerated component failure. They generally do not result in any increased polyethylene wear and overall can be effective in correcting recurrent dislocations.

Revision Total Hip Arthroplasty

Aseptic loosening of the femoral and acetabular components continues to be the most common indication for revision total hip surgery. The objectives of total hip revision surgery are to remove and replace loose components and bony defects with well-fixed, stable components that optimize hip biomechanics. In general, with hip revision surgery, the bone that remains after removal of the prosthetic components is sclerotic and does not provide optimal conditions for cement interdigitation. Therefore, cementless components are generally preferred in revision settings.

Recent literature has demonstrated that in general, only the loose components need to be revised. For example, in situations where patients have loose acetabulae with well-fixed, femoral components, the femur can be retained and only the acetabulum needs to be revised. Conversely, well fixed cementless acetabulae can be maintained and loose femoral components can be revised. Occasionally, a unique situation may arise in which a well-fixed, uncemented acetabular component with some minor bony defects is coupled with a worn polyethylene component that is no longer available. In such situations, it is acceptable to graft bony defects followed by the placement of a new cemented polyethylene into the cementless acetabulum.

Classification of Bony Defects. For both the femur and the acetabulum, bony defects are generally classified as either segmental or cavitary. Segmental acetabular defects are those in which there is lysis of the acetabular rim or medial wall. Cavitary defects occur when there exists volumetric defects within the acetabulum. Segmental femoral defects occur when there is loss of length of cortical femoral bone. Cavitary defects indicate loss of endosteal bone with preservation of cortical bone. Combination segmental and cavitary defects can occur in both the femur and acetabulum. The extent of cavitary and segmental defects determines the type of revision implants that should be used (Table 4.5).

Revision of the Acetabular Component. One of the most effective techniques of acetabular revision is the use of large, cementless acetabular components. When there is adequate bone present in the anterior and posterior columns such that the acetabular cup can achieve a rigid press-fit, such large components have functioned well. Bony defects that are present between the 2 columns can be filled with morcellized bone graft. Screws can be utilized for additional stability of the component. For a large cup to be successful, at least 50% to 66% of the cup must be in contact with native acetabular bone.

- Acetabular reconstruction or *protrusio* cages are useful when sufficient bone does not exist for an adequate press-fit of a large cementless cup.
- Bulk structural acetabular allografts may be necessary in situations with massive bone loss. A bulk allograft is a single, large piece of bone that is used to fill a native acetabular defect. Autograft can also be used for complex acetabular reconstructions.

Both of these techniques have demonstrated success in the short term, but in longer term follow-up, both techniques have demonstrated high rates of graft resorption and collapse, particularly when reconstruction cages are not used. Allografts have demonstrated particularly high failure rates within the first 5 years.

Indications for Acetabular Reconstruction Cages. Acetabular reconstruction cages are indicated in situations where there is massive acetabular bone loss that results in insufficient bone stock for the use of large cementless revision cups. In such situations, sufficient contact between the host bone and the large cementless cup cannot be achieved, thus necessitating the use of the cage construct. Such cages are also indicated when there exists a pelvic discontinuity between the ilium and ischium. In such situations, the cage can be used to bridge this pelvic defect. Pelvic defects that require cage reconstruction are best identified on plain x-ray by large amounts of ischial osteolysis.

Revision of Femoral Component. As with acetabular revision, revision of the femoral component can be performed with various techniques, including uncemented prostheses, cemented prostheses, impaction grafting, strut allografting, morcellized grafts, and bulk allografts. A frequently employed technique involves placement of a long-stem, extensively porous-coated,

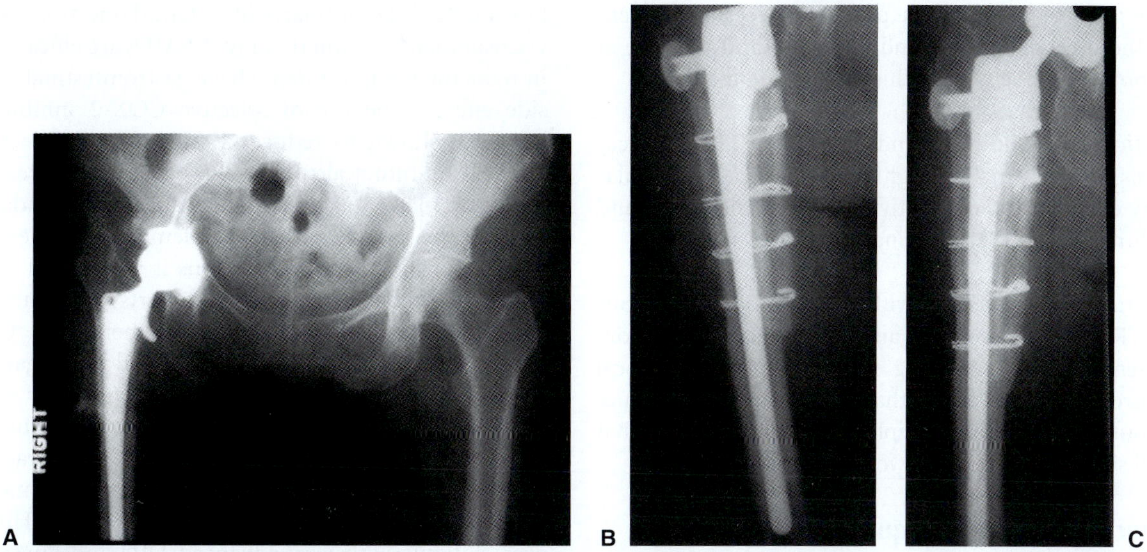

FIGURE 4.6 Radiography of onlay strut allograft. (*Source:* Emerson RH. Revision of the femoral component: Bulk allografts and struts. In: Callaghan JJ, Rosenberg AG, Rubash HE (eds.), The *Adult Hip*. Philadelphia: Lippincott-Raven, 1998;1498.)

uncemented stem. In order to provide prophylaxis against stress risers that may cause fractures at the site of the distal tip of the old femoral prosthesis, the revision stem should extend at least 2 to 3 cm past this old distal tip site. In cases where there is pronounced cortical disruption at the tip of the old prosthesis, the revision stem should extend the length of 2 femoral shaft diameters beyond the site of the old stem.

Onlay Strut Allograft. The technique of onlay strut allografts can be used to address large segmental femoral defects. The struts are secured to the native femur by cerclage wires or cables. They can be utilized with cemented or uncemented stems. Onlay grafts have the advantages that they provide more structural support than do morcellized grafts, while they also achieve better incorporation into the native host bone than do bulk segmental allografts (Fig. 4.6).

Impaction Grafting. A technique whereby morcellized allograft bone is used in combination with a cemented prosthesis to reconstitute bone stock. This technique has been used to fill cavitary defects in the proximal femur and proximal tibia for revision purposes. It is currently believed that the allograft bone undergoes some degree of incorporation and remodeling into native bone. The histology of impaction grafting demonstrates that 3 zones of bone develop: the inner zone consists of cement, necrotic trabecular bone, and fibrous tissue; the middle layer consists of living bone trabeculae; the outer zone is composed of viable cortical bone. Common complications of impaction grafting include stem subsidence and femur fracture. However, some degree of stem subsidence is critical to the success of impaction grafting. The technique does not demonstrate a higher infection rate than other revision techniques.

Segmental Bulk Allografts. In cases of massive femoral bone loss that precludes the use of techniques such as impaction grafting or onlay strut allografts, large, segmental, bulk femoral allografts may be required. In such situations, uncemented components are generally not preferred because the allograft bone has no potential to achieve biologic ingrowth into the component. In such settings, cementing of the femoral component to the allograft is preferred.

Removal of the Cement Mantle. Revision of cemented femoral components poses technical challenges associated with removal of the cement mantle. The technique of extended trochanteric osteotomy is highly effective in removing well-fixed, cemented femoral prostheses and the cement mantle.

II. KNEE RECONSTRUCTIVE SURGERY

Much like THA, total knee arthroplasty (TKA) has also been an extremely successful, efficacious operation for treating pain and deformity associated with advanced DJD of the knee. Many hundreds of thousands of TKAs are performed annually in the United States with good results. Survivorship of TKAs is presently estimated at 90% at 10 years and up to 75% at 20 years.

The goals of TKA include pain relief, reestablishment of the mechanical axis and joint line and Q angle at appropriate levels, and achieving ligament balance.

Indications. Similar to indications for THA, indications for TKA include significant knee pain, ambulatory dysfunction, correlative DJD by plain x-ray, and failure of conservative management.

Contraindications. As with THA, contraindications to TKA are relatively few and include active infection, absent or nonfunctioning extensor mechanism, local neurologic dysfunction that affects the musculature about the knee, and peripheral vascular disease that will significantly impede wound healing.

Specific Disorders Requiring TKA

Avascular Necrosis. Avascular necrosis of the knee can occur about the medial or lateral femoral condyles or the tibial plateau and most commonly occurs in women over age 60. The clinical history is usually one of sudden onset of knee pain. In advanced stages, plain radiographs demonstrate narrowing of the joint space and a defect in the lateral femoral condyle, along with sclerosis, a "crescent" sign, and femoral condyle flattening. Radionuclide bone scanning and MRI are useful for diagnosing this entity; these imaging modalities will demonstrate changes before they are evident by plain x-ray. This condition is often self-limiting and resolves with conservative management. However, in refractory, persistent cases of avascular necrosis, once there has been collapse of the articular surface, total knee replacement provides the most predictable result.

Paget Disease. In patients with Paget disease who require TKA, it is best to reduce the serum alkaline phosphatase level by at least 50% before the procedure. The pretreatment should commence 6 to 8 weeks before the TKA procedure.

TKA in Ankylosed or Fused Knees. The conversion of previously ankylosed or fused knees is technically challenging and is generally associated with poor outcomes. Patients can expect an ROM that lacks 5 to 10 degrees of extension to slightly greater than 60 degrees of flexion. The overall complication rate approaches 60%. The infection rate for such procedures is roughly 14%, while major complications such as extensor mechanism damage, loosening, or persistent pain requiring revision surgery is approximately 35%.

Nonarthroplasty Treatment of Knee Disorders

Conservative Modalities. Conservative modalities of alleviating knee DJD include weight loss, valgus bracing, NSAIDs, intraarticular steroid injections, and viscosupplementation therapy. NSAIDs are efficacious in reducing pain, but many have gastrointestinal (GI) side effects. The use of selective COX-2 inhibitors has been shown to reduce GI side effects. Selective COX-2 inhibitors also have the benefit of decreased effects on platelet aggregation, as do several standard, nonselective NSAIDs. Viscosupplementation therapy with hyaluronic acid preparations is being used with increasing frequency. Literature reports have demonstrated mixed results of viscosupplementation. One recent double-blind, placebo-controlled investigation indicated that patients aged 60 years and older with moderate to severe DJD would derive the greatest benefit from viscosupplementation therapy. Valgus bracing for medial compartment arthritis has been demonstrated in several studies to offer some benefit. However, patients with very advanced DJD and knees in greater than 20 degrees of varus are unlikely to benefit.

Autologous Chondrocyte Implantation (ACI) and Osteoarticular Allografts. These procedures are more aggressive surgical options for treating focal cartilage defects in the knee. However, they are not indicated for the treatment of generalized, multicompartmental knee DJD. The femoral focal cartilage lesions have demonstrated the best results with ACI. Osteoarticular allografts are an alternative to ACI for focal knee defects. This procedure involves harvesting full-thickness fragments of articular cartilage and subchondral bone from donors. The most common mode of failure of osteoarticular allografts is by graft collapse during the revascularization process. Other less frequent modes of failure include mechanical loosening of the graft, infection, and immune rejection.

Synovectomy. Synovectomy is currently indicated primarily for rheumatoid arthritis patients with painful synovitis that is unresponsive to medical management after 4 to 6 months and well-maintained ROM. The procedure has been demonstrated to relieve pain. Arthroscopic synovectomy is currently the preferred surgical technique.

High Tibial Osteotomy (HTO). An HTO can be effective for treating medial compartment gonarthrosis in the carefully selected patient. This procedure is generally considered appropriate for younger patients (under 60 years) with mild to moderate arthritis, preoperative ROM of 90 degrees or greater, between 10 and 15 degrees of varus deformity, and sufficient preoperative conditioning to complete the extensive rehabilitation program. Contraindications for HTO include the following:

1. Inflammatory arthritis
2. Multicompartment arthritis

3. Lateral tibial subluxation
4. Flexion contracture more than 15 degrees

However, for patients who have tibial deformities that are too large for HTO, a tibial osteotomy can be performed at or below the level of the tibial tubercle to achieve larger degrees of correction. Finally, for patients who have lateral compartment disease, a supracondylar femoral osteotomy can be performed. The indications for this procedure include single, lateral compartment arthrosis, less than 15 degrees of valgus deformity, less than 90 degrees ROM, and younger age.

Total Knee Arthroplasty

Total Knee Arthroplasty after HTO. In general, TKA after HTO is associated with inferior outcomes compared to TKA in a previously nonosteotomized knee. The major complication affecting TKA after HTO is patella infera. Patella infera can lead to decreased ROM of the TKA and can make intraoperative exposure of the joint more difficult. However, HTO has not been reported to increase rates of infection, postoperative manipulation under anesthesia, or loosening.

Primary TKA. Primary TKA demonstrates higher survival than revision TKA. Independent factors associated with improved survival of TKA include:

- Patients with a diagnosis of rheumatoid arthritis
- Patients who are older than 60 years
- The implantation of a condylar prosthesis with a metal-backed tibial component

Design and Biomechanics of TKA. Total knee reconstruction has as one of its primary goals the reestablishment of the mechanical axis of the lower extremity to one that passes through the center of the femoral head, the center of the tibial plateau, and the center of the tibiotalar articulation. This is accomplished by performing a valgus cut in the distal femur. Performing the valgus cut such that the femoral component is perpendicular to the mechanical axis of the femur results in balanced force transmission from the femoral head to the distal femur. Generally, the valgus cut angle utilized in the distal femur is between 5 and 7 degrees. This angle is the result of the difference between the anatomic axis and the mechanical axis of the femur. In patients who are very short, the valgus cut angle may need to be greater than 7 degrees, while very tall patients will require a valgus cut angle of less than 5 degrees to reestablish mechanical alignment.

Patellofemoral Tracking. The shape of the femoral component can significantly effect patellar tracking. Studies have demonstrated that a trochlear groove with a deep, anatomic configuration optimizes patellar tracking and minimizes contact stresses.

Conformity. The degree of conformity between the tibial and femoral component in TKA significantly effects the transmission of forces to the prosthesis and native bone. When there is greater conformity between components, there is also greater contact area between contact stresses between the femur and tibia; therefore, contact stresses are distributed over a larger area, which results in decreased peak contact stresses and a lower wear rate. However, greater conformity also leads to increased constraint; such constraint causes forces to be transmitted to the prosthesis–cement–bone interface, which can lead to accelerated component loosening. Conversely, decreased conformity has all the opposite effects on the prosthesis, with decreased contact surface area between components, increased peak stresses, increased component wear, and decreased force transmitted to the prosthesis–cement–bone interface. Consequently, rates of loosening are also less with decreased constraint.

Management of Joint Line. If the femoral or tibial components are incorrectly placed or sized, the patient's native joint line can be moved proximally or distally. Moving the joint line by more than 8 mm has been demonstrated to reduce ROM, impair patellar function, and reduce patellar stability.

Patellar Tracking. The patellofemoral articulation is one of the most challenging aspects of TKA, and complications related to it are currently the most common causes for revision. Patellar instability and maltracking can result from an excessively valgus knee, medially placed femoral or tibial components, or internally rotated femoral or tibial components. Additionally, errors in patellar management such as lateralization of the component or overstuffing of the patellar component can lead to maltracking. A lateral retinacular release can be performed to improve patellar tracking.

Patellar Resection. Another important aspect of patellar management is the amount of resection that is utilized. Reports have demonstrated that native patellar thickness should be maintained between 12 and 15 mm in order to decrease the risk of patellar stress fracture.

Metal-Backed Patellar Components. Metal-backed patellar components have been demonstrated in the literature to have higher failure rates. Conceptually, metal-backed patellae, similar to metal backed tibial components, should allow for more even force distribution across the patella. However, metal-backed patellae have been fraught with complications, including dissociation of the patellar button from the metal back, peg failure, poor bony ingrowth, and component fracture. Thus, currently, all polyethylene patellar components are considered the standard of care.

Postpatellectomy Patients. Patients who have previously undergone patellectomy are better served with a posterior cruciate–substituting TKA. An intact extensor mechanism provides a significant amount of anterior–posterior stability in a reconstructed knee; therefore, when the patella is absent, the posterior cruciate ligament (PCL) alone will not provide sufficient anterior–posterior stability and a posterior cruciate–substituting prosthesis is indicated.

Cementless TKA. Uncemented TKA has demonstrated survivorship comparable to cemented prostheses during the last 15 years. However, certain surgical and component design principles must be adhered to for successful outcome with such prostheses. The key surgical goal that must be accomplished for a successful uncemented TKA is stable, rigid fixation of the tibial component. The implant design must allow for minimal constraint at the femoral–tibial articulation.

Metal-Backed Tibial Components. A metal-backed tibial tray is an attempt to mimic the hard subchondral bone of the native knee. In healthy knees, the subchondral bone of the tibia does an excellent job of distributing the high forces experienced by the knee joint across the entire tibial plateau. A metal-backed tibial component attempts to mimic the function of the subchondral bone by evenly distributing loads across the entire surface of cancellous bone that is exposed when the tibial cuts are made. An all-polyethylene tibial component does not have the ability to load the cancellous tibial bone as evenly as can a metal-backed tibia.

Tibial Polyethylene During Primary TKA. Polyethylene wear is known to be a significant contributor to the failure of TKA. The thickness of the polyethylene insert for the tibial component significantly affects the wear rate of this component. Studies have demonstrated that the minimum thickness of the tibial polyethylene should be 6 to 8 mm in order to maintain acceptable wear rates.

Management of Flexion and Extension Gaps. Ligament balancing and management of flexion and extension gaps is critical to the success of TKA. In the sagittal plane, measures should be taken to balance the flexion and extension gaps. Strategies that can be utilized to balance flexion and extension gaps include increasing the amount of bone resected at the femur or tibia, changing the sizes of the tibial or femoral components, or altering the tension of the PCL. In general, when both the flexion and extension gaps are equally tight or loose, the solution lies in either increasing or decreasing the size of the tibial component. When there is laxity or tightness in only one position (i.e., flexion *or* extension), the solution generally lies in altering the size of the femoral component. When patients with posterior cruciate–retaining TKAs experience midflexion instability, the cause is often incompetence of the PCL. In such cases, the treatment is generally revision to a posterior-stabilized prosthesis.

Tight, Symmetrical Flexion and Extension Gaps. When both the flexion and extension gaps are tight, the goal is to reduce the height of the proximal tibia, which loosens both the flexion and extension spaces equally. Shortening the proximal tibia can be accomplished by either reducing the thickness of the tibial component or resection of additional proximal tibial bone.

Loose, Symmetrical Flexion and Extension Gaps. When both gaps are loose, the goal is to increase the height of the proximal tibia, which can be accomplished by adding metallic augmentation to the proximal tibia or by increasing the thickness of the tibial polyethylene component.

Asymmetric Flexion Gap Problems. If the flexion gap is tight and the extension gap is normal, several techniques can be used to address this asymmetry. If a PCL-retaining component is used, a tight flexion gap with an acceptable extension gap can be addressed by recessing the PCL. When a PCL-substituting or PCL-sacrificing prosthesis is used, other strategies that can be employed include increasing the amount of posterior slope of the tibial cut, resecting more posterior femoral condyle and downsizing the femoral component, and releasing a tight posterior capsule. When the flexion gap is loose and the extension gap is acceptable, the goal is to increase the size of the posterior condyles of the femur. This can be accomplished by adding cement or metal to the posterior femur. Subsequently, a larger femoral prosthesis can be inserted to increase the tightness of the flexion gap.

Asymmetric Extension Gap Problems. When the flexion gap is acceptable, but the extension gap is too rigid, resection of additionally distal femoral bone will achieve balance. Additionally, a posterior capsular release can improve the extension gap in such a situation. When the flexion gap is acceptable, but the extension gap is too loose, increasing the size of the *distal* femur by adding cement or metal augments will tighten the extension space. However, other potential strategies include downsizing the femoral component, which decreases the size of the flexion gap. At this point, the surgeon is faced with symmetrically loose flexion and extension gaps, which can then be addressed by increasing the size of the tibial component.

Management of Component Rotation. The rotational alignment of the femoral and tibial components is of critical importance in TKA. Internal rotation or medial placement of the tibial component effectively moves the tibial tubercle laterally, which increases the Q angle and possible lateral patellar subluxation. Similarly, internal rotation of the femoral component causes the patella to rest on the lateral aspect of the trochlear groove and increases the Q angle, resulting in subluxation.

Simultaneous Bilateral TKAs. Bilateral TKAs that are performed simultaneously have been shown to cause a higher 30-day postoperative mortality rate. However, other complications, such as bleeding, loosening, infection, and ROM, have not been shown to be significantly higher for simultaneous bilateral TKAs.

Complications of TKA

Early Postoperative Complications

Neurovascular Complications. Vascular injury after TKA is quite rare compared with other complications. Vascular insult can occur as a result of direct injury to the popliteal artery intraoperatively; additionally, thrombosis of the femoral or popliteal vessels can rarely occur. Tourniquet use has been implicated in thrombotic events during TKA in patients with preexisting vascular disease. Neurologic injury most commonly occurs to the peroneal nerve on the order of 0.3% to 4.0%. Patients with severe valgus deformities and severe flexion contractures that are corrected intraoperatively are at increased risk of peroneal nerve injury. The peroneal nerve may also suffer direct compression during TKA. Other risk factors for peroneal nerve palsy include prior lumbar laminectomy, epidural anesthesia, and prior HTO. When a peroneal nerve palsy is recognized postoperatively, the immediate treatment should include removal of all dressings and knee flexion. Symptoms of peroneal nerve injury include initial burning sensations on the dorsum of the foot followed by pain and subsequent weakness in foot dorsiflexion. Risk factors for neurologic injury during TKA are as follows:

1. Severe valgus deformity
2. Flexion deformity
3. Prior lumbar laminectomy
4. Epidural anesthesia
5. Prior HTO

Gastrointesintal Complications. GI complications including ileus and Ogilvie syndrome, are common after TKA. The incidence of ileus has been reported to be as high as 3%. Patients who are hypokalemic preoperatively are at increased risk of postoperative ileus. Additionally, extended periods of bedrest after TKA place patients at greater risk.

Range of Motion Difficulties. Patients may exhibit decreased ROM initially after TKA. Studies have shown that patients whose early postoperative ROM is less than 70 degrees have a significantly higher probability of requiring a manipulation under anesthesia than patients whose early postoperative ROM was 80 degrees. Patients can be expected to gain 33 degrees or more with a manipulation that is performed in 4 months or less after index TKA.

Wound Complications. Patients with prior surgical incisions about the knee, those who have received radiation, those who are morbidly obese, and those on chronic immunosuppressives for rheumatoid disease or transplantation are all at increased risk of wound complications after TKA. Additionally, TKAs that require extensive soft tissue dissection or that involve correction of large degrees of deformity are all at increased risk of wound complications. Studies have also demonstrated that more medial placement of skin incisions leads to lower oxygen tension in the lateral skin flap of the surgical wound. Therefore, anterior midline incisions are currently favored. Finally, the use of subcuticular polydioxanone sutures is associated with a higher rate of wound complications.

Late Postoperative Complications

Infection. Infection rates after TKA have been reported between 0.5% and 23%. The current infection rate is thought be on the order of 1% to 2%. Infections can be categorized in several ways. However, the most useful method of classification indicates the duration of the infection. Acute infections are those that have been present for 2 to 6 weeks. Acute infections can be the result of direct contamination of the surgical site during the index procedure. Acute hematogenous infections can be the result of transient bacteremia, such as that caused by dental instrumentation. Chronic infections are considered those that have been present for longer than 4 to 6 weeks. The duration of the infection is considered by many to be the most important factor guiding treatment.

Diagnosis of Infection. Aspiration of the knee is still considered the most reliable diagnostic tool for diagnosis of infection. Studies have demonstrated that aspiration can be 100% sensitive, specific, and accurate in diagnosing infection. Serial plain x-rays can be useful adjuncts to diagnosis, particularly if they demonstrate extensive and rapid loosening or periosteal reaction. Technetium Tc 99 bone scans and gallium scans are often not helpful because they will frequently show increased uptake for up to 3 years after index TKA. C-RP and ESR are also useful diagnostic tests.

Intraoperative Diagnosis of Infection. In recent years, the technique of using intraoperative frozen sections during revision TKA for diagnosis of infection has become more common. The presence of fewer than 5 polymorphonuclear leukocytes (PMNs) per high-power field (HPF) in the frozen section during revision surgery consistently indicates the absence of infection. More than 10 PMNs per high-power field is highly suggestive of infection.

Treatment of Infection. Acute hematogenous that is diagnosed and treated within 2 weeks can usually be treated with aggressive irrigation and débridement, polyethylene exchange, component retention, and an extended course of intravenous antibiotics. For late hematogenous and more chronic infections, the current treatment of choice is a 2-stage procedure, with removal of components and placement of antibiotic spacer with a prolonged course of intravenous antibiotics. Salvage rates of 90% have been reported with a 2-stage technique.

Chronic Antibiotic Suppression Therapy. In rare circumstances, the treatment of choice for patients with infected TKAs is chronic suppressive antibiotics with retention of the components. Patients who have severe medical comorbidities that preclude them from undergoing 2-stage revision surgery may be treated with chronic suppression. The success rate of such a treatment modality has been reported between 21% and 38%.

High-Risk Patients. Another rare circumstance encountered in infected TKA is that of a patient with significant risk of wound healing complications (e.g., diabetes mellitus or chronic immunosuppression), a nonfunctioning extensor mechanism, and a chronically infected TKA. In such situations, it is highly unlikely that a concurrent revision TKA with extensor mechanism reconstruction will remain infection free. In such situations, the preferred treatment may be component removal, eradication of infection via antibiotic spacer, and IV antibiotics followed by knee arthrodesis. Patients who are medically unfit for repeated surgery may be treated with resection arthroplasty or amputation.

Complications of Cementless TKAs. Patients who receive cementless TKAs may experience fibrous ingrowth of the porous-coated components. Such patients demonstrate lucencies around the tibial component with sclerosis around the tibial stem. Bone scan demonstrates increased uptake in areas of fibrous ingrowth. Clinically, patients experience pain with weight bearing but are relatively pain free at night and at rest. The most common complication after cementless TKA is osteolysis, which is often most prevalent around the tibial fixation screws. The incidence of osteolysis in cementless TKAs has been reported as high as 30%.

Patella Fracture. Fractures of the patella after TKA are most often stress fractures but can also occur as a result of maltracking, vascular compromise to the patella, trauma, excessive resection of patellar bone, and patient overactivity. Reports have demonstrated that patellar thickness less than 12 to 15 mm increases the risk of fracture. Treatment of patellar fracture is based on extensor mechanism function and component fixation. If the patient with a transverse fracture has an intact extensor mechanism with a well-fixed patellar component, nonsurgical treatment with cast immobilization for 6 weeks may be initiated. For vertical fractures, a shorter period of immobilization is acceptable. For fractures with loose components, the acceptable treatment is removal of the component with revision resurfacing if the residual patellar thickness is greater than 10 to 12 mm. If the remaining patella is very thin, then patellaplasty or partial patellectomy and extensor mechanism repair is the preferred treatment.

Patellar Clunk. Patellar clunk syndrome occurs after TKA when a fibrous nodule develops in the suprapatellar region. This nodule results in a painful clunk between 60 and 30 degrees of extension. This syndrome most often develops after implantation of a posterior-stabilized knee. Conservative treatment for patellar clunk includes exercise, physical therapy, and ROM therapy. If this treatment is ineffective, arthroscopic débridement of the suprapatellar nodule is often effective.

Periprosthetic Fracture. Fractures about TKAs can occur at the distal femur, in the supracondylar region, and at the proximal tibia. Distal femur fractures are associated with several factors, including anterior femoral notching of greater than 3 mm, osteopenia, rheumatoid arthritis, chronic steroids, and osteolysis. Such fractures can be treated operatively with blade plates, condylar screw plates, condylar buttress plates, antegrade or retrograde intramedullary nail fixation, or distal femoral replacement with tumor prosthesis. Surgical treatment methods are associated with increased incidence of infection and nonunion rates compared with nonsurgical treatments; however, surgical treatments do afford the ability to restore the distal femur to anatomic alignment. Fractures that are nondisplaced or minimally displaced with acceptable angulation and rotational alignment can be treated with immobilization. Proximal tibia fractures about prior TKA are rare. Loose tibial components with osteolytic breakdown can experience stress fractures. If the tibial fracture is distal to the implant, treatment is dependent on the status of the tibial component fixation. A well-fixed tibial component allows for treatment of the fracture only by internal fixation or nonoperative means. A loose tibial component usually necessitates revision to a longer stem prosthesis with possible allograft augmentation (Figs. 4.7, 4.8, and 4.9).

Polyethylene Wear. Similar to total hip replacement, polyethylene wear debris can affect the outcome of total knee replacement. Clinically, patients with significant wear particles can develop extensive synovitis that results in pain and swelling. Aspiration will demonstrate a cloudy fluid with a cell count of less than 30,000/ mm^3. Microscopic examination of this fluid may reveal polyethylene particles. Such patients usually have a normal C-RP and ESR. In such patients, the synovitis can progress to frank osteolysis. Treatment options include observation, irrigation and débridement with polyethylene exchange, or revision with component removal and possible bone grafting depending on the extent of bone loss.

Osteolysis. Osteolysis after TKA is much more common with cementless TKA than with cemented prostheses. When both femoral and tibial components are implanted without cement and supplemental screw fixation, the risk of osteolysis can be as high as 30%. When only the femur is uncemented, the risk is approximately 10%. If both components are cemented, the risk of osteolysis is very low. With cementless components, certain design features can reduce the rate of osteolysis. The use of monoblock tibial components with compression molding of the polyethylene to the tibial tray can significantly reduce lysis. Modular components allow motion to occur between the tibial polyethylene and metal tibial tray. The polyethylene particles generated from this motion result in osteolysis. Cemented components that utilize modular polyethylene inserts can also demonstrate wear and osteolysis. Finally, factors such as patient weight and activity level and oxidative degradation of the polyethylene components that were sterilized in air have also been suggested to cause osteolysis (Fig. 4.10).

Revision Total Knee Arthroplasty

As with total hip revision, revision of TKA has as its goals the removal of failing, loose components while minimizing bone loss; correction of bony defects, reestablishment of joint line and ligament balancing, and fixation of stable components to the remaining bone. The most common indications for revision TKA include patellofemoral problems such as instability,

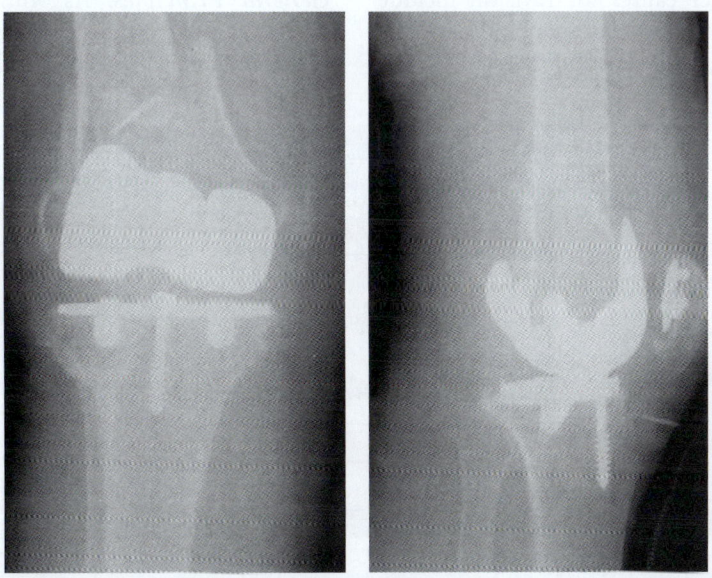

FIGURE 4.7 **(A) Anterior–posterior and (B) lateral radiographs of type I supracondylar fracture above a resurfacing total knee implant. (*Source:* McAlinden MG, Masri BA, Garbuz DS, et al. Periprosthetic fractures after total knee arthroplasty. In: Callaghan JJ, Rosenberg AG, Rubash HE, et al. (eds.), *The Adult Knee*. Philadelphia: Lippincott Williams & Wilkins, 2003;1364.)**

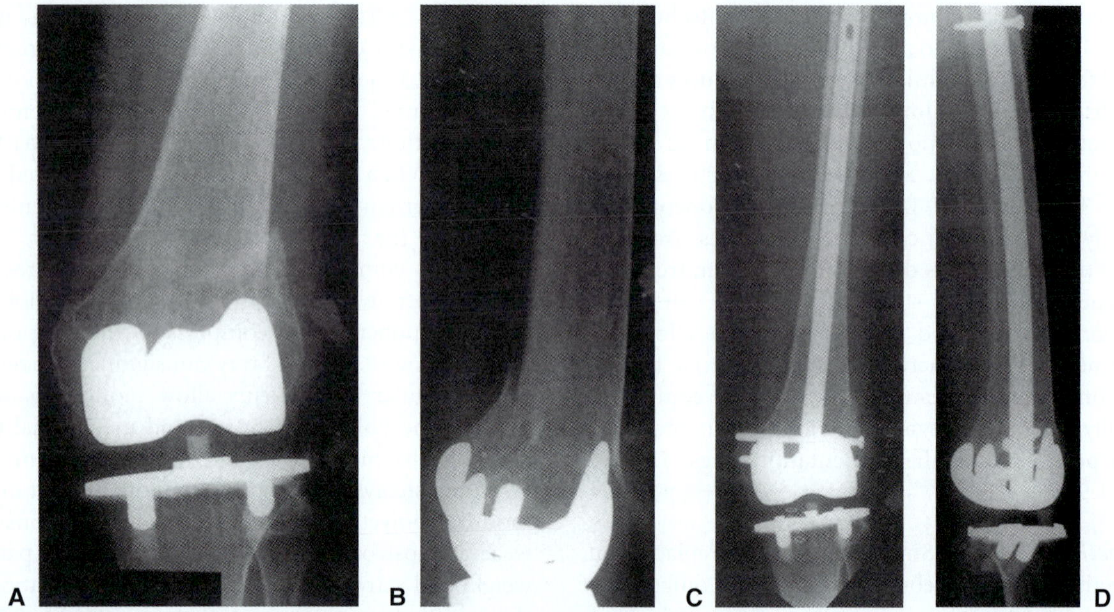

FIGURE 4.8 **Initial (A) Anterior–posterior and (B) lateral radiographs of type I supracondylar fracture above a cruciate-retaining total knee implant. (C) Anterior–Posterior and (D) lateral radiographs after closed reduction and fixation with a rigid intramedullary nail with interlocking screws proximally and distally. (*Source:* McAlinden MG, Masri BA, Garbuz DS, et al. Periprosthetic fractures after total knee arthroplasty. In: Callaghan JJ, Rosenberg AG, Rubash HE, et al. (eds.), *The Adult Knee*. Philadelphia: Lippincott Williams & Wilkins, 2003;1364.)**

maltracking, patella fracture, loosening, and anterior knee pain. Reports estimate that patellofemoral complications affect between 8% and 35% of patients after TKA. Other causes for revision include polyethylene wear, osteolysis, component malalignment, joint instability, and infection. In general, the tibial component fails and loosens more often than does the femoral component.

General Principles. As with THA revision, bony defects can be addressed in several ways during TKA revision. Smaller metaphyseal bony defects can be

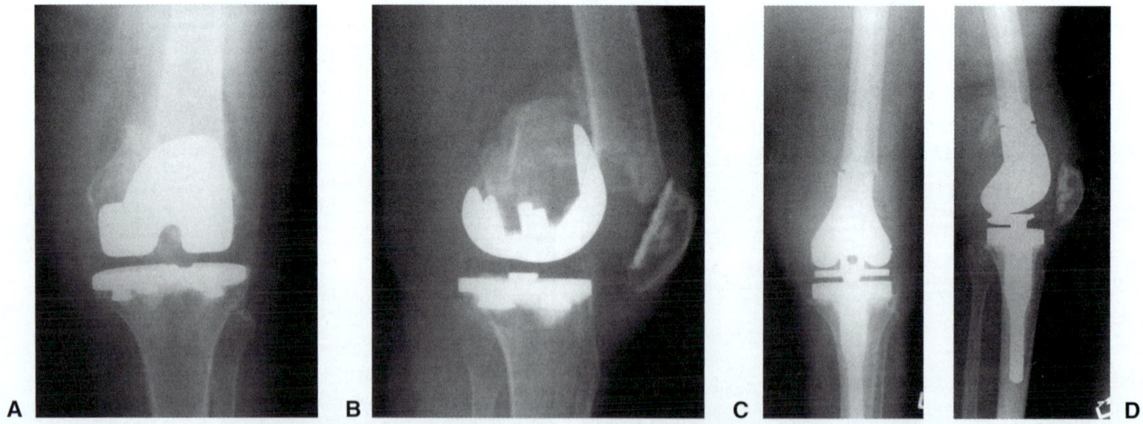

FIGURE 4.9 **(A) Anterior–posterior and (B) later radiographs of a type II supracondylar fracture above a cruciate-retaining total knee implant. (C, D) This fracture was treated with a revision total knee arthroplasty to an oncologic rotating-hinge prosthesis. (*Source:* McAlinden MG, Masri BA, Garbuz DS, et al. Periprosthetic fractures after total knee arthroplasty. In: Callaghan JJ, Rosenberg AG, Rubash HE, et al. (eds.), *The Adult Knee*. Philadelphia: Lippincott Williams & Wilkins, 2003;1365.)**

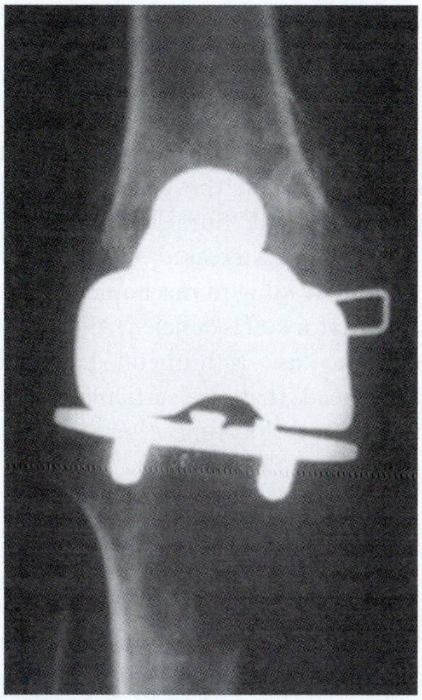

FIGURE 4.10 **Osteolysis after cementless total knee arthroplasty. An example of lytic bone resorption beneath the tibial baseplate. (*Source:* Muratoglu OK, Vittetoe DA, Rubash HE. Damage of implant surfaces in total knee arthroplasty. In: Callaghan JJ, Rosenberg AG, Rubash HE, et al. (eds.), *The Adult Knee.* Philadelphia: Lippincott Williams & Wilkins, 2003;302.)**

filled with cement or morcellized bone graft. For larger segmental bone loss, metal augments, allografts, large endoprosthetic implants, or impaction grafting can also be used. When significant bony defects are encountered, prostheses with longer stems should be used in both the femur and the tibia. Such prostheses can provide greater support and distribute forces to larger areas of the native bone.

Treatment of failed or painful TKA with simple polyethylene exchange only generally does not produce good results. The success rate of such procedures is only 50%, regardless of the presence or lack of osteolysis at the time of revision. The chances of success of polyethylene exchange are inversely proportional to the extent of preoperative polyethylene wear and undersurface wear.

Revision is generally best performed by first addressing the tibia. The appropriate height of the tibia to restore the joint line in revision settings can be estimated by using the top of the fibular head as a guide. Generally, the joint line is approximately 2 cm above the level of the fibular head. Once the tibia has been reconstructed and the joint line has been established, the femur can be revised to articulate with the tibia.

In revision settings, the surgeon has the option of introducing variable amounts of constraint into the prosthesis based on the stability of the native knee and the status of the native knee ligaments. If both the MCL and PCL are intact, a PCL-retaining revision system can be used. If the MCL is intact but the PCL is attenuated, a posterior-stabilized prosthesis is indicated. If both the PCL and one of the collateral ligaments are attenuated, a constrained device without a hinge is indicated. If the PCL and MCL are both completely absent and nonfunctioning, a hinged, rotating-platform device may be indicated. Use of constraint in revision TKA is described here:

1. *Intact PCL and MCL*—PCL-retaining *or* posterior stabilized
2. *Intact MCL and weak PCL*—Posterior-stabilized prosthesis
3. *One weak collateral ligament and weak PCL*—Constrained device without hinge
4. *PCL and MCL absent*—Hinged, rotating-platform device

Revision of Painful PCL-Retaining Knee. Patients may experience flexion instability after primary PCL-retaining TKA. Such patients complain of knee pain, effusion, and a feeling of instability without actual dislocation of the TKA.

Revision for Persistent Knee Pain. Patients with persistent knee pain after primary TKA with no identified cause may be candidates for revision surgery. In patients who demonstrate well-aligned TKA components with no evidence of loosening, lysis, infection, or malalignment, the success rate of revision surgery for pain is only 40%. Therefore, revision TKA should generally be avoided in such patients.

Revision Associated with Patellar Complication

Patellar Tendon Rupture. Patellar tendon rupture is a rare but serious complication of TKA. The incidence is reported to be between 0.17% and 1.4%. Patients with patellar tendon rupture after TKA demonstrate severe pain and inability to ambulate. Such patients are best treated with reconstruction of the extensor mechanism.

Massive Extensor Mechanism Failure. Patients who have massive anterior tibial cortical bone loss due to infection or other chronic condition after TKA are best treated with knee arthrodesis. In such patients, extensor mechanism reconstruction has a very high rate of failure, while 91% fusion rates can be expected.

Revision in Settings of Massive Bone Loss. Situations arise in which patients have massive tibial bone loss. Several techniques can be used to address such bony deficiencies. Large, structural bulk allografts often yield better results in such situations than do hinged prostheses, cement, or iliac crest bone graft. More recent reports have also demonstrated that impaction grafting can be used to restore bone stock during knee revision. However, longer term follow-up data is necessary to determine the utility of this technique in the knee.

Knee Arthrodesis for Failed Revision. On occasion, a previously chronically infected TKA may not be amenable to repeat prosthesis placement. In such situations, arthrodesis of the knee may be the only remaining viable option. Arthrodesis of previously infected TKA can be difficult because of the recurrence of infection in and around the internal fixation hardware used for fusion. Several methods can be used for knee arthrodesis, including external fixation, intramedullary nail fixation, and plate and screw fixation. External fixation has the disadvantage of potential pin tract infection. Intramedullary rods and dual knee plating leave metal hardware in the vicinity of the joint; this hardware can harbor persistent bacterial infection.

Revision of Cruciate Retaining Prostheses. Patients with cruciate-retaining prostheses may complain of flexion instability. Such instability can be a source of continued discomfort, pain, and dysfunction in patients after primary cruciate retaining TKA. Clinically, such patients will complain of pain, recurrent effusions, feelings of knee instability, and difficulty with stair climbing. Signs of flexion instability include pain in the pes anserine complex, positive posterior drawer, or posterior sag sign and greater-than-normal flexion. Radiography in such patients may demonstrate signs of PCL failure, including anterior subluxation of the femur on the tibia. The best treatment for such patients is revision of the prosthesis to a cruciate-substituting, posterior-stabilized prosthesis.

III. TOTAL SHOULDER REPLACEMENT SURGERY

The shoulder, compared to the hip and knee, has greater ROM, which, because of lower constraints, puts greater shear stresses on the implant and therefore increases risk of failure and osteolysis. Proper implant positioning and soft tissue tensioning are also critical to prevent mechanical failure. The two most critical factors to consider for a successful total shoulder replacement are the condition of the rotator cuff and the amount of glenoid stock for resurfacing. With a deficient rotator cuff, the glenoid should not be resurfaced because the humeral head will migrate superiorly and cause increased shear stresses on the superior glenoid, leading to mechanical loosening and failure. If the rotator cuff is deficient, the most common alternative is to use a humeral hemiarthroplasty with a large head that can articulate beneath the acromion without dislocating. Alternatively, a bipolar hemiarthroplasty could also work. These two methods still have limited ROM within the range of 60 to 80 degrees. More aggressive salvage techniques include superior subscapularis and teres advancement with closure of the rotator cuff deficiency followed by resurfacing of the humeral head with a similar or smaller sized head. In cases of a deficient glenoid, ensure to get an axillary lateral radiograph and/or CT scan preoperatively to assess the bone stock and glenoid version. Osteoarthritis predisposes to posterior glenoid erosion and hence relative retroversion. This retroversion can be corrected with anterior reaming of the glenoid or posterior bone grafting. The glenoid surface is replaced with an all-polyethylene component, preferably between 4 and 6 mm. Stem fixation can be cemented or uncemented, and the principles are similar to those of hip arthroplasty. A proximal porous-coated stem has an advantage for limiting osteolysis and avoiding excessive bone loss during extraction for revision surgery. The stem is positioned in 20 to 30 degrees of retroversion, but this position should be individualized and must correlate with the position of the glenoid to allow maximum articulation.

IV. GENERAL TOPICS IN TOTAL JOINT ARTHROPLASTY

Total Joint Arthroplasty After Organ Transplant. Patients who have undergone organ transplantation before total joint arthroplasty are at increased risk of infection. The risk has been reported to be as high as 19% in some series.

Anticoagulation. The postoperative management of deep venous thrombosis (DVT) is also a controversial topic in total joint replacement. Currently, popular agents for DVT prophylaxis include warfarin, low molecular weight heparin (LMWH), aspirin, unfractionated heparin, dextran, and mechanical devices such as sequential compression devices (SCD). There are advantages and disadvantages to each of these agents. Unfractionated heparin, despite its high efficacy in preventing thrombotic events, is associated with at least a 2.6% risk of major bleeding events, compared with only a 0.4% risk with aspirin, a 1.3% risk with warfarin, and a 1.8% risk with LMWH. Unfractionated heparin also results in a higher rate of thrombocytopenia. Unfractionated heparin exerts its effects by binding with antithrombin III to inactivate thrombin and factor Xa. LMWH acts at several sites in the coagulation pathway, with its major effects occurring on Factor Xa; additionally, it facilitates binding to antithrombin, which subsequently inactivates antithrombin III. LMWH offers the further advantage over unfractionated heparin in that it demonstrates improved bioavailability with a longer half-life and more consistent dose-response curve. LMWH has a lower incidence of thrombocytopenia than does unfractionated heparin. Both of these heparin-related agents have the disadvantage that they cannot be used with indwelling epidural anesthetic catheters. Warfarin functions by preventing the production of vitamin K–dependent clotting factors by the liver. These factors include II, VII, IX, and X. Warfarin has the disadvantage of requiring frequent international normalized ratio (INR) monitoring along with its very slow onset of action. Dextran functions through its dilutional effects on the blood, while SCDs improve venous return to the heart and stimulate endothelium to release fibrinolytic factors. Finally, aspirin functions by retarding thromboxane A_2 synthesis and inhibiting platelet aggregation.

Blood Management. Two areas of THA postoperative protocol that deserve special focus include management of blood loss and transfusions and anticoagulation. Because of the elective nature of THA, patients have the option to autodonate blood prior to surgery or undergo preoperative treatment with marrow-stimulating agents to increase preoperative hemoglobin levels. However, studies have shown that patients with normal preoperative hemoglobin levels (higher than 15 g/dl) rarely require transfusions postoperatively. Additionally, the preoperative autologous donation of blood in such patients increases the probability that such patients will require postoperative transfusions. Thus, recent literature has called into question the cost-effectiveness of predonation of blood in patients with normal preoperative hemoglobin. Overall, the preoperative hemoglobin is the most predictive factor in determining necessity of transfusion after THA/TKA. The overall risk of requiring a homologous transfusion after THA can be reduced by preoperative donation of autologous blood, intraoperative recycling and retransfusion of autologous blood, preoperative erythropoietin, and the use of spinal/epidural anesthesia. It is important to clarify that preoperative donation of autologous blood increases the likelihood of a patient requiring a transfusion of this same autologous blood after surgery. However, preoperative autodonation decreases the likelihood that patients will require a homologous, allogeneic transfusion. The use of uncemented THA components and postoperative vacuum drains have both been demonstrated to increase perioperative blood loss.

Erythropoietin. Preoperative use of marrow-stimulating agents such as erythropoietin has been shown to reduce postoperative transfusion requirements in prospective, randomized, controlled trials. Such agents can be particularly useful in patients whose preoperative hemoglobin levels are too low to tolerate autodonation. Erythropoietin use does entail small risks of increased thrombotic events and hypersensitivity. For these reasons, its use is not currently indicated in patients who have a preoperative hemoglobin of more than 13g/dl or who have recent history of DVT, MI, or stroke.

V. PROSTHETIC ARTICULAR BEARING SURFACES

The topic of articular bearings and the search for more durable bearing surfaces has been the subject of significant debate and research in recent years. Traditional surface couplings have included polyethylene acetabular liners with combinations of metal heads. These bearing surfaces are referred to as *hard-on-soft* combinations. Of these metals, the results have been least favorable for titanium heads because this metal is associated with higher rates of volumetric wear and the production of third-body wear particles. The problem with titanium is that its surface hardness is inferior to that of other alloys; therefore, it scratches more easily than other metals and is vulnerable to third-body abrasive wear. However, the traditional combination of cobalt-chromium on polyethylene has produced a record of predictable, long-term success. Despite this success, the search for improvements in the wear rate of hard-on-soft coupling continues. As discussed earlier, great enhancements have been made in the surface hardness of the polyethylene component. Ultra-high molecular weight polyethylene (UHMWPE), which has excellent wear properties, is now frequently used for acetabular liners. This polyethylene has increased surface hardness and wear properties in comparison to older generations of polyethylene. Recent advances in UHMWPE have included processes to achieve cross-linking of the polyethylene molecules to produce new, highly cross-linked (HCL) UHMWPEs. This newer generation of HCL UHMWPEs is produced when the polyethylene is gamma irradiated in an inert environment. Older versions of UHMWPEs were sterilized by gamma irradiation in air. This process resulted in the formation of free radicals that caused oxidation and compromised the wear properties of the material. Additionally, the packaging of the polyethylene in air-filled containers also resulted in oxidation of the material prior to its removal from the package and use. Newer generations of polyethylene are being packaged in more inert environments to reduce oxidation prior to use. Such HCL UHMWPEs have even better surface hardness and improved resistance to adhesive and abrasive wear. However, these improved wear properties come at the expense of decreased material properties, such as Young's modulus of elasticity and yield strength; these new components are more susceptible to fracture. Although HCL UHMWPE has been shown to perform well in THA, it may not be as desirable in TKA. Because the cross-linking process leads to decreased ductility and decreased resistance to fatigue, such HCL materials can succumb to early fatigue and fracture. The method by which the polyethylene is machined and processed into TKA components can also impact its long-term performance. In general, heat-pressed UHMWPE has demonstrated early failure, while polyethylene processed by ram extrusion or compression molding have not performed poorly.

Alumina, Ceramic, and Zirconium. Attempts to improve the femoral head component of the coupling have utilized new materials such as alumina, ceramic, and zirconium. Alumina components have the advantage of better scratch resistance than traditional cobalt-chromium heads and therefore demonstrate lower rates of third-body abrasive wear. Ceramic is a highly biocompatible, highly durable material that demonstrates excellent hardness and low roughness. The wear rates of ceramic–polyethylene couplings have been reported anywhere between 0 μm and 150 μm per year. This represents a 10% to 50% decrease in the wear rates that have been reported for traditional metal–polyethylene couplings (75 μm to 250 μm per year). However, ceramic components do have the disadvantage of increased susceptibility to fracture. Rates of fracture have been reported in the literature to be on the order of 0.004%.

Hard-on-Hard Bearings and Metal Heads Versus Ceramic Heads. In recent years, there has been increasing interesting in so-called hard-on-hard bearings, in which the "soft" polyethylene component of the coupling is replaced with a "hard" bearing such as ceramic or metal. The most common combinations of hard-on-hard bearings have been ceramic–ceramic and metal–metal bearings. A comparison is provided in Table 4.6. Both of these combinations have demonstrated significantly lower wear rates than those of hard-on-soft bearings. Ceramic–ceramic combinations have the best wear profile of currently available bearings, with annual wear rates of 0.5 μm to 2.5 μm per year. This ceramic coupling also has the lowest demonstrated frictional coefficient of currently available combinations. However, metal femoral heads have the advantage of larger numbers of neck-length options over ceramic heads. Metal–metal couplings also have extremely low wear rates on the order of 2.5 μm to 5.0 μm per year, with less than 0.6 mm^3 by volume of debris per year. Additionally, these hard-on-hard bearings are advantageous because the wear particles that are produced are on the order of 0.015 μm to 0.12 μm. These particles are significantly smaller than those produced by hard-on-soft combinations and are so small that they are believed to be immunologically inert, failing to activate the osteolytic pathway in the manner of larger polyethylene wear particles. Additionally, ceramic is highly resistant to scratching from third-body debris. However, these new hard-on-hard bearings are not without their disadvantages. As a material, ceramic is extremely brittle and therefore more susceptible to fracture than is metal or polyethylene. Therefore, concerns persist that catastrophic failure of ceramic–ceramic couplings can occur with component fractures. Overall, ceramic–ceramic bearings have superior tibological properties and lower wear rates than metal–metal articulations. However, metal–metal combinations allow for a greater number of neck-length options than do ceramic–ceramic couplings. With metal–metal couplings, the potential carcinogenic effects of metal wear particles that are produced is a concern. Although there have been no

TABLE 4.6 Comparison of ceramic–ceramic and metal–metal articulations in THA

Ceramic–Ceramic	*Metal–Metal*
1. Annual wear rate 0.5–2.5 μm/yr	1. Annual wear rate 2.5–5.0 μm/yr
2. Lower frictional coefficient	2. Higher frictional coefficient
3. Fewer neck-length options	3. More neck-length options
4. Fracture concern	4. Fracture risk not a concern
5. No carcinogenic concerns	5. Concern of carcinogenic effects
	6. Concern of metal hypersensitivity

reports that directly correlate metal–metal bearings with neoplasia, reports have demonstrated increased concentrations of metal ions in the urine and blood of patients with metal–metal THAs.

VI. PROPERTIES OF PROSTHETIC MATERIALS

Femoral Stem in THA. The design geometry of the femoral component in THA can significantly affect its physical properties. The stiffness of the femoral component is highly dependent on its shape and dimensions. The stiffness of the femoral stem is proportional to the fourth power of its diameter. Therefore, very small increases in stem diameter result in great increases in stiffness. The diameter of the stem and its modulus of elasticity increase proportionally in a linear fashion. Additions of hydroxyapatite or other surface coatings do not affect the stiffness of the stem unless such coatings greatly increase the diameter of the stem.

Modulus of Elasticity. Of the current commonly used materials for arthroplasty implants, alumina ceramic has the highest stiffness or modulus of elasticity, followed by cobalt-chromium, stainless steel, titanium, and PMMA. Thus, materials such as PMMA and titanium more closely approximate the elastic modulus of normal bone, while materials such as alumina and cobalt-chrome are significantly stiffer than normal bone. Modulus of elasticity of implant materials in descending order is provided here:

1. Alumina ceramic
2. Cobalt-chromium
3. Stainless steel
4. Titanium
5. Cortical bone
6. PMMA
7. Polyethylene
8. Cancellous bone
9. Ligament

VII. OSTEOLYSIS AND WEAR DEBRIS IN TOTAL JOINT ARTHROPLASTY

It is currently thought that wear particles generated from the acetabular or tibial polyethylene are the main inducers of the macrophage and histiocytic response that leads to osteolysis. However, there are other wear sources within the total joint arthroplasty construct, including the PMMA cement, the hydroxyapatite coating of the implants, and the metals of the implants such as cobalt, chromium, and titanium. Nonetheless, polyethylene is considered the major wear component that triggers the pathway for osteolysis. Wear particles are thought to be engulfed by macrophages. Macrophages excrete several osteolytic cytokines, which trigger the pathway of bony destruction and resorption.

Mechanisms of Wear. There are two main mechanisms by which wear particles are produced in the hip: adhesive wear and abrasive wear. Abrasive wear occurs when a rough surface contacts another surface, resulting in removal of particles from the less abrasive substance with less surface hardness. The mechanism is similar to the effect of sandpaper on wood. Abrasive wear can also be caused by third-body particles, which become entrapped between two closely contacting surfaces. Such third-body particles include cement, metal, and bone particles. Adhesive wear takes place at the femoral head–polyethylene articulation in THA and femoral condyle tibial–polyethylene articulation in TKA, when submicron polyethylene particles are sheared off and deposited within the joint space. These particles are then engulfed by macrophages and trigger the histiocytic osteolysis reaction. The size of the wear particles that induce the osteolytic response is on the order of 0.2 μm to 7 μm. UHMWPE that is predominantly used for acetabular liners produces particles of this size. Osteolysis is more often seen in THAs that have a polyethylene component that is less than 8.5 mm in thickness.

Reduction of Wear at the Head–Liner Interface. Reduction of adhesive wear at the head–liner interface has been addressed in several ways, one of which is by improving the wear properties of the polyethylene. During the last 20 years, it has been recognized that the process utilized for polyethylene sterilization and shelf packaging significantly impacts the wear rate of the acetabular liner. For many years, acetabular polyethylene had been sterilized with gamma irradiation in oxygen-rich environments. Such caustic environments compromised the wear profile of the polyethylene, leading to more rapid in vivowear rates and ultimately to greater osteolysis. Oxygen-rich environments result in the formation of free radicals, which cause damage to polyethylene. When polyethylene is irradiated, the end result on its wear and material properties is environment dependent; when irradiation occurs in an oxygen-rich environment, oxidation occurs, which produces delamination under the polyethylene surface, and cracking occurs on the surface. In an inert milieu such as gas plasma and ethylene oxide, cross-linking of the polyethylene occurs, which makes the substance less susceptible to abrasive and adhesive wear. However, this improved wear profile comes at the cost of increased brittleness and diminished mechanical properties. The sterilization of polyethylene in environments that do not cause high levels of oxidation such as gas plasma and ethylene oxide has significantly reduced the problem of oxidative degradation of polyethylene. The shelf-storage environment of the polyethylene after sterilization has also been recognized to affect the in vivowear profile of the acetabular liner. When such components are packaged and stored in oxygen-containing environments, the oxygen can further degrade the polyethylene. Thus, improvements in the intrapackage environment of the polyethylene components have further improved their wear properties.

Femoral Head Size. Other factors that were recognized to increase the rate of polyethylene wear included the use of larger femoral heads. Large heads increased the volumetric wear at the ball head–liner interface and ultimately led to increased wear debris and osteolysis. Although large heads reduced the linear wear that is more characteristic of smaller, 22-mm femoral heads, the increased volumetric wear resulted in an overall higher production of wear debris. In recent years, the use of polyethylene with improved wear properties has allowed the use of 32-mm femoral heads without the production of prohibitive amounts of wear debris. Finally, attempts to reduce the effective joint space in the total hip construct through elimination of holes in the metal shell have yielded mixed results. The effective joint space is a concept that describes the entire volumetric area within a hip joint construct that can be infiltrated by polyethylene wear particles and macrophages. Bone breakdown can occur anywhere within effective joint space. The theory implies that reductions in the effective joint space may reduce the amount of osteolysis that can occur. The use of bone screws for the fixation of metal shells is thought to create new voids in the acetabular bone that results in an increase in the effective joint space. Therefore, the elimination of bone screws for acetabular components could decrease the effective joint space and therefore decrease the osteolysis rate. Finally, the use of circumferential proximal porous coating for the femoral stem effectively seals off the diaphyseal component of the femoral canal from the effective joint space and therefore has been recognized to reduce osteolysis in the proximal femur.

Wear at the Shell–Liner Interface. It has been recognized in recent years that polyethylene wear debris can also be produced at the interface between the metal acetabular shell and the polyethylene liner. The mechanism by which this occurs is through motion between the shell and liner, which can result in wear particles being produced. This phenomenon is implant-specific and should become less problematic with new, better-designed locking mechanisms. This phenomenon is more prevalent when modular acetabular components are used because these components may have suboptimal locking mechanisms between the shell and liner, which allows relatively increased motion and therefore wear debris at this interface.

Treatment of Osteolysis. The treatment for osteolysis is variable, depending on the extent of bony destruction in both the acetabulum and the femur. However, it is possible for significant pelvic osteolysis to occur without causing loosening of the acetabular shell. In such cases, where there is pelvic osteolysis with a well-fixed acetabular shell, the treatment includes retention of the metal shell, bone grafting of the osteolytic defects, and exchange of the worn polyethylene liner. For more significant osteolysis with loosening of the acetabular and femoral components, more extensive revision surgery is required with replacement of loose components and grafting of bony defects.

References

1. Ayers DC, Dennis DA, Johanson NA, Pellegrini VD. Common complications of total knee arthroplasty. *J Bone Joint Surg Am* 1997;70:278–311.
2. Ayers DC. Supracondylar fracture of the distal femur proximal to a total knee replacement. In: Springfield DS (ed.), *Instructional Course Lectures 46*. Rosemont, IL: American Academy of Orthopaedic Surgeons, 1997;197–203.
3. Barnes CL, Scott RD. Patellofemoral complications of total knee replacement, In: Heckman JD (ed.), *Instructional Course Lectures 42*. Rosemont, IL: American Academy of Orthopaedic Surgeons, 1993;309–314.
4. Beaver RJ, Mahomed M, Backstein D, et al. Fresh osteochondral allografts for posttraumatic defects in the knee: A survivorship analysis. *J Bone Joint Surg Br* 1992;74:105–110.
5. Bellamy N, Campbell J, Robinson V, Gee T, Bourne R, Wells G. Viscosupplementation for the treatment of osteoarthritis of the knee. *Cochrane Database Syst Rev* 2005 Apr 18;(2):CD005321.
6. Berger RA, Jacobs JJ, Quigley LR, Rosenberg AG, Galante JO. Primary cementless acetabular reconstruction in patients younger than 50 years old: 7- to 11-year results. *Clin Orthop* 1997;344:216–226.
7. Berry DJ, Lewallen DG, Hanssen A, Cabanela ME. Pelvic discontinuity in revision total hip arthroplasty. *J Bone Joint Surg Am* 1999;81:1692–1702.
8. Bierbaum BE, Callaghan JJ, Galante JO, Rubash HE, Tooms RE, Welch RB. An analysis of blood management in patients having a total hip or knee arthroplasty. *J Bone Joint Surg Am* 1999;81:2–10.

9. Buckwalter JA, Einhorn TA, Simon SB. *Orthopaedic Basic Science*, 2nd ed. Rosemont, IL: American Academy of Orthopaedic Surgeons, 2000;182–215.
10. Callaghan JJ, Brand RA, Pedersen DR. Hip arthrodesis: A long-term follow-up. *J Bone Joint Surg Am* 1985; 67:1328–1335.
11. Casha JN, Hadden WA. Suture reaction following skin closure with subcuticular polydioxanone in total knee arthroplasty. *J Arthroplasty* 1996;11:859–861.
12. Cobb TK, Morrey BF, Ilstrup DM. The elevated rim acetabular liner in total hip arthroplasty: Relationship to postoperative dislocation. *J Bone Joint Surg Am* 1996;78:80–86.
13. Collier JP, Sutula LC, Currier BH, et al. Overview of polyethylene as a bearing material: Comparison of sterilization methods. *CORR* 1996;333:76–86.
14. Colwell CW, Spiro TE, Trowbridge AA. Use of enoxaparin, a low-molecular weight heparin, and unfractionated heparin for the prevention of deep venous thrombosis after elective hip replacement: A clinical trial comparing efficacy and safety. *J Bone Joint Surg Am* 1994;76:3–14.
15. Ecker ML, Lotke PA. Spontaneous osteonecrosis of the knee. *J Am Acad Orthop Surg* 1994;2:173–178.
16. Emerson RH Jr, Sanders SB, Head WC, Higgins L. Effect of circumferential plasma-spray porous coating on the rate of femoral osteolysis after total hip arthroplasty. *J Bone Joint Surg Am* 1999;81;1291–1298.
17. Engh CA, Massin P, Suthers KE. Roentgenographic assessment of the biologic fixation of porous-surfaced femoral components. *Clin Orthop* 1990;257:107–128.
18. Engh GA, Koralewicz LM, Pereles TR. Clinical results of modular polyethylene insert exchange with retention of total knee arthroplasty components. *J Bones Joint Surg Am* 2000;82:516–523.
19. Engh GA, Herzwurm PJ, Parks NL. Treatment of major defects of bone with bulk allografts and stemmed components during total knee arthroplasty. *J Bone Joint Surg Am* 1997;79:1030–1039.
20. Esler CN, Lock K, Harper WM, Gregg PJ. Manipulation of total knee replacements: Is the flexion gained retained? *J Bone Joint Surg Br* 1999;81:27–29.
21. Feagan BG, Wang CJ, Kirkley A, et al. Erythropoietin with iron supplementation to prevent allogeneic blood transfusion in total hip joint arthroplasty: A randomized, controlled trial. *Ann Intern Med* 2000;133:845–854.
22. Fitzgerald RH Jr. Infected total hip arthroplasty: Diagnosis and treatment. *J Am Acad Orthop Surg* 1995;3:249–262.
23. Garvin KL, Hanssen AD. Infection after total hip arthroplasty: Past, present, and future. *J Bone Joint Surg Am* 1995;77:1576–1588.
24. Gross AE et al. The use of allograft bone in revision of total hip arthroplasty. *CORR* 1985;197:115–122.
25. Guerra JJ, Steinberg ME. Distinguishing transient osteoporosis from avascular necrosis of the hip. *J Bone Joint Surg* 1995;77:616–624.
26. Hanssen AD, Rand JA. Evaluation and treatment of infection at the site of a total hip or knee arthroplasty. *J Bone Joint Surg Am* 1998;80:910–922.
27. Hartofilakidis G, Stamos K, Karachalios T, Ioannidis TT, Zacharakis N. Congenital hip disease in adults: Classification of acetabular deficiencies and operative treatment with acetabuloplasty combined with total hip arthroplasty. *J Bone Joint Surg Am* 1996;78:683–692.
28. Head WC, Emerson RH, Malinin TI. Structural bone grafting for femoral reconstruction. *CORR* 1999;369:223–229.
29. Hirsh J, Dalen JE, Anderson DR, et al. Oral anticoagulants: Mechanism of action, clinical effectiveness, and optimal therapeutic range. *Chest* 1998;114:445S–469S
30. Hsu HC, Luo ZP, Rand JA, An KN. Influence of patellar thickness on patellar tracking and patellofemoral contact characteristics after total knee arthroplasty. *J Arthroplasty* 1996;11:69–80.
31. Hurwitz DE, et al. Biomechanics of the hip. In: Callaghan JJ, Rosenberg AG, Rubash HE (eds.), *The Adult Hip*. Philadelphia: Lippincott-Raven, 1998;75–85.
32. Idusuyi OB, et al. Peroneal nerve palsy after total knee arthroplasty: Assessment of predisposing and prognostic factors. *J Bone Joint Surg Am* 1996;78:177–184.
33. Iorio R, et al. Heterotopic ossification after total hip and total knee arthroplasty: Risk factors, prevention, and treatment. *J Am Acad Orthop Surg* 2002;10:409–416.
34. Jaroszynski G, et al. Total hip replacement for the dislocated hip. *Instr Course Lect* 2001;50:307–316.
35. Jazrawi, et al. Alternative bearing surfaces for total joint arthroplasty. *J Am Acad Orthop Surg* 1998;6:198–203.
36. Joshi A, et al. Total hip arthroplasty in ankylosing spondylitis: An analysis of 181 hips. *J Arthroplasty* 2002;17:427–433.
37. Kelly MA. Nonprosthetic management of the arthritis knee. In: Callaghan JJ, et al (eds.), *Orthopaedic Knowledge Update: Hip and Knee Reconstruction*. Rosemont, IL: AAOS, 1995;245–249.
38. Lachiewicz, et al. Constrained components in total hip arthroplasty. *J Am Acad Orthop Surg* 2002;10:233–238.
39. Lachiewicz PF. Rheumatoid arthritis of the hip. *J Am Acad Orthop Surg* 1997;5:332–338.
40. Leopold SS, et al. Current status of impaction allografting for revision of a femoral component. *Instr Course Lect* 2000;49:111–118.
41. Lewallen DG, Berry DJ. Instructional Course Lectures, The American Academy of Orthopaedic Surgeons—Periprosthetic fracture of the femur after total hip arthroplasty. Treatment and results to date. *J Bone Joint Surg Am* 1997;79:1881–1890.
42. Lewallen DG. Instructional Course Lectures, The American Academy of Orthopaedic Surgeons—Neurovascular injury associated with hip arthroplasty. *J Bone Joint Surg Am* 1997;79:1870–1880.
43. Lindenfeld TN, et al. Joint loading with valgus bracing in patients with varus gonarthrosis. *Clin Orthop* 1997;344:290–297.

44. Lynch AF, et al. Extensor mechanism complications following total knee arthroplasty. *J Arthroplasty* 1987;2:135–140.
45. Maloney WJ, et al. Treatment of pelvic osteolysis associated with a stable acetabular component inserted without cement as a part of a total hip replacement. *J Bone Joint Surg Am* 1997;79:1628–1634.
46. Maloney WJ III. Primary cemented total hip arthroplasty. In: Callaghan JJ, et al (eds.), *Orthopaedic Knowledge Update: Hip and Knee Reconstruction.* Rosemont, IL: AAOS, 1995;179–189.
47. Maloney WJ III. The cemented femoral component. In: Callaghan JJ, et al (eds.), *The Adult Hip.* Philadelphia: Lippincott-Raven, 1998;959–979.
48. Mandelbaum BR, et al. Articular cartilage lesions of the knee. *Am J Sports Med* 1998;26:853–861.
49. Miller MD. *Review of Orthopaedics*, 3rd ed. Philadelphia: WB Saunders, 2000;560 (Anatomy, Table 11-8).
50. Millis MB, et al. Osteotomies about the hip for the prevention and treatment of osteoarthritis. *Instr Course Lect* 1996;45:209–226.
51. Mont MA, et al. Total knee arthroplasty after failed high tibial osteotomy. *Orthop Clin North Am* 1994;25:515–525.
52. Moskal JT, et al. The fate of stable femoral components retained during isolated acetabular revision: A six- to twelve-year follow-up study. *J Bone Joint Surg Am* 2002;84:250–255.
53. Naranja RJ Jr., et al. Total knee arthroplasty in a previously ankylosed or arthrodesed knee. *Clin Orthop* 1996;331:234–237.
54. Nelissen RG, Bauer TW, Weidenhielm LR et al. Revision hip arthroplasty with the use of cement and impaction grafting: Histological analysis of four cases. *J Bone Joint Surg Am* 1995;77:412–422.
55. Numair J, Joshi AB, Murphy JC, Porter ML, Hardinge KJ. Total hip arthroplasty for congenital dysplasia of dislocation of the hip: Survivorship analysis and long-term results. *J Bone Joint Surg Am* 1997;79:1352–1360.
56. O'Rourke M, et al. Osteolysis associated with a cemented modular posterior cruciate substituting total knee design. *J Bone Joint Surg Am* 2002;84:1362–1371.
57. Pagnano MW, Cushner FD, Scott WN. Role of the posterior cruciate ligament in total knee arthroplasty. *J Am Acad Orthop Surg* 1998;6:176–187.
58. Paprosky WG, Magnus RE. Principles of bone grafting in revision total hip arthroplasty: Acetabular technique. *CORR* 1994; 298:147–155.
59. Paterno SA, Lachiewicz PF, Kelly SS. The influence of patient-related factors and the position of the acetabular component on the rate of dislocation after total hip replacement. *J Bone Joint Surg Am* 1997;79:1202–1210.
60. Pellicci PM, et al. (eds.), *Orthopaedic Knowledge Update: Hip and Knee Reconstruction 2.* Rosemont, IL: American Academy of Orthopaedic Surgeons, 2000;265–274.
61. Pellicci PM, et al. (eds.) *Orthopaedic Knowledge Update: Hip and Knee Reconstruction 2.* Rosemont, IL: American Academy of Orthopaedic Surgeons, 2000;339–365.
62. Pellicci PM, et al. Posterior approach to total hip replacement using enhanced posterior soft tissue repair. *Clin Orthop* 1998;355L:224–228.
63. Peters PC, et al. Osteolysis after total knee arthroplasty without cement. *J Bone Joint Surg Am* 1992;74:864–876.
64. Petrera P, et al. Revision total hip arthroplasty: The acetabular component. *J Am Acad Orthop Surg* 1995;3:15–21.
65. Pitto RP, Hamer H, et al. Prophylaxis against fat and bone-marrow embolism during total hip arthroplasty reduces the incidence of postoperative deep vein thrombosis: A controlled, randomized clinical trial. *J Bone Joint Surg Am* 2002;84A(1):39–48.
66. Ranawat CS, Dorr LD, Inglis AE. Total hip arthroplasty in protrusion acetabuli of rheumatoid arthritis *J Bone Joint Surg* 1980;62:1059–1065.
67. Ranawat CS, Dorr LD, Inglis AE. Total hip arthroplasty in protrusion acetabuli of rheumatoid arthritis *J Bones Joint Surg* 1980;62:1059–1065.
68. Rand JA. The patellofemoral joint in total knee arthroplasty. *J Bone Joint Surg Am* 1994;76:612–620.
69. Rand JA. The patellofemoral joint in total knee arthroplasty. *J Bone Joint Surg Am* 1994;76:612–620.
70. Rinonapoli E, et al. Tibial osteotomy for varus gonarthrosis: 10- to 21-year follow-up study. *Clin Orthop* 1998;353:185–193.
71. Romness DW, Lewallen DG. Total hip arthroplasty after fracture of the acetabulum: Long-term results. *J Bone Joint Surg Br* 1990;72:761–764.
72. Santore et al. Intertrochanteric femoral osteotomies for developmental and traumatic conditions. *J Bone Joint Surg Am* 2004;86:2542–2553.
73. Schmalzried TP, Callaghan JJ. Wear in total hip and knee replacements. *J Bone Joint Surg Am* 1999;81:115–136.
74. Scifert CF, et al. A finite element analysis of factors influencing total hip dislocation. *Clin Orthop* 1998;355:152–162.
75. Sharkey PF, et al. The bearing surface in total hip arthroplasty: Evolution or revolution, In: Price CT (ed.), *Instructional Course Lectures 49.* Rosemont, IL: AAOS, 2000;41–56.
76. Sharkey PF, et al. Acetabular fracture associated with cementless acetabular component insertion: A report of thirteen cases. *J Arthroplasty* 1999;14:326–341.
77. Smith SE, et al. Total hip arthroplasty performed with insertion of the femoral component with cement and the acetabular component without cement: 10 to 13 year study. *J Bone Joint Surg Am* 1997;79:1827–1833.
78. Steinberg ME. *Early diagnosis, evaluation, and staging of osteonecrosis.* AAOS, 1994;513–518.
79. Tan V, et al. Carry it on the bad side! *Am J Orthop* 1998;27:673–677.
80. Tannenbaum DA, Matthews LS, Benson-Grady JC. Infection around total joint replacements in patients who have a renal or liver transplantation. *J Bone Joint Surg Am* 1997;79:36–43.

81. Tria AJ, et al. (eds). *Orthopaedic Knowledge Update: Hip and Knee Reconstruction 2*. Rosemont, IL: American Academy of Orthopaedic Surgeons, 1999;455–492.
82. Trousdale RT, et al. Periacetabular and intertrochanteric osteotomy for the treatment of osteoarthritis in dysplastic hips. *J Bone Joint Surg Am* 1995;77:73–85.
83. Urban RM, et al. The bone-implant interface of femoral stems with non-circumferential porous coating. *J Bone Joint Surg Am* 1996;78:1068–1081.
84. Vaccaro AR (ed.). *Orthopaedic Knowledge Update*, 8th ed. Chicago: AAOS;411–425.
85. Wasielewski RC, et al. Acetabular anatomy and the transacetabular fixation of screws in total hip arthroplasty. *J Bone Joint Surg Am* 1990;72:501–508.
86. White RE. Evaluation of the painful total hip arthroplasty. In: Callaghan JJ, et al. (eds.), *The Adult Hip*. Philadelphia: Lippincott-Raven, 1998;2:1377–1385.
87. Whiteside LA. Selection of the acetabular component. In: Steinberg ME, Garino JP (eds.), *Revision Total Hip Arthroplasty*. Philadelphia: Lippincott Williams & Wilkins, 1999;209–220.
88. Windsor RE. Knee arthrodesis. In: Insall JN, et al (eds.), *Surgery of the Knee*. New York: Churchill Livingstone, 1993;1103–1116.
89. Younger T, et al. Extended proximal femoral osteotomy: A new technique for femoral revision arthroplasty. *J Arthroplasty* 1995;10:329–338.

Key References

Numair J, Joshi AB, Murphy JCM, Porter ML, Hardinge K. Total hip arthroplasty for congenital dysplasia of dislocation of the hip: Survivorship analysis and long-term results. *J Bone Joint Surg Am* 1997;79:1352–1360.

The authors review the results of 230 cemented THAs in patients who had CDH or congenital dislocation with a mean follow-up of 9.9 years. The study demonstrates a higher failure rate for the acetabular component than the femoral component in this patient population; the study demonstrates satisfactory clinical results in this patient population at 10-year follow-up.

Trousdale RT, Ekkernkamp A, Ganz R, Wallrichs SL. Periacetabular and intertrochanteric osteotomy for the treatment of osteoarthritis in dysplastic hips. *J Bone Joint Surg Am* 1995;77:73–85.

The results of periacetabular osteotomy performed in 42 patients are reviewed with average 4-year follow-up. The average age of patients at time of index procedure was 37 years. The results were good to excellent in 32 of 33 hips.

Callaghan JJ, Brand RA, Pedersen DR. Hip arthrodesis: A long-term follow-up. *J Bone Joint Surg Am* 1985;67:1328–1335.

Twenty-eight patients with previous hip arthrodesis were examined at average postoperative follow-up of 35 years. Common findings at follow-up included ipsilateral knee pain (60%) and contralateral hip pain (25%). Patients whose hips were fused in abduction had more ipsilateral knee and back pain compared with those who were fused in neutral or adduction.

Berger RA, Jacobs JJ, Quigley LR, Rosenberg AG, Galante JO. Primary cementless acetabular reconstruction in patients younger than 50 years-old: 7- to 11-year results. *Clin Orthop* 1997:344;216.

Seventy-nine consecutive, cementless acetabular components in patients of average age 37 years at time of index procedure were analyzed with average follow-up of 106 months. The 10-year survival rate was 98.8%, with osteolysis being the most common problem encountered.

Smith SE, Harris WH. Total hip arthroplasty performed with insertion of the femoral component with cement and the acetabular component without cement: Ten to thirteen-year study. *J Bone Joint Surg Am* 1997;79:1827–1833.

Fifty-two consecutive hybrid total hip replacements were reviewed with 100% follow-up and average follow-up of 12.3 years. Average patient age at index procedure was 57 years. The dislocation rate was 13%. Eighty-five percent of patients had a good or excellent result, while 11% had a fair result.

Scifert CF, Brown TD, Pedersen DR, Callaghan JJ. A finite element analysis of factors influencing total hip dislocation. *Clin Orthop* 1998;355:152–162.

A validated three-dimensional finite element model was used to determine that increased head size resulted in increased resistance to dislocation, while a constant head–neck ratio with increasing head size did not increase the range of motion until impingement.

Pitto RP, Hamer H, Fabiani R, Radespiel-Troger M, Koessler M. Prophylaxis against fat and bone-marrow embolism during total hip arthroplasty reduces the incidence of postoperative deep vein thrombosis: A controlled, randomized clinical trial. *J Bone Joint Surg Am* 2002;84-A(1):39–48.

A randomized, controlled trial demonstrates that techniques can be utilized that reduce the rate of intraoperative bone marrow and fat embolism. The study further demonstrates that patients in whom these techniques are used demonstrate a lower rate of postoperative DVT and pulmonary embolism.

Lewallen DG, Berry DJ. Instructional Course Lectures, The American Academy of Orthopaedic Surgeons—Periprosthetic fracture of the femur after total hip arthroplasty. Treatment and results to date. *J Bone Joint Surg Am* 1997;79:1881–1890.

A review of the classification and treatment for periprosthetic femur fractures after total hip arthroplasty. The review concludes that critical factors guiding treatment decisions of these complex injuries include the classification of the fracture, the location of the fracture, the quality of the component fixation, and the quality of the bone around the component.

Bellamy N, Campbell J, Robinson V, Gee T, Bourne R, Wells G. Viscosupplementation for the treatment of osteoarthritis of the knee. *Cochrane Database Syst Rev.* 2005 Apr 18;(2):CD005321.

A systematic review of randomized clinical trials assessing the efficacy of viscosupplementation therapy for knee osteoarthritis. The review demonstrates that viscosupplementation can be effective in reducing knee pain and improving function. The greatest effect was observed in the 5 to 13 weeks after initial injection.

Ayers DC, Dennis DA, Johanson NA, Pellegrini VD: Common complications of total knee arthroplasty. *J Bone Joint Surg Am* 1997;79:278–311.

An exhaustive review of common complications observed after total knee arthroplasty. Complications discussed include wound complications, neurovascular injury, infection, fracture, extensor mechanism complications, and many others.

Crockarell JR, Hanssen AD, Osmon DR, Morrey BF. Treatment of infection with débridement and retention of the components following hip arthroplasty. *J Bone Joint Surg Am* 1998:80:1306–1313.

Forty-two patients who developed infection after primary total hip arthroplasty were treated with open irrigation and débridement, maintenance of components, and suppressive antibiotics. Only 14% of patients were successfully managed by this strategy. Authors conclude that early postoperative or acute infections are potentially managed with this strategy, but longer term, chronic infections will uniformly fail with this management.

Rand JA, Ilstrup DM. Survivorship analysis of total knee arthroplasty. Cumulative rates of survival of 9,200 total knee arthroplasties. *J Bone Joint Surg Am* 1991;73:397–409.

This study examines 9,200 consecutive knee arthroplasty operations that were performed between 1971 and 1987. It identified four factors associated with lower risk of failure: primary TKA, rheumatoid arthritis, age greater than 60 years, and the use of a condylar implant with a metal-backed tibial component.

Hirsh J, Dalen JE, Anderson DR, et al. Oral anticoagulants: Mechanism of action, clinical effectiveness, and optimal therapeutic range. *Chest* 1998;114:445S-469S.

An exhaustive review of current oral anticoagulants, their effectiveness, mechanisms of action, and complications.

Bierbaum BE, Callaghan JJ, Galante JO, Rubash HE, Tooms RE, Welch RB. An analysis of blood management in patients having a total hip or knee arthroplasty. *J Bone Joint Surg Am* 1999;81:2–10.

9482 patients who underwent either hip or knee replacement surgery were analyzed to determine patient related factors that were associated with requirements for allogeneic blood transfusions. The most important predictors of requirement for allogeneic transfusions included low preoperative hemoglobin, lack of pre-donated autologous blood, infection, fluid overload, and longer hospital stay. Revision total hip arthroplasty and bilateral total knee arthroplasty were associated with the greatest allogeneic transfusion requirement.

Refresher Questions

1. What design characteristic of uncemented, press-fit femoral components has been demonstrated to produce the greatest amount of distal femoral osteolysis?
   a) Fully circumferential proximal porous coating
   b) Extensively and fully porous coating (proximal and distal)
   c) Noncircumferential proximal porous coating
   d) Grit-blasted, fully, extensively coated stem

2. While performing a primary total knee arthroplasty, the surgeon notes that upon ligament balancing, the extension gap is tight, and the flexion gap is loose. Which of the following strategies will best address this problem?
   a) Resect more distal femur
   b) Use a smaller polyethylene insert
   c) Cut more proximal tibia
   d) Recess the posterior cruciate ligament

3. What is the most appropriate position for hip arthrodesis?
   a) 10 degrees of adduction, 0 degrees of rotation, 45 degrees of flexion
   b) 5 degrees of adduction, 5 degrees of external rotation, 30 degrees of flexion
   c) 15 degrees of abduction, 15 degrees of flexion, 15 degrees of external rotation
   d) 0 degrees of abduction, 0 degrees of flexion, 0 degrees of external rotation

4. Which of the following technical aspects of total knee arthroplasty can reduce patellar maltracking?
   a) Internal rotation of the femoral component
   b) Internal rotation of the tibial component
   c) Medialization of the femoral component
   d) Medialization of the patellar component

5. Which of the following acetabular quadrants is considered safest for the placement of acetabular screws?
   a) Posterior superior
   b) Anterior superior
   c) Anterior inferior
   d) Posterior inferior

6. Which of the following is not considered a key component of third-generation cement technique?
   a) Cement pressurization
   b) Vacuum porosity reduction of the cement
   c) Stem centralizer
   d) Antibiotic impregnation of cement

7. What is considered to be the optimum pore size to maximize biologic ingrowth of porous coated components?
   a) 25 to 50 microns
   b) 50 to 350 microns
   c) 350 to 450 microns
   d) 450 to 650 microns

8. Which of the following total hip arthroplasty component configurations has demonstrated the lowest wear rates?
   a) Metal-on-metal
   b) Ceramic-on-ceramic
   c) Metal-on-polyethylene
   d) Ceramic-on-polyethylene

9. Which of the following techniques is considered to be most sensitive and specific in diagnosing infection after total knee arthroplasty?
   a) Aspiration
   b) Technetium bone scan
   c) MRI
   d) ESR and CRP

10. Which of the following is not a mode of failure of a cemented femoral component?
   a) Cantilever bending
   b) Diaphyseal and calcar pivoting
   c) Subsidence of stem and cement within bone
   d) Osteolysis

Chapter 5

Foot and Ankle

SUDHEER C. REDDY, SELENE G. PAREKH, and
ENYI OKEREKE

I. ANATOMY

Muscular Anatomy of Leg

Anterior Compartment. For muscles of the anterior compartment (Table 5.1), the superior extensor retinaculum is a strong, broad band that holds down the tendons of the extensor compartment, preventing them from bowstringing during dorsiflexion of the ankle joint (Fig. 5.1). The inferior extensor retinaculum is a Y-shaped band of fascia, attaching laterally to the anterosuperior surface of the calcaneus, and it forms a loop around the peroneus tertius and extensor digitorum longus. The tibialis anterior is the strongest dorsiflexor and invertor of the foot and passes within its

TABLE 5.1 Muscles of the anterior compartment

Muscle	Proximal Attachment	Distal Attachment	Innervation	Action
Tibialis anterior	Lateral condyle and superior half of lateral surface of tibia	Medial and inferior surface of medial cuneiform, base of first metatarsal	Deep peroneal nerve	Dorsiflexes ankle and inverts foot
Extensor hallucis longus	Middle part of anterior surface of fibula and interosseous membrane (IOM)	Dorsal aspect of base of distal phalanx of hallux	Deep peroneal nerve	Extends great toe and dorsiflexes ankle
Extensor digitorum longus	Lateral condyle of tibia and superior three quarters of medial surface of fibula and interosseous membrane	Middle and distal phalanges of lateral four digits	Deep peroneal nerve (L5-S1)	Extends lateral four digits and dorsiflexes ankle
Peroneus tertius	Inferior third of anterior surface of fibula and IOM	Dorsum of base of fifth metatarsal	Deep peroneal nerve (L5-S1)	Dorsiflexes ankle and aids in eversion of foot

Source: Moore KL, Dalley AF. *Clinically Oriented Anatomy*, 4th ed. Philadelphia: Lippincott Williams & Wilkins, 1999.

own synovial sheath deep to the superior and inferior extensor retinaculum. The peroneus longus muscle opposes its motion.

Lateral Compartment. The peroneus brevis tendon can be identified at the level of the lateral malleolus because it is closest to the malleolus, whereas the peroneus longus tendon is located directly posterior to the brevis tendon (Table 5.2). Both the longus and brevis tendons are tethered down at the level of the lateral malleolus by the superior peroneal retinaculum, which is a band of deep fascia that extends from the tip of the lateral malleolus to the calcaneus (Fig. 5.2). Relevant to its location directly within the fibular groove, the most common location for longitudinal peroneus brevis tendon tears is at the fibular groove.

Posterior Compartment. The watershed area of the Achilles is approximately 4 cm from the insertion site (Table 5.3). The plantaris muscle is a vestigial muscle and has been proposed to act as an organ of proprioception for the gastrocnemius and soleus. It is commonly used as a tendon graft such as for medial collateral ligament reconstruction of the elbow or reconstruction of tendons of the hand. The popliteus muscle is a thin, triangular muscle that forms the floor of the popliteal triangle. When the knee is fully extended, the popliteus acts to rotate the femur laterally approximately 5 degrees on the tibial plateau to unlock the knee so that knee flexion can be initiated.

Muscular Anatomy of Foot

Muscles of the Dorsum and Sole. Muscles and tendons of the dorsum (Table 5.4) and sole (Table 5.5; Figs. 5.3 and 5.4) are arranged according to layers. On the plantar surface, the intrinsic muscles are mostly in the first and third, while the extrinsic tendons are mostly in the second and fourth layers. The knot of Henry is an important anatomic landmark in regards to the sole of the foot and represents the point at which the flexor digitorum longus (FDL) and the flexor hallucis longus (FHL) cross, with the FDL passing plantar to the FHL. An important point to remember is that the quadratus plantae inserts onto the tendon of the FDL distal to the Knot of Henry and is an agonist of FDL. An important mnemonic to remember is that the three plantar interossei adduct (PAD) digits arise from a single metatarsal. On the other hand, the four dorsal interossei abduct (DAB) digits arise from two metatarsals. The same mnemonic also applies to the interossei of the hand.

Arthrology of Foot and Ankle

Tibiofibular Joint. The medial aspect of the distal fibula and the lateral aspect of the distal tibia form the inferior tibiofibular joint. Four ligaments reinforce this joint: anterior and posterior tibiofibular ligaments, transverse tibiofibular ligament, and an interosseous ligament. The anteroinferior tibiofibular ligament is oblique and connects the bones anteriorly.

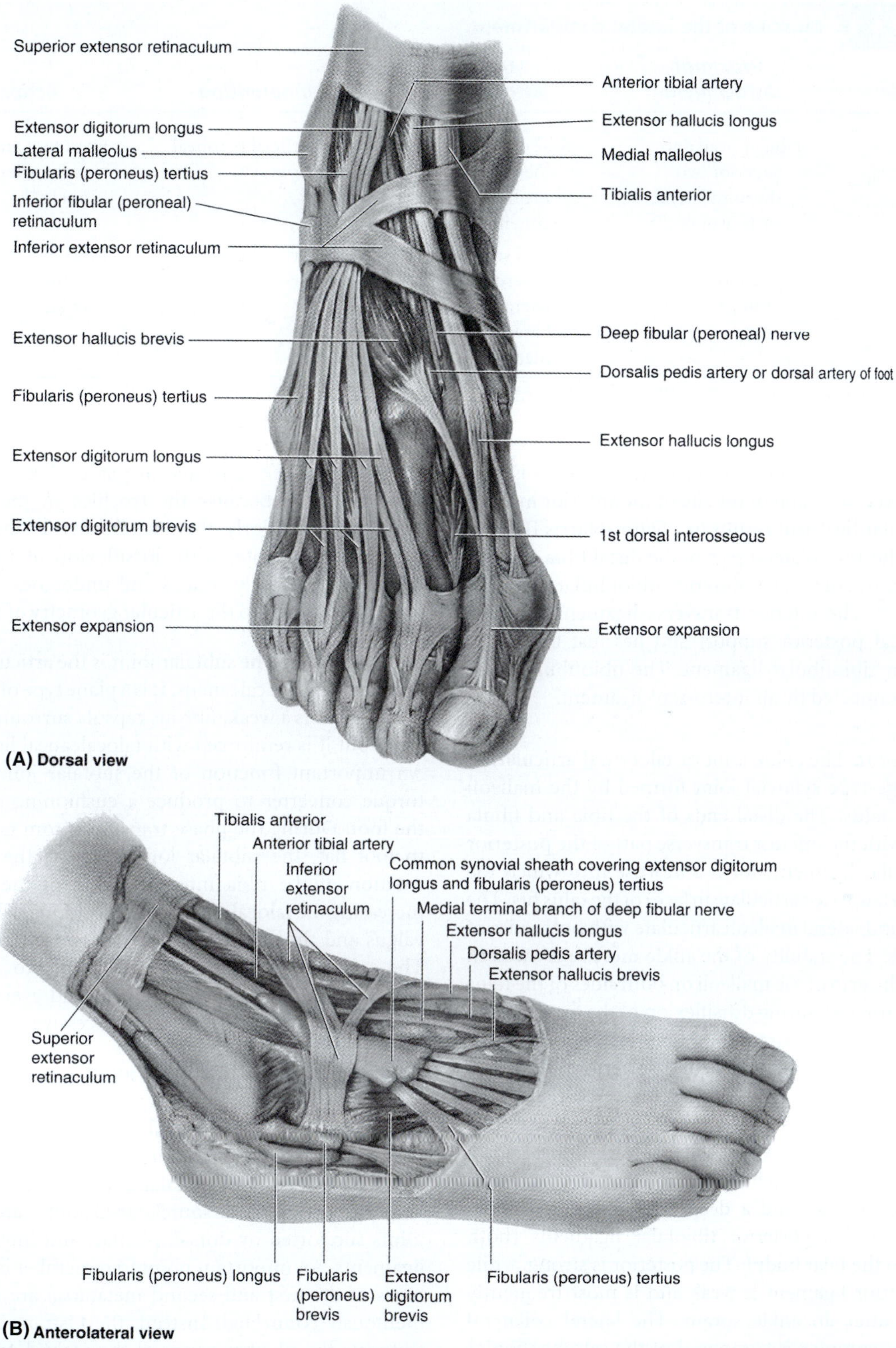

FIGURE 5.1 **Dissections of the right foot. Extensor and fibular retinacula of the ankle and the muscles and tendons of the dorsum of the foot are demonstrated. (A) The vessels and nerves are cut short. At the ankle, observe that the vessels and the deep fibular nerve lie midway between the malleolus and have tendons of two muscles on each side of them. (B) Observe the synovial sheaths of the tendons of the ankle. (*Source*: Moore KL, Dalley AF. *Clinically Oriented Anatomy*, 4th ed. Philadelphia: Lippincott Williams & Wilkins, 1999; 578 Fig. 5.34.)**

TABLE 5.2 Muscles of the lateral compartment

Muscle	Proximal Attachment	Distal Attachment	Innervation	Action
Peroneus longus	Fibular head and superior two thirds of lateral surface of fibula	Base of first metatarsal and medial cuneiform	Superficial peroneal nerve	Evert foot and weak plantarflexor of ankle
Peroneus brevis	Inferior two thirds of lateral surface of fibula	Dorsal surface of tuberosity on lateral side of base of fifth metatarsal	Superficial personal nerve.	Evert foot and weak plantarflexor of ankle

Source: Moore KL, Dalley AF. *Clinically Oriented Anatomy*, 4th ed. Philadelphia: Lippincott Williams & Wilkins, 1999.

In adolescents, in whom the distal tibial physes is partially closed, avulsion of the site of the anterior inferior tibiofibular ligament results in a Salter-Harris III fracture of the anterolateral part of the distal tibia, termed a Tillaux fracture. The posterior tibiofibular ligament is smaller. The inferior transverse ligament provides additional posterior support and lies just below the posterior tibiofibular ligament. The tibiofibular joint is also connected by an interosseus ligament.

Ankle Joint. The ankle joint or talocrural articulation is a hinge-type synovial joint formed by the malleoli and the talus. The distal ends of the tibia and fibula (along with the inferior transverse part of the posterior tibiofibular ligament) form a mortise into which the trochlea (superior articular surface) of the talus fits. The medial and lateral malleoli articulate with both sides of the talus. The stability of the ankle mortise is owed in part to the grip of the malleoli on both sides of the talus and is strongest during dorsiflexion of the foot because the wider anterior part of the talus is forced posteriorly, stretching the strong anterior and posterior tibiofibular ligaments (interosseous ligaments). Medially, the deltoid ligament is present and is composed of a superficial layer, the tibionavicular and tibiocalcaneal ligaments (that attach to the navicular, talar, and calcaneal bones), and a deep layer composed of an anterior and a posterior tibiotalar ligaments (both attach to the talar body). The posterior is strong, while the anterior ligament is weak and is most frequently injured after an ankle sprain. The lateral collateral ligament complex is composed of the calcaneofibular ligament, the anterior talofibular ligament (ATFL), and the posterior talofibular ligament (PTFL). The ATFL and the calcaneofibular ligaments are the most commonly sprained ligaments of the ankle joint. Inversion of the ankle in dorsiflexion stresses the calcaneofibular ligament, while inversion with the ankle in plantar flexion stresses the ATFL (Fig. 5.5). The ankle is relatively unstable in plantarflexion relative to dorsiflexion because the trochlea of the talus is narrower posteriorly than anteriorly, as mentioned previously. Of note, with dorsiflexion of the ankle, the fibula externally rotates and undergoes proximal translation owing to the articular geometry of the talus.

Subtalar Joint. The subtalar joint is the articulation of the talus with the calcaneus. It is a plane type of synovial joint. There is a weak, fibrous capsule surrounding the joint, but it is reinforced with talocalcaneal ligaments. An important function of the subtalar joint is as a torque converter to produce a cushioning effect on the foot. During the phase transition from heel strike to foot flat, the subtalar joint converts the internal rotation of the tibia into pronation of the foot by increasing the talocalcaneal angle, resulting in hindfoot valgus and thus unlocking the transverse tarsal joint. The subtalar joint also allows the foot to adapt to uneven surfaces through inversion and eversion and protects the tibiotalar joint from excessive stress.

Other Joints. Additional joints of the midfoot and forefoot include the transverse tarsal (Chopart) joint (calcaneocuboid and talonavicular), naviculocuneiform, intercuneiform, cuneocuboid, tarsometatarsal, metatarsophalangeal, and the interphalangeal joints. The tarsometatarsal joints are gliding joints supported by dorsal, plantar, and interosseous ligaments. An important point to remember is that the bases of the first and second metatarsal are not ligamentously connected. Instead, the Lisfranc ligament connects the plantar aspect of the second metatarsal base to the medial cuneiform and is an important soft tissue stabilizer of the midfoot. Also, it is important to note that anatomically the second metatarsal (often called the keystone of the tarsometatarsal complex) is recessed between the medial and lateral cuneiforms. The deep transverse metatarsal ligaments interconnect the metatarsal heads. Plantar and collateral ligaments

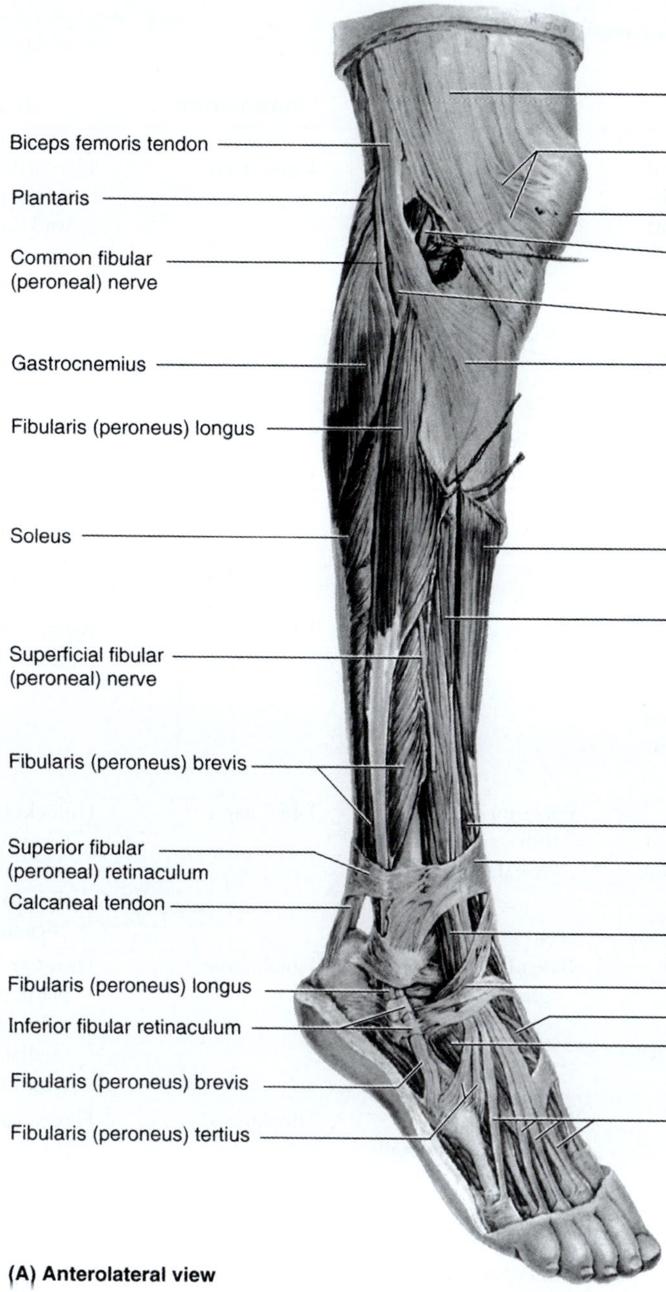

FIGURE 5.2 Dissections of the right leg. Muscles of the leg and foot. Observe the common fibular nerve in contact with the neck of the fibula (calf bone); here it is vulnerable to injury. Observe also the superior and inferior extensor and fibular retinacula. (*Source*: Moore KL, Dalley AF. *Clinically Oriented Anatomy*, 4th ed. Philadelphia: Lippincott Williams & Wilkins, 1999; 580, Fig. 5.35.)

support the metatarsophalangeal joints. The interphalangeal joints are supported by capsules.

Osteology of the Foot and Ankle

There are 26 bones in the foot: 7 tarsal and 5 metatarsal bones and 14 phalanges. The tarsus includes the talus, calcaneus, cuboid, navicular, and three cuneiforms.

Talus. The talus articulates with the tibia and fibula at the ankle mortise and with the calcaneus and navicular distally. It has a body, neck, and head. The body consists of a posterior process and three articular surfaces that include the trochlea, with surfaces for the malleoli articulations, and the posterior and middle calcaneal facets. The superior articular surface is wider anteriorly than posteriorly (the trochlea). It is the only tarsal

TABLE 5.3 Muscles of the posterior compartment

Muscle	Proximal Attachment	Distal Attachment	Innervation	Action
Gastrocnemius	*Lateral head:* lateral aspect of lateral condyle of femur *Medial head:* popliteal surface, superior to medial femoral condyle	Calcaneus (Achilles tendon)	Tibial nerve	Plantarflexes ankle, raises heel during walking, and flexes leg at knee joint
Soleus	Posterior aspect of head of fibula, superior to posterior surface of fibula	Calcaneus	Tibial nerve	Plantarflexes ankle, steadies leg on foot
Plantaris	Inferior end of lateral supracondylar line of femur and oblique popliteal ligament	Calcaneus	Tibial nerve	Assists gastrocnemius
Popliteus	Lateral surface of lateral condyle of femur and lateral meniscus	Posterior surface of tibia, superior to soleal line	Tibial nerve	Unlocks knee (externally rotates femur on tibia to initiate knee flexion)
Flexor hallucis longus (FHL)	Inferior two thirds of posterior surface of fibula and inferior part of IOM	Base of distal phalanx of hallux	Tibial nerve	Flexes great toe, plantarflexes ankle, supports medial longitudinal arch
Flexor digitorum longus (FDL)	Medial part of posterior surface of tibia inferior to soleal line, fibula	Base of distal phalanx of lateral 4 digits	Tibial nerve	Flexes digits 1–4, plantarflexes ankle, supports longitudinal arch of foot
Tibialis posterior	IOM, posterior surface of tibia inferior to soleal line, posterior surface of fibula	Tuberosity of navicular, cuneiform, cuboid, and bases of metatarsals 2–4	Tibial nerve	Plantarflexes ankle and inverts foot

Source: Moore KL, Dalley AF. *Clinically Oriented Anatomy*, 4th ed. Philadelphia: Lippincott Williams & Wilkins, 1999.

bone that does not have any muscular or tendinous attachments. The rounded talar head is directed anteromedially and rests on the sustentaculum tali of the calcaneus and articulates with the navicular distally. The calcaneonavicular (spring) ligament runs inferior to the talar head and serves to suspend it. The neck of the talus is oriented medially by approximately 10 to 44 degrees with reference to the axis of the talar body. It is highly susceptible to fracture. The tendon of the FHL runs in a groove within the posterior talar tubercle. Inferiorly also, the talus possesses posterior, middle, and anterior facets to articulate with the corresponding facets of the calcaneus. Between the middle and posterior facets is a transverse groove that, along

TABLE 5.4 Muscles of the dorsum of the foot

Muscle	Proximal Attachment	Distal Attachment	Innervation	Action
Extensor digitorum brevis	Superolateral calcaneus, sinus tarsi	Lateral capsule of MTP joint	Deep peroneal nerve	Assists in extension of digits

Source: Moore KL, Dalley AF. *Clinically Oriented Anatomy*, 4th ed. Philadelphia: Lippincott Williams & Wilkins, 1999.

with a similar grove on the dorsum of the calcaneus, forms the tarsal sinus. The talus also possesses a lateral and posterior process as well. The posterior process contains both a medial and lateral tubercle, with the FHL tendon running between the two tubercles. Of note, the underside of the tubercles comprises approximately 25% of the posterior facet of the subtalar joint. The lateral tubercle serves as the attachment site of the PTFL, while the medial tubercle serves as the attachment site for the posterior third of the deltoid ligament. The os trigonum is a frequently seen accessory bone found just posterior to lateral tubercle of posterior process and is joined to the lateral tubercle via a synchondrosis. A prominent lateral tubercle of the posterior process is known as a trigonal or Stieda process. The os trigonum can be clinically important because it can fracture, cause mechanical irritation of the FHL tendon, or can impinge against the tibial plafond during plantarflexion.

Calcaneus. The calcaneus is the largest and strongest bone in the foot and possesses three facets: the anterior, middle, and large posterior facets that articulate with the corresponding facets superiorly on the talus. There is a distal articular surface with the cuboid bone. The sustentaculum tali is an overhanging horizontal eminence on the anteromedial surface of the calcaneus and supports the talar head while allowing plantar vessels and nerves to pass below. Underneath the sustentaculum is a groove for the FHL. The calcaneal tuberosity lies posterior and is bonded by medial and lateral processes.

Cuboid. The cuboid is cubical in shape and is the lateral-most tarsal bone. Just anterior to the cuboid is a groove for the tendon of the peroneus longus muscle. It has four facets for articulation with the calcaneus, the lateral cuneiform, and the fourth and fifth metatarsals.

Navicular. The navicular is the most medial tarsal bone and is located anterior to the talar head with which it articulates. Distally, it also has three anterior facets for each of the three cuneiforms with which it also articulates. The tibialis posterior inserts on the medial aspect of the navicular.

Cuneiforms. The cuneiforms (medial, intermediate, and lateral) articulate with the navicular and posterior cuboid bones (lateral cuneiform) and the first three metatarsals. The intermediate cuneiform does not extend as far distally as the medial cuneiform, allowing the second metatarsal to recess between the medial and lateral cuneiforms.

Metatarsals and Phalanges. The five metatarsal bones number from medial to lateral and span the space between the tarsal bones and the phalanges. The first metatarsal is shorter and broader than the others; the second is the longest. The first metatarsal also possesses prominences on its plantar aspect with which it articulates with the sesamoids of the flexor hallucis brevis tendon. There are 14 phalanges in the foot, with the hallux possessing two phalanges and the remaining digits each possessing three phalanges.

Ossification. The calcaneus has two ossification centers, but the rest of the tarsal bones have only one each. Ossification centers for the calcaneus, talus, and usually the cuboid are present at birth. The center for the lateral cuneiform appears during the first year, the medial cuneiform during the second year, the intermediate cuneiform and navicular during the third year, and the posterior calcaneus during the eighth year. The first metatarsal and phalanges have secondary centers at their bases that first appear in the third or fourth year proximally and the sixth to seventh year distally. There are two ossification centers in the second through fifth metatarsals. The primary ossification is in the shaft, and the secondary is in the head, which appears between ages 5 and 8.

Ligamentous Anatomy of Foot and Ankle. The major ligaments of the foot are (1) the plantar calcaneonavicular ligament (spring ligament), (2) the long plantar ligament, and (3) the plantar calcaneocuboid ligament. The plantar calcaneonavicular ligament extends from the sustentaculum tali to the posteroinferior aspect of

TABLE 5.5 Muscles of the sole of the foot

Muscle	Proximal Attachment	Distal Attachment	Innervation	Action
First Layer				
Abductor hallucis	Medial tubercle of calcaneal tuberosity, flexor retinaculum, plantar aponeurosis	Medial side of base of proximal phalanx of first digit	Medial plantar nerve	Abducts and flexes first digit (hallux)
Flexor digitorum brevis	Medial tubercle of calcaneal tuberosity, plantar aponeurosis, intermuscular septae	Both sides of middle phalanges of lateral four digits	Medial plantar nerve	Flexes lateral 4 digits
Abductor digiti minimi	Medial and lateral tubercles of calcaneal tuberosity, plantar aponeurosis	Lateral side of base of proximal phalanx of fifth digit	Lateral plantar nerve	Abducts and flexes fifth digit
Muscle	**Proximal Attachment**	**Distal Attachment**	**Innervation**	**Action**
Second Layer				
Quadratus plantae	Medial surface of lateral margin of plantar surface of calcaneus	Posterolateral margin of tendon of FDL	Lateral plantar nerve	Assists flexor digitorum longus in flexing lateral 4 digits
Lumbricals	Tendons of FDL	Medial aspect of dorsal extensor expansion over lateral 4 digits	Medial plantar nerve (medial-most lumbrical), lateral plantar nerve (lateral 3 lumbricals)	Flex proximal phalanges, extend DIP joints of digits 2–5
Muscle	**Proximal Attachment**	**Distal Attachment**	**Innervation**	**Action**
Third Layer				
Flexor hallucis brevis	Plantar surface of cuboid and lateral cuneiforms	Both sides of base of proximal phalanx of first digit	Medial plantar nerve	Flexes proximal phalanx of first digit (has sesamoids of first MTP joint)
Adductor hallucis	*Oblique head:* bases of metatarsals 2–4 *Transverse head:* Plantar ligament of MTP joints (3–5)	Lateral side of base of proximal phalanx of 1st digit (plantar lateral plate)	Deep branch of lateral plantar nerve	Adducts first digit, maintains transverse arch of foot

TABLE 5.5 *(continued)*

Muscle	Proximal Attachment	Distal Attachment	Innervation	Action
Flexor digiti minimi brevis	Base of fifth metatarsal	Base of proximal phalanx of fifth digit	Superficial branch of lateral plantar nerve	Flexes proximal phalanx of fifth digit
Muscle	**Proximal Attachment**	**Distal Attachment**	**Innervation**	**Action**
Fourth Layer				
Plantar interossei	Bases and medial sides of metatarsals 2–5	Medial side of bases of proximal phalanges of digits 3–5	Lateral plantar nerve	Adducts digits 2–4, flex MTP joints
Dorsal interossei	Adjacent sides of metatarsals 1–5	*First:* Medial side of proximal phalanx of second digit *Second–Fourth:* Lateral sides of digits 2–4	Lateral plantar nerve	Abduct digits 2–4 and flex MTP joints

Source: Moore KL, Dalley AF. *Clinically Oriented Anatomy*, 4th ed. Philadelphia: Lippincott Williams & Wilkins, 1999.

the navicular. It is a crucial ligament in maintaining the longitudinal arch of the foot. The long plantar ligament extends from the plantar surface of the calcaneus to the cuboid groove. It also has fibers that extend to the base of the metatarsals and form a tunnel for the peroneus longus. The plantar calcaneocuboid (short plantar) is deep to the long plantar ligament and extends from the anterior aspect of the inferior surface of the calcaneus to the inferior aspect of the cuboid. The Lisfranc ligament is also an important structure and is a ligament that connects the plantar aspect of the second metatarsal base and the medial cuneiform. There is no intermetatarsal ligament between the first and second metatarsals (Fig. 5.6). The syndesmosis of the ankle is composed of the anterior inferior tibiofibular ligament (AITFL), the posterior inferior tibiofibular ligament (PITFL), and the interosseous membrane.

Blood Supply of the Foot and Ankle

Dorsal Blood Supply. One of the main arterial supplies to the foot is the dorsalis pedis, which provides blood to the dorsum of the foot along its branches: the lateral tarsal, medial tarsal, the arcuate, and first dorsal metatarsal branches. It is a direct continuation of the anterior tibial artery. It begins midway between the malleoli and runs anteromedially, deep to the inferior extensor retinaculum between the extensor digitorum longus (EDL) and extensor hallucis longus (EHL) tendons. It passes to the first interosseous space, where it divides into a deep plantar artery that passes to the sole of the foot and the first dorsal metatarsal artery (at risk during bunion surgery). The deep plantar artery is the largest branch and runs between the first and second metatarsals before contributing to the plantar arch. The lateral tarsal artery is a branch of the dorsalis pedis and runs laterally, supplying the extensor digitorum brevis muscle and the underlying tarsal bones.

Plantar Blood Supply. The blood supply of the sole of the foot is derived from the posterior tibial artery that divides deep to the abductor hallucis muscles to form the medial and lateral plantar artery. The medial plantar artery supplies the musculature of the hallux and skin on the medial side of the foot. The lateral plantar artery, which is the larger of the two terminal divisions of the posterior tibial artery, runs laterally and anteriorly deep to the abductor hallucis and flexor digitorum brevis muscles. It arches medially to form and anastomoses with the medial plantar artery to form the deep plantar arch in the fourth layer of the plantar foot. It also anastomoses with the deep plantar artery, which is a branch of the dorsalis pedis artery. The deep plantar arch gives off 4 plantar metatarsal arteries that divide distally to give off the plantar digital arteries.

Talus and Tarsal Blood Supply. The talus blood supply is illustrated in Figure 5.7. The artery of the

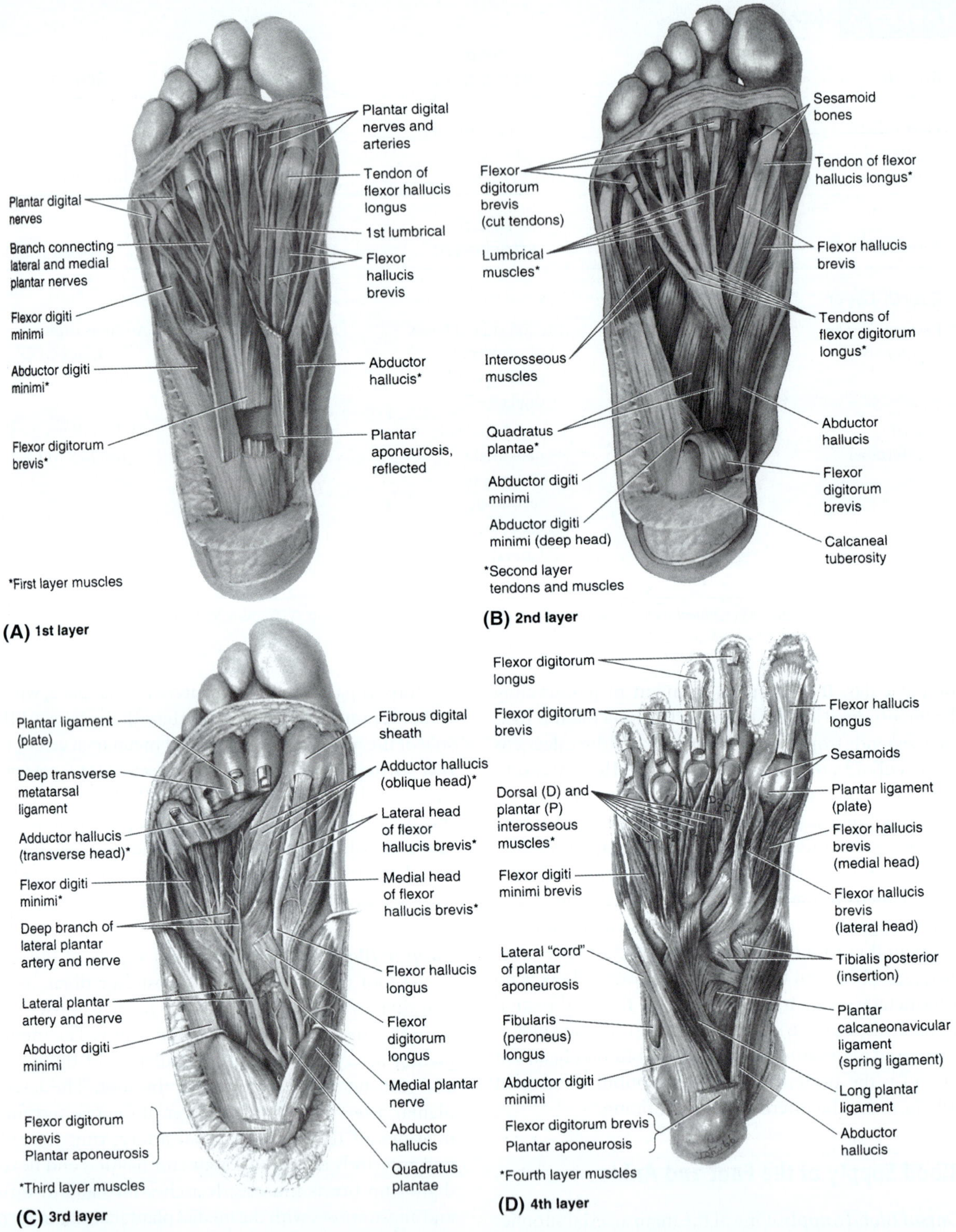

FIGURE 5.3 Layers of plantar muscles. (A) First layer, consisting of the abductors of the large and small toes and the short flexor of the toes. (B) Second layer, consisting of the long flexor tendons and associated muscles: four lumbricals and the quadratus plantae. (C) Third layer, consisting of the flexor of the small (little) toe and the flexor and adductor of the large (big) toe. (D) Fourth layer, consisting of the dorsal and plantar interosseus muscles. (*Source*: Moore KL, Dalley AF. *Clinically Oriented Anatomy*, 4th ed. Philadelphia: Lippincott Williams & Wilkins, 1999; 596-7. Fig. 5.43.)

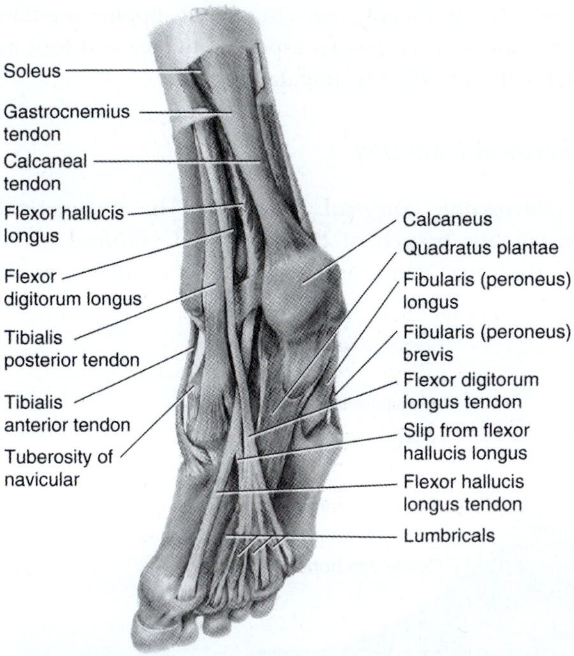

FIGURE 5.4 **Second layer of plantar muscles. This layer of foot muscles includes the tendons of the flexor hallucis longus and flexor digitorum longus, four lumbrical (*L. lumbricus*, earth worm) muscles, and the quadratus plantae. (*Source*: Moore KL, Dalley AF. *Clinically Oriented Anatomy*, 4th ed. Philadelphia: Lippincott Williams & Wilkins, 1999; 591. Fig. 5.39.)**

tarsal canal typically arises from the posterior tibial artery approximately 1 cm proximal to the origin of the medial and lateral plantar arteries. Passing between the sheaths of FDL and FHL, it enters the tarsal canal and is the primary blood supply to the talus. Calcaneal branches from the posterior tibial artery also supply the talus. Approximately 5 mm from the origin of the artery of the tarsal canal is the origin of the deltoid branch of the artery of the tarsal canal, which supplies the medial periosteal surface of the body of the talus and anastomoses with the dorsalis pedis artery or anterior tibial artery branches over the neck of the talus. The anterior tibial artery becomes the dorsalis pedis artery at the level of the ankle and supplies the superior surface of the neck of the talus. The sinus tarsi area is mainly supplied by the dorsalis pedis artery. The artery of the tarsal sinus is derived from an anastomotic loop between the lateral tarsal branch of the dorsalis pedis artery and the perforating peroneal artery. It partly supplies the talar head and body and then anastomoses with the artery of the tarsal canal within the tarsal canal.

Nervous Supply of the Foot and Ankle

The nervous supply to the foot and ankle is derived from the superficial and deep peroneal nerves as well as the terminal branches of the tibial nerve.

Common Peroneal Nerve. The common peroneal nerve splits into superficial and deep branches in the leg and terminates in the foot. The deep peroneal nerve supplies the interdigital space between the first and second toes and also supplies the extensor digitorum brevis (EDB). The medial and intermediate dorsal cutaneous nerves of the superficial peroneal nerve supply the sensation to the remainder of the dorsum of the foot. The superficial peroneal nerve lies between the fibular muscles and supplies cutaneous sensation to the inferior third of the lateral aspect of the leg and the majority of the skin on the dorsum of the foot. The dorsal medial cutaneous nerve crosses the EHL from lateral to medial and innervates the dorsomedial aspect of the great toe.

Tibial Nerve. The tibial nerve gives off the medial and lateral plantar nerves after splitting underneath the flexor retinaculum. Both the medial and lateral plantar nerves are in the second layer of the foot. The medial plantar nerve passes deep to the abductor hallucis and runs anteriorly on the lateral side of the medial plantar artery. The medial plantar nerve terminates at approximately the bases of the metatarsals by dividing into terminal sensory branches, supplying cutaneous innervation to the medial 3 1/2 digits of the foot and motor branches to the medial most lumbrical, the abductor hallucis, the flexor digitorum brevis (FDB), and the flexor hallucis brevis (FHB). The lateral plantar nerve is the smaller of the two tibial branches and runs obliquely under the cover of the quadratus plantae before it terminates in superficial and deep branches. The superficial branch divides into 2 digital branches that supply the lateral 1 1/2 digits. The distribution of the sensory and motor branches of the plantar nerves is similar to that in the hand. Therefore, like the median nerve in the hand, the medial plantar nerve supplies plantar sensation to the medial 3 1/2 digits and motor to the plantar muscles (FHB, abductor hallucis, FDB, and first lumbrical). Similar to the ulnar nerve, the lateral plantar nerve supplies plantar sensation to the lateral 1 1/2 digits and the remaining intrinsic muscles of the foot. The deep branch supplies the remainder of the musculature of the sole of the foot.

Sural Nerve. A union of branches of the tibial and common peroneal nerves forms the sural nerve.

It accompanies the small saphenous vein distally and courses posterior to the lateral malleolus. At approximately the level of the Achilles insertion into the calcaneus, it is 19 mm from the lateral border of the Achilles. It crosses the lateral border of the Achilles approximately 10 cm proximal to the calcaneus. This close relationship should be kept in mind when suturing the proximal part of the Achilles tendon. The saphenous nerve is a branch of the femoral nerve and is its largest cutaneous branch. It supplies the skin and fascia of the medial aspect of the leg and foot as far distally as the first metatarsal.

Surgical Anatomy

Arthroscopic Surgical Anatomy. The dorsolateral cutaneous branch of the superficial peroneal nerve is the most commonly injured nerve during ankle

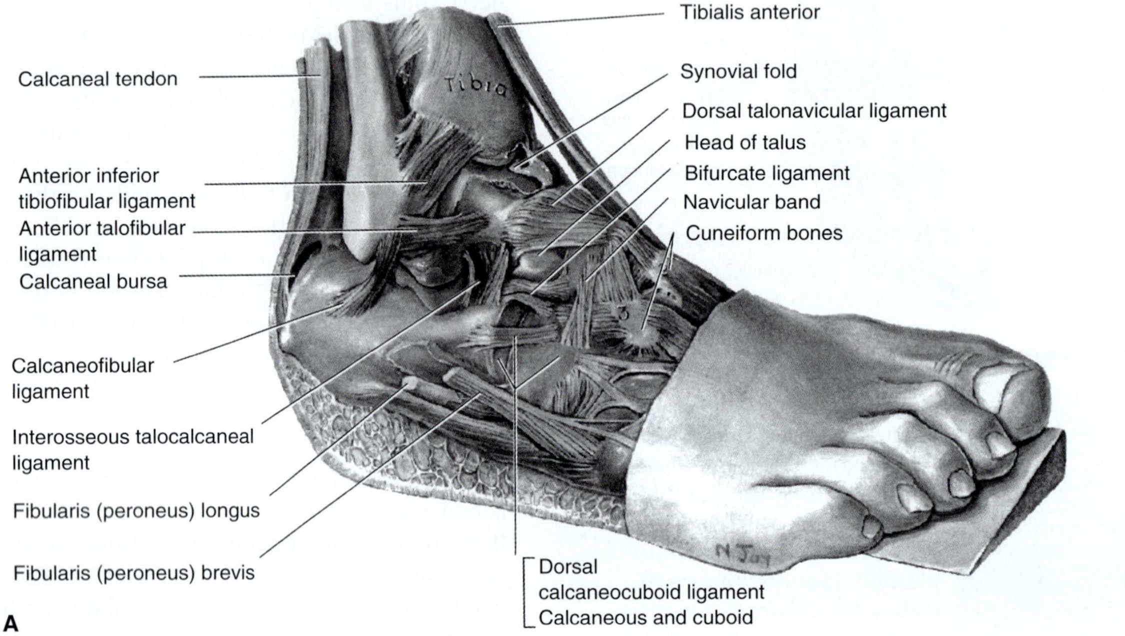

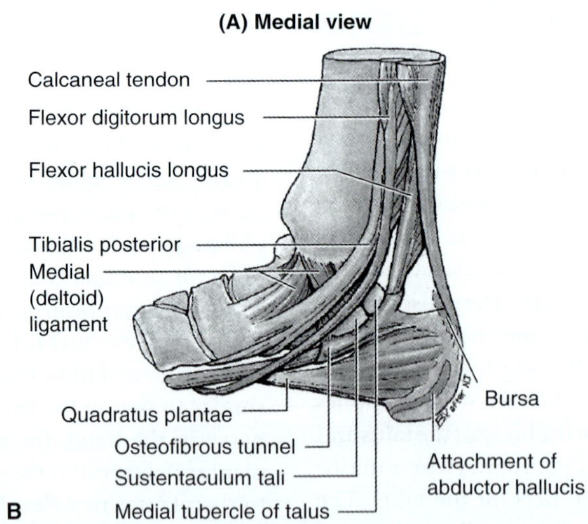

FIGURE 5.5 **(1) Dissection of the right ankle joint and the joints of inversion and eversion. Lateral view. The foot has been inverted to demonstrate the articular areas and the lateral ligaments that become taut during inversion of the foot. (2) Ankle and tarsal joints. Medial views. (A) Tendons of the medial aspect of the ankle. (B) Dissection of the ankle and tarsal joints. Observe the four parts of the medial ligament of the ankle. (*Source*: Moore KL, Dalley AF. *Clinically Oriented Anatomy*, 4th ed. Philadelphia: Lippincott Williams & Wilkins, 1999; 634–635, Figs. 5.64, 5.65.)**

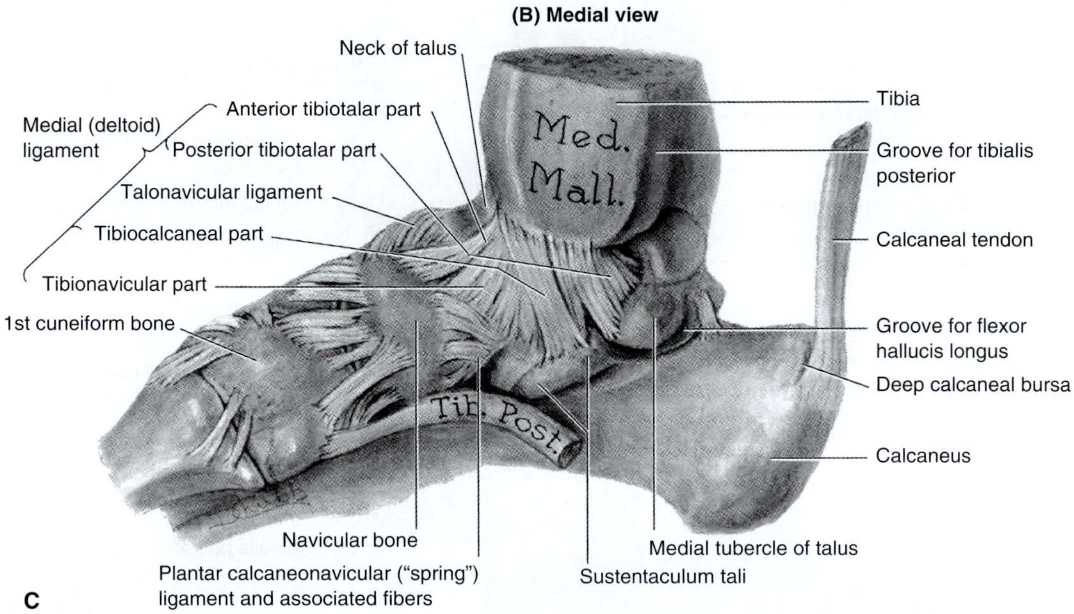

FIGURE 5.5 *(continued)*

arthroscopy because it is located adjacent to the lateral arthroscopic portal. The anteromedial portal places the greater saphenous vein at risk. Anterior central portals risks injury to the dorsalis pedis artery, and therefore these portals are not recommended. Posteromedial portals risks injury to the posterior tibial artery and are also not recommended, while posterior lateral portals can injure the sural nerves. Transachilles tendon portals are not recommended because of postoperative tendonitis.

Anterior Approach to the Ankle. An anterior approach is common for ankle fusion via the interval between the EHL and EDL. Protect the superficial peroneal nerve before incising the extensor retinaculum. Retract the deep peroneal nerve and anterior tibial artery medially along with the EHL.

Approach to the Medial Malleolus. This is the common approach used for medial malleolus fractures. The saphenous nerve and long saphenous vein are at risk with anterior approach. Posterior structures to the malleolus are at risk with posterior approaches such as the posterior tibial artery, vein, and nerve; the FDL; and the FHL.

Posteromedial Approach the Ankle and Foot. The posteromedial approach is commonly used for clubfoot release in pediatric surgery. It begins medial to the Achilles tendon, curving distally along the medial border of the foot. The posterior tibial neurovascular structures are at risk. The posterior tibialis tendon is a landmark for the location of the subluxated navicular in clubfoot surgery.

Lateral Approach to the Ankle. A lateral approach is commonly used for distal fibular fractures. The sural nerve is at risk posterolaterally and the superficial peroneal nerve anteriorly.

Lateral Approach to the Hindfoot. A lateral approach is commonly used for triple arthrodesis. The internervous plane is between the peroneal tertius (deep peroneal nerve) and peroneal tendons (superficial peroneal nerves). First, remove the fat pad covering the sinus tarsi, then reflect the EDB (lateral branch of deep peroneal nerve) from its origin to expose the joints. Protect the lateral branch of the deep peroneal nerve. The FHL is deep.

Anterolateral Approach to the Midfoot. An anterolateral approach is commonly used for resection of a calcaneonavicular bar. First, release the EDB. The calcaneal navicular (spring) ligament is at risk.

II. BIOMECHANICS OF THE FOOT AND ANKLE AND THE GAIT CYCLE

Gait Cycle

Determinants of Gait. There are 6 basic determinants of gait as defined by Saunders, Inman, and Eberhart: (1) pelvic rotation, (2) pelvic obliquity, (3) knee flexion in stance, (4) foot and ankle motion, (5) lateral displacement of the pelvis, and (6) axial rotations of

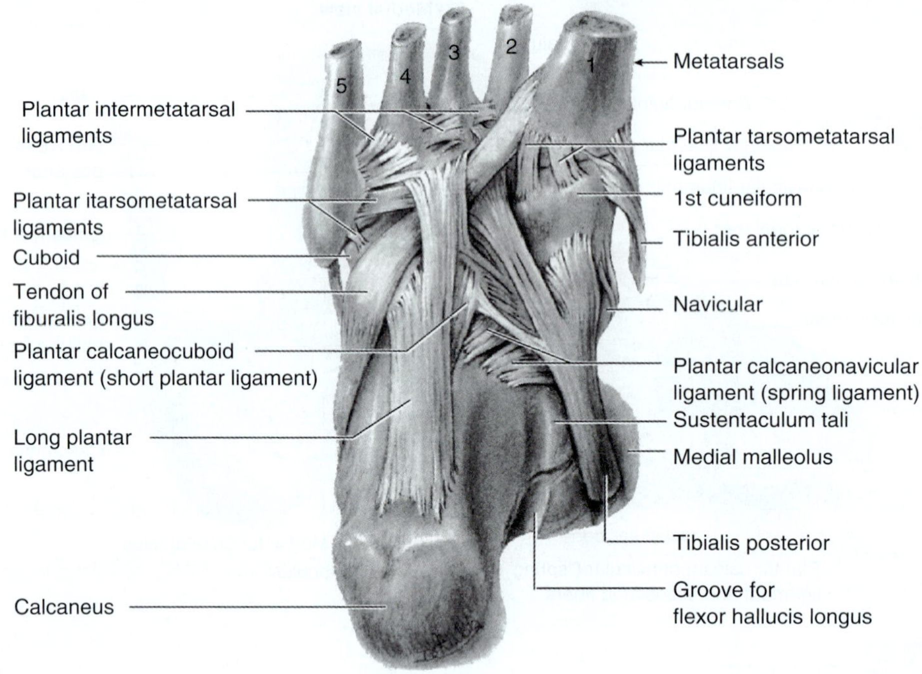

(A)

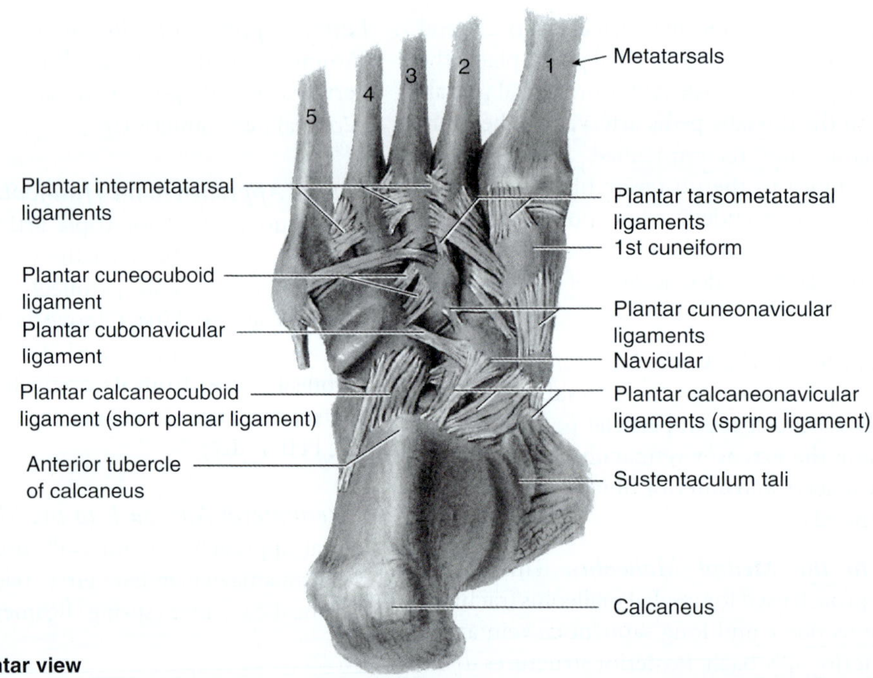

(B) Plantar view

FIGURE 5.6 **Plantar ligaments. Deep dissection of the sole of the right foot showing the attachments of the ligaments and the long tendons of the leg muscles. The main ligaments from this view are the plantar calcaneonavicular and the long and short plantar ligaments. (*Source*: Moore KL, Dalley AF. *Clinically Oriented Anatomy*, 4th ed. Philadelphia: Lippincott Williams & Wilkins, 1999; 639, Fig. 5.66.)**

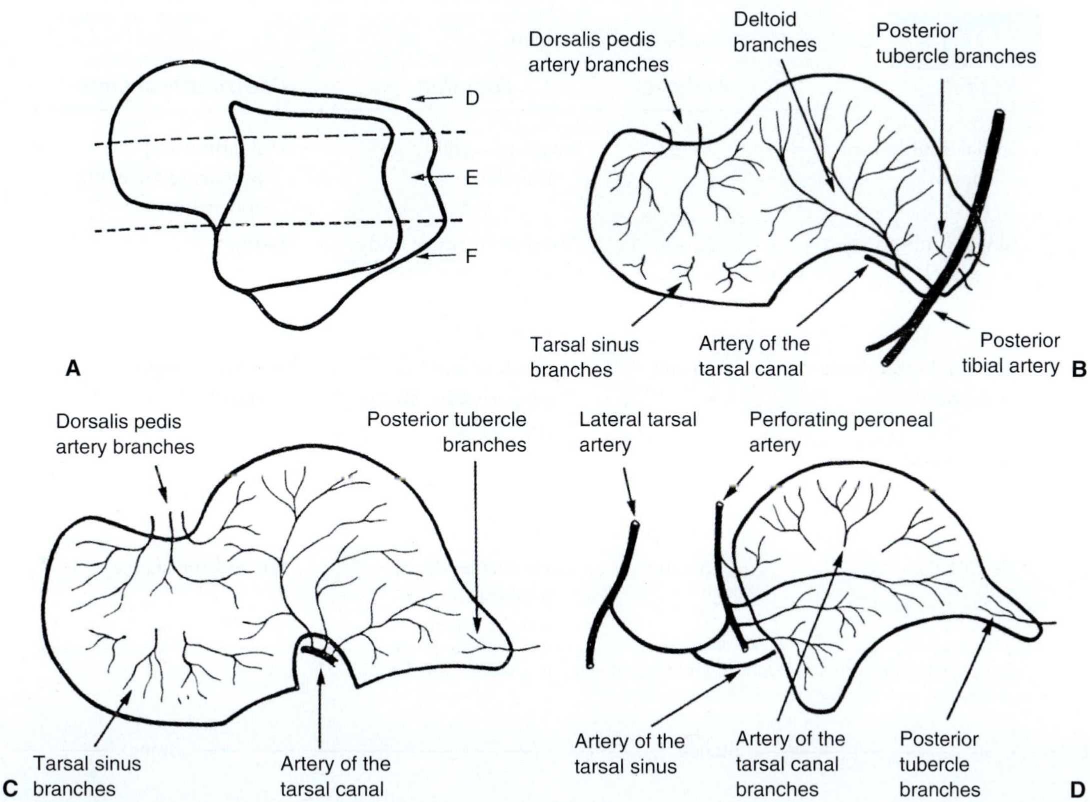

FIGURE 5.7 **Blood supply of the talus. (*Source*: Mulfinger G, Trueta J. The blood supply of the talus. *J Bone Joint Surg Br* 52-B(1):160–167,1970. Fig. 1.)**

the lower extremities. Abnormalities of 2 or more of these determinants can lead to inefficient gait.

Prerequisites of Gait. Based upon these determinants of gait, it is important to understand the 5 prerequisites of normal gait: (1) stability of the weight-bearing foot throughout the stance phase, (2) clearance of the nonweight-bearing foot during swing phase, (3) appropriate prepositioning during terminal swing of the foot for the next gait cycle, (4) adequate step length, and (5) energy conservation.

Periods and Functions. The gait cycle is typically broken into 6 distinct parts that define the functional periods and phases of the cycle (Table 5.6; Fig 5.8): (1) foot strike, (2) opposite toe-off, (3) reversal of fore shear to aft shear, (4) opposite foot clearance, (5) tibia vertical, and (6) successive foot strike. Historically, terms such as *heel strike* have been used to describe gait but should be avoided because these specific events could be absent or altered in individuals with a pathologic gait.

Stance Phase. Stance phase occurs when the foot is in contact with the ground from foot strike to toe-off. It constitutes approximately 62% of the gait cycle. The stance phase itself is divided into 3 distinct periods: (1) initial double-limb support (loading response), (2) single-limb stance, and (3) second double-limb support (preswing). The cardinal events for initial double-limb support are foot strike and opposite toe-off, while the defining events for single-limb stance are opposite toe-off and opposite foot strike. The double-limb support phase occurs when both feet are on the ground, and it lasts around 12% of the cycle, followed by a single support phase, which lasts about 50% of the cycle. Running produces a period of no weight bearing (float phase) on either extremity and ground reactive forces increase to almost 3 times body weight.

Swing Phase. The swing phase occurs when the foot is off the ground from toe-off to the next foot strike and constitutes 38% of the cycle. The swing phase is also divided into 3 stages: (1) initial swing, (2) midswing, and (3) terminal swing, with the defining events for initial swing being toe-off and foot clearance and terminal swing beginning with tibia vertical and completed with foot strike.

Ankle Axis of Rotation. During the gait cycle, the foot changes from a flexible structure at foot strike to a rigid structure at toe-off. The ankle joint functions

TABLE 5.6 Gait cycle: periods and functions

Period	*% Cycle*	*Function*	*Contralateral Limb*
Initial double-limb support	0–12	Loading, weight, transfer	Unloading and preparing for swing (preswing)
Single-limb stance	12–50	Support of entire body weight; center of mass moving forward	Swing
Second double-limb support	50–62	Unloading and preparing for swing (preswing)	Loading, weight transfer
Initial swing	62–75	Foot clearance	Single-limb stance
Midswing	75–85	Limb advances in front of body	Single-limb stance
Terminal swing	85–100	Limb deceleration, preparation for weight transfer	Single-limb stance

Source: Chambers HG. A practical guide to gait analysis. *JAAOS* 2002; 10: 222–231, Table 2.

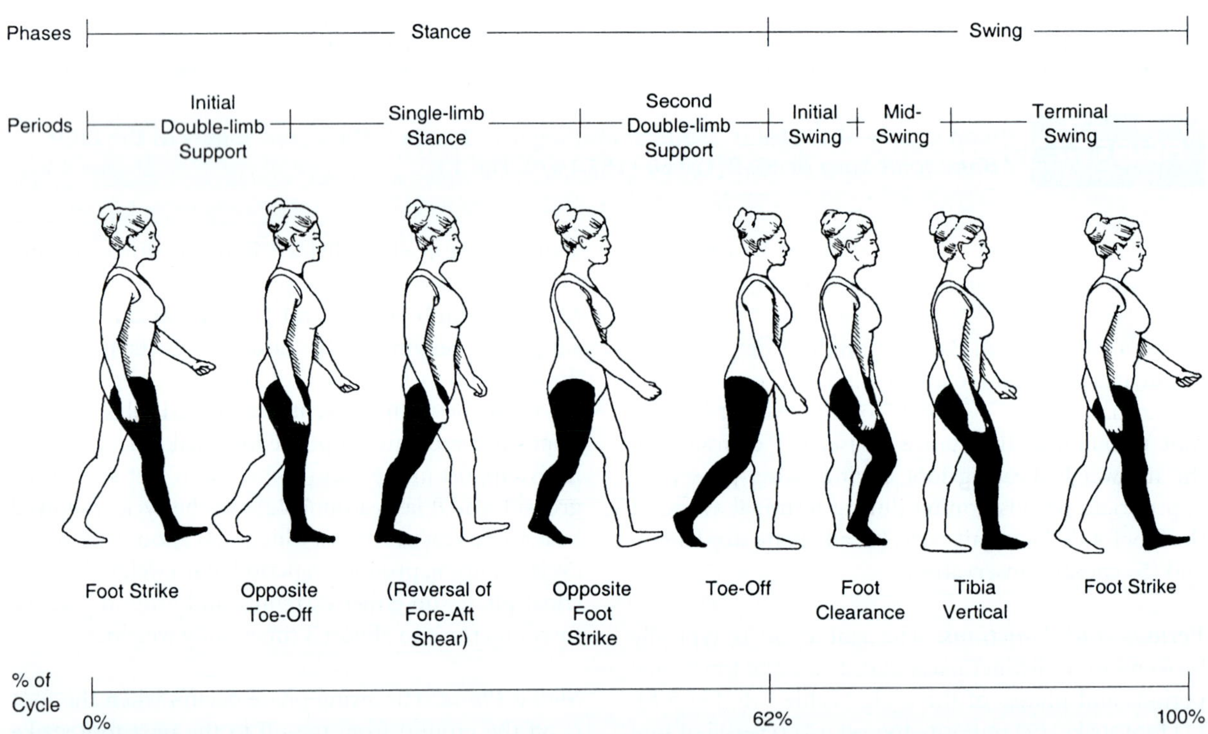

FIGURE 5.8 Typical normal gait cycle. (*Adapted with permission from* Sutherland DH, Kaufman KR, Moitoza JR. Kinematics of normal human walking. In: Rose J, Gamble JG (eds.), *Human Walking*, 2nd ed. Baltimore, MD: Williams & Wilkins, 1994; 23–44; from Chambers HG. A practical guide to gait analysis. *JAAOS* 10;2002,222–231, Fig. 1.)

as a mitered hinge: upon on foot strike, there is internal tibial rotation, hindfoot eversion, and a supple transverse tarsal (Chopart joint, which includes the talonavicular and calcaneocuboid joints). When foot strike occurs, the anterior muscles undergo eccentric joint contraction to control progression from foot strike to foot flat to absorb energy and stabilize the foot. During foot strike, the foot is pronated to unlock the Chopart joint. Unlocking the joint allows for a flexible midfoot that allows the foot to accept weight transfer during the transition from the foot strike to the foot flat stage. The foot is pronated as a result of internal rotation of the tibia and subsequent hindfoot valgus (hindfoot eversion). The tibialis posterior acts at the foot flat stage to prevent overpronation. During the foot flat stage, the leg externally rotates along with midfoot supination and hindfoot inversion. The latter two are accomplished by the action of the tibialis posterior, which initiates subtalar inversion. These actions then create a rigid transverse tarsal joint that allows the foot to serve as a platform for toe-off. At the end of the foot flat stage, the tibialis posterior and gastrocnemius-soleus complex are activated to effect heel rise. Of note, the supination of the foot during the transition from foot flat to toe-off is accomplished by both the external rotation of the leg and the windlass mechanism. The windlass mechanism is the tension placed on the plantar fascia as a result of dorsiflexion of the hallux that increases the midfoot arch height and locks the transverse tarsal joint.

Gait Velocity, Step Length, and Stride Length. Additional terminology that must be understood when analyzing gait are gait velocity, step length and stride length. Gait velocity is defined in units of centimeters per second, meters per minute, or cadence (number of steps per minute). The step length is the distance from the foot strike of one foot to the foot strike of the contralateral foot, while the stride length is the distance from the foot strike of one foot to the foot strike of the ipsilateral foot.

Ground Reactive Force. In characterizing the gait pattern of an individual, it is important to understand two critical components of gait: (1) characterization of the dynamic muscular control of the foot and ankle (seen on the electromyographic [EMG] report) and (2) the result of the sequential muscle activities on the mechanical characteristics of the foot and ankle during the gait cycle. Of note, the ground reaction force during walking reaches approximately 1.5 times body weight. In comparison, running, in which there is a float phase when neither limb is on the ground, generates approximately 3 times body weight.

III. PHYSICAL EXAMINATION OF THE FOOT AND ANKLE

Inspection. A complete examination starts with a thorough inspection of the foot. First, count the toes to make certain that there are 5. The toes should appear flat, straight, and in proportion to one another. Next, ask the patient to be seated to determine if the feet at rest are in a few degrees of plantarflexion and inversion. In evaluating the overall shape of the foot, the dorsum is domed because of the medial longitudinal arch of the foot that extends between the first metatarsal head and the calcaneus (arch is more prominent in the weight-bearing part of the foot). The arch may be abnormally high (pes cavus) or absent (pes planus). Also note changes in color in the weight-bearing and nonweight-bearing portions of the foot. As an example, if the foot is light pink when elevated but turns deep red when lowered (dependent rubor), it may indicate small-vessel vascular disease or arterial insufficiency. Finally, inspect the foot for unilateral or bilateral swelling. Swelling unilaterally indicates residual edema due to trauma; bilateral swelling may indicate cardiac pathology or lymphedema (Fig. 5.9).

Bony Palpation. Palpation of the foot should start with feeling for bony landmarks according to areas of the foot and the corresponding structures (Table 5.7).

Soft Tissue Palpation. Soft tissue palpation proceeds along a series of 10 zones that should be followed systematically to avoid potentially missing any pathology:

- *Zone I*—Head of the first metatarsal bone
- *Zone II*—Navicular tubercle and the talar head
- *Zone III*—Medial malleolus; evaluate the deltoid ligament, posterior tibial tendon, FDL, FHL, posterior tibial artery, tibial nerve, and saphenous vein (Fig. 5.10)
- *Zone IV*—Dorsum of the foot between the malleoli; evaluate the tibialis anterior tendon, EHL, EDL, and dorsalis pedis artery.
- *Zone V*—Lateral malleolus; evaluate the ATFL, calcaneofibular ligament, PTFL, peroneus longus, and brevis tendons
- *Zone VI*—Sinus tarsi and EDB muscles
- *Zone VII*—Head of the fifth metatarsal
- *Zone VIII*—Calcaneus and retrocalcaneal bursa area
- *Zone IX*—Plantar surface of foot
- *Zone X*—Toes; evaluate for claw toes, hammer toes, corns, and ingrown toenails

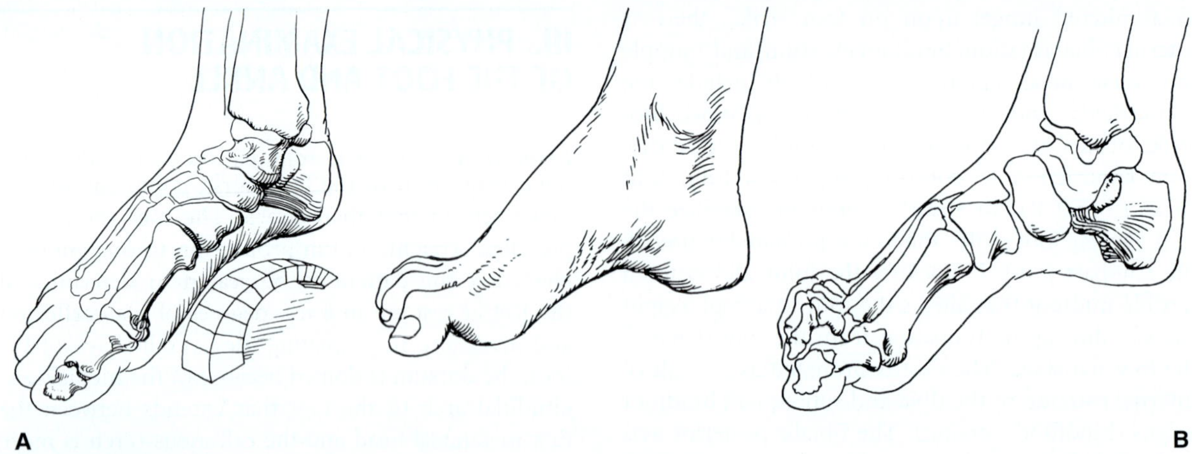

FIGURE 5.9 (A) The longitudinal arch of the foot. (B) An abnormally high arch (pes cavus). (*Source*: Hoppenfeld S. *Physical Examination of the Spine and Extremities*. Upper Saddle River, NJ: Prentice Hall, 1976, 198–199, Figs. 1 and 2.)

Ankle Instability. In testing for ankle joint stability, it is important to keep in mind that the ATFL is most commonly sprained. Applying an inversion stress to the ankle while in dorsiflexion will stress the calcaneofibular ligament. Performing an anterior drawer test with the ankle in plantarflexion will stress the ATFL. To adequately perform an anterior drawer test, make sure that the patient is sitting on the edge of the examination table with the legs dangling and the feet in a few degrees of plantar flexion. Place one hand on the anterior aspect of the tibia and grasp the calcaneus with the palm of the other hand. Then, pull the calcaneus anteriorly while pushing the tibia posteriorly. To test the stability of the deltoid ligament, stabilize the tibia and calcaneus and evert the foot. If the deltoid is torn, there will be gapping within the ankle mortise.

Joint Motion. Ankle dorsiflexion is 20 degrees, and plantarflexion is 40 degrees (Fig. 5.11). Subtalar inversion is 5 degrees, and eversion is 5 degrees. Forefoot motion is accomplished primarily at the transverse tarsal joints. Forefoot adduction is 20 degrees, and forefoot abduction is 10 degrees. The metatarsophalangeal (MTP) joints should also be assessed, with the first MTP joint allowing approximately 45 degrees of

TABLE 5.7 Palpation of the foot

Medial Aspect	Lateral Aspect	Area Sinus Tarsi	Area of the Hindfoot	Plantar Surface
Head of the first metatarsal bone and MTP joint	Fifth metatarsal bone; fifth MTP joint	Dome of talus	Dome of Calcaneus	Sesamoid bones
First MTC joint	Calcaneus	Inferior tibiofibular joint	Medial tubercle	Metatarsal heads
Navicular tubercle	Peroneal tubercle			
Head of talus	Lateral malleolus			
Medial malleolus				
Sustentaculum tali				
Medial tubercle of talus				

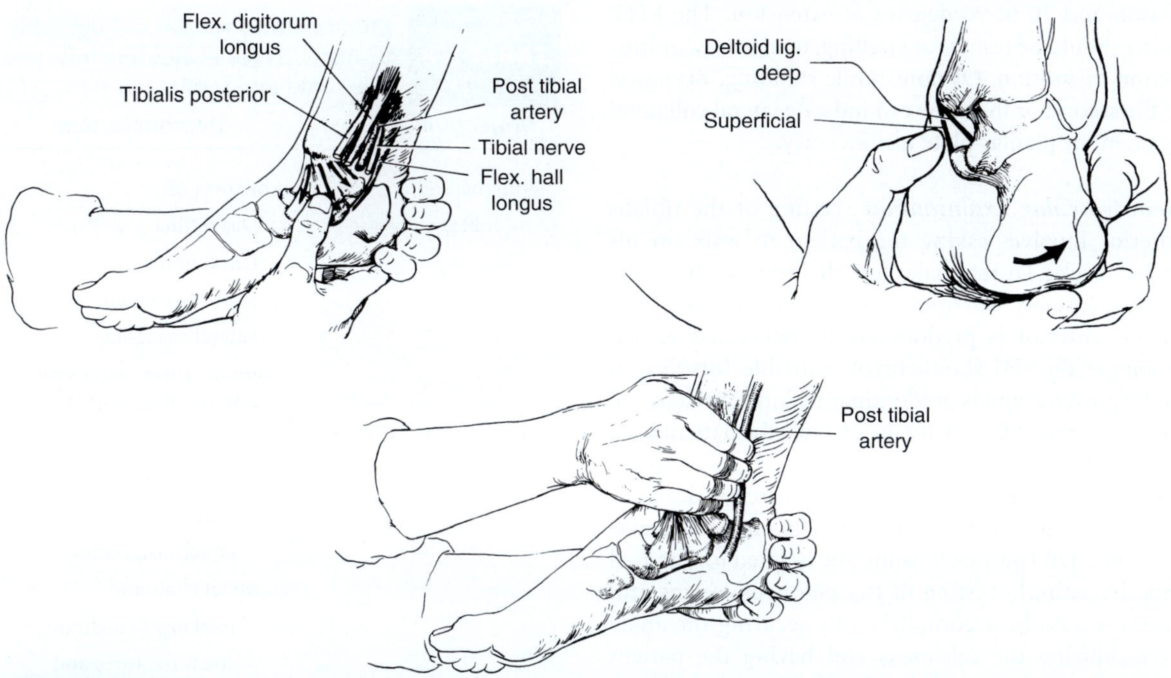

FIGURE 5.10 (A) The deltoid ligament. (B) Pain elicited upon eversion may be due to a sprain of the deltoid ligament. (C) Palpation of the posterior tibial artery, the main blood supply to the foot. (*Source*: Hoppenfeld S. *Physical Examination of the Spine and Extremities*. Upper Saddle River, NJ: Prentice Hall, 1976; 213, Figs. 38–40.)

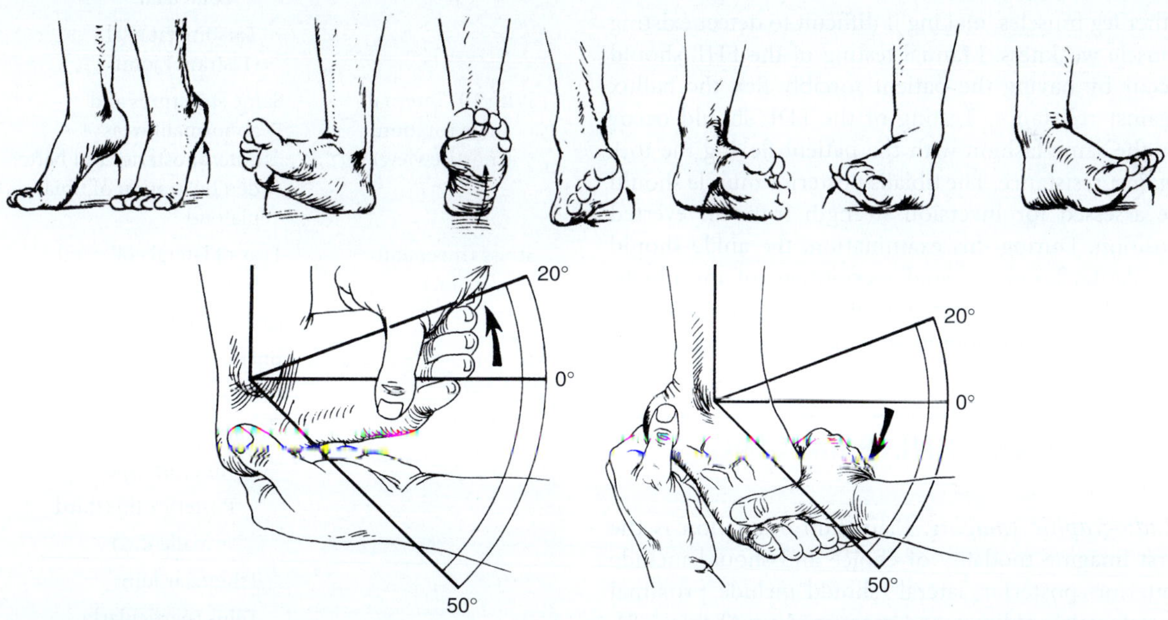

FIGURE 5.11 (A) Quick tests for foot and ankle range of motion. (B) Range of ankle dorsiflexion. (C) Range of ankle plantar flexion. (*Source*: Hoppenfeld S. *Physical Examination of the Spine and Extremities*. Upper Saddle River, NJ: Prentice Hall, 1976; 223 Figs. 65–67.)

flexion and 70 to 90 degrees of extension. The MTP joints should be tested for swelling, tenderness, or limitation of motion. Of note, while standing, deviation of the second or third toe can indicate lateral collateral ligament or plantar plate insufficiency.

Neurovascular Examination. Testing of the tibialis anterior involves asking the patient to walk on his or her heels. To manually test this muscle, have the patient forcibly dorsiflex and invert the foot. The tibialis anterior is predominantly innervated by L4. Testing of the EHL should involve forcible dorsiflexion of the great toe and is predominantly innervated by L5. Testing of the EDL also involves having the patient walk on his or her heels, and to manually test this muscle, the examiner should have the patient forcibly dorsiflex the toes. It is innervated by L5. This maneuver also tests the EDB (though it cannot be isolated for manual muscle testing). Testing of the peroneus longus and brevis should be accomplished by securing the ankle by stabilizing the calcaneus and having the patient plantarflex and evert the foot against resistance. These two muscles are innervated by L5 and S1. Testing of the gastrocnemius/soleus complex should commence with asking the patient to walk on his or her toes and then to jump up and down on the first MTP joints of the feet (balls of feet) one foot at a time. Manual muscle testing of this complex is difficult because it is stronger than all other leg muscles, making it difficult to detect existing muscle weakness. Manual testing of the FHL should occur by having the patient forcibly flex the hallux against resistance. Testing of the FDL should occur by the same fashion with the patient flexing the toes against resistance. The tibialis posterior muscle should be assessed for inversion strength from an everted position. During this examination, the ankle should be plantarflexed to avoid recruitment of the tibialis anterior. From an everted position, only the posterior tibial tendon functions as an invertor.

IV. FOOT AND ANKLE IMAGING

Radiographic Imaging. Plain film evaluation is the first imaging modality of choice and should include anterior–posterior, lateral (should include proximal metatarsals), oblique, and mortise views (Table 5.8). The mortise view should be performed with the foot in 15 degrees of internal rotation. With this view, the medial clear space can be evaluated to determine if there is lateral subluxation of the talus within the mortise. A medial clear space greater than 4 mm is considered abnormal. The lateral view of the foot should include the proximal metatarsals. Weight-bearing views should be obtained when indicated.

TABLE 5.8 Standard and special radiographic projections for evaluating injury to the ankle and foot

Projection	Demonstration
Anteroposterior (ankle)	Fractures of: Distal tibia Distal fibula Medial malleolus Lateral malleolus Pilon fractures (extension into tibiotalar joint)
(foot)	Fractures of: Distal portion of talus Navicular, cuboid, and cuneiform bones Metatarsals and phalanges (including stress fractures and accessory ossicles) Dislocations in: Subtalar joint Peritalar (anterior and posterior types) Total talar Tarsometatarsal (Lisfranc) joint
With 10° internal ankle rotation (mortise view)	Same structures and abnormalities as anteroposterior but better demonstration of tibial plafond
Stress (inversion, eversion)	Tear of lateral collateral ligament Ankle instability
Lateral (ankle and foot)	Boehler angle Fractures of: Distal tibia Anterior aspect Posterior lip (third malleolus) Tibiotalar joint Talus (particularly neck) Calcaneus (particularly in coronal plane) Posterior facet of subtalar joint Sustentaculum tali

TABLE 5.8 *(continued)*

	Accessory ossicles
	Cuboid bone
	Dislocations in:
	Subtalar joint
	Peritalar (anterior and posterior
	Tarsometatarsal (Lisfranc) joint
Stress (anterior-draw)	Tear of anterior talofibular ligament Ankle instability
Oblique	Fractures of:
Internal	Medial malleolus
External	Talus
	Tuberosity of calcaneus
	Metatarsais
	Phalanges
Posterior Tangential	Fractures involving:
(Harris-Beath)	Middle and posterior facets of sub joint
	Calcaneus (in axial plane)
Oblique Tangential	Fractures involving:
(Broden)	Posterior facet of subtalar joint
	Calcaneus
	Sustentaculum tali
Axial (sesamoid view)	Fractures of sesamoid bones

Source: Greenspan A. *Orthopaedic Radiology*, 3rd ed. Philadelphia: Lippincott Williams & Wilkins, 2000. Table 9.1, p. 295.

Stress views should also be obtained to evaluate for ligamentous instability. However, the main limitation of this study is the inability to properly evaluate soft tissue abnormalities. The Canale view allows for full visualization of the talar neck. It is performed with the foot in maximum plantar flexion and pronated 15 degrees, with the x-ray beam angled 75 degrees from horizontal in the anterior–posterior plane. The Broden view is obtained by internally rotating the foot 45 degrees and progressively angling the x-ray beam in 10-degree increments from vertical; it evaluates the posterior facet of the calcaneus. The Harris axial view allows for varus and valgus alignment to be appreciated with calcaneus fractures. Both Bohler angle and the critical angle of Gissane should be measured when evaluating a calcaneal fracture. Bohler angle represents the angle formed by the intersection of a line connecting the highest point of the anterior facet to the highest point of the posterior facet and a line connecting the highest point on the posterior facet to the most superior point on the calcaneal tubercle. The angle is normally within 25 to 40 degrees and decreases with a calcaneus fracture. The critical angle of Gissane is formed by the intersection of a line along the posterior facet and a line drawn anteriorly from this line toward the superior aspect of the anterior facet. An intraarticular fracture with collapse of the posterior facet will result in an increase in this angle (Fig. 5.12).

Nuclear Medicine. Both routine bone scans and labeled white blood cell (WBC) scan should be obtained to evaluate for infection, tumors, or stress fractures. The routine bone scan (such as a Tc 99m bone scan) is used to label areas of increased osteoblastic activity. A more accurate test to diagnose pathologies of the foot is the 3-phase bone scan. In this type of study, the first set of images is obtained immediately following the administration of the radioactive tracer and allows for assessment of the blood flow to the area. The second set of images is obtained typically within minutes of the first set and is used to assess soft tissue activity (to assess for hyperemia such as in cellulitis). The third set of images is obtained several hours after injection of the isotope to evaluate the distribution of the tracer within the osseous structures. A tagged (or labeled) WBC scan can be used to improve the specificity of the bone scan in diagnosing infection.

Computed Tomography (CT). CT scans are particularly useful in the ankle for evaluating talus and calcaneus fractures; fractures of the midfoot; pilon and trimalleolar fractures; navicular stress fractures; evaluation of osteochondral lesions of the talar dome; and tarsal coalitions. For calcaneus fractures, it is important to obtain CT scans that are perpendicular to the posterior facet.

Ultrasound. Particularly useful in evaluating the integrity of the Achilles tendon for rupture or tendinosis. Ultrasound is dependent on the expertise of the examiner, but it is noninvasive and inexpensive.

Magnetic Resonance Imaging (MRI). MRI allows for delineation of the soft tissues and the bone marrow within the foot; it has multiple applications, such as assessing the integrity of ligaments, tendons, osteochondral defects, stress fractures, and inflammatory disorders of the foot. Additional techniques such as fast spin echo (FSE) allow the rapid acquisition of data as well as pulse sequences such as spoiled gradient echo (SPGR), which can be used to evaluate cartilage. Magnetic resonance arthrography can be used to evaluate the osteochondral surface and stability of osteochondral fragments.

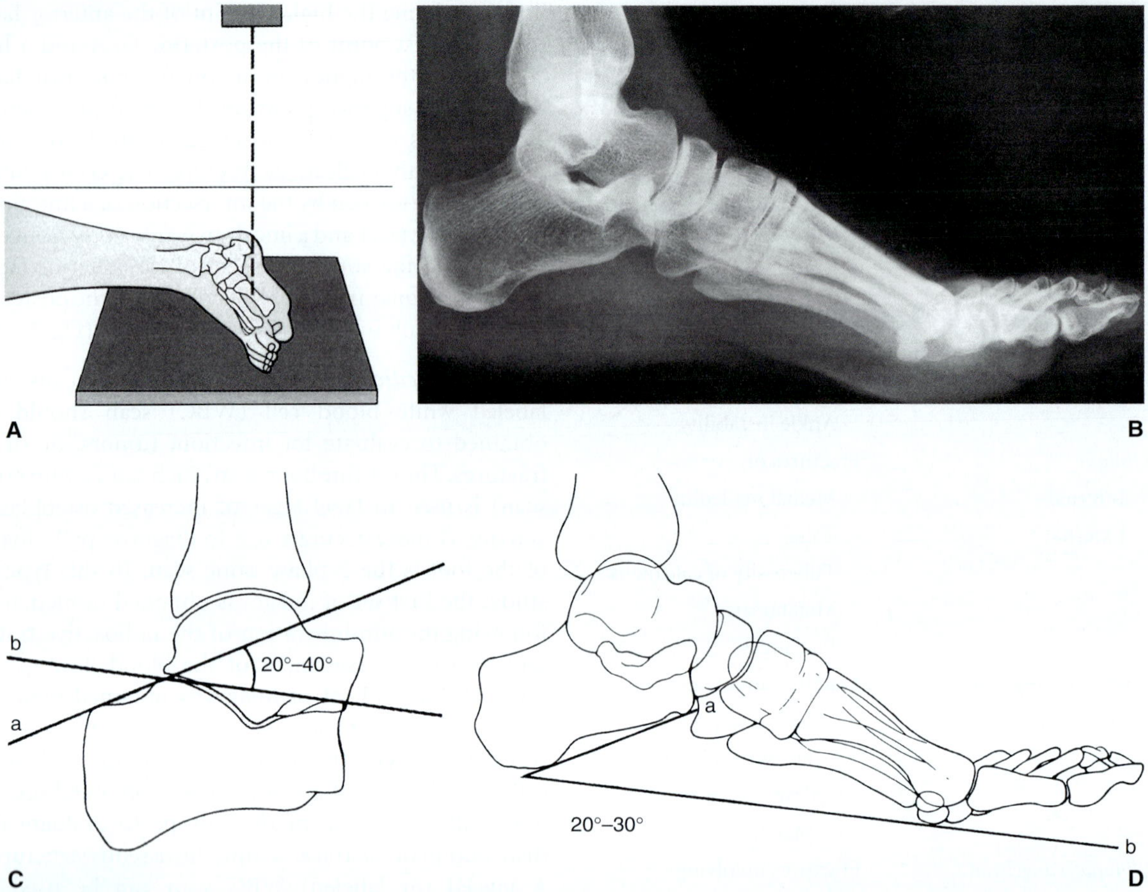

FIGURE 5.12 **(A) For the lateral view of the foot, the patient lies on his or her side with the knee slightly flexed and the lateral aspect of the foot against the film cassette. The central beam is directed vertically to the midtarsus. (B) The lateral radiograph demonstrates the bursal projection, the most prominent feature on the posterior aspect of the calcaneus; the posterior tuberosity where the Achilles tendon inserts; the medial tuberosity on the plantar surface where the plantar fascia inserts; the anterior tuberosity; the anterosuperior spine of the calcaneus; the posterior facet of the subtalar joint; the sustentaculum tali; and the talonavicular and calcaneocuboid articulations. The Chopart and Lisfranc joints are also well visualized. (C) The lateral view also allows evaluation of the angular relationship between the talus and the calcaneus—Boehler angle. This feature is determined by the intersection of a line (a) drawn from the posterosuperior margin of the calcaneal tuberosity (bursal projection) through the tip of the posterior facet of the subtalar joint, and a second line (b) drawn from the tip of the posterior facet through the superior margin of the anterior process of the calcaneus. Normally, this angle ranges between 20 and 40 degrees. (D) Calcaneal pitch is described by the intersection of a line drawn tangentially to the inferior surface of the calcaneus and one drawn along the plantar surface of the foot. (*Source*: Greenspan A. *Orthopaedic Radiology*, 3rd ed. Philadelphia: Lippincott Williams & Wilkins, 2000; 291, Fig. 9.21.)**

V. SHOES AND ORTHOSES

Shoes

Shoes are an important first-line treatment for common orthopedic foot problems. Evaluation of any patient with foot pathology should include an analysis of shoewear. Heels are typically worn on the posterolateral aspect of the shoe, and the insole of the shoe should be examined for forefoot pressure points that can reflect corns, calluses, and toe deformities such as hammer toes. There are 5 parts to the anatomy of a shoe (note: upper refers to the part of the shoe above the outsole): (1) toe box (anterior portion of a shoe's upper), (2) quarter (posterior aspect of a shoe's

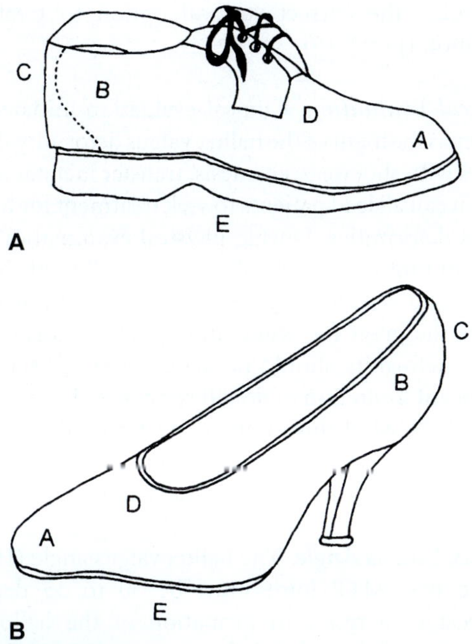

FIGURE 5.13 **Anatomy of the shoe: A, toe Box; B, quarter; C, counter; D, vamp; E, outsole. The insole is hidden inside the shoe and provides the surface on which the foot rests. (*Source: Orthopaedic Knowledge Update Foot and Ankle* 2. American Academy of Orthopaedic Surgeons, 1998; 56, Fig. 1.)**

upper), (3) counter (area at rear of shoe that encases heel and holds it in position), (4) vamp (anterior aspect of shoe's upper), and (5) outsole (bottom part of shoe that contacts ground).

Shoe Modifications. In addressing various foot pathologies, a number of shoe modifications can be made (Fig. 5.13). An orthopedic surgeon should be familiar with such modifications.

- *Rocker bar*—A piece of stiff material that is beveled at its anterior and posterior edges. The bar is placed parallel and slightly posterior to a line from the first to fifth metatarsal heads and extends approximately 0.5 to 1 cm below the level of the sole. This bar functions to shift the rollover point for the foot posterior to the metatarsal heads to transfer pressure away from the metatarsal heads.
- *Metatarsal bar*—A firm material fixed to the plantar aspect of the shoe, also posterior to the metatarsal heads but with a flatter plantar surface than the rocker bar, which is beveled. It provides broader contact with the floor but less resistance with rollover of the foot.

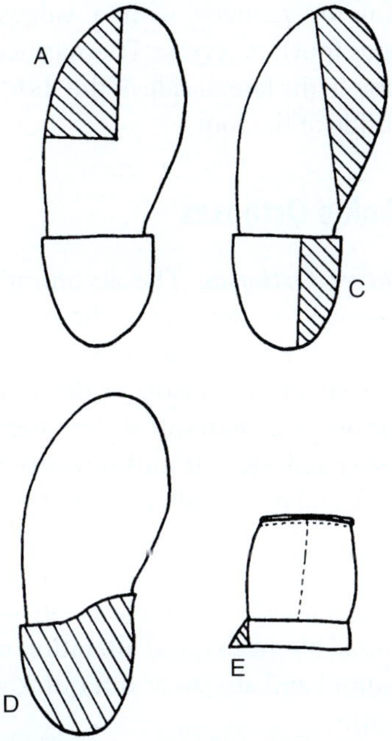

FIGURE 5.14 **Sole modifications. (A) lateral sole wedge shifts the weight from the lateral to medial side of the shoe. (B) medial toe wedge in combination with a medial heel wedge. (C) a Thomas heel. (D) supports the medial longitudinal arch. (E) a lateral heel flare resists eversion. (*Source: Orthopaedic Knowledge Update Foot & Ankle* 2. American Academy of Orthopaedic Surgeons, 1998; 60. Fig. 7.)**

- *Shoe wedge*—The function of a shoe can pronate or supinate the foot depending on if the shoe wedge is placed laterally or medially, respectively. Typically, patients cannot tolerate more than 5 degrees of hindfoot wedging (posting) (Fig. 5.14).
- *Shoe flare*—This sole modification provides a broader, enlarged, weight-bearing surface for the outsole in order to increase stability and resist inversion or eversion of the foot.
- *SACH (solid ankle cushion heel)*—A cushioned heel made of spongy material that is placed between the outer sole and bottom of the heel of the shoe above the outer sole. Its purpose is to reduce stress on the heel and ankle. It is beneficial for patients with tibiotalar arthritis or plantar fasciitis to provide pressure relief.
- *Thomas heel*—A 1-cm anterior extension of the medial border of the heel and can include a medial wedge to support the medial longitudinal arch.

It is useful for patients with a valgus hindfoot (planovalgus foot). A reverse Thomas heel provides an extension to the lateral side of the shoe to support the lateral side of the foot.

Foot and Ankle Orthoses

Accommodative Orthoses. The accommodative orthoses is designed to conform to the contour of the foot to maximize the contact area between the plantar aspect of the foot and the insole of the shoe. Accommodative orthoses are often soft and resilient to reduce contact pressure and shear at the bony prominences of the sole of the foot. They are often prescribed for diabetics or rheumatoid arthritis patients. Accommodative orthoses are often made of Plastazote. However, there are several disadvantages of the Plastazote inserts: they provide minimal biomechanical alteration of the forefoot and hindfoot and also wear out quickly (life span of 2 to 6 months).

Functional Orthoses. Functional orthoses control the way the foot meets the ground and can be used to correct a flexible deformity. They are often semirigid or rigid and are more stable but less flexible than accommodative orthoses. They can biomechanically alter the hindfoot and midfoot but, in the case of semirigid orthoses, can provide cushioning for a rigid deformity of the foot. The main disadvantage of the semirigid orthosis is that it requires skilled molding for fabrication. The materials often used for semirigid orthoses include cross-linked polyethylene foam, cellular rubber, and viscoelastic polymers. Rigid orthoses provide maximum tensile strength and firmness but have limited absorptive properties, potentially adding pressure to bony prominences. They require skilled molding as well.

VI. HALLUX VALGUS

Adult Hallux Valgus

Pathophysiology. Hallux valgus, along with hallux rigidus, are the two most common disorders affecting the first MTP joint. There is a possible maternal inheritance with this condition. A bunion deformity itself refers to a prominent medial eminence, while hallux valgus encompasses a broad range of pathologies that produce a valgus deformity of the great toe. The two are often seen concurrently. Hallux valgus resulting in a valgus deformity of the great toe is a complex deformity for which a multitude of surgical treatments are designed. The orthopedic surgeon must understand the nature of the deformity in order to determine the correct surgical option to treat the condition (Fig. 5.15).

Clinical Evaluation. Clinical evaluation initiates the proper assessment of the hallux valgus deformity. Difficulties with shoewear, cosmesis, transfer metatarsalgia, or pain can all lead patients to seek treatment for hallux valgus deformities. During physical examination, the range of motion (ROM) of the first MTP joint should be assessed, and the degree of restriction of dorsiflexion of the great toe while attempting to correct the valgus deformity should be determined. If there is a significant limitation of dorsiflexion, then it is unlikely that full ROM of this joint will be achieved. Also, the greater the severity of the deformity, the greater the degree of pronation and lateral deviation of the hallux.

Hallux Valgus Angle. The hallux valgus angle (HVA) of the first MTP joint must be 30 to 35 degrees or greater to result in pronation of the hallux. If present, pronation of the hallux will cause the abductor hallucis to move plantar to the flexion–extension axis, leaving the medial capsular structures as the only restraining medial structure preventing lateral deviation of the hallux. The adductor hallucis is unopposed by abductor hallucis once it has moved plantar to the flexion–extension axis, pulling the hallux farther into valgus. The medial capsular ligamentous structures are further stretched, creating a cycle resulting in progressive deformity of the hallux. Should the deforming forces continue, the first metatarsal head will drift medially because of the loss of the crista (the sesamoid ridge on the plantar aspect of the first metatarsal head is eroded because of the laterally directed force from the tibial sesamoid). The fibular sesamoid can displace into the first intermetatarsal space if the deformity is severe enough.

Radiographic Parameters in the Evaluation of Hallux Valgus. Angle, location, relative importance, and normal values are found in Table 5.9.

Conservative Treatment of Hallux Valgus. Most hallux valgus deformities can be treated conservatively with wide, soft shoes that provide an adequate toe box and sufficient insole padding to provide comfort. If concurrent hammer toe deformities exist, extra-depth shoes may be helpful. Stretching leather over bunion can also be beneficial. Only when nonsurgical options are exhausted without success should a surgical option be considered. Furthermore, the surgeon must have a distinct plan to approach the problem, as there are approximately 130 options available.

Surgical Treatment for Hallux Valgus Deformities. There are two main determining factors in deciding

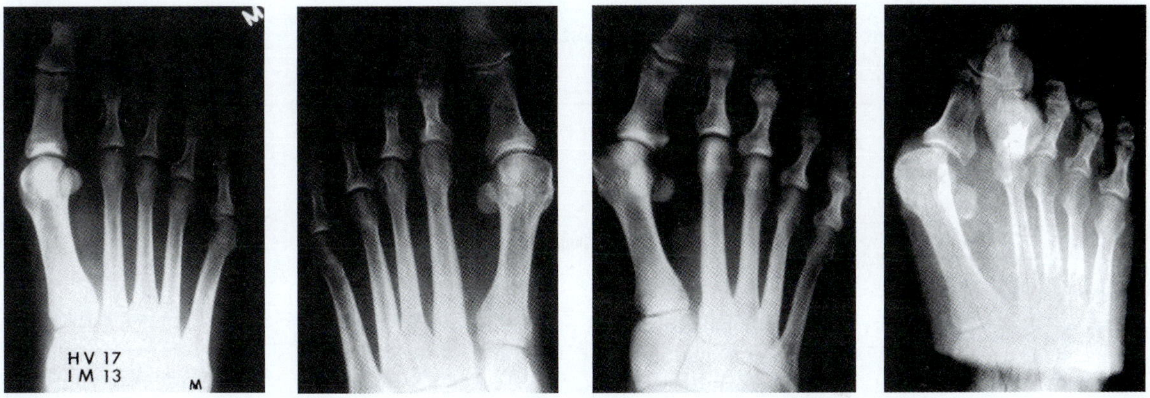

A B C D

FIGURE 5.15 **A spectrum of hallux valgus deformities. (A) Congruent joint with large medial imminence. (B) Mild subluxation of the metatarsophalangeal joint. (C) Moderate subluxation of the metatarsophalangeal joint. (D) Severe subluxation of the metatarsophalangeal joint. Note that as the deformity becomes more severe, the metatarsal head is pushed off the sesamoid sling. The hallux places increasing stress on the second toe as the severity of the deformity increases. (*Source: Orthopaedic Knowledge Update Foot & Ankle* 2. American Academy of Orthopaedic Surgeons, 1998; 123, Fig. 1.)**

the surgical approach to be used: (1) congruence of the MTP joint and (2) presence of arthrosis of the MTP joint (Fig. 5.16). A congruent MTP is defined as the absence of lateral subluxation of the proximal phalanx on the metatarsal head (Fig. 5.17), while an incongruent joint is one that exhibits lateral deviation (subluxation) of the proximal phalanx from the metatarsal head. In general, for patients with a congruent joint, a chevron osteotomy, medial eminence excision, the distal soft tissue procedure, and Akin procedure are all alternatives and are described in detail below. For the incongruent joint, the surgical procedure employed depends on the severity of the deformity as determined radiographically.

Treatment Options for a Congruent Joint. A congruent joint in reference to the MTP joint refers to a joint in which the articular surfaces of the proximal phalanx and metatarsal head are parallel. If the joints are not aligned, then surgical intervention should be targeted toward realigning the articular surfaces to recreate a congruent joint.

Distal Soft Tissue Procedure. This procedure is recommended for the treatment of mild hallux valgus disorders, especially in a middle-aged woman (40 to 50 yrs) who is clinically symptomatic and has an HVA of less than 30 degrees, an intermetatarsal angle (IMA) of less than 13 degrees, valgus of the interphalangeal joint of less than 15 degrees, no arthrosis at the MTP joint, and failed trials of nonoperative therapy. It involves the release of the lateral capsular structures and medial capsular plication. The conjoined adductor hallucis tendon is also released approximately 1.5 cm proximal to the musculotendinous junction, while the distal part of the tendon remains attached to its insertion on the base of the proximal phalanx. In performing the procedure, two incisions should be used with one in line with the first web space and the other along the medial aspect of the joint. A medial eminence, if present, should be excised in line with the first metatarsal. If the first and second metatarsals do not revert back to their original form after the distal soft tissue procedure, then a metatarsal osteotomy should be added. Postoperative care involves the use of a compression dressing that is changed weekly for 8 weeks, with the patient placed in a postoperative hard-soled shoe (wooden-soled shoe) and allowed to be weight bearing as tolerated. ROM exercises (both active and passive) are added at approximately 6 weeks after the operation. Contraindications to this procedure include (1) a deformity with an HVA more than 35 degrees and IMA more than 15 degrees, (2) a deformity with a distal metatarsal articulating (DMA) angle of more than 15 degrees, or (3) arthrosis at the MTP joint. Complications of this procedure include recurrence of the deformity, inadequacy of the lateral release, and poor tissue that results in a weak medial capsular repair.

Akin Procedure (Proximal Phalangeal). This procedure is also indicated for a congruent joint and is primarily used for those joints that have a prominent medial eminence with a DMA angle under 10 degrees. The major indication for the Akin is hallux valgus

TABLE 5.9 Radiographic parameters in the evaluation of hallux valgus

Angle	Location	Importance	Normal
Hallux valgus interphalangeus	Angle between long axis of first proximal phalanx and first distal phalanx	Identifies degree of deformity at IP joint	< 8 deg
Hallux valgus (HVA)	Angle between long axes of first proximal phalanx and first metatarsal, bisecting diaphyses of both bones	Identifies degree of deformity at MTP joint	< 15 deg
MPV (metatarsus primus varus)	Angle between long axes of first metatarsal and first cuneiform	Identifies obliquity vs. subluxation of MTC joint	< 25 deg
First intermetatarsal (IMA)	Angle between long axes of first and second metatarsal, bisecting the shafts of the first and second metatarsals	Not influenced by overresection of medial eminence. Not accurate for post-op evaluation of distal osteotomies	< 10 deg
Distal metatarsal articulating (DMA) angle	Angle of line bisecting metatarsal shaft with line through base of distal articular cartilage cap	Offset of angle is predisposing factor in development of hallux valgus	< 15 deg
Phalangeal articular	Articular angle of base of proximal phalanx in relation to longitudinal axis	Offset of angle is predisposing factor in development of hallux valgus	7–10 deg
Sesamoid position	Position of sesamoids in relation to metatarsal head	Lateral shift of sesamoids (fibular sesamoid can displace completely into first metatarsal space)	Positioned beneath first metatarsal head

interphalangeus, but it is often used as a secondary procedure in the treatment of hallux valgus deformities, often coupled with a distal soft tissue procedure or Chevron osteotomy if either of these two procedures did not correct the deformity adequately. This is especially the case if there is a large DMA angle or hallux valgus interphalangeus is present. The procedure is initiated with a longitudinal incision centered on the medial aspect of the joint from the interphalangeal joint to the distal metaphysis of the metatarsal. A capsular flap is then developed by the reflection of capsular tissue from the medial eminence. Care must be taken to protect the plantar and dorsal digital nerves while developing both the skin and capsular flaps. The medial eminence is resected, and osteotomy is then performed in the proximal metaphyseal region of the proximal phalanx. It is important to make the osteotomy distal to the concavity of the proximal phalanx to avoid violating the MTP joint. Contraindications for this procedure include an incongruent joint and a DMA angle of more than 15 degrees. The typical complication for this procedure is that the deformity will frequently recur, especially if the procedure was to treat an incongruent joint.

Chevron Procedure. The chevron is used to treat a mild deformity (HVA under 30 degrees with an IMA under 13 degrees) and can be performed in conjunction with a distal soft tissue procedure or an Akin, especially if the articular base of proximal phalanx has a lateral slope (large DMA) or if there is a hallux valgus interphalangeus associated with valgus

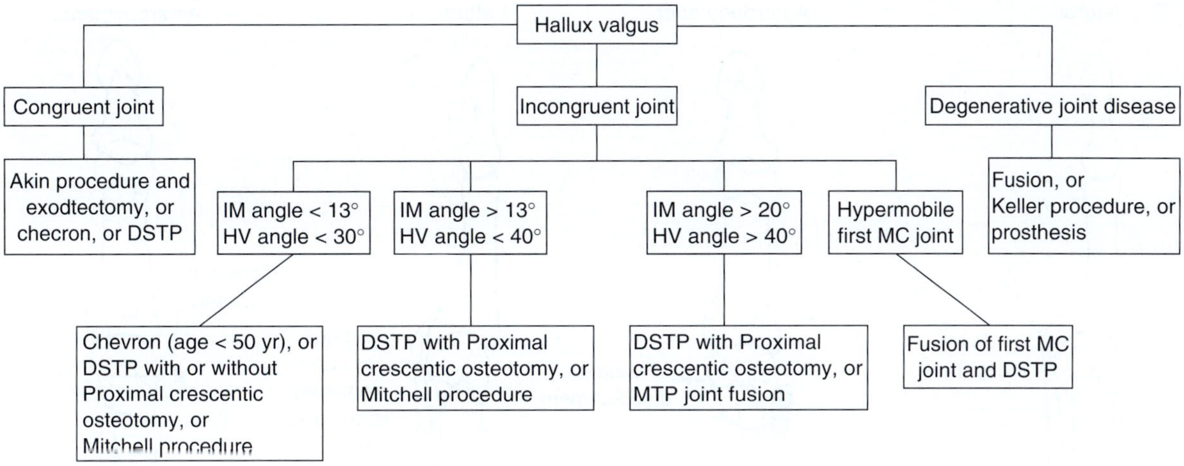

FIGURE 5.16 **Algorithm for selecting the operative approach to treatment of hallux valgus (HV). DSTP, distal soft-tissue procedure; MC, metatarsocuneiform. (*Adapted with permission from* Mann RA. Decision-making in bunion surgery. *Instr Course Lect* 1990;39:3–13; from Mann RA. Disorders of the First Metatarsophalangeal Joint, *JAAOS*, 3(1):34–43;1995, Fig. 6.)**

deformity at the MTP joint. The IMA should still be less than 13 degrees, but the HVA can be as high as 35 degrees, when employing both procedures. A biplanar chevron osteotomy is often employed to gain correction in the axial and coronal planes to treat a large DMA angle. There must be a congruent joint for this procedure to be successful, however (Fig. 5.18). The procedure is started with a medial incision to avoid the dorsal medial cutaneous and plantar cutaneous nerves with skin flaps. The medial eminence is resected, and then a medial-to-lateral drill hole is placed within the center of the metatarsal head to define the apex of the osteotomy. Next, an oscillating saw is used to make a V-shaped osteotomy in the coronal plane, with the angle of the osteotomy being 60 to 90 degrees to provide stability. Once the osteotomy is performed, the distal end is translated approximately 4 to 5 mm laterally and then stabilized to the metatarsal shaft with a 0.062-in Kirschner wire (Figs. 5.19, 5.20, and 5.21). Complications from this procedure involve a potential undercorrection if the deformity is too severe and avascular necrosis of the metatarsal head. Also, the FHL tendon is at risk because it is close to the base of the proximal phalanx. It is important not to do a lateral release to avoid devascularizing the metatarsal head during this procedure.

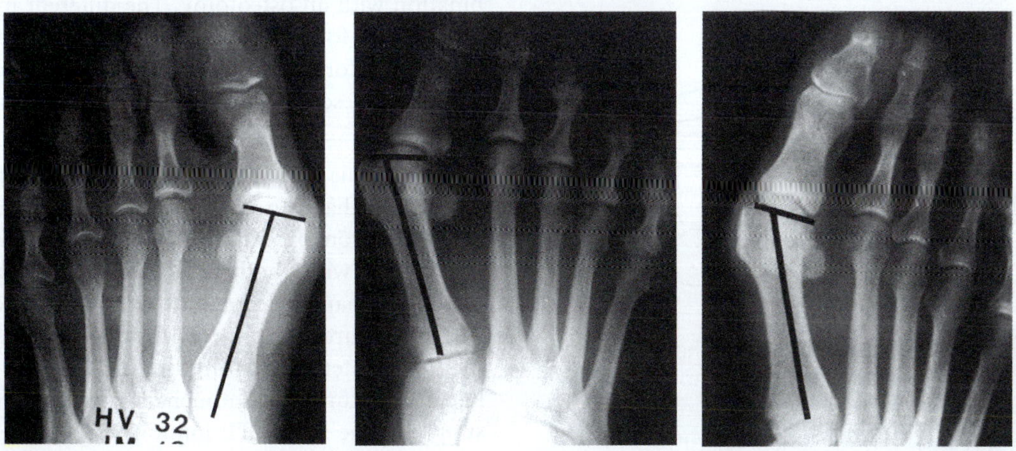

A B C

FIGURE 5.17 **Distal metatarsal articular angle (DMAA). (A) Normal DMAA. (B) Increased DMAA. (C) Increased DMAA with congruent joint. (*Source: Orthopaedic Knowledge Update Foot & Ankle 2,* American Academy of Orthopaedic Surgeons, 1998; 126, Fig. 6.)**

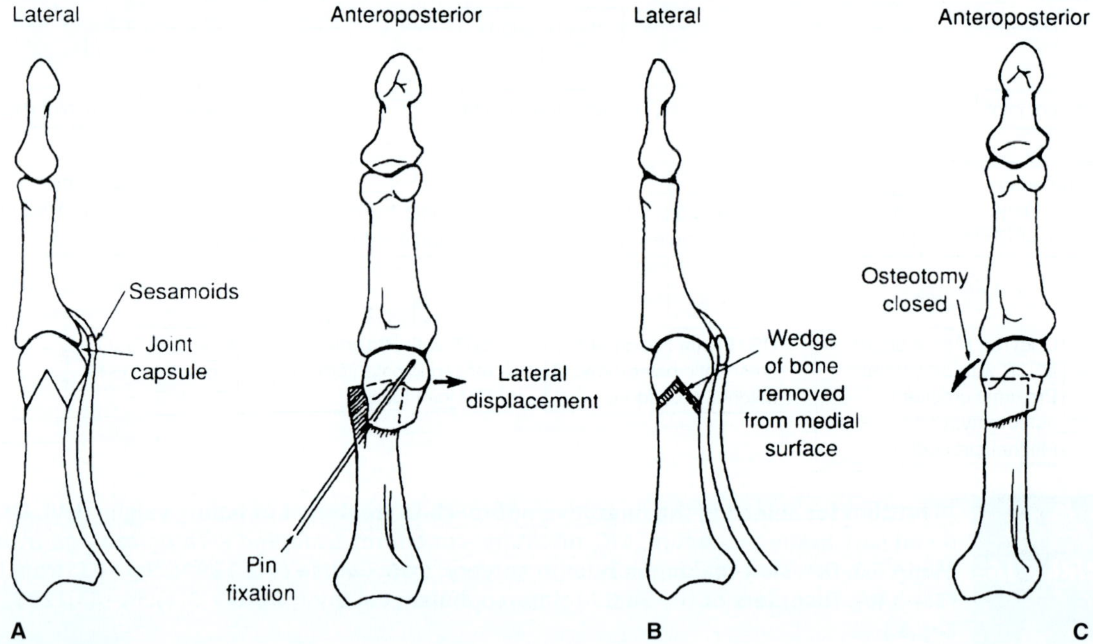

FIGURE 5.18 Biplanar chevron osteotomy to correct a laterally sloping distal metatarsal articular surface. (A) Placement of the normal chevron osteotomy. (B) Removal of medial bone wedge measuring 1 to 3 mm. This permits medial deviation of the articular surface of the metatarsal head, thereby correcting the DMA angle. (C) Distal articular surface after correction. The osteotomy site should be fixed with a pin. (*Source*: Mann RA. Disorders of the First Metatarsophalangeal Joint, *JAAOS* 3(1):34–43; 1995 Fig. 7.)

Treatment Options for Incongruent Joints. When using osteotomies to treat hallux valgus deformities, it is important to correct the intermetatarsal angle deviation while avoiding shortening of the metatarsal and providing stability at the osteotomy site. Primarily, metatarsal osteotomies are performed either proximally or distally; distal osteotomies provide less correction than proximal osteotomies. Generally, the distal osteotomy is used for mild or moderate deformities, and the proximal osteotomy is utilized for more severe deformities. The treatment of an incongruent joint should be directed toward restoring the normal anatomic relationship of the MTP joint and typically involves a distal soft tissue procedure in combination with an osteotomy. The different metatarsal osteotomies for more severe hallux valgus deformities that are performed in combination with a soft tissue release are described in the following sections.

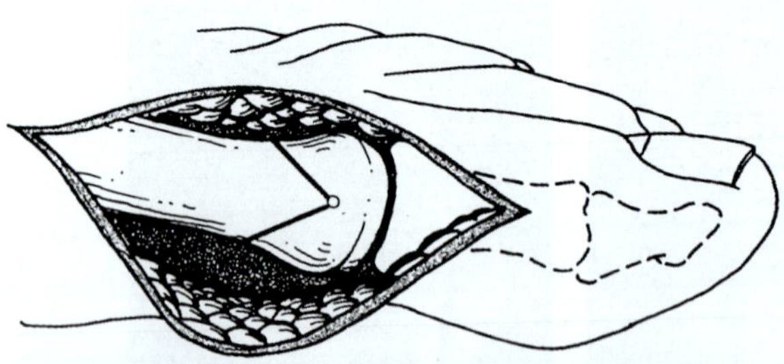

FIGURE 5.19 Illustration of the chevron osteotomy. A drill-hole in the center of the metatarsal head marks the apex of the osteotomy. The angle of the osteotomy cut is 60 to 90 degrees, providing a large, stable surface area. (*Source*: Coughlin MJ. Hallux valgus. *JBJS* 78-A(6):932–966,1996, Fig. 18.)

Mitchell. This is an extracapsular and more proximal osteotomy that can correct larger deformities than can a chevron procedure. The procedure indicated in patients with moderate hallux valgus deformity (HVA less than 40 degrees, IMA less than 20 degrees). The procedure is performed through a dorsomedial incision centered over the first MTP joint with the lateral structures left untouched to preserve the blood supply to the first MTP joint. The medial eminence is removed, and 2 dorsal-to-plantar drill holes are placed in the first metatarsal, with the first drill hole placed 1.5 cm proximal to the articular surface and the second drill hole placed 1 cm proximal and lateral to the first drill hole. A step-cut osteotomy is then performed midway between the two holes, and the

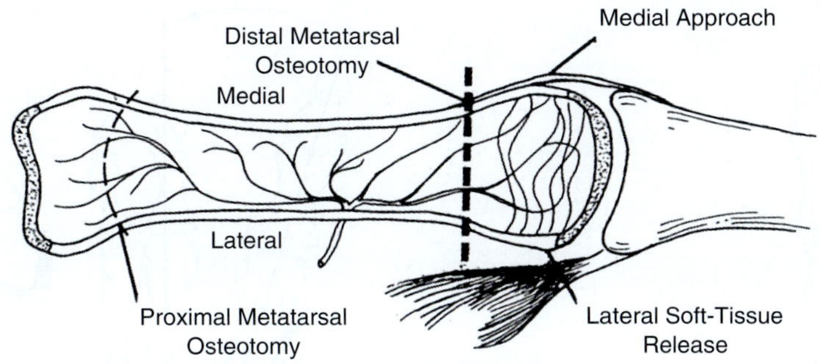

FIGURE 5.20 A dorsal view of the first metatarsal. The vascular supply to the head of the first metatarsal is through the medial and lateral soft tissue structures and medullary vessels. A proximal metatarsal osteotomy does not interrupt the intramedullary supply. A distal metatarsal osteotomy, when combined with an extensive lateral soft tissue release, may compromise the vascularity of the capital fragment. (*Source*: Coughlin MJ, Hallux valgus. *JBJS* 78-A(6):932–966,1996, Fig. 19.)

distal fragment is shifted laterally by 4 to 5 mm, lining up the two drill holes. The osteotomy is then stabilized with either suture through the drill holes and tied dorsally or through Kirschner wires. Malunion is a common complication with this procedure and leads to shortening with subsequent transfer metatarsalgia (Fig. 5.22).

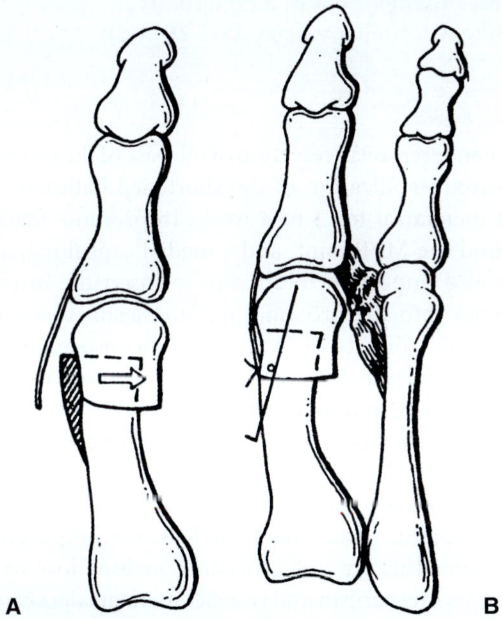

FIGURE 5.21 Illustrations of the chevron osteotomy. (A) The capital fragment is translated laterally (arrow). (B) The osteotomy is stabilized with a Kirschner wire, and the capsule is anchored with a suture through the metaphysis. (*Source*: Coughlin MJ. Hallux valgus. *JBJS* 78-A(6):932–966,1996, Figs. 20.)

Scarf, Ludloff, and Mau Osteotomies. These are also metatarsal osteotomies, with the Mau and Ludloff osteotomies being oblique osteotomies and the Scarf a step-cut osteotomy. The primary indications for these osteotomies are an increased IMA (14 to 18 degrees) with a normal or increased DMA angle.

Proximal Crescentic Osteotomy. This procedure is combined with medial eminence removal, first web-space lateral capsular release, and an adductor tendon release. It is contraindicated for a congruent joint. The osteotomy should be performed though a dorsal incision with the concavity of the osteotomy directed toward the heel followed by internal fixation of the osteotomy. The configuration of osteotomy should be of a dorsal semicircular (crescentic) shape. This procedure is designed to correct an incongruent severe hallux valgus deformity (IMA greater than 20 degrees, HVA of 50 degrees).

First Metatarsocuneiform Arthrodesis (Lapidus Procedure). This procedure can be combined with a distal soft tissue procedure to correct a hallux valgus deformity. It is recommended for patients who have subluxation of the MTP joint associated with a hypermobile MTC joint and a significantly medially slanted articular surface at the first MTC joint. It can also be used as a salvage procedure for a failed hallux valgus surgery. The contraindications for this procedure include a short first ray, arthrosis at the MTP joint, or juvenile hallux valgus with an open epiphysis. It can correct deformities with an IMA greater than 16 degrees and an HVA of at least 30 degrees. The procedure is performed in conjunction with a distal-soft tissue reconstruction. The first MTC joint is exposed through a 3-cm dorsal incision, directly medial to the EHL tendon. Next, a biplanar joint resection is performed to lateralize the first metatarsal (to reduce

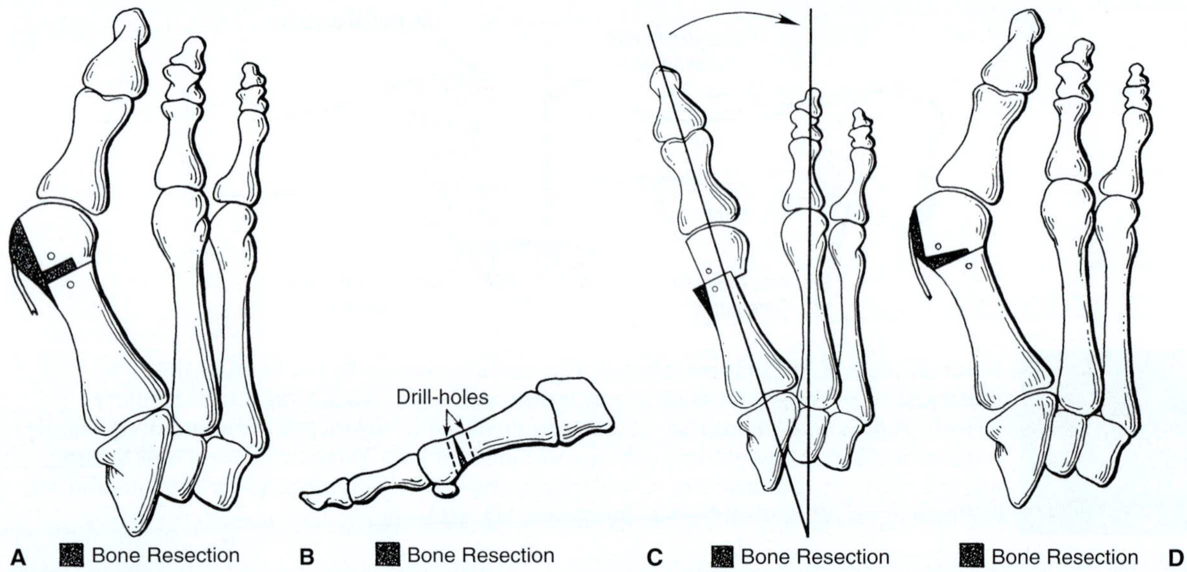

FIGURE 5.22 **Illustrations of a distal metatarsal osteotomy. (A) The proposed osteotomy for a moderate hallux valgus deformity. The width of the lateral shelf determines the amount of displacement of the capital fragment (the wider the shelf, the greater the displacement). (B) More plantar bone is resected at the site of the osteotomy to allow plantar flexion. This diminishes the prevalence of postoperative transfer lesions. (C) After shortening and displacement, the capital fragment is translated laterally (arrow). The medial metatarsal flare is resected. (D) With an increased distal metatarsal articular angle, a trapezoidal resection allows realignment of a congruous metatarsophalangeal joint. (*Source*: Coughlin MJ. Hallux valgus. *JBJS* 78-A(6): 932–966,1996, Figs. 23-A through D.)**

the IMA), along with flexing the first ray plantarly to reduce the likelihood of transfer metatarsalgia. The first metatarsal should then be aligned in neutral rotation to the medial cuneiform, with the joint bone grafted with autogenous cancellous bone from the distal tibia or iliac crest. The fusion can be fixed with 3.5-mm, fully threaded lag screws or 4.0-mm cancellous screws (typically two screws are used). The procedure is coupled with medial eminence removal, first web-space release of adductor hallucis, and lateral capsule release (Fig. 5.23).

Treatment Options for Arthritic Joints. With the presence of advanced arthritis, the treatment options change. The main goal with treatment in this condition is to relieve the pain of the arthritic deformity and secondarily to reduce the degree of the deformity. Simply realigning an arthritic joint will not treat the arthritis. Therefore, for advanced arthritis, MTP arthrodesis and in select cases, resection arthroplasty are advocated.

Resection Arthroplasty (Keller). This procedure is useful for patients with fewer functional demands who have an advanced hallux valgus deformity coupled with an arthritic joint. The procedure is coupled with medial eminence removal, resection of the base of the proximal phalanx, stabilization of the shortened hallux on the first metatarsal for 3 to 4 weeks to promote scarring around the MTP joint, and a medial capsulorrhaphy. It is also important to attempt to insert the intrinsic muscles into the proximal phalanx again to avoid a cock-up deformity of the hallux. This procedure will correct moderate to severe a hallux valgus (HVA of 30 to 45 degrees) and mild to moderate IMA (less than 14 degrees). A Keller can also be used to reduce the stress under the hallux by resecting the base of the proximal phalanx and shortening the toe and can be used to treat a neuropathic ulcer under the hallux. Complications seen after this type of procedure include loss of the windlass mechanism and transfer metatarsalgia caused by shortening of the hallux and recurrence of the deformity.

MTP Arthrodesis. MTP arthrodesis is an excellent pain-relieving procedure in patients who have a severe hallux valgus deformity, significant arthritis of the first MTP joint with articular symptoms, and possible dislocation of the MTP joint that is functionally incapacitating. It is an excellent procedure for patients with rheumatoid arthritis, those with severe hallux valgus deformities (HVA greater than

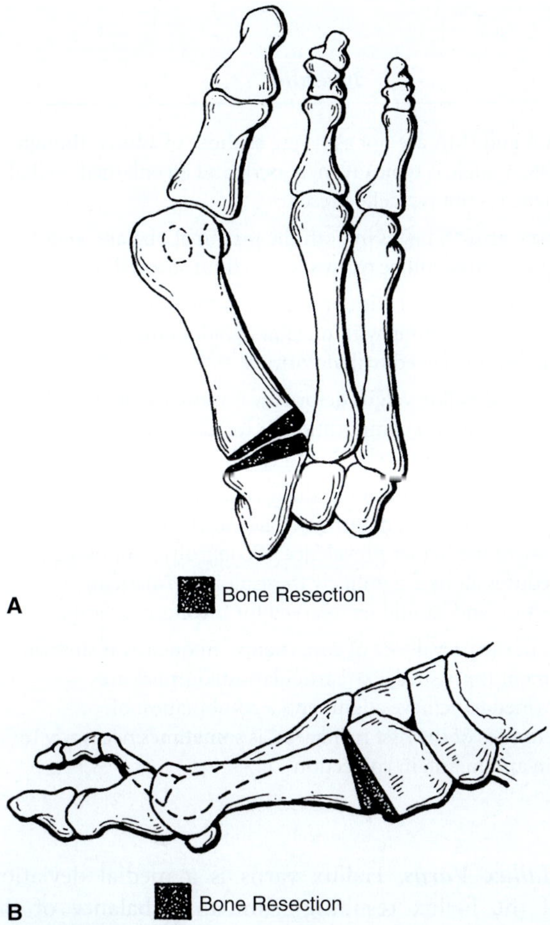

FIGURE 5.23 Illustrations of an arthrodesis of the first metatarsocuneiform joint. (A) Minimum resection of the articular surface and subchondral bone decreases the first–second intermetatarsal angle. (B) Slightly more bone is resected on the plantar surface to achieve plantar flexion at the site of the arthrodesis. (*Source*: Coughlin MJ. Hallux valgus. *JBJS* 78 A(6):932–966,1996, Figs. 29-A, B.)

40 degrees), a failed Silastic implant, and also in patients with neuromuscular disorders (cerebral palsy, Down syndrome). The IMA may spontaneously reduce a few degrees after arthrodesis (approximately 4 to 5 degrees). During this procedure, alignment is critical, and the joint should be placed in 15 degrees of dorsiflexion in relation to the floor, 15 degrees of valgus with no rotation. A dorsal plate should be used to maintain rigid internal fixation. Complications of this procedure include nonunion, transfer metatarsalgia, and malalignment of the arthrodesis.

Juvenile and Adolescent Hallux Valgus

The juvenile hallux valgus is different than the adult hallux valgus, and thus the treatment algorithms for this disorder are different. It is, by definition, a hallux valgus deformity that occurs during early adolescent or adolescent years. Generally, it is recommended that surgery be delayed until the patient reaches skeletal maturity. The factors involved that make it a distinct entity from adult hallux valgus are listed in Table 5.10.

Distal Soft Tissue Realignment. As stated previously, distal soft tissue realignment is an intraarticular procedure that is reserved for an incongruent joint. It is indicated for a mild hallux valgus deformity with an incongruent joint. Note that performing a distal soft-tissue procedure on a congruent joint can result in incongruency.

Chevron Distal First Metatarsal Osteotomy. This procedure is reserved for those with a mild hallux valgus deformity, typically with an HVA of less than 25 degrees and an IMA of less than 13 degrees. This osteotomy also affords the opportunity to correct excessive DMA angle by performing a medial closing-wedge osteotomy if a small (1 to 3 mm) wedge is removed medially to medialize the articular surface.

Mitchell Osteotomy. This procedure is not commonly used because of the risk of transfer metatarsalgia that can occur in up to 40% of cases. Shortening of the first metatarsal, which can be present in adolescents, can also be achieved. It is not commonly employed in adolescents, however.

Double and Triple First Metatarsal Osteotomies. These procedures have been advocated recently because of the high prevalence of congruency seen in juvenile hallux valgus deformities. They can correct an excessive DMA angle and are useful when the IMA is 13 to 14 degrees or more and the DMA angle is significant, especially 20 degrees or greater. As stated previously, to correct a significant DMA angle, a medial closing-wedge distal osteotomy should be performed.

First Cuneiform Osteotomy. This procedure has been advocated to treat a juvenile hallux valgus deformity with a large IMA in the presence of an open first metatarsal epiphysis along with medial cuneiform obliquity. Further indications include ligamentous laxity and a hypermobile first ray. It is an opening-wedge osteotomy that can achieve increased length in the first ray and can be performed in conjunction with shortening osteotomies of the proximal phalanx (Akin) or distal metatarsal.

TABLE 5.10 Adult versus juvenile hallux valgus

Adult	*Juvenile*
HVA and IMA are typically greater than in juveniles with an enlarged medial eminence	The HVA and IMA are not as severe as those of adults (though the DMA angle is typically increased) and an enlarged medial eminence is not typically present
Growth plates are closed	Epiphyseal growth plates in both the proximal phalanx and metatarsal may still be open and can limit surgical options
Hypermobile flatfoot is not frequently observed with adult hallux valgus	A hypermobile flatfoot with pronation of the foot during weight bearing, along with metatarsus adductus, is frequently associated with deformity
Recurrence is not as frequent as in the juvenile population	Recurrence of hallux valgus deformity is more frequent and is the most common complication in treating juvenile hallux valgus. It is thought to be due to epiphyseal overgrowth.
Incongruity is more of a factor and dictates treatment	Congruity is more common in the juvenile population, and as such, a hallux valgus deformity is less likely to progress; because of the higher prevalence of congruity, soft tissue procedures alone are unlikely to result in permanent correction and should be reserved for incongruent joints
Distal soft tissue procedures are more frequently employed owing to the higher prevalence of incongruity	Because of the prevalence of congruence, frequently if surgical treatment is pursued, extraarticular osteotomies are performed to achieve alignment; a combination of osteotomies of the first metatarsal is sometimes necessary to obtain and maintain correction

VII. GREAT TOE INJURIES

Sesamoid Injuries of the Hallux. The hallucal sesamoids (medial and lateral) are located within the tendon of the FHB muscle, and they absorb weight-bearing pressure, reduce friction, and protect tendons. The adductor hallucis brevis, metatarsal ligament, and FDB are attached to the fibular sesamoid. The abductor hallucis brevis and FDB are attached to the tibial sesamoid. The tibial sesamoid is the more frequently injured of the two because of its central location beneath first metatarsal head. The most common mechanisms of sesamoidal injury are hyperextension and axial loading that typically result in a fracture. Bipartite tibial sesamoid is present in 10% of population, and in 25% of these, it is bilateral. Patients complain of pain as the hallux extends in the terminal part of the stance phase of gait. The medial oblique (sesamoid) view is helpful for evaluating the tibial sesamoid, and axial sesamoid should be obtained if a pathological condition of the fibular sesamoid is suspected. The initial treatment should consist of NSAIDs, full-length shoe orthoses with a metatarsal pad, a metatarsal bar on the sole of the shoe, or cast immobilization. Excision of both sesamoids should be avoided.

Hallux Varus. Hallux varus is a medial deviation of the hallux resulting from an imbalance of the dynamic and static forces about the first MTP joint. Most commonly seen as a complication of hallux valgus surgery (excessive lateral soft-tissue release), it can also be inflammatory, neurogenic, or posttraumatic in origin as well. The deformity itself can range from mild to severe and can be flexible or fixed if advanced. Symptoms depend on the degree of severity of the disorder. Most commonly, however, the deformity is cosmetic and causes difficulties with footwear. Mild deformities can be treated with well-fitting shoes, taping, or bracing. Performing a medial capsular lengthening can also serve as a soft tissue reconstruction for more severe conditions due to soft tissue imbalance. Additional soft tissue procedures performed in conjunction with a capsular lengthening are an EHL transfer to the base of the proximal phalanx or rerouting the EHB tendon deep to the transverse metatarsal ligament and securing it to the metatarsal shaft. If the joint is arthritic, then an MTP fusion can be pursued.

Claw Hallux. Similar to a claw toe, a claw hallux is a hyperextension of the MTP joint with a concurrent flexion deformity of the interphalangeal joint, resulting in an intrinsic minus deformity. It is most commonly associated with neuromuscular disorders leading to a muscular imbalance between the intrinsic flexors and the extensors around the MTP joint. Treatment depends on the severity of the disorder, with nonsurgical treatment centered on footwear modification and surgical options involving EHL lengthening or EHB tendon release. Rigid deformities with arthritis should be fused.

Turf Toe. The mechanism for this condition is a hyperextension injury in which the plantar plate avulses from the proximal phalanx and the proximal phalanx is compressed against the dorsal aspect of the first metatarsal head. Football players have the highest incidence of turf toe. The treatment for this disorder includes taping, casting, and possible surgical repair of the plantar plate. Surgical repair is seldom indicated unless the joint is rendered unstable from the injury or a fracture is present.

VIII. LESSER TOE DEFORMITIES AND MTP JOINT DISORDERS

Hammer and Claw Toe Deformities. Both hammer toe and claw toe result from intrinsic and extrinsic muscle imbalance and have a multitude of causes (trauma, inflammation, neurologic disorders). These two entities are differentiated from each other by the fact that in a claw toe deformity, MTP joint hyperextension is the primary pathology, with any resultant deformity (namely flexion) at the proximal interphalangeal (PIP) or distal interphalangeal (DIP) joint secondary to chronic extension of the MTP joint (Fig. 5.24). Hammer toe deformity is primarily a flexion deformity of the PIP joint and can be accompanied by an extended MTP joint. However, there is always hyperextension of the MTP joint in claw toe, which is what differentiates it from a hammer toe. With the chronic extension at the MTP joint, the EDL tendon is unable to extend the PIP and DIP joints, allowing the FDS and FDP tendons to flex the DIP and PIP joints. However, in both claw and hammer toes, the extension of the MTP joint is accompanied by dorsal subluxation of the interossei, rendering them unable to flex the MTP joint and further exaggerating the deformity. A neurologic abnormality should be suspected if all four lesser toes have claw toe deformity.

Synovitis of the Second MTP Joint. Synovitis of the second MTP joint is the most common cause of a claw or hammer toe deformity, usually due to overuse but sometimes caused by an excessively long second metatarsal, a hypermobile first ray, or a varus stress from the first metatarsal that places an increased load on second MTP joint. Plantar plate insufficiency develops, leading to dorsal translation of the proximal phalanx, carrying the interossei and lumbrical tendons. This causes the intrinsic muscle–tendon units to migrate dorsal to the instant centers of rotation of the metatarsal head and results in the loss of the main flexion force on the MTP joint, leading to hyperextension.

Treatment. Treatment of both hammer and claw toes is geared toward accommodative shoewear, stretching exercises, and orthotic devices (such as metatarsal pads). In regards to surgical options, fixed hammer toes are treated with a DuVries resection arthroplasty of the proximal phalanx. Flexible hammer toes are secondary to contractures of the FDL. These are treated with a DuVries or release of the FDL. A Girdlestone flexor tendon transfer can also be considered. Claw toes can be treated with a release of the EDB and lengthening of the EDL and flexor-to-extensor tendon transfer if the deformity is flexible. If fixed, a resection arthroplasty of the proximal phalanx should be performed.

Cross-Over Toe Deformity. This deformity results from of incompetence of the plantar plate, which

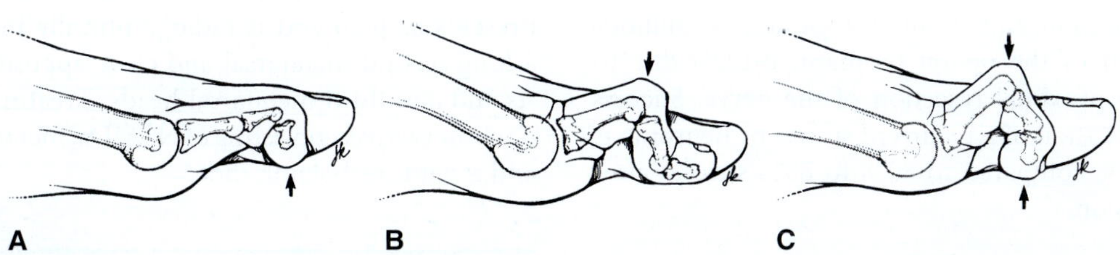

FIGURE 5.24 (A) Mallet toe. (B) Hammer toe. (C) Claw toe. (*Source*: Alexander IJ (ed.), *The Foot: Examination and Diagnosis*. New York: Churchill Livingstone, 1990; 68–71.)

causes dorsal instability of the PIP joint. Further imbalance is produced by the adduction moment of the dorsal interossei and the lumbrical that results in a net adduction moment and leads to attrition of the lateral capsular structures. If the deformity is mild, it can be treated with a flexor-to-extensor tendon transfer, but if severe, a metatarsal osteotomy or resection of the head of the proximal phalanx may be necessary.

Mallet Toe. Mallet toe is an isolated flexion deformity of the DIP joint. It can occur as an isolated lesser-toe deformity or in conjunction with claw toe. Typically, it is treated with resection of the condyles of the middle phalanx with or without an FDL release.

Interdigital Neuroma (IDN). The etiology of this lesion is likely that of degenerative changes with repetitive trauma to the interdigital nerve from the transverse intermetatarsal ligament. Perineural fibrosis has been seen in association with this condition. The common digital nerve to the third web space is anatomically enlarged because it receives contributions from the medial-most branch of the lateral plantar nerve and the lateral-most branch of medial plantar nerve (MPN) proximal to the deep transverse ligament. IDN are most commonly seen in the third web space. Removing shoewear and resting the foot often relieve the pain of an IDN. It is important to note that this is in contrast to hallux rigidus in which pain is exacerbated by removing the shoe (patients need a rigid surface such as a steel shank to prevent dorsiflexion of the arthritic joint). The most common physical finding is web space tenderness that is increased by palpation while also displacing metatarsals toward one another. Nonsurgical treatment includes the use of a wide toe box with a firm sole, a metatarsal pad, a metatarsal bar, and possibly steroids. Surgical treatment, if necessary, involves resection of the neuroma 2 to 3 cm proximal to the deep transverse ligament through a dorsal incision. Release of the deep transverse ligament has also been advocated but may not completely alleviate the condition. Recurrence of IDN is common and is often a glioma or bulbous enlargement of the neural remnant, usually due to inadequate proximal resection of the nerve. Success rate after excision of a recurrent stump or neuroma is 65% to 75% compared to 80% to 85% success after initial excision.

Hyperkeratotic Lesions. Hyperkeratotic lesions include the following:

- *Hard corns (heloma durum)*—Typically caused by poorly fitting shoes and toe deformities. Most commonly, they are located over the dorsolateral aspect of the fifth toe PIP.
- *Soft corns (heloma molle)*—Found between fourth and fifth toes deep in the interdigital web space and are soft because of the moist environment of this area.
- *Plantar foot corns*—Intractable plantar keratosis, discrete, under the plantar distal metatarsal condyles; initial treatment should consist of shaving of the callus and using an orthoses to reduce the pressure under the metatarsal condyle.
- *Seed corns*—Invagination of the epithelium.
- *Diffuse corns*—Secondary to short first or long second metatarsal shafts.

Bunionette/Tailor Bunion. A bunionette is an abnormal prominence of the fifth metatarsal head that is usually seen with medial deviation of the fifth toe. There are three types:

- *Enlarged fifth metatarsal head/lateral condyle*—Treat with resection or chevron.
- *Lateral bowing of the fifth metatarsal*—Treat with distal metatarsal osteotomy (chevron). Of note, the distal osteotomy (such as a chevron) will correct only about 1 degree in the IMA for every 1 mm of translation and cannot compensate for a large IMA. For deformities with a larger IMA, a more proximal diaphyseal shaft osteotomy should be performed.
- *Wide Fourth or Fifth Metatarsal angle*— Normal angle is approximately 6 to 8 degrees. Treat with fifth metatarsal osteotomy.

Freiberg Infarction. Freiberg infarction is an osteochondrosis of one of the lesser metatarsal heads, usually the second, that presents with activity-related pain. It is thought to be due to repetitive trauma with avascular necrosis (AVN) of the metatarsal head. Examination can reveal tenderness at the MTP joint. Treatment varies from metatarsal padding to a walking cast to allow healing to occur. Surgery (joint débridement and decompression) is recommended for severe conditions.

Second MTP Tenosynovitis. This condition often presents as pain and is radiographically indicated by a long second metatarsal and close apposition of the second and third metatarsal heads. Treatment should be conservative, consisting of NSAIDs, metatarsal pads, and a rigid steel-shank shoe.

IX. NEUROLOGICAL DISORDERS

Nerve Compression Disorders

Nerves of the foot and ankle are illustrated in Figure 5.25.

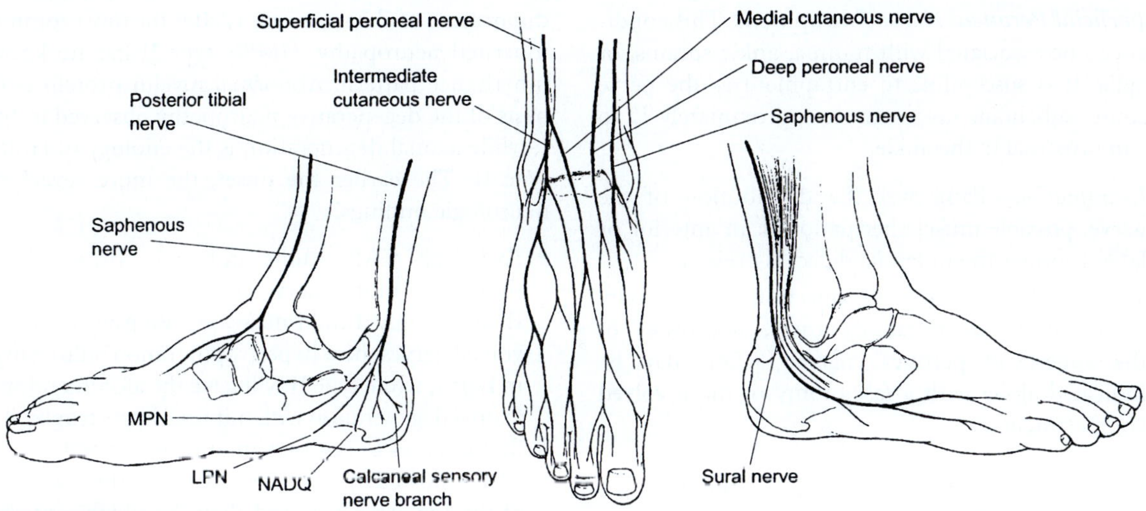

FIGURE 5.25 **Anatomy of the principal nerves crossing the ankle into the foot (LPN, lateral plantar nerve; MPN, medial plantar nerve; NADQ, nerve to abductor digiti quinti). (*Source*: Beskin JL. Nerve entrapment syndromes of the foot and ankle. *JAAOS* 595:261–269,1997, Fig. 1.)**

Tarsal Tunnel Syndrome (TTS). Any structure within the flexor retinaculum can cause TTS. Symptoms can be exacerbated by activity, but patients often state that pain is worse at night or at rest. Patients also frequently complain of a burning-type pain or radiation of pain proximally or distally into the sole of the foot. A patient with symptoms of an IDN should be examined for posterior tibial nerve (PTN) tenderness beneath the flexor retinaculum to assess for a reproduction of the pain, paresthesias, or to elicit tenderness, all of which could be present. Subtalar motion should be evaluated, and a middle facet coalition (tarsal coalition) should be suspected if TTS coexists with limitation of subtalar motion. TTS is a clinical diagnosis; however, if a space-occupying lesion is suspected, plain radiographs (for bony lesions) and/or MRI can be obtained.

- *Conservative treatment*—Should be employed for those patients without evidence of a space-occupying lesion. NSAIDs, immobilization, and local steroid injections and orthotics can be tried (the latter if there is a structural hindfoot abnormality). Patients with space-occupying lesions (tumor, ganglion, anomalous muscle), previous hindfoot trauma, a fixed valgus hindfoot deformity, positive EMG findings (those patients with a distal motor latency greater than 7.0 msec, prolonged sensory latency greater than 2.3 msec, or reduced EMG amplitudes in the abductor hallucis or abductor digiti minimi muscles) are the best candidates for surgery.
- *Surgical treatment*—Consists of release of the tarsal tunnel (flexor retinaculum) proximally over the PTN. Those with space-occupying lesions benefit most from surgery. It is important to release not only the flexor retinaculum but also the deep investing fascia of the lower leg that is contiguous with the superior border of the retinaculum and the deep fascia of the abductor hallucis brevis. However, while the extent of distal release has been debated, an inadequate distal release is a potential cause of failure for this operation.
- *Recurrence*—The most common etiology of recurrence of TTS is an inadequate release. Repeat tarsal tunnel release generally is not indicated unless there is a space-occupying lesion.

Anterior Tarsal Tunnel Syndrome. Anterior TTS is an entrapment neuropathy of the DPN by the distal margin of the inferior extensor retinaculum. The tendon of EHB, ganglia, and degenerative osteophytes are also sources of compression. Osteophytes and often ganglion cysts from degenerative and attritional ligamentous or capsular injury trap the nerve between the retinaculum and osteophyte and/or ganglion.

- *Examination*—Patients most commonly will have dysesthesias and paresthesias on the dorsum of the foot in the distribution of the DPN. Examination should involve palpation and percussion of the nerve.
- *Conservative treatment*—Should include the use of a well-padded tongue on the shoe or full-length rocker-sole steel shank, especially in patients with midfoot degenerative joint disease (DJD).
- *Surgery*—Locate the DPN distally lateral to the EHB tendon, trace proximally, and release all fascial and retinacular restraints.

Superficial Peroneal Nerve Entrapment. This condition can be associated with trauma, ankle sprains, or ganglia. It is susceptible to entrapment as the nerve becomes subcutaneous in nature approximately 12 to 15 cm proximal to the ankle.

- *Examination*—Pain over the distribution of the nerve, possible muscle herniation if an anterior or lateral compartment fascial defect is present.
- *Treatment*—Local steroid injection and activity modification. In refractory cases, neurolysis of the superficial peroneal nerve (SPN) may be indicated along with a fasciotomy of the involved compartments.

Sural Nerve Entrapment. Sural nerve entrapment is a rare entrapment disorder and can result from trauma (calcaneus, fifth metatarsal, or lateral malleolus) or ganglion. Nonsurgical therapy involves steroid injections and shoewear modification. Decompression of the nerve can also be performed.

Neuromuscular Disorders

Upper Motor Neuron Injury. CVA patients develop an equinovarus deformity of the ankle and foot and have resultant spasticity. As a result, spasticity management consisting of early splinting and physical therapy is indicated. EMG biofeedback has also been used to help improve spasticity. Pharmacologic therapy can also be pursued, with dantrolene or botulinum (Botox) injections often used to treat spasticity. Of note, CVAs occurring in the middle cerebral artery distribution tend to affect the distal extremities more significantly than CVAs in other distributions. In children, the most common upper motor neuron (UMN) injury is cerebral palsy. An important rule to remember regarding surgical intervention in patients with UMN injury–mediated spasticity is that surgery should not be performed for at least 6 months postinjury. For patients with severe spasticity, 12 to 18 months should be allowed for recovery before resorting to surgery. If TAL (tendoachilles lengthening) does not allow satisfactory bracing of the equinovarus deformity, a split anterior tibial tendon transfer (SPLATT) to the lateral aspect of midfoot is indicated. The posterior tibial tendon, although the strongest invertor of the hindfoot, rarely is overreactive in the stance phase of gait; if, however, this occurs, it should be transferred through the interosseous membrane and attached anteriorly to the midfoot. The SPLATT and posterior tibial tendon transfer should not be performed simultaneously.

Charcot-Marie-Tooth Disease (Hereditary Motor Sensory Neuropathy [HMSN]). The AD form of Charcot-Marie-Tooth disease is HMSN type I with a duplication of chromosome 17. It is the most common inherited neuropathy. HMSN type II has no known inheritance pattern. Abnormal myelin protein is the basis of the degenerative neuropathy observed in type I, while axonal degeneration is the etiology of HMSN type II. The earlier the onset, the more severe the neurologic findings.

- *Pathology*—EMG studies in type I show significant slowing of motor nerve conduction velocity (type II shows only a mild decrease). Biopsies of the involved nerves show hypertrophic onion bulb changes in type I, while type II will have the aforementioned axonal degeneration with minimal hypertrophy. The first muscles to atrophy are intrinsic muscles of the foot, followed by the peroneus brevis, then weakness of the toe extensors, and then the tibialis anterior. In addition, the EDB and EHB are atrophied. This atrophy leads to symmetrical elevation of the arches, a plantarflexed first ray, hindfoot varus, claw toes, decreased ankle jerks, and flatfoot or toe-heel gait. The claw toe deformity is due to the spasticity of the extrinsic flexor tendon, resulting in hyperflexion at the PIP and DIP joints. This results in the classic pes cavus deformity and, coupled with the unabated action of the posterior compartment, equinus develops also. The peroneus longus is spared. The cardinal muscle imbalance is between the tibialis anterior and peroneus longus, which leads to a plantarflexed first ray.
- *Examination*—Patients with Charcot-Marie-Tooth disease have an awkward gait (marionette gait), painful callosities beneath the metatarsal heads from clawed toes, and ankle instability (Fig. 5.26). Toe extensors are recruited in the swing phase of gait as ankle dorsiflexors due to weak tibialis anterior. The examiner must document flexibility of all components: hindfoot varus, forefoot pronation, adduction, and the plantarflexed first ray. Flexibility is assessed by the Coleman block test, which involves placing the patient's foot on a 1-inch thick wooden block, with the heel and lateral border of the foot placed on the block. The first through third metatarsals are allowed to pronate, and the plantarflexed first metatarsal is allowed to hang off the side of the block. If flexible, the hindfoot deformity will correct.
- *Conservative treatment*—Indicated for patients with minimal symptoms and consists of a molded orthoses with cushioning of the forefoot. Also, the plantarflexed first ray can be accommodated by using lateral forefoot and lateral heel wedges to allow flexion of the first metatarsal.
- *Surgical treatment*—
  - If the *varus heel* is correctable on the Coleman block test (indicating that the foot is supple), then a plantar fascia release along with elevation

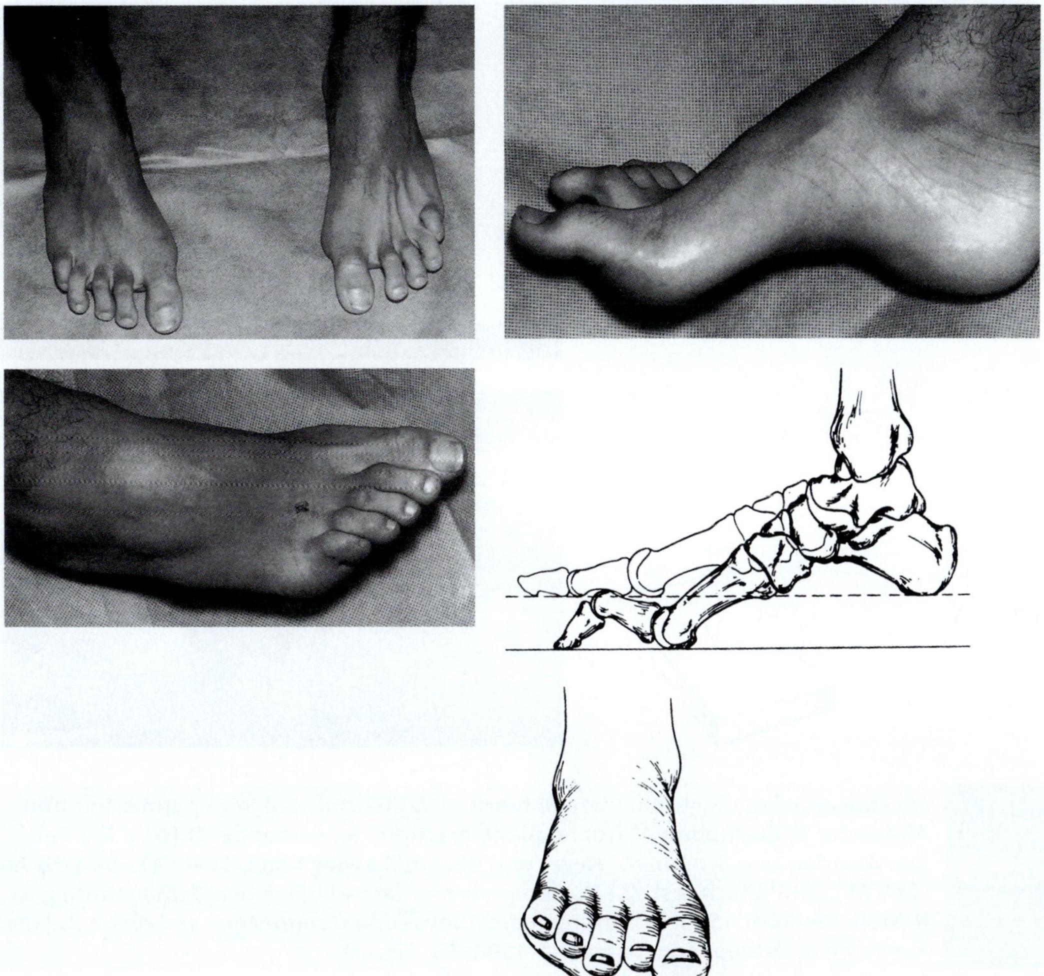

A B C D

FIGURE 5.26 **(A–C) Photographs of feet of young adult male with Charcot-Marie-Tooth disease, showing the cavus foot and claw toe deformities. Note the high arch associated with the cavus foot. There is also plantar flexion of the first ray. Claw toes are characterized by extension at the metatarsophalangeal joints and flexion at the proximal and distal interphalangeal joints. (D) Illustration of cavus foot with plantar flexion of the first ray and claw toes. (D modified from Richardson GE. Neurogenic disorders. In: Canale ST (ed.), *Campbell's Operative Orthopaedics*. St. Louis: Mosby, 1998:1828.) (*Source*: Thordarson DB. *Foot and Ankle*. Philadelphia: Lippincott Williams & Wilkins, 2004; 67 Fig. 3–18.)**

of the first metatarsal by a basilar closing-wedge osteotomy, transfer of the peroneus longus to the peroneus brevis (to compensate for the weakened peroneus brevis), and correction of the claw toes are performed (Fig. 5.27).

- Correction of the *claw toes* is performed using flexor-to-extensor tendon transfers (Girdlestone-Taylor procedure) and extensor tendon lengthenings, or tenotomy if the claw toes are flexible, or resection of the head and neck of the proximal phalanges if fixed.
- The *clawed hallux* can be treated with a Jones procedure (fusion of the interphalangeal joint with subsequent transfer of the EHL to the first metatarsal).
- A *fixed varus deformity* (does not correct with Coleman block test) with fixed cavus or equinocavovarus requires a hindfoot stabilization procedure such as a triple arthrodesis or closing-wedge calcaneal osteotomy with or without lateral translation of the calcaneal tuberosity and subsequent transfer of the tibialis posterior through interosseous membrane to the midfoot.
- The presence of significant *hindfoot arthritis* is also an indication to perform a triple arthrodesis.

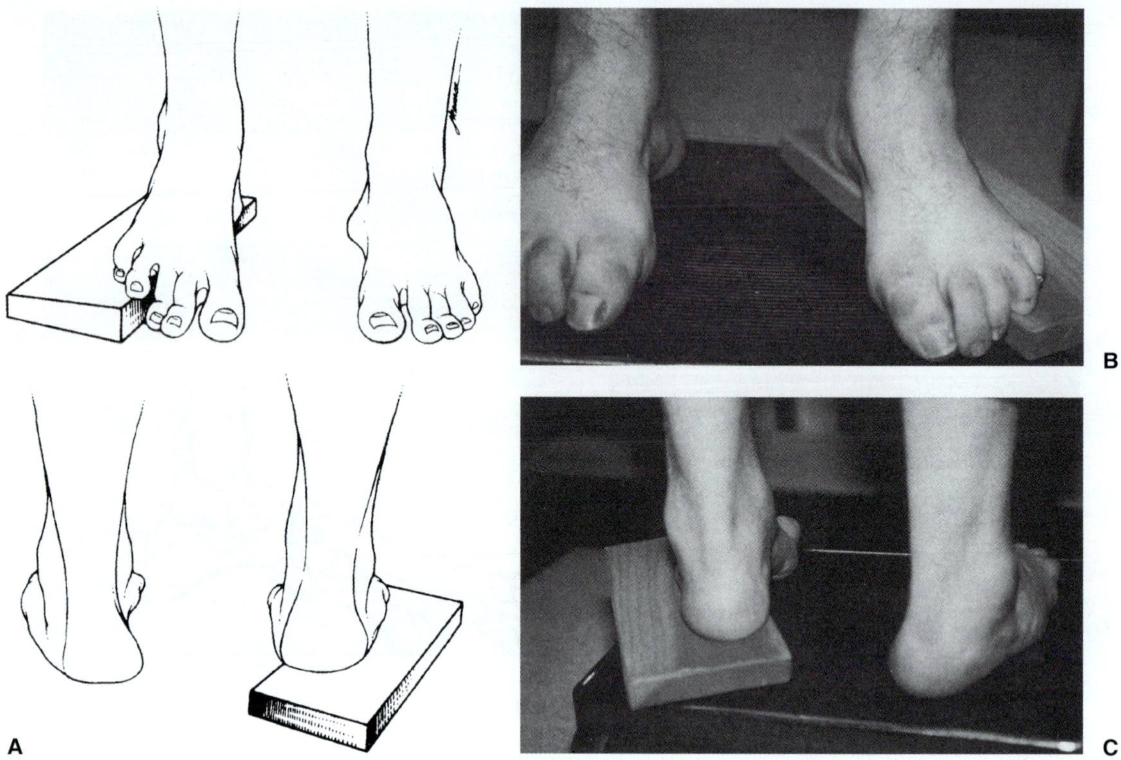

FIGURE 5.27 (A) Line drawing illustrating lateral block test. (Reproduced with permission from Alexander IJ. Evaluation of frontal plane mechacs. In: Alexander IJ (ed.), *The Foot: Examination and Diagnosis*. New York: Churchill Livingstone, 1990; 41–54.) (B) Anterior view of lateral block test. (C) Posterior view of lateral block test demonstrating a flexible hindfoot. (*Source: Orthopaedic Knowledge Update Foot and Ankle 2*. American Academy of Orthopaedic Surgeons, 1998; 92. Fig. 1.)

Typically, a TAL must be performed to achieve a plantigrade foot. The foot must be braced postoperatively to protect and maintain correction—use a full-length metal rocker sole in work boot attached to brace.

Postpolio Syndrome. The most likely etiology of this disorder is aging plus overuse of compensatory muscles, resulting in muscular weakness. Patients present with joint pain and muscle atrophy. Treatment of this disorder is usually nonoperative with exercise and activity modification. Intensive rehabilitation is not recommended.

X. ARTHRITIC DISORDERS OF THE FOOT

Inflammatory Arthritides: Rheumatoid Arthritis (RA)

Pathology. Foot involvement in patients with RA tends to be progressive with variable remissions. Approximately 85% of patients with long-standing RA have forefoot involvement. Women more affected than men, and it is associated with the serologic marker HLA-DR4. As with RA of other joints, synovitis is the inciting problem, which causes the release of proteinases and collagenases. These enzymes, in turn, impair periarticular ligamentous and capsular integrity and destroy hyaline cartilage. The lesser MTP joints are most commonly involved with a spectrum of disease that progresses from synovitis to plantar plate destruction with subsequent dorsal dislocation of the proximal phalanges on the metatarsal heads. The increased stress on the metatarsal heads leads to the development of plantar callosities. The midfoot is not commonly involved, but can RA involve the talonavicular and naviculocuneiform articulations. The hindfoot will most commonly develop a valgus deformity due to disruption of the talocalcaneal interosseous ligament that weakens the subtalar joint. The chronic hindfoot valgus deformity results in an effective shortening of the Achilles tendon.

Conservative Treatment. Conservative treatment of the forefoot deformities involves the use of metatarsal pads, extra-depth shoewear and, soft orthoses.

Surgical Treatment. The surgical treatment is most often directed to forefoot deformities. However, if the hindfoot deformity is marked (greater than 10 degrees), it should be addressed first.

- If the *valgus hindfoot deformity* is marked, a limited-motion or locked AFO with a valgus correcting T strap is added.
- For *fixed hindfoot deformity*, triple arthrodesis is usually necessary, along with a TAL (to achieve a plantigrade foot).
- If there are concomitant *deformities of the hip or knee*, these should be addressed before correcting any foot deformities.
- For rheumatoid *forefoot reconstruction*, the first MTP joint should be fused (even if the involvement is mild) in 15 degrees of valgus in the frontal plane, 10 degrees of extension in the sagittal plane, and neutral rotation in the axial plane as long as the interphalangeal joint of the hallux is stable. If the hallux joint is unstable, arthrodesis of joint and resection of the base of the proximal phalanx is recommended, but a hallux valgus deformity can occur subsequently.
- For the *lesser toes*, resection of the metatarsal heads at the neck-shaft level (the metatarsal heads should be resected in a cascade in a dorsal–distal to a plantar–proximal direction. The respective long extensor tendon should be interposed (interposition arthroplasty) and fixed with K-wires for immobilization.
- Correction of the *PIP joint deformity* is performed by resection of the head and neck of each proximal phalanx. Of note, attempting to perform a soft tissue procedure in RA foot deformities is not recommended.
- For *midfoot deformities*, a talonavicular (TN) arthrodesis can be combined with calcaneocuboid (CC) arthrodesis, which allows the patient to gain a stable, painless midfoot. A TAL, done percutaneously, restores the plantigrade nature of the foot.

Crystalline-Induced Arthropathies

Gout. The hallux MTP joint is most often involved (podagra) in gout. Treatment of an acute attack is with indomethacin or colchicine. Chronic gout is treated with allopurinol.

Pseudogout (Chondrocalcinosis). Pseudogout commonly affects the knee. The diagnosis is confirmed by joint aspiration revealing weakly positive birefringent crystals under polarized light microscopy. Radiographs will reveal intraarticular calcifications that are not characteristic of gout. Treatment is typically with NSAIDs.

Seronegative Spondyloarthropathies

Seronegative spondyloarthropathies have a predilection for involvement of the entheses (interface where ligament and tendon attach to bone). They are often called enthesopathies as well.

Psoriatic Arthropathy. The DIP joints are most commonly affected, but psoriatic arthropathy may also cause dactylitis (sausage digit) of a lesser toe (enlargement of the entire toe). Arthritis mutilans (severe destruction of synovial joints) is rare, most commonly seen in the DIP joints of digits with erosions of the proximal phalanx. Erosion produces the classic pencil-in-cup appearance seen in psoriatic arthropathy. Nail pitting is common. Treatment utilizes NSAIDs and methotrexate (MTX) for severe psoriasis. Strongest radiographic sign of psoriatic arthritis is evidence of arthritis mutilans with erosive arthritis of DIP joints. The MTP joints are not commonly involved. Surgery is not commonly indicated, but the procedures performed if the deformities are severe are similar to those for RA.

Reiter Syndrome. This entity clinically resembles psoriasis but is less symmetric and tends to have less interphalangeal joint involvement. There is usually a prodromal GI/GU infection or concomitant onset of arthritis. The HLA-B27 antigen is frequently seen with Reiter syndrome. The triad of uveitis, arthritis, and urethritis is infrequent but is a cardinal feature of the condition. Achilles tendonitis, retrocalcaneal bursitis, plantar fasciitis, and dactylitis are also seen in Reiter syndrome.

Ankylosing Spondylitis. This condition most commonly manifests in the foot as plantar fasciitis or Achilles insertional tendinitis but is not as common as the hallmark sacroiliitis that is seen in AS. There is a high association with HLA-B27. As with the other enthesopathies, surgery is not typically needed but consists of plantar fascia release or débridement of the Achilles insertion.

Lyme Disease. The knee is the joint most commonly affected by Lyme disease, but in the foot, Lyme disease presents as a diffuse inflammatory tendonitis. Infection is secondary to the spirochete: *Burgdorelli burgdorfi*. Treatment is with either doxycycline or amoxicillin, and articular destruction is rare.

Osteoarthritis

Osteoarthritis. Osteoarthritis commonly involves the naviculocuneiform, intercuneiform, metatarsocuneiform (MTC), and first MTP joints. Initial treatment is geared toward orthotic support (bracing), but

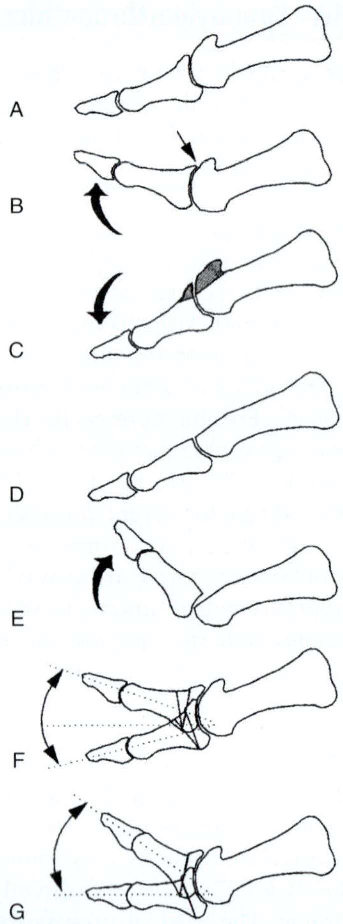

FIGURE 5.28 **(A) A hallux with joint space narrowing and dorsal osteophytes. (B) Dorsiflexion of proximal phalanx and impingement of dorsal osteophytes (small arrow). (C) Outline of bone to be removed with a cheilectomy. (D) Hallux status post cheilectomy. (E) Dorsiflexion without bony impingement following a cheilectomy. (F) A hallux with limited dorsiflexion and preserved plantarflexion with arc of motion identified by arrows. Segment of bone to be removed from proximal phalanx is outlined. (G) Hallux after Moberg dorsiflexion osteotomy of proximal phalanx. Note increased dorsiflexion without increase in arc of motion. (*Source: Orthopaedic Knowledge Update Foot and Ankle* 2. American Academy of Orthopaedic Surgeons, 1998; 152, Fig. 1.)**

if it fails, a limited arthrodesis using bone graft and open reduction with interval fixation (ORIF) can be employed. The medial (first or central (second and third) rays are most commonly involved and can be addressed surgically. The lateral two rays should not be arthrodesed but can be treated with a partial resection and interposition arthroplasty.

Hallux Rigidus. Degenerative arthritis of the first MTP joint results in the entity of hallux rigidus. There are two types: adolescent and adult. Focal chondral lesions in the first metatarsal head characterize the adolescent type. Generalized arthrosis with dorsal osteophytes characterizes the adult type. Adult hallux rigidus is described here. The etiology is multivariate, and hallux rigidus is thought to be caused by microtrauma, osteochondral defect (OCD) lesions, and possibly infection. Clinically, the patient will have pain and limited ROM with dorsal impingement. The earliest radiographic sign is a depression in the dome of the metatarsal head. Anterior–posterior views can show joint space narrowing and presence of osteophytes, while oblique images can show flattening of the metatarsal head (Fig. 5.28). Staging and treatment are shown in Table 5.11.

- *Nonoperative treatment*—Should consist of stiff-soled shoes with a wide toe-box and a rigid steel shank to prevent dorsiflexion of the hallux. Steroids can also be used but only conservatively.
- *Surgery*—Can be pursued if dorsiflexion is significantly limited and pain is severe. A cheilectomy, in which the dorsal impinging osteophytes are removed, can be performed (approximately 25% of the metatarsal head should be removed to allow 70 degrees of dorsiflexion). For end-stage hallux rigidus, an MTP fusion is the best option, but a Keller can also be performed for low-demand patients.

TABLE 5.11 Staging and treatment of hallux rigidus

Stage	*Description*	*Treatment*
I	Mild dorsal osteophyte formation, joint space preservation	Cheilectomy
II	Moderate osteophyte formation and joint space narrowing	Cheilectomy
III	Marked osteophyte formation, significantly diminished joint space	Arthrodesis/Keller resection arthroplasty

XI. ARTHRODESIS OF THE FOOT AND ANKLE

For terminal arthritis, fusion is an effective pain-relieving option. The following are common fusions for arthritis and deformities of the ankle and hindfoot.

Ankle. Ankle fusion is an option of last resort but is the standard treatment for disabling ankle arthritis. Posttraumatic arthritis is the most common indication for ankle arthrodesis. The position of the foot is important; and the following parameters should be kept in mind when performing this procedure: neutral dorsiflexion and plantarflexion, 5 to 10 degrees of valgus, 5 to 10 degrees of external rotation, and slight posterior translation of the talus in relation to the tibial plafond (to reduce the load transmitted to the midfoot during gait). There are a number of techniques to perform an ankle fusion, but the principles of removing the chondral surface, apposition of bleeding subchondral bone, and adequate compression across the articulation (using either 2 or 3 cancellous screws) remain the same.

Subtalar Arthrodesis. The subtalar joint should be fused in 3 to 5 degrees of valgus (replicating the degree of valgus observed in a normal joint). Fusion of the subtalar joint is approached through a lateral incision that extends from the tip of the fibula to the base of the fourth metatarsal. The internervous interval is between the sural nerve and the superficial peroneal nerve. The EDB is retracted medially to protect its innervation by the DPN, as is the fat of the sinus tarsi region by dissecting subperiosteally. A laminar spreader is inserted to open the subtalar joint. Cartilage and subchondral bone are removed, and the joint surfaces are prepared with an osteotome. Fixation of the subtalar joint is accomplished with a 7.0- or 7.3-mm cannulated screw that can be directed either in a superior-to-inferior (talus to calcaneus) or inferior-to-superior (calcaneus to talus) direction.

Triple Arthrodesis. This procedure fuses the subtalar, talonavicular, and calcaneocuboid joints. The transverse tarsal (talonavicular and calcaneocuboid) joints should be placed in neutral varus–valgus angulation and neutral abduction–adduction. The approach for fusion of the calcaneocuboid joint is the same as that for the isolated subtalar fusion. The cartilage and subchondral bone are removed, and the surfaces for fusion are prepared with an osteotome. A 4.5-mm cannulated screw is used for fixation. Fusion of the talonavicular joint is accomplished through a dorsomedial incision that is directed from the medial malleolar tip to the level of the naviculocuneiform joint. The interval between the anterior and posterior tibial tendons is utilized. The talonavicular joint is identified by abducting and adducting the forefoot. The joint surfaces are then decorticated with a curette and prepared in the same fashion. Fixation is identical to the calcaneocuboid joint (Fig. 5.29).

XII. TENDON DISORDERS OF THE FOOT AND ANKLE

Posterior Tibial Tendon

Posterior Tibial Tendon Insufficiency (PTTI). Diagnosis of PTTI is primarily a clinical one, and the condition is suspected in patients with long history of pes planus.

- *Pathology*—Patients often complain of pain medially and have tenderness posterior to the tip of the medial malleolus extending to the navicular tuberosity. It is in this zone where the posterior tibial tendon most commonly attenuates and ruptures. It is important to look for the "too many toes sign" (midfoot is abducted in relation to hindfoot), inability to perform a single heel raise, and hindfoot valgus deformity (Fig. 5.30). If the valgus deformity is excessive, the valgus force can lead to a stress fracture of the fibula.
- *Examination*—The inability to perform a single leg heel rise is due to the fact that the tibialis posterior is responsible for initiating hindfoot inversion to lock the transverse tarsal joint. Proper manual testing of the tibialis posterior should be conducted by having the patient invert the foot from an everted, plantarflexed position. The examiner should also evaluate possible Achilles tightness, possible fixed deformity of hindfoot or midfoot, and associated gait abnormalities. Radiographic evaluation should consist of weight-bearing anterior–posterior views of the ankles, both feet, and lateral views of both ankles and feet. Findings include a plantarflexed talus and collapse of the medial arch (through the naviculocuneiform and tarsometatarsal articulations).
- *Classification*—Classifying the type of PTTI allows for a more standardized approach to treatment. In general, treatment hinges upon the deformity being either rigid or flexible (Table 5.12).

Flexible Pes Planus (Flat Foot) Deformity. In flexible pes planus deformity, the arch is restored when the patient is not weight-bearing on the involved foot. The clinician must evaluate the ease of reduction of the midtarsal joint and also of reducing the forefoot (correction of supination). This condition can be

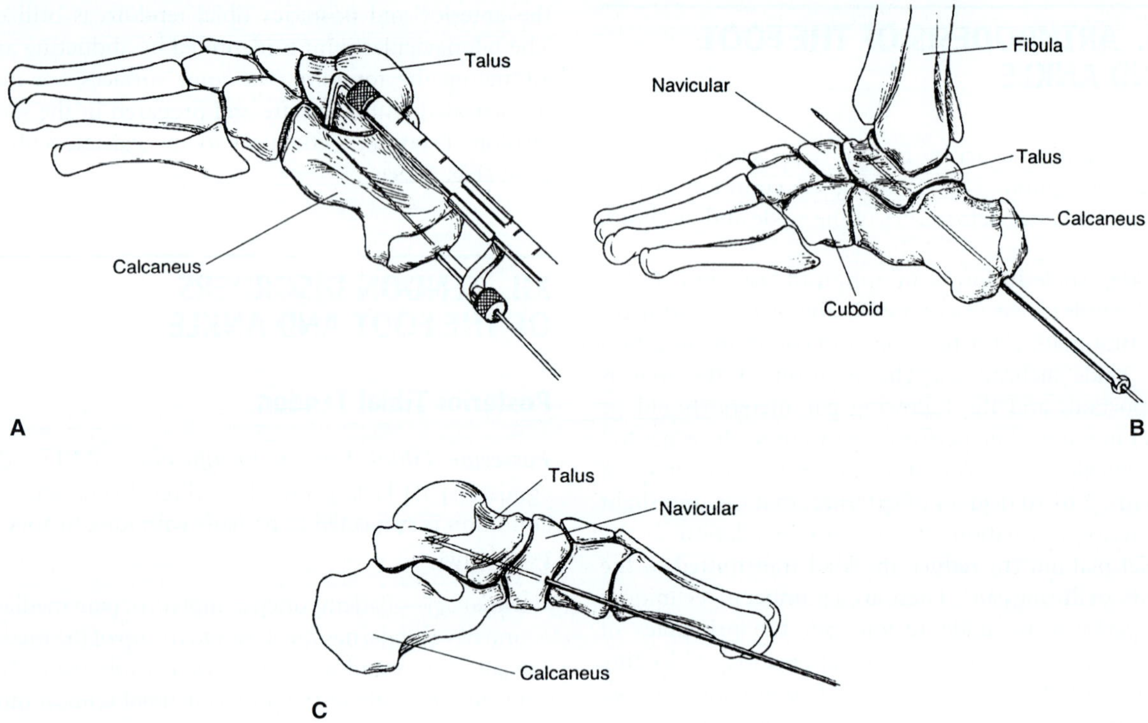

FIGURE 5.29 **(A) The drill guide is placed with the tip in the subtalar joint and the cannulated end over the calcaneus, off the weight-bearing surface of the foot. The guide is directed to allow the pin to cross the base of the talar neck after reduction of the subtalar joint. (B) After removal of the guide, the calcaneus is reduced, and the pin is drilled across the talus. The cannulated screw is placed after drilling and tapping. A washer is often used (not depicted). (C) The guide pin is placed across the talonavicular joint starting just proximal to the naviculocuneiform joint and is directed dorsally to enter the talar body. (*Source*: Wapner KL. Triple arthrodesis in adults. *JAAOS* 6(3):188–196,1998, Fig. 6.)**

treated with the use of a shoe with medial arch supports or heel wedges. Treatment should begin with immobilization for approximately 2 months to allow for symptom improvement and then graduating the patient to a stiff-soled shoe or AFO. A UCBL shoe insert with medial posting can be used to treat stage II PTTI. Stretching exercises of the gastrocnemius–soleus complex should be performed as well. Surgical treatment consists of tendon débridement for stage I and calcaneal osteotomy with FDL transfer for stage II.

Rigid Pes Planus Deformity. A rigid pes planus deformity occurs when the subtalar and midtarsal neutral positions cannot be passively reached. It can result from a congenital pes planus deformity that becomes rigid over time, unrecognized tarsal coalition, or it can be acquired as with posterior tibial tendon insufficiency. Patients often complain of pain in the tarsal sinus region. Peroneal muscle spasms can occur, resulting from pulling against a rigid hindfoot valgus deformity. Achilles tendon contracture can also be caused by the hindfoot valgus deformity. Initial treatment should include a rigid AFO, but once a rigid deformity develops, an arthrodesis (triple arthrodesis) along with a TAL is typically indicated.

Peroneal Tendon

Peroneus Brevis Tendinitis. This disorder can range from peroneal tendinitis to a longitudinal split in the peroneus brevis within the fibular groove. The disorder is one of attrition with the peroneus brevis becoming progressively mechanically abraded within the fibular groove because of an incompetent superior peroneal retinaculum. Treatment is conservative at first, involving a walking cast, NSAIDs to control inflammation, and possible débridement of the tendon if a longitudinal tear is present.

Peroneal Subluxation. This disorder involves the avulsion of the superior peroneal retinaculum (SPR) off of its fibular attachment, resulting in subluxation of the peroneal tendons. It is thought to occur because a strong and laterally directed contraction of the peroneal muscles causing an avulsion of the SPR. Nonoperative treatment is generally unsuccessful.

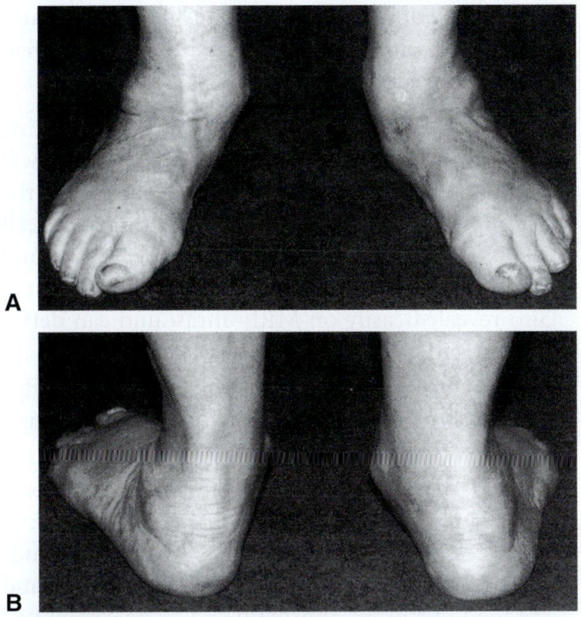

FIGURE 5.30 Views of a patient from the front and behind. Forefoot abduction, heel valgus, and "too many toes sign" are seen. (*Source*: Lin SS, Lee TH, Chao W, et al. Nonoperative treatment of patients with posterior tibial tendonitis. *Foot Ankle Clin* 1996;1:261–277.)

Surgical treatment in the acute setting involves repair of the SPR back to the fibula. Surgical options available include anatomic reconstruction, local soft tissue reinforcement (use of an Achilles tendon slip), fibular groove deepening (recession of the posterior cortex of the fibula), or substituting the calcaneofibular ligament (rerouting) to replace the attenuated SPR.

Anterior Tibial Tendon (ATT) Injuries

ATT Tenosynovitis. This disorder occurs most often in patients with an inflammatory arthritis. Rupture, however, of the ATT is most common in elderly patients who complain of poorly localized dorsal foot pain. Physical examination reveals tenderness in the region of the ATT insertion. Partial tears are treated by immobilization initially in a walking cast and if symptoms do not resolve in 6 to 8 weeks, then an AFO can be used until symptoms have resolved. Complete ruptures are difficult to treat because of the age of patients (most are elderly) and the quality of the degenerate tendon.

FHL Tendon Injuries

Tenosynovitis of the FHL. The FHL is susceptible to stenosing tenosynovitis that is caused by repetitive trauma (seen in dancers) that leads to inflammation of the tendon sheath and subsequent scarring. Patients typically present with posterior ankle pain associated with passive movement of the hallux interphalangeal joint. The presence of a nodule in the tendon can prevent full dorsiflexion of the hallux (similar to trigger finger). Surgery is typically needed and involves surgical exploration with possible tenolysis or tenosynovectomy.

Rupture of the FHL. Most ruptures are due to lacerations, but atraumatic ruptures can occur in elite athletes. Most atraumatic ruptures occur proximal to the distal phalanx and can occur underneath the sustentaculum or within the groove of the posterior process of the talus. The location of the rupture determines the treatment options, with primary repair indicated for distal ruptures (distal phalanx insertion or sesamoid region), while tenodesis to the FDL is

TABLE 5.12 Classification of PTTI

Stage	*Description*	*Treatment*
I	Tenosynovitis but no fixed deformity relative to contralateral side when standing, tenderness along PTT, can perform heel rise	Medial arch supports; immobilization in walking cast, and NSAIDs; tendon débridement only if conservative measures unsuccessful
II	Hindfoot flexible; cannot perform heel-rise because of loss of flexion of PTT with positive too-many toes sign; lateral ankle pain and obvious hindfoot valgus when standing; normal arc of subtalar motion is present	Medial heel wedge, hinged AFO; surgical options include calcaneal sliding osteotomy or arthrodesis of calcaneocuboid joint with a bone block (to correct valgus heel) and transfer of FDL to navicular with or without percutaneous TAL
III	Rigid valgus hindfoot deformity with lateral ankle, sinus tarsi pain, arthritic changes of subtalar joint	Rigid AFO; triple arthrodesis is best surgical option with TAL

indicated both proximally and distally for proximal ruptures (hindfoot or sustentaculum). Surgical repair can be difficult because of the vulnerability of the most medial branch of medial plantar nerve.

Achilles Tendon Injuries

Achilles Paratenonitis (Peritendinitis). This disorder is commonly seen in athletes, especially long-distance and middle-distance runners. Because of its vascularity, the paratenon is susceptible to inflammation, and peritendinitis often presents as diffuse discomfort and swelling of the tendon. Acutely, the Achilles can appear sausage-like because of its diffusely edematous condition. Tender nodules can often occur within the paratenon, reflecting localized hypertrophy of connective tissue. On physical examination, findings can vary depending on the degree of inflammation present within the paratenon. Decreased ankle dorsiflexion and hamstring tightness are commonly found in patients with Achilles pathology. Nodularity within the paratenon can be detected on palpation. There is often palpable tenderness on both sides of the tendon, with the medial side being more tender than the lateral. Conservative treatment is initially started and typically consists of modification of training regimens (such as a staged cross-training regimen), rest, ice massage, and NSAIDs. A small heel lift or a shock-absorbing orthotic can also help reduce acute symptoms. Brisement (injection of a dilute local anesthetic or saline solution under pressure) can also be performed to break up adhesions. Surgical therapy is considered for chronic cases that are resistant to conservative measures. A medial longitudinal incision is often utilized with full-thickness flaps of skin, subcutaneous tissue, and crural fascia developed. The anterior aspect of the paratenon is avoided to protect the blood supply to the Achilles tendon. Thickened paratenon is excised posteriorly, medially, and laterally around the tendon.

Achilles Tendinosis. Achilles tendinosis is a degenerative process in which there is little inflammation. It is asymptomatic because of the lack of inflammation and often presents as a frank rupture owing to its indolent nature. A distinguishing feature of tendinosis from paratenonitis is the mobility of the intratendinous nodule or thickening with the point of maximal tenderness during active ROM (painful arc sign). Conservative therapy should focus on pain relief, stretching exercises, and orthotics. If unsuccessful, surgical therapy is employed by removing the areas of degenerate tendon. Additionally, if the Achilles tendon is significantly attenuated because of extensive débridement, then an FHL augmentation can be performed.

Achilles Tendon Ruptures. Achilles tendon ruptures often present with a sharp pain, as if the patient had been hit in the leg with an object.

- *Clinical examination*—Examination reveals swelling and pain, with a palpable defect. The patient will be unable to perform a single heel raise, and the Thompson test will be positive (squeezing of the calf results in plantarflexion). Diagnosis by ultrasound will reveal a gap within the Achilles tendon that is also revealed easily on MRI; ultrasound can detect incomplete tendon ruptures as well.
- *Conservative treatment*—Treatment can be nonoperative, involving immobilization (short-leg cast) for 6 weeks and then passive ROM exercises.
- *Surgery*—Surgery is advocated for younger patients and those for whom nonoperative therapy is unsuccessful. For acute ruptures, the tendon ends can be exposed through a medial incision and the tendon stumps approximated using a modified Bunnell technique with a 2- or 4-suture technique. Surgical treatment for Achilles tendon ruptures is associated with a significantly lower rerupture rate but the most common complication is wound complications (Fig. 5.31).
    - **Chronic Achilles ruptures** can be treated with an FDL or FHL tendon transfer. The FHL is a safe tendon to transfer (it is away from the

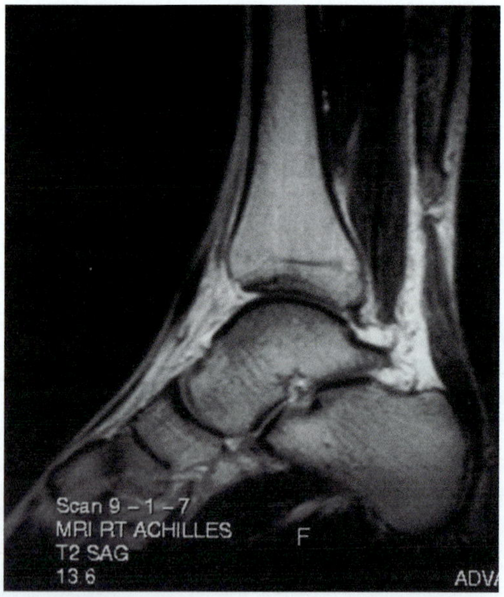

FIGURE 5.31 T2-weighted MRI of the ankle demonstrating acute Achilles tendon rupture. (*Source*: Thordarson DB. *Foot and Ankle*. Philadelphia: Lippincott Williams & Wilkins, 2004; 154. Fig. 8.3.)

neurovascular structures) and can directly be used to span Achilles gaps.

- Of note, *sural nerve injury* is a complication of ruptures of the Achilles tendon owing to its close anatomic relationship to the Achilles. At the Achilles tendon insertion, the sural nerve lies approximately 18.8 mm lateral to the lateral border of the Achilles. The proximal course of the nerve is more midline and crosses the lateral border of the Achilles approximately 9.8 cm proximal to the calcaneus.

XIII. HEEL PAIN

General Heel Pain

Plantar Fasciitis. This disorder usually occurs in overweight, middle-aged patients with heel pain. It presents with heel pain upon ambulation in the morning, and there is often localized tenderness at the plantar medial tuberosity of calcaneus. It is likely a degenerative process caused by microtears at the origin of the plantar fascia. There may also be entrapment of the first branch of the lateral plantar nerve. The treatment of plantar fasciitis is nonoperative for 6 to 12 months, using stretching and massage of the plantar fascia. If surgery treatment is required, only the medial third of the plantar fascia should be released to avoid medial longitudinal arch attenuation. The deep fascia of the abductor hallucis may need to be released if the first branch of the lateral plantar nerve is compressed.

Baxter Nerve Compression (Distal Tarsal Tunnel Syndrome). This condition is often seen in long-distance runners and results in compression of the first branch of the lateral plantar nerve to the abductor digiti minimi muscle as it passes between the fascial planes of the abductor hallucis and quadratus plantae. Treatment involves decompression of the abductor hallucis brevis and quadratus plantae.

Central Heel Pain

This entity represents a mild to moderate traumatic periostitis. Casting and/or cushioned heel pads are used to treat this condition.

Posterior Heel Pain

Retrocalcaneal Bursitis and Haglund Deformity. Retrocalcaneal bursitis is a distinct entity characterized by pain anterior to the Achilles tendon and involves inflammation of the retrocalcaneal bursa. It is often associated with prominence of the posterior–superior angle of the os calcis, which causes mechanical irritation of the bursa (Haglund deformity). Perhaps the best diagnostic sign for retrocalcaneal bursitis is the 2-finger squeeze test, in which pain is elicited by applying pressure medially and laterally anterior to the Achilles insertion.

- *Nonsurgical management*—Nonsurgical management should include rest, orthoses, and physical therapy (Achilles complex stretching maneuvers).
- *Surgery*—Those requiring surgical treatment for retrocalcaneal bursitis are usually long-distance runners (greater than 40 miles/week), are unwilling to discontinue running, and are willing to undergo surgery as a last resort in order to continue running. Partial calcaneal ostectomy is a successful procedure in this population and can often restore patients back to their original level of activity within 6 months.

Insertional Achilles Tendonitis. Insertional tendinitis is a true inflammatory process within the tendinous insertion of the Achilles. It is often associated with Haglund deformity and is frequently associated with hill running and interval training. Training errors such as improper stretching prior to exertion or excessive increases in training regimens can quickly exacerbate this condition. Like retrocalcaneal bursitis, insertional tendonitis presents with posterior heel pain thought to be caused by bony impingement from the calcaneus, local bursitis, or both. Most cases of insertional tendinitis improve with nonoperative intervention. Initial treatment should be guided toward NSAIDs, Achilles tendon stretching, and heel-lift orthotics. If unsuccessful, surgery can be pursued in which the tendon insertion is incised in its midline and any calcific or degenerate regions are removed. If more than 50% of the width of the tendon insertion is débrided, then tendon augmentation is required.

XIV. THE DIABETIC FOOT

Diabetic foot disease is dependent on two interlinked factors: diabetic neuropathy and an abnormal mechanical environment with neuropathy being the factor that most profoundly influences pathology.

Diabetic Foot Ulcers

Pathogenesis. It is important to realize that it is the neuropathy and not necessarily vascular insufficiency that contributes to the pathogenesis of diabetic foot ulcers. Classically, diabetic neuropathy presents with a "stocking-and-glove" distribution of neuropathy with diminished sensation being the hallmark of the disease.

The Semmes-Weinstein 5.07 monofilament represents the protective sensation threshold; patients who are able to feel this sensation are unlikely to develop ulcers. It is likely that the etiology of the neuropathy is neural damage caused by the accumulation of sorbitol (sorbitol theory) in which the excess glucose is converted to sorbitol by the enzyme aldose reductase. The overall result of sorbitol accumulation within the cell impairs fatty acid metabolism and subsequently reduces axonal transport. Additionally, other potential causes of the nerve injury include nonenzymatic glycosylation and an autoimmune response, with the latter playing a role in the autonomic component of diabetic neuropathy. Several mechanical factors contribute to the development of ulcers, including repetitive stress (overuse), shear and axial loading forces, and static deformities that increase pressure on any particular part of the foot. It is important to understand that high pressures or shear forces are not necessary to induce ulceration but instead can be due to repetitive exposure of the foot to a moderate or even mild stress experienced in daily activities.

Predictors. A thorough vascular evaluation should always be performed in a patient with a diabetic ulcer. The involved limb should be inspected for dependent rubor, shiny atrophic skin, pallor, and delayed capillary refill. If arterial insufficiency is suspected, then a Doppler arterial study is the best test to obtain. If ankle pressures are below 45 mmHg, it is likely that a foot ulcer due to arterial insufficiency will not heal without a revascularization. In predicting if a diabetic ulcer can heal, it is often important to determine the transcutaneous oxygen (TcO_2) pressure as well as the ankle–brachial ischemic index. An absolute toe pressure of at least 40 to 50 mmHg is required for healing along with an ischemic index of 0.6 or greater. If the TcO_2 is in the range of 30 to 40 mmHg and the ischemic index is between 0.5 and 0.6, the likelihood of healing is less predictable.

Wagner Classification. This classification is described in Table 5.13. An extra-depth shoe can be used for grade 0 ulcerations, while a total contact cast can be used for Wagner grade 1 and 2 ulcerations with limited bedside débridement and frequent examinations. Formal surgical intervention is often required for grade 3 lesions, while grade 4 and 5 lesions require amputation.

TABLE 5.13 Wagner classification of diabetic ulcers

Grade	Description
0	Ulcers have intact skin (bony deformities may be present)
1	Localized superficial ulcer
2	Deep ulcer to tendon, bone, ligament, or joint
3	Deep abscess or osteomyelitis
4	Gangrene of toes or forefoot
5	Gangrene of entire foot

Neuropathic Arthropathy (Charcot Foot)

Pathology. Charcot foot is a noninfective, destructive lesion of the bone and associated joints due to a fracture or dislocation in a patient with peripheral neuropathy, with diabetes being the most common cause of this particular lesion. The midfoot region is the most common area for neuropathic destructive changes to develop, leading to midfoot collapse. It is often caused by a minor initial injury such as a sprain. These resultant injuries can lead to deformities of the foot and ankle resulting in biomechanical alterations in load bearing and difficulties in shoe fitting, both of which can predispose to ulceration. The ulceration can lead to superficial infection or a deep infection with resultant osteomyelitis. It is, however, important to differentiate osteomyelitis from Charcot bony changes. Osteomyelitis will be focal or absent if present in a Charcot foot. A labeled WBC scan, such as an Indium-111 scan, is the most appropriate method of diagnosing osteomyelitis in the foot. The Eichenholtz classification of Charcot arthropathy is outlined in Table 5.14.

Treatment. The initial treatment is nonoperative for most Charcot deformities of the foot. A total contact cast (TCC) is used for stage I and II Charcot feet for immobilization and to allow healing. A Charcot restraining orthotic walker (CROW) can be used to maintain foot alignment during the healing phases as well. Additionally, if the hindfoot or ankle is involved, extended immobilization (approximately 12 to 18 months) in an ankle-foot orthoses is indicated. Operative intervention is indicated when the Charcot foot is deformed to a degree that precludes bracing or footwear or is susceptible to recurrent ulceration. Surgery should be limited to removing bony prominences, TAL to achieve a plantigrade foot, or selective arthrodeses to regain stability of the foot. Surgery is typically performed during stage III (resolution phase) after nonoperative treatment has failed.

TABLE 5.14 Eichenholtz classification of Charcot arthropathy

Stage	Radiographic Features	Clinical Features	Treatment
I (dissolution)	Demineralization of regional bone, periarticular fragmentation, joint dislocation	Acute inflammation, swelling, erythema, warmth	Total contact cast (used only for midfoot/forefoot surgery); minority need surgery
II (coalescence)	Absorption of osseous debris in soft tissues, organization and early healing of fracture fragments, periosteal new-bone formation	Less inflammation and swelling relative to stage I, increased stability at fracture site	Immobilization (AFO, TCC)
III (resolution)	Smoothing of edges of large fragments of bone, osseous ankylosis	Permanent enlargement of foot and ankle, with fixed deformity, minimum daily or activity-related swelling	Most likely to need surgery (type 3b)—neuropathic fracture of calcaneal tubercle, 2 degrees pes planus is uniformly nonoperative

Source: Johnson JE. Operative treatment of neuropathic arthropathy of the foot and ankle. *J Bone Joint Surg Am* 80-A(11):1700–1709,1998.

XV. FRACTURES, SPRAINS, AND DISLOCATIONS OF THE FOOT AND ANKLE

Ankle Sprains

Epidemiology and Grading. Lateral ankle sprains are the most frequent ankle injuries in sports. Eight-five percent of all sports-related ankle injuries are sprains. Sixty-six percent of all ankle sprains involve the ATFL, whereas 25% include the ATFL with the CFL. The grading system in Table 5.15 is useful for determining treatment.

Evaluation. Routine radiographic evaluation is not required unless patients demonstrate any of the Ottawa ankle rules. Examination should involve the entire ankle.

Lateral ankle

- Tenderness at the tip of the lateral malleolus
- Tenderness at the base of the fifth metatarsal
- Inability to bear weight

Medial ankle

- Tenderness at the tip of the medial malleolus
- Tenderness at the navicular
- Inability to bear weight

Nonoperative Treatment. Treatment for ankle sprains is initially nonoperative. Patients can be placed in an aircast for added support. They should be progressed to weight bearing as tolerated. Patients should be evaluated by a physical therapist for proprioception, gait and balance, and strength training. Persistent pain may entail a further workup, including radiographs and an MRI. A differential including neuropraxia of the superficial peroneal nerve (especially if the pain is burning in nature) synovitis, OCD, proximal fifth metatarsal fracture, fracture of the lateral process of

TABLE 5.15 Grading system for ankle sprains

Grade	Findings
I	Stretched fibers of the ligament; no laxity; no residual instability
II	Incomplete tear of ligament; mild laxity; mild instability; slight loss of function, strength, and proprioception
III	Complete disruption of the ligament; gross instability and laxity; potential for complete loss of function, strength, and proprioception.

Source: O'Donoghue DH. *Treatment of Injuries to Athletes.* Edited, 698–746, Philadelphia: WB Saunders, 1976.

the talus (snowboarder's ankle), peroneal subluxation or tear, and RSD must be entertained.

Surgical Treatment. Multiple methodologies are present for ligamentous reconstruction.

- *Brostrom procedure*—The peroneus brevis and plantaris tendons are used and the ligaments are tightened. The anatomic Brostrom is achieved with primary repair of the ends of the ATFL. This procedure is probably the most mechanically stable and favored in most primary reconstruction.
- *Gould modification*—This modification of the Brostrom procedure involves also reinforcing the ATFL repair with overlap of the nearby lateral talocalcaneal ligament plus the marginal ankle retinaculum.
- *Watson-Jones procedure*—The entire peroneus brevis tendon is isolated and passed through a drill hole in the fibula into the talus. This procedure recreates the ATFL only.
- *Evans procedure*—The entire peroneus brevis tendon is passed through a hole in the fibula and attached to the base of the fifth metatarsal to recreate the ATFL only.
- *Chrisman-Snook procedure*—The peroneus brevis is split longitudinally from the base of the fifth metatarsal. The tendon is used to recreate the ATFL and CFL.

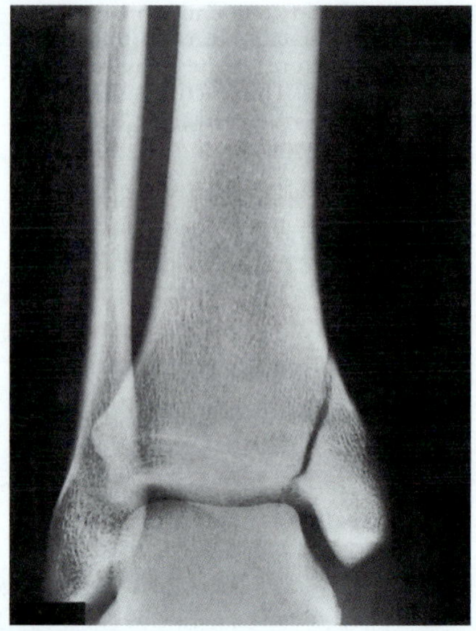

FIGURE 5.32 Anteroposterior radiograph of the ankle demonstrates the typical appearance of a unimalleolar fracture involving the medial malleolus. (*Source*: Greenspan A. *Orthopaedic Radiology*, 3rd ed. Philadelphia: Lippincott Williams & Wilkins, 2000; 299, Fig. 9.31.)

Ankle Fractures

Classification. There are many classification systems for ankle fractures to guide treatment. The classification systems are based on the mechanism of injury or the radiographic findings (Figs. 5.32 and 5.33). The Weber classification is radiographic, based on the level of the fibular fracture (Table 5.16). In the Lauge-Hansen classification, the first word defines the position of the foot at the time of the injury. The second word describes the direction of the deforming force (Table 5.17).

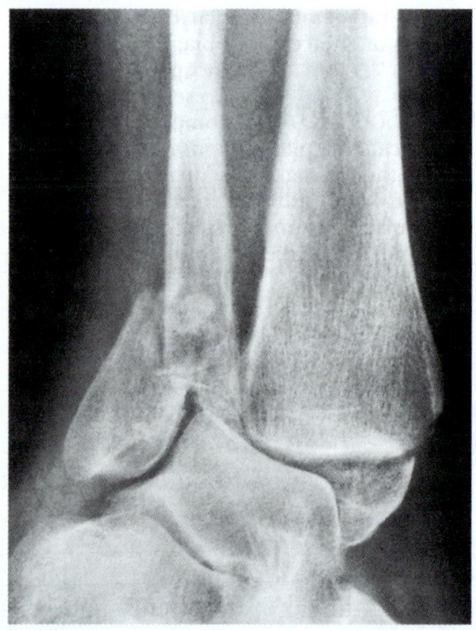

FIGURE 5.33 Oblique radiograph of the ankle shows a bimalleolar fracture involving both the tibial and fibular malleoli. (*Source*: Greenspan A. *Orthopaedic Radiology*, 3rd ed. Philadelphia: Lippincott Williams & Wilkins, 2000; 299, Fig. 9.32.)

Nonoperative Treatment. Nonoperative treatment is acceptable with nondisplaced fractures or fractures that can be stably reduced. Patients are placed in a straight-leg cast and are made nonweight bearing until clinical and radiographic healing of the fracture.

Operative Fixation of Ankle Fractures. Surgery is indicated if there is displacement or an unstable fracture pattern. Options include:

- ORIF with an interfragmentary screw and a 1/3 semitubular or dynamic compression plate on the fibula. Dynamic compression plates are preferred

TABLE 5.16 Weber classification of ankle fracture

Type	Location
A	Distal to the plafond (correlates to SAD)
B	At the plafond (correlates to SER, PAB)
C	Proximal to the plafond (correlates to PER)

for high Weber C fractures if there is adequate soft tissue coverage.

- Medial malleolar piece secured with 4.0 or 4.5 cancellous screws, tension banding, or Kirschner wires.
- Posterior malleolar piece, if present, may reduce on its own. Anterior-to-posterior screws are indicated if the fragment is greater than 25% of the articular surface.

Syndesmotic Injury

Patients with tenderness over the medial malleolus, proximal fibula, or interosseous membrane should be evaluated for a syndesmotic injury. Signs of injury include:

- Radiographic evidence present on the mortise view; greater than 4-mm medial joint space width.
- Intraoperative evidence using fluoroscopy. Cotton test looks at the presence of displacement at the distal joint with valgus stress on the distal fibula. The presence of displacement at the distal tibial–fibular joint with dorsiflexion and external rotation of the foot places the wider, anterior portion of the talus in the mortise and causes splaying of the distal tibial–fibular joint.
- Treatment with one or two 4.0 or 4.5 screws through either 3 or 4 cortices. Screws are removed at 3 months to allow for normal distal fibular motion.

Subtalar Dislocations

Subtalar dislocations tend to be associated with high-energy mechanisms and involve dislocation of the subtalar joint as well as the talonavicular joint. They are classified according to the direction of dislocation of the calcaneus as medial, lateral, anterior, and posterior. Anterior and posterior dislocations are very rare. Subtalar dislocations are frequently irreducible and require emergent open reduction, tendon relocation, and stabilization.

TABLE 5.17 The Lauge-Hansen classification of ankle fracture

Type	Direction of Force
SAD	Supination-adduction
SER	Supination-external rotation
PER	Pronation-external rotation
PAB	Pronation-abduction

Medial Dislocations. Medial dislocations are the most common and are associated with injury of the lateral ankle ligaments with medial dislocation of the calcaneus. The peroneal tendons (peroneus tertius) or the extensor retinaculum can block reduction. Impaction of the talus into the lateral aspect of the navicular can also block reduction. They are commonly associated with an osteochondral defect (OCD) of the talus.

Lateral Dislocations. The talar head and neck dislocate medially while the calcaneus dislocates laterally. In these dislocations, the posterior tibial tendon or FDL tendon or a small talar head fracture can block reduction.

Calcaneal Fractures

Posterior Facet Fractures. Approximately 75% of all calcaneal fractures are posterior facet fractures, and most have some degree of displacement. Displacement of the posterior facet of more than approximately 2 to 3 mm is an indication for ORIF. The Sanders classification (Table 5.18) is based on the number and location of the articular fragments as observed on CT as seen on the coronal image showing the widest surface of the inferior facet of talus. The posterior facet is divided into 3 fractures lines (denoted as A, B, and C) corresponding to lateral, middle, and medial fracture lines respectively. It is important to note that

TABLE 5.18 Sanders classification of calcaneal fractures

Type	Description
I	All nondisplaced regardless of number of fracture lines
II	2-pt fracture of posterior facet, subtypes IIA, IIB, IIC based on 1-degree fracture line
III	3-pt fracture in which have centrally displaced fragment
IV	4-pt articular fracture, comminuted

Source: Sanders R, Fortin P, DiPasquale T, Walling A. Operative treatment in 120 displaced intraarticular calcaneal fractures. Results using a prognostic computed tomography scan classification. *Clin Orthop* 290:87–95,1993.

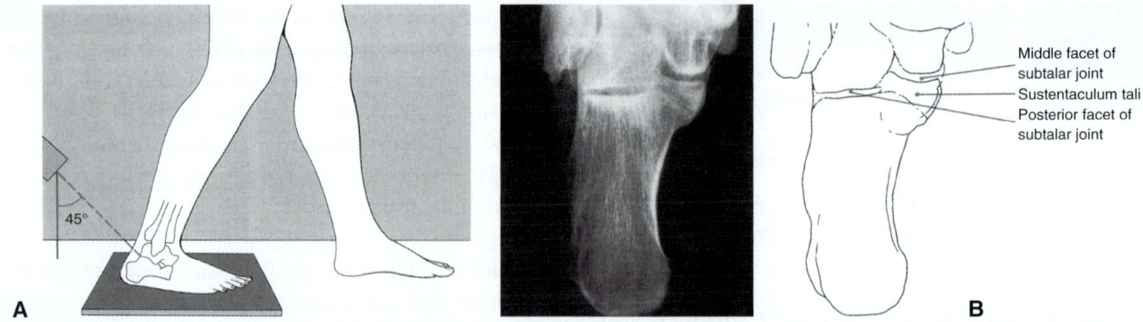

FIGURE 5.34 (A) For the posterior tangential (Harris-Beath) view of the foot, the patient is erect, with the sole of the foot flat on the film cassette. The central beam is usually angled 45 degrees toward the midline of the heel, but 35 or 55 degrees of angulation may also be used. (B) On the film in this projection, the middle facet of the subtalar joint is seen, oriented horizontally; the sustentaculum tali projects medially. The posterior facet projects laterally and is parallel to the middle facet. The body of the calcaneus is well demonstrated. (*Source*: Greenspan A. *Orthopaedic Radiology*, 3rd ed. Philadelphia: Lippincott Williams & Wilkins, 2000; 292–293, Fig. 9.23.)

the primary fracture line extends from anterolateral to posteromedial through the posterior facet.

Radiographic Evaluation. Radiographs should include anterior–posterior, lateral, and oblique views of the hindfoot; a Harris axial view; and a Broden view (Figs. 5.34 and 5.35). The Harris view is an axial view that provides visualization of the calcaneal tuberosity and the middle and posterior facets of the subtalar joint. Two radiographic measurements are also important when evaluating a calcaneus fracture.

- *Bohler angle*—The angle formed by a line drawn from the calcaneal tubercle posteriorly to posterior facet and from anterior tubercle to posterior facet. The normal angle is 25 to 40 degrees.
- *Angle of Gissane*—This crucial angle (normal range 120 to 145 degrees) is formed by confluence of two struts: one that extends along the posterior facet and the other extending anteriorly to the beak of calcaneus. An increase in this angle indicates a collapse of the posterior facet.

A CT scan should be routinely obtained because it provides the best visualization of intraarticular

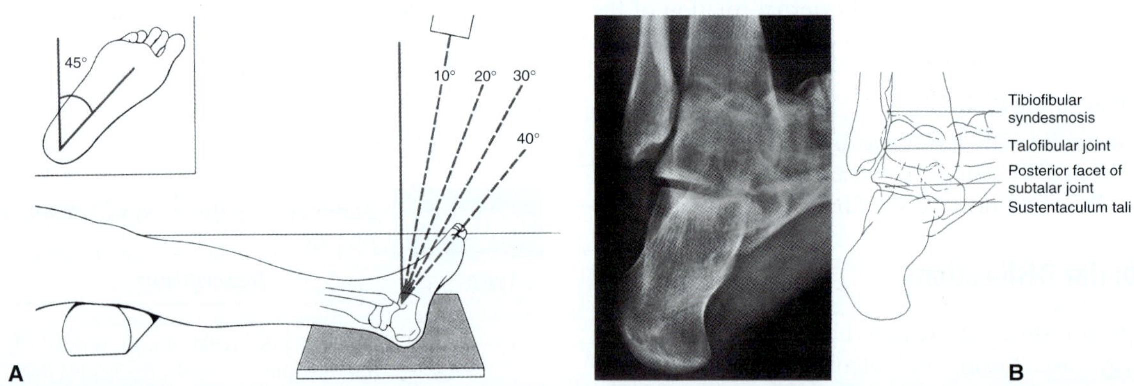

FIGURE 5.35 (A) For the Broden view of the foot, the patient is supine, with the knee slightly flexed and supported by a small sandbag. The foot rests on the film cassette, dorsiflexed to 90 degrees and together with the leg, rotated medially about 45 degrees (inset). The central beam is directed toward the lateral malleolus. Films may be obtained at 10, 20, 30, and 40 degrees of cephalad angulation of the tube. (B) A radiograph obtained at 30 degrees cephalad angulation demonstrates the posterior facet of the subtalar joint. Note also the good demonstration of the sustentaculum tali and the excellent visualization of the talofibular joint and tibiofibular syndesmosis. (*Source*: Greenspan A. *Orthopaedic Radiology*, 3rd ed. Philadelphia: Lippincott Williams & Wilkins, 2000; 292–293, Fig. 9.24.)

calcaneal fractures, and coronal and sagittal reconstructions (reformatted images) should be obtained.

Treatment. Treatment is often determined by the location of the fracture and the amount of comminution. Extraarticular fractures are treated surgically if the fragment is displaced more than 1 cm. Isolated sustentaculum fractures without concomitant posterior facet involvement are rare. Options for various types of calcaneus fractures as based on the Sanders classification are as follows: for type I fracture, the recommended treatment is no weight bearing for 4 to 6 weeks in a short-leg cast. Types II and III fractures are treated with ORIF. Type IV fractures generally tend to do poorly with surgical fixation, and many surgeons have resorted to nonoperative treatment or fusion. A long-term complication of comminuted calcaneal fractures (type IV) is a loss of heel height that leads to anterior ankle impingement. A value of less than 20 degrees is abnormal and suggestive of anterior impingement. Measurement of the talar declination angle is the angle formed by the longitudinal axis of the talus and the plane of support of the foot. Should this condition develop along with subtalar arthritis, a distraction bone-block arthrodesis of the subtalar joint to restore the talar declination angle and calcaneal pitch is appropriate.

Fractures of the Talus

Talar Neck Fractures. These fractures have a high risk of AVN if they are displaced, especially types II, III, and IV talar neck fractures (Fig. 5.36; Table 5.19). As stated previously, the artery of the tarsal canal from the posterior tibial artery is the primary blood supply to the talar body. The complications of talar neck fractures (namely AVN) are related to the degree of displacement. Following injury and treatment, the Hawkins sign is useful as a prognostic indicator for displaced talar neck fractures. A subchondral radiolucency (Hawkins sign) present in the talar dome on anterior–posterior radiographs approximately 6 to 8 weeks after a talar neck fracture suggests that there is an intact blood supply to this region and resorption of bone in this region.

Treatment of Talar Neck Fractures. The treatment options for talar neck fractures are as follows:

- *Type I*—Cast immobilization for 6 to 8 weeks (risk of AVN, 10%)
- *Type II*—Attempted closed reduction, then ORIF with posterior-to-anterior screw placement (provides greater mechanical strength) (risk of AVN, 30%)
- *Type III*—Open reduction, surgical fixation in same fashion as type II (urgent/emergent) (risk of AVN, 90%)
- *Type IV*—ORIF (urgent/emergent) (risk of AVN, approximately 100%)

Talar Body Fractures. These fractures are significant high-energy injuries, and complications such as AVN and posttraumatic arthritis of the subtalar or tibiotalar joints are frequent. If the talar body is extruded from the ankle mortise and is associated with a marginally displaced fracture, AVN develops in approximately 90% to 100% of patients. An important rule to remember is that talar body fractures with 2 mm of displacement or more are treated with ORIF. Caution must be used when using the medial approach to the talar neck because damage to the deltoid can adversely affect the talar blood supply as there is a branch of the artery of the tarsal canal that supplies the deltoid ligament and the medial talus.

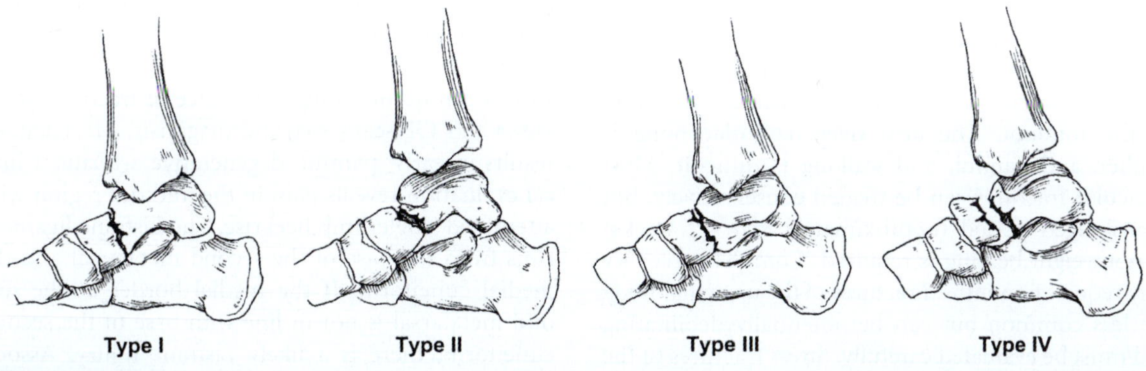

FIGURE 5.36 Classification of talar neck fractures. Type I, nondisplaced. Type II, fracture of neck and displacement of subtalar joint. Type III, fracture of neck and displacement of body from subtalar and ankle joints. Type IV, type III plus talonavicular dislocation. (*Source*: Fortin PT. Talus fractures: Evaluation and treatment. *JAAOS* 9(2):114–127, 2001; 117, Fig. 3.)

TABLE 5.19 Classification for talar neck fractures

Type	Description
I	Nondisplaced
II	Fracture of talar neck with subluxation/dislocation of subtalar joint
III	Fracture of talar neck with dislocation of subtalar and tibiotalar joints
IV	Type III with additional subluxation/dislocation of talar head from talonavicular joint

Source: Berlet GC, Lee TH, Massa EG. Talar neck fractures. *Orthop Clin North Am* 32(1):53–64,2001.

Talar Process Fracture. These fractures are lateral process fractures that are commonly seen in snowboarding and skateboarding.

Fractures of Tarsal Bones

The goals of treatment include maintaining the relative lengths of the medial and lateral columns of the foot. It is also important to maintain the integrity the medial longitudinal arch and the talonavicular joint.

Cuboid Fracture. "Nutcracker fracture" is a cuboid fracture with an associated avulsion of the navicular. It may not be apparent on standard anterior–posterior and lateral radiographs; it is best seen on a 30-degree medial oblique view of foot. Displaced fractures should be reduced anatomically to preserve the lateral column of the foot. Cuboid subluxations are most common in professional dancers with hypermobile joints that place excessive stress on the transverse tarsal joints.

Navicular Fracture. An avulsion fracture of the dorsal lip of the navicular is the most common type of navicular fracture, often due to a twisting-type injury of the midfoot. The area over navicular bone is swollen and painful, and walking is difficult. Most navicular fractures can be treated conservatively, but a prolonged period (approximately 8 to 12 weeks) of nonweight bearing is required. Complete recovery may require 6 months. Fractures of the navicular body are less common but can be potentially debilitating and must be evaluated carefully. Stress fractures of the navicular should be treated with cast immobilization for approximately 8 weeks.

Treatment of Navicular Fracture. Regardless of the type (Table 5.20), an anatomic/satisfactory reduction

TABLE 5.20 Sangeorzan classification of navicular fracture

Type	Description
I	Transverse fracture line
II	Dorsolateral to plantar medial fracture line with forefoot adduction
III	Central/lateral comminution with forefoot abduction

required, with at least 60% of the talonavicular joint surface restored. Navicular stress fractures are most common in athletes whose sports require sudden changes (track and field athletes). Diagnosis requires a high index of suspicion, and treatment is conservative (cast immobilization for 6 weeks). An accessory navicular is a common finding and can be symptomatic. Nonoperative treatment consisting of a semirigid orthosis with medial arch support is the best initial treatment. If this treatment fails, excision is usually curative.

Cuneiform Bone Fractures. Cuneiform bone fractures are unusual, and displaced medial cuneiform injuries require anatomic reduction and stable fixation to achieve a good functional outcome.

Fracture-Dislocation of Tarsometatarsal Articulation (Lisfranc Joint)

Etiology and Diagnosis. Lisfranc joint fracture-dislocations result from a direct injury to the foot, often caused by crushing force applied directly to the joint resulting in violent plantar or dorsiflexion of the foot, as in fall from a height. Fractures are associated with significant morbidity, including soft tissue injury and compartment syndrome. Radiographic evaluation includes anterior–posterior, 30-degree internal oblique, and lateral views of the affected foot. Lisfranc strains can occur without evidence of fracture. Stress views and CT scans may aid diagnosis. Misdiagnosis results in early, painful, degenerative arthritis. Clinical evaluation reveals pain in the midfoot region with attempted single-limb heel rise. The Lisfranc ligament runs from the base of the second metatarsal and the medial cuneiform. If the medial border of the second metatarsal is not in line with base of the second cuneiform, there is a likely Lisfranc injury. Associated fractures of the cuneiforms, cuboid, and second metatarsal are commonly seen as well. Dislocations of the tarsometatarsal articulation are classified into type A, total incongruity; type B, partial incongruity; and type C, divergent injury (Fig. 5.37).

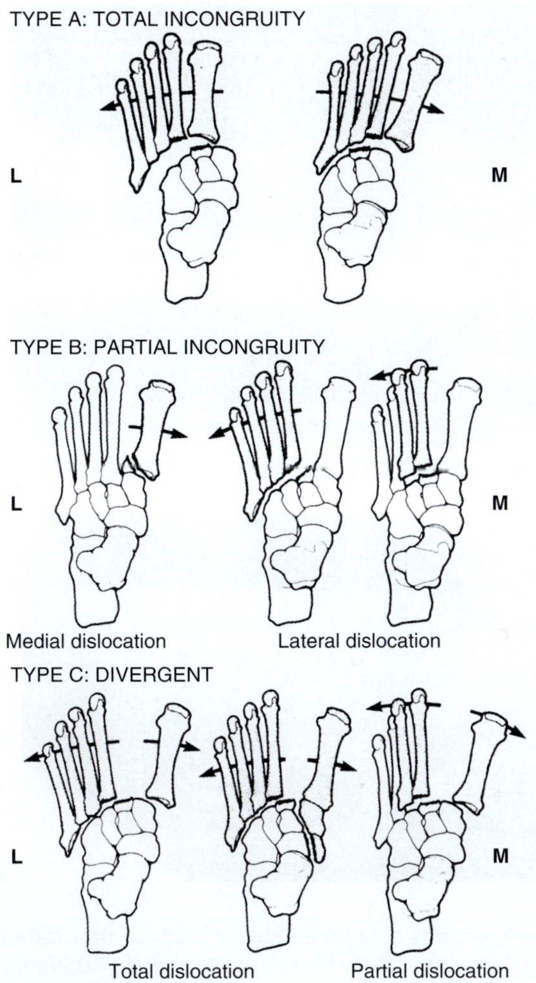

FIGURE 5.37 Diagram illustrating the classification of tarsometatarsal dislocations. L, lateral; M, medial. (Adapted from Hardcastle PH, Reschauer R, Kutscha-Lissberg E, Schoffmann W. Injuries to the tarsometatarsal joint: Incidence, classification and treatment. *J Bone Joint Surg* 1982;64B: 349–356; from DeLee JC. Fractures and dislocations of the foot. In: Mann RA, Coughlin MJ (eds.), *Surgery of the Foot and Ankle*, 6th ed. St. Louis, MO: Mosby, 1993; 1465–1703.)

Treatment. Anatomic reduction is the basis of treatment. Closed treatment and cast immobilization of TMT injuries is indicated when the joint is displaced less than 2 mm in any plane and there is no evidence of instability on stress views. Any instability (greater than 2 mm) in this joint requires anatomic reduction via surgical fixation. Most Lisfranc dislocations can be closed reduced with gentle axial traction. Fixation can be achieved with 3.5-mm screws to stabilize the medial column. The position of the second metatarsal must be restored first because it is the keystone to this joint. The remaining metatarsal can be fixed once the second metatarsal is stabilized. The screws are removed after healing has occurred usually after 3 months.

Fractures of Metatarsals

The metatarsals are common locations for stress fractures in which patients present with forefoot pain. Treatment is centered on activity modification and protective footwear. The fractures usually heal rapidly because the fractures occur primarily in metaphyseal bone.

Fractures of the Metatarsal Shaft. The first metatarsal is wider and shorter than the other four. There is no interconnecting ligament between the first and second metatarsals, which allows the hallux to be mobile. If there is no instability present, an isolated first metatarsal fracture can be treated with cast immobilization for 4 to 6 weeks. Any evidence of instability of the metatarsal head (either on weight-bearing or stress views) requires operative fixation. External fixation may be indicated for severely comminuted fractures with inadequate intact bone to allow lag screw or plate fixation. Fractures of central metatarsals can be treated nonoperatively using a hard-soled or stiff-soled shoe (cam walker). The indications for nonoperative management are less than 10 degrees of angulation and less than 4 mm of translation. It is important to note that excessive shortening of a shaft can lead to metatarsalgia, emphasizing the need for an accurate reduction.

Fractures of the Fifth Metatarsal. Avulsion fractures are most common in the fifth metatarsal and represent an avulsion of the lateral band of the plantar fascia/peroneus brevis. Such fractures are often confused with a Jones fracture. Treatment consists of a walking cast. Fractures of the metaphyseal–diaphyseal junction (area of poor vascularity) are termed Jones fractures, and in nonathletes, they are best treated with cast immobilization for 6 to 8 weeks (Fig. 5.38). If the patient is an athlete, intramedullary screw fixation is required to avoid nonunion. Proximal diaphyseal stress fractures also occur in athletes and are seen in the proximal 1.5 cm of the diaphyseal shaft of the metatarsal. They can be treated with no weight bearing in a short-leg cast for 6 to 8 weeks if acute. Delayed union or nonunion will require IM screw fixation and possible bone grafting.

MTP Joint Injuries. Loss of the normal cascade of the toes is suggestive of injury to MTP joint. Direct dorsal

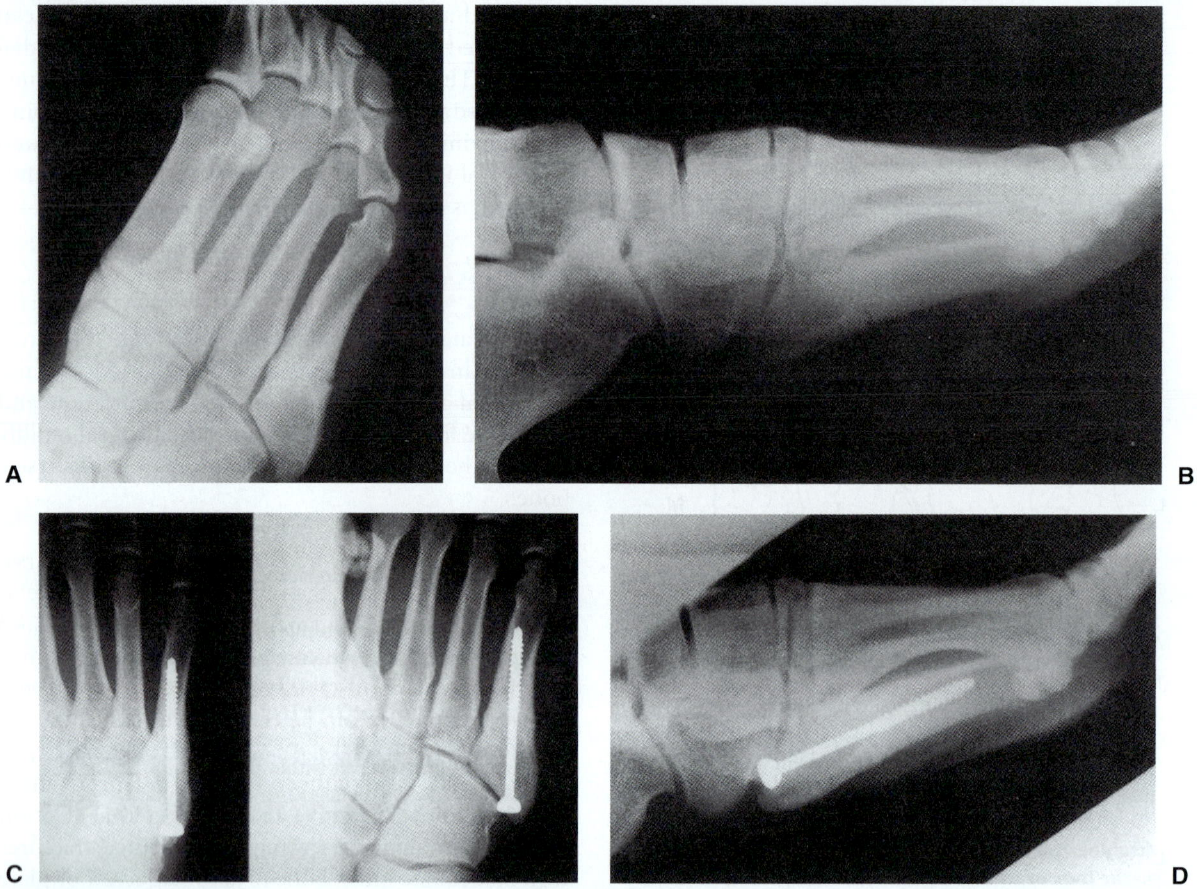

FIGURE 5.38 (A) Preoperative and (B) postoperative radiographs of a Jones stress fracture that failed to unite with conservative care. (C) and (D) Postoperative films approximately 10 weeks after surgery. (*Source: Orthopaedic Knowledge Update Foot and Ankle 2*. American Academy of Orthopaedic Surgeons, 1998, 249, Fig. 5, Chp. 19, Injuries to the midfoot and forefoot.)

stress testing of these joints can be used to evaluate for instability and detect a possible injury to the plantar plate (similar to evaluating the interphalangeal joints of the hand). If the joint is unstable, surgical fixation is often required to restore stability and function.

Sesamoid Injuries. Repetitive loading can result in a sesamoidal stress fracture. The medial sesamoid is injured more often than lateral. Patients often present with localized tenderness, swelling, and reduced plantarflexion strength at the hallux. The initial treatment of any isolated, stable sesamoidal injury is immobilization for 4 to 6 weeks, followed by use of a stiff-soled shoe for an additional 4 to 6 weeks.

Phalangeal Fractures. Phalangeal fractures are the most common injuries to the forefoot, with the proximal phalanx most commonly involved. All nondisplaced phalangeal fractures, regardless of articular involvement, can be treated with stiff-soled shoes and restricted weight bearing.

XVI. SOFT TISSUE TRAUMA AND COMPARTMENT SYNDROME

Soft tissue injuries may go unappreciated in the presence of fractures but can cause significant morbidity especially if compartment syndrome develops.

Acute Compartment Syndrome of the Leg. Most commonly, acute compartment syndrome is caused by muscle injury, leading to edema and bleeding that is often proportional to the degree of tissue damage. The fascial compartments within the leg itself are relatively nonyielding, leading to an increase in compartment pressures that can cause tissue ischemia and potentially permanent damage. Clinical evaluation of a patient with an impending compartment syndrome often reveals pain with palpation along the involved compartments and aggravation of pain with passive stretch of the muscles of the involved compartment(s).

Fasciotomies are usually recommended when the compartment pressure is within 30 mmHg of the diastolic blood pressure or within 30 mmHg of the mean arterial blood pressure. The fasciotomy of the leg can be performed with either a 1-incision or 2-incision approach. The 2-incision approach involves making an incision along the posterior aspect of the tibia, along the medial aspect of the leg. The superficial posterior compartment is then released, and the soleus is reflected posteriorly. Subsequently, the deep posterior compartment, which is subcutaneous in the distal part of the leg, is released. The anterolateral incision is made along the anterolateral aspect of leg. The incision must be approximately 7 cm away from the medial incision to avoid devitalizing the skin bridge between the two incisions. Care must be taken to avoid injuring the SPN, and then a subcutaneous dissection is carried out. The fascial covering of both the anterior and lateral compartments are then released.

The 1-incision (perifibular) approach involves making an incision directly over the fibula from the level of the fibular head to the level of the lateral malleolus. Care should be employed to avoid damaging the common peroneal nerve. The fascial plane between the soleus and FHL muscle is identified distally and extended proximally to the soleus origin. Both compartments are then released. The anterior edge of the incision is then retracted anteriorly to reveal the anterior and lateral compartments, which are then released.

Chronic Compartment Syndrome of the Leg. Often associated with repetitive exertion, chronic compartment syndrome is commonly seen in athletes in whom exercise elevates the intracompartment pressures within the involved compartments, resulting in pain. It typically affects the leg, thigh, and forearm. Patients often experience cramping, limited endurance, or fullness in the affected compartment when attempting to exercise. Criteria often used to diagnose chronic compartment syndrome include a resting pressure of 15 mmHg or more and/or 30 mmHg or more 1 minute following exercise or 20 mmHg or more 5 minutes following exercise. Treatment involves either activity modification or fasciotomy of the involved compartments in the same manner as described for acute compartment syndrome.

Acute Compartment Syndrome of the Foot. The foot is also susceptible to compartment syndrome because of the many separate compartments lined with inelastic fascial structures. Crush injuries and fractures are a common cause and result in increased compartment pressures from edema. Pulses are still maintained and should not be used to make the diagnosis. Pain with passive dorsiflexion of the foot (stretching of the intrinsics) is highly suggestive of acute compartment syndrome. Pressure measurements should be taken to confirm diagnosis. Keep the foot elevated at the level of the heart during evaluation. Fasciotomy is recommended if pressure is more than 30 mmHg. The approach is through 2 dorsal incisions and 1 medial incision. The pressure of the deep calcaneal compartment of the quadratus plantae is often the most elevated.

Chronic Compartment Syndrome of the Foot. This condition may result from a missed acute compartment. A common mistake is to place a patient in a cast without checking the foot during follow-up. Intrinsic muscles become ischemic and will necrose, resulting in lesser toe deformities with hyperdorsiflexion at the metatarsophalangeal joint and hyperplantarflexion deformities at the PIP and DIP joints due to the extrinsic muscles overcoming the remaining power of the intrinsics (claw toes). Sensory deficits are usually present because of concomitant local injuries to the nerves.

XVII. TUMORS OF THE FOOT AND ANKLE

Imaging

Radiographs. Any patient in whom a tumor of the foot is suspected should have plain radiographs. They can be used to evaluate the periosteal reaction in patients with a primary bone tumor, endosteal scalloping in patients with cartilaginous lesions, or osseous erosions or calcifications in patients with soft tissue lesions.

CT. CT is an excellent imaging modality to detect stress fractures, endosteal scalloping, or cortical destruction.

Nuclear Imaging. Radionucleotide scans, while not as informative in diagnosing primary tumors as radiographs or MRI, are useful in detecting skeletal metastases.

Angiography. Angiographic studies are most useful in delineating vascular tumors such as hemangiomas or arteriovenous malformations and can be used to plan a surgical resection or embolization.

MRI. MRI and plain radiographs are the modalities of choice to image most tumors of the foot and ankle. Administration of gadolinium can be used to define the vascularity of the tumor, and imaging in multiple planes can provide the location and orientation of the lesion.

Bone Tumors

Subungual Exostosis. Subungual exostosis is a benign lesion that arises from the dorsomedial aspect of the distal phalanx underneath the nail plate. It is thought to result from repetitive trauma and histologically can appear as hypercellular with a fibrous cap and underlying hyaline cartilage and cancellous bone. Treatment typically consists of complete excision.

Chondroblastoma. Chondroblastomas are always located juxtaposed to apophyseal or articular surfaces; they are lytic, expansile, and often painful. Most are found in either the subchondral bone of the talus or in the calcaneal apophysis. Large defects are treated with curettage and bone grafting.

Osteoblastoma. This lesion, while rare, can be seen in the foot and is commonly seen in the hindfoot (particularly the talar neck). If aggressive, however, osteoblastoma can cause extensive osseous destruction and a robust periosteal reaction. Most are lytic in nature and are larger than osteoid osteomas but are less expansile. Treatment is complete surgical resection with bone grafting depending on the size and location of the lesion.

Osteoid Osteoma. Osteoid osteomas are self-limited lesions that often present with nocturnal pain that is relieved with salicylates. They have a characteristic radiographic appearance with a radiolucent nidus surrounded by a rim of sclerotic bone. Nonsurgical treatment with nonsteroidal medication can be effective, but if necessary, intralesional curettage with complete excision of the nidus can be performed.

Enchondroma. As with enchondromas elsewhere in the body, enchondroma in the foot represents an abnormality of development of the physeal cartilage, in which the physeal cartilage is trapped within growing bone. It is often seen within the small, tubular bones of the foot and radiographically can present with endosteal scalloping, as is characteristic of cartilaginous tumors. Observation is the main treatment option, though if associated with a fracture, the fracture is immobilized for 6 weeks followed by curettage and bone grafting.

Unicameral Bone Cyst. This cyst is an abnormality of the growth plate whereby a cyst forms that eventually is found a certain distance away from the physeal scar and eventually consolidates. Virtually all unicameral bone cysts in the foot are located in the anteroinferior aspect of the calcaneus. The initial treatment is observation, as most are asymptomatic, but for those that are painful or have resulted in a pathologic fracture, curettage and bone grafting is appropriate (Fig. 5.39).

Intraosseous Lipoma. An intraosseous lipoma is a rare tumor found in the same location as a unicameral bone

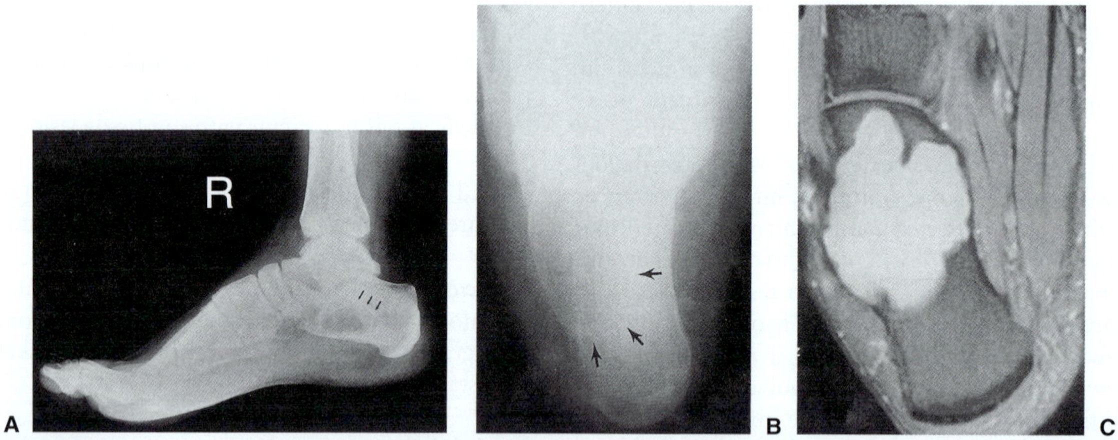

FIGURE 5.39 (A) A lateral radiograph of the foot and ankle showing a unicameral bone cyst in the anterior calcaneus with reinforced trabeculae superiorly. This 20-year-old male presented with heel pain. (B) Harris view demonstrates this laterally based, slightly expansile radiolucent abnormality with well delineated and sclerotic borders and no matrix production. (C) An axial T2 pulsed weighted MR sequence shows a homogeneous bright signal abnormality occupying the majority of the anterior calcaneus that is consistent with fluid. There are no fluid-fluid levels to suggest the presence of blood, and the cortices are intact circumferentially. (*Source: Orthopaedic Knowledge Update Foot and Ankle* 2. American Academy of Orthopaedic Surgeons, 1998; 17, Fig. 3, Chp. 2, Tumors.)

cyst in the foot, though it presents at an older age. The treatment is curettage; the recurrence rate is low.

Epidermal Inclusion Cyst. Primarily a soft tissue lesion that can subsequently involve bone (termed an epidermal bone cyst), epidermal inclusion cysts appear lytic on radiographs and expansile but have a well-defined sclerotic margin. The treatment method is curettage.

Giant Cell Tumor. This type of tumor is infrequently found within the foot, but the treatment is the same: curettage and adjuvant therapy (phenol or polymethylmethacrylate [PMMA] for structural support).

Chondrosarcoma. The most common malignant tumor of the foot, chondrosarcoma can be primary or secondary to a preexisting osteochondroma or enchondroma. Most are of low to intermediate grade, but high-grade ones can be found in the hindfoot. Radiographs will show endosteal scalloping with intense radionucleotide uptake on bone scan. T2-weighted imaging on MRI will be bright because of intralesional edema. Histologically, the tumor is relatively cellular, with sparse matrix and demonstrating invasion of bone. Low- and intermediate-grade tumors can be treated with wide local resection, but higher grade tumors of the hindfoot are treated with a below-knee amputation.

Soft Tissue Tumors

Ganglion Cyst. Ganglion cysts can occur in either the hand or foot and represent myxoid degeneration of collagen fibers of a joint capsule or tendon sheath, leading to cyst formation. Aspiration is both diagnostic and therapeutic. A steroid can be injected as well. Recurrent cysts are treated with excision.

Neurofibroma. Neurofibromas of the foot can be part of the systemic condition neurofibromatosis. They present as firm, painless, mobile masses that are found commonly along peripheral nerves. While it is a benign process, it is often interwoven with the surrounding nerve fibers.

Pigmented Villonodular Synovitis (PVNS). Most commonly seen in the knee, PVNS can also be seen in the various joints of the foot and ankle. It involves synovial proliferation, inflammation, and hemorrhage. It presents with subchondral erosions on plain film. Involvement is diffuse within the foot, often spreading to multiple joints. The initial treatment consists of synovectomy, but recurrence is high given the diffuse involvement. Radiation therapy has had some success as well. For those with severe arthritis due to multiple recurrences, fusion is a good salvage option (Fig. 5.40).

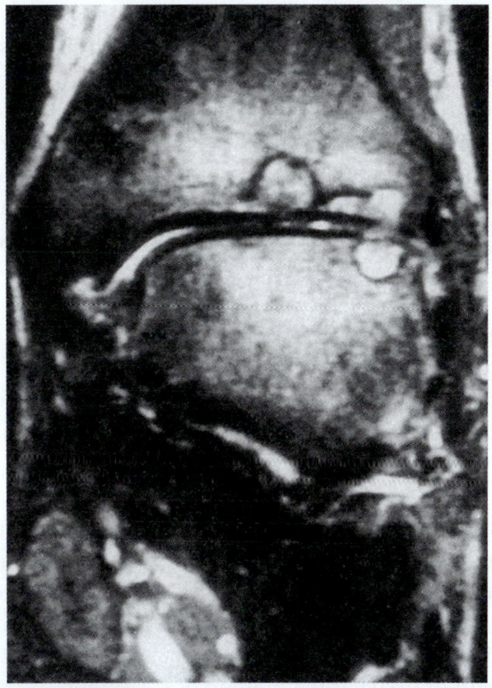

FIGURE 5.40 Patients with diffuse pigmented villonodular synovitis can develop subchondral bone erosions on both sides of the joint, as seen in this T2-weighted coronal MRI in a 60-year-old male with long-standing ankle pain and swelling. (From *Orthopaedic Knowledge Update Foot and Ankle 2*. American Academy of Orthopaedic Surgeons, 1998; 19, Fig. 6, Chp. 2, Tumors.)

Giant Cell Tumor of Tendon Sheath. Seen commonly in the forefoot, this tumor is a localized form of PVNS. The mass is generally fixed to a tendon or joint capsule and can cause subchondral erosions. Patients often complain of difficulty with footwear. Treatment consists of marginal excision.

Hemangioma. Hemangiomas are an abnormal collection of vessels, can be capillary or cavernous, and are occasionally symptomatic. These lesions can be managed by activity modification and nonsteroidal medication, though if resection is indicated, arteriography should be performed first.

Plantar Fibromatosis. Plantar fibromatosis is similar to Dupuytren disease of the hand with the offending cell being the myofibroblast. It can present with progressive toe contractures. Nonsurgical treatment consisting of modifying shoewear, inserts, and nonsteroidal medication should be attempted first. If surgical intervention is necessary, the plantar fascia can be resected from the calcaneus to its slips along the flexor tendons. However, the surgeon should be mindful of the potential loss of the windlass mechanism when performing this procedure.

Granuloma Annulare. Generally painless, granuloma annulare are benign, reactive dermal lesions that can grow rapidly. They are limited to the subcutaneous tissue but can extend into the underlying fascia. Treatment consists of excision.

Melanoma. Melanoma is the most common malignant tumor of the foot and has a poor prognosis because it is often at an advanced stage at the time of diagnosis. Pigmentation beneath the cuticle can be caused by malignant melanoma. Wide resection, with a 2-cm margin of tissue, is the method of treatment.

Clear Cell Sarcoma. A rare, deep-seated tumor that is highly malignant and can secondarily involve the underlying bones of the foot, clear cell sarcoma can appear dark on MRI owing to melanin deposition. It enhances with gadolinium because of its vascular nature. It is best treated with wide local excision and radiation.

Synovial Cell Sarcoma. This is the most common sarcomatous lesion of the foot and is also highly malignant in nature. Commonly seen in young adults (males more frequently), it often has characteristic soft tissue mineralization seen on CT or radiographs. Histologically, it appears either monophasic and spindled with intersecting fascicles or biphasic with both a spindled and a pseudoglandular (epithelioid) appearance. Treatment consists of wide resection with radiation or amputation (radical resection).

XVIII. INFECTIONS OF THE FOOT AND ANKLE

Bacterial Infections

Soft Tissue Infections. *Staphylococcus aureus* and β-hemolytic streptococci are most commonly responsible for soft tissue infections such as blisters, scratches, and other superficial infections. *Pasteurella multocida* are responsible for cat and dog bite infections. Penicillin alone can cover *Pasteurella multocida*, but a cephalosporin will cover *Pasteurella multocida* and *Staphylococcus aureus*. *Pseudomonas* is most commonly responsible for puncture wounds through sneakers. In other cases, *Staphylococcus aureus* is the most common organism. Puncture wounds can proceed to osteomyelitis, osteochondritis, and septic arthritis; therefore, evaluation and treatment should be aggressive. Consider bone scan and computed tomogram if an infection is noted. If septic arthritis or an abscess is present, aggressive surgical débridement through a dorsal approach should be done. Sesamoid bones should be excised if there is osteomyelitis.

Joint Infections. Joint infections are commonly caused by *Staphylococcus aureus*. In young adults, *Neisseria gonorrhoeae* should be considered. Parenteral antibiotics and serial aspirations are first-line treatment, but surgical débridement is recommended after a few days if the infection is not cured.

Bone Infections. Evaluate radiographically with bone scan, CT scans, and or MRI, bone infections usually require surgical débridement and parenteral antibiotics.

Diabetic Foot Infections. *Staphylococcus aureus* is the most common bacteria causing infection. Polymicrobial infections are, however, common. Infected feet account for 15% of diabetic hospital admissions. More than 5% of diabetic patients will need below-the-knee amputation. Superficial wound culture in diabetics may be inaccurate, and therefore deeper cultures or aspirations should be done when possible. Parenteral antibiotics for more serious infections and hyperbaric oxygen should be considered. Good prognostic factors for healing include brachial/anle systolic pressure ratio of 0.45 or higher, toe pressures greater than 30 mmHg, serum albumin greater than 3.5 mg/dL, and total lymphocyte count greater than 1500.

Mycobacterial Infections. Tuberculosis is rare in the foot. Atypical mycobacteria is also rare. Mycobacterium avium–intracellulare is seen in patients with AIDS. Mycobacterium marinum is seen in marine infections.

Fungal Infections

Tinea pedis. Tinea pedis is one of the most common fungal infections of the foot. It involves the skin and cuticles, often on the sole and interdigital spaces, and can present with scaling, itching, and blisters. Local skin infection can be treated with topical antifungal agents. Nail infections can be difficult to treat and may need oral griseofulvin. However, griseofulvin is not a favored treatment because of the long treatment period (8 months to a year) at significant risk of complications.

Other Fungal Infections. Other fungal infections include mycetoma, which can cause Madura foot. This is a chronic foot infection mostly seen in developing countries.

XIX. AMPUTATIONS OF THE FOOT AND ANKLE

General

Five thousand amputations are performed each year in the United States (Fig. 5.41). Eighty percent are vascular related, with diabetes a major cause for amputations. Tourniquets can be used in diabetic patients.

Great Toe Amputation. Amputation of the great toe significantly affects push-off. Save the proximal aspect of the proximal phalanx because it retains the attachment of the plantar fascia and maintains the windlass mechanism. A rocker-bottom prosthesis provides compensation for the lack of push-off. Parts of the lesser toes should be preserved to prevent adjacent toes from drifting toward each other.

Ray Amputation. The ray amputation can be a successful option in cases of infection, gangrene, or trauma. Minimal loss of function occurs with ray amputations of the lesser toes. Complications can occur with increased weight bearing on the remaining metatarsals.

Transmetatarsal Amputation. This is a well-tolerated amputation and allows ambulation in an off-the-shelf shoe with a forefoot filler. However, a custom-molded insole with a toe filler is the recommended prosthesis. The molded toe filler is used to prevent excess shear that can lead to **ulceration**, which is the most common complication.

Lisfranc Amputation. Through tarsometatarsal joints. The Lisfranc amputation results in significant equinovarus deformity with anterior weight bearing through the scar line, predisposing the wound to skin breakdown. Therefore, a TAL, and an early postoperative rigid dressing is preferred. A special shoe or a slipperlike prosthesis is the recommended prosthesis.

Chopart Amputation. The level of amputation is through the talonavicular and calcaneocuboid joints. It results in significant equinovarus deformity with anterior weight bearing through the scar line, predisposing the wound to skin breakdown. Therefore, an Achilles tendon lengthening and an early post-operative rigid dressing are preferred. A special shoe or a slipperlike prosthesis is the recommended prosthesis. An AFO is required for ambulation.

Boyd Amputation. The Boyd amputation excises all of the tarsal bones, except for the calcaneus. This procedure has fallen out of favor and is now primarily used for pediatric congenital amputees.

Symes Amputation. This amputation is the equivalent of an ankle disarticulation, with a heel flap securely attached to the distal tibia, which provides weight bearing for the residual limb. The Symes prosthesis extends to the distal limb.

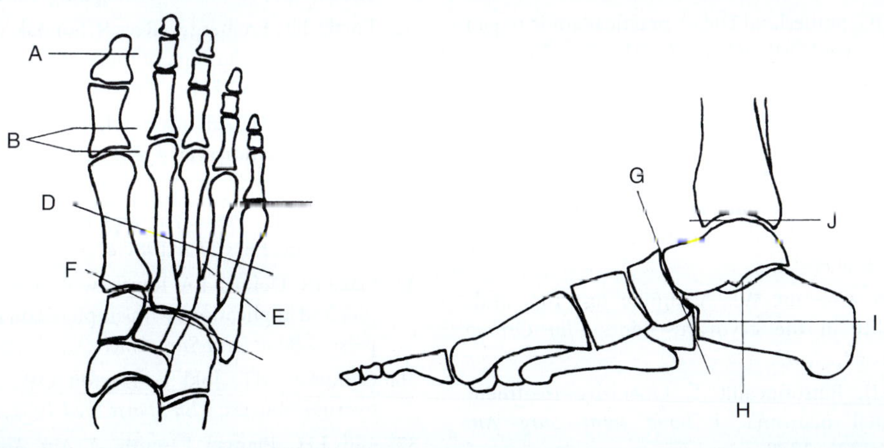

FIGURE 5.41 Levels of forefoot, midfoot, and hindfoot amputations. (A) Terminal Symes. (B) Great toe (at base of proximal phalanx preserves some function, or at metatarsophalangeal joint). (C) Lesser toe at MTP joint. (D) Transmetatarsal. (E) Ray(s). (F) Lisfranc. (G) Chopart. (H) Pirogoff (includes talectomy, 90 degree rotation, and fixation to distal tibia). (I) Boyd. (J) Symes. (*Source: Orthopaedic Knowledge Update Foot and Ankle 2*. American Academy of Orthopaedic Surgeons, 1998; 309. Fig. 1, Chp. 23, Amputations Below the Knee.)

References

1. Abidi NA, Gruen GS, Conti SF. Ankle arthrodesis: Indications and techniques. *J Am Acad Orthop Surg* 2000;8(3):200–209.
2. Anderson FC, Pandy MG. Individual muscle contributions to support in normal walking. *Gait Posture* 2003;17(2):159–169.
3. Astrom M, Rausing A. Chronic achilles tendinopathy. A survey of surgical and histopathologic findings. *Clin Orthop* 1995;16:151–164.
4. Baumhauer JF. Superficial peroneal nerve entrapment. *Foot Ankle Clin* 1998;3:439–446.
5. Beals TC, Pomeroy, GC, Manoli A. Posterior tibial tendon insufficiency. *J Am Acad Orthop Surg* 1999;7(2):112–118.
6. Bennett GL, Weiner DS, Leighley B. Surgical treatment of symptomatic accessory tarsal navicular. *J Pediatr Orthop* 1990;10(4):445–449.
7. Berlet GC, Lee TH, Massa EG. Talar neck fractures. *Orthop Clin North Am* 2001;32(1):53–64.
8. Beskin JL. Nerve entrapment syndromes of the foot and ankle. *J Am Acad Orthop Surg* 1997;5(5):261–269.
9. Brostrom L. Sprained ankles. VI. Surgical treatment of "chronic" ligament ruptures. *Acta Chir Scand* 1966;132(5):551–565.
10. Canale ST, Kelly FB Jr. Fractures of the neck of the talus. Long-term evaluation of seventy-one cases. *J Bone Joint Surg Am* 1978;60(2):143–156.
11. Caputo GM, Cavanagh PR, Ulbrecht JS, Gibbons GW, Karchmer AW. Assessment and management of foot disease in patients with diabetes. *N Engl J Med* 1994;331(13):854–860.
12. Carr JB, Hansen ST, Benirschke SK. Subtalar distraction bone block fusion for late complications of os calcis fractures. *Foot Ankle* 1988;9(2):81–86.
13. Chambers HG, Sutherland DH. A practical guide to gait analysis. *J Am Acad Orthop Surg* 2002;10:222–231.
14. Chou LB, Mann RA, Casillas MM. Biplanar chevron osteotomy. *Foot Ankle Int* 1998;19(9):579–584.
15. Chrisman OD, Snook GA. Reconstruction of lateral ligament tears of the ankle. An experimental study and clinical evaluation of seven patients treated by a new modification of the Elmslie procedure. *J Bone Joint Surg Am* 1969;51(5):904–912.
16. Coleman SS, Chesnut WJ. A simple test for hindfoot flexibility in the cavovarus foot. *Clin Orthop* 1977;123:60–62.
17. Coughlin MJ, Pinsonneault T. Operative treatment of interdigital neuroma. *J Bone Joint Surg Am* 2001;83A(9):1321–1328.
18. Coughlin MJ, Thompson FM. The high price of high-fashion footwear. In: Jackson D (ed.), *Instructional Course Lectures*. Rosemont, IL: American Academy of Orthopaedic Surgeons, 1995;371–377.
19. Coughlin MJ. Disorders of tendons. In: Mann RC, Coughlin MJ (ed.), *Surgery of the Foot and Ankle*. St. Louis: Mosby, 1999.
20. Coughlin MJ. Hallux valgus. *J Bone Joint Surg Am* 1996;78A(6):932–966.
21. Coughlin MJ. Treatment of bunionette deformity with longitudinal diaphyseal osteotomy with distal soft tissue repair. *Foot Ankle* 1991;11(4):195–203.
22. Dalakas MC, Elder G, Hallett M, et al. A long-term follow-up study of patients with post-poliomyelitis neuromuscular symptoms. *N Engl J Med* 1986;314(15):959–963.
23. Davis CA, Lubowitz J, Thordarson DB. Midtarsal fracture-subluxation: Case report and review of the literature. *Clin Orthop* 1993;292:264–268.
24. DeAsla RJ, Deland JT. *Anatomy and Biomechanics of the Foot and Ankle in Orthopaedic Surgery Essentials: Foot & Ankle*. In: Thordarson DB (ed.), Philadelphia: Lippincott Williams & Wilkins, 2004.
25. DiGiovanni BF, Partal G, Baumhauer JF. Acute ankle injury and chronic lateral instability in the athlete. *Clin Sports Med* 2004;23(1):1–19.
26. Donley B. Acquired hallux varus. *Foot Ankle Int* 1997;18(9):586–592.
27. Downs DM, Jacobs RL. Treatment of resistant ulcers on the plantar surface of the great toe in diabetics. *J Bone Joint Surg Am* 1982;64(6):930–933.
28. Evans DL. Recurrent instability of the ankle: A method of surgical treatment. *Proc R Soc Med* 1953;46(5):343–344.
29. Ferkel RD, Heath DD, Guhl JF. Neurological complications of ankle arthroscopy. *Arthroscopy* 1996;12(2):200–208.
30. Flynn JM, Skaggs DL, Sponseller PD, Ganley TJ, Kay RM, Leitch KK. The operative management of pediatric fractures of the lower extremity. *J Bone Joint Surg Am* 2002;84A(12):2288–2300.
31. Fortin PT, Balazsy JE. Talus fractures: Evaluation and treatment. *J Am Acad Orthop Surg* 2001;9(2):114–127.
32. Fortin PT, Freiberg A, Rees R, Sondak VK, Johnson TM. Malignant melanoma of the foot and ankle. *J Bone Joint Surg Am* 1995;77(9):1396–1403.
33. Fraipont MJ, Adamson GJ. Chronic exertional compartment syndrome. *J Am Acad Orthop Surg* 2003;11:268–276.
34. Franco AH. Pes cavus and pes planus. Analyses and treatment. *Phys Ther* 1987;67(5):688–694.
35. Gage JR, DeLuca PA, Renshaw TS. Gait analysis: Principles and applications with emphasis on its use in cerebral palsy. *J Bone Joint Surg Am* 1995;77A:1607–1623.
36. Galloway MT, Jokl P, Dayton OW. Achilles tendon overuse injuries. *Clin Sports Med* 1992;11(4):771–782.
37. Gill LH. Plantar Fasciitis. *J Am Acad Orthop Surg* 1997;5(2):109–117.
38. Greenspan A (ed.), *Orthopaedic Radiology: A Practical Approach*. Philadelphia: Lippincott Williams & Wilkins, 2000.
39. Guyton GP, Saltzman CL. The diabetic foot: Basic mechanisms of disease. *J Bone Joint Surg Am* 2001;83A(7):1084–1094.

40. Hardcastle PH, Reschauer R, Kutscha-Lissberg E, Schoffmann W. Injuries to the tarsometatarsal joint: Incidence, classification and treatment. *J Bone Joint Surg Br* 1982;64(3):349–356.

41. Heppenstall RB, Sapega AA, Scott R, et al. The compartment syndrome. An experimental and clinical study of muscular energy metabolism using phosphorus nuclear magnetic resonance spectroscopy. *Clin Orthop Relat Res* 1988;226:138–155.

42. Hoppenfeld S (ed.), *Physical Examination of the Spine and Extremities*. 276, Upper Saddle River, NJ: Prentice Hall, 1976.

43. Huang CK, Kitaoka HB, An KN, Chao EY. Biomechanical evaluation of longitudinal arch stability. *Foot Ankle* 1993;14(6):353–357.

44. Huefner T, Thermann H, Geerling J, Pape HC, Pohlemann T. Primary subtalar arthrodesis of calcaneal fractures. *Foot Ankle Int* 2001;22(1):9–14.

45. Hunter JC, Sangeorzan BJ. A nutcracker fracture: Cuboid fracture with an associated avulsion fracture of the tarsal navicular. *Am J Roentgenol* 1996;166(4):888.

46. Janisse D. Footwear prescriptions. *Foot Ankle Int* 1997;18(8):526–527.

47. Johnson JE. Operative treatment of neuropathic arthropathy of the foot and ankle. *J Bone Joint Surg Am* 1998;80A(11):1700–1709.

48. Jones D. Foot Orthoses. In: Heckman J (ed.), *Instructional Course Lecture*, Rosemont, IL: American Academy of Orthopaedic Surgeons, 1993:219–224.

49. Jones DC, James SL. Partial calcaneal ostectomy for retrocalcaneal bursitis. *Am J Sports Med* 1984;12(1): 72–73.

50. Keenan MA, Gorai AP, Smith CW, Garland DE. Intrinsic toe flexion deformity following correction of spastic equinovarus deformity in adults. *Foot Ankle* 1987;7(6):333–337.

51. Kirby EJ, Shereff MJ, Lewis MM. Soft-tissue tumors and tumor-like lesions of the foot. An analysis of eighty-three cases. *J Bone Joint Surg Am* 1989;71(4):621–626.

52. Kvist MH, Lehto MU, Jozsa L, Jarvinen M, Kvist HT. Chronic achilles paratenonitis. An immunohistologic study of fibronectin and fibrinogen. *Am J Sports Med* 1988;16(6):616–623.

53. Liu SH, Baker CL. Comparison of lateral ankle ligamentous reconstruction procedures. *Am J Sports Med* 1994;22(3):313–317.

54. Liu SH, Jason WJ. Lateral ankle sprains and instability problems. *Clin Sports Med* 1994;13(4):793–809.

55. Loucks C, Buckley R. Bohler's angle: Correlation with outcome in displaced intra-articular calcaneal fractures. *J Orthop Trauma* 1999;13(8):554–558.

56. Macey LR, Benirschke SK, Sangeorzan BJ, Hansen ST. Acute calcaneal fractures: Treatment options and results. *J Am Acad Orthop Surg* 1994;2(1):36–43.

57. Maffulli, N. Rupture of the achilles tendon. *J Bone Joint Surg Am* 1999;81(7):1019–1036.

58. Mann RA, Holmes GB Jr, Seale KS, Collins DN. Chronic rupture of the achilles tendon: A new technique of repair. *J Bone Joint Surg Am* 1991;73A(2):214–219.

59. Mann RA, Holmes GB Jr, Seale KS, Collins DN. Chronic rupture of the achilles tendon: A new technique of repair. *J Bone Joint Surg Am* 1991;73A(2):214–219.

60. Mann RA. Disorders of the first metatarsophalangeal joint. *J Am Acad Orthop Surg* 1995;3:34–43.

61. Mann RA. Flatfoot in adults. In: Coughlin MM, Mann RA (eds.), *Surgery of the Foot and Ankle*, St. Louis: Mosby, 1999;733–767.

62. McGarvey WC, Palumbo RC, Baxter DE, Leibman BD. Insertional achilles tendinosis: Surgical treatment through a central tendon splitting approach. *Foot Ankle Int* 2002;23(1):19–25.

63. Mehta JA, Brown C, Sargeant N. Charcot restraint orthotic walker. *Foot Ankle Int* 1998;19(9): 619–623.

64. Michelson JD, Checcone M, Kuhn T, Varner K. Intra-articular load distribution in the human ankle joint during motion. *Foot Ankle Int* 2001;22:226–233.

65. Mizel MS, Miller RA, Scioli MW (eds.), *Orthopaedic Knowledge Update Foot and Ankle 2*. Rosemont, IL: American Academy of Orthopaedic Surgeons, 1998.

66. Mizel MS, Yodlowski ML. Disorders of the lesser metatarsophalangeal joints. *J Am Acad Orthop Surg* 1995;3(3):166–173.

67. Moore KL, Dalley AF (eds.) *Clinically Oriented Anatomy*. Philadelphia: Lippincott Williams & Wilkins, 1999;1164.

68. Mulfinger G, Trueta J. The blood supply of the talus. *J Bone Joint Surg Br* 1970;52B(1):160–167.

69. Nawoczenski DA, Janisse DJ. Foot orthoses in rehabilitation—What's new. *Clin Sports Med* 2004;23:157–167.

70. O'Donoghue DH (ed.), *Treatment of Injuries to Athletes*. Philadelphia: WB Saunders, 1976;698–746.

71. O'Sullivan B, Cummings, B, Catton C. Outcome following radiation treatment for high-risk pigmented villonodular synovitis. *Int J Radiat Oncol Biol Phys* 1995;32(3):777–786.

72. Olmos PR, Cataland S, O'Dorisio TM, Casey CA, Smead WL, Simon SR. The Semmes-Weinstein monofilament as a potential predictor of foot ulceration in patients with noninsulin-dependent diabetes. *Am J Med Sci* 1995;309(2):76–82.

73. Perry J (ed.), *Gait Analysis: Normal and Pathological Function*. Thorofare, NJ: SLACK, 1992;524.

74. Peterson HA, Newman SR. Adolescent bunion deformity treated with double osteotomy and longitudinal pin fixation of the first ray. *J Pediatr Orthop* 1993;13:80–84.

75. Philbin TM, Leyes M, Sferra JJ, Donley BG. Orthotic and prosthetic devices in partial foot amputations. *Foot Ankle Clin* 2001;6(2):215–228..

76. Piggott, H. The natural history of hallux valgus in adolescents and early adult life. *J Bone Joint Surg Br* 1960;42B:749–760.

77. Plattner PF, Van Manen JW. Results of Akin type proximal phalangeal osteotomy for correction of hallux valgus deformity. *Orthopedics* 1990;13:989–996.

78. Saltzman CL, Tearse DS. Achilles tendon injuries. *J Am Acad Orthop Surg* 1998;6(5):316–325.

79. Sammarco GJ, DiRaimondo CV. Chronic peroneus brevis tendon lesions. *Foot Ankle* 1989;9:163–170.

80. Sanders R, Fortin P, DiPasquale T, Walling A. Operative treatment in 120 displaced intraarticular calcaneal fractures. Results using a prognostic computed tomography scan classification. *Clin Orthop* 1993;290:87–95.

81. Saunders JB, Inman VT, Eberhart HD. The major determinants in normal and pathological gait. *J Bone Joint Surg Am* 1953;35A:543–558.

82. Scaduto AA, Cracchiolo A 3rd. Lacerations and ruptures of the flexor or extensor hallucis longus tendons. *Foot Ankle Clin,* 2000;5(3):725–736.

83. Schepsis A, Jones H, Haas AL. Achilles tendon disorders in athletes. *Am J Sports Med* 2002;30(2):287–305.

84. Schepsis AA, Wagner C, Leach RE. Surgical management of achilles tendon overuse injuries. A long-term follow-up study. *Am J Sports Med* 1994;22(5):611–619.

85. Scranton PE, McMaster JG, Kelly E. Dynamic fibular function: A new concept. *Clin Orthop* 1976;118:76–81.

86. Shereff M, Baumhauer JF. Hallux rigidus and osteoarthrosis of the first metatarsophalangeal joint. *J Bone Joint Surg Am* 1998;80A(6):898–908.

87. Smith RW, Katchis SD, Ayson LC. Outcomes in hallux rigidus patients treated nonoperatively: A long-term follow-up study. *Foot Ankle Int* 2000;21(11):906–913.

88. Stephens HM, Walling AK, Solmen JD, Tankson CJ. Subtalar repositional arthrodesis for adult acquired flatfoot. *Clin Orthop Relat Res* 1999;365:69–73.

89. Stiell IG, Greenberg GH, McKnight RD, Nair RC, McDowell I, Worthington JR. A study to develop clinical decision rules for the use of radiography in acute ankle injuries. *Ann Emerg Med* 1992;21(4):384–390.

90. Thordarson DB, Schmotzer H, Chon J, Peters J. Dynamic support of the human longitudinal arch. A biomechanical evaluation. *Clin Orthop* 1995;316:165–172.

91. Torg JS, Pavlov H, Cooley LH, Stress fractures of the tarsal navicular: A retrospective review of twenty-one cases. *J Bone Joint Surg Am* 1982;64(5):700–712.

92. Trepman E, Yeo SJ. Nonoperative treatment of metatarsophalangeal joint synovitis. *Foot Ankle Int* 1995;16(12):771–777.

93. Vernino S, Low PA, Fealey RD, Stewart JD, Farrugia G, Lennon VA. Autoantibodies to ganglionic acetylcholine receptors in autoimmune autonomic neuropathies. *N Engl J Med* 2000;343(12):847–855.

94. Wagner FW. Transcutaneous doppler ultrasound in the prediction of healing and the selection of surgical level for dysvascular lesions of the toes and forefoot. *Clin Orthop Relat Res* 1979;142:110–114.

95. Wapner KL, Hecht PJ, Mills RH Jr. Reconstruction of neglected achilles tendon injury. *Orthop Clin North Am* 1995;26(2):249–63.

96. Wapner KL, Pavlock GS, Hecht PJ, Naselli F, Walther R. Repair of chronic achilles tendon rupture with flexor hallucis longus tendon transfer. *Foot Ankle* 1993;14(8):443–449.

97. Wapner KL. Triple Arthrodesis in Adults. *J Am Acad Orthop Surg* 1998;6(3):188–196.

98. Webb J, Moorjani N, Radford M. Anatomy of the sural nerve and its relation to the achilles tendon. *Foot Ankle Int* 2000;21(6):475–477.

99. Wetmore RS, Drennan JC. Long-term results of triple arthrodesis in Charcot-Marie-Tooth disease. *J Bone Joint Surg Am* 1989;71(3):417–422.

100. Whitesides TE Jr, Heckman MM. Acute compartment syndrome: Update on diagnosis and treatment. *J Am Acad Orthop Surg* 1996;4:209–218.

Key References

Canale ST, Kelly FB. Fractures of the neck of the talus. *J Bone Joint Surg Am* 60-A(2):143–156;1978.

The authors present a long-term review of 71 patients with talar neck fractures. Avascular necrosis occurred in 52% of the fractures, and the complications of avascular necrosis, malunion, subtalar arthritis, and infection resulted in 25 secondary procedures being performed.

Chambers HG, Sutherland DH. A practical guide to gait analysis. *J Am Acad Orthop Surg* 10:222–231;2002.

This review article that covers the fundamental topics of gait, gait analysis, and applications of gait analysis.

Coughlin MJ. Hallux valgus. *J Bone Joint Surg Am* 78-A (6):932–966;1996.

This article discusses the pathology, treatment options, and details of the various surgical therapies for treating hallux valgus disorders. Surgical procedures are detailed in a step-by-step fashion.

Guyton GP, Saltzman CL. The diabetic foot. *J Bone Joint Surg Am* 83-A(7):1084–1094;2001.

This review article covers the topics of diabetic neuropathy, pathogenesis of ulcers, and the abnormal wound healing of diabetics. Treatment options are discussed in detail along with an algorithm on treating Charcot arthropathy.

Mann RA. Disorders of the first metatarsophalangeal joint. *J Am Acad Orthop Surg* 3:34–43;1995.

This article presents a difficult topic in a manageable fashion. The pathology and etiology are covered in depth, and it also provides an algorithm that can be applied to treating any type of hallux valgus disorder.

Mann RA, Missirian J. Pathophysiology of Charcot-Marie-Tooth disease. *Clin Orthop* 234:221–228;1988.

This article presents the pathology and treatment options for Charcot-Marie-Tooth disease. Surgical treatment options are discussed in detail.

Mulfinger G, Trueta J. The blood supply of the talus. *J Bone Joint Surg Br* 52-B(1):160–167;1970.

This is a classic cadaveric study on 14 ankles to study the intraosseous and vascular pattern of the talus. The authors describe the vascular anastomoses around the talus and show that the main blood supply to the talus is through the artery of the tarsal canal.

Shereff MJ, Baumhauer JF. Hallux rigidus and osteoarthrosis of the first metatarsophalangeal joint. *J Bone Joint Surg Am* 80-A(6):898–908;1998.

This review article covers the entity of hallux rigidus, including the pathophysiology, etiology, clinical manifestations, and treatment modalities. Both nonoperative and operative treatment modalities are covered in depth, and controversies involving the treatment of this disorder are reviewed.

Refresher Questions

1. What is the main blood supply to the talus?
   a) dorsalis pedis artery
   b) posterior tibial artery
   c) anterior tibial artery
   d) artery of the tarsal canal
   e) medial tarsal

2. What nerve is at risk during surgical repair of Achilles tendon ruptures?
   a) saphenous nerve
   b) sural nerve
   c) medial plantar nerve
   d) lateral plantar nerve
   e) posterior tibial nerve

3. What is the correct progression of staging for Charcot arthropathy?
   a) resolution, dissolution, coalescence
   b) coalescence, resolution, dissolution
   c) dissolution, coalescence, resolution
   d) resolution, coalescence, dissolution
   e) coalescence, dissolution, resolution

4. A cheilectomy is used to treat what disorder?
   a) mallet toe
   b) hammer toe
   c) hallux valgus
   d) hallux rigidus
   e) Freiberg's infarction

5. The blood supply to the Achilles tendon is contained within what aspect of the Achilles tendon?
   a) anterior
   b) posterior
   c) medial
   d) lateral
   e) superior

6. The normal hallux valgus angle is:
   a) less than 5 degrees
   b) less than 10 degrees
   c) less than 15 degrees
   d) less than 20 degrees
   e) less than 25 degrees

7. Which of the following is not an indication for MTP arthrodesis?
   a) HVA greater than 40 degrees
   b) stage III osteoarthritis
   c) rheumatoid arthritis
   d) failed Silastic implant
   e) juvenile hallux valgus

8. What is the most common etiology of recurrent tarsal tunnel syndrome?
   a) poor-fitting footwear
   b) planovalgus foot
   c) peripheral neuropathy
   d) space-occupying lesion
   e) inadequate release of tarsal tunnel

9. What percentage of patients with rheumatoid arthritis have forefoot involvement?
   a) 10%
   b) 40%
   c) 50%
   d) 70%
   e) 90%

10. The Sanders classification of calcaneal fractures primarily evaluates what anatomic aspect of the calcaneus?
    a) anterior facet
    b) posterior facet
    c) middle facet
    d) calcaneal tubercle
    e) sustentaculum talus

11. The offending cell in plantar fibromatosis is:
    a) fibrocyte
    b) alveolar cell
    c) myofibroblast
    d) tenocyte
    e) squamous cell

12. The most common location in the foot for a unicameral bone cyst is:
    a) navicular
    b) midfoot
    c) talus
    d) cuboid
    e) calcaneus

13. What is the trajectory of the primary fracture line in posterior facet fractures of the calcaneus?
    a) superior to inferior
    b) inferior to superior
    c) medial to posterior

d) anterolateral to posteromedial
e) posterolateral to anteromedial

14. The Chrisman-Snook procedure utilizes what structure to repair the ATFL and CFL?
a) peroneus longus
b) peroneus brevis
c) flexor retinaculum
d) extensor digitorum brevis
e) abductor digiti minimi

15. Stance phase constitutes what percentage of the gait cycle?
a) 20%
b) 40%
c) 60%
d) 75%
e) 80%

Chapter 6

Hand and Microsurgery

SEPIDEH BAGHIAN

I. ANATOMY AND PHYSIOLOGY

Bone

Phalanges. There are 5 proximal, 4 middle, and 5 distal phalanges for a total of 14 phalanges in the hand. Primary ossification for the distal, middle, and proximal phalanges occurs during the ninth, tenth, and eleventh week of development, respectively. Secondary ossification centers develop around 2 to 3 years of age at the base of the phalanx, starting with the proximal phalanges. Physeal fusion occurs around 17 to 18 years in males and 15 to 16 years in females.

Metacarpals. There are 5 metacarpals in the hand, each with a head, neck, shaft, and base. In the shaft, the primary ossification center appears during the eighth week of development; the physis appears at 3 years at the junction of the head and neck. Because the thumb metacarpal resembles a phalanx, its physis appears at the base. The second metacarpal is the longest and has the widest base. The base of the third metacarpal bears a styloid process; the insertion of the extensor carpi radialis brevis is just distal to it. The metacarpal heads are roughened on each side with a tubercle that serves as the origin of the proper collateral ligaments of the metacarpophalangeal (MCP) joint.

Arthrology

Proximal and Distal Interphalangeal Joints. The proximal interphalangeal (PIP) and distal interphalangeal (DIP) joints are ginglymoid or uniaxial hinge joints. Congruity of the articular surfaces is an important contributor to the stability of the interphalangeal joints. Joint stability is also maintained by the capsule and extensor tendons dorsally, the collateral ligaments laterally, and the volar plate volarly. The collateral ligaments originate from the head and insert onto the volar plate and the volar aspect of the phalangeal base. They are the primary restraint to radial and ulnar deviation of the interphalangeal joint.

Metacarpophalangeal Joints. The MCP joints of the fingers are condyloid or biaxial joints, allowing for motion in the sagittal and coronal planes. Stability of the joint is achieved by its articular congruity, and the surrounding soft tissue: the extensor, flexor, and intrinsic tendons; sagittal bands; capsule; collateral ligaments; volar plate; and transverse intermetacarpal ligaments. The metacarpal head is wider in the anterior–posterior plane; as a result, it functions as a cam during flexion and extension of the MCP joint. In the sagittal plane, the distance from the center of rotation of the metacarpal head is greatest at the most volar aspect of the head and least at the most distal point of the head. As a result, the collateral ligaments become taut in flexion and lax in extension. The deep transverse metacarpal ligaments (TML) are fibrous bands that connect the palmar plates of the index to small finger metacarpals and prevent them from separating. The superficial TML or natatory ligaments are transverse bands of palmar fascia that run superficial to the flexor tendons at the level of the web space.

Thumb Metacarpophalangeal Joint. The MCP joint of the thumb is an ellipsoid joint that allows for flexion and extension and for limited abduction, adduction, and rotation. Range of motion (ROM) varies from thumb to thumb because of the differences in the curvature of the metacarpal head among individuals; more spherical heads have greater motion. Stability of the thumb MCP joint is dependent on its capsule, ligaments, and surrounding soft tissue; there is very little intrinsic stability from the congruency of the joint. Two sesamoid bones are attached to the volar plate; the radial and ulnar sesamoids serve as an attachment for the superficial head of the flexor pollicis brevis (FPB) and the adductor pollicis respectively. The collateral ligaments of the thumb MCP joint function similarly to those of the finger MCP joints; that is, they are taut in flexion and lax in extension as a result of the camlike effect of the metacarpal head. The ulnar collateral ligament (UCL) of the thumb MCP joint lies directly beneath the aponeurosis of the adductor pollicis. Gamekeeper's thumb is tearing of the UCL, usually at its base on the first phalanx of the thumb. Healing of this injury can be complicated by a Stener lesion, which is interposition of the adductor aponeurosis between the torn ligament and its point of insertion at the base of the proximal phalanx.

Innervation

Median Nerve. The median nerve enters the palm via the carpal tunnel, running between the flexor digitorum superficialis (FDS) and flexor carpi radialis (FCR). At the proximal border of the transverse carpal ligament (TCL), it gives off a palmer cutaneous branch (PCB) from its radial border running between the palmaris longus and FCR that provides sensation to the thenar skin. The PCB of the median nerve is at risk for injury during carpal tunnel surgery. At the distal border of the TCL, the median nerve divides into 5 or 6 branches: the recurrent motor branch to the muscles of the thenar eminence, a common digital nerve for the thumb, the proper digital nerve for the radial side of the index finger, and two common digital nerves for the adjacent areas of the index and long, and long and ring fingers respectively. The origin of the recurrent motor branch varies with respect to the TCL, with the majority being extraligamentous. It is responsible for innervating the superficial head of the FPB, the abductor pollicis brevis (APB), the opponens pollicis, and the two radial lumbricals.

Ulnar Nerve. The ulnar nerve enters the palm through Guyon canal, running medial to the ulnar artery. It divides into superficial and deep branches after passing the pisiform. The superficial branch innervates the palmaris brevis and then terminates into two branches: a proper digital branch for the ulnar side of the small finger and a common digital branch for the adjacent sides of the small and ring fingers. The deep branch dives dorsally between the heads of the abductor digiti minimi (ADM) and flexor digiti minimi (FDM), providing motor innervation to the muscles of the hypothenar eminence, the interossei, the ulnar two lumbricals, the deep head of the FPB, and the adductor pollicis.

TABLE 6.1 Intrinsic muscles of the hand

Muscle	Origin	Insertion	Function	Nerve
Lumbricals (4)	Arise from tendons of the flexor digitorum profundus	Join with interossei to form radial lateral bands	Extension of middle phalanges, flexion of proximal phalanges	Median to radial 2 lumbricals; ulnar to ulnar 2 lumbricals
Dorsal interossei (4)	Adjacent metacarpophalangeal	Proximal phalanx base/extensor apparatus	Abduction, flexion, extension of metacarpophalangeals	Ulnar
Volar interossei (3)	Adjacent metacarpophalangeal	Proximal phalanx base/extensor apparatus	Adduction of digits	Ulnar

Adapted from Doyle JR, Botte MJ. *Surgical Anatomy of the Hand and Upper Extremity.* Philadelphia: Lippincott Williams & Wilkins, 2003;182–183

Cutaneous Innervation of the Dorsal Hand. The dorsal branch of the ulnar nerve arises just distal to the middle of the forearm and courses distally to the hand. It innervates the ulnar border of the small finger, adjacent sides of the small and ring fingers, and adjacent sides of the ring and long fingers (Table 6.1).

Radial Nerve. The superficial branch of the radial nerve arises on the volar surface of the forearm just distal to the elbow. It travels down the forearm deep to the brachioradialis and divides into 5 dorsal digital nerves once it enters the hand. The terminal branch of the lateral antebrachial cutaneous nerve supplies the skin on the radial aspect of the thenar eminence and proximal phalanx of the thumb.

Blood Supply

Ulnar Artery. The ulnar artery enters the hand with the ulnar nerve superficial to the TCL through Guyon canal. The borders of Guyon canal are as follows:

- *Roof*— Volar carpal ligament (VCL) and palmaris brevis
- *Floor*— TCL, pisohamate and pisometacarpal ligaments, opponens digiti minimi (ODM)
- *Ulnar wall*— Flexor carpi ulnaris (FCU), pisiform, and ADM
- *Radial wall*— Extrinsic flexor tendons, TCL, hook of the hamate

In the canal, the deep branch of the ulnar artery emerges and descends between the flexor tendon sheath of the small finger and the FDM to join the main stem of the radial artery to form the deep palmar arch. The next branch that arises is the palmar digital artery to the ulnar side of the small finger. The main stem of the ulnar artery then courses radially across the palm to the superficial palmar arch. Three common digital arteries arise from the superficial palmar arch in the second through fourth web spaces that divide into proper digital arteries. The proper digital arteries run dorsal to the digital nerves in the fingers. The main trunk terminates by anastomosing with the superficial palmar branch of the radial artery. The superficial palmar arch is the primary blood supply to the hand.

Radial Artery. The radial artery enters the anatomic snuffbox and gives off dorsal and palmar carpal branches and a branch to the scaphoid before entering the palm through the two heads of the first dorsal interosseous muscle. The dorsal carpal branch forms part of the dorsal carpal arch, which gives off 3 dorsal metacarpal arteries. In the palm, the radial artery gives off the princeps pollicis artery and the artery to the radial side of the index finger. The main stem of the radial artery anastomoses with the deep branch of the ulnar artery to form the deep palmar arch, which is proximal to the superficial palmar arch.

Tendons

Extensor Tendons

Extensor Mechanism. The extensor mechanism consists of both the intrinsic and extrinsic extensor tendons. The intrinsic system is innervated by the ulnar and median nerves; the radial nerve (posterior interosseous branch) innervates the extrinsic system.

The index and small fingers have separate extrinsic tendons that are independent of the extensor digiti communis (EDC): the extensor indicis proprius (EIP) and the extensor digiti minimi (EDM) respectively. These tendons are located ulnar to their corresponding

EDC tendon as they insert into the extensor hood. The EDC tendon for the small finger is absent 50% of the time. The EIP tendon is often harvested for grafts.

Juncturae Tendinum. Juncturae tendinum are oblique bands that interconnect the tendons of the common extensor just proximal to the MCP joint. They are present between the index and long, long and ring, and ring and small fingers. Juncturae limit independent extension of these 3 digits and can mask the clinical presentation of a complete tendon laceration proximal to the juncture.

Relation to Axis of Rotation. At the MCP joint, the intrinsic muscles and tendons are palmar to the joint axis of rotation. At the PIP joint, they lie volar to the axis of rotation. At the PIP joint, the EDC tendon trifurcates into a central slip and two lateral slips. The central slip inserts at the dorsal base of the middle phalanx. Slips of tendons from the interossei and lumbricals emerge on either side of the PIP joint volarly and continue distally to merge with the two lateral slips of the EDC tendon. Together they form the conjoined lateral bands at the dorsum of the middle phalanx and continue distally to insert at the dorsal base of the distal phalanx as the terminal tendon. The primary function of the central slip and the terminal tendon is to extend the PIP and DIP joints respectively.

Auxiliary Ligaments. There are several auxiliary ligaments that assist in stabilizing the tendons and participate in digital motion.

- *Sagittal bands*—Sagittal bands arise from the volar plate to attach dorsally to the extensor tendon at the joint. These bands initiate extension at the MCP joint of a flexed finger. Injury to these bands can lead to subluxation of the extensor tendon. Incompetence of the radial bands can occur in patients with rheumatoid arthritis (RA) secondary to the extensive synovitis that develops at the MCP joint, causing flexion at this joint and ulnar deviation of the fingers.

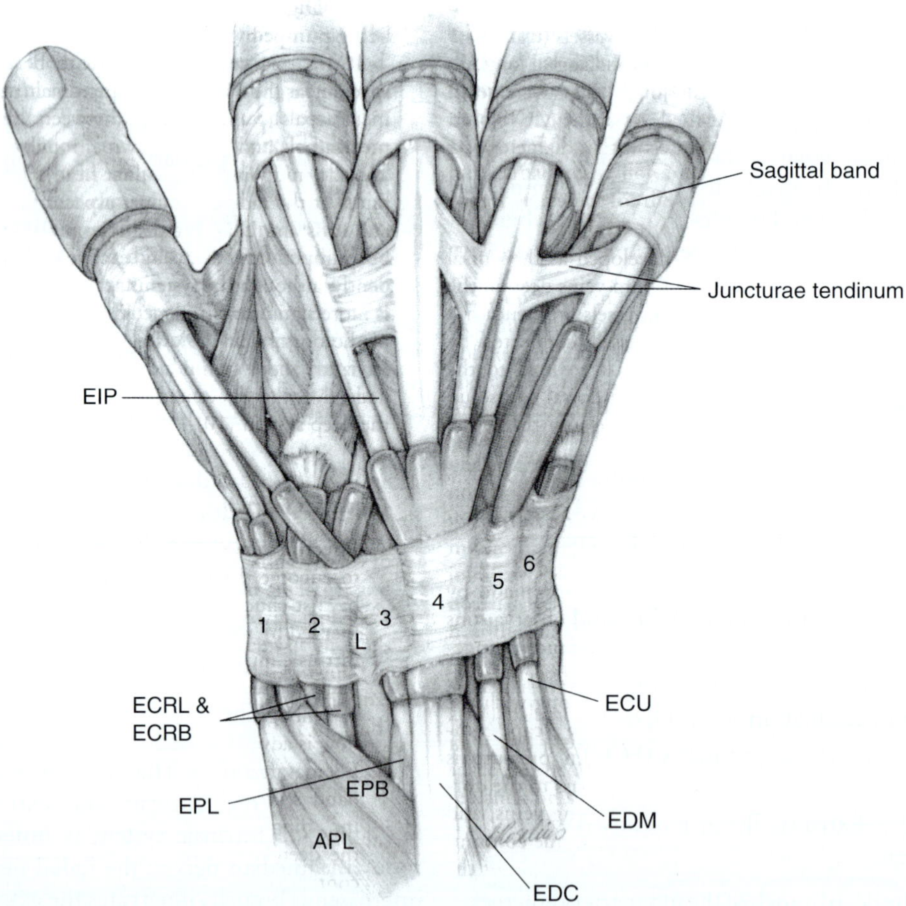

FIGURE 6.1 **Wrist extensor retinaculum and most common arrangement of the extensor tendons and juncturae. (*Source:* Doyle JR. Hand. In: Doyle JR, Botte M (eds.), *Surgical Anatomy of the Hand and Upper Extremity*. Philadelphia: Lippincott Williams & Wilkins, 2003;648, with permission.)**

The bands can rupture after acute trauma to an extended digit. The radial sagittal band of the long finger is the most frequently injured band.

- *Retinacular ligaments*
  - *Oblique retinacular ligament*—Fibers from the volar plate and flexor sheath at the PIP joint and travel distally and dorsally to insert in the terminal tendon. These fibers passively tighten with PIP extension to aid in DIP extension.
  - *Transverse retinacular ligament*—Fibers arise from the flexor sheath and lateral border of the middle phalanx and insert on the lateral border of the conjoined lateral bands; prevents dorsal displacement of the lateral bands.
- *Triangular ligament*—Fibers just distal to the central slip prevent subluxation of lateral bands.

Specific Extensor Tendons by Function. The extensor carpi radialis brevis (ECRB), extensor carpi radialis longus (ECRL), and extensor carpi ulnaris (ECU) are responsible for wrist extension. Thumb extension is provided by the extensor pollicis longus (EPL), extensor pollicis brevis (EPB), and abductor pollicis longus (APL). Finger extension occurs via the EDC, EIP, and EDM. With the exception of the EIP, the muscle bellies of the digital extensors terminate 3 to 4 cm proximal to the wrist joint. At this level, the tendons become enveloped by the extensor retinaculum (ER), which is an extension of fibers from the extensor muscle fascia. Septa divide the space deep to the ER into 6 compartments (Fig. 6.1). Table 6.2 lists the 6 dorsal extensor tendon compartments and associated pathology.

Flexor Tendons

Flexor Tendon Sheath. In the carpal canal, the FDS tendons run in two layers: the ring and long finger tendons lie superficial to the tendons of the small and index fingers. Before entering the carpal canal, the FDS and flexor digitorum profundus (FDP) tendons pass through the common flexor tendon sheath, also known as the ulnar bursa. The median nerve is sandwiched between the flexor retinaculum and the flexor tendon sheath. The flexor pollicis longus (FPL) tendon lies in its own sheath or radial bursa. The spread of infection from one bursa to the other can occur via the Parona space, which is a potential space bordered by the radial and ulnar bursae, the pronator quadratus, and the digital flexor tendons. It can serve as a channel for pus to spread between the bursae, leading to the formation of a horseshoe abscess. The common flexor tendon sheath ends in the middle of the palm. The tendons then enter the digital flexor tendon sheaths, which extend from the level of the metacarpal necks to the insertion of the FDP. Within the synovial sheath on the digit, the FDS tendon initially runs volar to the FDP tendon. At about the middle of the proximal phalanx, however, the FDS tendon splits into two bands. Prior to their insertion onto the base of the middle phalanx, the bands diverge to allow the FDP tendon to pass through to its insertion on the distal phalanx. This split in the FDS tendon is known as the Camper chiasm. The two slips of FDS tendon insert on the proximal half of the middle phalanx (Fig. 6.2).

Vincula. Vincula are derived from vascularized mesotenon that are adapted to serve as the blood supply to the digital flexor tendons in the confines of the digital sheath. A vinculum (singular) can be long or short, and each flexor tendon has one set of each. The vincula, paratenon, and the vessels from the synovial sheath form the blood supply to the flexor tendons (Fig.6.3).

Flexor Tendon Pulleys. Flexor tendon pulleys are thickenings of the digital sheath; their fibers cross tendons transversely or obliquely at the proximal and middle phalanges or at the joint level. They maintain the flexor tendons close to the joint axis to prevent bowstringing.

- *Palmar aponeurosis pulley*—Considered to be an accessory pulley that becomes important in the absence of the first or second annular pulley, the palmar aponeurosis pulley inserts into the deep transverse metacarpal ligament and is at risk for injury during fasciectomy for Dupuytren disease.
- *Annular pulley*—There are 5 annular pulleys; the odd-numbered pulleys A1, A3, and A5 are at the level of the MP, PIP, and DIP joints respectively and originate from the volar plate. The even-numbered pulleys A2 and A4 cross the body of the proximal and middle phalanges respectively. A2 and A4 are the most important.
- *Cruciform pulley*—There are 3 cruciform pulleys (C1, C2, and C3). This pulley is thinner and more narrow than its annular counterpart. It primarily facilitates sheath collapse and expansion during digital motion (Fig. 6.4).

Transverse Carpal Ligament and the Carpal Tunnel. The TCL functions as a flexor tendon pulley at the level of the wrist joint. It prevents bowstringing and subluxation during wrist flexion. The palmar aponeurosis pulley, digital flexor pulleys, and TCL are the three components of a system that functions to maintain a constant relationship between the joint axis and the flexor tendons, allowing for maximum joint movement within the limits of muscle tendon excursion.

Stenosing Flexor Tenosynovitis (Trigger Finger). Triggering occurs as a result of tendon entrapment

TABLE 6.2 Extensor tendon compartments and pathology

Compartment	Tendons	Important Features	Tendinopathy: Diagnosis and Treatment
1	APL EPB	APL has multiple slips; EPB has multiple slips that may run in separate sheaths	DeQuervain stenosing tenosynovitis—inflammation of compartment; Finkelstein provocative maneuver—ulnar deviation and wrist flexion with flexed thumb held in clenched fist causes pain over radial styloid; manage with splinting, NSAIDs, steroid injection; surgery involves release of tendon sheaths; important to release all slips of EPB
2	ECRL ECRB	ECRL inserts on radial aspect of second metacarpal base and provides radial deviation ECRB inserts on third metacarpal base and is main wrist extensor	Intersection syndrome—stenosing tenosynovitis causing pain on dorsal aspect of forearm, approximately 4 cm proximal to wrist; crepitus on exam; manage with splinting, NSAIDs, steroid injection; surgery involves release of compartment
3	EPL	Curves around Lister tubercle; passes ulnar to EPB	EPL tendonitis—pain, swelling, tenderness, and crepitus at Lister tubercle exacerbated by passive or active thumb interphalangeal joint flexion; early diagnosis and release decreases risk of rupture; rupture occurs most commonly in initially nondisplaced distal radius fractures; attritional rupture can also occur in conjunction with inflammatory or degenerative arthritis; surgery involves compartment release and tendon transposition to radial aspect of Lister tubercle
4	EDC EIP	EIP passes ulnar to EDC tendon to index finger	Tendonitis—common in patients with RA; typically involves EDC tendons to the index and small digits; isolated EIP tenosynovitis can also occur; tenderness and swelling over affected area that is worse with wrist flexion; manage with splinting, NSAIDs, steroid injection; surgery involves release of tendon sheaths
5	EDM	Passes ulnar to EDC tendon to small finger; EDC to small finger absent in 50%–60% of cases	Tendonitis—common in patients with RA; typically involves EDC tendons to the index and small digits; isolated EIP tenosynovitis can also occur; tenderness and swelling over affected area that is worse with wrist flexion; manage with splinting, NSAIDs, steroid injection; surgery involves release of tendon sheaths
6	ECU	Neutralizes radial deviation force of ECRL	ECU tendonitis—tenderness typically following twisting injury; dysesthesias of the dorsal sensory branch of ulnar nerve is common; subluxation of the ECU associated with TFCC injury; tendon subluxates with flexion and extension of wrist when held in supination and ulnar deviation; manage with splinting, NSAIDs, steroid injection; surgery involves release of sheath; reconstruct sheath if unstable and consider arthroscopic evaluation of TFCC

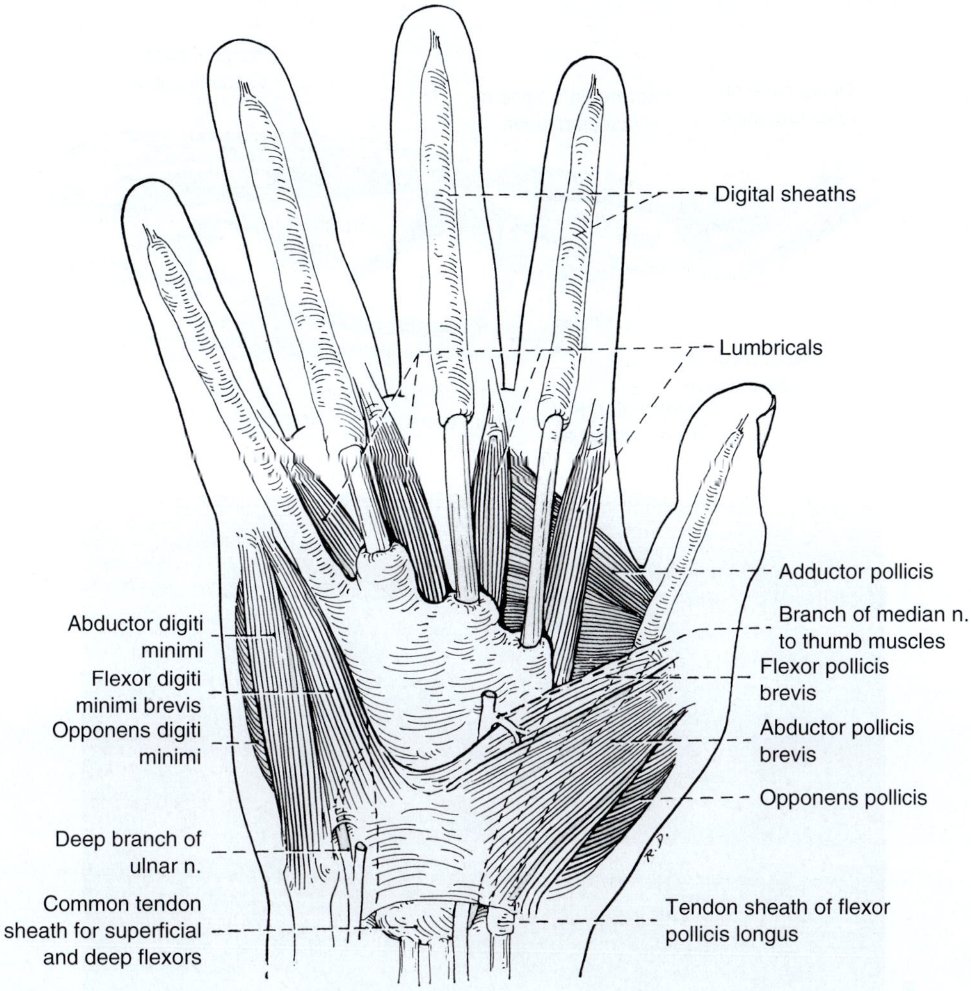

FIGURE 6.2 **Synovial tendon sheaths of the palm of the hand. (*Source:* Hollinshead WH. *Anatomy for Surgeons*, Vol. 3. New York: Harper & Row, 1968;501, with permission.)**

of the fingers and thumb. Patients typically present with painful snapping or catching of the involved flexor tendon as the patient attempts to flex and extend the digit. On occasion, locking of the digit in flexion may occur; extension can be achieved by passive digital manipulation. Tendon entrapment that results in triggering is the result of mechanical impingement of the digital flexor tendon as it attempts to glide through a stenosed pulley at the level of the metacarpal head. The triggering and locking is a result of an imbalance between the volume of sheath and its contents, and the condition prevents gliding of the tendon through the A1 pulley. Thickening secondary to inflammation occurs in a localized area of the involved flexor tendon; friction between the pulley and tendon can cause the development of a nodule, just distal to the A1 pulley, known as nodular tenosynovitis.

Diffuse Stenosing Tenosynovitis. When the inflammatory changes of the synovium extend beyond the A1 pulley, diffuse stenosing tenosynovitis develops. It is thought that stenosis of the pulley is secondary to repetitive compressive loading of the tendon. More than one digit may be affected; the most commonly involved digit is the thumb, followed by the ring, long, small, and index fingers respectively. Inflammatory changes of the synovium occur secondary to a systemic process. Prognosis following treatment is worse than for the primary type. In general, conservative management is successful in over 85% of cases and includes splinting, NSAIDs, and cortisone injections. In cases that have failed conservative treatment, surgical release, either open or percutaneous, entails the next level of treatment. Complications associated with surgical release include digital nerve transaction, injury to the A2 pulley, painful scars, and stiffness. Persistent pain is a complication following percutaneous release. Rupture of the A2 pulley is seen in rock climbers and is thought to occur following rapidly applied extension load to an acutely flexed finger, also known as crimping (Fig. 6.5).

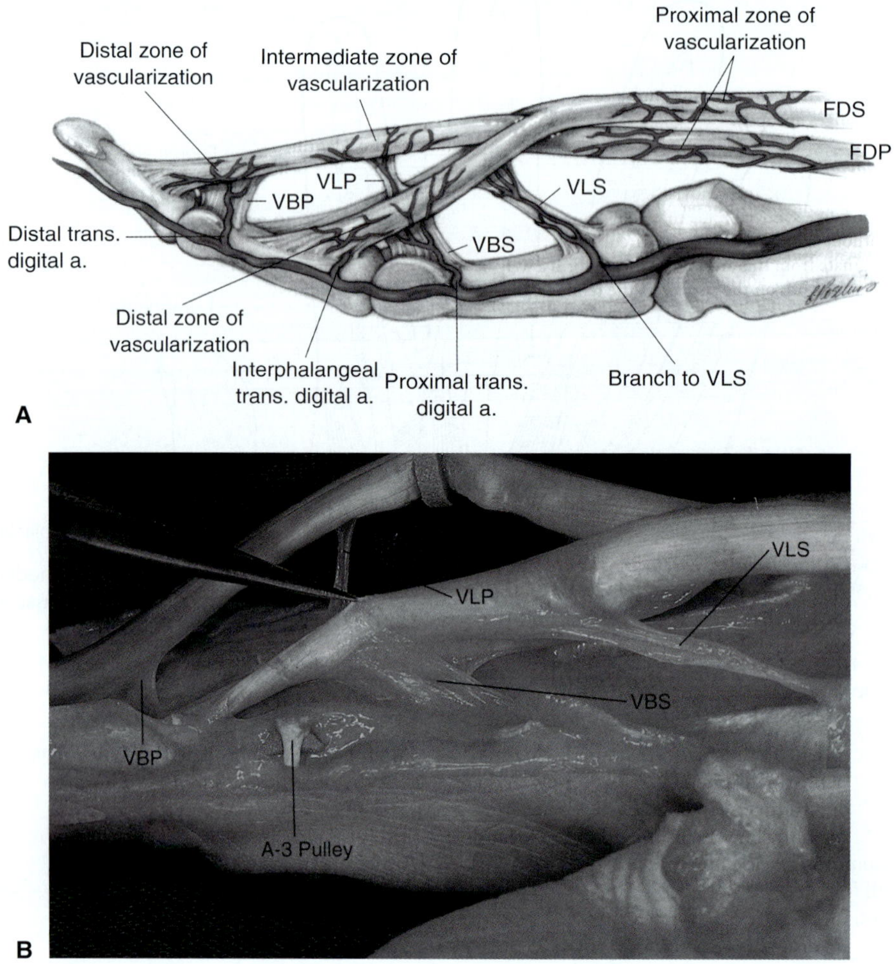

FIGURE 6.3 Vascular supply of the flexor tendons in their sheath: the vincular system. (A) A vinculum may be long and filamentous or short and mesentery-like. VBP and VLP, the short and long vinculum to the profundus tendon; VBS and VLS, the short and long vinculum to the superficialis. (B) Fresh cadaver dissection of right middle finger as viewed from the ulnar side. (*Source:* Doyle JR. Hand. In: Doyle JR, Botte M (eds.), *Surgical Anatomy of the Hand and Upper Extremity*. Philadelphia: Lippincott Williams & Wilkins, 2003;610, with permission.)

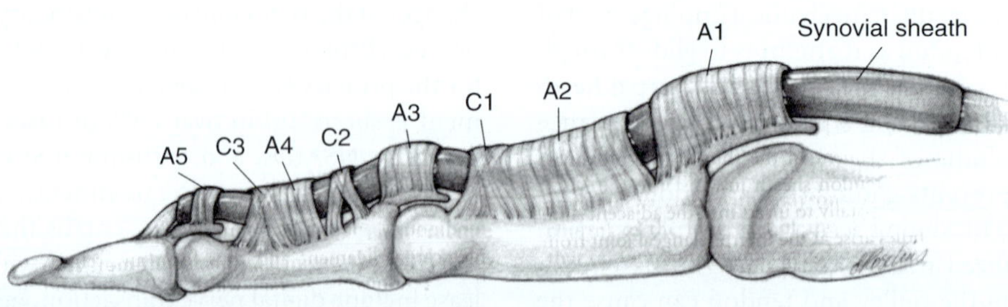

FIGURE 6.4 Digital flexor sheath. (*Source:* Doyle JR. Hand. In: Doyle JR, Botte M (eds.), *Surgical Anatomy of the Hand and Upper Extremity*. Philadelphia: Lippincott Williams & Wilkins, 2003;600, with permission.)

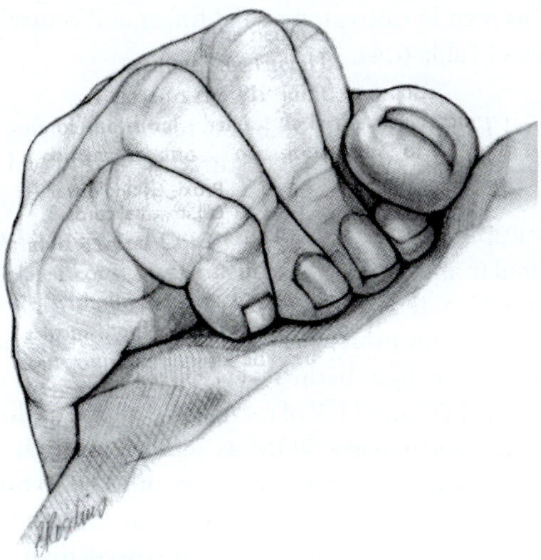

FIGURE 6.5 **The rock climber's technique of crimping, which may be associated with rupture of the second annular pulley. (*Source:* Doyle JR. Hand. In: Doyle JR, Botte M (eds.), *Surgical Anatomy of the Hand and Upper Extremity*. Philadelphia: Lippincott Williams & Wilkins, 2003;624, with permission.)**

Flexor Carpi Radialis (FCR) Tendonitis. The FCR tendon travels through a narrow tunnel in the distal forearm and wrist and turns a sharp corner over the ridge of the trapezium; this tight path makes the FCR prone to primary stenosing tenosynovitis and secondary injury resulting from traumatic or degenerative insults to the carpus. FCR tenosynovitis typically affects middle-aged females, who report an insidious onset. Patients typically present with tenderness and swelling at the distal palmar wrist over the scaphoid tubercle that is exacerbated with resisted flexion and radial deviation. Linburg syndrome is tenosynovitis secondary to intertendinous connection between the FPL and FDP to the index finger and is present in 25% of cadavers; it must be ruled out. An injection with lidocaine can confirm the diagnosis. Initial management includes immobilization, activity modification, and NSAIDs; a cortisone injection may be considered in cases that are not associated with neighboring arthritis. Surgical release and débridement of local sharp edges or osteophytes is performed when conservative management fails.

Flexor Carpi Ulnaris (FCU) Tendonitis. FCU tendonitis can be calcific or a result of repetitive trauma. Degenerative changes of the pisotriquetral joint must be ruled out. Management includes splinting, activity modification, NSAIDs, and cortisone injection. Refractory cases are treated with débridement of calcium deposits and release.

Intrinsic Muscles

The intrinsic muscles of the hand consist of 4 lumbricals and 7 interossei; together they make up the intrinsic half of the extensor mechanism. They work in concert with the extrinsic long extensors via the dorsal aponeurosis to control digital motion. The lumbricals run volar to the deep transverse metacarpal ligament, and the interossei lie dorsal to it.

Lumbricals

Lumbricals function as the main extensors of the interphalangeal joints. They form the FDP tendons in the palm and insert into the lateral band of the dorsal aponeurosis on the radial side of the 4 fingers. Lumbricals run volar to the MCP joint and dorsal to the interphalangeal joints, making them MCP joint flexors, interphalangeal joint extensors, and antagonists of their corresponding FDP tendon. Lumbrical contraction relaxes FDP flexion, thereby enhancing extension at the interphalangeal joint. Conversely, FDP contraction relaxes the corresponding lumbrical, thereby enhancing flexion at the interphalangeal joint. The ulnar 2 lumbricals are innervated by the ulnar nerve and are bipennate; the radial 2 lumbricals are innervated by the median nerve and are unipennate.

Interossei

There are 4 dorsal and 3 volar interosseous muscles that are responsible for finger abduction and adduction respectively. The third metacarpal is the axis for this motion.

Dorsal Interossei. Dorsal interossei arise from adjacent sides of the metacarpals and are abductors of the index, long, and ring fingers. They are larger than the volar interossei, consisting of a superficial and deep belly. The tendon of the deep belly is called the lateral tendon. From its origin, it runs volar to the axis of the MCP joint to insert into the dorsal aponeurosis of the extensor hood at the proximal phalanx. It functions as an abductor and flexor of the MCP joint and extensor of the interphalangeal joints.

Volar Interossei. Volar interossei arise from the metacarpals of the index, long, and ring fingers to insert into the adductor side of the lateral bands of the dorsal aponeurosis. They, like the deep belly of their dorsal counterparts, are part of the extensor mechanism and function as adductors and flexors of the MCP joint and extensors of the interphalangeal joint.

II. TENDON INJURIES

Extensor Tendon Injury. Classification and management of extensor tendon injuries are based on the anatomic zone of injury (Fig. 6.6 and Table 6.3). There are 9 zones; odd-numbered zones are over joints, and even-numbered zones are over bones. The thumb is considered separately because of the smaller number of phalanges. In general, closed tendon injuries are managed conservatively; open tendon injuries are treated with formal débridement and repair. Nonabsorbable suture is utilized using suture technique that consists of a core stitch such as the modified Kessler. Partial tendon injuries that are open are repaired if more than 50% of the tendon width is disrupted. Proximal tendon injuries typically have a better outcome than more distal injuries. Because the extensor mechanism is linked, tendon discontinuity causes an imbalance of forces that can lead to deformity at an adjacent finger joint as seen in untreated mallet finger and central slip injuries (Table 6.4).

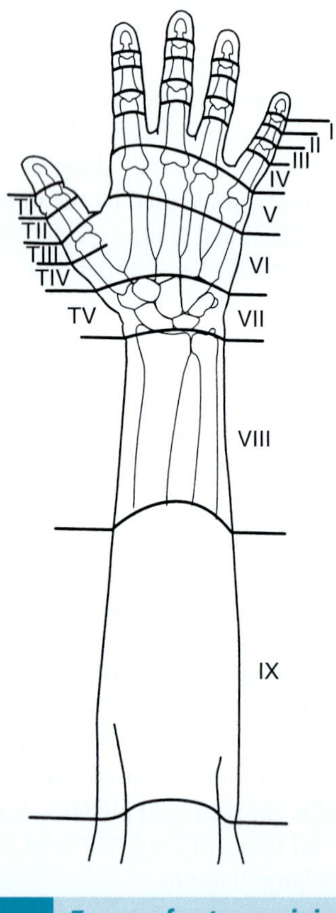

FIGURE 6.6 **Zones of extensor injury. (*Source:* Doyle JR. Hand. In: Doyle JR, Botte M (eds.), *Surgical Anatomy of the Hand and Upper Extremity*. Philadelphia: Lippincott Williams & Wilkins, 2003;649, with permission.)**

Flexor Tendon Injury. Flexor tendon injuries can result from spontaneous rupture, avulsion, and lacerations and can range from partial tendon injury to multiple tendon involvement with associated neurovascular and osseous injuries. After a neurovascular examination, tendon integrity is assessed. A digit with a flexor tendon injury will disrupt the normal resting cascade of the digits because it is more extended. Function of the FDS and FDP of each digit must be evaluated for active and passive ROM as well as strength. The FDS is isolated by holding all of the uninvolved fingers in full extension. The FDP is isolated by immobilizing the MCP and PIP joints of the involved digit. It is important to keep in mind that laceration of the skin does not necessarily correlate with the level of tendon injury. Once tendon injury has been confirmed, repair must be performed within a few days following injury; in the interim, the forearm and wrist must be immobilized in a forearm-based dorsal splint with the wrist in approximately 20 degrees of flexion, the MCP joints in 50 degrees of flexion, and the interphalangeal joints in extension. Classification of injury is based on the zone or location along the flexor mechanism. There are 5 zones; zones of the thumb are different from zones of the fingers. In general, intrasynovial flexor tendon repairs should be performed within 10 to 14 days of injury utilizing a core and epitendinous suture technique. The number of sutures crossing the repair is directly proportional to the strength of the repair.

Several other important factors must be taken into consideration when repairing tendons.

- Four to 6 strands is optimal.
- The diameter of suture is also directly proportional to the strength of the repair; 3–0 or 4–0 caliber nonabsorbable suture is recommended.
- Locking suture technique does not increase repair strength.
- Failure of the repair frequently occurs at the knot.
- Repair supplemented with a running circumferential epitendon suture technique increases the strength of the core stitch up to 50% and minimizes gapping.
- Suture technique must withstand gap formation of 3 mm at the repair site during the initial 3 weeks following repair.

Following are factors that affect prognosis following tendon injury:

- Guillotine lacerations have a better outcome than crush injuries.
- Zone II injuries have the poorest outcome.
- Children typically have a better outcome than adults.

TABLE 6.3 Finger extensor injuries

Zone	Anatomic Level	Disorder	Treatment
I	DIP	Mallet finger	
		Type I: closed/blunt	Stack splint 6–8 weeks; night splint and wean for 2 weeks
		Type II: laceration	Repair skin and tendon in single layer; splint
		Type III: abrasion with skin loss	Repair skin and tendon in single layer; splint
		Type IV	
		A: transepiphyseal	Splint
		B: hyperflexion injury (20%–50% of articular surface)	Splint-fix
		C: hyperextension injury (> 50% of articular surface; usually with subluxation)	Fix if large enough (over button or tension band); pin DIP if subluxated
II	Middle phalanx	Usually lacerations	Under 50% involvement: splint for 2 weeks then begin protected ROM
			Over 50% involvement: repair with nonabsorbable suture; splint DIP in extension for 6 weeks and allow active PIP flexion
III	PIP	Boutonniére lesion (rule out pseudoboutonniére injury)	Splint PIP in neutral; allow active DIP motion
		Laceration	Repair with modified Kessler, 4-0 nonabsorbable suture
IV	Proximal phalanx	Usually partial lacerations	Repair with modified Kessler, 4-0 nonabsorbable suture; repair isolator lateral band lesions
V	MCP	Human bite (fight bite)	Open irrigation and débridement; delayed repair of extensor mechanism in 7–10 days
		Laceration	Repair with modified Kessler, 4-0 nonabsorbable suture; repair sagittal bands
		Closed sagittal band; dislocation of EDC usually ulnar to MP	Within 2 weeks of injury, splint with MCP at 20 degrees, interphalangeal joints free
VI	Metacarpal	Laceration	Repair with core stitch
VII	Extensor retinaculum (carpus)	Laceration; rule out rheumatoid arthritis in closed atraumatic cases	Repair laceration; splint wrist in 45 degrees of extension for 4–5 weeks; fingers free
VIII	Distal forearm	Closed injury rare	Splint incomplete injuries; repair complete lacerations
IX	Mid to proximal forearm	Penetrating injury	Must explore to rule out radial or posterior interosseous nerve injury versus tendon laceration; repair muscle belly and nerve

Adapted from Tan V, Daluiski A. Tendon. In: Beredjiklian PK, Bozentka DJ (eds.), *Review of Hand Surgery*. Philadelphia: Saunders, 2004;27–47.

TABLE 6.4 Finger flexor tendon injuries

Zone	Anatomic Level	Injury	Treatment
I	Distal to FDS insertion for digits; FPL insertion for thumb	FDP avulsion (Jersey finger) Leddy classification based on level of tendon retraction Type I: palm Type II: PIP joint (held by vinculum longum); most common Type III: A4 pulley (held by bony avulsion fragment) A: profundus avulsed off of fracture fragment	Repair within 7–10 days Repair within 3 months ORIF of fracture Treat according to level of tendon retraction
II	Between metacarpal neck and zone I for fingers; neck of proximal phalanx to metacarpal neck for thumb	Typically involves injury to FDS and FDP; historically known as no man's land because of poor results after injury in this zone FDS avulsion is not common; limited PIP motion and mass at A1 pulley	Repair FDS and FDP tendons; repair digital nerve/artery; tendon excision and tenolysis
III	Between distal palmar crease and distal edge of transverse carpal ligament for fingers; region of the thenar eminence in thumb	Tendon repair in this zone less likely to impede motion because the injury is proximal to the digital flexor sheath	Exploration and repair of tendons and neurovascular structures
IV	Carpal tunnel	Injury typically involves tendons and neurovascular structures such as the median nerve	Exploration and repair of tendons and neurovascular structures; recovery is guarded
V	Distal forearm (proximal edge of transverse carpal ligament to musculotendinous junction of flexor tendons)	Injury can involve digital and wrist flexors and neurovascular structures (spaghetti wrist)	Exploration and repair of tendons and neurovascular structures; good prognosis in the absence of neurovascular injury

- Most common complication is stiffness and contracture secondary to adhesion formation.
- Factors associated with adhesion formation include severity of injury, surgical technique (Fig. 6.7), disruption of tendon blood supply, gapping at the repair site, and prolonged immobilization following surgical repair.

Contraindications to primary tendon repair include extensive soft tissue injury to the finger and palm, significant skin loss over the flexor tendon, and contaminated wounds. Partial tendon lacerations do not require repair if injury involves less than 60% of the tendon width. Injuries involving more than 60% of the tendon width require repair to minimize risk of complete rupture, entrapment, and triggering.

Rehabilitation. The goal of rehabilitation following surgery is to initiate early controlled motion in order to optimize tensile strength, function, and excursion as well as to minimize adhesion formation and increase gliding and diameter of collagen fibrils. Most rehabilitation protocols are designed to immobilize the upper extremity with the wrist and MCP joints in flexion, and the interphalangeal joints are in extension during periods of rest. The patient must refrain from use of the hand for at least 6 to 8 weeks. The more popular early controlled-motion protocols include the modified Louisville or Kleinert and the modified Duran. The modified Louisville protocol has popularized a dynamic wrist splint consisting of an elastic outrigger attached to a dorsal blocking splint with the wrist and MCP joints in flexion and the interphalangeal joints in extension. Active extension is allowed up to the limit of the splint. The wrist splint is synergistic because it maximizes the degree of intrasynovial tendon excursion as a result of the tenodesis effect of the

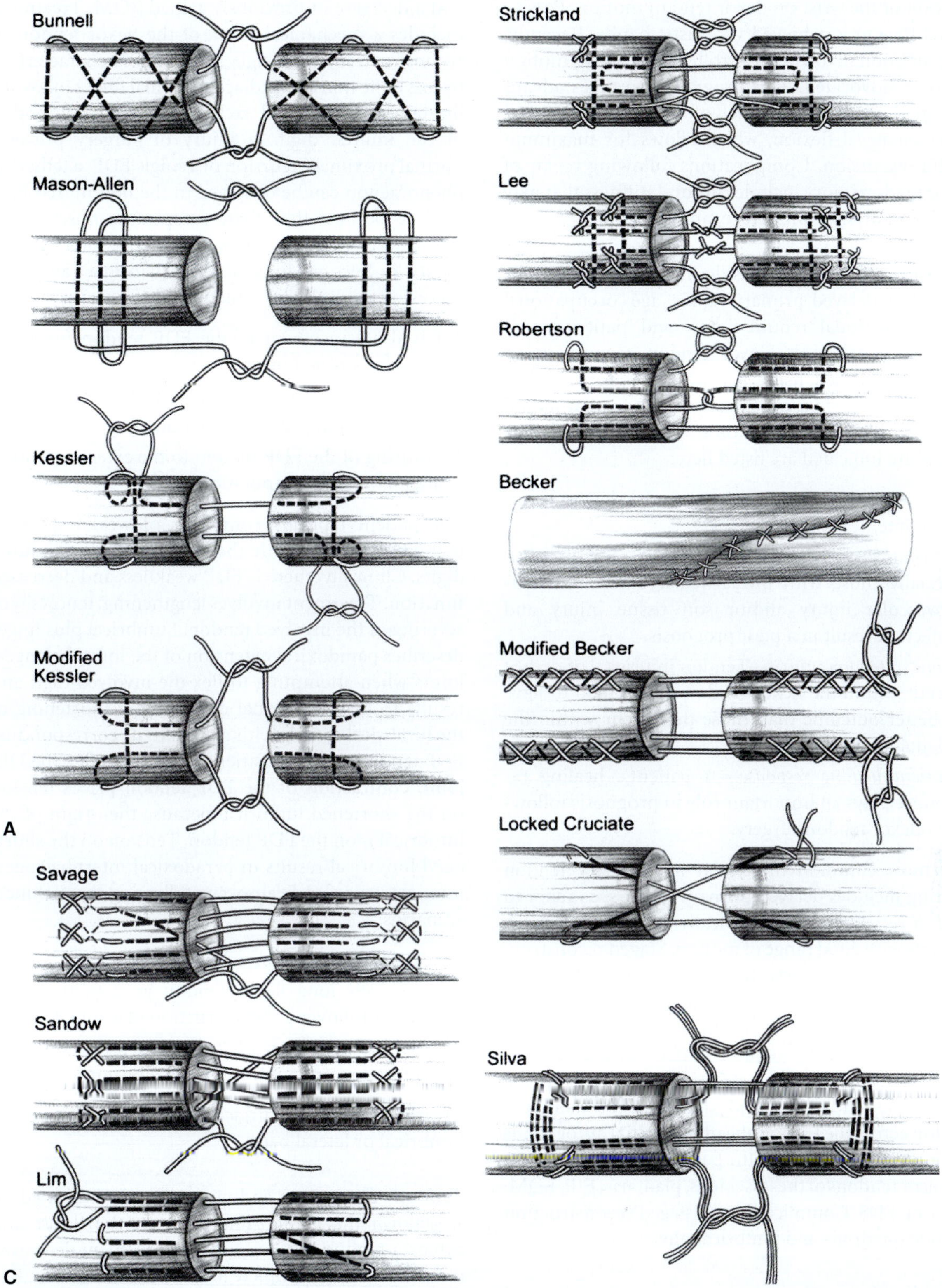

FIGURE 6.7 Core repair techniques. (*Source:* Berger RA, Weiss A-PC (eds.), *Hand Surgery*, Vol. 1. Philadelphia: Lippincott Williams & Wilkins, 2004;686.)

position of the wrist on flexor tendon motion. Passive digital flexion is achieved via elastic bands. Recently, rehabilitation involving controlled early active motion has been advocated. This program also takes advantage of the synergistic effect of wrist extension and interphalangeal flexion, which allows for maximum tendon excursion. Complications following repair of flexor tendon injury include rupture, stiffness that may require tenolysis, contracture, and quadrigia.

Reconstruction. When considering salvage surgery for a failed or delayed primary repair, age, occupational status, functional requirements, and patient needs must be considered. Flexor tendon reconstruction can be performed using a primary tendon graft or may require staged reconstruction. Factors that should be considered in determining the type of salvage procedure indicated are listed here:

- *Patient age*—Younger patients tend to have a better outcome.
- *Mechanism of injury*—Crush injuries; fractures, especially those with intraarticular extension; neurovascular injury and/or soft tissue injury and infection result in a poor prognosis.
- *Zone of tendon injury*—Tendon injuries that do not occur within the flexor tendon sheath tend to have a better outcome than those that occur within the digital tendon sheath.
- *Patient healing response*—A patient's healing response plays an important role in prognosis following flexor tendon surgery.

The most common indication for primary tendon grafting includes delayed primary repair secondary to tendon retraction and is typically reserved for young patients with good range of motion. Staged reconstruction consists of 2 parts: the purpose of the first part is to prepare a healthy bed for tendon gliding within a reconstructed tendon sheath, including placement of a silicone Hunter tendon implant and pulley reconstruction. The second stage involves attaching the autogenous tendon graft and passing the reconstructed tendon across the tendon sheath. Potential autogenous tendon graft sites include the palmaris longus, the long extensor tendons of the lesser toes, plantaris, EIP, EDM, and ring FDS. Complications of staged reconstruction include quadrigia and lumbrical plus.

Complications. The most common complication following flexor tendon grafting is adhesion formation at the level of the proximal juncture or along the surface of the graft. This complication can be minimized by gentle handling of the tissues intraoperatively and a good hand therapy program postoperatively. Pulley disruption results in bowstringing of the tendon graft and a decrease of previously gained ROM. Treatment includes a mechanical block of the flexor tendon or reconstruction. Quadrigia syndrome is characterized by loss of flexion of an adjacent normal finger following limitation of proximal excursion of the FDP tendon of the injured digit. If injury or surgery prevents normal proximal excursion of a single FDP, a tethering phenomenon can be observed in the noninjured FDP tendons because they share a common muscle belly. The adjacent FDP tendons are then limited in their ability to become fully flexed. Quadrigia can occur following these clinical situations:

- Distal advancement of the FDP tendon following repair of a zone I injury
- Scarring of the FDP tendon following amputation
- Excess tension placed on a tendon graft
- Suturing of the FDP tendon to the extensor tendon after a fingertip amputation

The patient typically complains of weakness in an inability to grasp with the injured and noninjured digits. Clinically, there is FDP weakness and decreased function. Treatment involves lengthening, tenolysis, or severing of the involved tendon. Lumbrical plus finger describes paradoxical extension of the interphalangeal joints when attempting to flex the involved digit and results from a functional or anatomic shortening of the lumbrical muscle with respect to its corresponding FDP tendon. When a patient attempts to flex the DIP joint, contraction of the FDP tendon places tension on the shortened lumbrical because the origin of the lumbrical is on the FDP tendon. Tension on the shortened lumbrical results in paradoxical interphalangeal joint extension and can occur following these clinical scenarios:

- Scarring of the lumbrical muscle
- Excessively long flexor tendon graft to the distal phalanx following reconstruction of a zone I injury
- Proximal migration of the FDP tendon following amputation or an unrecognized avulsion

Treatment includes surgical release of the involved lumbrical or lateral band.

Tendon Transfer. Tendon transfer is indicated to reestablish the equilibrium between the flexor and extensor tendon systems and to supplement decreased muscle power or complete loss of motor function. Key points and principles of tendon transfer are as follows.

- Contracture correction
- Adequate strength of donor tendon—the donor muscle–tendon unit must have a minimum strength of grade 4 because there will be a loss of one grade following transfer

- Degree of tendon excursion between the donor and recipient sites should be comparable; in general, wrist flexors and extensors require 33 mm of excursion; finger and thumb extensors require 50 mm, and digital flexors require 70 mm of excursion
- Optimal function is achieved when the donor tendon is transferred to restore one function; multiple recipient sites results in decreased strength and excursion
- Motion is improved when the recipient site is close to a joint's axis of rotation, although strength is decreased
- Harvest of the donor tendon should not result in severe loss of function
- Optimal transfers are synergistic; for example, a wrist flexor is transferred to restore digital extension
- Selection of tendon transfers depends on the deficits present and the availability of possible donors; Table 6.5 lists transfers that are typically performed following nerve paralysis

Stiffness. Digital stiffness can result from joint contracture, imbalance between the flexor and extensor tendon systems, or tendon scarring. Stiffness secondary to joint contracture is characterized by decreased active and passive range of motion regardless of the position of the adjacent joints, whereas joint stiffness resulting from scarring or imbalance is dependent on the position of the adjacent joints. Imbalance results in intrinsic or extrinsic tightness.

- *Intrinsic tightness*—Intrinsic tightness is often a result of trauma such as burns, upper motor neuron injury, or incorrect immobilization of the hand. Patients typically complain of pain and stiffness and have a positive Bunnell intrinsic tightness test as a result of the seesaw effect that a nonarticular contracting structure has as it spans two joints. Flexion of one joint allows for extension of another, and vice versa. The intrinsic tightness test is based on this observation and examines interphalangeal joint motion with the MCP joints passively flexed and in full extension. Passive flexion of the MCP joints relaxes the intrinsics; extension places tension on the intrinsics. The intrinsic tightness test is positive if there is limitation of interphalangeal joint flexion with the MCP joints in extension versus when they are in flexion. Management consists of aggressive ROM exercises; intrinsic muscle release with or without joint arthroplasty or arthrodesis is indicated if conservative treatment fails.
- *Extrinsic tightness*—Typically a result of trauma or tendon shortening following repair of extensor or flexor tendons, extrinsic extensor tightness is tested with the wrist and MCP joints in flexion; if there are extensor tendon adhesions or tightness, there will be limited flexion of the interphalangeal joints. If there is limited interphalangeal extension with the wrist and MCP joints in extension, then extrinsic flexor tightness may be present. Treatment includes therapy and possible surgical release.

III. WRIST

Osteology

Distal Radius. The distal radius forms the distal radioulnar joint (DRUJ) at its articulation with the distal ulna at the sigmoid notch and it forms the radiocarpal joint at its articulation with the scaphoid and lunate. The tendon of the EPL runs radially around Lister tubercle. This important surgical landmark is situated approximately 0.5 cm proximal to the dorsal lip of the articular surface of the distal radius. The EPL is at risk for rupture with distal radius fractures. The lunate and scaphoid fossae form the distal articular surface of the distal radius.

- *Palmar tilt*—The angle formed between the plane of the distal articular surface and the plane that is perpendicular to the longitudinal axis of the distal radius on a lateral x-ray. It measures 11 degrees in most individuals.
- *Radial height*—The distance measured from the most ulnar aspect of the distal radius to the tip of the radial styloid on an anterior–posterior x-ray. It typically measures around 12 mm.
- *Radial inclination*—The angle formed by a line perpendicular to the longitudinal axis of the radius and the tangential of the distal articulating surface on an anterior–posterior x-ray (Fig. 6.8). On average, it measures 22 degrees. The distal radial physis appears around the age of 2 years and fuses between 17 and 20 years.

Distal Ulna. The distal ulna consists of the ulnar head and styloid. The styloid process is approximately 1 cm proximal to the radial styloid. The distal ulna physis appears at the age of 5 years and fuses at 20 years. Ulnar variance refers to the relative lengths of the radius and ulna at the DRUJ (see Fig. 6.8).

- *Ulnar neutral*—Equal length of the radius and ulna in the anterior–plane
- *Ulnar negative*—Ulna is 1 to 6 mm shorter than the radius.
- *Ulnar positive*—Ulna is 1 to 5 mm longer than the radius; may play a role in the pathology behind Kienbock disease and ulnolunate joint arthritis.

Carpal Bones. There are 8 carpal bones: scaphoid, lunate, triquetrum, pisiform, trapezoid, trapezium,

TABLE 6.5 Common tendon transfers following nerve palsies

Palsy	*Deficit*	*Transfer*	*Alternative Transfer*	*Key Points*
Radial	Wrist extension	PT to ECRB	FCR to ECRB	Requires at least 1 wrist flexor (excluding PL)
	Finger extension	FCU to EDC II–V	FDS III–IV to EDC II–V FCR to EDC II–V	Limits ability to make fist and flex wrist simultaneously
	Thumb extension	PL to EPL	FDS III to EPL	
PIN	Finger extension	FCR to EDC II–V	FDS III to EPL	FCR then FCU to minimize radial deviation of the wrist
	Thumb extension	PL to EPL		
Low median	Thumb opposition	FDS IV to AbPB	EIP to AbPB AbDM to AbPB PL to AbPB	Opposition requires thumb adduction and short flexors; opposition may be preserved with ulnar-innervated FPB; pulley should be in close proximity to pisiform
High median	Thumb IP flexion	BR to FPL		FDS and PL unavailable for transfer
	Index and long finger flexion	FDP IV–V to FDP II–III	ECRL to FDP II–III	AIN palsy: BR to FPL, FDP IV-V to FDP II-III
	Thumb opposition	EIP to AbPB	EDQ to AbPB	
Low ulnar	Interossei and ulnar lumbricals	FDS to lateral bands	ECRL to lateral bands EDQ and EIP to lateral bands FCR plus graft to lateral bands	Transfer to lateral bands may lead to swan-neck deformity
	Thumb adduction	ECRL plus graft to AdP	BR plus graft to AdP	Transfer grafts to flexor tendon sheaths
	Index finger abduction	EIP to first DIO	AbPL to first DIO ECRL to first DIO	
High ulnar	Low ulnar nerve deficits (plus)	EIP to first DIO		
	Ring finger and small finger FDP	FDP II–III to FDP IV–V		
Low median and ulnar	Thumb adduction	BR plus graft to abductor tubercle of thumb		
	Thumb abduction	EIP to AbPB		
	Index finger abduction	AbPL to first DIO		
	Clawed fingers	ECRL or BR plus graft to A2 pulleys		

TABLE 6.5 *(continued)*

High median and ulnar	Low median and ulnar deficits (plus)	Same as above except for clawed fingers	
	Thumb IP flexion	BR or EIP to FPL	
	Finger flexion	ECRL to FDP	
	Clawed fingers	Tenodesis of MCP joints	
	Wrist flexion	ECU to FCU	
Brachial plexus	Elbow flexion	Steindler flexorplasty*	Bipolar latissimus transfer; pec major transfer; triceps transfer; SCM† transfer

*Steindler flexorplasty involves proximal transfer of flexor pronator mass

†SCM, sternocleidomastoid muscle

Adapted from Tan V, Daluiski A. Tendon. In: Beredjiklian PK and Bozentka DJ (eds), *Review of Hand Surgery*. Philadelphia: Saunders, 2004;27–47.

capitate, and hamate. They are arranged in 2 rows between the bases of the metacarpals distally and the distal radius and ulna proximally. The scaphoid is part of both the proximal and distal rows. The pisiform is a sesamoid bone that lies in the FCU tendon. The hook of the hamate serves as a point of insertion for the TCL, the hypothenar muscles, and the fascia comprising the floor of Guyon canal. It lies between the Guyon canal and the carpal canal. The ulnar neurovascular bundle lies just ulnar to the hook of the hamate. Ossification of the carpal bones begins with the capitate and continues in a counterclockwise direction on a posterior–anterior radiograph of the right wrist with the palm up.

Blood Supply

The primary blood supply of the carpus stems from branches of the radial, anterior interosseous, and ulnar arteries via the dorsal and palmar transverse arches. The blood supply to the scaphoid is provided by a branch of the radial artery that enters the bone at its dorsal ridge. As a result, the vascular supply to the proximal pole of the scaphoid is retrograde and can lead to avascular necrosis after injury (Fig. 6.9).

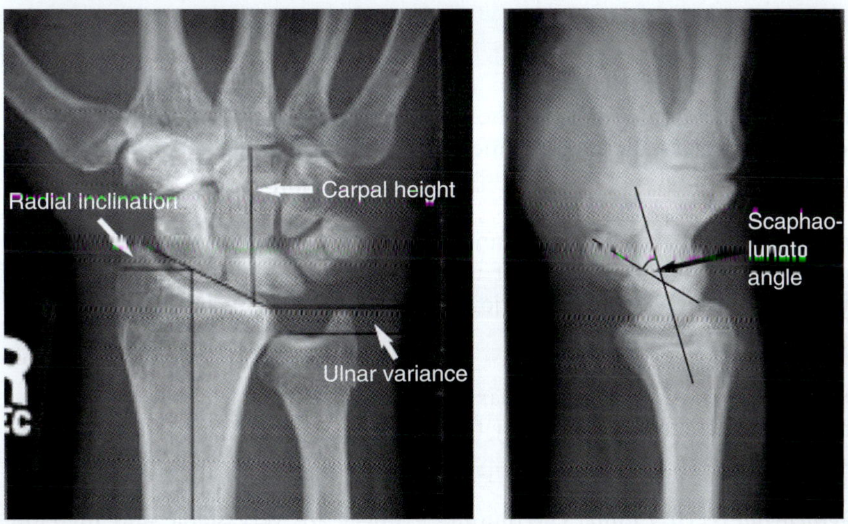

FIGURE 6.8 Radiographic measurements of the wrist. (*Source:* Allan CH, Joshi A, Lichtman DM. Kienbock's disease: Diagnosis and treatment. *J Am Acad Orthop Surg* 2001;9:128–136.)

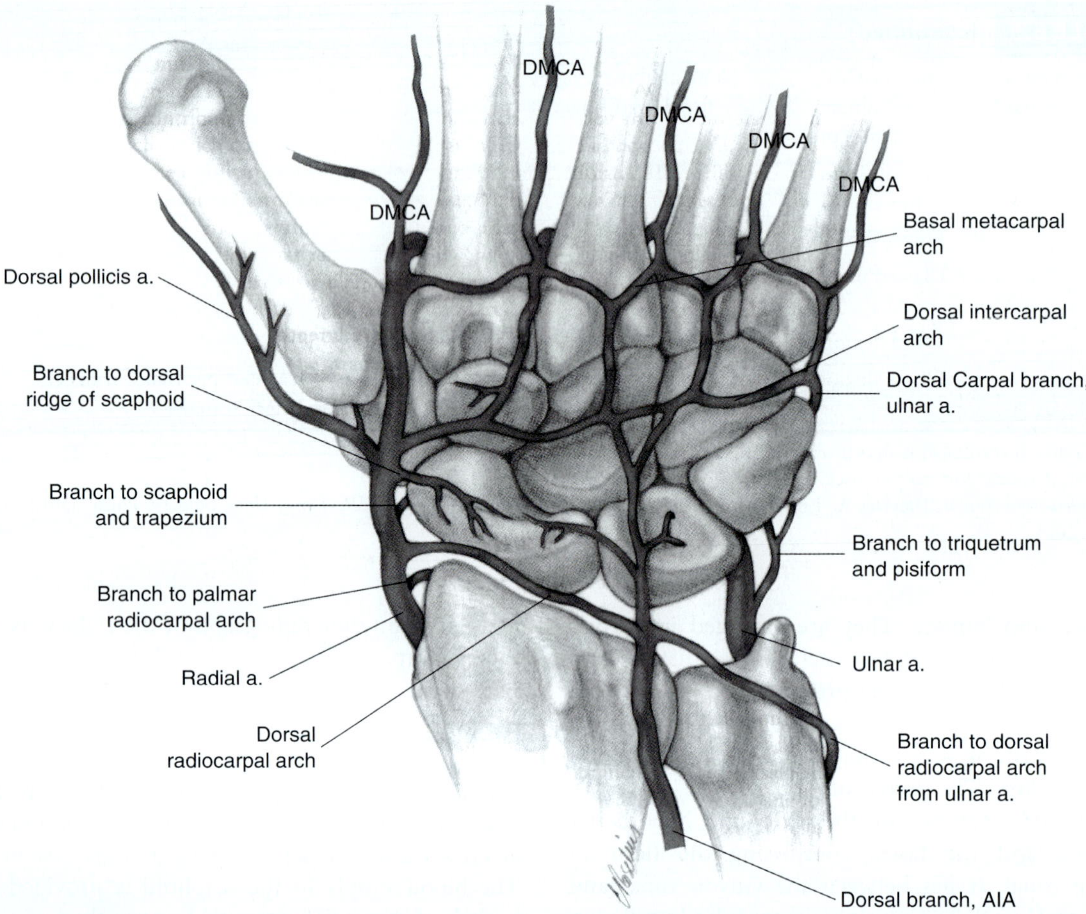

FIGURE 6.9 **Schematic drawing of the arterial supply of the dorsal wrist. (*Adapted from* Gelberman RH, Panagis JS, Taleisnik J, et al. The arterial anatomy of the human carpus. Part I: The extraosseous vascularity. *J Hand Surg [Am]* 1983;8:367–375.)**

Arthrology

Radiocarpal Joint. The radiocarpal joint is an ellipsoid joint composed of the distal radius, scaphoid, lunate, and triquetrum. The volar radiocarpal ligament provides the majority of structural support.

Intercarpal Joint. The intercarpal joint is formed by the articulation between the distal aspect of the proximal row and the distal row. The midcarpal joint lies between the proximal and distal carpal rows.

Distal Radioulnar Joint. The DRUJ is a uniaxial trochoid joint; its primary stability is provided by the triangular fibrocartilage complex (TFCC).

Thumb Carpometacarpal (CMC) Joint. The thumb CMC joint is a saddle or double-hinge joint formed by the articulation between the thumb metacarpal base and trapezium. The configuration of the joint allows for flexion–extension, abduction–adduction, and pronation–supination. Joint stability is provided by the capsule, intermetacarpal, anterior and posterior oblique, ulnar collateral, and dorsoradial ligaments. The beak or deep anterior oblique ligament is the primary stabilizer of the thumb CMC joint. It is an intraarticular ligament that serves as a pivot point for rotation. Attenuation of this ligament is thought to contribute to degenerative changes associated with basal joint arthritis.

Small to Index Finger CMC Joints. The small and ring finger CMC joints are hinge joints, making them the two more mobile of the four CMC joints. On average, they have 30 degrees of flexion and extension, which is important in power grip. Unlike the small and ring fingers, the CMC joints of the index and middle finger are very stable and therefore have very little mobility. Three types of ligaments are responsible for CMC joint stability: the dorsal (strongest), palmar, and interosseous ligaments. The middle finger metacarpal acts as a rigid spine that supports movement of the thumb and adjacent fingers.

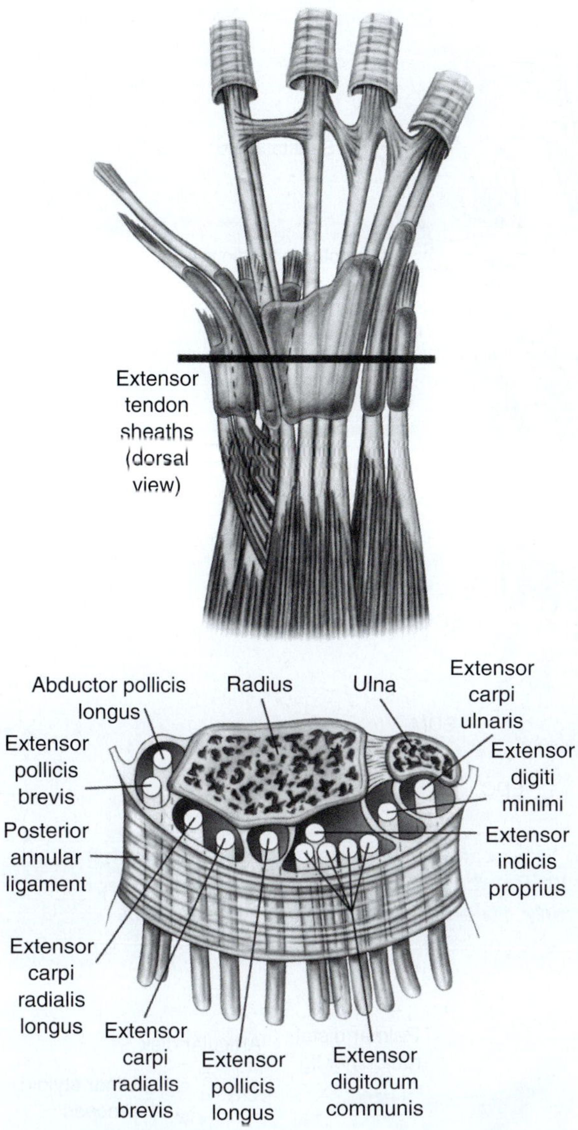

FIGURE 6.10 **(A) Extensor tendon sheaths. (B) Dorsal compartments. (*Source:* Berger RA, Weiss A-PC (eds.). *Hand Surgery*, Vol. 1. Philadelphia: Lippincott Williams & Wilkins, 2004:780.)**

Extensor Tendons. The extensor tendons of the thumb, digits, and wrist are enclosed in synovial sheaths as they course along the dorsal distal radius through a series of 6 tunnels (Fig. 6.10). Anatomic snuffbox is a triangular space between the tendons of the first and third dorsal compartments. The radial artery courses through it just before it enters the hand.

Extensor Retinaculum. The tendons gain entrance to the hand after passing beneath the extensor retinaculum (ER). The ER is a wide, fibrous band that prevents tendon bowstringing at the wrist joint by holding the tendons snugly to the distal radius. The compartments are separated by septa formed from that arise from the ER and insert onto the distal radius (Fig. 6.11).

Extensor Compartments. The EPB is always ulnar to the APL. The APL often has two slips of tendon. The ECRL tendon lies radial to the ECRB tendon; these wrist extensors insert onto the bases of the second and third metacarpals respectively. The ECRB is the main extensor of the wrist. The posterior interosseous nerve (PIN) and artery lie on the floor of the fourth compartment. The propius tendons of the index and small fingers are ulnar to their corresponding extensor digitorum communis tendons.

Ligaments

Wrist stability is a result of the integrity of the extrinsic and intrinsic ligaments. The extrinsic ligaments of the wrist are connections between carpal bones and forearm or metacarpal bones. Intrinsic ligaments connect carpal bones to each other.

Extrinsic Ligaments. The extrinsic ligaments comprise both palmar and dorsal components. The palmar extrinsic ligaments include the radial collateral ligament, palmar radiocarpal ligament, and ulnocarpal complex. The components of the palmar radiocarpal ligaments are the radioscaphocapitate, radiolunate, and radioscapholunate ligaments. The radioscaphocapitate ligament crosses the waist of the scaphoid and is subsequently transected in a volar approach to the scaphoid. The radiolunate ligament passes from the radius to the triquetrum before inserting on the lunate. It consists of a long and short component, which function as the primary restraint to lunate dislocation in perilunate dislocation. The radioscapholunate ligament is also known as the ligament of Testut and is a vascular remnant of the carpus. The ulnocarpal complex consists of the ulnolunate and ulnotriquetral ligaments and the triangular fibrocartilage complex (TFCC). The ulnolunate and ulnotriquetral ligaments help maintain DRUJ and ulnocarpal stability during forearm rotation. The TFCC is the primary stabilizer of the DRUJ. The complex consists of the articular disk, the dorsal and palmar radioulnar ligaments, the meniscus homologue, and the ulnar collateral ligament (ECU sheath). The dorsal and palmar radioulnar ligaments originate from the sigmoid notch and insert onto the base of the ulnar styloid. They aid in stabilizing the DRUJ during pronation and supination. The dorsal and palmar radioulnar ligaments and the peripheral 15% to 20% of the articular disk are well vascularized. The central 80% to 85% is completely avascular; tears in this area will not heal. The dorsal extrinsic ligaments

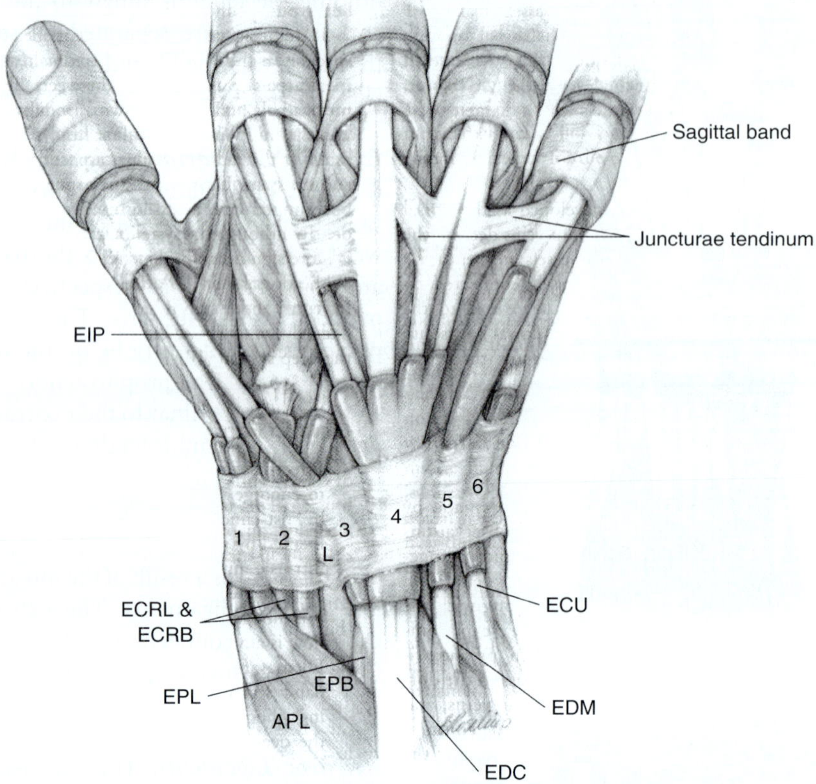

FIGURE 6.11 The wrist extensor retinaculum and the most common arrangement of the extensor tendons and juncturae. (*Source:* Doyle JR. Hand. In: Doyle JR, Botte M (eds.), *Surgical Anatomy of the Hand and Upper Extremity*. Philadelphia: Lippincott Williams & Wilkins, 2003;648, with permission.)

consist of three ligaments that originate on the dorsal lip of the distal radius and insert onto their corresponding carpal bones: the radiotriquetral, radiolunate, and dorsal radioscaphoid ligaments. The dorsal radiocarpal and intercarpal ligaments prevent dorsal subluxation of the scaphoid by stabilizing its proximal pole. Incompetence of the radiotriquetral ligament can lead to a static volar intercalated segment instability (VISI) (Fig. 6.12).

Intrinsic Ligaments. Intrinsic ligaments include the scapholunate and lunotriquetral ligaments.

- *Scapholunate ligament*—The scapholunate ligament (SLL) is a C-shaped structure that connects the dorsal, palmar, and proximal surfaces of the scaphoid and lunate. The dorsal portion of the ligament is the strongest and provides the bulk of the ligament's resistance to widening between the proximal pole of the scaphoid and lunate. It is the primary stabilizer of the scapholunate joint.
- *Lunotriquetral Ligament*—Like the SLL, the lunotriquetral ligament (LTL) is also C-shaped, spanning

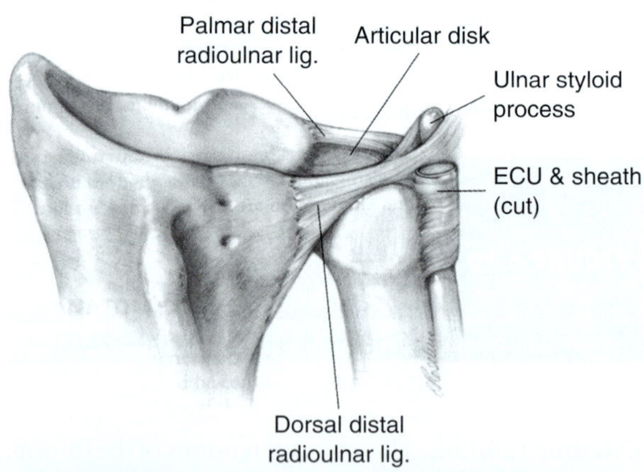

FIGURE 6.12 Dorsal and palmar distal radioulnar ligaments and the triangular fibrocartilage. (*Source:* Doyle JR. Hand. In: Doyle JR, Botte M (eds.), *Surgical Anatomy of the Hand and Upper Extremity*. Philadelphia: Lippincott Williams & Wilkins, 2003;496, with permission.)

the dorsal, palmar, and proximal surfaces of the lunate and triquetrum. Contrary to the SLL, the palmar region of the LTL is the thickest and strongest and is the main stabilizer of the lunotriquetral joint.

IV. FOREARM

Osteology

The forearm contains 2 long bones, the radius and ulna, that articulate with the distal humerus at the elbow (trochlea/ulna, capitellum/radial head), with the carpus distally at the wrist, and with each other at the elbow and the wrist.

Radius. Proximally, the radius consists of radial head and neck and the radial tuberosity, which is the insertion of the biceps tendon. The tuberosity always faces the direction opposite the thumb; that is, it is lateral in pronation and medial in supination. The radial shaft has a bow that is convex laterally. It is important to restore the radial bow so that forearm rotation is maintained. Distally, the radius comprises the styloid process, the radiocarpal articular surface, the ulnar or sigmoid notch, and the Lister tubercle. The growth plate of the proximal radius appears at the age of 5 years and fuses between 15 and 18 years.

Ulna. The ulna comprises the olecranon, trochlear notch, and coronoid process proximally, and gradually tapers to end distally as the ulnar head and styloid process. The apophysis of the olecranon appears at the age of 10 years and fuses at 16 years.

Arthrology

Pronation and supination of the forearm occurs as a result of the radius rotating and translating about the ulna via the proximal and distal radioulnar joints. The longitudinal axis of the forearm starts at the center of the radial head proximally and continues distally to the head of the ulna. The proximal radioulnar joint consists of the radial head articulating with the semilunar notch of the ulna. The rotational stability of the joint is provided primarily by the annular ligament.

Nerves

Median Nerve. The median nerve contains fibers from all levels of the brachial plexus: C5 to T1. It enters the forearm medial to the brachial artery, running on the anterior surface of the brachialis. It passes between the two heads of the pronator teres and then the two heads of the FDS, running between this muscle and the FDP until the distal third of the forearm. At the level of the wrist, the median nerve lies radial to the tendon of the palmaris longus (PL) and medial to the FCR as it enters the carpal canal. The muscular branches of the median nerve in the forearm supply the pronator teres, FCR, PL, and FDS. The anterior interosseous nerve (AIN) is the largest motor branch of the median nerve. It originates from the posterior surface of the median nerve between 2 and 8 cm distal to the level of the medial epicondyle and continues distally between the FPL and the FDP. It supplies the radial half of the FDP, FPL, and the pronator quadratus.

Ulnar Nerve. The ulnar nerve is composed of fibers from C8 to T1 (occasionally C7). A potential point of compression in the arm is at the arcade of Struthers, which is a fascial band between the medial intermuscular septum and the medial head of the triceps muscle. It gains entrance to the forearm after passing behind the medial epicondyle, where it is tethered by Osborne ligament. It continues between the ulnar and radial heads of the FCU and courses between this muscle and the FDP. The ulnar artery joins the nerve at the middle of the forearm, the nerve running ulnar to the artery. The dorsal ulnar cutaneous nerve branches off of the ulnar nerve approximately 7 cm proximal to the pisiform. The ulnar nerve proper and artery continue distally to enter the hand via the Guyon canal. The FCU is the only muscle to receive motor branches from the ulnar nerve in the forearm.

Radial Nerve. The radial nerve contains fibers from C5 to T1. It enters the forearm anterior to the lateral epicondyle, between the brachialis and brachioradialis. It divides into the superficial radial and posterior interosseous branches approximately 1 to 3 cm distal to the lateral epicondyle. Before its division, it distributes motor branches to the ECRL and brachioradialis. Branches to the ECRB can be from the radial, superficial radial, PIN, or the bifurcation point. The superficial radial branch is purely sensory. It continues caudally between the brachioradialis and ECRL, emerging on the ulnar border of the brachioradialis tendon at the junction of the middle and distal thirds of the forearm. It provides sensory branches to the skin on the dorsoradial aspect of the wrist and hand. The PIN is the deep motor branch of the radial nerve. This branch travels under the ECRB and passes between the two heads of the supinator. The proximal edge of the supinator is the arcade of Frohse, which can be a point of compression of the PIN. The nerve provides motor branches (proximal to distal) to the supinator, the EDC, ECU, EDM, APL, EPL, EPB, and EIP (Table 6.6).

Cutaneous Innervation. Cutaneous innervation of the forearm is provided by 3 nerves: the posterior, medial, and lateral antebrachial cutaneous nerves.

TABLE 6.6 Muscles of the wrist and hand

Muscle	Origin	Insert	Function	Nerve
		Thenar		
Abductor pollicis brevis	Transverse carpal ligament, scaphoid, trapezoid	Radial side, base of proximal phalanx of thumb	Adduction of thumb	Median
Opponens pollicis	Trapezium	Radiopalmar surface of thumb	Palmar abduction, pronation of thumb	Median
Flexor pollicis brevis	Trapezium, capitate	Base of proximal phalanx of thumb	Flexion of proximal phalanx of thumb	Median
Adductor pollicis	Capitate, second and third MCP	Ulnar side, base of proximal phalanx of thumb	Adduction of thumb, assistance with opposition	Ulnar
		Hypothenar		
Palmaris brevis	Transverse carpal ligament, palmar aponeurosis	Ulnar palm	Corrugation of skin on ulnar palm	Ulnar
Abductor digiti minimi	Pisiform, tendon of flexor carpi ulnaris	Ulnar side, base of proximal phalanx of little finger, aponeurosis of extensor digiti minimi	Abduction of little finger from palm	Ulnar
Flexor digiti minimi	Transverse carpal ligament, hamate	Ulnar side, base of proximal phalanx of little finger	Flexion of proximal phalanx of middle finger	Ulnar
Opponens digiti minimi	Transverse carpal ligament, hamate	Ulnar side of metacarpal of little finger	Opposition of little finger to thumb, flexion of metacarpal of little finger	Ulnar

Adapted from Doyle JR, Botte MJ. *Surgical Anatomy of the Hand and Upper Extremity.* Philadelphia: Lippincott Williams & Wilkins, 2003;182

Anastomoses. The Martin-Gruber anastomosis describes anastomotic motor fiber connections between the median and ulnar nerves in the forearm. The extent of injury to the ulnar nerve can be underappreciated because of motor branches from the median nerve supplying muscles that are typically innervated by the ulnar nerve. The incidence of the Martin-Gruber anastomosis is 10% to 25%. The Riche-Cannieu anastomosis describes connections between motor branches of the median and ulnar nerves that occur in the hand.

Blood Supply

The brachial artery divides into the radial and ulnar arteries at the level of the radial neck in the cubital fossa. The radial artery runs posterior to the brachioradialis and emerges just lateral to the FCR tendon at the wrist. The ulnar artery runs between the FDS and FDP muscles in the proximal forearm. Distally, it courses between the FDP and FCU tendons alongside the ulnar nerve.

Interosseous Membrane

The interosseous membrane of the forearm extends from the radius to the ulna. The interosseous ligament is the central band of the interosseous membrane and is an important stabilizer against proximal migration of the radius after radial head excision.

Compartments

The forearm is divided into 3 compartments. The mobile wad of Henry consists of the brachioradialis, ECRB, and ECRL. The dorsal compartment contains the extensor musculature. The volar compartment contains the flexor musculature. All 3 compartments must be released when decompressing compartment syndrome of the forearm.

TABLE 6.7 Classification systems for nerve injuries

Seddon Classification	*Sunderland Classification*	*Pathology*
Neuropraxia	Grade I	Myelin injury or ischemia
Axonotmesis		Axons disrupted, variable stromal disruption
	Grade II	Axons disrupted, endoneurial tubes intact, perineurium intact, epineurium intact
	Grade III	Axons disrupted, endoneurial tubes disrupted, perineurium intact, epineurium intact
	Grade IV	Axons disrupted, endoneurial tubes disrupted, perineurium disrupted, epineurium intact
Neurotmesis	Grade V	Axons disrupted, endoneurial tubes disrupted, perineurium intact, epineurium disrupted

Source: Edstrom LE, Karacaoglu E. Chronic nerve injuries and treatment of neuromas. In: Berger RA, Weiss CA-P (eds.), *Hand Surgery*, Vol. 1. Philadelphia: Lippincott Williams & Wilkins, 2004:848.

Tendon

Tendons are composed of type I collagen, which equals 85% of the tendon's dry weight. The fibrils of collagen are organized into parallel rows or fascicles.

V. COMPRESSIVE NEUROPATHIES

Pathophysiology

The pathophysiologic changes associated with chronic nerve compression are part of a continuum of changes occurring in the nerve; the degree of change is directly proportional to the force and duration of compression. Histologically, the first of the series of pathologic changes that occur with chronic nerve compression is breakdown of the blood–nerve barrier. The endoneurial edema that follows leads to thickening of the perineurium and increased endoneurial pressure (higher than 30 mmHg). The increase in endoneurial pressure alters the microvasculature of the nerve, which leads to ischemia. Chronic ischemia results in demyelination and subsequent axonal degeneration. Patient symptoms are a direct reflection of the histopathologic neural changes that the affected nerve is undergoing at a particular phase of nerve compression: early, intermediate, or late (Tables 6.7 and 6.8).

Epidemiology and Risk Factors

There is an increased incidence of compressive neuropathy in patients with certain systemic or inflammatory diseases. Disruption of hemodynamic equilibrium, anatomic variations, tobacco smoking, and the presence of a mass have also been associated with compressive neuropathy. Repetitive or work-related activity has not been determined to be a risk

TABLE 6.8 Phases of nerve compression

Phase	*Symptoms*	*NCV**	*EMG***	*Pathology*	*Treatment*
Early	Intermittent paraesthesia	Normal or - sensory latency	Normal	Endoneurial edema	Splint, steroid injection, activity modification
Intermediate	Constant numbness	+		Endoneurial edema	Surgical decompression
Advanced	Sensory and motor loss	+	+	Endoneurial fibrosis with axonal degeneration	Surgical decompression; irreversible changes have occurred

EMG, electromyography; NCV, nerve conduction velocity.

TABLE 6.9 Risk factors for compression neuropathy

Systemic Conditions	*Inflammatory Disease*	*Anatomic Variation*	*Neoplasm/Mass*	*Personal Traits*
Diabetes mellitus	Rheumatoid arthritis	Anomalous tendon/ muscle	Ganglion	Middle age
Alcoholism	Infection	Persistent median artery	Lipoma	Female gender
Tobacco smoking	Gout	Trauma (e.g., wrist fracture)	Hematoma	
Obesity	Tenosynovitis	Synovial fibrosis		
Pregnancy				
Hypothyroidism				
Mucopolysaccharidosis/ mucolipidosis				
Renal failure				
Hereditary motor and sensory neuropathy				
Degenerative cervical spine				

factor in compressive neuropathies; however, extremes of flexion and extension can significantly increase canal pressure. (Table 6.9).

Double-Crush Phenomenon. The double-crush phenomenon describes the concept that disruption of synthesis or blockage of transport along an axon may increase susceptibility of axons to compression along the same nerve, proximal and/or distal to the initial site of injury.

Physical Examination

Provocation testing utilizes joint movement or direct pressure to increase compression on the nerve, thereby reproducing or increasing the patient's symptoms in the corresponding neural distribution.

Sensory Evaluation. There are 4 sensory receptors that are distinguished by the size of the receptive field and response qualities (Table 6.10). Meissner and Pacinian corpuscles are quickly adapting receptors that respond to moving touch. Merkel cells and Ruffini end organs have slowly adapting receptors that respond to static touch. Threshold testing is the minimum stimulus required to evoke a response; it is determined using vibration thresholds for the quickly adapting receptors and cutaneous pressure thresholds for the slowly adapting receptors. Tactile discrimination refers to the number of innervated sensory receptors and is evaluated using static and moving 2-point discrimination; it reflects late stages of chronic nerve compression. Early changes occurring with chronic nerve compression are reflected by changes in vibration

TABLE 6.10 Sensory evaluation

Fiber population	*Fast Adapting*		*Slow Adapting*	
Receptor type	Meissner corpuscle	Pacinian corpuscle	Merkel cell	Ruffini end organ
Sensation	Moving touch	Vibration	Constant touch	Constant touch
Clinical test	Moving 2-point discrimination	Tuning fork	Static 2-point discrimination	Cutaneous pressure (Semmes-Weinstein monofilaments)
Type of test	Innervation density	Threshold	Innervation density	Threshold

and cutaneous pressure thresholds, making threshold testing more sensitive. It is the earliest abnormal finding that can be clinically detected. The first sensory nerve function to return after injury is protective sensation and the last to return is 2-point discrimination.

Motor Evaluation. Motor testing for compressive neuropathy is gauged by strength and is graded on a scale of 1 to 5 (5 is full strength). There is no clinically measurable decrease in strength in the early phase of compression. Motor strength in the intermediate and advanced phases is characterized by weakness and muscle wasting respectively.

Testing

Electrodiagnostic Testing. Electrodiagnostic testing includes electromyography (EMG) and nerve conduction studies (NCS). The results of these tests are operator dependent; they serve as adjuvants to the physical examination. EMG uses needlelike electrodes placed into the muscle to evaluate spontaneous and volitional electrical activity of individual muscle fibers and motor units. It aids in distinguishing between primary nerve versus muscle dysfunction and partial versus complete nerve dysfunction. EMG measures insertional activity, rest activity, and number of motor unit potentials. Insertional activity describes the brief burst of electrical activity that a healthy muscle generates with insertion of the needle electrode. Abnormal insertional activity includes positive sharp waves (early denervation) or electrical silence (advanced motor degeneration). During rest, healthy muscle is electrically silent. Muscle innervated by an injured nerve demonstrates spontaneous activity with fibrillation potentials, the earliest sign of muscle denervation. Fibrillation potentials are generated after a minimum of 2 weeks of muscle denervation and are the most sensitive indicator of motor axon loss. They represent action potentials from individual muscle fibers and are present in compression neuropathies long before there is any clinical evidence of motor weakness. Volitional muscle contraction normally generates so many motor action potentials (MAPs) that single MAPs cannot be seen, creating a full interference pattern. After nerve injury, MAPs activation is incomplete and the number of MAPs that are recruited decreases.

Nerve Conduction Studies. NCS can evaluate motor, sensory, and mixed nerves. During motor conduction studies, motor nerves are indirectly assessed via compound muscle action potentials, which represent the muscle response after motor nerve stimulation. The amplitude of compound muscle action potentials is directly related to the number of muscle fibers that are recruited, giving an approximation of the number of functional axons and motor fibers. Latency reflects the time between the application of stimulus to the first deflection recorded by the electrode measured in milliseconds. Sensory nerve function is assessed by evaluating the amplitude, latency, area of recorded response, duration, and conduction velocity of sensory nerve action potentials (SNAPs). Demyelination interrupts normal conduction of the action potential, resulting in increased latency of nerve conduction velocity (NCV). As axonal injury progresses, the SNAPs and compound MAPs decrease in amplitude.

Management

Management of a compressive neuropathy depends on the type of deficit (sensory or motor), and the duration of symptoms. In general, for a purely sensory deficit, conservative management lasts for at least 6 months; surgery can be considered if symptoms are not alleviated or if they progress. On the other hand, for motor or combined motor and sensory deficits, surgery should be considered if symptoms progress or fail to resolve after 3 to 6 months of nonoperative management.

Median Nerve

Carpal tunnel syndrome is the most common compression neuropathy of the upper extremity. It is caused by compression of the median nerve by the TCL at the wrist. (Table 6.11; Fig. 6.13). In addition to the median nerve, the carpal canal contains 9 digital flexor tendons: the 4 tendons of both the FDP and FDS and the FPL tendon. There are several anatomic variations of the motor branch of the median nerve with respect to the TCL, the most common being extraligamentous. This branch is at risk of iatrogenic injury during carpal tunnel release. Failure to completely release the TCL is the most common cause of persistent symptoms after surgery. Other

TABLE 6.11 Borders of the carpal canal

Border	Structure
Radial	Scaphoid tubercle
	Trapezium
Ulnar	Hook of the hamate
	Pisiform
Roof	TCL
Floor	Capitate
	Hamate

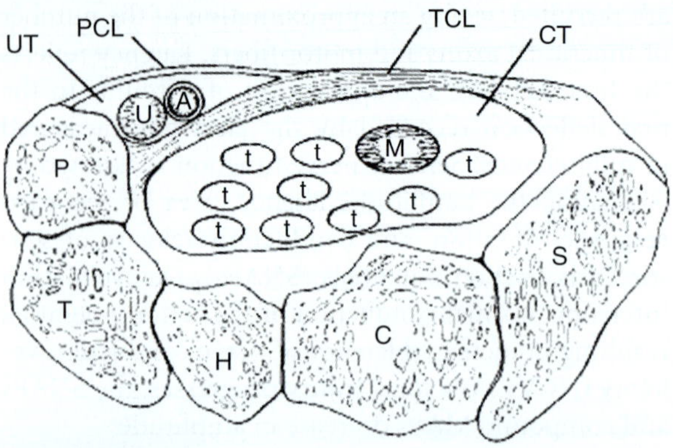

FIGURE 6.13 Cross section of the wrist demonstrating the relationship of the carpal tunnel (CT) and the ulnar tunnel (UT). A, ulnar artery; C, capitate; H, hamate; M, median nerve, P, pisiform; PCL, palmar carpal ligament; S, scaphoid; t, flexor tendon; T, triquetrum; TCL, transverse carpal ligament; U, ulnar nerve. (*Source:* Szabo RM, Steinberg DR. Nerve entrapment syndromes in the wrist. *J Am Acad Orthop Surg* 1994;82:115–123.)

compressive neuropathies of the median nerve include pronator and AIN syndromes (Table 6.12).

Ulnar Nerve

Compression neuropathy of the ulnar nerve (Table 6.13) occurs at the wrist in the Guyon canal (Tables 6.14 and 6.15) and at the elbow in the cubital tunnel (Table 6.16; Fig. 6.14). Cubital tunnel syndrome is the second most common compression neuropathy of the upper extremity; compression most commonly occurs between the two heads of the FCU and less commonly in the epitrochlear groove. Weakness of the ulnar nerve as a result of compression at the elbow can be appreciated with the presence of Froment sign, which is compensatory FPL flexion secondary to weakness of the adductor pollicis with pinch. Wartenberg sign describes abduction of the small finger due to weakness of the third palmar interosseous muscle. Compression of the ulnar nerve at the elbow can be distinguished from compression in the Guyon canal by examining the sensibility of the dorsal ulnar aspect of the hand. If there is a sensory deficit in this area, then compression of the nerve is proximal to the Guyon canal, because the dorsal cutaneous branch of the ulnar nerve originates 5 to 6 cm proximal to the ulnar styloid. It is responsible for cutaneous sensation over the dorsal ulnar aspect of the hand. Compression of

TABLE 6.12 Compressive neuropathies of the median nerve

Syndrome	*Sites of Compression*	*Symptoms*	*Provocative Test*	*EMG/NCS*	*Treatment*
Carpal tunnel (most common)	TCL	Pain/paraesthesias in palmar radial $3\frac{1}{2}$-digits Night pain Numbness Weakness Clumsiness	Direct compression (most sensitive); Phalen Tinel	Gold standard	Early NSAIDs Splint Steroid injection Intermediate to advanced carpal tunnel release
Pronator	Pronator teres Ligament of Struthers FDS origin Bicipital aponeurosis	Pain/paraesthesias in palmar radial $3\frac{1}{2}$-digits and palm and forearm	Palpable supracondylar process Pressure over pronator teres with forearm supinated Resisted elbow flexion, pronation, and flexion of PIP joint of long finger	Nondiagnostic	Activity modification NSAIDs Splint Global release
AIN	Pronator teres FDS arcade Lacertus fibrosus Bicipital bursa Accessory FPL	Vague forearm pain Weak thumb interphalangeal flexion Weak index/long DIP flexion	Pronator quadratus weakness	Diagnostic	Activity modification NSAIDs Splint Global release if no improvement by 3–6 mos.

TABLE 6.13 Compressive neuropathies of the ulnar nerve

Syndrome	Site of Compression	Symptoms	Provocative Test	EMG/NCS	Treatment
Ulnar tunnel	Mass/structure compressing ulnar nerve in one of the zones of Guyon canal: Ganglion cyst (most common in zones I and II) Lipoma Hook of hamate fracture Ulnar artery thrombosis or aneurysm (most common in zone III) Fibrous/congenital bands Zones of Guyon canal: I: proximal to bifurcation of ulnar nerve (both motor and sensory) II: deep motor branch III: superficial sensory branch	I: pain/paraesthesia over dorsal and ulnar _ digits; intrinsic motor weakness II: intrinsic motor weakness III: pain/paraesthesia over ulnar _ digits	Reverse Phalen Direct pressure proximal to Guyon canal Decreased grip strength if motor branch involved Allen test	Diagnostic but supplement with MRI to rule out mass, Doppler for vascular etiology	Padded gloves Activity modification NSAIDs Splint Decompression with excision of mass and release of hypothenar muscle origin
Cubital tunnel (second)	Heads of FCU Arcade of Struthers Osborne ligament Medial epicondyle Medial head triceps Medial intermuscular septum Flexor-pronator aponeurosis Mass Malunion	Pain/paraesthesias in ulnar dorsal hand Weakness of intrinsics FCU weakness Clawing of ring and small fingers	Tinel Froment sign: using FPL to compensate for weak adductor pollicis DIP flexion weakness of small and ring fingers Wartenberg sign	Supplement to clinical exam	Activity modification NSAIDs Splint Global release with transposition of ulnar nerve

the nerve in the Guyon canal would cause a sensory deficit along the ulnar 11/2 digits.

Radial Nerve

Compression neuropathies involving the radial nerve can occur in the arm and forearm. In the arm, compression is usually due to trauma or fibers from the lateral head of the triceps or trauma such as humeral shaft fractures. The current indication for immediate exploration of the radial nerve after a humeral shaft fracture is if there is a nerve palsy in the presence of an open fracture. Compression neuropathy of the radial nerve in the forearm include radial tunnel, PIN, and Wartenberg syndromes (Tables 6.17, 6.18, and 6.19). Symptoms of radial tunnel and Wartenberg syndrome are purely sensory; PIN syndrome involves motor deficits only.

TABLE 6.14 Borders of guyon's canal

Border	Structure
Radial	Hook of hamate
Ulnar	Pisiform
	Abductor digiti minimi
Roof	Volar carpal ligament
	Palmaris brevis
Floor	Transverse carpal ligament
	Hypothenar muscles

Thoracic Outlet Syndrome

Thoracic outlet syndrome (TOS) refers to the signs and symptoms that result from compression of the neurovascular structures of the upper extremity in the costoclavicular and shoulder regions. The thoracic outlet contains 3 sites of potential compression: the interscalene triangle, the costoclavicular junction, and the subcoracoid spaces. The etiology of TOS is either

TABLE 6.15 Zones of Guyon's canal

Zone	Anatomic Region	Neurologic Deficit	Most Common Causes of Compression
I	Proximal to ulnar nerve division	Motor and sensory	Ganglion cyst Hook of the hamate fracture
II	Surrounds deep motor branch	Motor	Ganglion cyst Hook of the hamate fracture
III	Surrounds sensory branch	Sensory	Ulnar artery thrombosis Ulnar artery aneurysm

Source: Szabo RM, Steinberg DR. Nerve entrapment syndromes in the wrist. *J Am Acad Orthop Surg* 1994; 2:115–123.

TABLE 6.16 Borders of cubital tunnel

Border	Structure
Radial	Olecranon
Ulnar	Medial epicondyle
Roof	Osborne ligament
Floor	Medial collateral ligament

Source: Posner MA. Compressive ulnar neuropathies at the elbow: I. Etiology and diagnosis. *J Am Acad Orthop Surg* 1998;6:282–288.

neurogenic or vascular in nature. Vascular type can be arterial or venous and is due to pathology of the subclavian vasculature such as stenosis, aneurysm, or thrombosis. Patients typically present with venous congestion, ischemia, and Raynaud phenomenon. Diagnosis is based on clinical examination findings and angiography. The neurogenic type is not as common; diagnosis is based on physical examination. Provocative maneuvers such as Wright, Adson, and hyperabduction are often performed on physical examination; the specificity of these maneuvers is low. EMG and NCS are nondiagnostic. Plain radiographs of the cervical spine and chest should be taken to rule out cervical rib and Pancoast tumor respectively. Other potential sites of compression include congenital fibrous bands, the anterior scalene muscle, transverse process of vertebrae, clavicular malunion, and sternocleidomastoid muscles. Treatment includes activity modification and physical therapy. Surgical indications include intractable pain, neurologic deficit, or arterial insufficiency.

VI. INFECTIONS

Infections of the hand can be acute or chronic. The majority of acute hand infections require emergent surgery. Host factors strongly influence the severity

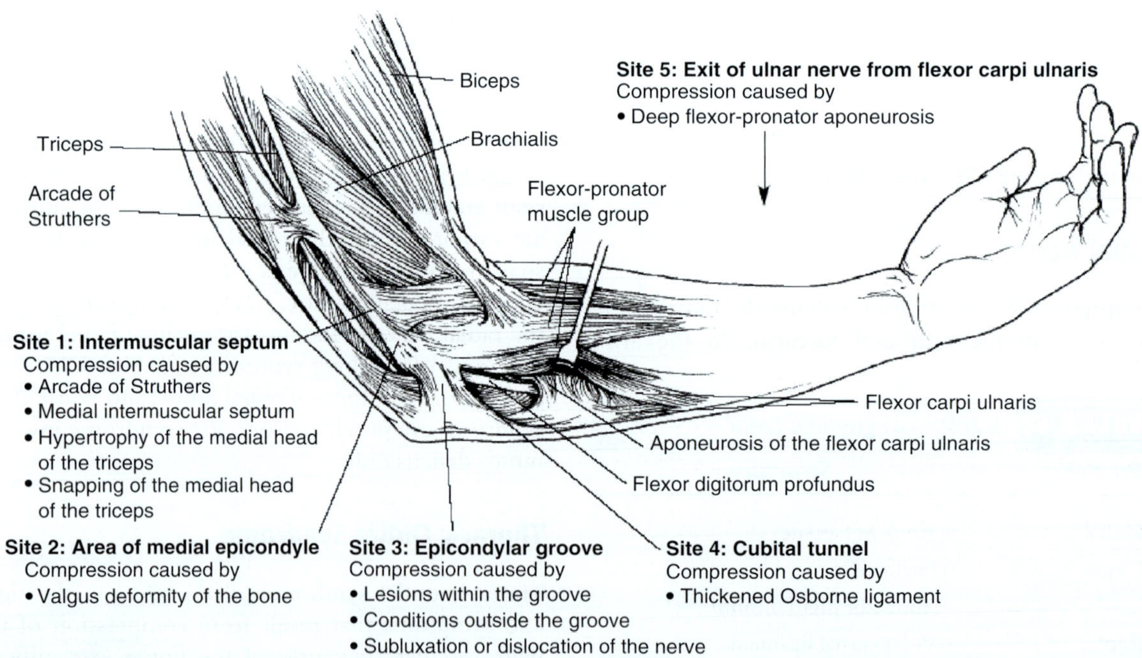

FIGURE 6.14 The five sites for potential ulnar nerve compression and the causes of compression at each site. (*Adapted from* Amadio PC. Anatomical basis for a technique of ulnar nerve transposition. *Surg Radiol Anat* 1986;8:155–161.)

TABLE 6.17 Compressive neuropathies of the radial nerve

Syndrome	Sites of Compression	Symptoms	Clinical/Provocative Test	EMG/NCS	Treatment
Radial nerve compression in the arm	Fibrous arch of lateral head of triceps Postural compression Humeral shaft fracture Tourniquet palsy	Weakness of thumb, finger, and wrist extension	Weakness with resisted extension of thumb, fingers, and wrist	Diagnostic	Activity modification NSAIDs Splint Decompression Explore radial nerve palsy in the presence of open humeral shaft fracture
Posterior Interosseous	Arcade of Frohse (most common) Recurrent leash of Henry ECRB Distal border of supinator Fibrous bands anterior to radial head Trauma Mass	Weakness of thumb, finger, and wrist extension No sensory changes	Pain at lateral elbow Weakness and ulnar drift with wrist extension	Diagnostic	Activity modification NSAIDs Splint Global release
Radial tunnel	Arcade of Frohse (most common) Recurrent leash of Henry ECRB Distal border of supinator Fibrous bands anterior to radial head	Pain from lateral elbow to dorsal wrist	Tenderness in mobile wad; pain with resisted supination with elbow and wrist in extension	Nondiagnostic	Activity modification NSAIDs Splint Global release
Sensory radial nerve Wartenberg syndrome	Forearm pronation elicits scissorlike action between ECRL and brachioradialis (BR)	Pain/paraesthesia dorsal-radial hand, wrist, and forearm	Tinel Forceful forearm pronation	Nondiagnostic	Activity modification NSAIDs Splint Release of fascia between ECRL and BR (only after at least 1 yr of conservative treatment)

and duration of infection. The host's ability to successfully illicit an immune response can be stunted by chronic immunosuppressive drug therapy (e.g., corticosteroids), alcoholism, intravenous drug abuse, malnutrition, human immunodeficiency virus (HIV) infection, autoimmune disease, and diabetes, which is the most prevalent of the immunosuppressive diseases. The peripheral neuropathy and the small vessel disease associated with diabetes contribute to potential delays in diagnosis and treatment, inability to clear the infection, and the need for multiple surgical débridements. Nonhost-related factors that influence the outcome of hand infections include the timing of diagnosis and treatment, the organism causing the infection, the location of the infection, the adequacy of surgical débridement, and the efficacy of antibiotic therapy. Common hand infections are described in Table 6.20.

Paronychia and Eponychia. Paronychia and eponychia are infections of the soft tissue fold surrounding the nail. Paronychias typically do not require formal incision and débridement in the operating room; they can be treated in the emergency department or outpatient clinic.

TABLE 6.18 Anatomic structures in compressive neuropathies

Structure	Description	Clinical Relevance
Ligament of Struthers	Spans from supracondylar process of distal humerus to medial epicondyle	Site of medial nerve compression in pronator syndrome
Arcade of Struthers	Band with fascial fibers from medial intermuscular septum and medial head of triceps that attaches to medial intermuscular septum	Site of ulnar nerve compression in cubital tunnel syndrome
Arcade of Frohse	Proximal edge of supinator muscle	Site of PIN compression in PIN syndrome
Recurrent leash of Henry		Site of PIN compression in PIN syndrome
Osborne ligament or Osborne fascia	Leading edge of FCU; fibers medial epicondyle and olecranon and roof of cubital tunnel	Site of ulnar nerve compression in cubital tunnel syndrome

Felon Subcutaneous Abscess. This type of abscess involves the palmar pad of the distal phalanx (pulp) of a finger or thumb. This area is made of multiple compartments that are divided by septae. Infection of these compartments can lead to compartment syndrome of the distal phalangeal pulp. Clinically, a patient with a felon will present with tense swelling and throbbing pain that does not extend proximal to the DIP flexion crease. Felons typically do not require formal incision and débridement in the operating room; they can be treated in the emergency department or outpatient clinic.

Septic Flexor Tenosynovitis. Septic flexor tenosynovitis is an infection of the flexor tendon sheath of the fingers or thumb. The digital flexor tendon sheath is typically inoculated after penetrating trauma (from a foreign body or animal bite) over the palmar aspect of the PIP or DIP joint. The flexor tendon gliding mechanism is destroyed by the purulence that accumulates in the flexor tendon sheath. Pyogenic flexor tenosynovitis rarely develops from hematogenous spread; disseminated gonococcal infections are the most common cause of this mechanism of inoculation. Diagnosis is primarily clinical; Kanavel described 4 cardinal signs of flexor tenosynovitis:

1. Fusiform swelling of the involved digit (sausage digit)
2. Semiflexed position of the finger
3. Severe tenderness with palpation along the course of the tendon sheath
4. Excruciating pain with passive extension of the finger that is felt along the course of the tendon sheath

Pain with palpation along the flexor tendon sheath and with passive extension are the most reliable and reproducible signs. The flexor tendon sheath consists of a double-layered tube with a visceral and parietal wall. The visceral layer is adjacent to the tendon and is the epitenon. The parietal layer is adherent to the flexor pulley system. The sheaths begin at the level of the metacarpal neck and extend distally to just proximal to the DIP joint. The high pressure that develops within the sheath as a result of the infection can inhibit the tendon's supply of nutrients, leading to tendon necrosis and subsequent rupture. The thumb and small finger sheaths are often continuous with the radial and ulnar bursae respectively. The two bursae can communicate proximally through the Parona space, which is a potential space that lies between the pronator quadratus and FDP tendon sheath. A horseshoe abscess develops when infection within the thumb or small finger sheaths tracks proximally via the radial or ulnar bursa respectively and tracks to the flexor sheath of the opposite side of the hand.

TABLE 6.19 Borders of the radial tunnel

Border	Structure
Radial	ECRL
	ECRB
Ulnar	Biceps tendon
	Brachialis
Roof	Brachioradialis
Floor	Radiocapitellar joint capsule

Deep Space Infections. Deep space infections occur as a result of inoculation of a potential space in the hand or forearm. These septated spaces are located between the fascial planes of muscles. There are 4

TABLE 6.20 Common hand infections

Type	Location	Pathogen	Antibiotic	Treatment	Comment
Paronychia eponychia	Eponychium	Acute: *S. aureus* Chronic: *C. albicans*	Acute: oral or IV first-generation cephalosporin or Staph-specific penicillin Chronic: oral antifungal	Soaks Acute: bedside I&D Chronic: eponychial marsupialization	Most common hand infection Can extend to the pulp
Felon	Distal pulp	*S. aureus*	Oral or IV first generation cephalosporin or Staph-specific penicillin	Bedside I&D	15%–20% of hand infections; can lead to compartment syndrome of distal pulp
Flexor tenosynovitis	Digital flexor tendon	Acute: *S. aureus; Pasturella multocida* (animal bites) Chronic: *Mycobacterium marinum*	Acute: IV first-generation cephalosporin or Staph-specific penicillin or Unasyn Chronic: minocycline	If immunocompromised or more than 12 hours since onset: formal I&D	Kanavel signs: swollen digit, pain with passive extension, pain along the flexion tendon sheath, fusiform digit
Deep space infection	Midpalmar, thenar hypothenar, Parona	*S. aureus*	IV first-generation cephalosporin or Staph-specific penicillin or Unasyn	Formal I&D	
Deep subfascial space infection Collar button abscess	Dorsal subcutaneous and subaponeurotic web space, interdigital web space	*S. aureus*	IV first-generation cephalosporin or Staph-specific penicillin or Unasyn	Formal I&D with dorsal and palmar incisions for web space abscess	
Dog bites	Most common animal bite	alpha-hemolytic *Streptococcus* most common; *P. multocida*	First-generation cephalosporin, penicillin, or amoxicillin/clavulanate	Formal I&D	24% infection rate
Cat bites		*P. multocida*	IV first-generation cephalosporin, penicillin or Unasyn	Formal I&D	76% infection rate
Human bites	Adjacent to 3rd and 4th MC heads	*S. aureus* most common; *Eikenella corrodens*	Amoxicillin/clavulanate and penicillin with Staph-specific penicillin or first-generation cephalosporin and penicillin	Formal I&D	
Herpetic Whitlow	Index and thumb most common	Herpes simplex virus 1 or 2	Antiviral medication (e.g., acyclovir)	Conservative management; no surgery	Most common hand infection in children and dentists
Cellulitis		*Streptococcus* and *S. aureus*	First-generation cephalosporin or Staph-specific penicillin or amoxicillin/clavulanate		

(*continued overleaf*)

TABLE 6.20 *(continued)*

Type	*Location*	*Pathogen*	*Antibiotic*	*Treatment*	*Comment*
IV drug abuse		Methicillin-resistant *S.aureus*, Gram-positive or Gram-negative or polymicrobial	Nafcillin and gentamycin		
Necrotizing fasciitis	Develops after soft tissue insult	Group A beta-hemolytic *Streptococcus* most common			Most common findings on presentation: erythema pain edema induration fluctuance fever soft tissue gas on radiography
Diabetic infection					
Osteomyelitis		*S. aureus*	First-generation cephalosporin or Staph-specific penicillin or amoxicillin/clavulanate		Open fractures most common cause
Septic arthritis		*S. aureus*			

palmar spaces: the midpalmar, thenar, and hypothenar spaces are located in the hand, and the Parona space is in the forearm. Most deep palmar space infections involve the thenar space. Clinically, a patient presents a diffusely edematous hand, especially over the dorsum of the hand. Extensive dorsal swelling can also result from an infection involving dorsal subcutaneous or subaponeurotic space. Palpation of the affected region is very painful. Once the diagnosis has been established, the area must be urgently débrided in the operating room. The wound is packed open, and IV antibiotics are administered.

Collar Button Abscess. A collar button abscess is an infection of the web space. It is named after the hourglass shape characteristic of vintage collar buttons. Patients present with the adjacent fingers in abduction as a result of the accompanying swelling, pain, and erythema. The abscess usually develops from a callus, crack, or blister in the skin of laborers.

Bites. Penetrating injuries, either from a bite or a foreign body, warrant an update of tetanus immunization. The immunization status against rabies of an animal should be determined. Empirical broad spectrum antibiotic treatment should be initiated upon presentation. Wounds are left to close by secondary intention following formal incision and débridement. Human bites are usually the result of a fist fight after an individual strikes another in the mouth with a closed fist. The MCP joint becomes directly inoculated with oral flora of the human mouth. The most common organism that is cultured is *S. aureus*. *Eikenella corrodens* is cultured in 7% to 29% of cases. *Bacteroides* is the most common anaerobe that is isolated from human bites. Dog bites are the most common type of animal bite in the United States. Alpha-hemolytic streptococcus is the organism most frequently cultured from these wounds. *Pasturella multocida* may be cultured as well but is more often present in cat bites. Cat bites are much more susceptible to infection than dog bites (76% and 24% respectively) because of the deep, penetrating inoculation capability of the cat's long, sharp teeth.

Necrotizing Fasciitis. Necrotizing fasciitis describes infection of the superficial fascial layers of the extremity. Group A streptococcus is the organism most frequently isolated; however, more often than not, the infection is polymicrobial with Gram-negative, Gram-positive, aerobic, and anaerobic bacteria. It typically develops from a seemingly innocuous soft tissue injury such as an insect bite, contusion, or minor burn that spreads rapidly and can lead to multiple organ failure, adult respiratory distress syndrome, and death. Rapid diagnosis and treatment with broad spectrum IV antibiotics along with prompt, aggressive surgical débridement are essential in minimizing the high morbidity and mortality associated with these limb- and life-threatening infections. The currently reported mortality rate from necrotizing fasciitis is 26%.

Risk factors for increased mortality include obesity, diabetes, advanced age, malnutrition, immunocompromise, intravenous drug abuse, and peripheral vascular disease. Death is a result of the multiple organ failure, ARDS, and/or sepsis as a result of the host's immune response to streptococcal pyogenic exotoxins. These exotoxins illicit a massive T-cell response, which in turn leads to the release of cytokines such as tumor necrosis factor and several kinds of interleukins; cytokines are responsible for the septic shock and tissue necrosis.

VII. TUMORS

Guidelines for the management of neoplasms of the hand and upper extremity are based on the following key features:

- Location of the lesion
- Histologic grade and clinical behavior
- Likelihood of metastasis

The location of the lesion determines if the tumor is resectable and if the involved region is salvageable. A lesion is typically resectable if it is confined within a single anatomic compartment (i.e., intracompartmental vs. extracompartmental). Histologic grading and the aggressiveness of tumor invasion and spread are based on the malignant features noted by the pathologist on the tissue obtained from a biopsy.

Diagnosis and Staging. Histologic staging and subsequent treatment of benign neoplasms of the musculoskeletal system are based on the degree, if any, of local invasion of surrounding tissue.

With the aid of clinical and radiographic features as well as the presence or absence of metastasis, the pathologist and surgeon can determine the final tissue diagnosis and surgical stage. Lymph node metastasis is not the typical means of spread for sarcomas. Less than 5% of patients with sarcomas develop lymph node metastasis; sarcomas that are known to spread to the lymph nodes include rhabdomyosarcoma, epithelioid sarcoma, clear cell sarcoma, and angiosarcoma. In the presence of lymph node involvement, carcinomas and melanomas must also be included in the differential diagnosis of neoplasms of the extremity.

Radiographic Studies. The best imaging study for evaluating an extremity tumor is magnetic resonance imaging (MRI) with and without gadolinium. Total body bone scans and computerized tomography (CT) scans of the chest, abdomen, and pelvis are important in the work-up for metastasis. CT scans are also helpful in delineating bony and/or lesions involving a joint.

Bone and Cartilage Neoplasms. Only 2% to 4% of all bone tumors arise in the hand or wrist. Approximately 87% of all hand bone tumors are benign. Benign (Table 6.21; Figs. 6.15, 6.16, and 6.17) and malignant (Table 6.22; Figs. 6.18, 6.19, and 6.20) bone and cartilage tumors are described in the figures and tables noted.

Soft Tissue Neoplasms. Benign (Table 6.23, Figs. 6.21 to 6.25) and malignant (Table 6.24; Fig. 6.26) soft tissue tumors are described in the figures and tables noted.

Cutaneous Lesions. Cutaneous lesions are described in Table 6.25 and Figures 6.27 and 6.28.

VIII. VASCULAR DISORDERS

Types of vascular disorders are listed by category in Table 6.26, and vascular anatomy is shown in Figure 6.29. Vascular disorders of the hand and upper extremity are described using the following terminology:

- Critical vascular events lead to tissue death and necrosis without treatment.
- Noncritical vascular events describe vascular injury with enough collateral circulation to avoid tissue ischemia.
- Vascular competency is the ability to adjust physiologic thermoregulation and nutritional arterial flow to maintain core temperature and to satisfy metabolic needs.
- Arterial insufficiency refers to blood flow that cannot adequately meet the metabolic needs of the surrounding tissue.
- Thermoregulatory flow refers to blood supply that is not involved in cellular metabolism.
- Nutritional flow is blood supply that is involved in cellular metabolism.

Arterial Supply. The blood supply to the hand and forearm is composed of a network of interconnections between the radial and ulnar arteries that provides an excellent source of collateral circulation. In most patients, the superficial and deep palmar arches serve as the major blood supply. The ulnar artery is the main contributor to the superficial palmar arch and is the

TABLE 6.21 Benign bone and cartilage tumors

Lesion/Syndrome	Epidemiology/Unique Features	Clinical Presentation	Imaging	Treatment
Enchondroma (see Fig. 6.15)	Most common primary bone tumor of the hand Most common in proximal phalanges 40% of lesions occur in hand 10–40 years of age Less than 1% risk of malignant transformation if solitary	Localized swelling Pathologic fracture	X-ray: central, lytic, expansile intramedullary lesion with cortical thinning, stippled calcification	Biopsy, curettage—bone graft; let fracture heal before curettage
Ollier	Multiple enchondromatosis 30% risk of malignant transformation	Polyostotic	Multiple enchondromas	Continue growth after skeletal maturity and onset of pain should raise suspicion for malignant transformation
Maffucci	Multiple enchondromatosis and multiple hemangiomas 75%–100% risk of malignant transformation	Polyostotic Continues to grow after skeletal maturity	Multiple enchondromas with phleboliths (calcified thrombi within hemangiomas)	Continued growth after skeletal maturity and onset of pain should raise suspicion for malignant transformation
Osteo-chondroma	Rare in the hand Most common at distal aspect of proximal phalanx Form at tendon insertions or growth plates 20–30 years of age	May cause rotational deformity or mechanical block	Medullary cavity of lesion is continuous with that of the shaft	Excise lesions that impair function or cause progressive deformity or pain
Subungual exostosis	May be result of trauma or infection Fibrocartilaginous cap	Subungual exostosis causes nail deformity		Nail removal and excision of exostosis
Osteoid osteoma (see Fig. 6.17)	5%–15% occur in hand/wrist Most common in proximal phalanx and carpus Late 20s–30s	Local swelling with or without constant dull ache, worse at night, relieved with NSAIDs	Central radiolucent nidus (< 1 cm) surrounded by reactive sclerosis; cortical, medullary, or subperiosteal	Curettage of nidus or en bloc excision (must completely excise nidus to minimize risk of recurrence)
Fibrous dysplasia	Monostotic or polyostotic	Pain/swelling Pathologic fracture	Expansile "soap bubble" metaphy-seal–diaphyseal lesion with sclerotic rim and ground glass matrix	
Unicameral bone cyst	Cystic lesion of unknown etiology Rare in hand/forearm	Asymptomatic unless pathologic fracture	Well-circumscribed septated lytic metaphyseal lesion	Treat if deformity or fracture exists Cyst aspiration Corticosteroid injection En bloc excision Curettage and bone graft

TABLE 6.21 *(continued)*

Lesion/Syndrome	*Epidemiology/Unique Features*	*Clinical Presentation*	*Imaging*	*Treatment*
Aneurysmal bone cyst	3%–5% incidence in hand Second decade Most common in metacarpals	Pain/swelling Pathologic fracture	Asymmetric expansile lytic lesion with thin rim of cortex; fluid–fluid levels	Curettage and bone graft with cryosurgery High recurrence rate
Giant cell tumor of bone (see Fig. 6.16.)	2% incidence in hand Locally aggressive with 2% rate of metastasis to lungs Higher incidence of metastasis (18%) and recurrence (50%) with lesions in the hand Third to fourth decade Distal radius third most common location	Pain/swelling Pathologic fracture	Expansile, lytic epiphyseal lesion with geographic margin	Curettage and bone graft with adjuvant therapy and bone graft or bone cement; wide resection with soft tissue extension to minimize risk of recurrence

dominant artery in 88% of hands. The radial artery is the major contributor to the deep palmar arch and is dominant in only 12% of cases. A persistent median or large interosseous artery may be present also. The arches are complete if there is a major connection to a branch from a separate artery. The superficial palmar arch is completed by branches from the deep palmar arch, radial artery, or median artery in 78.5% of hands and is incomplete in 21.5% of cases; it is the more variable of the 2 arches. The deep palmar arch is completed by the superior and/or inferior deep branches of the ulnar artery 98.5% of hands. The digital blood supply in the majority of hands receives flow from both the superficial and deep arches.

Evaluation. Proper evaluation of a vascular disorder requires a thorough history and physical. Several key points must be addressed in the patient's history:

- Account of a traumatic event
- Repetitive injury

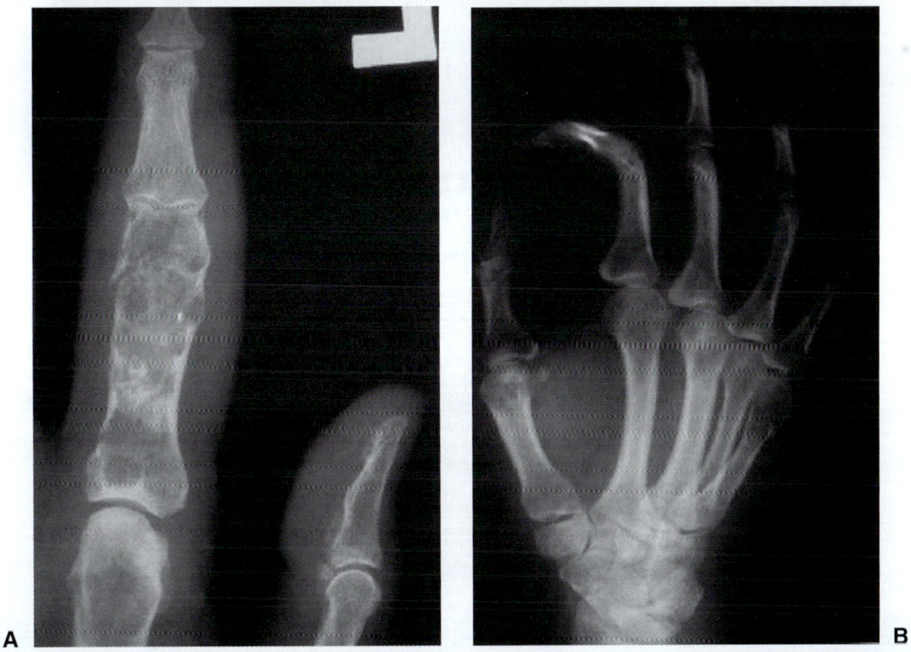

FIGURE 6.15 **Enchondromas of the (A) proximal phalanx and of the (B) fifth metacarpal head. (*Source:* Bickels J, Wittig JC, Kollender Y, Kellar-Graney K, Mansour KL, Meller I. Enchondromas of the hand: Treatment with curettage and cemented internal fixation. *J Hand Surg* 2002;27A:870–875, Fig. 4.)**

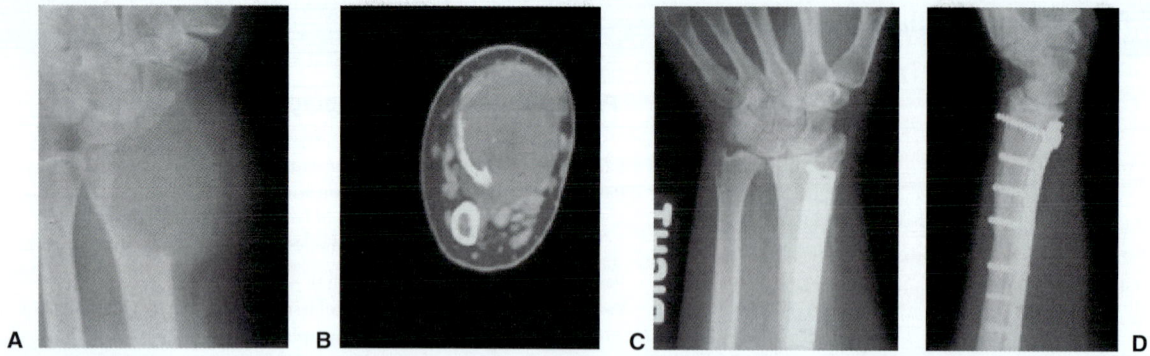

FIGURE 6.16 (A) An extensive and destructive stage-3 giant cell tumor of the right distal radius. (B) The lesion as seen on computed tomography. Note the extent of the tumor and the cortical destruction on the lateral side (C, D). (*Source:* Plate AM, Lee SJ, Steiner G, Posner MA. Tumorlike lesions and benign tumors of the wrist and hand. *J Am Acad Orthop Surg* 2003;11:1529–141.)

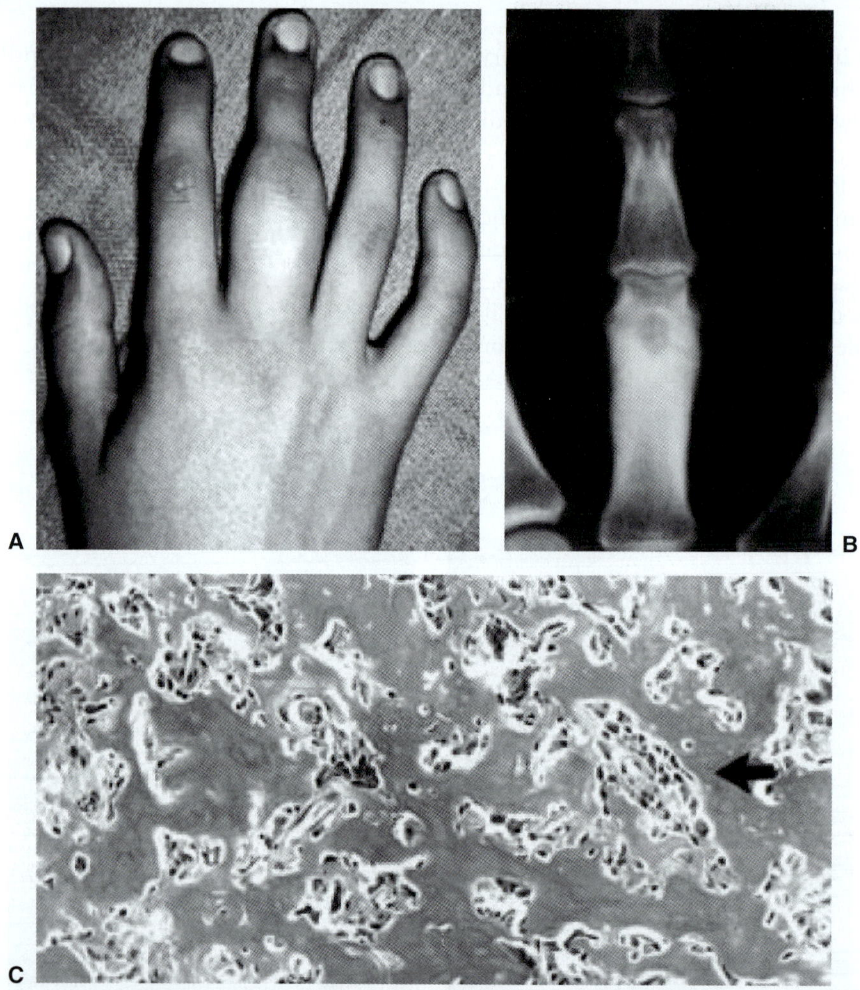

FIGURE 6.17 (A) Osteoid osteoma of the proximal phalanx of the middle finger. (B) Posteroanterior radiograph showing a radiolucent lesion or nidus surrounded by sclerotic bone. (C) Photomicrograph of the nidus showing irregular trabeculae of woven bone (arrow) bordered by osteoblasts (left of arrow) and osteoclasts, separated by blood vessels. (H&E staining, original magnification × 120.) (*Source:* Harness NG, Mankin HJ. Giant-cell tumor of the distal forearm. *J Hand Surg* 2004;29A:188–193.)

TABLE 6.22 Malignant bone and cartilage tumors

Lesion/Syndrome	Epidemiology/Unique Features	Clinical Presentation	Imaging	Treatment
Chondrosarcoma (see Fig. 6.18)	Most common primary malignant bone tumor of the hand Most common in proximal phalanges and metacarpals Over 60 years of age Can arise de novo or from preexisting enchondroma or osteochondroma	Slow-growing, firm, painful mass Localized swelling	Intralesional lysis, cortical thinning and expansion, endosteal scalloping, and stippled calcification	Wide en bloc excision Digit/ray amputation No role for chemotherapy or radiation therapy
Osteogenic sarcoma (see Fig. 6.19)	Rare as primary lesion in the hand (0.18% incidence) Most common in proximal phalanges and metacarpals Fourth to sixth decades	Rapidly growing, firm, painful mass	Expansile, sclerotic lesion with new bone formation/destruction; soft tissue expansion Periosteal reaction	Wide en bloc excision Digit/ray amputation Adjuvant chemotherapy
Ewing sarcoma (see Fig. 6.20)	Rare in the hand First to second decade Most common in proximal phalanges and metacarpals	Presents like an infection with pain, swelling, and erythema Fever, elevated white blood cells and ESR	Expansile, lytic, destructive with large soft tissue component Mixed sclerotic and lytic pattern Periosteal reaction	Wide en bloc excision Digit/ray amputation Adjuvant chemotherapy and radiation therapy
Metastasis	Rare in the hand with 0.3% incidence Distal phalanx is most common site in the hand Bronchogenic carcinoma most common primary malignancy (50%) followed by breast, renal, and colon Predilection for dominant hand Median survival with hand metastasis is 6 months	May present like an infection with pain, swelling, and erythema Pathologic fracture	Destructive lytic or sclerotic lesion	Radiation therapy for multiple or inoperable lesions Curettage and cement lesions that impair function or cause progressive deformity or pain Amputation effective for local control or palliative treatment

- Presence of soft tissue swelling
- Medical or family history of blood dyscrasias or disorders
- Drug or tobacco use
- Presence and frequency of Raynaud phenomenon
- Severity and extent of numbness, sensitivity to cold, numbness, weakness, and pain

A complete physical examination of the upper extremity and neck is essential and should address these areas:

- Skin integrity
- Capillary refill
- Quality of distal pulse
- Skin turgor
- Presence of fungal infection of the nails

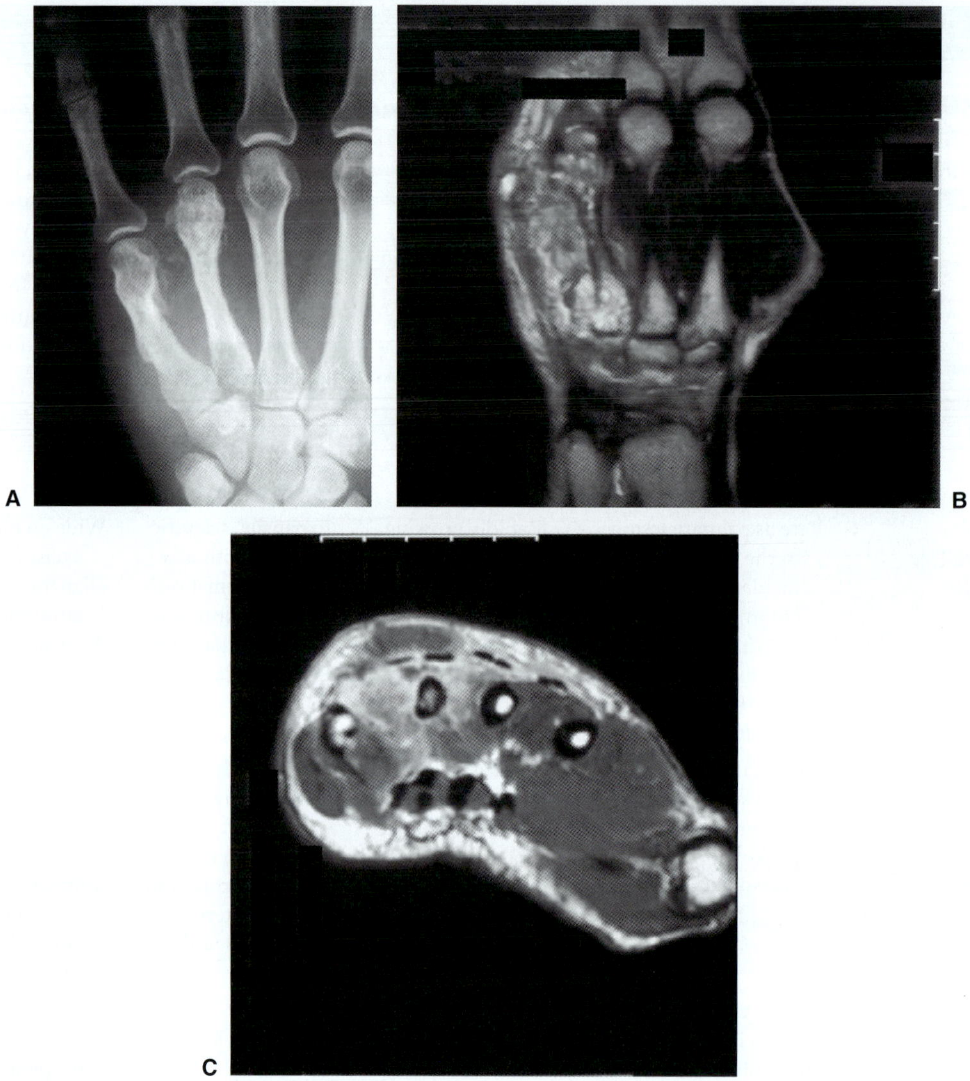

FIGURE 6.18 **(A) Plain radiograph showing chondrosarcoma involving the fourth metacarpal and adjacent intraosseous musculature. (B) Coronal MRI. (C) Axial MRI better shows the extent of soft tissue involvement. (*Source:* Athanasian EA. Malignant bone and soft-tissue sarcomas. *J of the Amer Soc for Surg of the Hand* 2004;4:60–72.)**

- Palpation/auscultation of bruits/masses
- Allen test is used to examine the competency of palmar arch anastomoses between the radial and ulnar artery. Both vessels are occluded at the wrist. The hand is exsanguinated by repeated opening and closing of the hand. Digital perfusion is assessed after pressure on 1 of the 2 vessels is released; reperfusion time should be within 3 seconds. The test is repeated by releasing the second vessel. Prolonged reperfusion suggests an incomplete arch.

The history and physical examination can be enhanced with diagnostic testing and imaging.

Acute Vascular Injury. Arterial trauma of the upper extremity occurs as a result of blunt or penetrating trauma or iatrogenic and accounts for 30% to 50% of all peripheral vascular injuries. Most vascular injuries involve the brachial artery; 80% are penetrating in nature. Signs and symptoms may be delayed or masked and can lead to thrombosis, hemorrhage, aneurysms, compartment syndrome, and embolization distally. Vascular injury can occur in conjunction with a fracture or innocuous wound. Penetrating trauma usually presents with exsanguination that may result in hypotension. Findings on physical examination that have a high correlation with arterial trauma include absent or diminished peripheral pulses, hypotension, a thrill or bruit, and associated neurologic deficits. Vascular integrity cannot be based on the presence of a peripheral pulse, distal

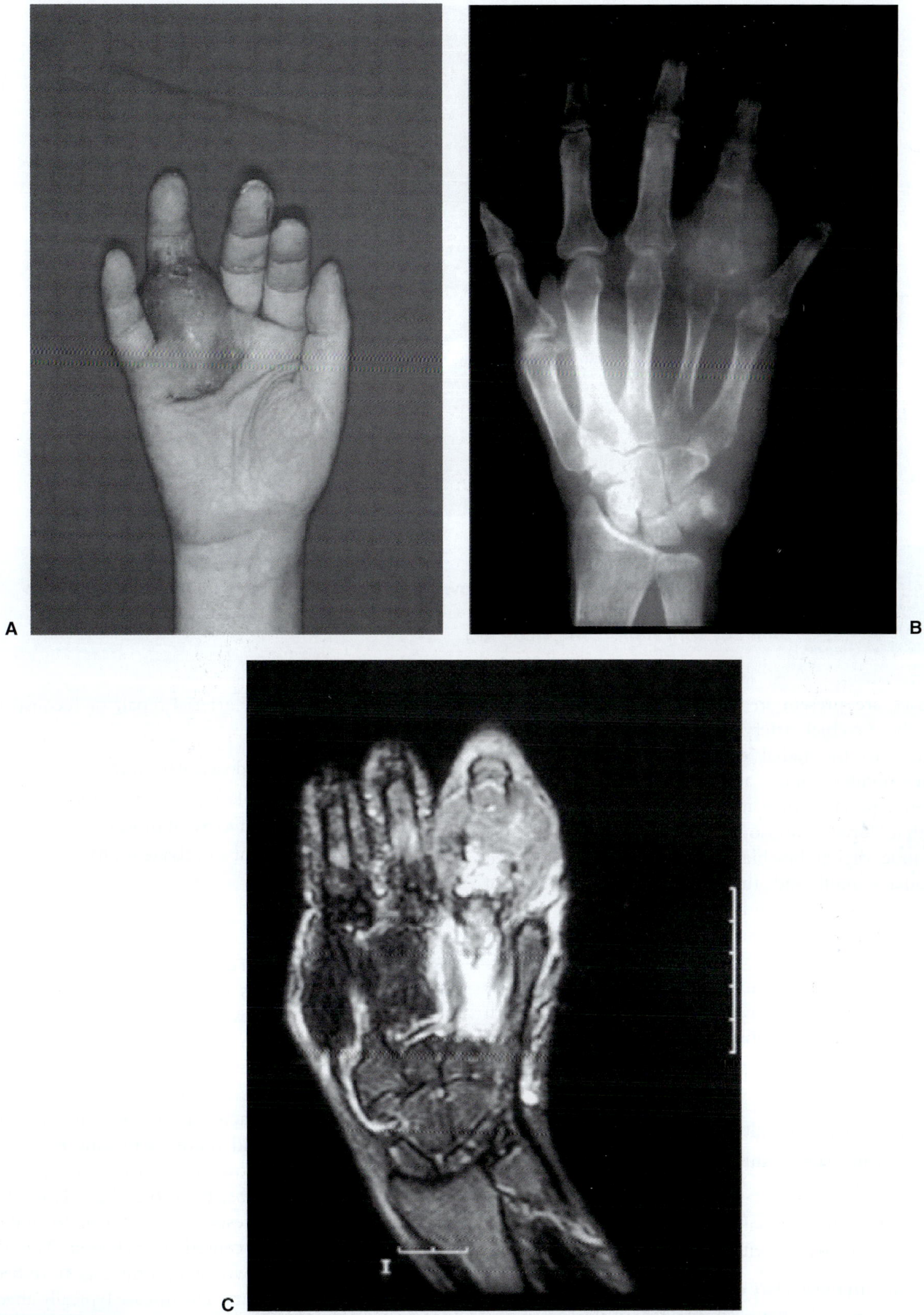

FIGURE 6.19 (A) Proximal phalanx osteogenic sarcoma of the ring finger. (B) Radiograph shows extensive bone destruction and soft tissue extension. (C) Coronal MRI shows extensive edema. (*Source:* Athanasian EA. Malignant bone and soft-tissue sarcomas. *J Am Soc Surg Hand* 2004;4:60–72.)

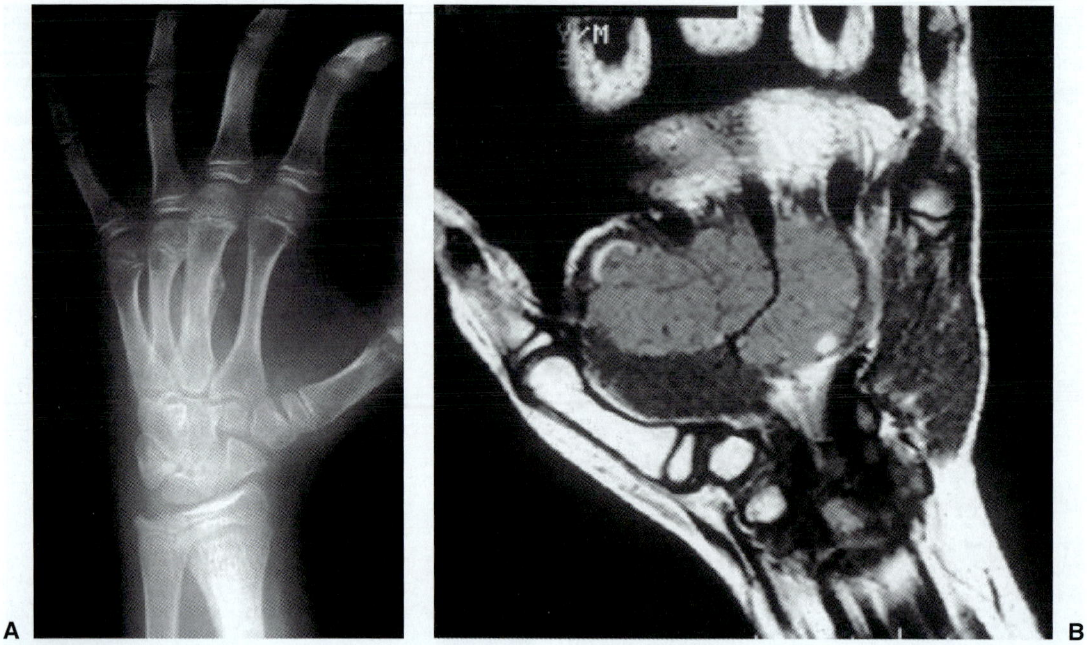

FIGURE 6.20 (A) Oblique radiograph of a third metacarpal Ewing sarcoma showing periosteal new bone formation. (B) Coronal MRI showing extensive soft tissue mass commonly seen with Ewing sarcoma. (*Source:* Athanasian EA. Malignant bone and soft-tissue sarcomas. *J Am Soc Surg Hand* 2004;4:60–72.)

pulses are present in 25% of patients with injury to the brachial artery and 50% of patients with injury to the radial or ulnar arteries. The Allen test provides a more accurate assessment of arterial flow, especially when it is performed in conjunction with a Doppler ultrasound. Clinical signs of ischemia include digital brachial index of $\leq$ 0.7, decreased capillary refill and turgor, and an Allen test of longer than 6 seconds after release. The role of arteriography in assessing acute vascular injury is controversial.

Once clinically significant arterial disruption has been recognized, surgical exploration is indicated with the following exceptions:

- Direct assessment may further compromise the limb or the patient
- The presence of multilevel vascular injury
- Clinically significant thrombosis or embolism is possible

Indications for arterial repair or reconstruction via end-to end repair or with a graft include the following:

- Injury to the axillary or brachial artery
- Injury to the radial or ulnar artery in the absence of adequate collateral circulation
- Injury to both the radial and ulnar arteries

Relative indications for arterial repair or reconstruction are listed here:

- Combined neural and vascular injury
- Technically achievable repair without significantly increasing the patient's risk of morbidity
- Presence of significant soft tissue injury

Vasospastic Disease

Raynaud Phenomenon and Disease. Raynaud disease is paroxysmal cyanosis of the digits caused by vasospasm of small arteries and arterioles. It is a result of an exaggerated sympathetic response to cold temperature or other stresses that cause intense vasospasm. The digits undergo 3 stages reflected by sequential color changes that are characteristic of Raynaud disease: blanching, cyanosis, and rubor. Blanching is a result of cessation of bloodflow followed by venous stasis, which produces the subsequent blue hue. The rubor of the third phase is a result of reperfusion secondary to reactive hyperemia caused by ischemia. There is bilateral involvement with symptoms that have been present for at least 2 years. The disease typically affects 20% to 30% of premenopausal females and follows a benign course; there are no ischemic changes such as ulceration and gangrene. Excessive pain due to cold

TABLE 6.23 Benign soft tissue tumors

Lesion/Syndrome	Epidemiology/Unique Features	Clinical Presentation	Imaging	Treatment
Ganglion cyst (see Fig. 6.21)	Most common soft tissue tumor of the hand (50%–70% of hand masses) F greater than M by 3:1 Second to fourth decades May be in close proximity to osteoarthritic joint Not associated with malignancy Dorsal: 70%; most common along capsule over scapholunate ligament Volar: 20%; most common along capsule over radiocarpal joint Filled with clear, gelatinous mucin Intraosseous ganglia most commonly occur in scaphoid or lunate	Slow-growing, firm, painful mass Cosmetic deformity Localized swelling that fluctuates in size Weakness if impinging on nerve Transilluminates	Degenerative joint changes often present with cysts at the DIP or CMC joints Communication between cyst and joint on arthrogram	Most resolve without treatment Aspiration/ corticosteroid injection 13%–100% recurrence after aspiration Excision (including stalk) 10% recurrence rate after excision Volar ganglia more likely to recur than dorsal ganglia Must evaluate arterial blood supply to hand prior to excision of volar ganglia
Giant cell tumor of tendon sheath (pigmented villonodular synovitis) (see Fig. 6.22)	Second most common hand tumor Volar surfaces of radial 3 digits and DIP joint region most common	Slow-growing, firm, nodular, fixed, painless mass Does not transilluminate	Soft tissue mass with or without pressure erosion of underlying bone	Marginal excision Risk of recurrence 5%–50% because of incomplete excision or satellite lesion
Epidermal inclusion cyst (see Fig. 6.23)	Posttraumatic invagination of epithelial cells into underlying soft tissue or bone Third most common tumor of the hand Most common lesion of distal phalanx Most common in left long finger and thumb in males between third and fourth decades	Slow growing and painless Well circumscribed	Well-demarcated lytic lesion	Marginal excision or curettage and bone graft Recurrence rare
Mucous cyst	Ganglion cyst on dorsum of DIP joint Fifth to seventh decades		Degenerative joint changes often present with cysts at the DIP joint	Aspiration Excision and include osteophyte
Carpometacarpal boss	Degenerative bony prominence or spur Base of second or third CMC joints F > M Third to fourth decades 30% associated with ganglion cyst	Firm, palpable, tender mass at base of CMC joints Readily visible with wrist flexion	30–40 degrees supination and 20–30 degrees ulnar deviation provides "carpal boss view" Osteophytic spur May have degenerative changes of the adjacent joint	Excision of spur and ganglion

Note: F = female; M = male.

(continued)

TABLE 6.23 (continued)

Lesion/Syndrome	Epidemiology/Unique Features	Clinical Presentation	Imaging	Treatment
Schwannoma	Most common benign nerve tumor Arises from Schwann cell Most common on volar forearm or hand Fourth to fifth decades	Slow-growing, painless mass Neurologic deficit may be present Positive Tinel sign	Eccentric, well-circumscribed, encapsulated mass	Marginal excision with 4% risk of postoperative neurologic deficit Recurrence rare
Pyogenic granuloma (see Fig. 6.24)	Associated with trauma	Rapidly growing, pedunculated red mass that bleeds easily		Cauterize with silver nitrate Excision
Lipoma		Subcutaneous or intramuscular soft nontender Neurologic deficit if compressing on nerve	Well-circumscribed homogenous mass	Marginal excision if symptomatic or cosmetic deformity
Glomus tumor (see Fig. 6.25)	Tumor of glomus bodies, with smooth muscle and vascular tissue Glomus bodies thermoregulators within the skin 65% subungual/fingertip Solitary or multiple lesion	Dark red or blue nodules; bluish hue to nail bed Triad of cold hypersensitivity, paroxysmal pain, and pinpoint pain Nail ridging common	Well-demarcated, dark on T1 and bright on T2 MRI	Excision if symptomatic 25% recurrence due to multiple lesions
Vascular malformation	Common in children Usually on dorsum Hemangiomas grow rapidly within first few years of life; more than 70% involute by age 7	Soft, painless, palpable, compressible mass		
Fibromatosis (Dupuytren disease)	Dupuytren disease is fibromatosis of palmar fascia Garrod node is fibromatosis of dorsal PIP joints (knuckle pads); present in 20%–40% patients with Dupuytren	Nontender nodules in the palm with or without flexion deformity		Release if deformity is present
Calcifying aponeurotic fibroma	Rare	Slow-growing, painless mass	Soft tissue mass with stippled calcifications	Wide excision if symptomatic High recurrence rate (> 50%) due to local aggressiveness of tumor No malignant transformation

sensitivity is the most frequent presenting symptom. The defining characteristics of Raynaud disease are as follows.

- Bilateral hand involvement
- Absence of occlusive disease
- Absence of gangrenous or trophic changes
- Absence of systemic disease
- Female predominance
- Symptoms for 2 years
- Triphasic color changes

Diagnostic work-up should aim to distinguish a vasospastic from a vaso-occlusive state, to examine the effects of structural and/or functional deficits, and to distinguish primary Raynaud disease from secondary

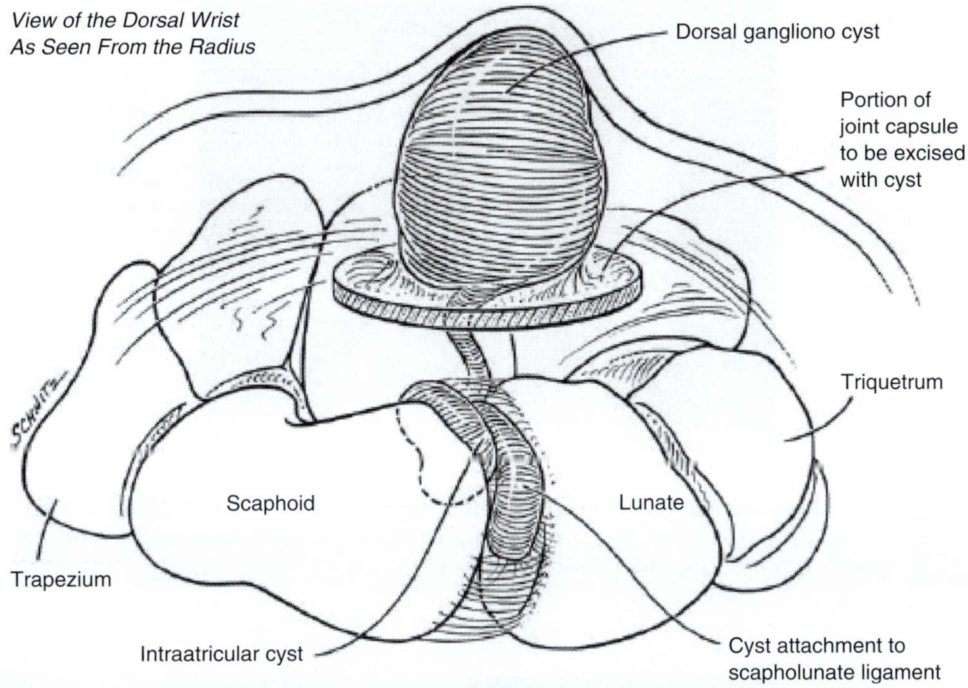

FIGURE 6.21 Ganglion cyst with pedicle attachment to the scapholunate ligament. (*Source:* Minotti P, Taras JS. Ganglion cysts of the wrist. *J Am Soc Surg Hand* 2002;2:102–107.)

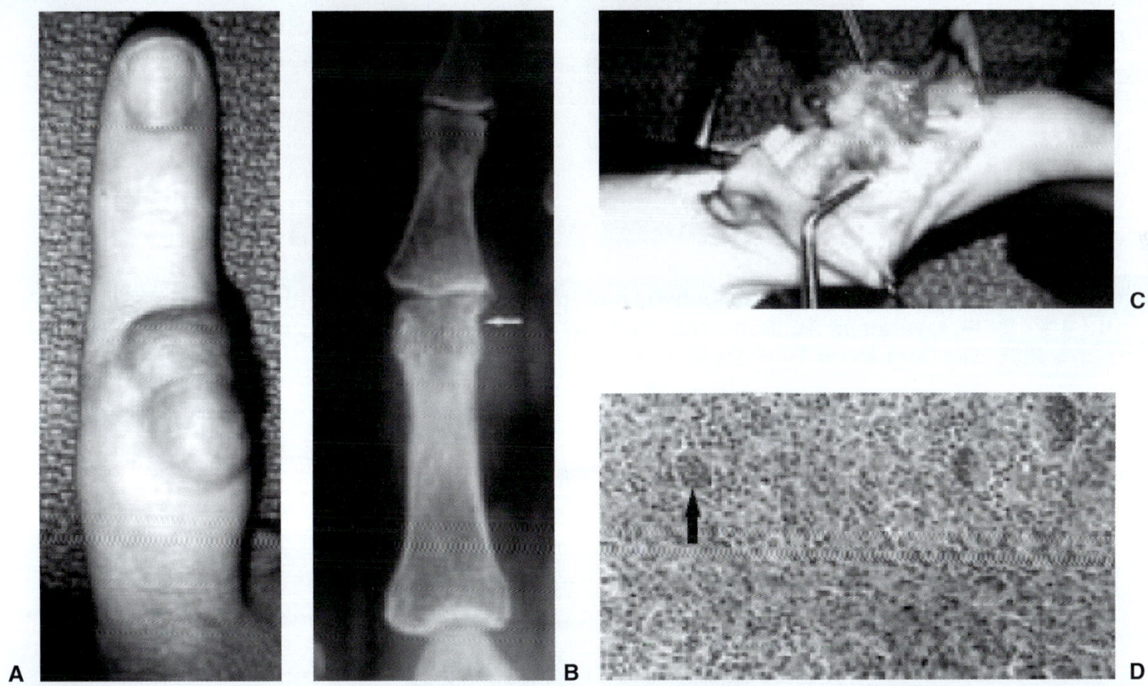

FIGURE 6.22 (A) Giant cell tumor of the tendon sheath. (B) Posteroanterior radiograph. (C) At surgery, the nodular lesion was found to be attached to the tendon, and there was a small intracapsular extension into the proximal interphalangeal joint (tip of probe). (D) Photomicrograph showing sheets of round to ovoid mononuclear cells and osteoclastlike giant cells (arrow) with thin bands of collagenous stroma. (H&E stain, original magnification × 125.) (*Source:* Plate AM, Lee SJ, Steiner G, Posner MA. Tumorlike lesions and benign tumors of the wrist and hand. *J Am Acad Orthop Surg* 2003; 11:1529–141.)

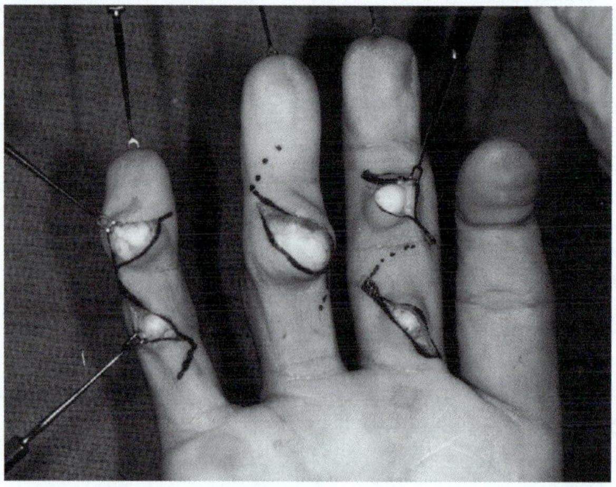

FIGURE 6.23 Multiple epidermal inclusion cysts of the right hand. (*Source:* Goebel SX, Rasi LM, Stern PJ. Multiple epidermal inclusion cysts in a patient with rheumatoid arthritis: A case report. *J Hand Surg* 2000;25A:768–771.)

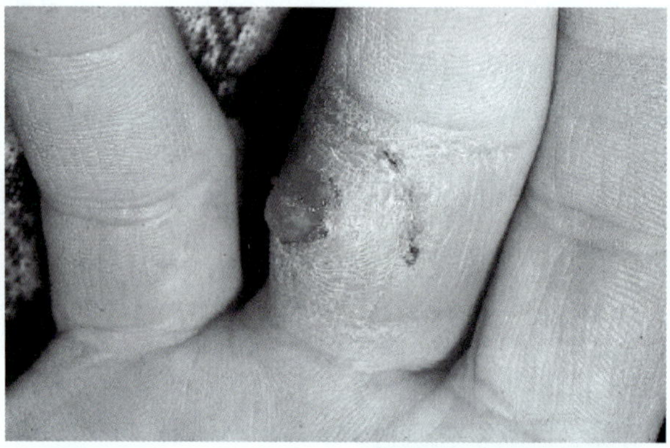

FIGURE 6.24 Pyogenic granuloma. Exophytic pink-red glistening papule with ulceration. (*Source:* Gray JP, Jayaraman AG, Robinson-Bostom L. Cutaneous conditions of the hands: Part 2. *J Am Soc Surg Hand* 2003;3:66–77.)

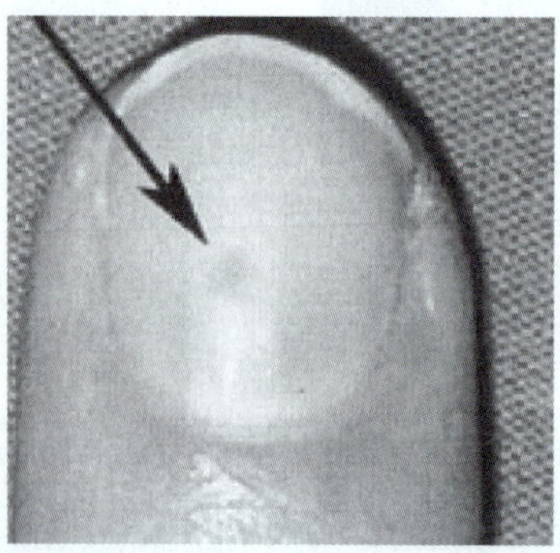

FIGURE 6.25 Glomus tumor. (*Source:* Tuncali D, Yilmaz AC, Terzioglu A, Aslan G. Histologic types of the glomus tumor. *J Hand Surg* 2005;30A:161–164.)

TABLE 6.24 Malignant soft tissue tumors

Lesion/Syndrome	Epidemiology/Unique Features	Clinical Presentation	Imaging	Treatment
Epithelioid sarcoma	Most common soft tissue sarcoma of the hand and forearm High-grade sarcoma Spreads via lymphatics, fascial planes, tendons	Slow-growing, painless nodule on palmar aspect of the hand or digit May ulcerate	Degenerative joint changes often present with cysts at the DIP or CMC joints Communication between cyst and joint on arthrogram	Wide resection Digit/ray amputation High rate of recurrence Adjuvant radiation therapy Chemotherapy for metastatic disease
Synovial sarcoma (see Fig. 6.26)	Arises adjacent to joints and tendons or bursae High-grade sarcoma Most commonly occurs in the carpus Regional lymph node metastasis	Slow-growing, painless mass on dorsum of hand or in palm	Soft tissue calcifications on x-ray 20%–30%	Wide resection Digit/ray amputation High rate of recurrence Adjuvant radiation therapy Chemotherapy for metastatic disease
Malignant fibrous histiocytoma (MFH)	19% of MFH occur in upper extremity, especially the forearm Fifth to seventh decades	Slow growing and painless Well circumscribed	Well-demarcated lytic lesion	Wide excision or radical resection Digit/ray amputation Adjuvant chemotherapy and radiation therapy
Malignant peripheral nerve sheath tumor	More than 50% arise from neurofibromas 30% occur in upper extremity			Wide excision or radical resection Digit/ray amputation Not chemo- or radiosensitive High rate of recurrence

A B

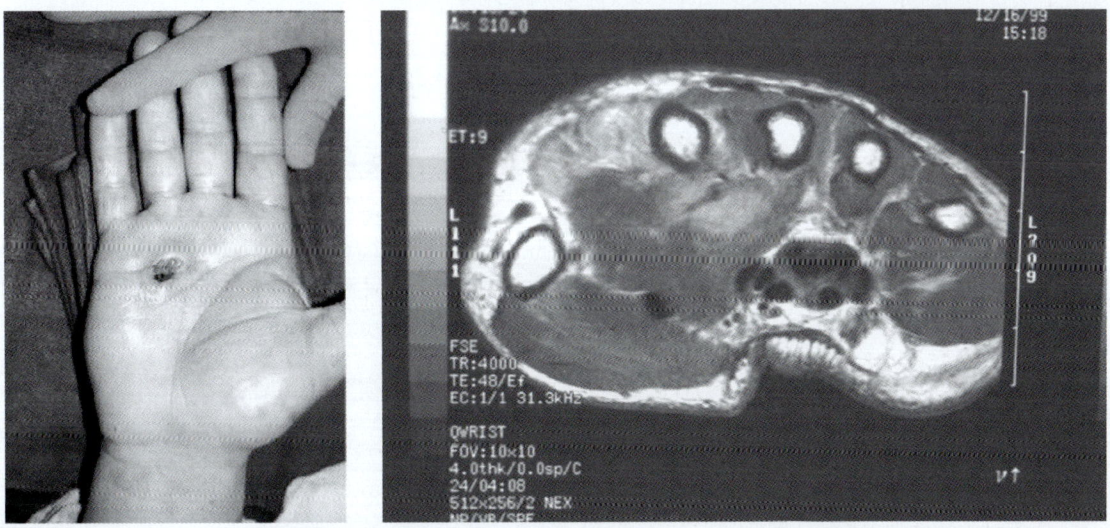

FIGURE 6.26 (A) Synovial sarcoma. (B) Axial MRI of a synovial sarcoma surrounding the index metacarpal. (*Source:* Athanasian EA. Malignant bone and soft-tissue sarcomas. *J Am Soc Surg Hand* 2004;4:60–72.)

TABLE 6.25 Cutaneous lesions

Lesion/Syndrome	Epidemiology/Unique Features	Clinical Presentation	Treatment
Melanoma (see Fig. 6.27)	Third most common malignant tumor of the epidermis of the hand Spreads via hematogenous and lymphatic routes Most commonly spreads to lungs and liver Types Lentigo maligna: superficial spreading (most common) Nodular: acral-lentiginous Clinical staging based on depth of invasion, presence of lymphocytes, lymph node involvement, mitotic index, ulceration or bleeding Curable if treated before the start of vertical growth	Superficial spreading arises within or contiguous with a pigmented nevus; radial growth phase can last months to years	Local resection if < 1 mm thick with 1-cm margin Wide resection if 1–4 mm with 2-cm margin Wide resection if > 4 mm with 3 cm margin; lymph node biopsy indicated Digit/ray amputation Chemotherapy for distant metastasis
Squamous cell carcinoma (see Fig. 6.28)	Most common skin cancer of the hand Radiation is risk factor Usually on dorsal forearm and hand Spreads via lymphatics Can arise from chronic ulcers, burn scars (Marjolin ulcer), or previous sites of radiation	Papules or plaques that are skin-colored or pink, smooth or hyperkeratotic	Wide resection Digit/ray amputation High rate of recurrence Adjuvant radiation therapy Chemotherapy for metastatic disease
Basal cell carcinoma	Second most common skin cancer of the hand Locally aggressive Rarely metastasizes	Slow-growing and painless nodular or ulcerating nodule with telangiectatic vessels	Cryosurgery Electrodesiccation Curettage Radiation for recurrent lesions

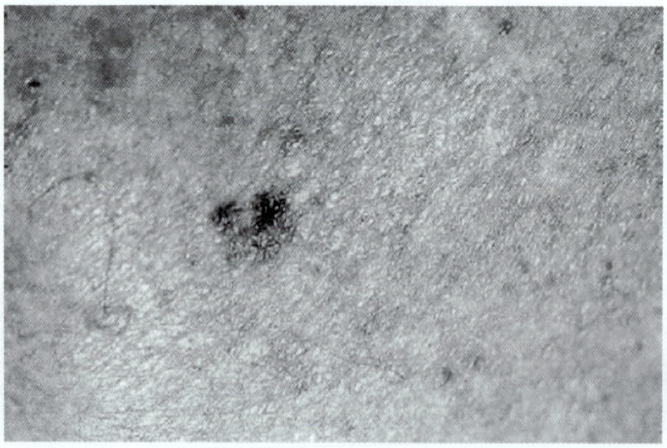

FIGURE 6.27 Macule characteristic of lentigo maligna melanoma *in situ*. (*Source:* Gray JP, Jayaraman AG, Robinson-Bostom L. Cutaneous conditions of the hands: Part 2. *J Am Soc Surg Hand* 2003;3:66–77.)

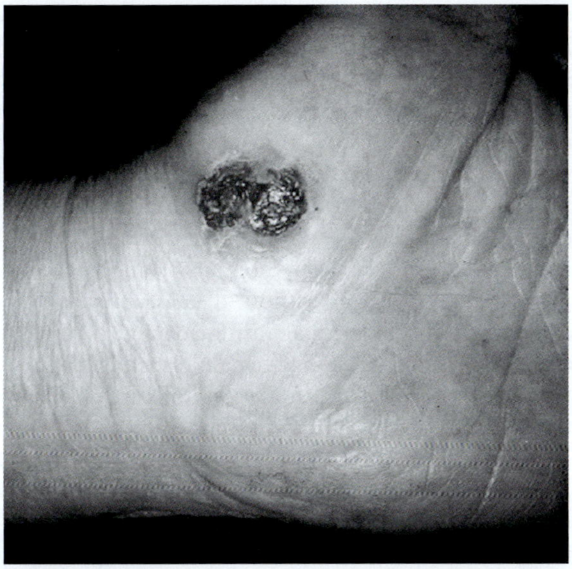

FIGURE 6.28 **Squamous cell carcinoma. (*Source:* From Gray JP, Jayaraman AG, Robinson-Bostom L. Cutaneous conditions of the hands: Part 2. *J Am Soc Surg Hand* 2003;3:66–77.)**

TABLE 6.26 Types of vascular disorders

Acute/Traumatic Injury
Arteries
Veins
Iatrogenic Injury
Cannulation injury
Vascular access
Chronic Disease
Occlusive disease
Thrombosis
Aneurysm
Embolism
Vasospastic disease
Vaso-occlusive disease
Congenital/Hereditary Disease
Connective tissue disorders
Ehlers-Danlos (aneurysms)
Disorders of coagulation
Arteriovenous malformations

Adapted from Koman LA, Ruch DS, Smith BP, Smith TL. Vascular disorders. In: Green DP, Hotchkiss RN, Pederson WC, Wolfe SW (eds.), *Green's Operative Hand Surgery*, 5th ed. Philadelphia: Elsevier, 2005;2265–2313.

Raynaud phenomenon (Table 6.27). Raynaud phenomenon refers to vascular insufficiency of the extremities as a result of arterial constriction that is stimulated by another condition such as scleroderma, systemic lupus erythematosus, Buerger disease, or atherosclerosis. Contrast arteriography or MRA are the diagnostic studies of choice; they can provide information on both structure and function of the vessels of interest. Patients with Raynaud disease respond to conservative treatment. Patients with systemic illnesses and Raynaud phenomenon may require surgery, depending on the adequacy of collateral circulation.

Occlusive Vascular Disease

Hypothenar Hammer Syndrome. Arterial occlusion in the upper extremity secondary to trauma most commonly involves the ulnar artery and superficial palmar arch. Ulnar artery thrombosis or hypothenar hammer syndrome describe occlusion or thrombosis of the ulnar artery as it courses through the Guyon canal. This phenomenon most commonly occurs in middle-aged male laborers with a history of concomitant hammering with the palm of the hand and tobacco use. Repetitive trauma results in the disruption of the internal elastic lamina, leading to the development of mural thrombus, complete occlusion, embolic events distally, or aneurysmal dilatation. Patients typically present with symptoms of cold sensitivity and pain, numbness, and weakness. Findings on physical examination include the absent flow of the ulnar artery based on the Allen test, changes in the nail bed, ulnar hypoesthesia, presence of a pulseless or pulsatile mass, prolonged capillary refill, and decreased turgor. Although rare, skin ulceration and gangrene may be present in severe cases. Aneurysms and thrombosis have been observed in body builders, wrestlers, golfers, and baseball players.

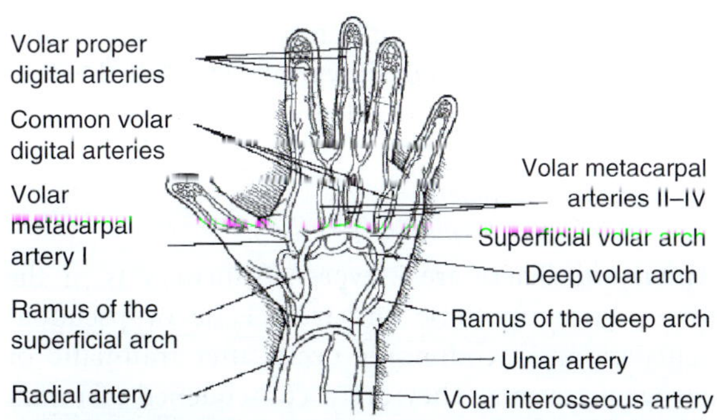

FIGURE 6.29 **Vascular anatomy. (*Source:* Phillips CS, Murphy MS. Vascular problems of the upper extremity: A primer for the orthopaedic surgeon. *J Am Acad Orthop Surg* 2002;10:401–408.)**

TABLE 6.27 Raynaud disease versus Raynaud phenomenon

Characteristic	Disease	Phenomenon
History		
Triphasic color change	Yes	Yes
Age > 40	No	Yes
Rapid progression	No	Yes
Underlying disease	No	Yes
Female predominance	Frequent	Occasional
Physical examination		
Trophic findings	Infrequent	Frequent
Abnormal Allen test	No	Common
Asymmetrical findings	Infrequent	Frequent
Laboratory tests		
Blood chemistry	Normal	Frequently abnormal
Microangiology	Normal	Frequently abnormal
Angiography	Normal	Frequently abnormal

Treatment options include the following:

- Behavior and environmental modifications
- Cessation of tobacco use
- Biofeedback
- Oral medication
- Thrombolysis
- Ligation or resection of the involved segment
- Reconstruction
- Cervicothoracic sympathectomy

Radial Artery Thrombosis. Thrombosis of the radial artery occurs less frequently than ulnar artery thrombosis; when it does occur, it typically involves the deep branch as it passes through the anatomic snuffbox. The radial artery may be resected or ligated if collateral circulation is sufficient.

Aneurysm. There are 2 types of aneurysms in the upper extremity: false and true. False or pseudoaneurysms most commonly occur after traumatic or iatrogenic events. They are a consequence of injury to the arterial wall with subsequent hemorrhage with extravasation, leading to the formation of a hematoma. The hematoma can organize and recanalize, forming a false lumen that is continuous with the lumen of the vessel. The false lumen can be differentiated from the true lumen because it lacks an endothelial layer. False aneurysms usually involve the axillary, brachial, radial, and anterior interosseous arteries and are typically located in the antecubital fossa, the volar wrist, and anatomic snuffbox. True aneurysms result after injury to a vessel allows gradual expansion of the vessel lumen and can be distinguished from false aneurysms by their uniform shape and by the presence of an endothelial lining. A true aneurysm occurs in an area of arterial circulation that is subject to repetitive trauma.

An aneurysm classically presents as an expanding, pulsatile mass with or without distal ischemia. Signs and symptoms of arterial insufficiency are rare; an aneurysm usually presents as a painless, palpable mass. Soft tissue pain and/or neural symptoms are secondary to mass effect; signs and symptoms of distal ischemia are often a result of embolic phenomena. Both types of aneurysms progress slowly over time, eventually leading to thrombosis and/or emboli. Doppler ultrasonography can detect aneurysms; however, angiography remains the gold standard for diagnostic imaging.

Management of aneurysms fall into four categories:

1. Resection and ligation
2. Resection and reanastomosis
3. Resection with graft interposition
4. Excision of the defective area followed by "patch" grafting

Choice of treatment is dependent on vasomotor tone and the adequacy of collateral circulation.

Arteriovenous Fistula. Acquired arteriovenous fistulas are the result of penetrating injury, infection, or surgery for hemodialysis access. An arteriovenous fistula occurring as a result of infection or trauma may result in a "steal" phenomenon, leading to further ischemic and neural events. Dialysis-associated steal syndrome occurs in 1% of patients who undergo radiocephalic fistulas, which may lead to shunting and subsequent high-output cardiac failure. Treatment options include observation, banding or narrowing of the shunt, and ligation.

Atherosclerosis. Symptomatic atherosclerosis in the upper extremity typically involves the subclavian and innominate arteries, with symptomatic left subclavian disease occurring 3 times more frequently than the right. Diagnosis can be confirmed by Duplex or arteriography; management is similar to the management of posttraumatic occlusive disease.

Arteritis. Buerger disease or thromboangiitis obliterans is an inflammation and occlusion involving small and medium-sized vessels. The disease most commonly afflicts young male smokers. Patients often present with symptoms of cold intolerance, claudication, pain at rest, Raynaud phenomenon, and digital ischemia and necrosis. Buerger disease can be diagnosed by arteriography and can be distinguished from atherosclerosis by the extent of peripheral vessel involvement. Histologically, arterial and venous thrombosis with infiltration of lymphocytes and polymorphonuclear leukocytes into the thrombus and vessel wall is seen. Treatment begins with cessation of smoking, which can decrease progression and the need for amputation.

- *Takayasu arteritis*—Also known as pulseless disease, Takayasu arteritis typically involves the axillary and subclavian arteries of young females. It is a granulomatous vasculitis involving medium and large arteries. The clinical syndrome is characterized by ocular changes and significant waning of peripheral pulses, numbness, and sensitivity to cold in the upper extremity. The decrease in distal pulses is a result of fibrosis and stenosis of the arch of the aorta with narrowing of the origins or distal parts of the great vessels that arise from the arch. Treatment involves corticosteroids and arterial reconstruction.
- *Giant cell arteritis*—Giant cell or temporal arteritis is the most common of the vasculitides. It is heralded by acute and chronic, granulomatous inflammation of the medium and small arteries, particularly those in the head, subclavian, and axillary arteries. The disease typically afflicts females after the fifth decade of life; clinical symptoms often include severe unilateral headaches or facial pain, typically along the course of the temporal artery. Ocular involvement can lead to permanent blindness. If symptoms include arthralgias and myalgias, the disease is referred to as polymyalgia rheumatica. Diagnosis is established with a biopsy of the temporal artery. Treatment includes steroids and arterial reconstruction.

Polyarteritis Nodosa. Polyarteritis nodosa is characterized by necrotizing inflammation of small and medium muscular arteries. Patients present with symptoms of general malaise, hypertension, fever, weight loss, and myalgias. Diagnosis is established by tissue biopsy. Treatment includes steroids and cyclophosphamide.

Vascular Neoplasms

Vascular Malformation. Vascular malformations occur when blood flows across a low-resistance fistula instead of a high-resistance capillary bed, leading to scarring, toricity, dilatation, and early degeneration of the vessels. The flow potential becomes greater than that of the afferent arteries, causing reversal of flow in the arteries that are distal to the fistula and eventually ischemia in the distal capillary bed. Proximal and distal collateral circulation is initiated to satisfy the low-resistance shunt. Recipient veins are forced to dilate, causing a net increase in flow and an increased cardiac output in order to supply both systems. Vascular malformations can be classified into 2 categories: slow-flow or fast-flow lesions. Slow-flow lesions are painless, red, cutaneous, and compressible. Fast-flow lesions are painful, warm, and noncompressible; there is often an associated thrill and/or bruit. Distal ischemia and high-output cardiac failure are associated with fast-flow lesions.

Vascular malformations are present at birth and are associated with several congenital syndromes, including Klippel-Trenaunay-Weber, Proteus, and Maffucci syndromes. They are typically quiescent until stimulated by trauma, infection, hormonal changes, or iatrogenic causes. Signs and symptoms include increased hair growth and body temperature, hyperhidrosis, pain due to the increased proximal flow, and ischemia distal to the malformation. They rapidly decompress when the limb is elevated. Patients typically present with sudden pulsatile bleeding and pain. Doppler studies can assess size and activity. MRI or MRA or angiography delineate the lesion. Treatment of slow-flow lesions include compression garments, low-dose aspirin, sclerotherapy, embolization, and excision.

Hemangiomas. Hemangiomas are vascular tumors that are present at birth and are the most common vascular tumors of the hand. They have a growth cycle consisting of an early proliferative phase followed by involution; 50% involute by the age of 5 years, and 70% regress by the age of 7 years. Hemangiomas are firm and are consistent in size and turgor with limb elevation; they are compressible but do not change in size or compressibility when the limb is elevated. Depending on their depths, they are bright blue, red, or flesh colored. Doppler ultrasound can distinguish hemangiomas from vascular malformations; MRA or angiography can further delineate the lesion. Treatment is supportive: local or systemic steroids, sclerotherapy, and excision.

IX. WRIST PAIN

Avascular Necrosis

Kienbock Disease. Kienbock disease is avascular necrosis of the lunate and is a source of chronic wrist pain. Anatomic variations of blood supply and bone geometry combined with trauma or repetitive loading are possible etiologic factors. The lunate's blood supply originates from both dorsal and palmar arteries. Potential causes of loss of blood supply include traumatic disruption, primary circulatory dysfunction, or ligamentous injury resulting in bone necrosis. The subsequent changes that ensue are sclerosis, collapse, and fragmentation of the lunate, which leads to decreased carpal height, proximal migration of the capitate, and hyperflexion of the scaphoid. Degenerative changes of the radiocarpal joint and carpus occur as a result of abnormal carpal motion and mechanics. It has been postulated that certain variations in bone geometry, such as flattened radial inclination, small lunate, or negative ulnar variance, could increase the risk of developing Kienbock disease.

Kienbock disease is often unilateral and most commonly afflicts males between the ages of 20 and 40 years. Patients typically have a history of wrist trauma months to years prior to seeking treatment. The most common symptoms are dorsal wrist pain and decreased ROM secondary to reactive synovitis. The Lichtman classification of Kienbock disease describes 4 radiographic stages based on changes noted on x-rays and bone scan or MRI (Table 6.28; Fig. 6.30).

Treatment of Kienbock disease is based on the stage at presentation. Management of stages II to IIIA depends on ulnar variance; the goal of surgery is to level the joint and unload the lunate so that it has a chance to revascularize and also to prevent collapse. Joint-leveling procedures that aid in unloading the lunate include radial shortening and ulnar lengthening. The ulnar-minus wrist with Kienbock disease is unloaded via radial shortening. Scaphocapitate (SC) or scaphotrapeziotrapezoid (STT) fusion can also decrease the forces transmitted across the radiolunate joint. Proximal row carpectomy is best indicated for stage IIIB. The foundation of treatment for stage IV Kienbock disease consists of proximal row carpectomy and wrist arthrodesis.

Avascular Necrosis of the Scaphoid (Preiser Disease). Avascular necrosis of the scaphoid, or Preiser disease, is a rare condition; its etiology has been attributed to collagen vascular disorders, trauma, steroid use, and idiopathic reasons. Patients present with wrist pain and have symptoms similar to those of Kienbock disease: tenderness over the dorsal wrist, decreased ROM and grip strength, and swelling. Radiographs may be normal or depict sclerosis, fragmentation with collapse of the proximal pole, and radioscaphoid arthritis (Fig. 6.31). MRI and CT scan can further delineate changes within the scaphoid. Treatment of Preiser disease includes observation, revascularization, arthroscopic débridement, scaphoidectomy, proximal row carpectomy, and silicone arthroplasty. Avascular necrosis can occur in other carpal bones, but it is rare. Idiopathic AVN can be seen involving the capitate, but it should be distinguished from AVN of the capitate head that is caused by capitate neck fracture commonly associated with scaphoid fractures. Risk factors include trauma, Gaucher disease, steroid use, and gout. Most of the idiopathic cases occur in women. The vascular anatomy places the capitate at risk because the vessels entering the distal portion extend proximally to supply

TABLE 6.28 Lichtman stages of Kienbock's disease

		Treatment		
Stage	**Radiographic Features**	**Ulnar Negative**	**Ulnar Neutral**	**Ulnar Positive**
I	Normal radiographs; changes in signal intensity on MRI; abnormal bone scan	Cast 3 months Radial shortening ± revascularization	Cast 3 months Radial shortening or revascularization	Cast 3 months Capitate shortening or STT/SC arthrodesis
II	Sclerotic changes of the lunate with or without fracture lines on radiographs	Radial shortening ± revascularization	Radial shortening or revascularization	Capitate shortening or STT/SC arthrodesis
IIIA	Lunate collapse with normal carpal alignment and height	Radial shortening	Radial shortening	Capitate shortening or STT/SC arthrodesis
IIIB	Lunate collapse with proximal migration of capitate, decreased carpal height, fixed rotation of scaphoid (signet ring sign)	Capitate shortening STT arthrodesis or proximal row carpectomy	Capitate shortening STT arthrodesis or proximal row carpectomy	Capitate shortening STT arthrodesis or proximal row carpectomy
IV	Lunate collapse with degenerative changes at the midcarpal joint, radiocarpal joint or both	Wrist arthrodesis	Wrist arthrodesis	Wrist arthrodesis

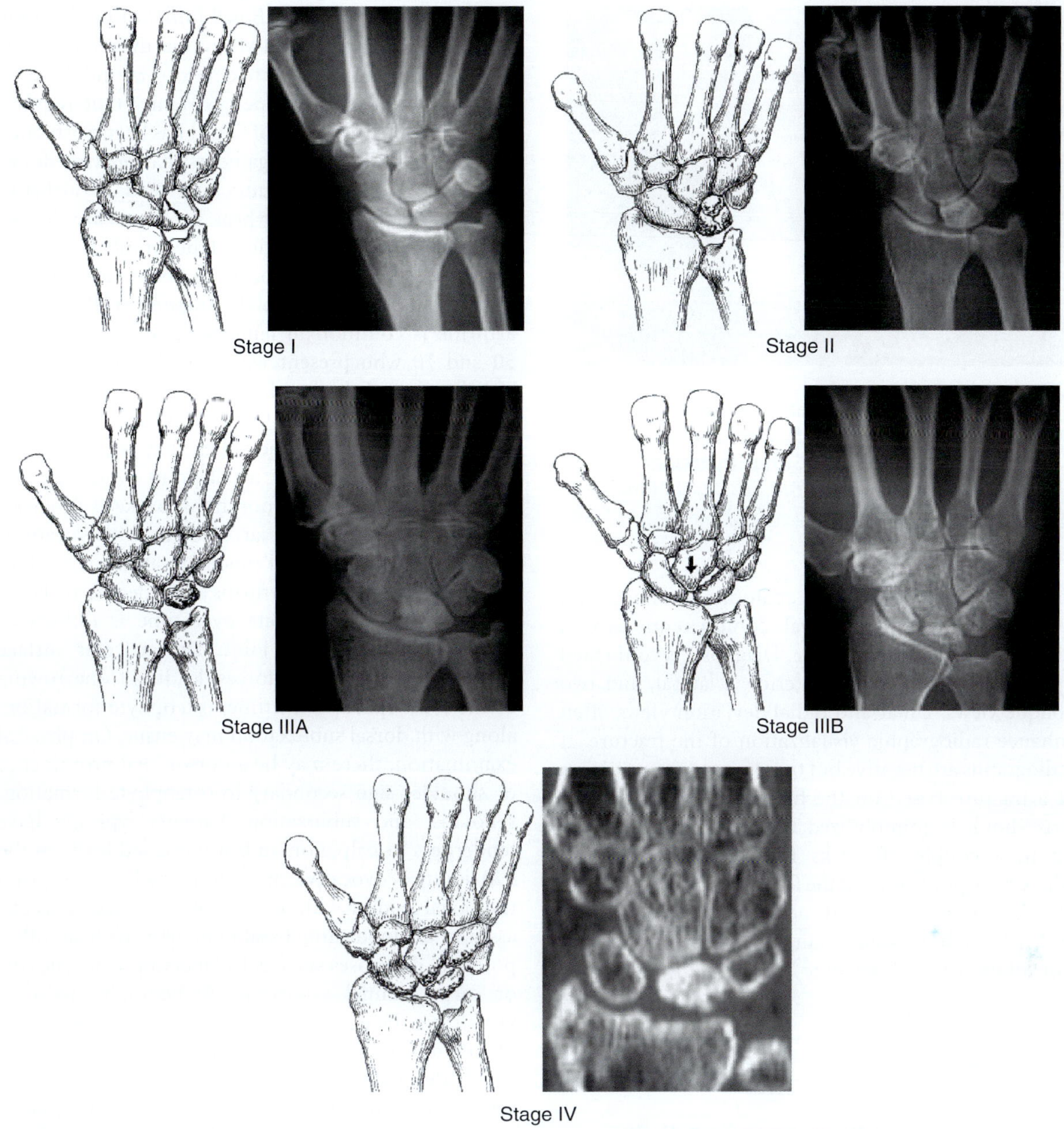

FIGURE 6.30 **Lichtman stages of Kienbock disease. (*Source:* Allan CH, Joshi A, Lichtman DM. Kienbock's disease: Diagnosis and treatment. *J Am Acad Orthop Surg* 2001;9:128–136.)**

the neck and head. AVN of the metacarpal head (Dietrich disease) is also rare but commonly affects the middle finger and uncommonly affects the thumb. The relative prominence of the third metacarpal and its increased vulnerability to trauma may explain the increased incidence.

Scaphoid Fractures. The scaphoid is the most frequently fractured carpal bone, accounting for 60% of carpal fractures and 11% of fractures of the hand. Eighty percent of fractures occur at the scaphoid waist. Eighty percent of scaphoid fractures occur in males between the ages of 20 to 30. The injury is often a result of falling on an outstretched hand, with the wrist in dorsiflexion and radial deviation.

The blood supply to the scaphoid is provided by a dorsal and volar source. The proximal third of the scaphoid is a watershed area; fractures in this area require 6 to 11 weeks longer to heal than fractures of the middle third and have a 14% to 40% incidence of avascular necrosis.

Diagnosis of a scaphoid fracture is based on initial signs and symptoms, the mechanism of injury, and the age of the patient. Pain with palpation over

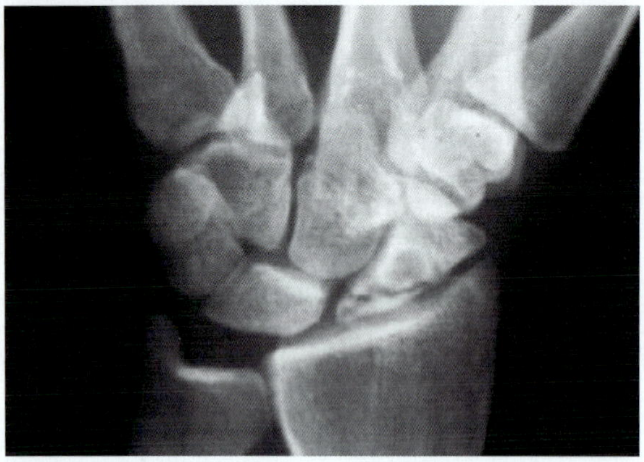

FIGURE 6.31 **Avascular necrosis of the scaphoid. (*Source:* Sokolow C, Theron P, Saffar P. Preiser's disease. *J Am Soc Surg Hand* 2004;4:103–108.)**

the scaphoid tubercle and anatomic snuffbox and tenderness with longitudinal compression have a diagnostic sensitivity of 100%. Diagnosis is confirmed by radiographs: a posteroanterior, a lateral, and two oblique views. Ulnar and radial deviation views often enhance radiographic visualization of the fracture. If radiographs are negative but there is a strong suspicion of a fracture based on the history and physical, the wrist should be immobilized; the patient should follow up in a couple of weeks for repeat radiographs, where resorption around the fracture line will facilitate identifying the fracture. If radiographs are equivocal, an MRI or a bone scan obtained at 72 hours from the time of injury can determine if a fracture is present.

X. ARTHRITIS

Osteoarthritis and Posttraumatic Arthritis of the Hand

Arthritis of the joints of the hand, wrist, and forearm develops from one of these conditions: inflammatory arthritis, posttraumatic arthritis, septic arthritis, and osteoarthritis (OA). Osteoarthritis describes the degeneration of articular cartilage that occurs without an obvious etiology. Radiographic diagnosis of osteoarthritis include asymmetric decrease of the joint space, sclerosis, and the development of subchondral cysts and osteophytes. The prevalence of OA in the general population increases with age and is more common in males than in females until menopause. The most commonly involved joints of the hand are the DIP joint, the CMC joint of the thumb, and the PIP joint.

Carpometacarpal Joint (Basal Joint) of the Thumb. The trapeziometacarpal (TM) joint is the second most common joint of the hand to develop OA and the most common joint of the upper extremity that requires surgery for the treatment of OA. It has been postulated that excess laxity of the ligaments that provide dorsal stability of the basal joint could lead to arthritis. The dorsoradial and volar beak ligaments are the key restraints to dorsal translation of the thumb metacarpal (Fig. 6.32). The volar beak ligament anchors the base of the metacarpal to the trapezium. Basal joint arthritis is common in females between the ages of 50 and 70 who present with pain in the thumb or radial aspect of the hand. The onset is insidious and the duration can range from months to years. The pain is exacerbated by activities that require lateral pinch, such as writing, needlepoint work, cutting with scissors, turning doorknobs or keys in locks, and turning the lid of a jar. Patients with vocations requiring frequent lateral pinch are at greater risk of developing basal joint arthritis. The degree of laxity that the joint can tolerate over time is influenced by forces that load the joint. The articular surface becomes worn by shear forces, leading to narrowing of the joint space. With time, osteophyte formation, along with dorsal subluxation may ensue. On physical examination, there may be a dorsoradial prominence or shoulder sign secondary to osteophyte formation, synovitis, and subluxation. Patients typically have tenderness to palpation and/or increased laxity at the TM joint. Provocative maneuvers such as the grind test (axial loading with rotation of the metacarpal) can assist in distinguishing basal joint arthritis from other potential diagnoses such as DeQuervain tenosynovitis or carpal tunnel syndrome. Radiographs assist in visualizing the extent of arthritic changes; stress views can demonstrate the degree of laxity present. Eaton and Littler describe 4 radiographic stages of basal joint arthritis (Fig. 6.33); treatment, however, is ultimately determined by the severity of the patient's symptoms (Table 6.29).

Treatment of basal joint arthritis begins with conservative measures such as NSAIDs, activity modification, and immobilization with a thumb spica splint. Steroid injections may provide additional relief if noninvasive treatment has been exhausted. Surgical treatment is considered if conservative modalities fail to alleviate symptoms and is based on clinical and radiographic features. Involvement of the MCP joint of the thumb is characterized by a hyperextension deformity. Arthrosis of the MCP joint must be treated in order to minimize stress across the CMC joint.

Interphalangeal Joints. The DIP joint is the most common joint of the hand to develop OA. PIP joint involvement is less frequent (Table 6.30).

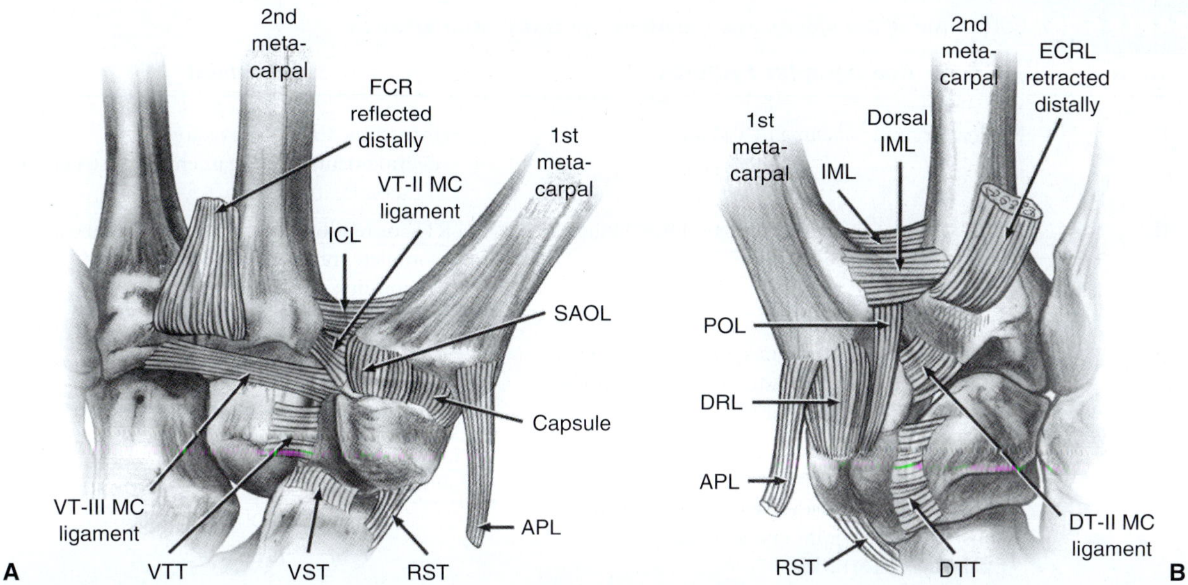

FIGURE 6.32 (A) Deep volar ligaments of the carpometacarpal joint. (B) Dorsal ligaments of the carpometacarpal joint. APL, abductor pollicis longus; DRL, dorsoradial ligament; DT-II MC, dorsal trapezio-second metacarpal; DTT, dorsal trapeziotrapezoidal ligament; ECRL, extensor carpi radialis longus; FCR, flexor carpi radialis; ICL, intercarpal ligament; IML, intermetacarpal ligament; POL, posterior oblique ligament; RST, radial scaphotrapezial ligament; SAOL, superficial anterior oblique ligament (beak ligament); VST, volar scaphotrapezial ligament; VT-II MC, volar trapezio-second metacarpal, VT-III MC, volar trapezio-third metacarpal; VTT, volar trapeziotrapezoidal ligament. (*Source:* Berger RA, Weiss APC (eds.). *Hand Surgery*, Vol. 2. Philadelphia: Lippincott Williams & Wilkins, 2003;1280.)

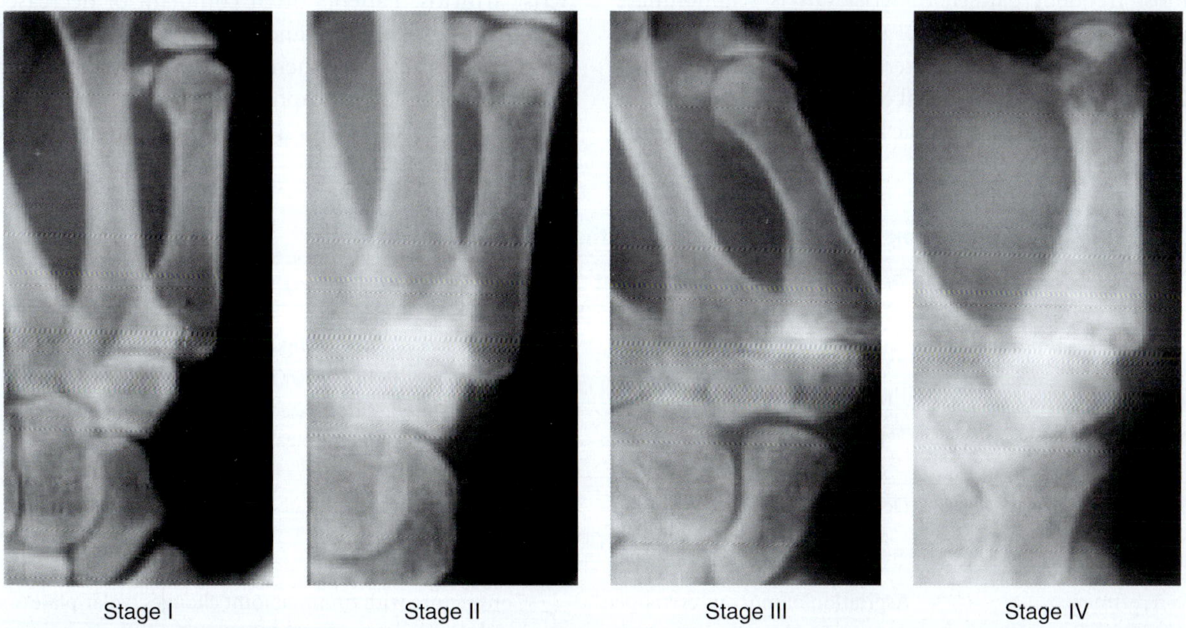

FIGURE 6.33 Eaton and Littler stages of basal joint arthritis. (*Source:* Barron AO, Eaton RG. Save the trapezium: Double interposition arthroplasty for the treatment of stage IV disease of the basal joint. *J Hand Surg* 1998;23A:196–204.)

TABLE 6.29 Eaton and littler stages and treatment of basal joint arthritis

Stage	Radiographic Features	Treatment
I	Normal or mild widening of TM joint	Arthroscopic CMC synovectomy and débridement; volar ligament reconstruction if excess laxity present
II	Decreased joint space, osteophytes/loose bodies < 2 mm; normal ST joint	LRTI† or tendon interposition—partial or complete trapeziectomy; metacarpal osteotomy; prosthetic arthroplasty; trapeziometacarpal arthrodesis*††
III	Significantly decreased joint space with subchondral sclerosis; osteophytes/loose bodies > 2 mm; normal ST joint	Partial trapeziectomy with tendon interposition; LRTI with complete trapeziectomy; prosthetic arthroplasty; trapeziometacarpal arthrodesis
IV	Significantly decreased joint space with subchondral sclerosis, cysts and osteophytes/ loose bodies; ST joint involvement (pantrapezial arthritis)	Complete trapeziectomy and LRTI

*CMC, carpometacarpal; LRTI, ligament reconstruction with tendon interposition; ST, scaphotrapezial; TM, trapeziometacarpal
*†† See Table 6.33 for optimal position of fusion.

Wrist

Scapholunate Advanced Collapse. The most common site of OA in the wrist is at the radiocarpal joint. It is typically a result of abnormal wrist mechanics due to chronic scapholunate dissociation or rotary subluxation of the scaphoid. OA of the radiocarpal joint most frequently affects middle-aged male laborers. The most frequent pattern of wrist OA is scapholunate advanced collapse (SLAC). The proximal carpal row functions as a mobile, intercalated unit that bridges 2 rigid structures: the distal carpal row and the radius. As a result, disruption of the ligaments in the proximal row leads to instability. Disruption of the scapholunate interosseous ligament (SLIL) leads to dorsiflexion of the lunate, creating a dorsiflexed intercalated segment instability (DISI) pattern of injury. SLIL discontinuity causes the scaphoid to flex palmarly, leading to abnormal distribution of load and increased contact forces. This alteration in the mechanics of wrist function and motion leads to the SLAC pattern of wrist arthritis. Patients often complain of decreased pinch and grip strength and stiffness in the wrist. On physical examination, there is focal tenderness with palpation of the radioscaphoid joint. The progression of a SLAC wrist follows a predictive pattern. There

TABLE 6.30 Comparison of OA in distal and proximal interphalangeal joints

Joint	Distal Interphalangeal Joint	Proximal Interphalangeal Joint
Clinical Symptoms	Progressive pain, swelling, deformity, and stiffness	Progressive pain, swelling, deformity, and stiffness with or without contracture
Physical Exam	Heberden nodes, decreased ROM, bone spurs, mucous cysts	Bouchard nodes, decreased ROM; joint contracture 2 degrees to collateral ligament fibrosis; mucous cysts not as common
Radiographs	Decreased joint space, subchondral sclerosis and cysts, osteophytes	Decreased joint space, subchondral sclerosis and cysts, osteophytes
Treatment	Aspiration of mucous cyst; open excision of mucous cyst with joint débridement; DIP joint arthrodesis or arthroplasty	Contracture with minimal joint changes: volar plate release, collateral ligament excision, and osteophyte débridement; arthroplasty or arthrodesis*

* See Table 6.33 for optimal position of fusion.

TABLE 6.31 Watson stages of SLAC wrist

Stage	Radiographic Features	Treatment
I	Degenerative changes between radial styloid and distal pole of scaphoid	Splint, NSAIDs, cortisone injections; radial styloidectomy; proximal row carpectomy (PRC)
II	Involvement of proximal pole of scaphoid and scaphoid fossa	PRC; SLAC procedure*
III	Proximal migration of the capitate with degeneration of the capitolunate joint	SLAC procedure; total wrist arthrodesis

*Scaphoid excision with lunate-capitate-hamate-triquetrum (four corner) fusion.

TABLE 6.32 Optimal position for arthrodesis

Joint	Position
DIP	10–20° flexion
PIP	30–45° flexion, cascading from the index to the small fingers in increments of 5°
Thumb MP	15° flexion
	10° pronation
Thumb CMC	30–40° palmar abduction
	35° radial abduction
	15° pronation
	10° extension
Wrist	10° dorsiflexion neutral deviation

Source: Naidu S, Temple JD. Arthritis. In: Beredjiklian PK, Bozentka DJ (eds.), *Review of Hand Surgery*. Philadelphia: Saunders, 2004;171–187.

is early degeneration at the tip of the radial styloid and distal scaphoid. The next stage involves the entire radioscaphoid joint. The capitolunate joint becomes involved, which leads to proximal migration of the capitate. The radiolunate joint is still preserved at this stage. The SLAC wrist can be radiographically divided into 3 progressive stages (Table 6.31). Treatment is based on severity of symptoms and radiographic stage. Patients who undergo a proximal row carpectomy or the SLAC procedure often lose approximately 50% of wrist motion and grip strength. The ideal position for a total wrist arthrodesis is neutral deviation and 10 degrees of dorsiflexion (Table 6.32).

Scaphoid Nonunion Advanced Collapse. The pattern of wrist arthritis that evolves from chronic scaphoid nonunion is similar to the SLAC wrist and has been described as scaphoid nonunion advanced collapse (SNAC). Over time, chronic nonunion of a scaphoid fracture leads to collapse of the scaphoid, and the carpus develops a fixed DISI pattern. The resulting change in carpal mechanics progresses to a pattern of wrist arthritis that is similar to the SLAC wrist. There are 4 radiographic stages that describe the progressive pattern of SNAC wrist arthrosis (Fig. 6.34). Management is based on the patient's symptoms and the extent of degenerative changes (Table 6.33).

Scaphotrapezial-Trapezoidal Joint. The scaphotrapeziotrapezoid (STT) joint is the second most common area of wrist OA. It is postulated that change

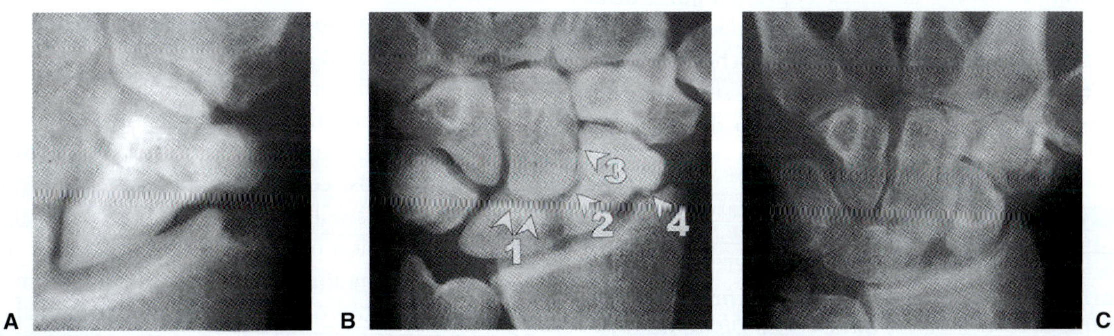

FIGURE 6.34 Watson SNAC wrist stages. (A) Stage I SNAC arthrosis. (*Source:* Ruch DS, Chang DS, Poehling GG. The arthroscopic treatment of avascular necrosis of the proximal pole following scaphoid nonunion. *Arthroscopy* 1998;14:747–752.) (B) Stage II SNAC arthrosis. (*Source:* Trumble TE. Arthritis. In: Trumble TE [ed.], *Principles of Hand Surgery and Therapy*. Philadelphia: Saunders, 2000:401–43.) (C) Stage III SNAC arthrosis. (*Source:* Tomaino MM, Miller RJ, Cole I, Burton RI. Scapholunate advanced collapse wrist: Proximal row carpectomy or limited wrist arthrodesis with scaphoid excision? *J Hand Surg Am* 1994;19:134–142.)

TABLE 6.33 Watson stages of SNAC wrist

Stage	Radiographic Features	Treatment
I	Arthritic changes and osteophyte formation (beaking) of radial styloid	Radial styloidectomy and ORIF of scaphoid nonunion with bone graft or excision of distal pole of scaphoid
II	Radioscaphoid arthrosis	PRC; SLAC procedure; total wrist arthrodesis
III	Midcarpal joint involvement (scaphocapitate and capitolunate joints)	SLAC procedure and total wrist arthrodesis
IV	Pancarpal arthrosis	SLAC procedure and total wrist arthrodesis

of the mechanics of the STT joint occurs as a result of ligamentous injury of the scaphoid. Palmar flexion of the scaphoid progresses until the articular surfaces of the trapezium and trapezoid are dorsal to the distal scaphoid. Abnormal distribution of forces across the STT joint leads to arthritic changes of the STT joint. Treatment includes STT arthrodesis if there is no associated basal joint arthrosis. Pantrapezial arthritis is treated with a trapeziectomy and ligament reconstruction with tendon interposition (LRTI).

Ulnar Impaction Syndrome. Ulnar impaction syndrome is the degenerative process that results from chronic overloading of the ulnocarpal joint. Shear forces across the articular surfaces and tensile forces from the soft tissues contribute to this process. Ulnocarpal impingement is the painful convergence of a resected ulnar stump against the distal metaphysis of the radius. Ulnar-positive variance increases ulnocarpal loading and is therefore a known risk factor of ulnar impaction syndrome. Common causes of acquired ulnar-positive variance include radial shortening following an Essex-Lopresti injury, distal radius fracture, or physeal injury. Congenital causes include Madelung deformity and dyschondroplasia. Load transmission between the distal radius and ulna is dependent on ulnar variance (Table 6.34).

TABLE 6.34 Affect of ulnar variance load distribution

Variance (mm)	% Load Across the Distal Ulna	% Load Across the Distal Radius
0	20	80
+1	30	70
+2	40	60
−1	10	90
−2	5	95

Symptoms associated with ulnar impaction syndrome include ulnar wrist pain, swelling, and decreased ROM. On examination, there is local tenderness to palpation at the ulnar head; pain is exacerbated by ulnar deviation during power grip. It is important to differentiate between ulnar impaction syndrome and DRUJ arthritis, which has a similar presentation. Radiographs are obtained to measure ulnar variance and to evaluate the DRUJ and carpus for arthritic changes. Treatment is initiated with activity modification, NSAIDs, splinting, and corticosteroid injections. Surgery is reserved for patients with clinical and radiographic evidence of ulnocarpal impaction without DRUJ arthritis who fail conservative management. In the negative or neutral variance wrist, arthroscopic débridement of the joint, lunotriquetral interosseous ligament, and articular disk is an option. The load across the ulnocarpal joint in the ulnar-positive variant wrist can be decreased by ulnar shortening osteotomy or partial distal ulnar resection (wafer procedure).

Distal Radioulnar Joint Arthritis. Degenerative changes of the DRUJ can occur as a result of inflammatory arthritis, OA, posttraumatic arthritis, or chronic DRUJ instability. It is essential to differentiate DRUJ arthritis from ulnocarpal impaction syndrome; in some cases, the two conditions may coexist. Symptoms of DRUJ arthritis are similar to ulnocarpal impaction syndrome. The most common symptoms include ulnar wrist pain and swelling, decreased grip strength, and stiffness. Palpation over the DRUJ elicits pain, which is exacerbated by forearm rotation. Radiographs may reveal early signs of arthritis in the proximal part of the joint. Osteophytes develop along the proximal border of the ulnar head, sparing the sigmoid notch. Management of DRUJ arthritis begins with conservative measures such as activity modification, NSAIDs, splinting, and corticosteroid injections. The goal of surgery is to eliminate the DRUJ by resection of all or part of the distal ulna, arthrodesis, or ulnar head replacement (Table 6.35; Fig. 6.35).

TABLE 6.35 Surgical options for DRUJ arthritis

Procedure	Description	Key Points
Darrach (Fig. 6.51)	Distal ulnar resection	Distal ulnar stump instability
Bowers hemiresection-interposition arthroplasty	Excision of articular surface of ulnar head	Preserve ulnar attachments to TFCC, minimizing postoperative instability
Sauve-Kapandji (Fig. 6.52)	Radioulnar joint fusion	Retains support of the ulnar carpus, decreasing risk of ulnar translation; complications include instability and decreased ROM 2 degrees regeneration of the resected portion
Ulnar head replacement arthroplasty	Metal alloy implant with modular head and stem	TFCC ligaments can be sutured to the implant
Wide distal ulnar resection	Similar to Darrach	Salvage procedure
One-bone forearm	Radioulnar fusion	Salvage procedure—complete loss of forearm motion

XI. RHEUMATOID ARTHRITIS

RA is a chronic, systemic autoimmune disease that affects 1% of the population; the female-to-male ratio is 2.5:1, and prevalence increases with age. Genetic and environmental factors may play a role in the etiology of the disease; HLA-DR4 occurs in 70% of RA patients. The disease is characterized by destructive, proliferative synovitis involving multiple joints. The joint destruction and deformity that ensue are a result of hypertrophied rheumatoid synovium. The pathologic synovial tissue erodes articular cartilage and invades the underlying subchondral bone, expanding the supporting soft tissue structures that help stabilize the joint. Treatment of RA consists of medical and surgical management. Medications used for the treatment of RA include antiinflammatory and immunosuppressive medication such as methotrexate and TNF inhibitors (e.g., etanercept and infliximab). Many patients with RA have upper extremity manifestations of the disease. The disease attacks the extensor and flexor tendons, resulting in loss of normal structure and balance of flexion and extension forces across adjacent joints of the hand and wrist.

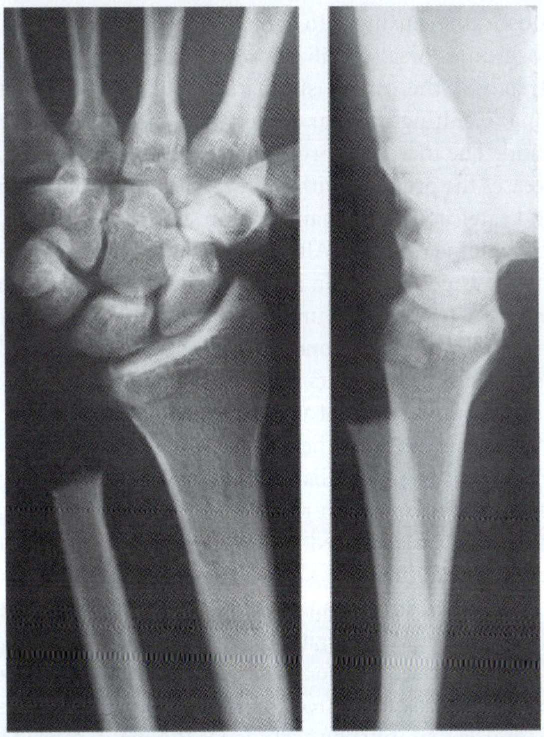

FIGURE 6.35 Distal ulnar resection (Darrach). (*Source:* van Schoonhoven J, Fernandez DL, Bowers WH, Herbert TJ. Salvage of failed resection arthroplasties of the distal radioulnar joint using a new ulnar head prosthesis. *J Hand Surg Am* 2000;25A:438–446.)

The main goals of surgical treatment in patients with RA are to alleviate pain, restore function, slow disease progression, and improve appearance of the hand. If the patient has multiple joint involvement, lower extremity surgery should be performed before upper extremity procedures; proximal joints should be assessed before distal joints. Preventive procedures should be considered before reconstructive surgery. Planning and timing of surgery should be coordinated with the patient's rheumatologist after the patient's medical treatment has been established. Other clinical manifestations of RA must be evaluated prior to surgery. Surgical treatment for RA can be divided into 5 categories: synovectomy, tenosynovectomy, tendon procedures, arthroplasty, and arthrodesis. Determining the type of surgery indicated depends on the pattern of disease. Synovectomy is performed in cases with mild disease that is controllable with medication and is limited to 1 or 2 joints; it is contraindicated in patients with rapidly progressive arthritis. Patients with rapidly progressive disease may require early tenosynovectomy to avoid tendon rupture.

Tenosynovitis

RA can involve the synovium that line the extensor and flexor tendons of the wrist and hand. The resulting tenosynovitis is often painful and deforming and can ultimately lead to tendon rupture. The 3 most common areas of tendon sheath involvement are the dorsal wrist and the volar wrist and digits. Dorsal or extensor tenosynovitis presents as swelling of the dorsal wrist; it is often the first sign of RA. The hypertrophic synovium adheres to and infiltrates the tendon, leading to weakening and potential rupture of the tendon. If the process does not resolve after 4 to 6 months of medical treatment, dorsal synovectomy should be considered in order to avoid rupture.

The proliferative synovium that develops within the flexor tendon sheaths at the wrist can cause median nerve compression that often presents as carpal tunnel syndrome. As the tenosynovitis progresses, the gliding motion of the tendons is disrupted, leading to decreased active and passive ROM of the digits and possible tendon rupture. Patients may complain of morning stiffness, decreased grip strength, and symptoms of carpal tunnel syndrome. Early decompression of the median nerve and flexor tendon tenosynovectomy can avoid irreversible injury to the median nerve and flexor tendons.

Digital flexor tenosynovitis in patients with RA occurs when rheumatoid nodules develop in the digital flexor tendons within the sheath. The size of the nodules and their location with respect to the annular pulleys establish the severity of digital dysfunction. Clinical presentation includes swelling along the volar aspect of the digit, triggering, and locking; passive ROM is greater than active ROM. Treatment includes tenosynovectomy and nodule excision; partial release of the A2 and A4 pulleys is performed if additional release is required. If left untreated, digital flexor tenosynovitis may result in tendon rupture.

Tendon Rupture

Extensor Tendon. Tendon ruptures in the hand are common in patients with RA; they are often painless and occur following mild activity. Tendon ruptures are a result of attrition or direct tendon invasion or ischemic necrosis secondary to compression of the tendon's blood supply from the proliferative synovium. Rupture secondary to attrition occurs when the tendon moves over bony spurs or becomes eroded by the chronic synovitis. The cause of a single tendon rupture is typically responsible for subsequent ruptures if left untreated.

Attrition rupture of the extensor tendons most typically occurs at the Lister tubercle and the distal ulna. Patients with extensor tendon rupture present with failure to maintain digital extension after the digit has been passively extended. The most commonly ruptured extensor tendon is the EDM, followed by the EDC tendon to the ring and small fingers. The EPL is the fourth most common extensor tendon to rupture; it is often secondary to chronic abrasion as the tendon moves over bony spicules at the Lister tubercle. Vaughan-Jackson syndrome is multiple extensor tendon rupture secondary to attrition or ischemic necrosis; it is the most common pattern of tendon rupture in RA patients. Attrition rupture of the extensor tendons occurs as they become worn over bony spurs at the distal end of the ulna. Rupture begins with the EDM and progresses in an ulnar to radial direction. Multiple extensor tendon rupture can also be a result of caput ulnae syndrome. Chronic DRUJ synovitis leads to articular injury and capsular and ligamentous attenuation. These changes distend the ECU subsheath, causing it to subluxate in a volar and ulnar position. Dorsal stabilizers of the carpus continue to stretch as the carpus supinates away from the distal ulna, resulting in volar subluxation of the carpus and hand. The increased prominence of the ulnar head increases the pressure within the extensor compartments and can lead to Vaughan-Jackson syndrome secondary to ischemic necrosis. Although the most likely cause of loss of finger extension in patients with RA is multiple extensor tendon rupture, 3 other potential diagnoses that can mimic this condition must be excluded. MCP joint dislocation results in a flexed and ulnarly deviated digit. The presence of visible or palpable tendons on the dorsal aspect of the hand and the lack of passive MCP joint extension distinguish MCP joint dislocation from extensor tendon rupture. The second condition that must be excluded is dislocation of the extensor tendons into the valleys between metacarpal heads due to attritional stretching of the radial sagittal band. The ability to maintain digital extension after the finger is passively placed into extension differentiates extensor tendon subluxation from tendon rupture. The third diagnosis that must be excluded is PIN palsy caused by proliferative synovitis at the elbow. PIN compression can result in paralysis of the wrist and finger extensors. Patients with this condition often present with radial deviation of the wrist and lack active finger extension. Presence of MCP joint extension with wrist flexion is a result of the tenodesis effect. A negative tenodesis effect indicates discontinuity of the extensor tendons, thereby excluding PIN palsy. Treatment options for extensor tendon ruptures are described in Table 6.36.

TABLE 6.36 Treatment of extensor tendon ruptures

Number of Ruptures	Treatment
Single	Primary repair Suture to adjacent tendon Tendon graft
Double (usually EDC to ring finger and EDM or EDC to small finger)	Same as single rupture with EIP transfer
Triple	Same as double rupture with FDS tendon transfer
Quadruple	Same as triple with an additional FDS
All extensor tendons	Dorsal tenosynovectomy with excision of bony spicules and retinacular transfer to prevent tendon abrasion from underlying bone

Adapted from Feldon P, Terrono AL, Nalebuff EA, Millender LH. Rheumatoid arthritis and other connective tissue diseases. In: Green DP, Hotchkiss RN, Pederson WC, Wolfe SW (eds.), *Green's Operative Hand Surgery*, 5th ed. Philadelphia: Elsevier, 2005;2049–2136.

Flexor Tendon. Flexor tendon rupture in patients with RA most commonly occurs in the wrist. Attrition rupture of the flexor tendons most frequently occurs at the volar aspect of the wrist, just over the scaphoid. Rupture of the FPL secondary to RA is known as a Mannerfelt lesion; it is the most common tendon to rupture. The FPL tendon typically ruptures from an osteophyte at the level of the STT joint. Treatment of FPL tendon rupture includes osteophyte débridement and repair with a free tendon graft or FDS transfer. Interphalangeal arthrodesis is done if there is significant involvement of the interphalangeal joint of the thumb. FDP rupture in the wrist may be camouflaged by an intact superficialis. Treatment includes repair with a free tendon graft or tenorrhaphy to an adjacent FDP tendon. DIP fusion is indicated if there is extensive arthritis of the DIP joint. Flexor tendon rupture in the palm or digit is uncommon; rupture in the palm is treated like rupture in the wrist. Rupture in the digital sheath is managed with tenosynovectomy and DIP arthrodesis. Rupture of the FDS tendons does not cause functional deficits.

Wrist

Wrist synovitis typically begins in the ulnar portion of the wrist; the ulnar head ulnar carpal ligaments, resulting in supination of the carpus, dorsal dislocation of the distal ulna, and volar subluxation of the ECU tendon. This process is known as caput ulnae syndrome; it is characterized by DRUJ instability, prominence of the distal ulna, and supination of the carpus. Volar subluxation of the ECU tendon leads to radial deviation of the wrist and places the extensor tendons at risk for rupture. Synovitis involving the radiocarpal joint attenuates the extrinsic and intrinsic carpal ligaments, causing the scaphoid to assume a volar-flexed position. Rotary instability of the scaphoid, volar subluxation of the ulnar carpus, and dorsal dislocation of the distal ulna lead to carpal collapse similar to the SLAC pattern and imbalance of the extensor tendons (Fig. 6.36). The metacarpals drift radially, causing ulnar shift of the MCP joints. The goal of treatment is prevention or reconstruction. Synovectomy of the DRUJ and radiocarpal joint is considered in the presence of unsuccessful 6-month trial of medical management. DRUJ instability can be treated with DRUJ reconstruction,

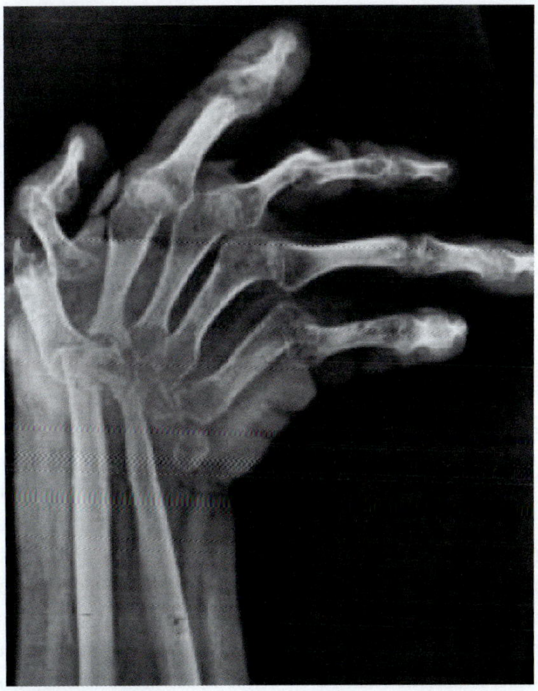

FIGURE 6.36 Rheumatoid wrist. (*Source:* Herren DB, Simmen BR. Limited and complete fusion of the rheumatoid wrist. *J Am Soc Surg Hand* 2002;2:21–31.)

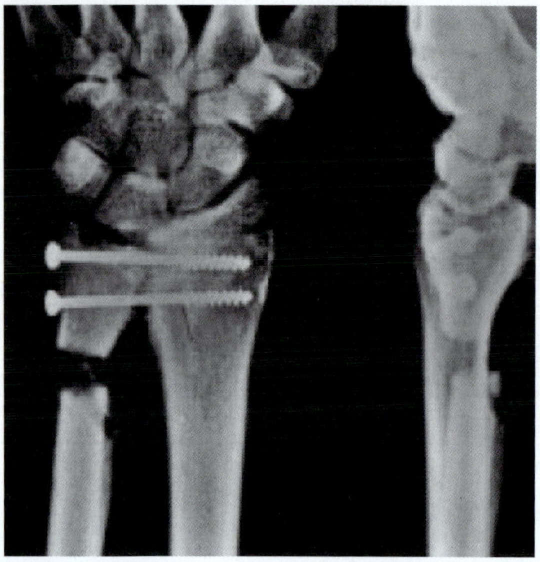

FIGURE 6.37 Sauve-Kapandji procedure. (*Source:* Lamey DM, Fernandez DL. Results of the modified Sauve-Kapandji procedure in the treatment of chronic posttraumatic derangement of the distal radioulnar joint. *J Bone Joint Surg Am* 1998;80:1758–69.)

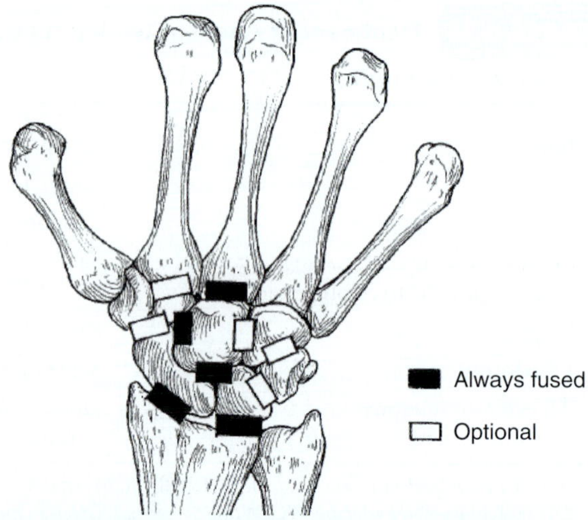

FIGURE 6.38 Articular surfaces involved in total wrist arthrodesis. (*Source:* Jebson PJL, Adams BD. Wrist arthrodesis: Review of current techniques. *J Am Acad Orthop Surg* 2001;9:53–60.)

the Sauve-Kapandji procedure, or distal ulnar resection (Fig. 6.37). The Sauve-Kapandji procedure consists of an ulnar osteotomy with resection of 10 to 12 mm of the distal ulnar metaphysis. The ulnar head is then fused to the sigmoid notch with pins or screws. Partial arthrodesis of the radiocarpal or radiolunate joint is reserved for patients with moderate disease and can restore function in patients with progressive ulnar translocation of the carpus. The treatment of choice for the rheumatoid wrist is total wrist arthrodesis, with a 90% success rate (Fig. 6.38). Position of fusion is 10 to 20 degrees of dorsiflexion and neutral deviation. Methods of fixation include intermedullary rods, staples, pins, or plate and screws. Complications include poor wound healing, hardware migration, painful hardware, infection, tendon adhesion, and pseudarthrosis (most common). Total wrist arthroplasty is a motion-preserving procedure and is indicated in patients with minimal deformity, intact extensor tendons, and good bone stock. Complications include implant loosening and infection. In patients with bilateral wrist involvement, bilateral fusions or total wrist arthroplasty and total wrist fusion are treatment options.

Metacarpophalangeal Joint

Multiple factors are responsible for the deformity that occurs in the MCP joints of patients with RA.

- Asymmetric shape of the metacarpal head contributes to ulnar deviation of the MCP joint with flexion.
- Carpal collapse leads to radial deviation of the wrist and metacarpals and ulnar deviation of the fingers.
- Proliferative synovitis causes stretching of the radial sagittal band, leading to ulnar subluxation of the extrinsic extensor tendons.
- Rupture or volar dislocation of the extensor tendons leads to increased flexion forces, causing volar subluxation of the proximal phalanx.
- Proliferative synovitis stretches the volar plate and accessory collateral ligaments, causing volar displacement of the flexor tendon and disruption of the balance forces at the proximal phalanx.
- Proliferative synovitis causes contracture of the interosseous muscles, which contributes to volar subluxation of the MCP joint.
- Radial deviation of the rheumatoid wrist contributes to MCP deformity.

Treatment of rheumatoid MCP joint depends on the stage of disease present, as classified by Millender and Nalebuff (Table 6.37). The most common complication following reconstructive surgery of the MCP joint is recurrent deformity.

Proximal Interphalangeal Joint

Swan Neck Deformity. The prevalence of swan neck deformity in patients with RA is 14%. This deformity

TABLE 6.37 Classification and treatment of MP joint deformity

Stage	Features	Treatment
I	Synovial proliferation	Splinting
II	Synovitis without deformity	Synovectomy
III	Articular erosion with ulnar and volar deviation of digits that is passively correctable	Synovectomy with soft tissue realignment (extensor tendon relocation, radial collateral ligament reconstruction, intrinsic release)
IV	Severe articular destruction with fixed deformity	Resection arthroplasty with or without silicone spacer and extensor tendon relocation with radial collateral ligament reconstruction

is characterized by PIP joint hyperextension with DIP joint flexion (Fig. 6.39). The PIP joint is the major site of deformity. Proliferative synovitis results in loss of static (volar plate, collateral ligaments) and dynamic (FDS tendon) joint stabilizers. Forces from the extensor mechanism are unopposed and cause the PIP joint to hyperextend and the DIP joint to flex. Intrinsic tightness has also been implicated in the development of deformity. The DIP can also be the main site of deformity, often presenting as a mallet finger secondary to terminal tendon rupture and subsequent PIP hyperextension. Rupture of the terminal tendon secondary to DIP joint synovitis can result in DIP joint flexion and PIP joint hyperextension. Rupture of the FDS may occur as a result of synovitis, causing PIP joint hyperextension. Subluxation of the lateral bands dorsal to the axis of rotation of the PIP joint with contracture of the triangular ligament and attenuation of the transverse retinacular ligament can result in deformity. There are 4 types of swan neck deformities; treatment depends on the type of deformity, with fusion of the DIP joint and either soft tissue reconstruction of the PIP joint, arthroplasty, or arthrodesis.

Boutonnière Deformity. Boutonnière deformity is also a result of soft tissue imbalance secondary to attenuation caused by proliferative synovitis and has a prevalence of 36% among RA patients. The deformity has 3 features: PIP joint flexion, DIP joint hyperextension, and MCP joint hyperextension (Fig. 6.40). In rheumatoids, synovitis of the PIP joint stretches the central slip and capsule, resulting in increased flexion at the PIP joint. Volar subluxation of the lateral bands lead to DIP hyperextension. The oblique retinacular ligament becomes contracted and contributes to the extension contracture of the DIP joint. In contrast to swan neck deformity, boutonnière deformity always starts at the PIP joint: synovitis of the PIP joint results in attenuation of the extensor mechanism (transverse retinacular ligament, triangular ligament, and central slip). The lateral bands migrate volarly, subsequently becoming PIP joint flexors. Over time, the capsular tissues contract, resulting in a fixed joint deformity. Treatment depends on the type of boutonnière deformity present. In all cases, an extensor tenotomy is performed on the DIP joint. The PIP joint undergoes either soft tissue correction if the joint is passively correctable or fusion if the deformity is fixed.

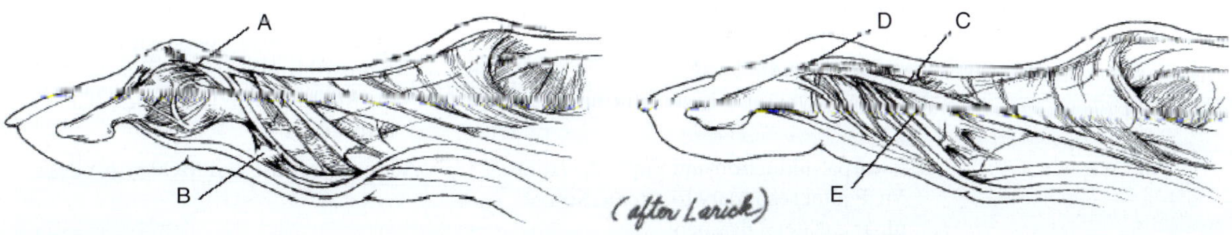

FIGURE 6.39 Swan neck deformity. Left: Rupture of terminal tendon secondary to DIP joint synovitis, resulting in DIP joint flexion and PIP joint hyperextension (A). Rupture of the FDS may occur as a result of synovitis, causing PIP joint hyperextension (B). Right: Subluxation of the lateral bands dorsal to the axis of rotation of the PIP joint (C) with contracture of the triangular ligament (D) and attenuation of the transverse retinacular ligament (E). (*Source:* Boyer MI, Gelberman RH. Operative correction of swan-neck and boutonnière deformities in the rheumatoid hand. *J Am Acad Orthop Surg* 1999;7:92–100.)

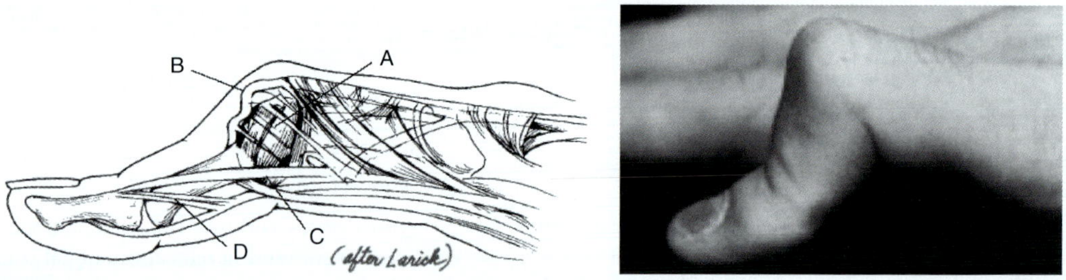

FIGURE 6.40 Boutonnière deformity. Left: Synovitis of the PIP joint (A) stretches the central slip (B) and capsule, resulting in increased flexion at the PIP joint. Volar subluxation of the lateral bands lead to DIP hyperextension (C). Oblique retinacular ligament contracture contributes to the extension contracture of the DIP joint (D). Right: Boutonnière deformity demonstrating flexion of the PIP joint and hyperextension of the DIP joint. (*Source:* Boyer MI, Gelberman RH. Operative correction of swan-neck and boutonnière deformities in the rheumatoid hand. *J Am Acad Orthop Surg* 1999;7:92–100.)

Thumb

Deformities of the rheumatoid thumb have been classified into 6 types. Treatment depends on the type of deformity and includes synovectomy, tendon transfer, tenodesis, arthroplasty and arthrodesis (Table 6.38).

Juvenile Rheumatoid Arthritis

Juvenile rheumatoid arthritis (JRA) is the most common connective tissue disease affecting children. The disease evolves at or before the age of 16 years, with a mean age between 1 and 3 years of age. The

TABLE 6.38 Classification and treatment of thumb deformities

Type	*Characteristics*	*Treatment*
I Boutonnière	MCP flexion and IP hyperextension Stage 1: MCP and IP joint deformities are passively correctable Stage 2: Fixed MCP joint deformity and passively correctable IP joint Stage 3: Fixed MCP and IP joint deformity	Stage 1: splinting; synovectomy with extensor realignment Stage 2: MCP arthrodesis or arthroplasty and IP joint release Stage 3: MCP arthroplasty and IP arthrodesis
II Boutonnière with CMC involvement	Rare	MCP arthrodesis and CMC hemiarthroplasty
III Swan neck	MCP joint hyperextension and IP joint flexion Stage 1: CMC joint synovitis, MCP joint not involved Stage 2: CMC joint synovitis and subluxation with MCP joint hyperextension that is passively correctable Stage 3: CMC joint destruction and dislocation with fixed MCP joint hyperextension deformity	Stage 1: CMC hemiarthroplasty; resection arthroplasty with LRTI and MCP arthrodesis Stage 2: MCP capsulodesis with CMC hemiarthroplasty; resection arthroplasty with LRTI Stage 3: MCP arthrodesis with CMC hemiarthroplasty; resection arthroplasty with LRTI and MCP arthrodesis
IV Gamekeeper's	Metacarpal adduction and radial deviation of MCP joint secondary to attenuation of ulnar collateral ligament	Adductor release and MCP arthrodesis
V Swan neck without MCP and CMC joint involvement	MCP joint synovitis attenuates volar plate, causing MCP joint hyperextension; IP joint develops secondary flexion deformity from increased tension on flexor tendon	Volar capsulodesis or MCP arthrodesis
VI Arthritis mutilans	Severe articular destruction and bone resorption of the MCP and IP joints	Arthrodesis of MCP and IP joints

CMC, carpometacarpal; IP, interphalangeal; LRTI, ligament reconstruction tendon interposition arthroplasty; MCP, metacarpophalangeal

TABLE 6.39 Types of juvenile rheumatoid arthritis

Feature	*Systemic (Still's)*	*Polyarthritis*	*Pauciarthritis*
Frequency	10%	30%	60%
Number of joints involved	Variable	‡5 (symmetric)	†4 (asymmetric)
Female–male ratio	1:1	3:1	5:1
Extraarticular manifestations	Extensive: rash, myalgia serositis,organomegaly, anemia, leukocytosis, thrombocytosis, and arthritis	Moderate	None
Chronic uveitis	Rare	5%	5%–15%
RF	Rare	10%	Rare
ANA	10%	40%–50%	75%–85%
Clinical course	Systemic disease is self-limited; 50% develop severe chronic arthritis	Systemic disease is mild; arthritis may be unremitting	No systemic disease; uveitis is the primary morbidity
Prognosis	Moderate	Moderately good to guarded	Excellent except for risk of blindness

female-to-male ratio is 2:1 except in cases of systemic disease, which has a 1:1 male-to-female ratio. Etiology of the disease is unclear; there is a strong association of HLA-A2, HLA-DR, HLA-DQ, and HLA-DP genotypes. There are 3 subtypes of JRA: systemic (Still disease, 10%), polyarticular (30%), and pauciarticular (60%; Table 6.39). Although JRA primarily involves large joints, there are small joint manifestations, especially with the polyarticular type of the disease. Patients with polyarticular disease may initially present with isolated swelling of the fingers. Unlike its adult counterpart, JRA is not associated with rheumatoid factor and subcutaneous nodules. Seropositivity for antinuclear antibodies (ANA) is a hallmark of the disease; approximately 40% of children test positive for ANA. Seventy percent to 90% of patients with JRA begin adulthood without any serious disability.

Clinically, hand and wrist deformities include ulnar deviation and flexion of the wrist and metacarpals and radial deviation and extension of the fingers. In contrast, the deformity characterized by adult RA involves radial deviation of the wrist and ulnar deviation of the digits. Radiographic changes associated with JRA include periarticular soft tissue swelling, juxtaarticular osteoporosis, and decreased bone growth secondary to premature epiphyseal closure (Fig. 6.41). Periosteal new bone formation causes widening of the phalanges, a common feature of JRA.

Treatment of JRA is primarily medical. NSAIDs and methotrexate are the two most common pharmacologic agents. Hydroxychloroquine, gold compounds, D-penicillamine, anti-TNF-α agents, and systemic steroids are also used to treat patients with JRA. Splinting, physical therapy, and intraarticular steroid injections play important roles in the management of JRA. Synovectomy can provide relief in patients with mechanical impairment of joint motion. Tenosynovectomy can be considered to decrease the risk of tendon rupture over the dorsum of the wrist or for adhesive tenosynovitis and a trigger finger. Reconstructive joint surgery is usually reserved for skeletally mature patients who enter the late teenage years or adulthood with severe disability.

Other Systemic Inflammatory Arthritides

A summary of other inflammatory arthritides and connective tissue disorders is provided in Table 6.40.

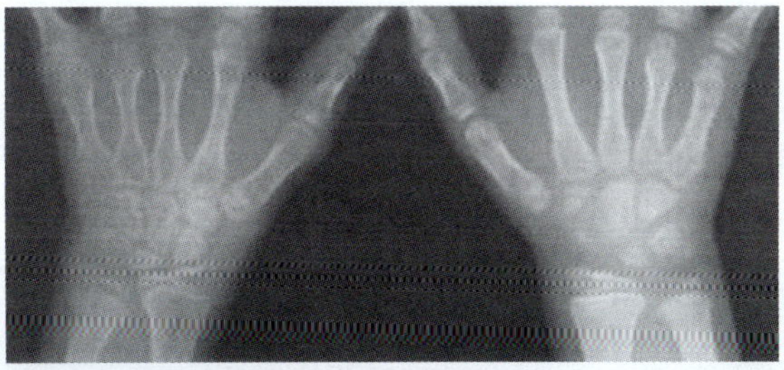

FIGURE 6.41 Bilateral hand radiographs of juvenile rheumatoid arthritis. (*Source:* Cassidy JT. Juvenile rheumatoid arthritis. In: Harris ED Jr, Budd RC, Genovese MC, Firestein GS, Sargent JS, Sledge CB (eds.), *Kelley's Textbook of Rheumatology*, 7th ed. Philadelphia: Elsevier, 2005;1579–1618.)

TABLE 6.40 Inflammatory arthritides and connective tissue disorders

Disease	*Features*	*Clinical Presentation*	*Imaging*	*Treatment*
Gout	Primary type is idiopathic; secondary type is a result of hyperuricemia from another disease; affects males more than females; usually between fourth and sixth decades of life; 1%–15% incidence; definitive diagnosis: joint aspirate reveals negative birefringent uric acid crystals under polarized microscope	Can mimic septic arthritis; acutely warm, swollen, erythematous joint	Tophi (soft tissue densities); intra- and extraarticular erosions	Colchicine or indomethacin for acute attacks; allopurinol for chronic therapy; excision of gouty tophi, tenosynovectomy and fusion for severe arthritic joints
Pseudogout (calcium pyro-phosphate deposition disease), chondro-calcinosis	Deposition of calcium pyrophosphate crystals into articular cartilage; definitive diagnosis: joint aspirate reveals positive bifringent calcium pyrophosphate crystals under polarized microscope	Morning stiffness and flexion contractures of fingers; can mimic septic arthritis	Calcium deposits visible in TFCC and menisci of the knee	Splint/immobilize joints during acute inflammatory attack; NSAIDs and intraarticular steroid injections alleviate the inflammation
Systemic lupus erythematosus (SLE)	Multisystem autoimmmune disease affecting musculoskeletal, cardiovascular, pulmonary, and renal systems; female–male ratio is 9:1; more common in black females; mean age of onset is 15–25 years; most common hand manifestation is joint deformity characterized by tendon subluxation, ligamentous and volar plate laxity leading to imbalance of forces across the joint; no erosive changes in joints	85% present with malar rash on face; maculopapular rash on hands, Raynaud phenomenon; symmetric joint synovitis with morning stiffness and painful ROM; most common joints involved are fingers, thumb, and wrist; volar subluxation and ulnar deviation of the MCP joints with secondary metacarpal deviation; dorsal subluxation of the distal ulna	Joint deformity without erosive articular changes	Maintain ROM in passively correctable deformities by splinting, stretching, and ROM exercises; consider surgery before deformities become fixed; high recurrence rate with soft tissue reconstruction; therefore, fusion and/or arthroplasty are procedures of choice
Psoriatic arthritis	Scaly, erythematous rash on extensor surfaces of extremities; 5% of patients develop inflammatory arthritis; rash precedes arthritis in 75%–80% of patients; 80% have nail changes: pitting is most common; 95% of patients with arthritis have peripheral joint involvement; 25% have polyarthritis and 5% have isolated DIP joint disease with erosion of terminal phalanges, DIP joint destruction, oncolysis and nail pitting; associated with HLA-B27, HLA-DR4, and HLA-DR7	Hand involvement is asymmetric; sausagelike swelling of the digits; shortening of fingers secondary to collapse (opera glass hand); most common deformity is flexion deformity of the PIP joint and MCP hyperextension	Osteolysis is most common radiographic finding in the hand and leads to joint space widening; pencil-in-cup appearance secondary to osteolytic tapering of proximal bone; spontaneous ankylosis 3 types of hand deformities based on radiographs: I. Spontaneous fusion of DIP and PIP joints II. Osteolysis III. RA-like stiffness and deformity	NSAIDs, systemic steroids, or immunosuppressive pharmacotherapy; UV light improves skin rash; osteotomy and arthrodesis with bone graft or arthroplasty are the mainstays of treatment

TABLE 6.40 *(continued)*

Disease	Features	Clinical Presentation	Imaging	Treatment
Scleroderma	Systemic disease involving the skin, lungs, heart, GI tract, kidneys, and hands; CREST (calcinosis, Raynaud, esophageal dysfunction, sclerodactyly, and telangiectasia) describes the disease's manifestations Thought to be a connective tissue and vascular disorder that leads to fibrosis; more common in females Raynaud phenomenon is a common early manifestation and can result in gangrene of the fingers; circulation improves distal to proximal; diagnosis confirmed with seropositivity for antinuclear and anticentromere antibodies	Most common digital deformity is progressive PIP flexion contracture with skin blanching; compensatory MCP hyperextension with extensor tendon rupture and ulceration of the skin over the joints; contracture of first web space decreases thumb mobility; calcinosis can be intracutaneous or subcutaneous	Soft tissue calcifications	Protective splinting of ulcerations with dressing changes; Raynaud treated with heated gloves and calcium channel blockers; débridement of calcium deposits; DIP joint is fused or amputated; PIP joint is fused; MCP joint hyperextension deformity treated with resection arthroplasty; first web space contracture treated with soft tissue release and IP or MCP fusion of the thumb

XII. SOFT TISSUE AND MICROVASCULAR SURGERY

Nail

Anatomy. The nail includes the following structures.

- *Perionychium/nail complex*—Comprises nail fold, nail bed, hyponychium, paronychium, and eponychium
- *Nail fold*—Most proximal aspect of the perionychium; composed of dorsal roof and ventral floor (germinal matrix)
- *Nail bed*—Soft tissue beneath nail; consists of sterile and germinal matrices
- *Nail plate*—Actual nail
- *Nail wall*—Dorsal skin over the fold
- *Germinal matrix*—Floor of the nail fold; creates 90% of nail plate thickness; does not adhere to nail plate
- *Sterile matrix*—Region of the nail bed distal to the germinal matrix; adheres to the nail plate
- *Hyponychium*—Skin distal to the nail bed
- *Paronychium*—Skin along the sides of the nail
- *Eponychium*—Skin proximal to the nail; covers the nail fold
- *Nail vest (cuticle)*—Extension of the eponychium onto the nail
- *Lunula*—Distal aspect of germinal matrix that appears as a white arc located on the nail distal to the eponychium
- *Blood supply*—Terminal branches of the radial and ulnar volar digital branches
- *Sensation*—Branches of the volar ulnar digital nerve and both dorsal and volar radial digital nerve branches

Trauma. Examination of injuries to the perionychium includes evaluation of possible associated injuries such as fractures of the distal phalanx; 50% of nail bed injuries include injury to the underlying bone. The most common cause of trauma to the perionychium is from doors, followed by crushing of the finger between two surfaces and lacerations from tools. The most distal aspect of the nail bed is the most common area of the perionychium that is injured. Nail bed injuries can be classified into 5 types (Table 6.41); treatment depends on the type of injury.

Surgical Repair. Nail bed repairs should be done using fine absorbable suture (e.g., 6-O or 7-O chromic). Once the repair is completed, the nail or a silicone sheet is used to protect the repair and to maintain the nail fold. Nail bed exploration can be done up to 1 week after initial injury. Approximately 50% of nail bed injuries are associated with fracture of the distal phalanx. Posttraumatic complications of nail bed injuries include nonadherence (most common), ridging, splitting, cornification of the nail bed, and nail

TABLE 6.41 Classification and treatment of nail bed injuries

Type of Injury	Features	Treatment
Subungual hematoma	Bleeding from a laceration beneath the nail; pressure builds within this confined space, causing severe throbbing pain	Evacuation of the hematoma with microcautery or heated paperclip; removal of the nail and repair of the nail bed is indicated if the nail is broken or the edges are disrupted or if the hematoma undermines > 50% of the nail
Simple laceration	Caused by compression of the nail by a sharp object	Removal of the nail and repair of the nail bed
Stellate laceration	Pattern of nail bed laceration seen after crush injury; visible after nail is removed	Removal of the nail and repair of the nail bed
Severe crush	Often associated with fracture of the underlying distal phalanx	After repair of the nail bed, the nail can be used as a splint; displaced fractures can be reduced and stabilized with longitudinal or crossed K-wires
Avulsion	Avulsion of the germinal matrix; typically presents as a laceration of the nail bed within the nail fold and an intact nail bed distally; may present as a Salter I fracture in children	Radiographic evaluation; repair of the nail bed; avulsed fragments of nail bed can be replaced as grafts; split-thickness sterile matrix grafts can be harvested from the injured digit, an unsalvageable digit, or the great toe

cysts and spikes. These deformities result from scar development in the nail bed or matrices or incomplete excision of the germinal matrix. These deformities can be treated with excision of the offending scar or matrix. Hooked nail deformity occurs when the nail bed has been stretched over a distal finger amputation during primary repair. Bone loss at the distal phalanx leads to inadequate structural support for the overlying nail bed, resulting in a hooked nail deformity. A local or regional flap with bone graft or a free vascularized toe transfer are options to correct a hooked nail deformity. Partial amputation of the soft tissue of the fingertip without exposed bone can be left to close by secondary intention if the wound is less than 1 cm^2. Full-thickness skin grafts from the hypothenar region of the palm should be considered for larger defects. If the bone is exposed, the bone is shortened; coverage is obtained by primary closure or by using a soft tissue flap.

Skin Grafting

Skin consists of two layers: the epidermis and the dermis. The epidermis represents 5% of skin thickness, but thickness varies depending on the region of the body. Proper hand motion and function is dependent on skin that is elastic and mobile and densely populated by epidermal appendages. Skin of the dorsum of the hand is thin, elastic, and mobile. Palmar skin is thick and glabrous and lacks sebaceous glands and hair follicles. These characteristics must be kept in mind when considering options for replacing the skin of the hand.

Types of Grafts. The two main types of skin grafts are split-thickness and full-thickness grafts. The main characteristic that differentiates the two types is the mechanism of harvest.

- *Split-thickness grafts*—Involve the harvest of the superficial layer of skin with a dermatome or a knife. The average thickness of split-thickness grafts is 0.015 inch, with a range of 0.008 to 0.020 inch, and the surface area of the graft can be extended by running the graft through a mesher. The holes in the graft minimize hematoma formation and increase the expandability. The donor site is left to reepithelialize on its own. The disadvantages of split-thickness grafts are that they contain few epidermal appendages and have a greater chance of contracting. A split-thickness graft is indicated for coverage of a simple wound with adequate soft tissue beds or a marginal wound that will undergo extensive delayed reconstruction.
- *Full-thickness grafts*—Consist of the entire layer of skin and are harvested through an incision that must be closed primarily. These grafts have the advantages of greater structural support, protection, sensibility, and epidermal appendages. Full-thickness grafts are also less likely to contract. Disadvantages of these grafts include higher chance of failure or infection, the need for well-vascularized soft tissue beds, and limited availability. A full-thickness graft is indicated for an area where it is essential to obtain maximum

skin thickness and epidermal appendages with minimal postoperative contracture, such as the palmar skin of the hand. Causes of graft failure include inadequate débridement with residual layers of devitalized tissue, hematoma formation underneath the graft, insufficient dressing, and secondary infection.

Flaps. A flap is skin and underlying soft tissue that is harvested for tissue defects and that receives its vascular supply from a source other than the tissue on which it is transferred. The pedicle refers to the area of the flap that contains its vascular supply. Flaps can be classified according to their vascular supply. Random-pattern flaps receive their blood supply from multiple minute vessels within the subdermal or subcutaneous network. Axial-pattern flaps receive their vascular supply from a single, constant vessel that is substantially larger than those within the subdermal plexus. The region of skin and soft tissue that is supplied by the axial vessel is called the vascular territory of the vessel. The vessel of an axial-pattern flap may supply skin alone or skin and underlying tissue. These types of axial flaps are known as composite flaps and are referred to as cutaneous, fasciocutaneous, musculocutaneous, and osteocutaneous. Flaps consisting of bone, muscle, or fascia can be harvested without the overlying skin. Flaps can be divided into 3 groups based on location. A local flap is tissue that is transferred from tissue adjacent to the defect. The main advantages of the local flap are that it maintains length; the donor site does not need a skin graft; and the quality, color, and texture of the donor tissue resembles that of the recipient site. An additional benefit is that ROM can be initiated early. There are 3 types of local flaps: transposition, rotation, and advancement. In transposition and rotation types, the flap is transferred laterally relative to its pedicle to cover the defect. Transposition flaps require closure or grafting of the secondary defect, whereas that of the rotational flap can be closed primarily. An advancement flap is characterized by a pedicle that lies opposite the primary defect. Regional flaps are harvested from another part of the limb. The primary disadvantages of these flaps is that their use requires a 2-stage procedure: one for harvest and one for division of the flap. The prolonged immobilization that is necessary postoperatively may result in stiffness. Regional flaps are contraindicated in patients with systemic disease such as RA, diabetes, and vasospastic conditions and in patients with arthritic changes in the involved digits. Distant flaps are harvested from another part of the body; unless it is a free flap, distant flaps typically require a 2-stage procedure. The type of flap indicated depends on the angle and level of amputation. Tables 6.42 and 6.43 describe the types of flaps and indications for their use. The main cause of flap failure is insufficient arterial supply, usually secondary to thrombosis caused by vasospasms. Other factors that may compromise flow include hematoma, edema, hypotension, hypothermia, infection, and compression.

XIII. BURNS

More than 80% of patients with severe burns have involvement of the hand. Early and aggressive treatment is essential in minimizing the devastating functional and cosmetic deformities that result from burns to the hand.

Treatment Principles. The basic principles of treatment of hand burns are as follows:

- Assess size and depth of the burn
- Escharotomy if indicated
- Proper wound care and dressing application
- Early hand therapy and splinting
- Decision about nonoperative or operative treatment
- Surgical treatment: escharectomy, skin grafting, and flap coverage if needed
- Early postoperative therapy and functional rehabilitation
- Secondary and tertiary surgery if needed

Postburn Deformities. Common postburn deformities of the hand are as follows:

- First web space adduction contractures
- Web space contractures
- Dorsal skin contractures
- Burn syndactyly
- Digital flexion contracture
- Boutonnière deformity
- Dorsal skin deficiency
- Loss of digit secondary to ischemia
- Median and ulnar nerve compression syndrome

Prognosis. The cause of a burn is one of the most useful factors in predicting healing prognosis. Scalds consist of a mixed pattern of injury and have a high chance for spontaneous healing, especially in younger patients. Flames cause the most extensive injury and often result in partial- or full-thickness burns. Depth of injury is a common method of classifying burns and often determines the type of treatment required. Superficial, first-degree burns are those in which cells of tissue are injured. They are self-limited and heal without scarring. Superficial partial-thickness, second-degree burns involve destruction of the entire epidermis and some of the dermis. These burns are the most painful

TABLE 6.42 Flap types and indications for their use

Flap Type	Description	Indication/Recipient Site
Local		
V-Y advancement	Can be advanced 1 cm; triangular flap with a base at the distal margin of the wound and apex in the midline of the DIP crease	Dorsal oblique or transverse fingertip amputation
Kutler or lateral V-Y advancement	Two triangular flaps that are advanced from each side of the fingertip; base of the triangle is the distal wound edge	Transverse fingertip amputation
Axial flag	Based on dorsal digital or proper digital artery within the web space of the donor digit (index or long finger)	MCP joint of index or long finger or dorsal or volar proximal phalanx of the index finger
Digital artery island	Based on ulnar or radial digital artery	Fingertip amputation
Moberg	Volar advancement flap based on the proximal phalanx of the thumb; preserves tactile gnosia; donor site may require skin graft	Thumb tip amputations through the distal phalanx; covers defects ≤ 2.5 cm
Dorsal metacarpal artery	Based on first or second metacarpal artery and branches of the radial nerve; based on the first interosseous space to the PIP joint of the index finger	Thumb and first web space defects; proximal defects of the long and ring fingers
Regional		
Flap Type	***Description***	***Indication/Recipient Site***
Cross-finger	Rectangular flap from the dorsum of the middle phalanx of the donor digit, which is radial to the injured finger; index finger donor is the long finger; donor site requires full-thickness skin graft	Volar defect of the fingertip that is not suitable for coverage with an advancement flap
Reversed cross-finger	Similar to cross-finger	Dorsal defect of the fingertip that is not suitable for coverage with an advancement flap
Thenar flap	Donor site is the thenar eminence with the base located proximally; maximum width of flap is 2 cm; donor site requires full-thickness skin graft	Used for transverse and volar oblique fingertip amputations
Neurovascular island	Donor site is based on digital neurovascular bundle and can be harvested from any digit; ideal for areas where restoration of sensibility is critical; donor site requires full-thickness skin graft	Loss of soft tissue at the pulp of the thumb or index finger
Cross-thumb	Harvested from the dorsum of the thumb's proximal phalanx; donor site requires full-thickness skin graft	Radial defects of the index finger
Fillet flap	Based on the neurovascular bundle of a digit that is not salvageable or that is going to be sacrificed secondary to extensive bony, nerve, and/or soft-tissue damage	Considered when bone and soft tissue loss is so severe that reconstruction is not option
Radial artery forearm	Fasciocutaneous or osteocutaneous flap that can be harvested if there is adequate blood supply from the ulnar artery (Allen test); leaves large donor site defect that is cosmetically suboptimal; requires split-thickness skin graft	Wounds dorsum of the hand, forearm, or elbow

TABLE 6.42 *(continued)*

Flap Type	Description	Indication/Recipient Site
Local		
Ulnar artery forearm	Fasciocutaneous flap that can be harvested if the blood supply from the radial artery is adequate (Allen test); donor site can be closed primarily and skin has less hair than radial artery forearm flap	Defects at the hand and elbow
Reversed posterior interosseous artery	Fasciocutaneous flap that is harvested from the lateral epicondyle to the DRUJ with the forearm in pronation	Dorsal first web space or dorsum of MCP joint
Lateral arm	Fasciocutaneous flap based on posterior radial collateral artery; transection of the posterior brachial cutaneous nerve leads to hypoesthesia at the posterolateral elbow; graft can be as large as 8 × 15 cm; donor site usually requires split-thickness skin graft	Anterior or posterior elbow, rotational flap for the shoulder, or free tissue transfer
Scapular	Cutaneous flap based on cutaneous branch of circumflex scapular artery; lateral border of the scapula can be used as vascularized bone graft	Combined dorsal hand and metacarpal bony defect
Distant		
Flap Type	**Description**	**Indication/Recipient Site**
Latissimus dorsi	Rotational musculocutaneous flap; based on thoracodorsal artery; requires harvest and transfer can be done in one procedure	Used for coverage or functional restoration of soft tissue (e.g., elbow flexion); reconstructive shoulder, breast, head, and neck; and abdominal procedures
Groin	Fasciocutaneous flap based on superficial circumflex iliac artery; donor site defects up to 12 cm can be closed primarily; 2-stage procedure: first for harvest and transfer followed by division of the flap 3–4 weeks later	Any soft tissue defect along distal two thirds of forearm volar and/or dorsal hand defects

type. They have the potential to heal, although not without a scar. Deep partial-thickness, second-degree burns appear moist and mottled. The skin blanches with pressure, bleeds after a needle prick, and contains nerve endings in the vital layers. Full-thickness, third-degree burns are distinguished by death of the germinal components of the epidermis, dermal appendages, and nerve endings. These burns cannot heal on their own. A fourth degree burn is characterized by necrosis of tissue that is deep to the subcutaneous layer (e.g., tendons, muscle and bone). These types of burns are typically a result of contact or high-voltage burns.

Management. Initial treatment includes immobilization, elevation, tetanus immunization, and neurovascular monitoring.

Specific Burn Types

Electrical Burns. Seventy-five percent of electrical injuries involve the upper extremity and are typically a result of occupational exposure. The rate of amputation is between 40% and 70%; mortality rate is between 8% and 14%. Over 50% of patients continue to experience neurologic deficits, and 85% of patients are permanently disabled following a high-voltage injury in work-related accidents. The extent of injury is determined by current, voltage, duration of contact, tissue resistance, and the course of flow through the body. Electrical burns can be divided into high voltage (more than 1000 v) and low voltage (less than 1000 v) injuries. The amount of voltage is directly proportional to the extent of injury, which occurs

TABLE 6.43 Preferred techniques for specific cases

Region	Palmar	Dorsal-Larger Defects
Distal to PIP joint	Loss more dorsal: V–Y advancement Loss more palmar: middle/ring—digital artery island flap < 40: Female, thenar; male, cross-finger > 40: Important—neurovascular island; not important—revise amputation	Reversed cross-finger
PIP joint	Cross-finger	Reversed cross-finger
Proximal phalanx	Small defect: transposition from lateral aspect Large defect Palmar only: cross-finger Palmar and lateral: index/middle—axial flag; ring/small—vascular island	Reversed cross-finger
MCP joint	Index/middle: axial flag Ring/small: vascular island	Index/middle: axial flag Ring/small: vascular island
Metacarpus or several fingers syndactylized	Worthless digit: fillet Small defect: vascular island or SDMA Large defect: (free lateral arm) or forearm fascia and skin graft	Worthless digit: fillet (free lateral arm)
Thumb	More dorsal loss: V–Y advancement Palmar but < 2/3 of pulp: Moberg Palmar but > 2/3 pulp: Neurovascular island (e.g., toe) or FDMA/SDMA	FDMA† from index Forearm (preferably PIA††) No donor digit, no vessel Male: infraclavicular Female: iliac

FDMA,† first dorsal metacarpal artery; PIA,†† posterior interosseous artery; SDMA, second dorsal metacarpal artery
Adapted from Browne EZ, Pederson WC. Skin grafts and skin flaps. In: Green DP, Hotchkiss RN, Pederson WC, Wolfe SW (eds.), *Green's Operative Hand Surgery*, 5th ed. Philadelphia: Elsevier, 2005;1629–1713.

when the electrical energy is converted into thermal energy. High-voltage injuries are often life threatening; initial treatment consists of cardiac and respiratory monitoring because the most common causes of death are ventricular fibrillation and respiratory arrest. Injury to the kidneys from myoglobinuria can be minimized with aggressive hydration. Contact burns can be deep, with areas of erythema, edema, blistering, and/or charring. The upper extremity is typically in a fixed, flexed position secondary to severe muscle contraction and necrosis, and there is usually an associated compartment syndrome. Because of the high incidence of compartment syndrome, treatment should begin with fasciotomies of all compartments, escharotomies, and serial débridement of nonviable tissue. Initial coverage can be obtained with split-thickness grafts until definitive reconstructive surgery can be performed. Amputation is considered if injury is too extensive for salvage or the patient's life is in jeopardy; absolute indications for amputation include life-threatening sepsis, unsalvageable limb injury, or an insensate extremity. Complications resulting from electrical burns include vascular occlusion, wound infection from nonvital tissue, multiorgan failure, systemic sepsis, failure to reconstruct or salvage the limb, pulmonary abnormalities, cerebral hemorrhage, peripheral neuropathy, and muscle fibrosis.

Chemical Burns. Burns from hazardous agents are responsible for over 60% of admissions from work-related chemical injuries. Damage is usually limited to the skin, but unlike thermal burns, some chemicals may remain active and continue destroying tissues. Degree of injury depends on the surface area exposed to the agent, length of contact, and local characteristics of the skin. Treatment begins with removal of the noxious agent by removing affected clothing and diluting or neutralizing the agent. Copious lavage with water for 1 to 2 hours decreases the concentration of chemical on the skin and slows its rate of reaction. Once the offending agent has been removed, nonviable tissue, blisters, and bullae are débrided. As with thermal burns, neurovascular monitoring is essential for detecting an impending compartment syndrome. Topical antibacterial ointment should be applied. Table 6.44 lists features of burns from common

TABLE 6.44 Injury characteristics of common chemical agents

Agent	*Commercial Use*	*Injury Characteristics*	*Treatment*
Phenol	Cleaning detergents, cosmetics, plastics	Protein denaturation, rapidly absorbed	Water irrigation, remove with glycerol or polyethylene glycol
Phosphorus (white)		Highly fat soluble	Water irrigation, copper sulfate stains particles for identification, excision
Lyes	Cement, oven cleaners	Liquefaction necrosis with saponification, dehydrates cells	Water irrigation
Hydrofluoric acid	Rust removers	Painful, deep ulcerations below tough coagulum	Local infiltration of calcium gluconates
Hydrochloric acid	Pool cleaners	Shallow ulcers form with coagulated eschar and base	Water irrigation, magnesium oxide, soap, soda lime
Muriatic acid	Toilet bowl cleaners	Hard eschar with indolent ulcer	Water irrigation
Sodium hydrochloride	Bleach	Coagulation of proteins	Water irrigation
Elemental sodium			**AVOID WATER** (contact with water causes violent exothermic reaction); Apply mineral oil

Adapted from Bentivegna PE, Deane LM. Chemical burns of the upper extremity. *Hand Clin* 1990;6:253–259; Reilly DA, Garner WL. Management of chemical injuries to the upper extremity. *Hand Clin* 2000;16:215–224.

chemical agents. Injection injuries to the hand from paint guns may appear benign on presentation but are actually extensive and require wide incision and débridement in order to remove the hazardous material, which typically is injected into a digital sheath.

Frostbite. Frostbite results from crystal formation within soft tissue after exposure to cold temperature for over an hour; temperatures below −2°C increase the risk for developing frostbite. In addition to the ambient temperature, the severity of frostbite injury depends on wind chill factor, duration of exposure, altitude, wetness of the tissue, the patient's vascular integrity, and history of cold exposure injury. Cold exposure causes an increase in viscosity and slowing of blood flow within the capillaries. Vascular insult causes extravasation of fluid and formation of thrombi from red blood cell aggregation. Within 1 hour, thrombi can develop in the terminal arterioles and lead to cell death and tissue necrosis. Frostbite injury can be classified into 4 degrees based on the depth of soft tissue injury. First-degree injuries cause erythema, edema, and hyperemia of the superficial skin. Second-degree injuries are full-thickness and present with erythema, blister, and bulla formation with skin sloughing; there is no necrosis of the underlying tissue. Third-degree frostbite injuries involve the skin and subcutaneous tissue. These injuries are characterized by a grayish hue to the skin; there is edema of the surrounding tissue with skin loss down to the subcutaneous level. Fourth-degree frostbite results in cyanosis without blistering or swelling. Necrosis extends to the subcutaneous layer with involvement of the underlying muscle, tendon, and bone. Management of acute frostbite is initiated by elevation and immobilization of the extremity and administration of tetanus prophylaxis. Technetium 99m bone scans or MRI is performed within the first few days after injury to evaluate circulation and viability of the exposed soft tissue and bone and define the level of amputation. Specific guidelines for management of acute frostbite are as follows.

- Restoration of core body heat
- Rapid rewarming of the frozen extremity in a 40°C to 44°C water bath
- Analgesia
- Triple-phase bone scan or MRI
- Tetanus prophylaxis
- Open dressing
- Physical therapy
- Antibiotics in cases of infection
- Incision and débridement or amputation only after level is demarcated

XIV. REPLANTATION

Replantation describes surgical reattachment of a fully amputated part and must be differentiated from revascularization, which is the repair of a partially amputated part that still has some soft tissue attachment to the body but has no perfusion. Advances in microsurgery are responsible for the over 85% to 90% survival rate of replanted limbs worldwide. Viability, however, does not correlate with function. The function of a replanted part is anticipated to be equal to or better than function following revision amputation with or without the use of a prosthesis. Multiple factors influence the outcome of a replanted part, the most important being location, level, and mechanism of injury. Ischemia time (Table 6.45), the degree of wound contamination and personal characteristics of the patient also play a significant role in determining the success rate following replant surgery. Ring avulsion injuries have been classified by Urbaniak on the basis of the degree of injury (Table 6.46).

Traumatic amputations arrive at level-one trauma centers by air. Evaluation and initial treatment of these injuries are as follows:

- *Primary survey*—Assess airway, breathing, and circulation; control hemorrhage; administer tetanus prophylaxis and intravenous antibiotics
- *Secondary survey*—Wrap amputated part in gauze moistened with saline or lactated Ringer solution, store in specimen bag and place on ice

Indications for reimplantation:

- Thumb
- Single digit distal to zone II
- Multiple digits
- Partial hand
- Risks associated with surgery
- Wrist or proximal to wrist
- Children

Contraindications for replantation:

- Prolonged ischemia time
- Single border digit

TABLE 6.45 Duration of ischemia

Level of Injury	Warm Ischemia Time	Cold Ischemia Time (4°C)
Digits	< 12 hours	< 24 hours
Proximal to wrist	< 6 hours	< 10 hours

TABLE 6.46 Urbaniak classification of ring avulsion injuries

Class	Characteristics
I	Adequate circulation; standard bone and soft tissue treatment is sufficient
II	Inadequate circulation; vessel repair preserves viability and permits immediate or delayed repair of other tissue
	IIa: bone, tendons, nerves, and veins intact
	IIb: bone, tendon, or nerve injury
	IIc: venous compromise only
III	Complete degloving or amputation; these injuries have the worst prognosis

- Avulsion
- Frostbite
- Multilevel/segmental
- Single digit zone II
- Crush/mangling
- Contamination
- Prior impaired function
- Life-threatening injury
- Severe medical problems
- Poor anesthesia candidate
- Major psychiatric disorder

Patient factors to consider:

- Age (children have better outcomes, especially if younger than 9 years old)
- Associated injuries (life over limb)
- High risk for anesthesia
- Preexisting comorbidity such as severe arthritis, diabetes, coronary artery disease, peripheral vascular disease, or psychiatric illness
- Vocation
- Motivation
- Tobacco, alcohol, drug abuse
- Cost of care
- Religious or cultural beliefs

Risks associated with replant surgery:

- Infection
- Metabolic disturbance (hyperkalemia, metabolic acidosis, and myoglobinuria)
- Preexisting comorbidity such as severe arthritis, diabetes, coronary artery disease, peripheral vascular disease, or psychiatric illness
- Hemorrhage
- Need for transfusion

- Compartment syndrome
- Risk of anesthesia

Determining Candidates. The mechanism of injury is an important factor in determining if an amputated part is replantable. Guillotine amputations are ideal for replantation because there is minimal damage to the soft tissue and bone. Crush, mangled, or avulsion injuries are suboptimal for replantation or revascularization because of the difficulty in repairing the arterial supply. Close inspection of the amputated part may reveal the red-line and ribbon signs secondary to excessive traction on the neurovascular bundle. Stretching of the digital artery causes tearing of branches along the course of the vessel; the resulting hemorrhage creates a red line or streak on the lateral border of the digit. Traction on the digital artery can also result in elastic recoiling of the vessel, creating the ribbon sign. These signs are contraindications to replantation. Segmental or multilevel injuries are associated with poor outcomes.

Surgery. The operative sequence of repair and reconstruction during replant surgery can be remembered using the mnemonic BEFAN V: bone, extensor tendon, flexor tendon, artery, nerve, vein, and skin. Postoperative management of the replant patient includes the following:

- Continuous monitoring in the surgical intensive care unit
- Intravenous antibiotics
- Anticoagulation with dextran, aspirin, and Thorazine
- Patient should be warm, well hydrated, and calm
- Avoid caffeine and tobacco

Postoperative Management. Surface temperature is the most reliable and noninvasive means of assessing perfusion. Blood flow is compromised if the temperature of the replanted part drops below 30°C or greater than 2°C per hour. Replant failure most often occurs within the first 5 to 7 days following surgery. Initial management of the failing patient begins by placing the limb in a more dependent position, loosening the dressing, increasing hydration, and administering a heparin bolus. Medical leeches can be used to decrease venous congestion and can be used continuously within the first postoperative week. Leeches may infect patients with *Aeromonas hydrophila*, a Gram-negative anaerobic rod. The patient should return to the operating room for a second look with possible revision surgery if the part continues to fail. The most common cause of early replant failure is arterial thrombosis secondary to vasospasm followed by venous congestion. The most common complications following replant surgery include infection and cold intolerance. Success rates of replantation surgery are listed in Table 6.47.

TABLE 6.47 Success rates with replantation surgery

Part	Survival Rate
Thumb	75%–85% with TPD of 9–11 mm for sharp amputations; 50% for avulsions
Digits	75%–85% with TPD of 8 mm for sharp amputations
Hand and distal forearm	70% but poor TPD and absent or weak pinch and grasp strength; cold intolerance is common
Proximal forearm	65%
Transarticular level	70%–85%
Transhumeral	50%

Soft Tissue Reconstruction Ladder. Management of tissue injury is based on the soft tissue reconstruction ladder and is applicable to acute or chronic soft tissue injury with or without bony involvement, limb salvage oncologic resection, osteomyelitis, and nonunions. The reconstruction ladder begins with thorough débridement of nonvital tissue; serial débridements may be necessary in order to obtain a bed of healthy, viable tissue. Table 6.48 lists the hierarchy of managing soft tissue defects, beginning with the most basic technique and leading to the most complex of reconstructive procedures.

Timing of Treatment. Timing of free tissue transfer is essential in order to minimize the exposure of vital structures and the risk of infection. In traumatic cases, the timing of definitive wound management depends on type of fracture and soft tissue injury, the structures that are exposed, contamination, and overall health of the patient. In severe upper extremity trauma, wound coverage within 5 to 7 days from time of injury is associated with a good prognosis. Risk of postoperative infection, flap failure, osteomyelitis, and nonunion are significantly minimized with early, aggressive wound débridement and flap coverage within 5 days. Wounds that have undergone tumor resection after irradiation have a high rate of complications. Free tissue transfer is recommended immediately following tumor resection in order to decrease patient morbidity and increase the success rate of limb salvage.

Postoperative Flap Management. Types of flaps are described in Table 6.49. Postoperative management of flaps is similar to management of replants. Patients

TABLE 6.48 Reconstructive ladder for soft tissue injury

Procedure	Indications	Example
Primary wound closure	Minor trauma; may be delayed depending on the degree of contamination and soft tissue insult	Grade I open fracture
Delayed primary wound closure	24–48 hours after initial débridement, (e.g., open fracture)	Grade II, IIIA, and some IIIB open fracture
Healing by secondary intention	Wound is left open; eventually heals and closes by granulation and epithelialization (e.g., donor sites for skin grafts)	Abscess
Skin grafts	Indicated for coverage of wounds that cannot be closed primarily and cannot be left to heal by secondary intention; recipient site must be a clean bed of well-vascularized granulation tissue; can be applied to fat, paratenon, fascia, muscle, and periosteum	Third-degree thermal burns
Flaps (local or distant)	Indicated for intricate wounds with exposed neurovascular structures, bone stripped of periosteum, or inadequate blood supply or soft tissue; type of flap depends on wound location or inadequacy of donor site	Gastrocnemius flap for IIIB and IIIC open fractures of the proximal tibia
Free tissue transfer	Summit of the reconstructive ladder; may be used in conjunction with a lower level procedure such as skin graft or rotational flap; can be functional	IIIB and IIIC open fractures of the distal tibia or free vascularized fibula bone graft for fracture nonunion or avascular necrosis of the femoral head

should be under continuous monitoring in the intensive care unit. The flap should be checked for color, temperature, turgor, capillary refill, and ability to bleed. Acute postoperative complications occur within the first 48 hours following surgery and include arterial insufficiency (the most common cause of failure), venous congestion, hematoma, hemorrhage, and flap edema. Late flap failure is most commonly a result of error in technique and includes improper harvest, compromise of the pedicle during harvest, poor microsurgical technique, increased tissue tension or edema secondary to poor insetting technique, or pedicle avulsion from excessive extremity motion. Treatment options for flap failure include delayed débridement (in the absence of infection, the flap can be used as a biologic dressing, allowing for granulation of the wound bed), skin grafting, second free flap transfer, and amputation.

XV. CONGENITAL ANOMALIES

The incidence of congenital deformities of the upper extremity is 1 in 626 live births or 1% to 2% of newborns; approximately 10% of cases require surgical attention. Most of these deformities are associated with systemic abnormalities involving the cardiovascular, renal, neurologic, craniofacial, and musculoskeletal systems. The etiology of congenital hand anomalies is unknown in 40% to 50% of cases. Potential causes include genetic abnormalities or exposure to teratogens in the environment during embryologic development. Development of the upper extremity begins around 4 weeks of gestation, when the limb bud appears on the lateral body wall arising from the eight through tenth somites. The limb bud consists of undifferentiated mesenchymal tissue; it grows and differentiates under the guidance of the apical ectodermal ridge that overlies it. At week 5 of gestation, the hand paddle appears; separation of the fingers occurs by apoptosis of the cells between the digits and is complete by week 8. Skin creases develop when hand movement begins, which is around 9 weeks' gestation.

Classification

The most widely used classification of congenital deformities of the upper extremity is based on embryonic malfunction. Failure of formation occurs in 1 of 2 directions: transverse or longitudinal.

TABLE 6.49 Types of flaps

Flap	Vascular Anatomy	Comments
	Fascial and Fasciocutaneous Flaps	
Radial forearm	Pedicle: radial artery	Radial artery is sacrificed; complications most commonly due to skin graft problems at donor site; can be innervated by the medial and lateral antebrachial cutaneous nerves
Posterior interosseous	Pedicle: posterior interosseous artery (septocutaneous perforators between ECU and EDM); anastomoses between posterior and anterior interosseous arteries at the level of the DRUJ maintain viability	Useful for defects of the dorsum of hand; advantage over radial forearm flap is that a large artery is not sacrificed; elevation of flap limited by posterior interosseous nerve branch to ECU
Lateral arm	Pedicle: posterior radial collateral artery (pedicle length is 7–8 cm)	Can be used for coverage after severe thumb web space contracture release; harvest leads to numbness in posterolateral elbow due to transaction of posterior cutaneous nerve of forearm; can be innervated by posterior cutaneous nerve of forearm
Ulnar artery	Pedicle: ulnodorsal artery (arises 2.5 cm proximal to pisiform); (pedicle length up to 20 cm)	Cause of paresthesias in the hand after flap elevation due to transient ischemia of ulnar nerve
Brachioradialis	Pedicle: anterior recurrent radial artery	Can be innervated by radial nerve
Temporoparietal fascial	Pedicle: superficial temporal artery	
Scapular	Pedicle: circumflex scapular artery	
Groin	Pedicle: superficial circumflex iliac artery	Superficial circumflex iliac artery runs 2.5 cm distal to inguinal ligament; thigh numbness after groin flap secondary to meralgia paresthetica (lateral femoral cutaneous nerve)
Anterolateral thigh	Pedicle: lateral femoral circumflex artery (descending branch between rectus and vastus lateralis)	Can be innervated by medial and lateral cutaneous nerves of thigh
Lateral thigh	Pedicle: profunda femoris artery (third perforator)	Can be innervated by medial and lateral cutaneous nerves of thigh
Dorsalis pedis	Pedicle: anterior tibial-dorsalis pedis artery	
	Muscle and Myocutaneous Flaps	
Latissimus dorsi	Pedicle: thoracodorsal artery (pedicle length up to 11.2 cm)	Release of tendon insertion has greatest effect on axis of rotation of a pedicled latissimus flap; can be innervated by the thoracodorsal nerve and can serve as functional muscle transfer
Vastus lateralis	Pedicle: lateral femoral circumflex artery (proximal); profunda femoris artery (distal)	
Serratus anterior	Pedicle: thoracodorsal artery	No scapular winging occurs if only lower muscle slips are harvested; can serve as functional muscle transfer; can be innervated by long thoracic nerve

(continued overleaf)

TABLE 6.49 (continued)

Flap	Vascular Anatomy	Comments
Rectus abdominis	Pedicle: inferior epigastric artery	
	Pedicle: lateral femoral circumflex artery (proximal); profunda femoris artery (distal)	
Gracilis	Pedicle: medial femoral circumflex artery	Can serve as functional muscle transfer
	Osseous and Osteocutaneous Flaps	
Fibula and osteocutaneous fibula	Pedicle: peroneal artery	Can be transferred as an osteocutaneous flap by including fasciocutaneous perforators in the middle to distal third of fibula; vascularized fibular graft remodels and hypertrophies more rapidly than nonvascularized grafts
Iliac crest and osteocutaneous iliac crest	Pedicle: Superficial circumflex iliac artery	Can be harvested as an osteocutaneous flap with iliac crest bone
	Composite Tissue Flaps	
Great toe, second toe	Pedicle: first dorsal metatarsal artery	First dorsal metatarsal artery runs superficial to first dorsal interosseous muscle in 78% of cases
Toe wraparound	Pedicle: first dorsal metatarsal artery	

Transverse Failure of Formation

Transverse arrest deformities are also known as congenital amputations and are named according to the level of involvement: complete arm, midarm, proximal forearm, wrist, midhand, and fingers. The proximal third of the forearm amputation is the most common of the congenital amputations. The proximal portion of the limb is abnormal, and the segment distal to the amputation level is either underdeveloped or absent. Most cases occur sporadically and are unilateral. It is thought that these deformities are a result of disruption of the blood supply to the apical ectodermal ridge. Treatment begins with family education and prosthesis fitting between 6 to 9 months of life; fitting prior to the age of 2 years increases the rate of its acceptance. Transition to a body-powered device typically occurs between 15 to 24 months of life. Surgery is not indicated in proximal forearm deficiency unless a rudimentary spicule of bone or nubbin is irritating the stump. The Krukenberg procedure involves separation of the radius and ulna in order to establish pincer function. This procedure is indicated in cases of bilateral amputations with long forearms or in patients from underdeveloped countries who cannot obtain prosthetic appliances.

Longitudinal Failure of Formation

Longitudinal deficiencies can be divided into preaxial (radial), postaxial (ulnar), and central types. The central type consists of absence of the second, third, and fourth rays.

Phocomelia. Phocomelia is abnormal proximal-to-distal limb growth and is characterized by an intercalary or intersegmental deficiency. The incidence of phocomelia is 1% of all upper extremity congenital deformities. There are 3 main types: complete, proximal, and distal. The complete type refers to a hand that is attached to the trunk. The proximal type is characterized by absence of the arm, with the forearm articulating directly with the trunk. The distal type is described as direct articulation between the hand and arm secondary to absence of the forearm. The absent portion of the limb varies but typically involves a segment between the hand and shoulder. In the past, ingestion of the teratogen thalidomide during the first trimester of pregnancy was linked to phocomelia; recent cases are sporadic. Phocomelia is associated with radial-ray deficiency of the opposite extremity, cleft lip, and cleft palate. Management is nonsurgical.

Radial Deficiency. Radial deficiency or radial club hand is a preaxial deformity that results from partial or complete absence of the radius. It is the most common type of longitudinal failure of formation and is characterized by a radially deviated wrist and a short forearm (Fig. 6.42). Partial or complete absence of the thumb and radial wrist may be present as well. The ulnar is typically short and bowed. Incidence of radial club hand is

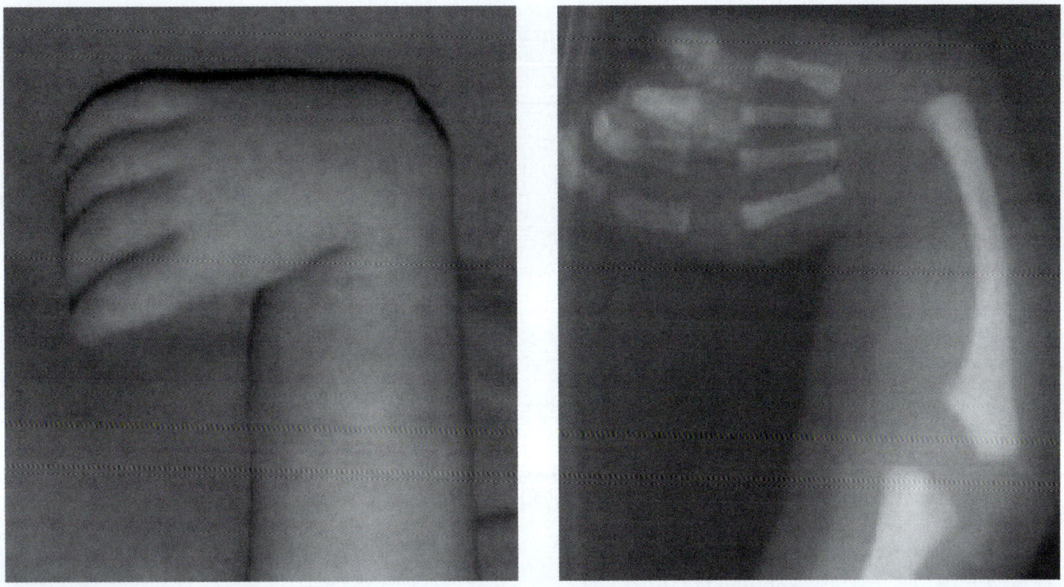

FIGURE 6.42 **Radial club hand. (A) Clinical and (B) radiographic appearance of type 4 radial club hand. (*Source:* Gallant GC, Bora FW Jr. Congenital deformities of the upper extremity. *J Am Acad Orthop Surg* 1996;4:162–171.)**

1 in 30,000 births; 50% of cases are bilateral, and there is a slightly higher occurrence in males. Familial cases occur in patients with Holt-Oram syndrome, thrombocytopenia absent syndrome, Fanconi anemia, and VACTERL (Table 6.50). Severity is graded 1 through 4 and is based on radiographic findings (Table 6.51). Distinguishing between complete and partial absence cannot occur until the age of 3 years because in radial deficiency, ossification of the radius is delayed.

The goals of surgery are to balance the wrist on the forearm, maintain motion of the wrist and digits, enhance forearm growth, correct radial deviation of the wrist, reconstruct the thumb, and improve overall function of the forearm. Procedures that aim to improve both function and cosmesis include forearm lengthening, thumb reconstruction, index pollicization, and carpal centralization. Prior to any surgery, management must begin with serial casting and stretching of the soft tissues. For type 1 deformity, thumb reconstruction is the primary goal of surgery. For types 2, 3, and 4, treatment includes carpal centralization, thumb reconstruction, and lengthening of the ulna via distraction osteosynthesis.

Ulnar Deficiency. Ulnar deficiency is a postaxial deformity that is partial or complete absence of the ulna.

TABLE 6.50 Syndromes associated with radial deficiency

Syndrome	*Associated Anomalies*	*Inheritance*
VACTERL	Vertebral, anal, cardiac, tracheoesophageal, renal/radial, limb	Sporadic
Holt-Oram	Cardiac; other upper extremity deformities	Autosomal dominant
Fanconi anemia	Pancytopenia	Autosomal recessive
TAR	Thrombocytopenia, anemia; radius absent but thumb present	Autosomal recessive
Trisomy 13	Multiple	Sporadic
Trisomy 18		
Nager, Rothmund-Thomson	Craniofacial	Variable depending on syndrome

TAR, thrombocytopenia-absent-radius

Adapted from James MA, Bednar M. Deformities of the wrist and forearm. In: Green DP, Hotchkiss RN, Pederson WC, Wolfe SW (eds.), *Green's Operative Hand Surgery*, 5th ed. Philadelphia: Elsevier, 2005;1469–1526.

TABLE 6.51 Bayne classification of radial deficiency

Type	Thumb	Carpus	Distal Radius	Proximal Radius
1	Hypoplastic or absent	Absent, hypoplastic or coalition	> 2 mm shorter than ulna	Normal, radioulnar synostosis, or congenital dislocation of the radial head
2	Hypoplastic or absent	Absent, hypoplastic or coalition	Hypoplasia	Hypoplasia
3	Hypoplastic or absent	Absent, hypoplastic or coalition	Physis absent	Variable hypoplasia
4	Hypoplastic or absent	Absent, hypoplastic or coalition	Absent	Absent

Adapted from James MA, Bednar M. Deformities of the wrist and forearm. In: Green DP, Hotchkiss RN, Pederson WC, Wolfe SW (eds.), *Green's Operative Hand Surgery*, 5th ed. Philadelphia: Elsevier, 2005;1469–1526.

With an incidence of 1 in every 100,000 live births, it is much less common than radial club hand. Unlike radial deficiency, ulnar deficiency occurs sporadically and is not associated with systemic disorders. It is, however, associated with other musculoskeletal abnormalities such as phocomelia, proximal femoral focal deficiency, fibular deficiency, and scoliosis. Unilateral involvement is more common than bilateral deficiency. Ulnar deficiency is characterized by hypoplasia of the entire upper extremity and deformity of the elbow, wrist, and hand. Missing digits occurs in 90% of hands; 70% have thumb deformities and 30% have an associated syndactyly. Thumb abnormalities include narrowing of the first web space to complete absence of the thumb and represent a strong predictor of function. There are 4 types, the most common being partial absence of the ulna (Table 6.52). A recently proposed classification is based on abnormalities of the first web space.

Management of ulnar deficiency depends on forearm stability, function, and ROM; children with ulnar club hand have better function than those with radial club hand. Mild deformity is managed with stretching and serial casting. Elbow instability or restricted ROM secondary to radial head dislocation can be treated by excising the proximal radius and creating a 1-bone forearm with the distal radius and proximal ulna. Forearm rotation is compensated for by shoulder motion. Derotational osteotomy of the humerus may improve forearm position in patients with radiohumeral synostosis and an internal rotation deformity. Other treatment options address existing codeformities such as thumb hypoplasia and syndactyly.

TABLE 6.52 Classification of ulnar deficiency

Type	Features
1	Hypoplastic ulna
2	Partial absence of the ulna
3	Complete absence of the ulna
4	Radiohumeral synostosis

Central Hand Deficiency. Central hand deficiency or cleft hand is characterized by failure of formation of at least one central ray of the hand: the index, long, or ring finger. During fetal development, central ray differentiation does not occur at the time of the radial and ulnar rays (thumb and small finger respectively). Cleft hand is traditionally divided into 2 main types: typical and atypical. Currently there is some controversy regarding the mechanism of failure between the 2 types. Typical cleft hand is thought to be a result of digital ray fusion. Atypical cleft hand is thought to be a result of the body's attempt to regenerate structures after necrosis of mesenchymal tissue has arrested their development. The incidence of cleft hand is 4% of all congenital upper extremity deformities.

Typical cleft hand can be clinically described as a V-shaped defect of the hand, most frequently due to absence of phalanges. It is usually bilateral and is passed on as an X-linked dominant trait with incomplete penetrance. Syndactyly of the thumb–index web space or ring–small web space may also be present, and the foot may be involved as well. Other associated anomalies include cleft lip and cleft palate. Atypical cleft hand is actually a type of symbrachydactyly that affects the central 3 rays. Symbrachydactyly includes hand deformities ranging from short digits (brachydactyly) that may be joined (syndactyly) to the absence of the central fingers or rays. In atypical cleft hand, the index, long, and ring metacarpals are present, but the fingers are not, resulting in a U-shaped cleft. Atypical cleft hand deformities are unilateral, occur sporadically, do not involve the foot, and are not associated with systemic disorders. Symbrachydactyly and subsequently atypical cleft hand are, however, associated with Poland syndrome. Poland syndrome is characterized by an ipsilateral thoracic wall defect, most commonly absence of the sternocostal part of the pectoralis major muscle.

The deficiencies in symbrachydactyly and Poland syndrome are thought to result from inadequacy of the blood supply during fetal limb development. Poland syndrome is associated with proximal arterial insufficiency involving the subclavian or axillary artery; distal arterial insufficiency affects development of the apical ectodermal ridge, resulting in symbrachydactyly. Treatment is typically nonoperative; correction of syndactyly followed by surgical closure is indicated in patients with severe deformity.

Failure of Differentiation

Syndactyly. Syndactyly is defined as failure of digital separation secondary to abnormal interconnections between adjacent fingers. It is one of the most common congenital hand anomalies, with an incidence of 2 to 3 per 10,000 live births. Fifty percent of cases are bilateral. The most common site of involvement is between the long and ring fingers. Eighty percent of cases are sporadic, although familial inheritance does occur. Associated anomalies include polydactyly, constriction bands, brachydactyly, cardiac abnormalities, toe webbing, and spine deformities. Etiology is thought to be secondary to failure of separation of the apical ectodermal ridge. Classification is based on the degree of interconnections present and the extent of their involvement. Complete syndactyly occurs when the interconnection extends the entire length of the adjacent fingers. Incomplete syndactyly describes interconnections that end proximal to the fingertip. Simple syndactyly involves soft tissue; complex syndactyly refers to additional bony involvement. Complicated syndactyly occurs in conjunction with other congenital anomalies such as Apert or Poland syndrome. Apert syndrome is characterized by severe syndactyly in conjunction with craniosynostosis, ankylosis of the interphalangeal joints, hypertelorism, flattened facies, and mental retardation. Early treatment minimizes progressive bone deformity. Surgical correction is done over several sequential surgeries that require full-thickness skin grafts. Guidelines are as follows:

- *Timing*—Border digits and digits of unequal length early (3 to 6 months of age)
- *Commissure reconstruction*—Avoid skin graft
- *Number of digits separated*—Never operate on both sides of digit during single setting
- *Skin graft*—Almost always necessary except in incomplete syndactyly
- *Dressings*—Bulky dressing above the elbow reinforced with plaster

Because of potential abnormalities of the neurovascular bundles, only one side of a digit is corrected at each procedure in order to minimize vascular insult. Subsequent separation of the opposite side is done 3 to 6 months after the original procedure.

Symbrachydactyly. Symbrachydactyly refers to patterns of digital loss that share certain features but also have characteristics similar to simple transverse absence of digits. The main difference between symbrachydactyly and transverse absence of digits is the presence of digital remnants or nubbins in the former. Symbrachydactyly can occur sporadically or in conjunction with syndromes such as Poland syndrome. The central deficiency form of symbrachydactyly is known as atypical cleft hand. Treatment is conservative; in cases of severe functional impairment, digital reconstruction via microvascular toe transfer is considered.

Symphalangism. Symphalangism is the failure of interphalangeal joint development. Patients with symphalangism lack skin creases and motion at the interphalangeal joints, and radiographically, they appear as decreased joint space or ankylosed joints. The incidence of symphalangism is 1% of all congenital upper extremity deformities and primarily affects Caucasians. It is passed as an autosomal dominant trait and is associated with syndactyly and anomalies of the foot. Management is nonsurgical. In cases of severe functional deficits, patients may benefit from an arthrodesis in a more functional position.

Camptodactyly. Camptodactyly describes a painless, progressive flexion contracture of the proximal interphalangeal joint of the small finger (Fig. 6.43). The distal interphalangeal and MCP joints are not involved but may develop compensatory deformities. Incidence is less than 1% of the population; most cases are sporadic, and two thirds of cases are bilateral. Treatment begins with splinting and stretching of the finger. If the flexion deformity at the proximal interphalangeal joint is greater than 60 degrees, surgery may be an option and typically involves release of contracted volar soft tissue structures.

Clinodactyly. Clinodactyly is deviation of a finger in the coronal plane and is more common than camptodactyly. It typically involves radial deviation of the

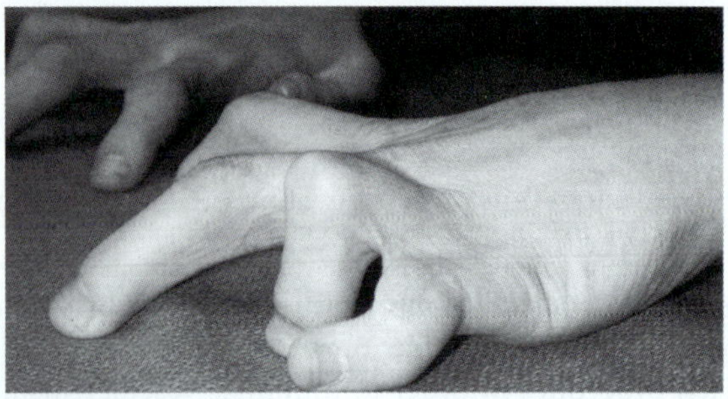

FIGURE 6.43 Severe ring-finger camptodactyly. (*Source:* Berger RA, Weiss A-PC (eds.). *Hand Surgery*, Vol. 2. Philadelphia: Lippincott Williams & Wilkins, 2004;1478.)

middle phalanx of the small finger, which causes the distal interphalangeal joint to appear angulated. Clinodactyly can involve multiple digits and is often associated with delta-shaped middle phalanges. Incidence in healthy children is from 1% to 20%. It is more common in males and is often bilateral. It is often passed as an autosomal dominant trait but can also occur sporadically. Familial clinodactyly does not occur in conjunction with systemic disorders. Clinodactyly can be a clinical manifestation of many chromosomal abnormalities and genetic disorders; the prevalence of clinodactyly in patients with Down syndrome ranges from 35% to 79%. Clinodactyly of the thumb is a common manifestation of Apert syndrome, diastrophic dwarfism, triphalangeal thumbs, and Rubinstein-Taybi syndrome. Treatment is conservative.

Kirner Deformity. Kirner deformity refers to volar curvature of the distal phalanx. It most commonly involves the small finger but is not clinically apparent until 8 to 12 years of age; it is usually bilateral and can be sporadic or transmitted as an autosomal dominant trait. Incidence is 1 in 410 live births and more common in females. Kirner deformity has been associated with Silver, Turner, and Cornelia de Lange syndromes. Osteotomy is reserved for severe deformities.

Delta Phalanx. A delta phalanx is a triangular bone with a C-shaped epiphysis. The abnormal shape of the physis leads to progressive angular deformity. It typically appears as an extra phalanx of the thumb or the middle phalanx of the small finger. The involved small finger or thumb typically angulates toward the central axis of the hand. The incidence of delta phalanx is unclear. It is often bilateral and is more common in males. It can occur in conjunction with polydactyly and syndactyly. Surgery is considered only in cases of severe cosmetic or functional deformity and consists of a closing-wedge osteotomy and partial excision of the physis.

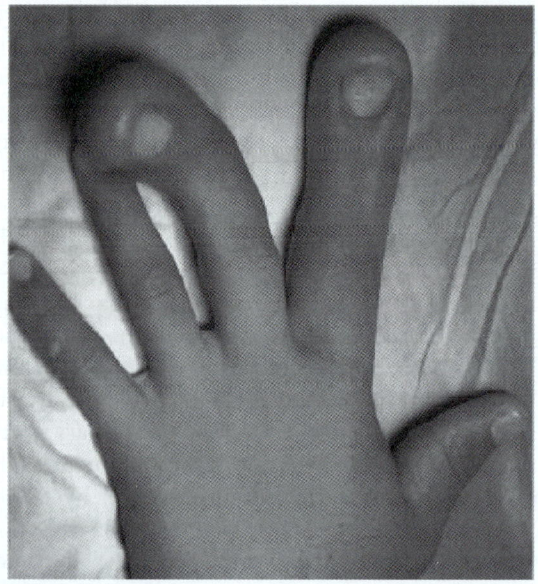

FIGURE 6.44 Macrodactyly of the left index and long fingers. (*Source:* Metin A, Sadan A, Ercetin O. Surgical treatment of macrodactyly in older children and adults. *J Hand Surg Am* 2004;29: 1010–1019.)

Macrodactyly. Macrodactyly occurs as a result of excessive growth of the soft tissue and osseous structures of the involved digit and can involve one or multiple digits (Fig. 6.44). It is often an isolated deformity but is also associated with Klippel-Trenaunay-Weber syndrome and neurofibromatosis. Klippel-Trenaunay-Weber syndrome is characterized by varicose veins, hemangiomas, and limb hypertrophy. Macrodactyly may be progressive or static. Progressive macrodactyly is more common and is apparent during childhood. The affected finger or fingers stiffen as they enlarge. Growth ceases when the child has reached skeletal maturity. Static macrodactyly occurs when there is an abnormally large digit at birth that grows proportionately until skeletal maturity. Treatment consists of observation.

Synostosis. Fusion of bones that normally divide is described as synostosis. It can present as an isolated abnormality or as a manifestation of a syndrome or disorder such as ulnar deficiency; it is, however, not usually associated with systemic disorders with the exception of fetal alcohol syndrome and trisomy 13 and 21. Synostosis most frequently occurs at the elbow and can present as an isolated entity or in conjunction with

TABLE 6.53 Blauth classification and treatment of thumb hypoplasia

Type	Features	Treatment
I Short thumb	Minor generalized hypoplasia; associated with Fanconi and Holt-Oram syndromes	Augmentation
II Adducted thumb	Absence of intrinsic thenar muscles Narrowing of first web space Ulnar collateral ligament insufficiency	Opponensplasty Release of first web space Ulnar collateral ligament reconstruction
III Abducted thumb	Similar to type II plus extrinsic muscle and tendon abnormalities A. Stable CMC joint B. Unstable CMC joint	A. Contracture release, reconstruction B. Pollicization
IV Pouce flottant	"Floating thumb" is short and unstable and connected to the hand by a stalk that contains the neurovascular bundle	Pollicization
V Absent thumb	Absence	Pollicization

Adapted from Kozin SH. Current concepts review: Upper extremity congenital anomalies. *J Bone Joint Surg Am* 2003;85:1564–1576; Gallant GC, Bora FW Jr. Congenital deformities of the upper extremity. *J Am Acad Orthop Surg* 1996;4:162–171.

a radial head dislocation. Patients with ulnar deficiency may have a concomitant radiohumeral synostosis. Metacarpal transverse synostosis is bilateral in 60% to 80% of cases and occurs most frequently between the small and ring fingers. Clinical presentation is often delayed because of compensatory motion at the wrist and shoulder. Rotational osteotomy is reserved for patients with deformities that significantly restrict function.

Polydactyly. Polydactyly can present on the radial or ulnar side of the limb. Radial or preaxial polydactyly occurs more frequently in Caucasians; postaxial polydactyly is more common among blacks and is often passed as an autosomal dominant trait. The supernumerary digit can be rudimentary and pedunculated or well developed. The former can be removed by strangulating its vascular supply with a suture tied around its base; a well-developed digit must be removed in the operating room. Duplications of the thumb tends to occur in Caucasians; most cases are sporadic, unilateral, and do not occur in conjunction with other systemic conditions. Preaxial polydactyly most frequently presents as a duplication of the proximal and distal phalanges that simultaneously articulate with a bifid metacarpal head. Surgical correction involves using the spare osseous and soft tissue structures to reconstruct a functional thumb with normal alignment.

Thumb Hypoplasia. The incidence of thumb hypoplasia is 4%. Occurrence can be sporadic, genetic, or part of a syndrome, especially those of the cardiovascular system, the gastrointestinal tract, and the spine. Thumb hypoplasia most commonly occurs in conjunction with radial deficiency and can be divided into 5 types (Table 6.53; Fig. 6.45). A hypoplastic or short thumb does not reach the level of the proximal interphalangeal joint of the index finger. Treatment is based on the type of deformity present. The key structure that defines if a thumb is reconstructable is the presence of a stable basal joint. Thumb reconstruction is contraindicated in the absence of the CMC joint; in this case, thumb restoration is best achieved by pollicization.

Thumb Duplication. The incidence of thumb polydactyly is approximately 8 per 100,000 births. It affects Caucasian and Asian populations, is typically unilateral, and occurs more commonly in males. Most cases are sporadic, although there is an autosomal dominant variant associated with the triphalangeal thumb. Both the radial and ulnar duplicates are hypoplastic. Wassel classified thumb polydactyly into 7 types, the most common being type IV: duplication of the proximal phalanx (Fig. 6.46). Treatment depends on the type of deformity present.

Treatment of the type IV thumb requires reconstruction of the ulnar collateral ligament.

Trigger Thumb. The incidence of trigger thumb is approximately 2%, and roughly 30% of cases resolve by 12 months of age. The majority of cases are bilateral and sporadic. Trigger thumb is caused by contracture of the A1 pulley, thus limiting the gliding of the FPL. Trigger thumbs are not congenital; they are a result of an acquired discrepancy between an enlarged FPL tendon and a tight flexor tendon sheath. Patients typically present with a fixed flexion contracture of the interphalangeal joint and pain at the volar aspect of the MCP joint. Attempted extension may produce a

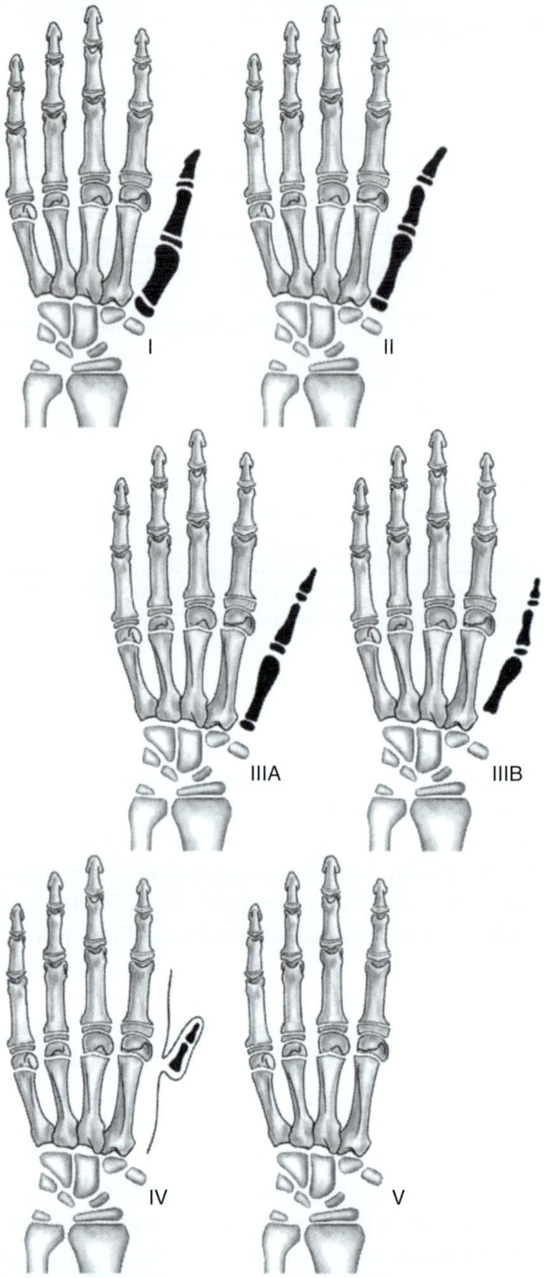

FIGURE 6.45 Classification of thumb hypoplasia. (*Source:* Berger RA, Weiss A-PC (eds.). *Hand Surgery*, Vol. 2. Philadelphia: Lippincott Williams & Wilkins, 2004;1446.)

palpable click. If triggering continues beyond 1 year of age, release of the A1 pulley is recommended.

Constriction Bands. A constriction band is an amniotic band that forms a circumferential skin crease around a digit, forearm, or arm that can lead to vascular and lymphatic insufficiency. Incidence of constriction bands is 1 in 15,000 births and is often sporadic. Most cases are associated with other congenital upper extremity anomalies, including brachydactyly, syndactyly, and hypoplastic digits; 40% of patients have congenital abnormalities involving other regions of the skeleton, such as cleft lip and cleft palate and clubfoot. There are 4 types of constriction bands; distal constriction bands are the most common and most frequently involve the central digits.

Madelung's Deformity. Madelung deformity is a growth disturbance of the volar and ulnar distal radial epiphysis. The resulting deformity is characterized by volar and ulnar angulation of the articular surface of the distal radius, premature fusion of the ulnar half of the radial physis, a short ulna, and a short, bowed radius. The carpus subsequently becomes lodged between the ulna and distal radius, and the ulnar head subluxates dorsally. The majority of patients present between the ages of 6 to 13 years. The incidence is 2% of all congenital upper extremity deformities. It is more common in females and is often bilateral. Although the etiology of the deformity is unclear, it has been shown that it can be passed as an autosomal dominant trait. Symptoms include pain and limited ROM secondary to ulnocarpal impingement. Treatment is indicated only in the presence of pain and begins with splinting, which may permanently alleviate symptoms. Surgery is indicated in patients with persistent pain and involves radial osteotomy in conjunction with an ulnar shortening osteotomy or radial osteotomy with distraction lengthening.

Congenital Radial Head Dislocation. Congenital radial head dislocation (CRHD) is the most common congenital deformity of the elbow and is typically bilateral. The etiology of CRHD is not known, and occurrence can be sporadic or familial. Clinical presentation is often delayed because the lack of forearm rotation is well compensated by the shoulder and wrist. Patients typically present after a perceived elbow injury and complain of restricted motion and prominence. Unilateral CRHD can be difficult to distinguish from chronic traumatic dislocation. Diagnosis is confirmed with radiographs. The radial head is not aligned with the capitellum, the radial head is misshapen, the capitellum is dysplastic, and ulnar variance is positive. Ultrasound can be used to visualize the unossified dislocated radial head in infants. Classification of CDRH is based on the direction of dislocation. Most dislocations are anterior (47%); 43% are posterior, and 10% are lateral.

CDRH is associated with congenital radioulnar synostosis, Klinefelter, Cornelia de Lange, Ehlers-Danlos, and nail-patella syndromes. Most children are asymptomatic. Pain secondary to degenerative changes

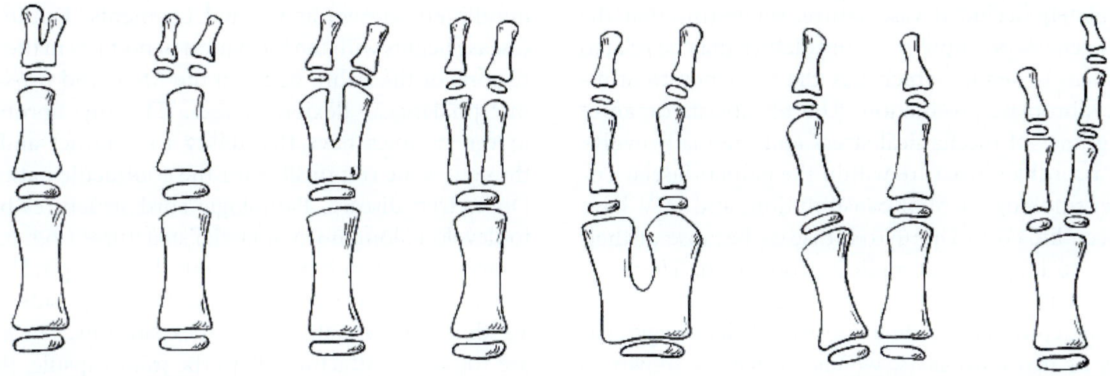

FIGURE 6.46 Wassel classification of thumb polydactyly. (*Source:* Gallant GG, Bora FW Jr. Congenital deformities of the upper extremity. *J Am Acad Orthop Surg* 1996;4:162–171.)

may develop in adolescence or adulthood, which can be treated with radial head excision.

Trigger Finger. Trigger finger is significantly less common than trigger thumb and usually does not resolve with release of the A1 pulley. This deformity is thought to result from abnormal associations and connections between the FDP and FDS or thickening of the A2 and A3 pulleys.

Arthrogryposis. Arthrogryposis is a congenital syndrome of nonprogressive joint contractures secondary to failure of motion in utero. The etiology of arthrogryposis is not known but is thought to be due to neurologic or muscular abnormalities, vascular compromise, maternal morbidity, or restricted space in utero. Arthrogryposis varies in presentation, number of joints affected, and severity. Classic arthrogryposis or amyoplasia is the most common form of the condition and is distinguished by symmetric limb positions. The upper extremities are internally rotated and adducted at the shoulder and extended at the elbows. The forearms are pronated, the wrists are flexed, and the hands are in ulnar deviation. The digits are characterized by flexion contractures, and the thumb is flexed and adducted in the palm. Distal arthrogryposis is limited to the distal part of the extremities. The hand is in a clenched fist, and the digits deviate ulnarly. Distal arthrogryposis responds to early therapy and splinting. Arthrogryposis can also occur in conjunction with other syndromes, including Larsens, multiple pterygium, Beal (contractual arachnodactyly), and Freeman-Sheldon (whistling face syndrome).

Treatment must be individualized, with the goal of independent self-feeding and perineal care. Early therapy includes alternating between passive joint motion and splinting. Static progressive splinting has been successfully used to decrease the degree of contracture. Surgery includes a combination of soft tissue release, tendon transfer, and osteotomies.

XVI. DUPUYTREN CONTRACTURE

Epidemiology. Dupuytren disease occurs sporadically or can be inherited as an autosomal dominant trait. Severity of disease and age at presentation may be a result of variable penetrance of gene expression in familial cases. It is prevalent in certain Caucasian populations, particularly Scottish, Irish, Scandinavian, and Australian. It is more common in males than females (7:1 ratio) and typically presents after the age of 40; less than 10% of patients are under the age of 40 years. Patients present upon noticing a nodule or development of a progressive palmar cord. Dupuytren disease is not associated with pain; patients often seek medical attention only when joint motion has been significantly compromised. There is often pitting of the skin and nodule formation near the distal palmar crease. As the nodule enlarges, cords become palpable. The ring and small fingers are often the first digits affected, and the process typically begins in the palm and spreads distally to involve the digits.

Pathogenesis. The pathogenesis of Dupuytren disease is based on 2 types of cells that are present in the diseased tissue: the myofibroblast and the fibroblast. The myofibroblast is primarily responsible for the development of Dupuytren disease. It has characteristics of a smooth muscle cell and a fibroblast and can be found in the palmar fascial nodules that are characteristic of Dupuytren disease. Dupuytren fascia has a high concentration of type III collagen, a high type-III-to-type-I collagen ratio, and increased amounts of total collagen. Fibroblasts are abundant in Dupuytren tissue, especially around partially or completely occluded vasculature, suggesting that the pathogenesis of Dupuytren contracture may be related to tissue ischemia, which has the tendency to stimulate fibroblast production. The fibroblasts organize along lines of mechanical stress and gradually evolve into a cordlike structure within the palmar fascia. Tobacco smoking, alcohol consumption, and HIV have all been linked to Dupuytren disease because of their ability to increase free radical production. There are 2 forms of diseased tissue that develop: the nodule and the cord. The nodule consists of dense aggregations of myofibroblasts, which have been shown to actively contract. Cords are composed of highly organized collagen, much like tendons, and do not contain myofibroblasts.

Anatomy of the Palm. The palmar aponeurosis is a thin sheet of fascia that organizes distally into pretendinous bands that run toward the digits. Part of the pretendinous bands bifurcate into 2 parts that dive deep into the palm and simultaneously wrap around the metacarpal head and twist 90 degrees. These woven extensions of the pretendinous band are known as the spiral bands. The natatory ligaments have fibers that attach to the flexor tendon sheath at the MCP joint; other fibers run in the coronal plane to weave into the skin and fascia of the web space. Fibers passing volar to the neurovascular bundle are called Grayson ligaments. Fibers that run dorsal to the neurovascular bundle are known as Cleland ligaments. Dupuytren disease begins with the formation of nodules in the fatty regions of the palm, between the MCP and proximal interphalangeal flexion creases. The myofibroblasts in the nodules have the ability to contract and are thought to be responsible for the contractile nature of Dupuytren disease. Pathologic cord structures begin to develop along normal fascial structures (Fig. 6.47). Pretendinous bands become central cords, spiral bands become spiral cords. Dupuytren disease spreads along a 3-dimensional path of fascial expansions. The cords are rooted by attachments to the joint capsule, flexor tendon sheath, interosseous fascia, periosteum, and skin. These fascial attachments blend together and intertwine within the neurovascular bundle of an involved finger or web space. As the pathologic cords contract, the pathway becomes more linear, causing a flexion contracture of the adjacent joints; the entrapped neurovascular bundle spirals around the Dupuytren cord and is pulled toward the midline of the finger. The spiral cord runs underneath the neurovascular bundle and raises it to a more superficial plane, making it susceptible to injury during surgery. The greatest indicator of superficial and central displacement of the neurovascular bundle is contracture at the PIP joint. The pretendinous cord causes contracture at the MCP joint; the spiral cord is anchored to the middle phalanx and causes severe PIP contractures. The natatory cord is responsible for web space contracture, and the

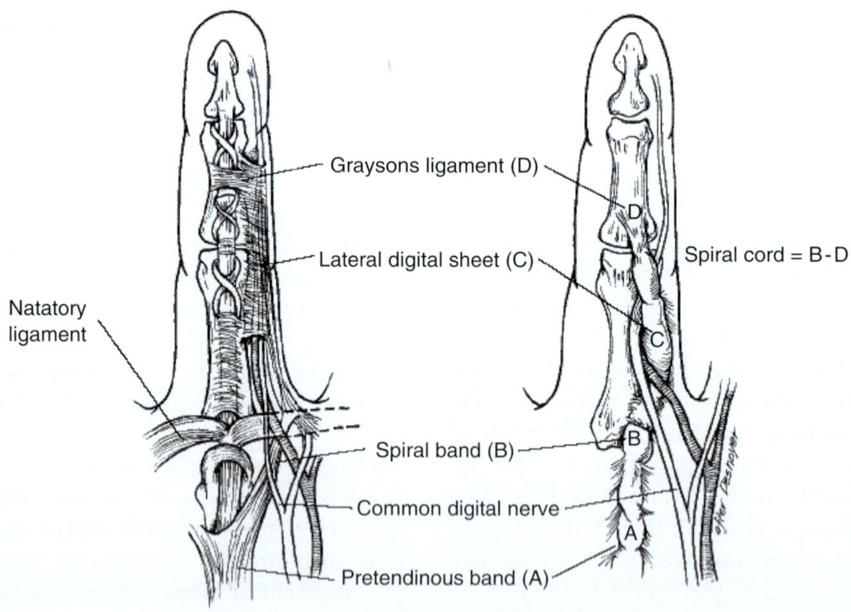

FIGURE 6.47 **Normal and pathologic anatomy of the digital palmar fascia. Left: Normal anatomy. Right: Development of a spiral cord from 4 palmar fascial structures: the pretendinous band, the spiral band, the lateral digital sheet, and the Grayson ligament. The involved digital nerve winds around the cord and is drawn toward the midline of the finger. (*Source:* Benson LS, Williams CS, Kahle M. Dupuytren's contracture. *J Am Acad Orthop Surg* 1998;6:24–35.)**

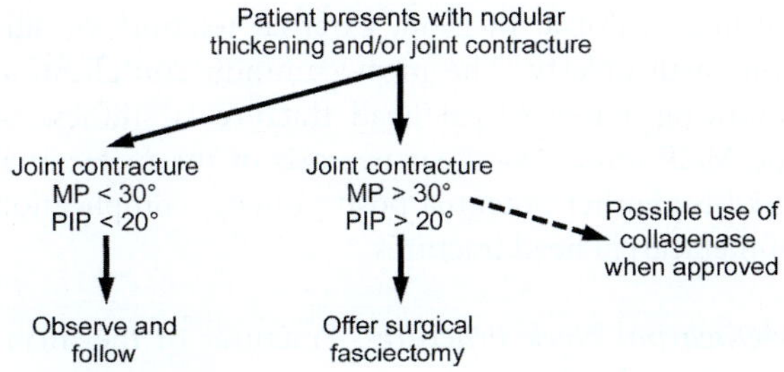

FIGURE 6.48 **Algorithm for evaluation and treatment of Dupuytren contracture. (*Source:* Berger RA, Weiss A-PC (eds.). *Hand Surgery*, Vol. 2. Philadelphia: Lippincott Williams & Wilkins, 2004;1097.)**

retrovascular cord contributes to contractures at the DIP and PIP joints.

Surgery. The goal of surgery for Dupuytren disease is to improve hand function by excising pathologic tissue. Nonoperative management with splints, corticosteroid injections, and therapy has been anecdotal. Surgery is indicated when contractures cause functional impairment. The "table top" test is a good guideline for determining if surgical intervention is necessary (Fig. 6.48). A positive test is when the patient cannot place the palm of the involved hand completely flush against a flat, hard surface. The test correlates with MCP joint contractures greater than 30 to 40 degrees. An MCP joint contracture greater than 40 degrees warrants surgery. Surgery is recommended when there is any PIP joint contracture because correction and maintenance of PIP joint flexion deformity is difficult. Surgery for Dupuytren disease involves selective fasciectomy where all diseased fascia in the palm and finger are resected. Skin is either excised and replaced with a full-thickness skin graft, closed primarily, or left open to close by secondary intention. Therapy is initiated within 2 to 5 days postoperatively. The most common complication following this complex procedure is hematoma formation, which can result in recurrence or complex regional pain syndrome, also known as a "flare" reaction. The overall success rate is approximately 80% with a recurrence rate of 10% per year.

XVII. FRACTURES AND DISLOCATIONS

Compartment Syndrome. The forearm consists of three compartments (Fig. 6.49): dorsal, volar, and mobile wad. These compartments have interconnections between them; therefore, release of the volar compartment may decompress the dorsal compartments as

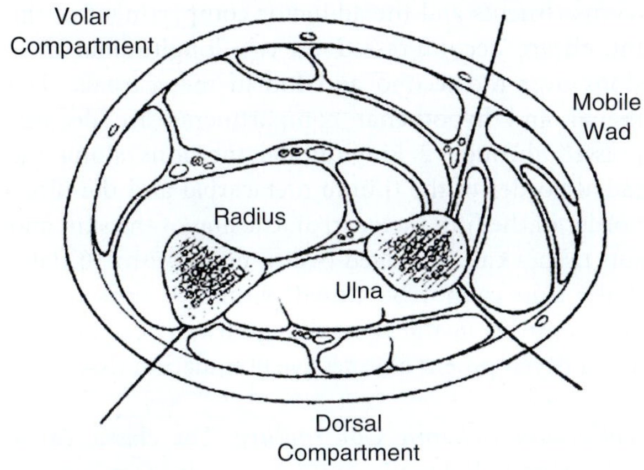

FIGURE 6.49 **Compartments of the forearm. (*Source:* Seiler JG III, Olvey SP. Compartment syndrome of the hand. *J Am Soc Surg Hand* 2003;3:184–198.)**

well. It is important to release both the superficial and deep volar compartments. After volar decompression of the forearm, pressures of the dorsal compartment and mobile wad are remeasured and dorsal fasciotomy is performed only if pressures remain elevated. Volar forearm decompression begins just proximal to the medial epicondyle and across the antecubital fossa. It extends distally the volar ulnar forearm and ends with a carpal tunnel release. The dorsal forearm incision begins just distal to the lateral epicondyle and extends down to the midline of the wrist. There are 10 compartments in the hand (Fig. 6.50): 4 dorsal interosseous, 3 volar interosseous, thumb adductor, thenar, and hypothenar. The carpal tunnel is not a true fascial compartment but must be included in the volar decompression. The dorsal and volar interosseous muscle

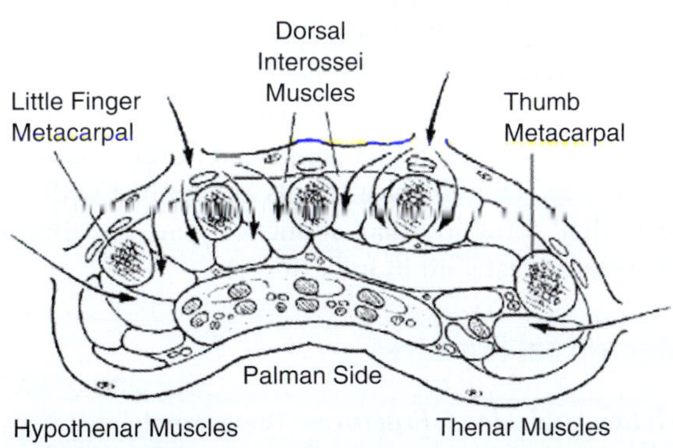

FIGURE 6.50 **Compartments of the hand. (*Source:* Seiler JG III, Olvey SP. Compartment syndrome of the hand. *J Am Soc Surg Hand* 2003;3:184–198.)**

compartments and the adductor compartment of the thumb are decompressed via two longitudinal incisions over the second and fourth metacarpals. The thenar and hypothenar compartments are decompressed through 2 longitudinal incisions along the radial border of the thumb metacarpal and the ulnar border of the fifth metacarpal. Closing of the skin and soft tissues can be staged over a period 5 to 10 days; if the skin cannot be closed within 10 days of the fasciotomy, split-thickness skin graft can be applied to avoid development of excessive granulation tissue.

Volkmann Ischemic Contracture. The classic cause of Volkmann ischemic contracture is displaced supracondylar humerus fractures in children. The sharp, jagged edge of the distal humerus displaces anteriorly and can potentially injure the brachial artery or median nerve by direct contact or by trapping of the neurovascular structures between the bone and surrounding soft tissue. Bleeding and soft tissue swelling can impede venous outflow and lead to elevated compartment pressures and subsequent ischemia if it is not recognized. Direct trauma to the main vessels can lead to ischemia secondary to insufficient arterial supply. Volkmann ischemic contracture can also be a result of tightly or improperly applied dressings and casts, snake bites, prolonged compression, crush injuries, and burns. The classic deformity that develops is a result of ischemic insult to the structures in the deep volar compartment of the forearm. The hand has an intrinsic minus deformity, and the wrist is held in flexion. Sensory abnormalities involving the median and/or ulnar nerves may also be present. Treatment includes skin and soft tissue releases, tendon lengthenings, resection of scarred muscles, nerve exploration and/or reconstruction, muscle slides, and tendon transfers.

Functional Splinting. Fractures of the hand and wrist should be splinted in the position of function and allow for maximum ROM of uninvolved joints. The wrist is immobilized in 20 to 30 degrees of extension, the MCP joints are flexed to 60 to 70 degrees of flexion, and the interphalangeal joints are placed in full extension or left free. Thumb spica splints are applied with the first MCP joint in volar abduction and the thumb interphalangeal joint in full extension.

Metacarpal Fractures

Metacarpal Head Fractures. Metacarpal head fractures are uncommon and usually involve the articular surface. They are usually the result of direct trauma or an axial load and most commonly involve the index finger. Most fractures are comminuted. Intraarticular fractures can also occur in conjunction with dorsal MCP joint dislocations. Management includes ORIF through a dorsal incision, external fixation, or silicone arthroplasty. The most common complication following a metacarpal head fracture is stiffness of the MCP joint. Avascular necrosis of the metacarpal head is another potential posttraumatic complication of metacarpal head fractures.

Metacarpal Neck Fractures. Fractures of the metacarpal neck (boxer fractures) are common and frequently involve the ring and small metacarpals (Fig. 6.51). They are usually the result of altercations or punching a clenched fist into a wall. The fracture usually results in apex dorsal angulation. Management is based on the extent of angulation in the sagittal plane, presence of a rotational deformity, and the metacarpals involved. Sagittal plane angulation can be radiographically determined by measuring the angle between a line along the longitudinal axis of the metacarpal shaft and a line from the center of the metacarpal head to the fracture site or by measuring the angle formed by the intersection of the tangentials to the proximal and distal fragments. Presence of a rotational deformity is indicated if there is a disruption in the natural cascade of the nails toward the scaphoid when the fingers form a fist.

The CMC joints of the small and ring digits have 20 to 30 degrees of motion and can compensate for angulation of 30 degrees following a metacarpal neck fracture. The index and long finger CMC joints are not as mobile; as a result, angulation greater than 10 or 15 degrees requires reduction of the index and long metacarpals. No degree of rotational deformity

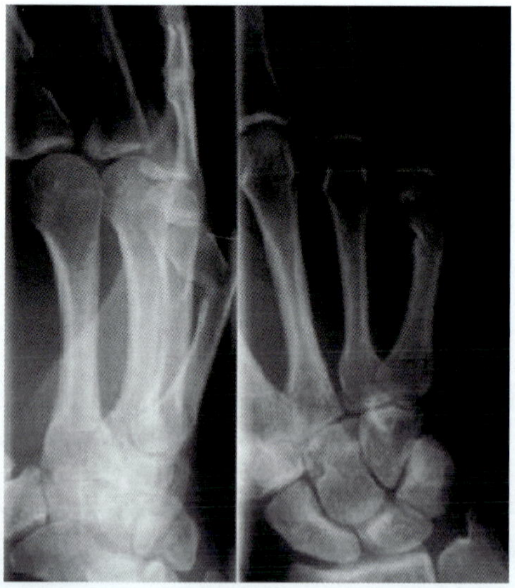

FIGURE 6.51 Metacarpal neck fracture involving the small finger. (*Source:* Weinstein LP, Hanel DP. Metacarpal fractures. *J Am Soc Surg Hand* 2002;2:168–179.)

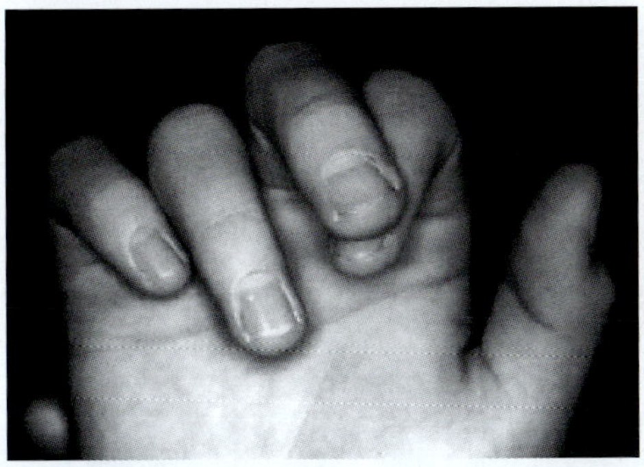

FIGURE 6.52 **Rotational deformity resulting from a metacarpal neck fracture. (*Source:* Morgan WJ, Slowman LS. Acute hand and wrist injuries in athletes: Evaluation and management. *J Am Acad Orthop Surg* 2001;9:389–400.)**

is acceptable because it can lead to overlapping of the digits with digital flexion (Fig. 6.52.). Most injuries can be managed by closed reduction and casting. The technique for closed reduction is described by Jahss and consists of longitudinal traction to disimpact the fracture, followed by flexion of both the MCP and PIP joints to 90 degrees. The proximal phalanx acts as a joystick for manipulation of the fractured head because of the tautness of the MCP joint collateral ligaments during flexion. Reduction is established by applying a dorsally directed force with or without a derotational component. Surgery is reserved for grossly displaced, unstable, or open fractures (e.g., fight bite).

Metacarpal Shaft Fractures. Metacarpal shaft fractures occur in 3 patterns: transverse (Fig. 6.53), oblique, and comminuted. Minimally displaced or nondisplaced fractures can be treated with immobilization for 4 to 6 weeks. Displaced or unstable fractures can be treated with closed reduction and casting or pinning, external fixation, or ORIF. Fractures that require reduction include those with excessive apex dorsal angulation (more than 20 degrees for the index and long fingers; more than 30 degrees for the ring and small fingers) and shortening of more than 5 mm flexion. Oblique and comminuted fractures are usually unstable and should be closely monitored with radiographs if treated with closed reduction. Operative management through a dorsal approach is indicated in open fractures, multiple metacarpal fractures, and unstable fracture patterns. Fixation can be achieved via external fixators, Kirschner pins, compression screws, or plating. Common complications include malunion and malrotation, both of which can be treated with corrective osteotomies.

Thumb Metacarpal Fractures. Fractures of the thumb metacarpal shaft most commonly occur at the proximal metaphyseal–diaphyseal junction or involve the articular surface of the thumb metacarpal base. Extraarticular fractures can be successfully managed with closed reduction and immobilization. Reduction is indicated in fractures with more than 30 degrees of angulation or more than 4 mm of shortening. Pinning or ORIF is reserved for grossly displaced and unstable fractures. Intraarticular fractures can subdivided into Bennett and Rolando fractures. Bennett fracture describes an intraarticular thumb metacarpal base fracture with an associated subluxation of the CMC joint (Fig. 6.54). Axial rotation of the basal joint of the thumb is restrained by ligaments, extrinsic tendons, the joint capsule, and geometry of the articular surface. Stability of the CMC joint is provided by 5 ligaments: the anterior (volar) and posterior oblique ligaments, the anterior and posterior intermetacarpal ligaments, and the dorsal radial ligament. Joint compressive forces are high during simple pinch and grasp; therefore, any disruption of the congruency between the articular surfaces following an intraarticular fracture or injury to the soft tissue restraints will result in posttraumatic arthritis. A Bennett fracture occurs when a flexed metacarpal is axially loaded, resulting in a Bennett fragment. The Bennett fragment consists of the volar-ulnar portion of the metacarpal base that remains attached to the anterior oblique ligament. This ligament inserts on the trapezium and maintains the Bennett fragment in place while the remainder of the metacarpal subluxates in a proximal and dorsoradial direction as a result of forces from the adductor pollicis (metacarpal head displaced into palm) and APL (displaced metacarpal rotated into supination). The goal of treatment is to restore joint stability by reattaching the Bennett fragment and to restore the congruity of the articular surface. A Bennett fragment less than 15% to 20% of the articular surface can be managed by closed reduction and pinning. If the fragment involves more than 20% of the joint surface or there is a stepoff of greater than 1 to 2 mm, ORIF is preferred. Rolando fracture classically refers to a T- or Y-shaped fracture-subluxation of the basal joint of the thumb; currently, it includes any comminuted intraarticular fracture in volving the base of the first metacarpal. Treatment goals are similar to those for Bennett fracture. In cases of severe comminution, external fixation and/or bone graft are potential treatment options. Complications of Bennett and Rolando fractures include malunion and posttraumatic arthritis.

Metacarpal Base and CMC Fracture-Dislocations

Small Finger. A reversed Bennet fracture pattern is an intraarticular fracture of the volar-radial base of the small finger metacarpal with an associated dislocation

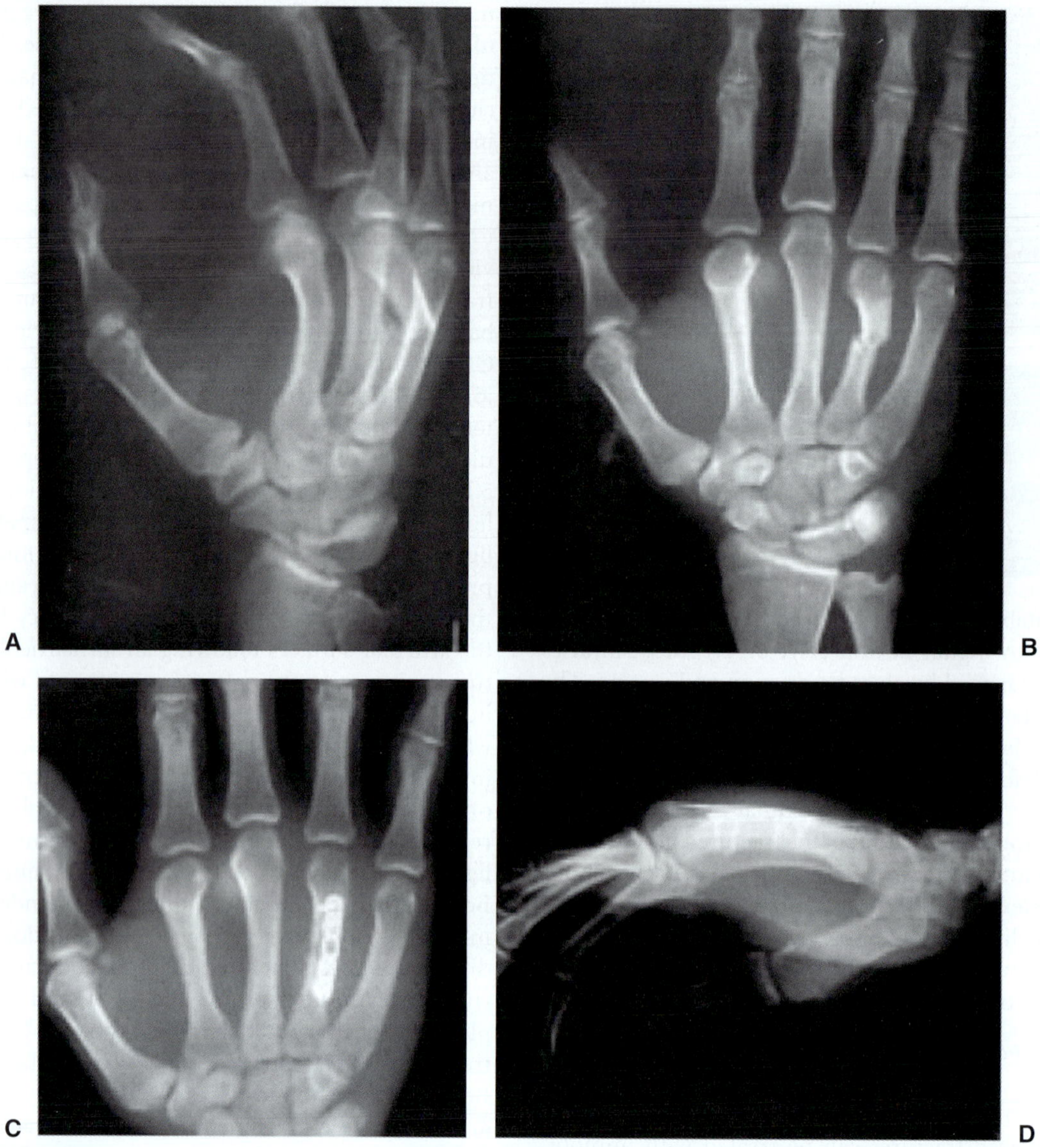

FIGURE 6.53 **(A) Oblique radiograph shows transverse metacarpal shaft fracture and apex dorsal angulation. (B) Posteroanterior film reveals slight comminution and ulnar displacement. (C) Postoperative posteroanterior film obtained after reduction and internal fixation with a plate and screw construct. (D) Lateral radiograph after fixation shows correction of preoperative angulation and appropriate screw length. (*Source:* Kozin SH, Thoder JJ, Lieberman G. Operative treatment of metacarpal and phalangeal shaft fractures. *J Am Acad Orthop Surg* 2000;8:111–121.)**

of the remainder of the metacarpal. This pattern of injury is best visualized with an anterior–posterior radiograph with the forearm pronated 30 degrees from the fully supinated position. Treatment includes closed reduction and pinning or ORIF.

Multiple. Multiple CMC fracture-dislocations occur as a result of a high-energy axial load across the CMC joints that typically require ORIF. Fixation can be achieved with longitudinal pinning extending from the metacarpals into the carpal bones.

Proximal and Middle Phalangeal Fractures

Extraarticular Phalangeal Base Fractures. Extraarticular phalangeal base fractures occur at the metaphyseal–diaphyseal junction and are characterized by dorsal comminution, impaction, and apex volar angulation. Reduction is recommended if angulation is more than 25 degrees and can be maintained with immobilization or pinning. ORIF is reserved for irreducible fractures and fractures that occur in conjunction with other injuries.

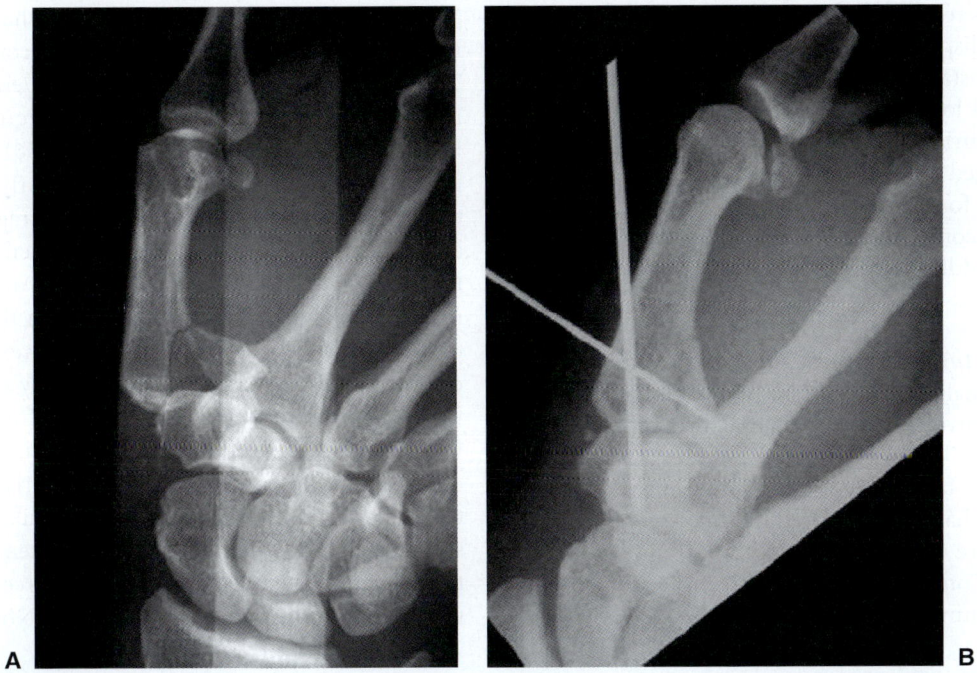

FIGURE 6.54 **Intraarticular fracture of thumb metacarpal base. (A) Fracture-subluxation of a Bennett fracture. (B) Closed reduction and percutaneous fixation. (*Source:* Weinstein LP, Hanel DP. Metacarpal fractures. *J Am Soc Surg Hand* 2002;2:168–179.)**

Intraarticular Phalangeal Base Fractures. Intraarticular fractures occurring at the base of the phalanx fall into 4 categories: nondisplaced, volar/lateral, dorsal lip, and comminuted (pilon). Nondisplaced fractures are managed conservatively with buddy taping. Avulsion fractures of the dorsal base of the middle phalanx (dorsal lip) are a result of detachment of the central slip and typically occur after a PIP joint dislocation following a hyperflexion injury of the PIP joint. Involvement of the articular surface is less than 25% in most cases. The injury can be treated in an extension splint if the fracture is nondisplaced and the joint is congruent and reduced. If the avulsed fragment is displaced more than 2 mm, ORIF is recommended to avoid extensor lag and boutonnière deformity. Fractures of the volar base of the middle phalanx are more common and may be a result of a hyperextension or axial load injury. Hyperextension injuries typically involve less than 30% of the articular surface with little comminution. Axial load injuries often involve most of the articular surface and are comminuted. Volar lip fractures usually result in an unstable PIP joint, depending on the percentage of articular involvement. If there is less than 30% of the articular surface involved, they are typically stable. Fractures with $\geq$ 50% involvement usually result in an unstable joint that subluxates dorsally. Dorsal subluxation is represented by the "V" sign (opening of the joint space) on a lateral radiograph of the PIP joint (Fig. 6.55).

The goal of treatment is restoration of joint stability, which can be accomplished by extension block splinting or pinning, external fixation, or ORIF. Lateral volar lip fractures occur as a result of collateral ligament avulsion injuries.

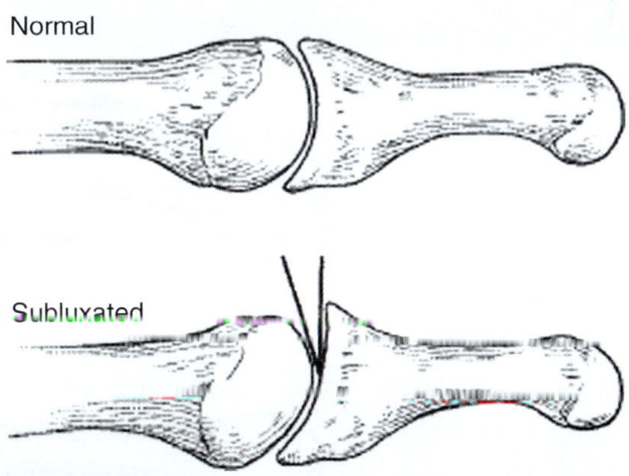

FIGURE 6.55 **Light's dorsal V sign on a lateral radiograph suggests PIP joint subluxation because the articular surfaces are not congruent or parallel. (*Source:* Blazar PE, Steinberg DR. Fractures of the proximal interphalangeal joint. *J Am Acad Orthop Surg* 2000;8:383–390.)**

ORIF is recommended for injuries with more than 2 mm of displacement, more than 25% involvement, or joint instability. Pilon fractures occur as a result of an axial load that causes central depression of the articular surface. Treatment of these fractures varies from hinged external fixation to limited ORIF with bone graft for elevation of the joint surface. The most common complication following articular fractures of the middle phalangeal base is PIP joint flexion contracture.

Base Fractures. Fractures occurring at the base of the proximal phalanx can be nondisplaced, avulsion fractures involving the collateral ligament, T or Y pattern, or pilon. Nondisplaced fractures can be treated with buddy taping. Avulsion injuries of the collateral ligament that are displaced by more than 2 mm may require open reduction with pinning or internal fixation. Comminuted fractures can be treated with joint-spanning hinged external fixators.

Shaft Fractures. Patterns of phalangeal shaft fractures include transverse, oblique or spiral, and comminuted. Transverse fractures occur more frequently in the middle phalanx, whereas spiral and oblique fractures involve the proximal phalanx (Fig. 6.56). Proximal phalangeal fractures tend to angulate volarly secondary to the flexion force of the proximal fragment and an extension force on the distal fragment from the insertion of the central slip (Fig. 6.57). Angulation of middle phalangeal fractures depends on the location of the fracture relative to the FDS. Fractures that occur distal to the FDS insertion angulate volarly as a result of the FDS insertion forcing the proximal fragment into flexion and the extension force of the terminal tendon on the distal fragment. Fractures that arise proximal to or at the insertion of the FDS angulate dorsally secondary to the extension force of the central slip on the proximal fragment and the flexion force exerted by the FDS insertion on the distal fragment. Nondisplaced

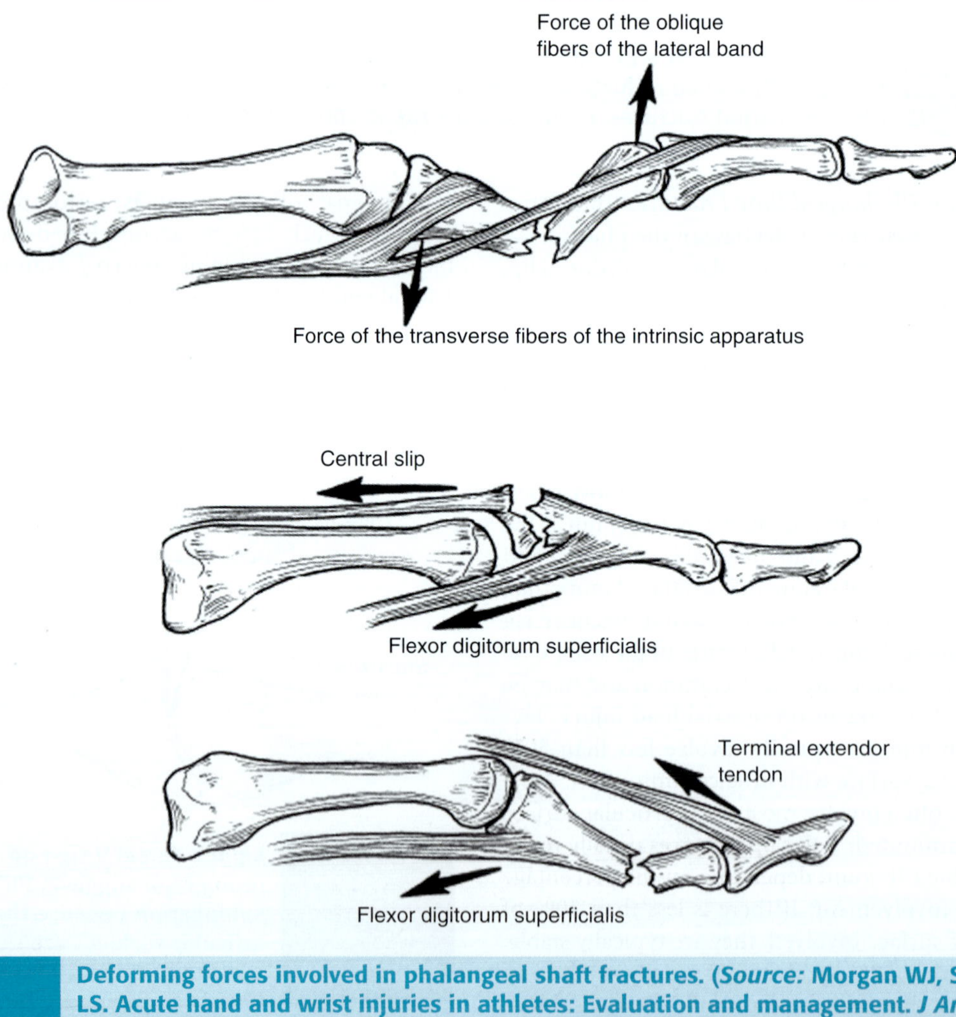

FIGURE 6.56 **Deforming forces involved in phalangeal shaft fractures. (*Source:* Morgan WJ, Slowman LS. Acute hand and wrist injuries in athletes: Evaluation and management. *J Am Acad Orthop Surg* 2001;9:389–400; *adapted from* Breen TF. Sports related injuries of the hand. In: Pappas AM, Walzer J (eds.), *Upper Extremity Injuries in the Athlete.* New York: Churchill Livingstone, 1995;475.)**

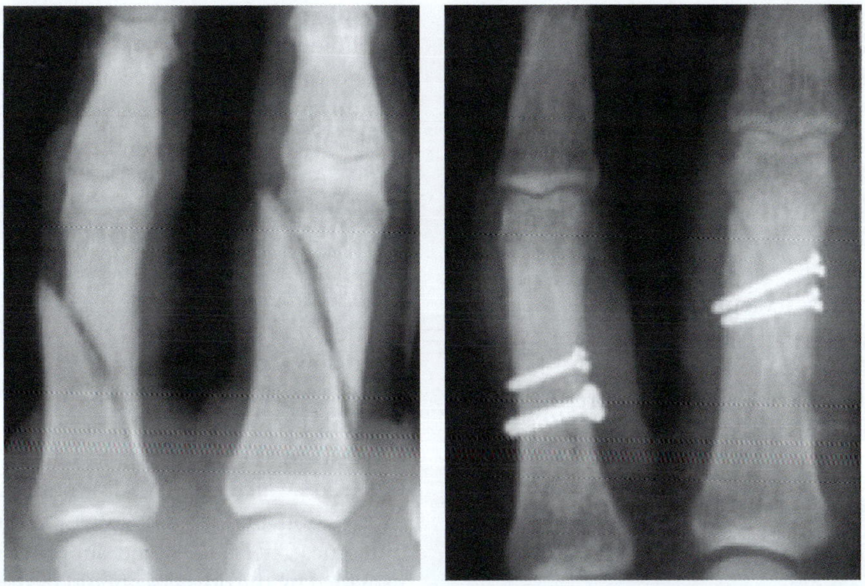

FIGURE 6.57 **(A) Posteroanterior radiograph of displaced long- and ring-finger spiral proximal phalanx fracture. (B) Radiograph obtained after ORIF with multiple lag screws. (*Source:* Kozin SH, Thoder JJ, Lieberman G. Operative treatment of metacarpal and phalangeal shaft fractures. *J Am Acad Orthop Surg* 2000;8:111–121.)**

fractures can be managed conservatively by buddy taping or immobilization. Displaced fractures that are stable following closed reduction can also be managed with immobilization in a cast. Acceptable reduction is one with no rotational deformity, less than 2 mm of shortening, more than 50% bone apposition, and less than 10 degrees of angulation. Surgery is required for unstable fractures such as the spiral and oblique types, irreducible fractures, comminuted fractures with associated soft tissue injury such as tendon laceration, fractures with extensive bone loss, and multiple fractures. ORIF via a dorsal or midaxial approach can be achieved by compression screws, plates, or pinning. External fixation is indicated for open or highly comminuted fractures or those with concomitant soft tissue injury. Complications include malunion, nonunion, stiffness, and PIP joint extensor lag.

Neck Fractures. Phalangeal neck fractures are uncommon in adults and are managed with closed reduction and cast immobilization or percutaneous pinning.

Condylar Fractures. Phalangeal condylar fractures are intraarticular injuries that are common in athletes. These fractures are inherently unstable, and nonoperative treatment requires close follow-up. Fractures can be unicondylar, bicondylar, comminuted, or triplane. Displaced unicondylar fractures require ORIF with multiple Kirschner pins or lag screws. Bicondylar and comminuted fractures are challenging to fix and have been treated with minicondylar plates, dynamic traction, and external fixation. A triplane fracture involves the transverse, sagittal, and coronal planes of the head of the proximal phalanx and can be treated with 2 interfragmentary screws. Phalangeal head fractures can also result from collateral ligament avulsion. These injuries should be managed surgically if there is greater than 2 mm of displacement. Complications following phalangeal condylar fractures include flexion contracture and posttraumatic arthritis.

Distal Phalanx Fractures

Fractures of the distal phalanx are the most frequently occurring fractures of the hand and usually involve the thumb and middle finger because these fingers are the most distally extending digits during manual activity.

Tuft Fractures. Fractures of the tuft are often a result of a crush injury and occur in conjunction with a nail bed laceration. Closed fractures can be managed by decompression of the subungual hematoma by piercing the nail with a large-gauge needle and splinting for 2 weeks. Open fractures are managed with irrigation and débridement followed by repair of any injury to the nail bed in the emergency room. A short course of oral antibiotic therapy is recommended to minimize risk of infection. Complications include cold sensitivity, nail deformity, and abnormal sensibility.

Shaft Fractures. Distal phalangeal shaft fractures can be divided into 2 types: longitudinal and transverse;

the latter can be subdivided into stable and unstable patterns. Nondisplaced transverse fractures do not require internal fixation because the surrounding soft tissue provides adequate stabilization. Displaced transverse fractures may be open and occur in conjunction with a nail bed laceration. Management includes débridement followed by stabilization with retrograde Kirschner pin fixation.

Articular Fractures. Fractures involving the volar articular surface of the base of the distal phalanx often occur in conjunction with an FDP avulsion. Management of these injuries includes reattachment of the tendon and/or avulsed bone.

Carpal Bone Fractures

Fractures of the carpal bones are common and often occur as a result of falling on an outstretched hand. The scaphoid is the most frequently fractured carpal bone and accounts for 60% of carpal bone fractures. The triquetrum is the second most commonly fractured carpal bone and accounts for about 14% of carpal bone fractures.

Scaphoid Fractures

The scaphoid is the most commonly fractured carpal bone. Scaphoid fractures typically occur following a fall on an outstretched hand that is in ulnar deviation and more than 90 degrees of extension. The majority of the load is concentrated in the radial half of the palm. Approximately 80% of the scaphoid surface consists of articular cartilage. It articulates with the lunate, capitate, trapezium, trapezoid, and distal radius, thus making it a major link between the proximal and distal carpal rows.

Diagnosis of a scaphoid fracture is considered by presenting signs and symptoms, mechanism of injury, patient age, and radiographs. Physical findings, including tenderness over the anatomic snuffbox and scaphoid tubercle and pain with axial compression of the thumb metacarpal toward the wrist, have a diagnostic sensitivity of 100%. Initial radiographs have a false-negative incidence of 2% to 25%; therefore, if there is a strong clinical suspicion of a scaphoid fracture in the absence of radiographic findings, the patient can be splinted and radiographically reevaluated in 1 to 3 weeks. Alternatively, to avoid delay in diagnosis, the patient can undergo a bone scan 72 hours following the time of injury, an MRI, or CT scan. Bone scans have been shown to have a sensitivity of 100% and specificity of 98%. MRI has a sensitivity and specificity of 100% and can be obtained immediately if radiographs are negative in the setting of a high clinical suspicion. Fracture is ruled out if MRI or bone scan is negative.

Location of the injury has an important role in outcome. The main blood supply of the scaphoid is provided by the dorsal scaphoid branches of the radial artery (Fig. 6.58). These branches enter the bone via the dorsal ridge and distal tubercle and provide 70% to 80% of the blood supply to the bone. As a result of this retrograde blood flow, AVN and nonunion are associated with fractures of the proximal pole. The distal 20% to 30% of the scaphoid receives its blood supply from the volar scaphoid branches of the radial artery. With proper treatment, almost all distal pole fractures, 80% to 90% of scaphoid waist, and 60% to 70% of proximal pole fractures progress to bony union.

Pattern of injury, stability, and displacement also play important roles in determining prognosis following a scaphoid fracture. Horizontal oblique and transverse fractures are described as stable patterns that will heal, whereas a vertical oblique fracture has been described as inherently unstable. Criteria for unstable fractures include more than 1 mm of displacement, a scapholunate angle greater than 60 degrees (normal is 30 to 60 degrees), or a capitolunate or radiolunate angle greater than 15 degrees (normal is 0 to 15 degrees). Any displaced or angulated fracture is considered unstable and will likely need surgery. Other factors that affect

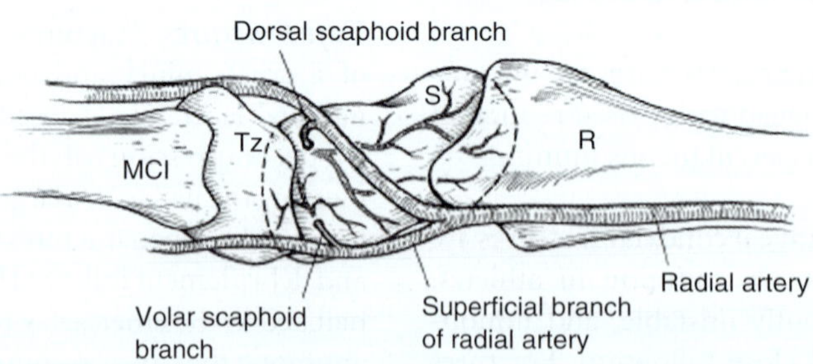

FIGURE 6.58 **Primary blood supply to the scaphoid is through the dorsal branch of the radial artery. MCI, first metacarpal; R, radius, S, scaphoid; Tz, trapezium. (*Source:* Trumble TE, Salas P, Barthel T, Robert KQ III. Management of scaphoid nonunions. *J Am Acad Orthop Surg* 2003;11:380–391.)**

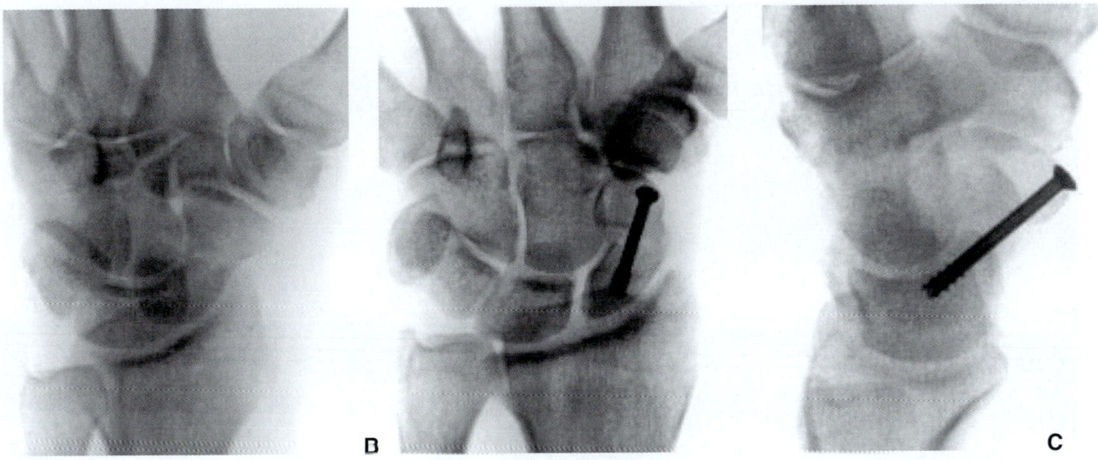

A B C

FIGURE 6.59 **(A) Oblique view of the wrist demonstrates a nondisplaced scaphoid waist fracture. Posteroanterior (B) and lateral (C) radiographs depict fracture percutaneous internal fixation with a 3.0-mm screw. (*Source:* Ring D, Jupiter JB, Herndon JH. Acute fractures of the scaphoid. *J Am Acad Orthop Surg* 2000;8:225–231.)**

the stability of an acute fracture are degree of comminution and the presence of any associated carpal instability such as a scapholunate dissociation. Failure to recognize these injuries will lead to abnormal wrist mechanics during load-bearing. The most common pattern of instability following a scaphoid fracture is dorsal intercalated segment instability (DISI).

Nondisplaced fractures of the distal pole or middle waist that are stable have been traditionally treated with immobilization in a thumb spica cast for 8 to 12 weeks. Nondisplaced proximal pole fractures are difficult to treat and may require immobilization for as long as 20 weeks. Operative fixation of a nondisplaced fracture is useful for managing injuries in athletes and manual laborers; studies have reported return to play or work within 5 to 7 weeks following internal fixation (Fig. 6.59).

For displaced or unstable fractures, treatment is operative; methods of fixation include closed reduction and percutaneous pinning, closed reduction and fixation with a compression screw, arthroscopically assisted reduction, and fixation or ORIF with a compression screw. Distal pole fractures are typically treated using a dorsal approach; fractures of the waist and proximal pole can be managed using a volar incision.

Nonunion of a scaphoid fracture occurs as a result of a delay in diagnosis and treatment or if a fracture fails to heal within 6 months of cast immobilization. The rate of nonunion increases from 19% to 88% in patients with unrecognized injuries. Even with proper treatment, the rate of scaphoid nonunion has been reported as high as 15%; 20% of these nonunions occur following fractures of the proximal third of the scaphoid. Patients typically present with pain and decreased ROM. Diagnosis can be confirmed with plain radiographs, CT scan, or MRI. CT scans define osseous anatomy and can provide precise measurement of intrascaphoid angles and quantify the extent of cortical contact. MRI can be used to assess vascularity and patients with nonunions that have failed previous surgery to evaluate the extent of avascular necrosis (Fig. 6.60). Treatment includes ORIF and bone graft in cases of nondisplaced fractures or proximal pole fractures without fragmentation. Vascularized distal radius bone grafts can be used to treat nonunions complicated by AVN. Injuries with fragmentation and collapse secondary to AVN typically progress to a SNAC pattern of wrist arthrosis. Treatment includes salvage procedures such as excision of the fragment, radial styloidectomy, intercarpal fusion, proximal row carpectomy, 4-corner fusion, and complete wrist arthrodesis.

Triquetral Fractures

The triquetrum is the second most commonly fractured carpal bone. Triquetral fractures can occur through the body or the dorsal rim; body fractures result from impaction of the ulnar border of the wrist or can be part of a perilunate greater arc injury. Rim fractures are often a result of an avulsion of the dorsal radiocarpal, dorsal intercarpal, or lunotriquetral ligaments or following impaction from the ulnar styloid. Nondisplaced body fractures and dorsal rim fractures can be managed with cast immobilization. Displaced body fractures typically require ORIF.

Hamate Fractures

Fractures of the hamate represent 7% of carpal fractures. Fractures typically involve the body or,

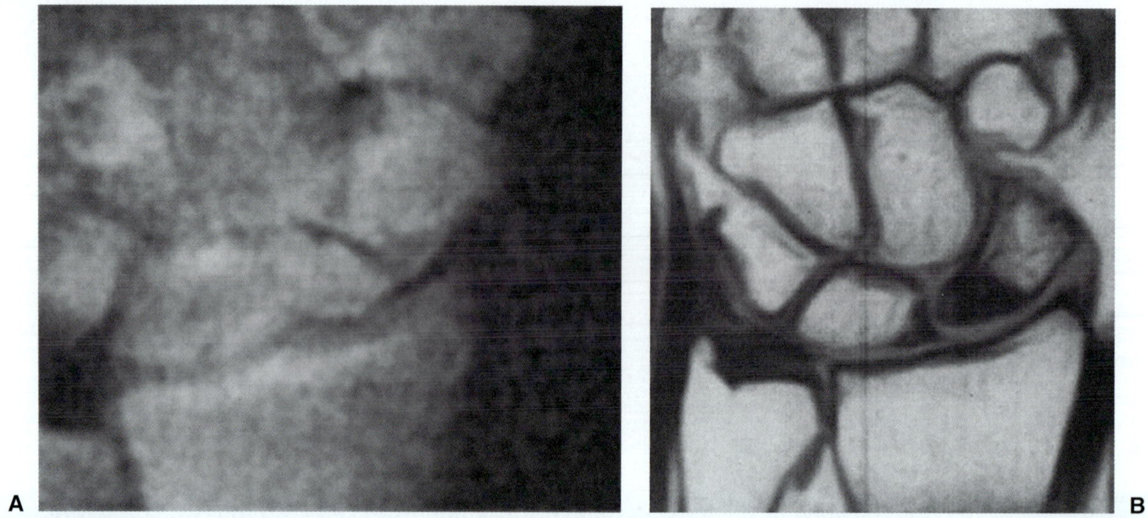

FIGURE 6.60 **(A) Radiograph of avascular proximal pole. (B) MRI depicting avascular necrosis of the proximal pole of the scaphoid following fracture. (*Source:* Segalman KA, Graham, TJ. Scaphoid proximal pole fractures and nonunions. *J Am Soc Surg Hand* 2004;4:233–249.)**

less commonly, the hook (Fig. 6.61). Body fractures are often part of significant trauma to the hand or wrist such as dorsal fracture-dislocations involving the fourth and/or fifth CMC joints or part of a greater arc perilunate injury. Hook fractures are typically isolated injuries resulting from direct impact by the base of a bat, or hammer, racquet, or golf club. Both body and hook fractures have been associated with ulnar neuropathy. The retinaculum flexorum joins the hook of the hamate and the trapezium and therefore fracture can affect both bones at the same time. On physical examination, patients with body fractures typically have dorsoulnar swelling and deformity as well as tenderness at the CMC joints. In patients with hook fractures, there may be pain with resisted DIP flexion of the ring and small fingers with the wrist in ulnar deviation. Body and hook fractures can be diagnosed with standard radiographs; hook fractures are best visualized on a carpal tunnel view. CT scans can outline fractures that are not evident on radiographs. Nondisplaced body and hook fractures can be managed with cast immobilization. ORIF is often required for body fractures that occur in conjunction with diffuse hand and wrist injury. Untreated hook fractures can progress to painful nonunion and associated chronic ulnar neuropathy and/or attritional rupture of the digital flexor tendons of the ring and small fingers.

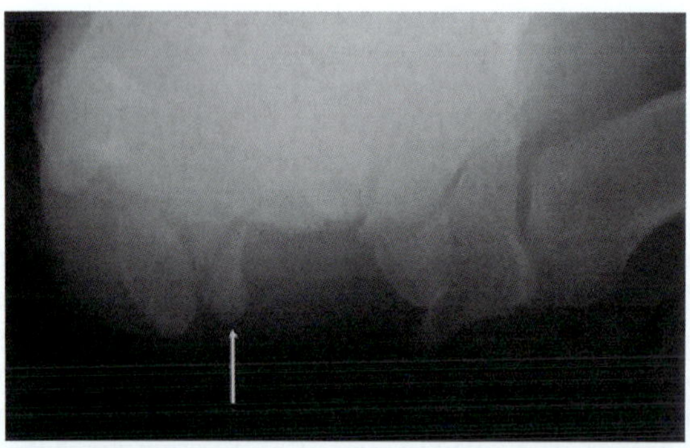

FIGURE 6.61 **Carpal tunnel view reveals a fracture through the hook of the hamate that was not detected on standard views of the hand. (*Source:* Shah MA, Viegas SF. Fractures of the carpal bones excluding the scaphoid. *J Am Soc Surg Hand* 2002;2: 129–140.)**

Trapezium Fractures

Fractures of the trapezium make up about 3% of carpal fractures and typically involve the body or the ridge. Body fractures occur with axial loading of the wrist during excessive dorsiflexion and radial deviation, causing it to become crushed between the radial styloid and the thumb metacarpal base. They can occur in conjunction with fracture-dislocations of the thumb CMC joint. Patients with fractures of the body may present with an abnormal dorsoradial prominence at the base of the thumb metacarpal and tenderness of the basal joint or distal portion of the anatomic snuffbox. Fractures involving the ridge are often isolated injuries that occur following trauma or transverse carpal ligament avulsion. Patients may have point tenderness just distal to the scaphoid tuberosity or the distal aspect of the snuffbox. Diagnosis can be confirmed with plain radiographs or CT scan. Ridge fractures can be managed with cast immobilization. Displaced, intraarticular body fractures are treated with ORIF.

Pisiform Fractures

Fractures of the pisiform comprise 2% of all carpal bone fractures. This sesamoid bone is tethered by the FCU tendon, the pisohamate, pisometacarpal, and pisotriquetral ligaments. It is also attached to the transverse carpal ligament and ADM. The ulnar neurovascular bundle lies just radial to the pisiform in the Guyon canal. Fractures usually occur following impact from a fall on an outstretched hands and forceful contraction of the FCU. Approximately 50% of pisiform fractures are associated with other wrist injuries such as a perilunate dislocation or fractures involving the distal radius or other carpal bones. Patients typically exhibit tenderness over the pisiform and may have symptoms of ulnar nerve injury. Pisiform fractures can be delineated on lateral wrist and carpal tunnel view radiographs. The majority of these fractures can be treated with splint immobilization. Complications include nonunion or posttraumatic arthritis, which can be treated with enucleation of the pisiform and FCU reconstruction.

Distal Radius Fractures

Fractures of the distal radius comprise approximately 20% of all fractures evaluated in emergency rooms across the United States and occur most frequently in adolescents and the elderly. Approximately 50% of distal radius fractures extend into the radiocarpal and/or DRUJ. Although most of these fractures are managed by closed reduction and cast immobilization, those that compromise joint stability and/or articular congruity frequently require additional stabilization with Kirschner pins, external fixation, bone graft, and/or internal fixation.

The distal radius plays a crucial role in wrist biomechanics during motion and loading. The dorsal cortex of the distal radius is convex and, along with the Lister tubercle, serve as a fulcrum for the extensors as they cross the wrist joint.

The articulating area of the distal radius is comprised of 3 concave articular surfaces: the scaphoid and lunate fossae and the sigmoid notch. These surfaces articulate with the scaphoid, lunate, and ulnar head respectively. The scaphoid and lunate fossae are divided by an anterior–posterior ridge. Although the weakest osseous region of the distal radius occurs at the metaphyseal flare, there are regions of cortical thickening along the metaphysis that are typically resistant

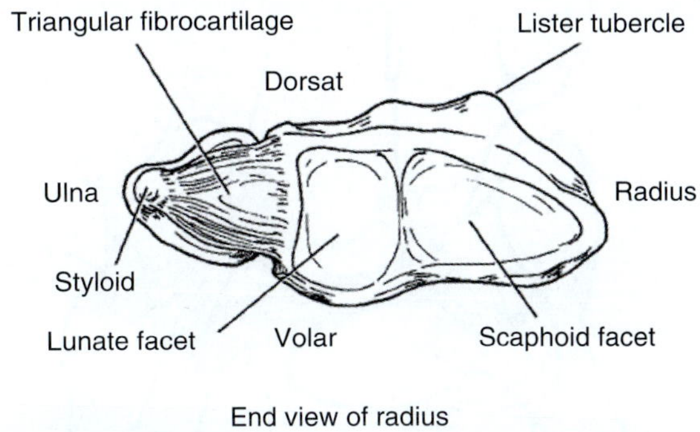

FIGURE 6.62 Axial view of articular surface of distal radius and DRUJ. (*Source:* Trumble TE, Culp R, Hanel DP, Geissler WB, Berger RA. Intraarticular fractures of the distal aspect of the radius. In: *Instructional Course Lectures: The American Academy of Orthopaedic Surgeons.* Rosemont, IL. 1998;80A:582–600.)

to fracture-yielding forces, resulting in predictable fracture patterns that often propagate between the scaphoid and lunate fossae. Other compressive loads will propagate in the coronal plane or result in central depression and fragmentation. The sigmoid notch provides a concave surface that articulates with the head of the ulna at the DRUJ (Fig. 6.62). During forearm supination and pronation, the distal portion of the ulna translates palmarly and dorsally respectively. Stability of the DRUJ is provided primarily by the TFCC. The TFCC originates from the base of the ulnar styloid and inserts at the ulnar margin of the lunate facet. A large ulnar styloid fracture or peripheral disruption of the TFCC can lead to DRUJ instability. The dorsal and palmar borders of the TFCC form the dorsal and palmar radioulnar ligaments, which tend to rotate the fracture fragments of the lunate fossa.

Dorsal extrinsic radiocarpal ligaments that originate from the dorsal cortex of the distal radius include the radiotriquetral and radioscaphoid ligaments; these ligaments do not contribute to the malalignment of fracture fragments. The palmar aspect of the distal radius serves as an attachment for the extrinsic radial palmar wrist ligaments: the radioscaphocapitate, radial collateral, short and long radiolunate, and radioscapholunate ligaments (Fig. 6.63). These stout palmar ligaments are responsible for displacement of the volar lip into extension.

The brachioradialis is the only tendon to insert on the distal radius and is responsible for displacing the radial styloid.

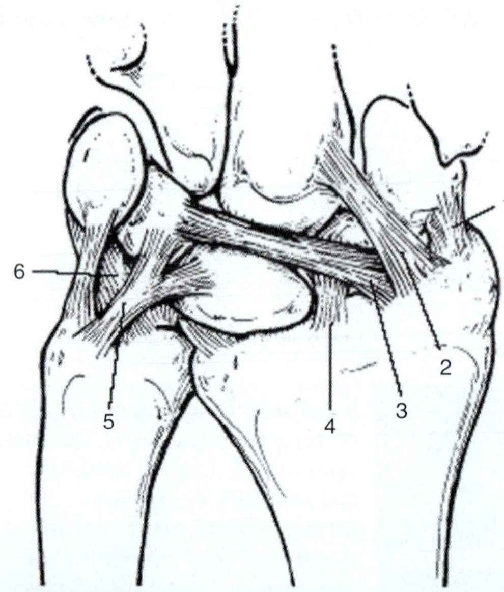

FIGURE 6.63 **Palmar extrinsic wrist ligaments. 1, radial collateral ligament; 2, radioscaphocapitate ligament; 3, radiolunatotriquetral ligament; 4, radioscapholunate ligament; 5, ulnolunate ligament; 6, meniscus homologue. (*Source:* Jupiter JB. Complex articular fractures of the distal radius: Classification and management. *J Am Acad Orthop Surg* 1997;5:119–129.)**

Additional stability of the radiocarpal joint is provided by the interosseous carpal ligaments such as the scapholunate and lunotriquetral ligaments, which stabilize the bones of the proximal carpal row that articulate with the distal radius and the TFCC. The integrity of the carpal bones is defined by their osseous shape and ligamentous attachments. An axial load can be transmitted across the carpus and result in interosseous ligament injury and/or fracture of the carpal bone. The scapholunate ligament is the most frequently injured interosseous ligament, and the scaphoid is the most commonly fractured carpal bone (Fig. 6.64).

The entire articular surface of the distal radius has a radial inclination of approximately 22 degrees in the coronal plane and a palmar tilt averaging 11 degrees in the sagittal plane. Radial inclination is determined radiographically by measuring the angle formed between a line tangential to the distal radial articular surface and a line perpendicular to the radial shaft on a posteroanterior view. Palmar tilt is measured as the angle formed by the plane of the articular surface and the plane perpendicular to the radial shaft on a lateral

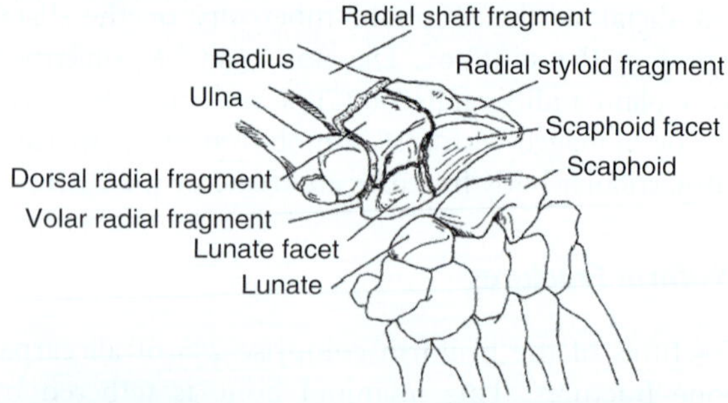

FIGURE 6.64 **Fracture line propagation in distal radius fractures. (*Source:* Trumble TE, Culp R, Hanel DP, Geissler WB, Berger RA. Intraarticular fractures of the distal aspect of the radius. In: *Instructional Course Lectures: The American Academy of Orthopaedic Surgeons.* Rosemont, IL. 1998;80A:582–600.)**

radiograph. Radial height is the distance measured from the most ulnar aspect of the distal radius to the tip of the radial styloid on an anterior–posterior x-ray. It typically measures about 12 mm.

Functional outcome is determined by a combination of factors, including the restoration of hand and carpus alignment with the forearm, the severity of the injury, and associated injuries and complications. Most patients who sustain distal radius fractures are elderly; these patients tend to do well with conservative management as a result of a low-energy mechanism and a low functionally demanding lifestyle; they are also at an increased risk of mortality from other existing comorbidities.

On the other hand, the number of healthy, active patients over the age of 60 years is growing; in this population, the age of the patient should not be the main determinant of treatment. Instead, the goals of management should be influenced by the patient's functional status and activity level and should focus on restoring ROM and function of the digits, hand, and forearm, while minimizing the risk of potential complications. The treatment of unstable distal radius fractures in the elderly population with rigid internal fixation has been shown to allow for early return to function with a low rate of potential postoperative morbidity and complication.

Classification. There are several different classification systems for fractures of the distal radius.

- *Eponyms*—Common eponymic descriptions for fractures of the distal radius are listed in Table 6.54 and described in the following sections.

TABLE 6.54 Common eponyms for distal radius fractures

Eponym	*Fracture Description*
Colles	Distal radius fracture with dorsal angulation (apex volar), dorsal comminution, dorsal displacement, and radial shortening
Smith	Distal radius fracture with volar displacement/translation; extraarticular or intraarticular extension
Barton	Dorsal or volar articular shear fracture-subluxation that is unstable; carpus shifts with the fracture fragment
Chauffeur	Avulsion fracture of the radial styloid with translation of the carpus
Lunate load/die punch	Central depression of the lunate fossa following impaction of the lunate

- *Frykman*—Frykman classification differentiates between extraarticular and intraarticular involvement of the distal radius fracture and the presence or absence of an associated ulnar styloid fracture.
- *AO*—The AO classification categorizes distal radius fractures into 3 main types: extraarticular, partial articular, and complete articular. These 3 types are subdivided into groups and subgroups based on the extent of articular and metaphyseal comminution, yielding 27 distinct fracture patterns. AO classification stresses the importance of an intact metaphysis in reduction of the articular surface. Significance of the metaphysis has been emphasized by Trumble, who compared the metaphysis to a 4-sided box; each side represents a column. Marked comminution of the metaphysis of the distal radius is defined as involvement of more than 50% of the diameter of the metaphysis as visualized on any radiographic view, comminution of at least 2 cortices of the metaphysis, or more than 2 mm of shortening of the distal radius. Loss of integrity of $\geq$ 2 sides or cortices is also associated with malalignment.

Initial Evaluation and Management. The severity of injury to the bone and soft tissue depends on the mechanism of injury and quality of the patient's bone stock and adjacent soft tissue. Open distal radius fractures are rare, but it is not uncommon for patients to present with small soft tissue defects or shearing of the skin resulting from sharp edges of fracture fragments or gross deformity. The most common type of open fracture of the distal radius is Gustilo I, which most frequently involves the volar-ulnar region of the wrist. Patients with open fractures of the distal radius should receive antibiotic and tetanus prophylaxis and should be taken to the operating room for emergent irrigation and débridement.

A thorough neurovascular exam should be documented on presentation and following any manipulation or stabilization. Patients who present with acute median neuropathy in the setting of a distal radius fracture should undergo immediate closed reduction; the majority resolve following reduction in low-energy injuries. However, patients who have sustained high-energy trauma should be closely monitored for the development of acute carpal tunnel syndrome and/or possibly forearm compartment syndrome, especially within the first 48 to 72 hours of injury or surgery. Symptoms that fail to resolve within 24 to 48 hours following reduction or that worsen warrant early open reduction with or without internal fixation and carpal tunnel release. Acute tendon disruption is rare but has been reported. Integrity of the tendons, especially the EPL and FPL, should be assessed.

Closed reduction under local or regional anesthesia and/or conscious sedation is not necessary if the patient has acceptable alignment and will ultimately undergo surgery; these patients can be managed with a sugar tong splint for temporary stabilization. The importance of elevation of the affected extremity and ROM of the digits must be emphasized to patients and their caretakers in the immediate preoperative and postoperative periods.

Radiographic Evaluation. Premanipulation radiographs are one of the best predictors of stability following closed reduction; postreduction radiographs are helpful in delineating fracture fragments. Preoperative assessment of distal radius fractures involving the articular surface or a complex pattern of injury can be facilitated with CT. CT imaging provides superior detail of the articular surface, including the integrity of the lunate facet and sigmoid notch, presence of central depression or impaction, and degree of comminution of the dorsal and volar rims. The detail provided by CT images can facilitate planning the surgical approach, the need for arthroscopic evaluation, capsulotomy, method of reduction, and type of fixation.

Disruption of the SLIL can be assessed in the operating room following induction of anesthesia. Radiographic visualization of the wrist under traction can be obtained with an image intensifier. Fernandez described the Shenton sign of the wrist or the axial scaphoid shift sign to evaluate the integrity of the scapholunate ligament. A traction view of the wrist that reveals a stepoff of the proximal carpal arc is consistent

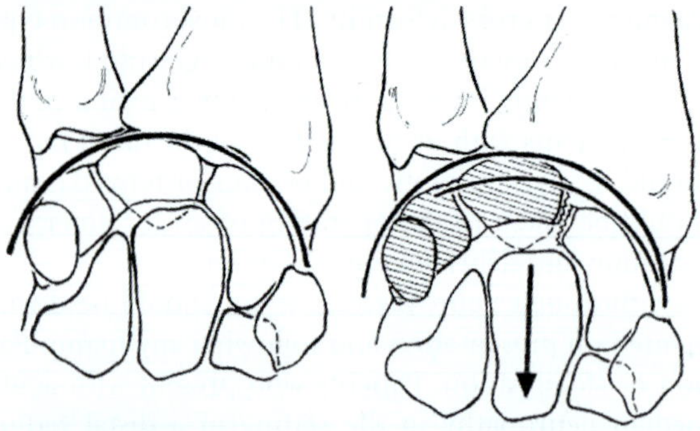

FIGURE 6.65 **Shenton sign of the wrist. (*Source:* Jupiter JB. Complex articular fractures of the distal radius: classification and management. *J Am Acad Orthop Surg* 1997;5:119–129.)**

with complete disruption of the SLL. Disruption of the proximal carpal arc after traction has been applied is indicative of SLL disruption (Fig. 6.65).

Nondisplaced Fractures. Nondisplaced stable fractures of the distal radius can be managed with a combination of a sugar tong splint for 3 weeks and immobilization in a long-arm cast with the wrist in slight flexion and ulnar deviation for 3 weeks followed by 3 weeks of immobilization with a removable splint.

Displaced Fractures. Anatomic reduction of distal radius fractures is indicated with any of the following parameters: intraarticular stepoff of more than 1 to 2 mm (especially the lunate facet), loss of palmar tilt of $\geq$ 10 degrees, loss $\geq$ 2 mm of radial height, radial inclination change $\geq$ 5 degrees, and disruption of the DRUJ. Surgery is warranted when acceptable closed reduction cannot be achieved or is too unstable to maintain.

Knirk and Jupiter and Catalano and colleagues have both reported that displacement of more than 1 to 2 mm of the articular surface results in posttraumatic arthritis. Sequelae of posttraumatic arthritis include pain, stiffness, carpal instability, and decreased grip strength. Malunion resulting in an increase of dorsal tilt or shortening of the distal radius by 2.5 mm leads to a significant shift of axial load from the radius to the ulna as well as change in the transmission of load across the carpus, leading to midcarpal instability. Increased dorsal tilt also restricts forearm rotation by increasing the tension of the interosseous membrane. Indications for ORIF of distal radius fractures are as follows:

- Articular stepoff
- > 5 mm of shortening
- > 20 degrees of dorsal angulation
- DRUJ dislocation
- Ulnar fracture
- Radiocarpal instability
- Comminution

Closed Reduction and Percutaneous Kirschner Wire Fixation. Closed reduction and percutaneous pinning is ideal for unstable extraarticular fractures. Kirschner wire fixation may also be used in conjunction with external or internal fixation. Wires may be placed into distal fragments to act as joysticks or placed within the radial styloid. Kapandji describes placement of the wires within the fracture site to serve as buttresses. Kirschner wires can also be placed across the DRUJ if it is unstable.

External Fixation. External fixation is indicated for open fractures and for severe comminution of the metaphysis and/or articular surface. Traction from the device minimizes the need for an intact metaphysis to support the articular surface and to align the joint with the radial shaft, especially in cases with comminution $\geq$ 2 cortices. Reduction of the fracture fragments is achieved by longitudinal traction and volar shift of the fracture and is maintained via ligamentotaxis. Augmentation with Kirschner wires has been shown to significantly increase the stability of an unstable extraarticular distal radius fracture. External fixators are typically removed after 4 to 6 weeks. Complications associated with external fixation includes pin track infections and associated osteomyelitis, fracture through a pin site, loosening, stiffness, and injury to the superficial radial sensory nerve.

Internal Fixation. Other potential surgical approaches include limited open and arthroscopically assisted internal fixation. Limited open reduction and internal fixation may provide slightly greater postoperative ROM in comparison to standard open reduction and internal fixation; however, accurate restoration of articular congruency may be compromised because of inadequate direct visualization of the articular surface. Improved visualization of the articular surface and assessment of the integrity of the interosseous carpal ligaments and the TFCC can be achieved arthroscopically.

The approach for traditional open reduction and internal fixation with plate and screws is determined by the initial displacement of the fracture. Large fragments can be captured with screws, while smaller fragments can be stabilized with wire loops or suture. A dorsally displaced fracture or die-punch fracture may benefit from a dorsal approach; a volarly displaced fracture may benefit from a volar approach. Both approaches provide extended exposure that is suitable for fixation of a distal radius fracture with metaphyseal comminution using a buttress or distraction plate. Combined dorsal and volar plating is useful for stabilizing complex fractures with extensive articular, dorsal, and volar metaphyseal comminution. The volar approach of Henry begins with a longitudinal incision along the FCR tendon. The FCR is retracted ulnarly, while the radial artery is taken radially. Dissection is carried to the pronator quadratus, which is incised along its radial border. The distal radius can then be visualized following subperiosteal elevation of the pronator quadratus. The dorsal approach to the distal radius begins with a longitudinal incision centered over the Lister tubercle. The extensor retinaculum is incised over the third compartment, which holds the EPL. The second and fourth compartments are mobilized to expose the distal radius. During closure, the deep layer of the retinaculum is repaired to minimize tendon contact with the hardware. The EPL remains in the subcutaneous tissue during closure. Dorsal plating may mandate removal of hardware following fracture healing in order to minimize tendon irritation and possible rupture.

Bone Graft. Use of autogenous cancellous bone graft can accelerate the healing of metaphyseal defects and serve as a scaffold for elevated articular fragments. Bone graft substitutes can be used in order to minimize the risk and morbidity associated with harvesting autogenous bone graft. Reconstitution of bone stock in cases that involve large defects of the metaphysis can be reliably achieved using autogenous bone graft.

Complications. Distal radius fractures are associated with a high rate of complications directly related to the extent of injury to the articular surface, metaphysis, and adjacent structures. Injury to the median and/or ulnar nerves, compartment syndrome, and DRUJ instability are complications that can develop during the immediate postinjury period. Late adverse sequelae following distal radius fractures include tendon irritation and eventual rupture secondary to irritation from hardware; the most commonly involved tendons are the EPL and the common extensor tendons. Flexor tendon adhesion can be prevented by stressing the importance of digital ROM exercises during and following the treatment period. Alteration of the normal biomechanics of the radiocarpal and radioulnar joints occurs in the setting of a malunion, leading to pain, stiffness, arthrosis, and midcarpal and/or DRUJ instability. Treatment of extraarticular malunion includes corrective radial osteotomy with or without resection of the distal ulna and is indicated for younger patients with $\geq$ 15 degrees of dorsal angulation or for painful wrist deformity in older patients. A stepoff of more than 2 mm involving the articular surface is regarded as an indication for corrective surgery. Delayed union or nonunion is defined as failure to demonstrate radiographic evidence of healing after 4 months from the time of injury and has been related to a history of tobacco smoking, overdistraction, and insufficient immobilization. Treatment includes débridement of the nonunion site, fragment realignment with rigid fixation, and autogenous iliac crest cancellous bone graft. Severe posttraumatic arthritis can be treated with arthrodesis or arthroplasty of the wrist.

Ulnar Styloid Fractures. Fifty percent of distal radius fractures are associated with a concomitant ulnar styloid fracture. Injury to the TFCC and subsequent DRUJ instability is a concern because the ulnar styloid serves as an attachment site for several of the structures that comprise the TFCC, including the dorsal and volar radioulnar ligaments, the tendon subsheath of the ECU, and the UCL. Acute DRUJ instability is defined as gross dislocation of the DRUJ resulting in scaphopisiform overlap on a lateral radiograph, increased anteroposterior translation in comparison to the contralateral wrist, and evidence of subluxation of the DRUJ on CT images. Chronic DRUJ instability can be defined by ulnar-sided symptoms and abnormal rotation of the forearm in conjunction with 1 of the aforementioned radiographic findings. Ulnar styloid fractures that involve the base or are displaced by more than 2 mm are important clinical risk factors for the development of DRUJ instability. Treatment includes reduction of the ulnar styloid and repair of the TFCC.

XVIII. INSTABILITY

Dislocations and Ligament Injuries of the Joints of the Digits

Proximal Interphalangeal Joint

Stability of the PIP joint results from its articular congruence, capsule, proper and accessory collateral ligaments, volar plate, and the central slip. The collateral ligaments are the primary restraints to radial and ulnar joint translation. The volar plate is suspended by the collateral ligaments and inserts at the volar aspect of the base of the middle phalanx. The majority of PIP joint stability to varus–valgus stress is provided by the proper collateral ligaments; the volar plate is the primary stabilizer against dorsal translation and a secondary stabilizer against lateral deviation. PIP joint dislocation occurs in 1 of 2 planes: radioulnar or dorsovolar. The direction of dislocation is in reference to the position of the middle phalanx. The most common direction of dislocation is dorsal. Table 6.55 describes 3 grades of injuries following dorsal displacement.

TABLE 6.55 Patterns of PIP joint injury following dorsal dislocation

Type	Description of Injury
I	Hyperextension injury with volar plate avulsion and incomplete disruption of the collateral ligaments
II	Dorsal dislocation with complete rupture of the volar plate and complete split in the collateral ligaments
III	Dorsal dislocation with associated avulsion fracture of the volar base of middle phalanx; stable injuries involve < 40% of the articular surface; unstable injuries occur following > 40% of the articular surface and must undergo ORIF

TABLE 6.56 Types of collateral ligament injury

Type	Description of Injury
I	Microscopic tearing of the ligament but clinically stable with stress
II	Mild ligament disruption with < 20° of lateral deviation and firm endpoint with stress testing
III	Complete ligament disruption with > 20° of lateral deviation and no endpoint with stress testing

Dorsal PIP Dislocation. Acute dorsal PIP joint dislocations are often the result of hyperextension in conjunction with axial compression; this mechanism of injury occurs frequently in sports that involve handling of a ball such as basketball. Fracture of the volar lip of the middle phalanx can occur in cases involving a large load. Injury to the collateral ligaments can result in varus–valgus instability. Failure typically occurs proximally and often involves the radial collateral ligament. The most frequently injured digit is the index finger. Disruption of the volar plate typically occurs distally from the base of the middle phalanx and can result in dorsal dislocation; combined disruption of the collateral ligaments and volar plate results in lateral translation of the proximal phalangeal joint.

Radiographic evaluation should include plain radiographs; CT scan is helpful in cases involving avulsion or fracture of the articular surface. Physical examination reveals tenderness, swelling and increased laxity with lateral stress. Integrity of the collateral ligaments is assessed actively and passively. If the patient is able to voluntarily complete a full ROM without any displacement or deviation, then the joint is stable and requires only a brief period of immobilization. Passive stability is assessed by applying lateral force to the joint in full extension and in 30 degrees of flexion; the angle of deviation is measured as the degree of translation of the middle phalanx from the longitudinal axis. Lateral translation of more than 20 degrees correlates with collateral ligament disruption.

Lateral PIP Dislocation. Lateral PIP dislocations occur following complete rupture of one collateral ligament with partial disruption of the volar plate from the middle phalanx. Table 6.56 lists the 3 types of injury that have been observed. Presence of dorsovolar instability is assessed by comparing the degree of joint translation to a noninjured digit following application of a dorsovolar shearing force. On occasion, the volar plate may rupture and/or an osteochondral fragment or flexor tendon may become interposed between the articular surfaces, resulting in an irreducible dislocation that warrants open reduction. Most dorsal dislocations of the PIP joint can be reduced by manipulation. Stability of the joint in the coronal and sagittal planes should be assessed following reduction. Joints that are stable following reduction are treated with buddy taping; isolated hyperextension instability is treated with an extension block splinting for 1 month. Unstable joints must undergo ORIF or volar plate arthroplasty. Patients with open injuries should receive tetanus prophylaxis and antibiotics and undergo irrigation and débridement with or without internal fixation. The most important points of treatment are patient education and early mobilization. Complications include stiffness and flexion contracture.

Volar PIP Dislocation. Volar dislocations of the PIP joint are rare; a rotatory component may be present, resulting in volar rotatory subluxation. The mechanism of injury is axial compression combined with a rotatory force on a partially flexed middle phalanx that results in partial rupture of the volar plate and unilateral disruption of a collateral ligament; this mechanism of injury occurs, for example, when a digit becomes caught in a dryer that is spinning. The involved condyle will rupture through the extensor mechanism and may buttonhole between the central slip and the lateral band, making the injury unamenable to closed reduction. The central slip usually remains intact. Treatment often requires open reduction and brief immobilization or ORIF if there is an associated fracture or avulsion of the dorsal lip of the base of the middle phalanx that is displaced more than 1 mm.

DIP Joint of the Fingers and Thumb Interphalangeal Joints

DIP joint anatomy and associated stability is analogous to that of the PIP joint of the finger with the exception that the lever arm of the distal phalanx is shorter and there is added stability provided by the insertions of the extensor and flexor tendons. Therefore, DIP joint dislocations are rare; when they occur, displacement is typically dorsal and a result of hyperextension. This injury often occurs as an open injury. Evaluation and treatment are analogous to PIP joint dislocations. Most joints are amenable to closed reduction and stable afterward; unstable joints are immobilized for a couple of weeks in slight flexion using a dorsal extension block splint. Digital DIP joint and thumb interphalangeal joint dislocations are usually reducible via manipulation. Irreducible (complex) dislocations are rare and are most commonly a result of proximal volar plate disruption and subsequent interposition. Flexor tendons, fracture fragments and a sesamoid bone may also be interposed between the articular surfaces. Fracture-dislocations typically involve the volar lip of the distal phalanx. ORIF should be considered if there is DIP joint instability, if the fragment involves more than 50% of the articular surface, and if there is a concomitant FDP tendon avulsion.

MCP Joint

Stability of the MCP joint is provided by congruence of the articular surfaces of the metacarpal head and the base of the proximal phalanx, joint capsule, the flexor and extensor tendons, volar plate, and accessory and proper collateral ligaments. The sagittal bands and intrinsic muscle tendons serve as secondary stabilizers. The volar plates of the fingers are interconnected by the deep transverse metacarpal ligament and serve as the primary stabilizer against dorsal translation. The collateral ligaments are under tension in flexion and lax in extension because the nonspherical shape of the metacarpal head creates a cam effect; therefore, the MCP joint is inherently more congruent and more stable to varus–valgus stress in flexion exceeding 70 degrees than in extension.

Collateral ligament injuries are rare; they typically involve the radial side of the index finger and the ulnar side of the small finger and occur in conjunction with an avulsion fracture. Evaluation and examination is similar to that for PIP joint dislocation. Lateral stability is assessed by stress testing the collateral ligaments with the MCP joint in flexion. Stable injuries are treated with buddy taping; slightly unstable injuries with a solid endpoint are treated with splinting and buddy taping. Grossly unstable joints with or without an associated avulsion fracture are treated with ORIF.

Dorsal and Complex MCP Joint Dislocation. Dislocation of the MCP joint is typically dorsal and can be simple or complex (irreducible). The index finger is the most commonly involved digit, and the mechanism is usually hyperextension. Simple dislocations are amenable to closed reduction and splinting for 2 weeks in 60 to 70 degrees of flexion. Joints that are not stable after reduction may require ORIF. Complex dislocations are irreducible by closed means secondary to interposition of the volar plate and/or osteochondral fragments; the index and small finger metacarpal necks become entrapped by a noose formed by the lumbrical and flexor tendons. Complex dislocations are radiographically characterized by bayonet apposition of the articular surfaces. The metacarpal head may cause dimpling of the palmar skin. Complex dislocations must be treated with open reduction, which typically involves longitudinal division of the volar plate through a volar or dorsal incision.

Volar MCP Joint Dislocation. Volar dislocations of the MCP joint are rare and may be the result of a hyperflexion injury. There may be a rotatory component to the deformity. These injuries are characterized by disruption of at least 1 of the 2 collateral ligaments in addition to the volar plate. They are usually not amenable to closed reduction and will require repair of the involved collateral ligament to restore lateral stability. Complications include recurrent instability, stiffness, flexion contracture, degenerative arthritis, traumatic open reduction, iatrogenic injury to the neurovascular bundle during open reduction, and osteonecrosis of the metacarpal head.

Thumb MCP Joint

Stability of the MCP joint of the thumb is a result of its soft tissue attachments; there is little support from the osseous structures. These soft tissue stabilizers include the capsule, volar plate, proper collateral ligaments, and accessory collateral ligaments. The proper collateral ligaments are the primary stabilizers to varus–valgus stress when the joint is flexed to $\geq$ 30 degrees. The volar plate is the main stabilizer against hyperextension and a secondary stabilizer to varus–valgus stress in extension.

Injury to the UCL of the thumb can be acute or chronic. An acute injury occurs following forced hyperabduction and extension that results in ligament injury with or without a concomitant avulsion. Acute injuries are referred to as skier's thumb, because this is commonly seen in skiers who fall on an outstretched hand while gripping onto a ski pole. Ligament injuries are either incomplete or complete; the latter is disruption of the UCL with associated instability. A Stener lesion consists of interposition of the adductor aponeurosis between the proximal aspect of the ligament, which is displaced superficial and proximal to the adductor aponeurosis; the distal portion of the ligament lies deep to the aponeurosis. The aponeurosis acts as a mechanical barrier that prevents healing of a ligament injury and can progress to chronic instability. Chronic laxity of the UCL is also known as gamekeeper's thumb resulting from repeated hyperextension and adduction. Once the diagnosis has been confirmed radiographically, the stability of the joint is assessed by stressing it in full extension and at 30 degrees of flexion in order to isolate the UCL. Laxity is compared to the contralateral side; complete disruption is present if there is $\geq$ 30 degrees to 35 degrees of translation in extension or $\geq$ 15 degrees in 30 degrees of flexion. Presence of a painful mass on the ulnar aspect of metacarpal head–neck junction suggests a Stener lesion.

Partial disruptions are treated with immobilization for 4 to 6 weeks. Complete disruption of the ulnar collateral ligament often requires repair and/or internal fixation of concomitant avulsion fractures. Ligament reconstruction with tendon graft is indicated in patients with chronic symptomatic instability.

CMC Joint

The CMC joints of the index and long fingers are inherently very stable with very little motion because of the multiple articulations and ligamentous attachments of the bases of the index and long metacarpals. The CMC joints of the ring and small fingers are more mobile than their radial counterparts, allowing for approximately 10 and 40 degrees of motion in the sagittal plane respectively.

Interpretation of standard radiographs of the CMC joints of the fingers can be enhanced by obtaining a Bora view, which is a lateral view taken with the forearm in 30 degrees of pronation.

Fracture-dislocations of the radial three fingers typically result from high-energy trauma that involves multiple joints. Reduction may be closed or open; stabilization must be maintained by pinning the joint or internal fixation of fractures. Isolated CMC dislocations of the small finger typically occur in conjunction with a fracture (baby or reverse Bennett fracture-dislocation). Please refer to the metacarpal fracture section of this chapter to review reverse Bennett fracture.

Wrist Joint

The wrist is composed of 8 carpal bones in two rows, with the scaphoid acting as a link between the two rows. In the wrist, the muscles that act on the carpi do not insert on or arise from any of the carpal bones (one exception is the FCU on the hamate); therefore, the wrist has very little constraint on motion. For example, motion of the proximal carpi occurs only from pressure from the distal carpi or through tension from the ligaments. Overall wrist function is the result of the combination of carpal bone motion on each other, with stability provided by ligamental attachments and indirect tendinous action.

Wrist motion is centered on the head of the capitate, and in general, there is little motion between the carpal bones and the metacarpals, with each row of individual bones acting as one unit. However, the proximal row is much less constrained then the distal row and as a result can show more intercarpal motion. Instability of the wrist is described in many ways and may be *static* (no wrist action required to reveal instability) or *dynamic* (may be normal on single-view x-ray, but with wrist action, instability may reveal itself on radiograph). Dissociative carpal instability describes instability of the carpi within a row resulting from a tear in an intrinsic ligament, while nondissociative carpal instability describes instability between the rows resultant of a tear in supporting extrinsic ligaments. A combined intrarow and interrow instability is known as combined carpal instability. Four patterns of instability are clinically described: dorsiflexion instability, palmar flexion instability, ulnar translocation, and midcarpal instability.

Dorsiflexion Instability

The most common pattern of carpal instability, dorsiflexion instability is a dissociative instability in which there is disruption of the scapholunate ligament. The result is movement of the scaphoid into volar flexion with the rest of the proximal row moving into extension. Overall, a "zigzag" radiolunatecapitate alignment (with a dorsally rotated lunate) and increase of the scapholunate angle to greater than 30 to 60 degrees is produced and is known as a *dorsal intercalated segment instability*.

Palmar Flexion Instability

The second most common instability is palmar flexion, a dissociative instability that is opposite of the dorsiflexion instability. In this case, damage to the ligaments supporting the lunate and triquetrum result in volar rotation of the lunate and extension of the triquetrum and scaphoid. This pattern is known as a *volar intercalated segment instability*, and a scaphoidlunate angle less then 30 degrees may be seen.

Ulnar Translocation

Commonly seen in wrists affected by RA, ulnar translocation is a nondissociative instability in which the carpus translates ulnarly on the distal radius. Radiolunate fusion is reliable in RA patients.

Carpal Instability

Anatomy. The wrist is composed of the bases of the 5 metacarpal bones, the proximal and distal carpal rows, and the distal aspects of the radius and ulna;

it serves as the link between the hand and the forearm. The distal row consists of the trapezium, trapezoid, capitate, and hamate. The scaphoid, lunate, triquetrum, and pisiform make up the proximal row. The pisiform is a sesamoid and functions primarily as a lever arm for the FCU. The scaphoid serves as the link between the proximal and distal carpal rows. There are no musculotendinous attachments to the carpus; as a result, carpal bone stability must rely on ligamentous attachments and articular anatomy. There are 2 major groups of carpal ligaments: extrinsic ligaments, which are extracapsular and extend from the radius or metacarpals to insert on the carpal bones, and intrinsic ligaments, which are intracapsular and arise from and insert on adjacent carpal bones.

The extrinsic system comprises of dorsal and palmar divisions. The palmar division (Table 6.57) consists of the palmar radiocarpal ligaments, the radial collateral ligament, and the ulnocarpal complex. The palmar radiocarpal ligaments include the radioscaphocapitate ligament, the radiolunate ligament, and the radioscapholunate ligament (ligament of Testut). The ulnocarpal complex consists of the ulnolunate ligament, the UCL, the dorsal and palmar radioulnar ligaments, and the TFCC. The dorsal extrinsic ligaments consist of 3 ligaments that arise from the dorsal rim of the distal radius and include the radiolunate ligament, the dorsal radioscaphoid ligament, and the radiotriquetral ligament.

The intrinsic ligaments are divided into groups according to their length. The short intrinsic ligaments attach bones of the distal carpal row and typically do not fail secondary to injury. The intermediate ligaments include the scapholunate ligament, the lunotriquetral ligament, and the ligaments of the scaphotrapezial joint. There are 2 long intrinsic ligaments. The dorsal intrinsic intercarpal ligament runs from the scaphoid to the capitate and triquetrum. The long palmar intrinsic

TABLE 6.57 Palmar, Dorsal, and intrinsic carpal systems

Palmar System	
Ligament	***Important Features***
Palmar radiocarpal	
Radioscaphocapitate	Runs across the waist of the scaphoid; may play a role in scaphoid waist fractures
Long radiolunate	
Short radiolunate	Prevents dorsal dislocation of lunate in hyperextension injuries
Radioscapholunate	Neurovascular conduit (ligament of Testut) acts as check on motion of the proximal pole of the scaphoid
Radial collateral	
Palmar ulnocarpal (ulnocarpal ligamentous complex)	
Dorsal and palmar radioulnar	
Ulnolunate	
Ulnar collateral	
TFCC	
Dorsal System	
Ligament	***Important Features***
Radiolunate	
Dorsal radioscaphoid	
Radiotriquetral	Important stabilizer against VISI
Intrinsic Carpal	
Short intrinsic	
Intermediate Intrinsic	
Scapholunate (SLIL)	Consists of dorsal and palmar parts; dorsal SLIL consists of strong, thick fibers; important dorsal carpal stabilizer
Lunotriquetral (LTIL)	Consists of dorsal and palmar parts; dorsal LTIL consists of strong, thick fibers; important volar carpal stabilizer
Long Intrinsic	
Long palmar/deltoid	Important stabilizer of midcarpal joint

ligament, which is also known as the V, or deltoid, ligament, arises from the scaphoid and inserts distally on the capitate. The V ligament is one of the main stabilizers of the midcarpal joint.

Classification. Larsen and colleagues proposed a classification system for carpal instability that is based on the following 6 characteristics.

- *Chronicity*—Duration of injury can be acute, subacute, or chronic. With the exception of ligament avulsions, the potential for primary ligamentous healing after 6 weeks is little.
- *Severity*—The degree of resulting instability is graded as predynamic (partial ligament tears without malalignment after loading), dynamic (complete injury with carpal malalignment under certain loads), and static (complete injury with permanent carpal malalignment).
- *Etiology*—Not all causes of instability are traumatic; diseases such as RA can lead to ligament rupture.
- *Location*—The area of abnormal function may not always coincide with the location of initial injury. It is important to identify the number of joints involved also.
- *Direction*—The direction of malalignment must be identified. Several patterns of malalignment have been described; the most common type is DISI. Intercalated segment refers to the middle third of a 3-part system that is under compression. The system loses stability if connection between the middle third and proximal or distal third is lost. The proximal carpal row represents the intercalated segment between the forearm and hand. DISI pattern of injury occurs when the lunate, which acts as an intercalated segment, falls into hyperextension. VISI refers to excessive hyperflexion of the lunate. Passive abnormal ulnar or radial displacement of part of or the entire proximal row is referred to as ulnar or radial translocation respectively. Dorsal translocation refers to dorsal subluxation or dislocation of the carpal condyle, which typically occurs following a distal radius malunion.
- *Pattern*—Patterns of carpal instability can be divided into 4 major types.
    - *Carpal instability dissociative (CID)* occurs following disease or injury that leads to abnormal function of a joint between bones in the same row. Examples of CID include scapholunate dissociation, lunotriquetral dissociation, scaphoid nonunion or malunion, and advanced stages of Kienbock disease.
    - *Carpal instability nondissociative (CIND)* refers to abnormal function between the radius and proximal row and/or between both carpal rows without disruption between bones in the same row.
    - *Carpal instability complex (CIC)* has features of both CID and CIND types.
    - *Carpal instability adaptive (CIA)* refers to malalignment involving areas proximal or distal to the wrist.

Carpal instability can also be described as static versus dynamic instability—static instability can be visualized on plain radiographs. Dynamic instability can only be appreciated on stress radiographs.

Carpal Kinematics and Mechanics. Motion at the carpus occurs in 2 planes: flexion–extension and radial–ulnar deviation. Roughly half of flexion–extension occurs at the radiocarpal joint and half occurs at the midcarpal joint. Approximately 60% of radial–ulnar deviation occurs at the midcarpal joint and 40% at the radiocarpal joint. The center of rotation for motion of the carpus is within the head of the capitate. The midcarpal and radiocarpal joints translate in various directions during motion. During radial–ulnar deviation, the proximal row moves from flexion to extension and from extension to flexion with radial deviation. It is believed that this rotation is a result of pressure on the scaphoid's distal pole, which rotates into flexion with radial deviation. Flexion of the scaphoid leads to subsequent flexion of the lunate via the scapholunate ligament.

Etiology and Groupings. Instability occurs when there is disruption of the normal soft tissue and osseous constraints of the wrist. Instability is particularly obvious when a compressive force loads the wrist. Carpal instability can be grouped into 2 broad categories: dissociative and nondissociative.

- *CID* is instability secondary to intrinsic ligament injury.
- *CIND* is instability following extrinsic ligament injury, resulting in midcarpal or radiocarpal instability.

Instability can also be categorized into 4 main patterns: dorsiflexion instability, palmar flexion instability, ulnar translocation, and midcarpal instability.

- *Dorsiflexion instability*—Occurs following disruption of the scapholunate ligament, resulting in volar flexion of the scaphoid. The lunate and triquetrum rotate into extension because they are no longer connected to the scaphoid. The carpus becomes shortened, and the capitate migrates proximally and shifts dorsal to the longitudinal axis of the radius. Radiolunatocapitate alignment becomes zigzagged as a result of this injury and is known as DISI,

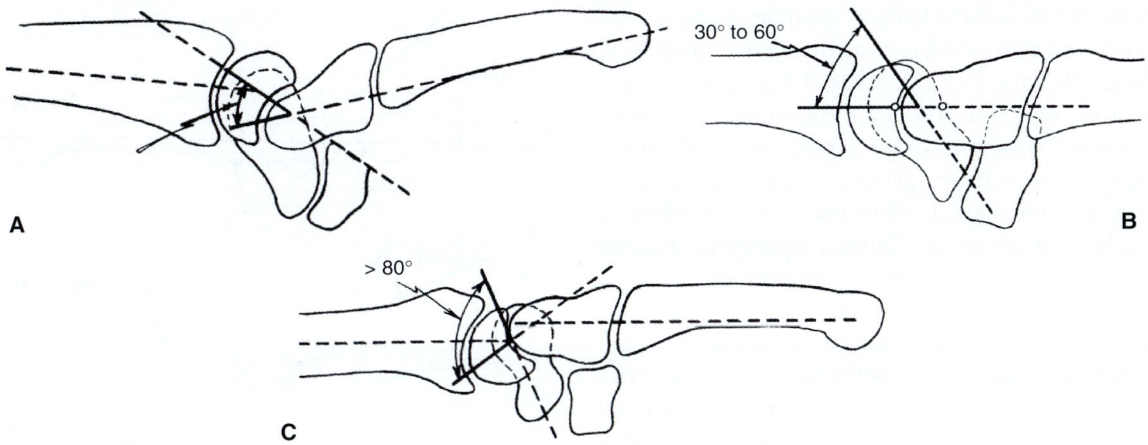

FIGURE 6.66 **(A) VISI deformity. (B) Normal carpal alignment. (C) DISI deformity. (*Source:* Cooney WP, Linscheid RL, Dobyns JH. Fractures and dislocations of the wrist. In: Rockwood CA, Green DP, Bucholz RW, Heckman JD (eds.), *Rockwood and Green's*, 4th ed. Philadelphia: Lippincott-Raven, 1996;762.)**

dissociative (Fig. 6.66). DISI is the most common pattern of carpal instability.

- *Palmar flexion instability*—Occurs following disruption of the lunotriquetral ligament. Disruption of this ligament leads to volar flexion of the lunate and extension of the triquetrum. This pattern of injury is known as VISI, dissociative.
- *Ulnar translocation*—Refers to abnormal ulnar displacement of the carpus and is typically seen in patients with inflammatory arthritis.
- *Midcarpal instability*—Can occur following ligamentous injury or malunion of a distal radius fracture where the normal palmar tilt becomes reversed, leading to carpal subluxation.

Mechanism of Injury. Carpal instability results from extension, ulnar deviation, and supination of the wrist; this is typically the mechanism injury following a fall on an outstretched hand with the wrist in dorsiflexion, ulnar deviation, and supination. Mayfield describes 4 stages of progressive perilunate instability that were observed in cadavers following this mechanism of injury (Table 6.58 and Fig. 6.67). The space of Poirer is the area formed by the diverging RSC and long RL ligaments and is a weak zone that is often violated in perilunate dislocations. The force vector and location

TABLE 6.58 **Mayfield stages of perilunate instability**

Stage	*Description*
I	Scapholunate diastasis
II	Dorsal dislocation of the capitate
III	Lunotriquetral dissociation
IV	Dislocation of the lunate

Source: Bednar JM, Osterman AL. Carpal instability: Evaluation and treatment. *J Am Acad Ortho Surg* 1993:1;10–17.

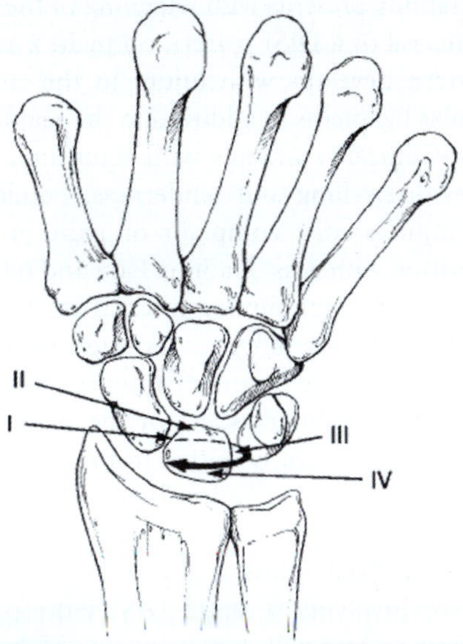

FIGURE 6.67 **Mayfield stages of progressive perilunate instability. I. Scapholunate diastasis. II. Dorsal dislocation of the capitate. III. Lunotriquetral dissociation. IV. Dislocation of the lunate. (*Source:* Bednar JM, Osterman AL. Carpal instability: Evaluation and treatment. *J Am Acad Ortho Surg* 1993:1;10–17.)**

and the position of the hand at the time of impact will determine if there will be a fracture, carpal instability, or both. Patients with carpal instability typically have a history of falling on an outstretched arm with subsequent symptoms of pain, snapping of the wrist with repetitive activity, giving way, and weakness. On physical examination, patients may exhibit tenderness to palpation along the injured ligaments, painful clicking, and pain at extremes of motion.

Scapholunate dissociation refers to abnormal carpal mechanics that results following rupture of the scapholunate ligament. It is the most common type of CID problem and can occur as an isolated injury or in conjunction with distal radius fractures or displaced scaphoid fractures. There is a spectrum of injuries, from scapholunate ligament sprains to perilunate dislocations; most scapholunate dissociations represent the initial stage of progressive carpal instability about the lunate, typically resulting from an indirect mechanism of injury that involves hyperextension, ulnar deviation, and midcarpal supination of the wrist. The ligament is usually disrupted from its scaphoid attachment. The dorsal portion of the ligament is responsible for most of the stability between the proximal pole of the scaphoid and lunate and is also responsible for providing the flexion moment across the lunate. Scapholunate dissociation can be static or dynamic; static instability presents with widening of the scapholunate interval or a DISI pattern on plain x-rays. The DISI pattern develops with injury to the surrounding capsular ligaments in addition to the scapholunate ligament. Clinically, patients with acute injuries may present with swelling and tenderness. Patients with chronic injuries may complain of pain or a popping sensation with wrist loading. Pain and tenderness over the dorsal scapholunate interval is characteristic. The Watson instability test is often positive and is performed with the examiner's thumb maintaining pressure on the palmar aspect of the distal pole of the scaphoid. The wrist is shifted from ulnar to radial deviation, resulting in a painful clunk caused by dorsal subluxation of the proximal pole of the scaphoid on the rim of the distal radius.

In cases involving a static DISI pattern, posterior–anterior x-rays will show widening of more than 3 mm of the scapholunate interval (Terry Thomas sign) and the cortical ring sign, which represents the cortex of the distal pole in a volarly flexed scaphoid. Lateral radiographs demonstrate an increase in the scapholunate angle, flexion of the scaphoid, and extension of the lunate. The scapholunate angle normally measures about 47 degrees (range 30 to 60 degrees) and increases to more than 70 degrees in cases of scapholunate instability (Fig. 6.68). Dynamic instability can be radiographically demonstrated with a posterior–anterior view of an ulnarly deviated, clenched fist that reveals widening of the scapholunate interval (Fig. 6.69).

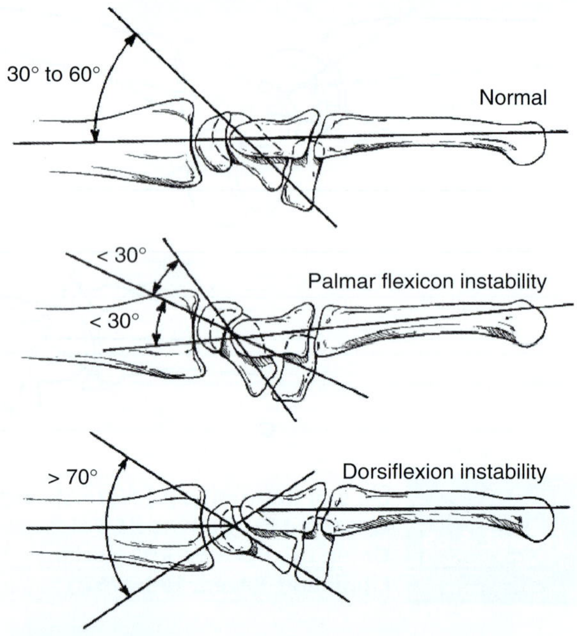

FIGURE 6.68 **Radiographic measurement of scapholunate angle in normal wrist and carpal instability. (*Source:* Bednar JM, Osterman AL. Carpal instability: Evaluation and treatment. *J Am Acad Ortho Surg* 1993:1;10–17.)**

An example of a static VISI pattern is lunotriquetral dissociation, the second most common type of carpal instability pattern. Anatomic studies have demonstrated that the palmar portion of the lunotriquetral ligament is the strongest and most stout. This region of the ligament is responsible for transmitting an extension moment across the triquetrum to balance the flexion moment of the scapholunate ligament. Patients typically complain of ulnar-sided wrist pain and/or weakness; unlike scapholunate injuries, there may not be a history of trauma. Symptoms are exacerbated when the wrist is axially loaded in ulnar deviation and pronation. The shear test for lunotriquetral instability is performed with the wrist in neutral. The examiner supports the lunate by placing his or her contralateral thumb over the dorsal lunate. The ipsilateral thumb is placed on the pisotriquetral joint and a load is applied in the anteroposterior plane. This load places a shear force across the lunotriquetral joint and results in pain, clicking, or both in the presence of instability. The ballottement test involves stabilizing the pisotriquetral joint between the thumb and index finger of one hand and the lunate in the opposite hand. The lunotriquetral joint is then loaded in an anterior to posterior direction. A test is positive if there is pain

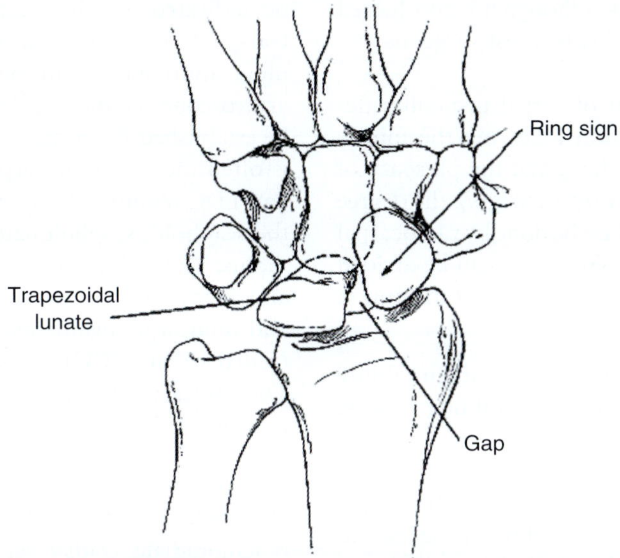

FIGURE 6.69 **Scapholunate dissociation. (*Source:* Bednar JM, Osterman AL. Carpal instability: Evaluation and treatment. *J Am Acad Ortho Surg* 1993:1;10–17.)**

and increased laxity in comparison to the contralateral wrist. Lunotriquetral instability can be differentiated from a TFCC tear by pain at the DRUJ on palpation and with forearm rotation. On radiographs, this injury will demonstrate the cortical ring sign, shortening of the scaphoid, and triangular appearance of the lunate on a posterior–anterior view but no widening of the scapholunate interval. Disruption of the Gilula arcs can be noted. The lateral radiograph demonstrates a palmarly flexed lunate and a scapholunate angle of less than 30 degrees (Fig. 6.70). Fluoroscopy and MRI may provide additional information; however, arthroscopy is both diagnostic and therapeutic.

Ulnar translocation is a CIND pattern of instability in which the carpus shifts ulnarly on the distal radius as a result of attenuation or disruption of the volar capsular and radiocarpal ligaments. This injury can be radiographically demonstrated by measuring the distance between a line extending from the long axis of the ulna and the head of the capitate divided by the length of the third metacarpal (ulnar carpal alignment). This ratio is normally 0.30 : 0.03. Also, if there is less than 50% of the lunate articulating with the radius on a posterior–anterior with the wrist in neutral, an increase in the distance between the radial styloid and scaphoid can also be noted.

Midcarpal instability is another type of CIND pattern of instability that can result after trauma as in cases of distal radius malunions that are dorsally angulated or in patients with ligamentous laxity. Patients may complain of mechanical symptoms and may or may not have pain. On examination, a clunk is appreciated when the wrist is loaded and translated from radial to ulnar deviation with the forearm in pronation. There may also be palmar sagging along the ulnar aspect of the wrist. Plain radiographs are usually normal; fluoroscopy often reveals a mechanical shift between the carpal rows. In general, fluoroscopy and MRI are additional imaging modalities that can delineate ligamentous injury for all types of injuries. Wrist arthroscopy is the most sensitive but also is a more

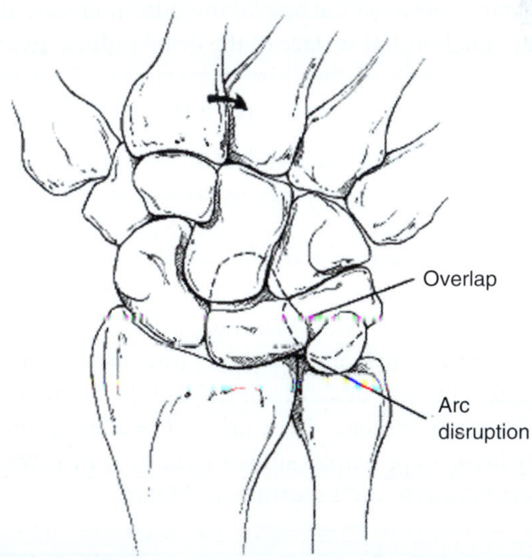

FIGURE 6.70 **Lunatotriquetral dissociation. (*Source:* Bednar JM, Osterman AL. Carpal instability: Evaluation and treatment. *J Am Acad Ortho Surg* 1993:1;10–17.)**

invasive method of diagnosis, although it is considered to be the best imaging modality by most surgeons.

Management. Management of carpal instability depends on time of presentation following the injury, the extent of ligamentous injury, and the presence of degenerative changes in the carpus. Staging the degree of a ligamentous injury can best be done by radiocarpal and midcarpal arthroscopy. Treatment can be divided into 3 categories based on the chronicity of the injury: acute, subacute, or chronic.

- *Acute*—Patients with acute scapholunate instability often present with symptoms resembling a wrist sprain that is treated with immobilization; the degree of injury can be assessed with diagnostic imaging. Partial tears can typically be treated by arthroscopic pinning for 6 to 8 weeks to avoid tear progression. Acute complete tears of the scapholunate ligament are best treated by open reduction and pinning with primary repair of the ligament.
- *Subacute*—Subacute scapholunate injuries present over 2 months following time of initial injury but are without degenerative changes; diagnosis is made with dynamic wrist imaging or arthroscopy. Treatment includes reconstruction via dorsal capsulodesis, tenodesis, bone-ligament-bone composite grafts, or intercarpal fusion.
- *Chronic*—Chronic injuries with associated degenerative changes lead to SLAC wrist due to the changes in mechanics and kinematics of the wrist. Carpal collapse is a result of chronic instability and leads to a decrease in the carpal height ratio. This ratio is the distance between the base of the third metacarpal to the subchondral surface of the distal radius, divided by the length of the third metacarpal. The carpal height ratio in a normal wrist is 0.54.

Treatment of lunotriquetral injuries with no gross instability or deformity begins with immobilization. Surgery is indicated in cases that require reestablishment of the rotational stability of the proximal row and the lunocapitate axis and may consist of ligament repair or reconstruction, arthrodesis of the lunotriquetral and midcarpal joint, proximal row carpectomy, or ulnar lengthening or shortening osteotomy, depending on the ulnar variance. Treatment of midcarpal instability involves principles similar to those for treatment of scapholunate and lunotriquetral injuries.

XIX. SELECTED EXPOSURES

Wrist Arthroscopy. Wrist arthroscopy is indicated for patients with mechanical wrist pain that has not been diagnosed via other modalities and that is retractory to conservative management. Operative arthroscopy may be indicated for the treatment of certain ligament tears, TFCC tears, articular cartilage injuries, and ulnar abutment syndrome. Using a 2.5- or 3.0-mm arthroscope, 3 radiocarpal and 3 midcarpal portals can be established for surgery. The first portal established is often the 3–4 radiocarpal portal between the EPL and EDC tendons. This portal allows visualization of the scaphoid, scapholunate (SL) ligament, and distal radius. The 4–5 radiocarpal portal between the EDC and EDM tendons allows visualization of the TFCC and ulnocarpal ligaments. The 6R radiocarpal portal (radial to the ECU) is used for inflow or outflow. The midcarpal portals include the midcarpal radial, midcarpal ulnar, and scaphotrapezial-trapezoid.

Anterior Approach to the Forearm. The Henry approach (anterior) utilizes the interval between the brachioradialis (radial nerve) and the pronator teres (median nerve). Proximally, it is necessary to isolate and ligate the leash of Henry and subperiosteally to strip the supinator from its insertion. During this approach, the superficial branch of the radial nerve is at risk and should be protected by isolating it laterally. Supination of the forearm displaces the PIN ulnarly.

Posterior Approach to the Forearm. The dorsal approach of Thompson utilizes the interval between the ECRB (radial nerve) and EDC (PIN). The PIN must be isolated and protected during this approach. Extensive retraction of the supinator will result in a traction injury to the PIN.

The dorsal and volar approaches to the wrist are covered under distal radius fractures.

References

1. Abboud JA, Beredjiklian PK, Bozentka DJ. Metacarpophalangeal joint arthroplasty in rheumatoid arthritis. *J Am Acad Orthop Surg* 2003;11:184–191.
2. Abrams RA, Botte MJ. Hand infections: Treatment recommendations for specific types. *J Am Acad Ortho Surg* 1996;4(4):219–230.
3. Adams BD. Distal radioulnar joint instability. In: Green DP, Hotchkiss RN, Pederson WC, Wolfe SW (eds.), *Green's Operative Hand Surgery*, 5th ed. Philadelphia: Elsevier, 2005;605–644.
4. Allan CH, Joshi A, Lichtman DM. Kienbock's disease: Diagnosis and treatment. *J Am Acad Orthop Surg* 2001;9:128–136.
5. Amadio PC, Botte MJ. Treatment of malunion of the distal radius. *Hand Clin.* 1987;3:541–561.
6. Amadio PC, Moran SL. Fractures of the carpal bones. In: Green DP, Hotchkiss RN, Pederson WC, Wolfe SW (eds.), *Green's Operative Hand Surgery,* 5th ed. Philadelphia: Elsevier, 2005;711–768.
7. Anderson GA. Ulnar nerve palsy. In: Green DP, Hotchkiss RN, Pederson WC, Wolfe SW (eds.), *Green's*

Operative Hand Surgery, 5th ed. Philadelphia: Elsevier, 2005;1161–1196.

8. Ashmead D IV, Rothkopf DM, Valton RL, Jupiter JB. Treatment of hand injuries by external fixation. *J Hand Surg Am* 1992;17:956–964.
9. Athanasian EA. Bone and soft tissue tumors. In: Green DP, Hotchkiss RN, Pederson WC, Wolfe SW (eds.), *Green's Operative Hand Surgery,* 5th ed. Philadelphia: Elsevier, 2005;2211–2263.
10. Athanasian EA. Malignant bone and soft-tissue sarcomas. *J Am Soc Surg Hand* 2004;4:60–72.
11. Baratz ME, Schmidt CC, Hughes TB. Extensor tendon injuries. In: Green DP, Hotchkiss RN, Pederson WC, Wolfe SW (eds.), *Green's Operative Hand Surgery,* 5th ed. Philadelphia: Elsevier, 2005;187–217.
12. Barron AO, Eaton RG. Save the trapezium: Double interposition arthroplasty for the treatment of stage IV disease of the basal joint. *J Hand Surg Am* 1998;23: 196–204.
13. Barron AO, Glickel SZ, Eaton RG. Basal joint arthritis of the thumb. *J Am Acad Orthop Surg* 2000;8:314–323.
14. Bednar JM, Osterman AL. Carpal instability: Evaluation and treatment. *J Am Acad Orthop Surg* 1993;1:10–17.
15. Benson LS, Williams CS, Kahle M. Dupuytren's contracture. *J Am Acad Orthop Surg* 1998;6:24–35.
16. Bentivegna PE, Deane LM. Chemical burns of the upper extremity. *Hand Clin* 1990;6:253–259.
17. Berger RA, Weiss APC (eds.), *Hand Surgery.* Philadelphia: Lippincott Williams & Wilkins, 2003;1280.
18. Bickels J, Wittig JC, Kollender Y, Kellar-Graney K, Mansour KL, Meller I. Enchondromas of the hand: Treatment with curettage and cemented internal fixation. *J Hand Surg* 2002;27A:870–875.
19. Blazar PE. Dislocations and instability. In: Beredjiklian PK, Bozentka DJ (eds.), *Review of Hand Surgery.* Philadelphia: Saunders, 2004;127–154.
20. Blazar PE, Steinberg DR. Fractures of the proximal interphalangeal joint. *J Am Acad Orthop Surg* 2000;8:383–390.
21. Bond CD, Shin AY, McBride MT, Dao KD. Percutaneous screw fixation or cast immobilization for nondisplaced scaphoid fractures. *J Bone Joint Surg Am* 2001;83:483–488.
22. Bora FW Jr, Didizian NH. The treatment of injuries to the carpometacarpal joint of the little finger. *J Bone Joint Surg Am* 1974;1459–1463.
23. Bora FW, Osterman AL, Thomas VJ, et al. The treatment of ruptures of multiple finger extensor tendons at the wrist level by a free tendon graft in the rheumatoid patient. *J Hand Surg Am* 1987;12:1038–1040.
24. Boyer MI. Acute flexor tendon injury. In: Green DP, Hotchkiss RN, Pederson WC, Wolfe SW (eds.), *Green's Operative Hand Surgery,* 5th ed. Philadelphia: Elsevier, 2005;219–240.
25. Boyer MI, Gelberman RH. Operative correction of swan-neck and boutonniere deformities in the rheumatoid hand. *J Am Acad Orthop Surg* 1999;7:92–100.
26. Browne EZ, Pederson WC. Skin grafts and skin flaps. In: Green DP, Hotchkiss RN, Pederson WC, Wolfe SW (eds.), *Green's Operative Hand Surgery,* 5th ed. Philadelphia: Elsevier, 2005;1629–1713.
27. Cassidy JT. Juvenile rheumatoid arthritis. In: Harris ED Jr, Budd RC, Genovese MC, Firestein GS, Sargent JS, Sledge CB (eds.), *Kelley's Textbook of Rheumatology,* 7th ed. Philadelphia: Elsevier, 2005;1579–1618.
28. Cassidy JT, Levinson JE, Bass JC, et al. A study of classification criteria for a diagnosis of juvenile rheumatoid arthritis. *Arthritis Rheum* 1986;29:274.
29. Catalano LW, Cole RJ, Gelberman RH, Evanoff BA, Gilula LA, Borrelli J. Displaced intra-articular fractures of the distal aspect of the radius. Long-term results in young adults after open reduction and internal fixation. *J Bone Joint Surg Am* 1997;79A:1290–1302.
30. Chidgey LK. The distal radioulnar joint: Problems and solutions. *J Am Acad Orthop Surg* 1995;3:95–109.
31. Chin KR, Jupiter JB. Treatment of triplane fractures of the head of the proximal phalanx. *J Hand Surg Am* 1999;24:1263–1268.
32. Chin KR, Jupiter JB. Wire-loop fixation of volar displaced osteochondral fractures of the distal radius. *J Hand Surg Am* 1999;24A:525–533.
33. Chou KH, Sarris I, Papadimitriou NG, Sotereanos D. Fractures of the hand, wrist, and forearm axis. In: Beredjiklian PK, Bozentka DJ (eds.), *Review of Hand Surgery*. Philadelphia: Saunders, 2004;101–125.
34. Davis TRC. Median nerve palsy. In: Green DP, Hotchkiss RN, Pederson WC, Wolfe SW (eds.), *Green's Operative Hand Surgery,* 5th ed. Philadelphia: Elsevier, 2005;1131–1159.
35. Dias JJ, Wray CC, Jones JM, Gregg PH. The value of early mobilisation in the treatment of Colles' fractures. *J Bone Joint Surg Br.* 1987;69:463–467.
36. Dingman P. Resection of the distal end of the ulna (Darrach operation): An end result study of twenty-four cases. *J Bone Joint Surg Am* 1965;34:893–900.
37. Doi K, Hattori T, Otsuka K, Abe T, Yamamoto H. Intra-articular fractures of the distal aspect of the radius: Arthroscopically assisted reduction compared with open reduction and internal fixation. *J Bone Joint Surg Am* 1999;81A:1093–1110.
38. Donthineni-Rao R. Tumors. In: Beredjiklian PK, Bozentka DJ (eds.), *Review of Hand Surgery*. Philadelphia: Saunders, 2004;189–205.
39. Doyle JR, Botte MJ (eds.), *Surgical Anatomy of the Hand and Upper Extremity*. Philadelphia: Lippincott Williams & Wilkins, 2003.
40. Doyle JR. Palmar and digital flexor tendon pulleys. *Clin Orthop* 2001;383:84–96.
41. Elliott DC, Kufera JA, Myers RA. Necrotizing soft-tissue infections: Risk factors for mortality and strategies for management. *Ann Surg* 1996;224:672–683.
42. Enneking WF. Staging of musculoskeletal neoplasms. In: Uhtoff HK, Stahl E (eds.), *Current Concepts of Diagnosis and Treatment of Bone and Soft Tissue Tumors*. New York: Springer-Verlag, 1984;1–21.

43. Feldon P, Terrono AL, Nalebuff EA, Millender LH. Rheumatoid arthritis and other connective tissue diseases. In: Green DP, Hotchkiss RN, Pederson WC, Wolfe SW (eds.), *Green's Operative Hand Surgery,* 5th ed. Philadelphia: Elsevier, 2005;2049–2136.
44. Fernandez DL, Geissler WB. Treatment of displaced articular fractures of the radius. *J Hand Surg Am* 1991;16A:375–384.
45. Fernandez DL, Ring D, Jupiter JB. Surgical management of delayed union and nonunion of distal radius fractures. *J Hand Surg Am* 2001;26A:201–209.
46. Fernandez DL, Wolfe SW. Distal radius fractures. In: Green DP, Hotchkiss RN, Pederson WC, Wolfe SW (eds.), *Green's Operative Hand Surgery,* 5th ed. Philadelphia: Elsevier, 2005;645–710.
47. Finkelstein H. Stenosing tendovaginitis at the radial styloid process. *J Bone Joint Surg Am* 1930;12:509–540.
48. Fontes RA, Ogilvie CM, Miclau T. Necrotizing soft-tissue infections. *J Am Acad Orthop Surg* 2000;8:151–158.
49. Freeland AE, Sud V. Unicondylar and bicondylar proximal phalangeal fractures. *J Am Soc Surg Hand* 2001;1:14–24.
50. Frykman GK. Fracture of the distal radius including sequelae: Shoulder-hand-finger syndrome, disturbance in the distal radioulnar joint and impairment of nerve function: A clinical and experimental study. *Acta Orthop Scand* 1967;108:5–153.
51. Gallant GC, Bora FW Jr. Congenital deformities of the upper extremity. *J Am Acad Orthop Surg* 1996;4:162–171.
52. Garcia-Elias Marc, Geissler WB. Carpal instability. In: Green DP, Hotchkiss RN, Pederson WC, Wolfe SW (eds.), *Green's Operative Hand Surgery,* 5th ed. Philadelphia: Elsevier, 2005;535–604.
53. Geissler WB, Fernandez DL, Lamey DM. Distal radioulnar joint injuries associated with fractures of the distal radius. *Clinical Orthop* 1996;327:135–146.
54. Gelberman RH, Menon J. The vascularity of the scaphoid bone. *J Hand Surg Am* 1980;5:508–513.
55. Gelberman RH, Panagis JS, Taleisnik J, et al. The arterial anatomy of the human carpus. Part I: the extraosseous vascularity. *J Hand Surg Am* 1983;8:367–375.
56. Gelberman RH, Wolock BS, Siegel DB. Fractures and non-unions of the carpal scaphoid. *J Bone Joint Surg Am* 1989;58:453.
57. Gellman H, Botte M, Shankwiler J, Gelberman RH. Arterial patterns of the deep and superficial palmar arches. *Clin Orthop* 2001;383:41–46.
58. Germann G, Philipp K. The burned hand. In: Green DP, Hotchkiss RN, Pederson WC, Wolfe SW (eds.), *Green's Operative Hand Surgery* 5th ed. Philadelphia: Elsevier, 2005;2159–2190.
59. Glickel SZ, Barron OA, Catalano LW III. Dislocations and ligament injuries in the digits. In: Green DP, Hotchkiss RN, Pederson WC, Wolfe SW (eds.), *Green's Operative Hand Surgery,* 5th ed. Philadelphia: Elsevier, 2005;343–388.
60. Glowacki K. Giant cell tumors. *J Am Soc Surg Hand* 2003;3:100–107.
61. Goebel SX, Rasi LM, Stern PJ. Multiple epidermal inclusion cysts in a patient with rheumatoid arthritis: A case report. *J Hand Surg* 2000;25A:768–771.
62. Goldfarb CA, Gerlberman RH, Boyer MI. Flexor tendon reconstruction: Current concepts and techniques. *J Am Soc Surg Hand* 2005;5:123–131.
63. Gray H. *Gray's Anatomy*. New York: Bartleby, 2000.
64. Gray JP, Jayaraman AG, Robinson-Bostom L. Cutaneous conditions of the hands: Part 2. *J Am Soc Surg Hand* 2003;3:66–77.
65. Green DP. Radial nerve palsy. In: Green DP, Hotchkiss RN, Pederson WC, Wolfe SW (eds.), *Green's Operative Hand Surgery,* 5th ed. Philadelphia: Elsevier, 2005;1113–1129.
66. Gulgonen A. Compartment syndrome. In: Green DP, Hotchkiss RN, Pederson WC, Wolfe SW (eds.), *Green's Operative Hand Surgery,* 5th ed. Philadelphia: Elsevier, 2005;1985–2013.
67. Gupta R. Nerve. In: Beredjiklian PK, Bozentka DJ (eds.) *Review of Hand Surgery*. Philadelphia: Saunders, 2004;79–100.
68. Gupta R, Bozentka DJ, Bora FW. The evaluation of tension in an experimental model of external fixation of distal radius fractures. *J Hand Surg Am* 1999;24A:108–112.
69. Gustilo RB. Current concepts in the management of open fractures. *AAOS Instr Course Lects* 1987;36:359–366.
70. Gustilo RB, Anderson JT. Prevention of infection in the treatment of 1025 open fractures of the long bones. *J Bone Joint Surg Am* 1976;58:453.
71. Haddad FS, Goddard NJ. Acute percutaneous scaphoid fixation: A pilot study. *J Bone Joint Surg Br* 1998;80:95–99.
72. Harness NG, Jupiter JB, Orbay JL, Raskin KB, Fernandez DL. Loss of fixation of the volar lunate facet fragment in fractures of the distal part of the radius. *J Bone Joint Surg Am* 2004;86A:1900–1908.
73. Harness NG, Mankin HJ. Giant-cell tumor of the distal forearm. *J Hand Surg* 2004;29A:188–193.
74. Henry AK. *Extensile exposure,* 2nd ed. Edinburgh: Churchill Livingstone, 1973.
75. Heppenstall RB. Compartment syndrome: Pathophysiology, diagnosis, and treatment. *Tech Orthop* 1997; 12:92–108.
76. Heppenstall RB, McCombs PR, Delaurentis DA. Vascular injuries and compartment syndromes. In: Bucholz RW, Heckman JD (ed.), *Rockwood, and Green's Fractures in Adults,* 5th ed. Philadelphia: Lippincott Williams & Wilkins, 2001;318–352.
77. Herren DB, Simmen BR. Limited and complete fusion of the rheumatoid wrist. *J Am Soc Surg Hand* 2002;2:21–31.
78. Hollinshead WH. *Anatomy for Surgeons,* Vol. 3. New York: Harper & Row, 1969.

79. Howard RF. Hand and microsurgery. In: Miller MD (ed.), *Review of Orthopaedics,* 4th ed. Philadelphia: Saunders, 2004;358–414.

80. Hresko MT, Rosenberg BN, Pappas AM. Excision of the radial head for congenital dislocation resulted in patients younger than 18 years. *J Pediatr Orthop* 1999;19:106–113.

81. James MA, Bednar M. Deformities of the wrist and forearm. In: Green DP, Hotchkiss RN, Pederson WC, Wolfe SW (eds.), *Green's Operative Hand Surgery,* 5th ed. Philadelphia: Elsevier, 2005;1469–1526.

82. Jebson PJL, Adams BD. Wrist arthrodesis: Review of current techniques. *J Am Acad Orthop Surg* 2001;9:53–60.

83. Jones KJ. Thoracic outlet compression syndrome. In: Green DP, Hotchkiss RN, Pederson WC, Wolfe SW (eds.), *Green's Operative Hand Surgery,* 5th ed. Philadelphia: Elsevier, 2005;1047–1073.

84. Jupiter JB. Complex articular fractures of the distal radius: Classification and management. *J Am Acad Orthop Surg* 1997;5:119–129.

85. Jupiter JB, Fernandez DL, Whipple TL, Richards RR. Intra-articular fractures of the distal radius: Contemporary perspectives. *AAOS Instr Course Lect* 1998;47:191–202.

86. Jupiter JB, Fernandez DL. Complications following distal radial fractures. *J Bone Joint Surg Am* 2001;83:1244–1265.

87. Jupiter JB, Ring D, Weitzel PP. Surgical treatment of displaced fractures of the distal radius in patients older than 60 years. *J Hand Surg* 2002;27A:714–723.

88. Kaempffe FA, Wheeler DR, Peimer CA, Hvisdak KS, Ceravolo J, Senall J. Severe fractures of the distal radius: Effect of amount and duration of external fixator distraction on outcome. *J Hand Surg Am* 1993; 18A:33–41.

89. Katarincic JA. Cleft hand. *J Am Soc Surg Hand* 2003;3:108–116.

90. Katz MA, Levin LS, Goldner RD, Urbaniak JR. Microvascular hand surgery. In: Beredjiklian PK, Bozentka DJ (eds.), *Review of Hand Surgery*. Philadelphia: Saunders, 2004;155–170.

91. Kay SP, McCombe D, Kozin SH. Deformities of the hand and fingers. In: Green DP, Hotchkiss RN, Pederson WC, Wolfe SW (eds.), *Green's Operative Hand Surgery,* 5th ed. Philadelphia: Elsevier, 2005;1381–1444.

92. Kienbock R, Peltier L (trans-ed). Concerning traumatic malacia of the lunate and its consequences: Degeneration and compression fractures [classic reprint]. *Clin Orth* 1980;149:4–8.

93. Kihara H, Palmer AK, Werner FW, Short WH, Fortino MD. The effect of dorsally angulated distal radius fractures on distal radioulnar joint congruency and forearm rotation. *J Hand Surg Am* 1996;21:40–47.

94. Knirk JL, Jupiter JB. Intra-articular fractures of the distal end of the radius in young adults. *J Bone Joint Surg Am* 1986;68A:647–659.

95. Koman LA, Ruch DS, Smith BP, Smith TL. Vascular disorders. In: Green DP, Hotchkiss RN, Pederson WC, Wolfe SW (eds.), *Green's Operative Hand Surgery,* 5th ed. Philadelphia: Elsevier, 2005;2265–2313.

96. Koval KJ, Zuckerman JD. *Handbook of Fractures,* 2nd ed. Philadelphia: Lippincott Williams & Wilkins, 2002;10–15.

97. Kozin SH. Current concepts review: Upper extremity congenital anomalies. *J Bone Joint Surg Am* 2003;85:1564–1576.

98. Kozin SH. Deformities of the thumb. In: Green DP, Hotchkiss RN, Pederson WC, Wolfe SW (eds.), *Green's Operative Hand Surgery,* 5th ed. Philadelphia: Elsevier, 2005;1445–1468.

99. Kozin SH. Pediatric hand surgery. In: Beredjiklian PK, Bozentka DJ (eds.), *Review of Hand Surgery*. Philadelphia: Saunders, 2004;223–245.

100. Kozin SH. Syndactyly. *J Am Soc Surg Hand* 2001;1:1–13.

101. Kozin SH, Kay SP, Griffin JR, Ezaki M. Congenital contracture. In: Green DP, Hotchkiss RN, Pederson WC, Wolfe SW (eds.), *Green's Operative Hand Surgery,* 5th ed. Philadelphia: Elsevier, 2005;1507–1526.

102. Kozin SH, Thoder JJ, Lieberman G. Operative treatment of metacarpal and phalangeal shaft fractures. *J Am Acad Orthop Surg* 2000;8:111–121.

103. Laffert RD. Thoracic outlet syndrome. *J Am Acad Orthop Surg* 1994;2:317–325.

104. Lamey DM, Fernandez DL. Results of the modified Sauve-Kapandji procedure in the treatment of chronic post-traumatic derangement of the distal radioulnar joint. *J Bone Joint Surg Am* 1998;80:1758–1769.

105. Leung YL, Beredjiklian PK, Monaghan BA, Bozentka DJ. Radiographic assessment of small finger metacarpal neck fractures. *J Hand Surg Am* 2002;27:443–448.

106. Light TR. Buttress pinning techniques. *Orthop Rev* 1981;10:49–55.

107. Linscheid RL. Kienbock's disease. *Instr Course Lect* 1992;41:45–53.

108. Mackinnon SE, Novak CB. Compression neuropathies. In: Green DP, Hotchkiss RN, Pederson WC, Wolfe SW (eds.), *Green's Operative Hand Surgery,* 5th ed. Philadelphia: Elsevier, 2005;999–1045.

109. Marcus AM, Hunt TR III. Infection. In: Beredjiklian PK and Bozentka DJ (eds.), *Review of Hand Surgery*. Philadelphia: Saunders, 2004;207–222.

110. May MM, Lawton JN, Blazar PE. Ulnar styloid fractures associated with distal radius fractures: Incidence and implications for distal radioulnar joint instability. *J Hand Surg Am* 2002;27A:965–971.

111. McFarlane RM. Patterns of the diseased fascia in the fingers in Dupuytren's contracture. *Br J Plast Surg* 1964;17:271–280.

112. McFarlane RM. Patterns of the diseased fascia in the fingers in Dupuytren's contracture. *Plast Reconstr Surg* 1974;54:31–44.

113. McFarlane RM. Dupuytren's disease. *J Hand Surg Br* 1996;21:566–567.

114. McGrouther DA. Dupuytren's contracture. In: Green DP, Hotchkiss RN, Pederson WC, Wolfe SW (eds.), *Green's Operative Hand Surgery,* 5th ed. Philadelphia: Elsevier, 2005;159–185.

115. Melone CP. Articular fractures of the distal radius. *Orthop Clin North Am* 1984;15:217–236.

116. Melone CP. Open treatment for displaced articular fractures of the distal radius. *Clin Orthop* 1988;202:103–111.

117. Metin A, Sadan A, Ercetin O. Surgical treatment of macrodactyly in older children and adults. *J Hand Surg Am* 2004;29:1010–1019.

118. Mih AD. Congenital clasped thumb. *Hand Clin* 1988;14:77–84.

119. Mills WJ Jr. Frostbite: A method of management including rapid thawing. *Northwest Med* 1966;65:119–125.

120. Minotti P, Taras JS. Ganglion cysts of the wrist. *J Am Soc Surg Hand* 2002;2:102–107.

121. Miura T, Suzuki M. Clinical differences between typical and atypical cleft hand. *J Hand Surg Br* 1984;9:311–315.

122. Miyake T, Hashizume H, Inoue H, Shi Q, Nagayama N. Malunited Colles' fracture. Analysis of stress distribution. *J Hand Surg Br.* 1994;19:737–742.

123. Monaghan BA. Anatomy. In: Beredjiklian PK, Bozentka DJ (eds.), *Review of Hand Surgery*. Philadelphia: Saunders, 2004;1–26.

124. Morgan WJ, Slowman LS. Acute hand and wrist injuries in athletes: Evaluation and management. *J Am Acad Orthop Surg* 2001;9:389–400.

125. Muller ME, Nazarian S, Koch P, Schatzker J. *The Comprehensive Classification of Fractures of Long Bones*. Berlin: Springer-Verlag, 1990.

126. Naidu S, Temple JD. Arthritis. In: Beredjiklian PK, Bozentka DJ (eds.), *Review of Hand Surgery*. Philadelphia: Saunders, 2004;171–187.

127. Newport ML. Extensor tendon injuries in the hand. *J Am Acad Orthop Surg* 1997;5:59–66.

128. Newport ML, Lane LB, Stuchin SA. Treatment of trigger finger by steroid injection. *J Hand Surgery Am* 1990;15:748–750.

129. Olson SA, Finkemeier CG, Moehring HD. Open fractures. In: Bucholz RW, Heckman JD (eds.), *Rockwood and Green's Fractures in Adults*, 5th ed. Philadelphia: Lippincott Williams & Wilkins, 2001;285–315.

130. Orbay JL, Fernandez DL. Volar fixed-angle plate fixation for unstable distal radius fractures in the elderly patient. *J Hand Surg* 2004;29A:96–102.

131. Patterson T. Congenital ring-constrictions. *Br J Plast Surg* 1961;14:1–31.

132. Phillips CS, Murphy MS. Vascular problems of the upper extremity: A primer for the orthopaedic surgeon. *J Am Acad Orthop Surg* 2002;10:401–408.

133. Plate AM, Lee SJ, Steiner G, Posner MA. Tumorlike lesions and benign tumors of the wrist and hand. *J Am Acad Orthop Surg* 2003;11(2):129–141.

134. Posner MA. Compressive ulnar neuropathies at the elbow: I. Etiology and diagnosis. *J Am Acad Orthop Surg* 1998;6:282–288.

135. Quitkin MH, Rosenwasser MP, Strauch RJ. The efficacy of silver nitrate cauterization for pyogenic granuloma of the hand. *J Hand Surg* 2003;28A:435–438.

136. Reilly DA, Garner WL. Management of chemical injuries to the upper extremity. *Hand Clin* 2000;16:215–224.

137. Rettig AC, Kollias SC. Internal fixation of acute stable scaphoid fractures in the athlete. *Am J Sports Med* 1996;24:182–186.

138. Richards RA, Wilson RL. Management of extensor tendons and the distal radioulnar joint in rheumatoid arthritis. *J Am Soc Surg Hand* 2003;3:132–144.

139. Richards RR. Current concepts review—Chronic disorders of the forearm. *J Bone Joint Surg Am* 1996;78:916–930.

140. Ring D. Intra-articular fractures of the distal radius. *J Am Soc Surg Hand* 2002;2:60–77.

141. Ring D, Jupiter JB, Herndon JH. Acute fractures of the scaphoid. *J Am Acad Orthop Surg* 2000;8:225–231.

142. Ring D, Prommersberger K, Jupiter JB. Combined dorsal and volar plate fixation of complex fractures of the distal part of the radius. *J Bone Joint Surg Am* 2004;86:1646–1652.

143. Rizzo M, Beckenbaugh RD. Results of biaxial total wrist arthroplasty with a modified (long) metacarpal stem. *J Hand Surg Am* 2003;28:577–584.

144. Rozental TD, Beredjiklian PK, Steinberg DR, Bozentka DJ. Open fractures of the distal radius. *J Hand Surg* 2002;27A:77–85.

145. Rozental TD, Bozentka DJ, Katz MA, Steinberg DR, Beredjiklian PK. Evaluation of the sigmoid notch with computed tomography following intra-articular distal radius fracture. *J Hand Surg* 2001;26A:244–251.

146. Rozental TD, Branas CC, Bozentka DJ, Beredjiklian PK. Survival among elderly patients after fractures of the distal radius. *J Hand Surg* 2002;27A:948–952.

147. Ruch DS, Chang DS, Poehling GG. The arthroscopic treatment of avascular necrosis of the proximal pole following scaphoid nonunion. *Arthroscopy* 1998;14:747–752.

148. Ruch DS, Ginn TA, Yang CC, Smith BP, Rushing J, Hanel DP. Use of a distraction plate for distal radius fractures with metaphyseal and diaphyseal comminution. *J Bone Joint Surg Am* 2005;87A:945–954.

149. Ruch DS, Koman LA, Smith TL. Chronic vascular disorders of the upper extremity. *J Am Soc Surg Hand* 2001;1:73–83.

150. Schneider LH. Fractures of the distal phalanx. *Hand Clin* 1988;4:537–547.

151. Schoen FJ, Cotran RS. Blood vessels. In: Cotran RS, Kumar V, Collins T (eds.), *Robbins Pathologic Basis of Disease,* 6th ed. Philadelphia: Elsevier, 1999;493–541.

152. Segalman KA, Graham TJ. Scaphoid proximal pole fractures and nonunions. *J Am Soc Surg Hand* 2004;4:233–249.

153. Seiler JG III, Olvey SP. Compartment syndrome of the hand. *J Am Soc Surg Hand* 2003;3:184–198.

154. Shah MA, Viegas SF. Fractures of the carpal bones excluding the scaphoid. *J Am Soc Surg Hand* 2002;2:129–140.

155. Shea K, Fernandez DL, Jupiter JB, Martin C. Corrective osteotomy for malunited, volarly displaced fractures of the distal end of the radius. *J Bone Joint Surg Am* 1997;79A:1816–1826.

156. Shin AY, Amadio PC. Stiff finger joints. In: Green DP, Hotchkiss RN, Pederson WC, Wolfe SW (eds.), *Green's Operative Hand Surgery,* 5th ed. Philadelphia: Elsevier, 2005;417–459.

157. Shin AY, Battaglia MJ, Bishop AT. Lunotriquetral instability: Diagnosis and treatment. *J Am Acad Orthop Surg* 2000;8:170–179.

158. Short WH, Palmer AK, Werner FW, Murphy DJ. A biomechanical study of distal radial fractures. *J Hand Surg Am.* 1987;12:529–34.

159. Shuler FD. Anatomy. In: Miller MD (ed.), *Review of Orthopaedics,* 4th ed. Philadelphia: Saunders, 2004;621.

160. Simic PM, Weiland AJ. Fractures of the distal aspect of the radius: Changes in treatment over the past two decades. Instructional course lectures. *J Bone Joint Surg Am* 2003;85A:552–564.

161. Simonian PT, Trumble TE. Scaphoid nonunion. *J Am Acad Orthop Surg* 1994;2:185–191.

162. Smith RJ. Intrinsic muscles of the fingers: Function, dysfunction and surgical reconstruction. *AAOS Instr Course Lect* 1975;24:200–220.

163. Sokolow C, Theron P, Saffar P. Preiser's disease. *J Am Soc Surg Hand* 2004;4:103–108.

164. Steiner GC. Benign cartilage tumors. In: Taveras JM, Ferrucci JT (eds.), *Radiology*. Philadelphia: Lippincott, 1986;7.

165. Stern PJ. Fractures of the metacarpals and phalanges. In: Green DP, Hotchkiss RN, Pederson WC, Wolfe SW (eds.), *Green's Operative Hand Surgery,* 5th ed. Philadelphia: Elsevier, 2005;277–341.

166. Stevanovic MV, Sharpe F. Acute infections in the hand. In: Green DP, Hotchkiss RN, Pederson WC, Wolfe SW (eds.) *Green's Operative Hand Surgery,* 5th ed. Philadelphia: Elsevier, 2005;55–93.

167. Strickland J. Flexor tendon injuries: I. Foundations of treatment. *J Am Acad Orthop Surg* 1995;3:44–54.

168. Strickland J. Flexor tendon injuries: II. Operative technique. *J Am Acad Orthop Surg* 1995;3:55–62.

169. Strom PC, Muller CA, Boll T, Pfister U. Two procedures for Kirschner wire. *J Bone Joint Surg Am* 2004;86A:2621–2628.

170. Su CW, Lohman R, Gottlieb LJ. Frostbite of the upper extremity. *Hand Clin* 2000;16:235–247.

171. Szabo RM, Steinberg DR. Nerve entrapment syndromes in the wrist. *J Am Acad Orthop Surg* 1994;82:115–123.

172. Taleisnik J, Watson HK. Midcarpal instability caused by malunited fractures of the distal radius. *J Hand Surg Am* 1984;9(3):350–357.

173. Tan V, Daluiski A. Tendon. In: Beredjiklian PK, Bozentka DJ (eds.), *Review of Hand Surgery*. Philadelphia: Saunders, 2004;27–47.

174. Taras JS, Kaufmann RA. Flexor tendon reconstruction. In: Green DP, Hotchkiss RN, Pederson WC, Wolfe SW (eds.), *Green's Operative Hand Surgery,* 5th ed. Philadelphia: Elsevier, 2005;241–276.

175. Terrono AL. The rheumatoid thumb. *J Am Soc Surg Hand* 2001;1:81–92.

176. Tomaino MM, Miller RJ, Cole I, Burton RI. Scapholunate advanced collapse wrist: Proximal row carpectomy or limited wrist arthrodesis with scaphoid excision? *J Hand Surg Am* 1994;19:134–142.

177. Trumble TE, Culp R, Hanel DP, Geissler WB, Berger RA. Intra-articular fractures of the distal aspect of the radius. Instructional course lectures. *J Bone Joint Surg Am* 1998;80A:582–600.

178. Trumble TE, Salas P, Barthel T, Robert KQ III. Management of scaphoid nonunions. *J Am Acad Orthop Surg* 2003;11:380–391.

179. Trumble TE, Schmitt SR, Vedder NB. Factors affecting functional outcome of displaced intraarticular distal radius fractures. *J Hand Surg Am* 1994;19:325–40.

180. Trumble TE, Vo D. Proximal pole scaphoid fractures and nonunion. *J Am Soc Surg Hand* 2001;1:155–171.

181. Trumble TE, Wagner W, Hanel DP, Vedder NB, Gilbert M. Intrafocal (Kapandji) pinning of distal radius fractures with and without external fixation. *J Hand Surg Am* 1998;23:381–394.

182. Trumble TE. Arthritis. In: Trumble TE (ed.), *Principles of Hand Surgery and Therapy.* Philadelphia: Saunders, 2000;401–435.

183. Tuncali D, Yilmaz AC, Terzioglu A, Aslan G. Histologic types of the glomus tumor. *J Hand Surg* 2005;30A:161–164.

184. Uroskie JA, Baratz ME, Schmidt CC. Vascular disorders of the hand and upper extremity. In: Beredjiklian PK, Bozentka DJ (eds.), *Review of Hand Surgery*. Philadelphia: Saunders, 2004;63–77.

185. Ursprung PS und Verlauf des R. Muscularis des nervus digitalis palmaris communis I (*N. medianus*). *Chir Praxis* 1974;18:471–474.

186. van Schoonhoven J, Fernandez DL, Bowers WH, Herbert TJ. Salvage of failed resection arthroplasties of the distal radioulnar joint using a new ulnar head prosthesis. *J Hand Surg Am* 2000;25A:438–446.

187. Von Schroeder HP, Botte M. The dorsal aponeurosis, intrinsic, hypothenar and thenar musculature of the hand. *Clin Orthop* 2001;383:97–107.

188. Wagner WF Jr, Tencer AF, Kiser P, Trumble TE. Effects of intra-articular distal radius depression on wrist joint contact characteristics. *J Hand Surg Am* 1996;21:554–560.

189. Walsh JJ, Berger RA, Cooney WP. Current status of scapholunate interosseous ligament injuries. *J Am Acad Orthop Surg* 2002;10:32–42.

190. Wassel HD. The results of surgery for polydactyly of the thumb. A review. *Clin Orthop* 1969;125:175–193.

191. Watson HK, Ballet FL. The SLAC wrist: Scapholunate advanced collapse pattern of degenerative arthritis. *J Hand Surg* 1984;9:358–365.

192. Weber ER. Biomechanical implications of scaphoid waist fractures. *Clin Orthop* 1980;149:83–89.

193. Weber ER, Chao EYS. An experimental approach to the mechanism of scaphoid waist fractures. *J Hand Surg Am* 1978;3:142–148.

194. Weckesser EC, Reed JR, Heiple KG. Congenital clasped thumb (congenital flexion-adduction deformity of the thumb): A syndrome, not a specific entity. *J. Bone Joint Surg* 1968;50A:1417–1428.

195. Weinstein LP, Hanel DP. Metacarpal fractures. *J Am Soc Surg Hand* 2002;2:168–179.

196. Wigart CR, Wolfe SW. Limited incision open techniques for distal radius fracture management. *Orthop Clin North Am* 2001;32:317–327.

197. Wolfe SW. Tenosynovitis. In: Green DP, Hotchkiss RN, Pederson WC, Wolfe SW (eds.), *Green's Operative Hand Surgery,* 5th ed. Philadelphia: Elsevier, 2005;2137–2158.

198. Wolfe SW, Austin G, Lorenze M, Swigart CR, Panjabi MM. A biomechanical comparison of different wrist external fixators with and without K-wire augmentation. *J Hand Surg Am* 1999;24A:516–524.

199. Wyrick JD. Proximal row carpectomy and intercarpal arthrodesis for the management of wrist arthritis. *J Am Acad Orthop Surg* 2003;11:277–281.

200. Young BT, Rayan GM. Outcome following nonoperative treatment of displaced distal radius fractures in low-demand patients older than 60 years. *J Hand Surg* 2000;25A:19–28.

201. Young SD, Mikola. Thumb carpometacarpal arthrosis. *J Am Soc Surg Hand* 2004;4:73–93.

202. Zalavras CG, Patzakis MJ. Open fractures: Evaluation and management. *J Am Acad Orthop Surg* 2003;11:212–219.

203. Zhao C, Amadio PC, Momose T, Couvreur P, Zobitz ME, An KN. Effect of synergistic wrist motion on adhesion formation after repair of partial flexor digitorum profundus tendon lacerations in a canine model *in vivo*. *J Bone Joint Surg Am* 2002;84:78–84.

Key References

Carpal Instability

Mayfield JK, Johnson RP, Kilcoyne RK. Carpal dislocations: Pathomechanics and progressive perilunar instability. *J Hand Surg Am* 1980;5:226–241.

This classic article presents the pathomechanics of progressive perilunate instability following a hyperextension and ulnar deviation injury and the principles of treatment.

Distal Radius Fractures

Jupiter JB, Ring D, Weitzel PP. Surgical treatment of redisplaced fractures of the distal radius in patients older than 60 years. *J Hand Surg Am* 2002;27:714–723.

This paper establishes criteria for early operative fixation of displaced distal radius fractures in patients 60 years of age.

Scaphoid Fractures

Filan SL, Herbert TJ. Herbert screw fixation of scaphoid fractures. *J Bone Joint Surg Br* 1996;78:519–529.

Dr. Herbert presents his experience treating over 400 scaphoid fractures with the revolutionary screw that he developed and popularized. Postoperative changes that are reported include hypertrophic scarring and STT joint changes on radiographs.

Anatomy

Gelberman RH, Menon J. The vascularity of the scaphoid bone. *J Hand Surg Am* 1980;5:508–513.

This is one of three landmark papers that elegantly describes the intricate blood supply to the scaphoid bone. The authors emphasize that the majority of the blood supply is provided by the branch of the radial artery that enters the dorsal ridge of the scaphoid and recommend a volar approach to the scaphoid in order to minimize disrupting the vascularity of the proximal pole.

Nerve

Gelberman RH (ed.). *Operative Nerve Repair and Reconstruction*. Philadelphia: JB Lippincott, 1991.

Dr Gelberman provides a well-referenced, comprehensive text that reviews clinical and surgical points of nerve injury and repair.

Infection

Kanavel A. *Infections of the Hand*, 4th ed. Philadelphia: Lea & Febiger, 1921.

This classic text presents Dr. Kanavel's ground-breaking work on the pathoanatomy of hand infections and stresses the importance of the potential spaces of the hand with respect to the collection and spread of microbial disease in the hand.

Tendon

Gelberman RH, VandeBerg JS, Lundborg GN, Akeson WH. Flexor tendon healing and restoration of the gliding surface: An ultrastructural study in dogs. *J Bone Joint Surg Am* 1983;65:70–80.

This landmark study examines tendon healing in canines by comparing total immobilization with early mobilization. It provides objective evidence that the intrasynovial gliding surface is restorable and that good results can be obtained with early mobilization after flexor tendon repair of zone II injuries.

Littler JW, Eaton RG. Redistribution of forces in the correction of boutonnière deformity. *J Bone Joint Surg Am* 1967;49:1267–1274.

This article describes boutonnière deformity and proposes a method of reconstruction that involves release and transfer of the lateral bands to the insertion site of the central slip.

Dupuytren Contracture

McFarlane RM. Patterns of the diseased fascia in fingers in Dupuytren's contracture. *Plas Reconstr Surg* 1974;54:31–44.

This classic article defines the pathoanatomy of Dupuytren contracture by identifying the specific ligaments and structures that are affected by the disease.

Congenital Deformity

Bora FW Jr, Osterman AL, Kaneda RR, et al. Radial club-hand deformity. Long-term followup. *J Bone Joint Surg Am* 1981;63:741–745.

This article provides reports from a long-term follow-up for the treatment of radial club-hand deformity on a large series of patients.

Refresher Questions

1. A woman injures the MCP joint of her thumb while skiing. Examination reveals tenderness along the ulnar aspect of the MCP joint. Radially directed stress of the joint in full extension produces 5 degrees of angulation. When the MCP joint is flexed 30 degrees, a radially directed stress produces 45 degrees of angulation. Radiographs are otherwise normal. Management should consist of
   a) a thumb spica cast and reassessment in 3 weeks.
   b) a thumb spica cast and reassessment in 3 weeks.
   c) repair of the ulnar collateral ligament of the MCP joint.
   d) adductor pollicis advancement on the proximal phalanx.
   e) repair of the MCP joint dorsal capsule

2. A partial laceration of the flexor tendon should be repaired when the percentage of tendon lacerated is more than
   a) 10%
   b) 20%
   c) 40%
   d) 60%
   e) 90%

3. What is the preferred type of graft for skin loss on the palmar aspect of the hand?
   a) unmeshed split-thickness
   b) meshed split-thickness
   c) multiple pinch
   d) full-thickness
   e) full-thickness with attached subcutaneous fat

4. A 48-year-old laborer sustains a traumatic amputation of his ring finger at the level of the proximal interphalangeal joint. Treatment the day of injury consists of primary closure after the FDP tendon is first sutured over the end of the remaining phalanx. What is the most likely complication?
   a) lumbrical-plus deformity to the ring finger
   b) intrinsic-plus deformity to the hand
   c) extrinsic-plus deformity to the hand
   d) extrinsic-minus deformity to the hand
   e) quadregia effect to the hand

5. Successful reconstruction of a hypoplastic thumb, excluding pollicization, is most dependent on which of the following factors?
   a) presence of the EPL tendon
   b) presence of the thenar muscles
   c) presence of the FPL tendon
   d) stability of the MCP joint
   e) stability of the CMC joint

6. What type of cell is associated with the pathogenesis of Dupuytren contracture?
   a) atypical macrophage
   b) myofibroblast
   c) tenocyte
   d) dermatocyte
   e) fibroblast

7. Following open carpal tunnel release, grip strength is expected to return to preoperative levels by how many weeks?
   a) 4
   b) 6
   c) 8
   d) 12
   e) 20

8. What is the most common infection occurring in a toddler's and preschooler's hand?
   a) paronychia
   b) felon (pulp infection)
   c) thenar space abscess
   d) herpetic whitlow
   e) septic flexor tenosynovitis

9. What is the most common congenital hand anomaly?
   a) symbrachydactyly
   b) camptodactyly

c) Syndactyly
d) polydactyly
e) constriction ring syndrome

10. What is the major advantage of allowing early active motion of a repaired zone II flexor tendon injury?

a) increased tendon excursion
b) greater repair strength
c) less postoperative pain
d) better patient compliance
e) faster tendon healing

Chapter 7

Adult Spine

TODD A. MICHENER AND KINGSLEY R. CHIN

I. ANATOMY

Knowledge of spinal anatomy is critical to the evaluation of the spine patient and understanding spinal pathology, imaging studies, and surgical approaches.

Column Theory. Denis classified the spine into three columns to help determine stable versus unstable fractures (Fig. 7.1):

1. *Anterior column*—Consists of the anterior longitudinal ligament (ALL) and anterior half of the vertebral body, disk, and annulus fibrosis.
2. *Middle column*—Consists of the posterior half of the vertebral body, posterior longitudinal ligament (PLL), disk, and annulus fibrosis.
3. *Posterior column*—Consists of the posterior elements: the pedicles, facets, lamina, ligamentum flavum, spinous processes, and interspinous and supraspinous ligaments.

Bones. Table 7.1 shows the bony anatomy of the spine.

Plumb Line. The sagittal plumb line in stance goes from the odontoid process through C7-T1 intervertebral disks and anterior to the thoracic vertebrae before crossing the spinal column again at the T12-L1 disk space. It travels posterior to the lumbar spine and finally crosses the spine again at the posterosuperior corner of S1, then travels anterior to the sacrum (Fig. 7.2). The coronal plumb line should bisect C1 and the sacrum.

Intervertebral Disk. Found between vertebral bodies from C2-3 to L5-S1 and rarely between the upper sacral vertebra, the intervertebral disk is relatively avascular. Only the outermost layers receive nutrients

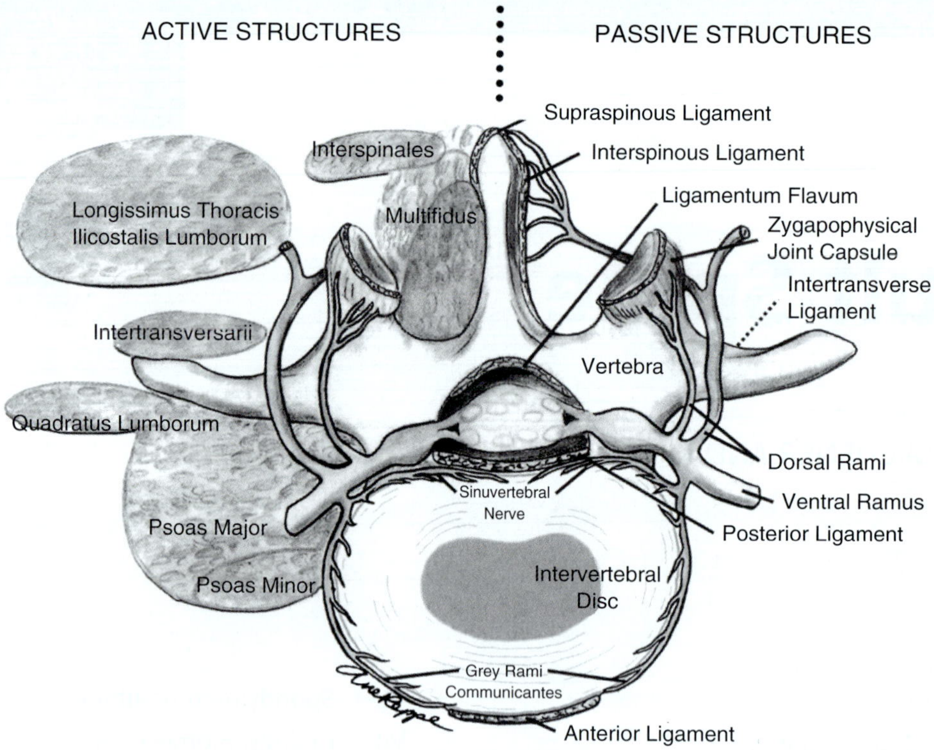

FIGURE 7.1 **Lumbar level (axial) showing muscles and nerves. (*Source*: Herkowitz H, Dvorak J, Bell GR, Nordin M, Grob D (eds.), *The Lumbar Spine*, 3rd ed. Philadelphia: Lippincott Williams & Wilkins, 2004;32.)**

from peripheral vascularization, while the central portion (nucleus pulposus) receives nutrients through diffusion from the vertebral endplates. The disks combine to make up approximately 1/4 of the length of the spinal column, but this measurement may change with position. Disks account for approximately 25% of spinal height. When an individual is lying flat, nutrients and fluid enter the disk and increase height, but the opposite happens with prolonged stance. The nucleus pulposus is made of predominantly type II collagen and is a remnant of the primitive notochord. The outer layers constitute the annulus fibrosis and are made of predominantly type I collagen. This multilayered fibrocartilaginous lattice of overlapping sheets runs in opposite directions, which adds strength especially in rotation. The thickest layers are anterior; the thinnest are posterolaterally. The outermost layers are continuous with the anterior and posterior longitudinal ligaments. The thinner posterolateral sections of the annulus and PLL are the most common sites for disk herniations. The annulus acts as a shock absorber by converting radially directed forces from the nucleus into hoop stresses at the disk periphery, where the fibers are attached firmly to the endplates by hyaline cartilage.

Smoking affects the disks by reducing solute exchange capacity and oxygenation, leading to impaired nutrition to the disk. Smoking reduces the cellular uptake rate of nutritional substances and has been shown to reduce metabolite production within pig disks. Smokers are noted to have a greater rate of disk degeneration.

Ossification Centers. Each vertebra has three primary ossification centers: 2 in the centrum/body and 1 cartilaginous center for each arch. The arches unite at the third month of fetal life. The 5 secondary ossification centers appear after puberty: 2 transverse processes, 1 spinous process, and 2 vertebral body endplates. The axis (C2) ossifies from 5 primary and 2 secondary centers. The dens is formed from 2 primary growth centers that originate from the centrum/body of the atlas (C1). Mammillary processes arise from ossification centers in the lumbar vertebrae. The arches fuse with the centrum during the seventh year in order from thoracic, cervical, lumbar, and sacrum. Spina bifida results from failure of arch formation.

Ligaments. Ligamentous anatomy of the spine is described in Table 7.2.

Musculature. Musculature of the spine is described in Table 7.3.

TABLE 7.1 Bony Anatomy of the Spine

Region (Mean spinal length = 71 cm)	No. (33 vertebrae)	Alignment	Angles	Features	Facet Orientation
Cervical	7	Lordosis	1. 20–40 degrees (50% flexion-extension between Occiput–C1; 50% rotation between C1–C2)	Foramina for vertebral artery C1 (atlas): no vertebral body or spinous process C2 (axis): dens (odontoid process) articulates with atlas Bifid spinous process and anterior tubercle except C7	45 degrees sagittal 0 degrees coronal Superior articular facet is anteroinferior to the above inferior facet
Thoracic	5	Kyphosis (Increases with age)	1. 20–50 degrees (mean 35) 2. T10 – L2 = 5 degrees 3. T12 – L2 = 3 degrees	Ribs (costal) facets present on T1 – L2 bodies and transverse processes Rounded foramen	60 degrees sagittal 20 degrees coronal Superior facet is anterior to above inferior facet
Lumbar	5	Lordosis (decreases with age)	1. 40–80 degrees (mean 60 degrees) 2. 60%–70% between L4 and S1	Largest vertebrae bears 80% axial load while facets bear 20% Mammilary processes project posteriorly from the superior articular facets L3 endplate and pedicles are parallel to floor while standing	Sagittal = 90 Coronal = 45 anterior Superior facet is anterolateral to inferior facet above
Sacrum	5	Kyphosis		Fusion of 5 spinal elements Promontory is anteroposterior portion of S1 Four pairs of anterior and posterior sacral foramina with respective branches of sacral nerves; the anterior foramina are larger Sacral canal opens caudally into sacral hiatus	
Coccyx	4	Kyphosis		Fusion of lowest 4 spinal elements Attachment site for muscles of the pelvic floor Attaches dorsally to gluteus maximus, external anal sphincter, and coccygeal muscles	

Blood Vessels. The aorta supplies spinal blood flow via branches of the vertebral, deep cervical, intercostals, and lumbar arteries. The segmental and radicular arteries branch from the aorta and provide additional blood flow to the spinal elements. The dorsal branches supply the dura and posterior elements; the ventral branches supply the vertebral body via ascending and descending branches, delivered underneath the PLL in 4 separate ostia. The aorta lies on the left; the azygos vein and inferior vena cava lie on the right.

- *Spinal Cord*—The arteries of the spinal cord include the anterior spinal artery, which lies in the anterior median fissure, and the 2 posterior spinal arteries, which run along the posterolateral sulci. Arterial supply to the spinal cord occurs from anterior and posterior spinal arteries and segmental branches of the vertebral artery and dorsal arteries that travel via the dorsal and ventral rootlets to the respective portions of the cord. The most significant radicular artery to the cervical spine originates from the deep cervical artery and accompanies the left C6 spinal nerve root.
- *Vertebral Artery*—The vertebral artery branches off the subclavian artery and ascends through the transverse foramina of C6 to C1. In less than 5% of cases, it may enter at C7. The vertebral artery travels posterior to the longus colli muscles, anterior to the nerves, and anteromedial to the lateral mass until, at C2, it goes laterally to enter the C1 foramen. It then curves medially along the superior border of the C1 grove to within 1.5 cm of midline before diving vertically through the foramen magnum to become the basilar artery. The vertebral artery is at risk 12 mm from the midline posterior aspect of C1 laterally and 8 mm from the superior aspect of C1. Anteriorly, the distance between the vertebral arteries decreases cephalad from 27.4 to approximately 2.3 mm at C6 and from 22.6 to approximately 1.8 mm at C3. The distance between the lateral border of the uncinate process and the medial border of the transverse foramen also decreases from a mean of 3.3 to approximately 1 mm at C6 and from 1.7 to approximately 0.8 mm at C4. Vertebral veins travel medial to the artery and are more likely to be injured first.

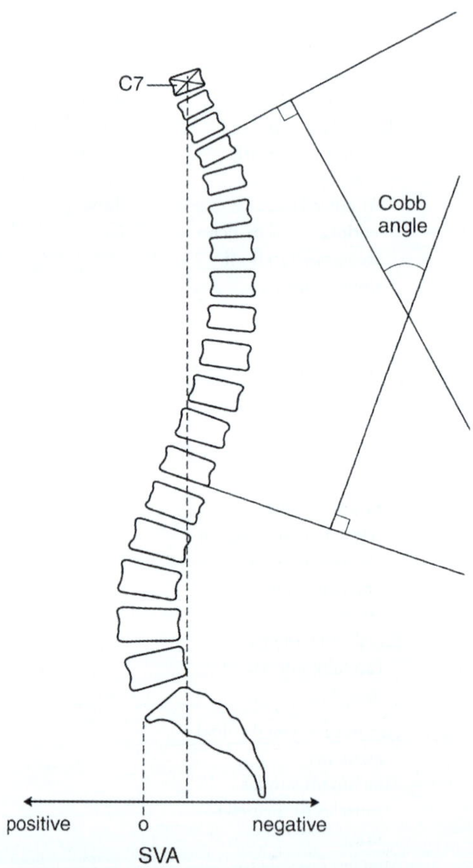

FIGURE 7.2 **Sagittal vertical axis (plumb line). Cobb angle. (*Source:* Herkowitz H, Dvorak J, Bell GR, Nordin M, Grob D (eds.), *The Lumbar Spine*, 3rd ed. Philadelphia: Lippincott Williams & Wilkins, 2004;611.)**

Innervation of the Spinal Canal. Superior and inferior branches of the sinuvertebral nerve innervate the articular connective tissue, periosteum, meninges, and vascular structures within the spinal canal.

Artery of Adamkiewicz. Also called the great anterior medullary artery, the artery of Adamkiewicz makes a major contribution to the anterior spinal artery and is the main blood supply to the lower spinal cord. It originates from the left side in 80% of people and accompanies the ventral roots of T9-11 but can originate from T5 to L5. It originates close to the foramen and costotransverse articulation, so ligation of the segmentals should be done at the level of the vertebral bodies to avoid injury. It is the largest of the medullary arteries and is also called the arteria radicularis magna. It supplies the caudal two thirds of the spinal cord.

Venous Drainage. Venous drainage of the vertebral bodies occurs through the central sinusoid located on the dorsum of each vertebral body. Epidural veins drain the neural elements, but spinal stenosis decreases this drainage and precipitates claudication.

Nerves. There are 8 cervical, 12 thoracic, 5 lumbar, 5 sacral, and 1 coccygeal nerve roots (Fig. 7.3). The dorsal and ventral roots join to form the spinal nerve. The ventral root and dorsal root ganglion are located

TABLE 7.2 Ligamentous Anatomy of the Spine

Ligament	*Features*
Anterior longitudinal ligament (ALL)	Limits hyperextension and supports the annulus fibrosis Begins at the basion as the anterior occipital membrane and ends on the anterior sacrum Thickest opposite the disk spaces and widens as it descends to the sacrum Separate fibers extend from 1 to 5 levels (deepest fibers span 1 level; intermediate fibers 2 to 3 levels; most superficial span 4 to 5)
Posterior longitudinal ligament (PLL)	Limits hyperflexion Hourglass-shaped with wider (thinner) sections over the disks posterolaterally Herniated disks occur lateral to thinner portions Consists of 2 layers (superficial layer lies adjacent to dura; deep layer connects to the annulus fibrosis centrally and extends into the foramen) Weaker than ALL Extends from occiput to the posterior sacrum Begins at posterior border of basion as the tectorial membrane and ends on sacrum Separated from center of vertebral body by space, allowing passage of dorsal branch of spinal artery
Intertransverse ligament	Runs between transverse processes Limits lateral bending, and in the lumbar spine acts as a border between the anterior and posterior structures (floor for bone graft during posterolateral fusion)
Ligamentous capsule	Overlay the zygapophyseal (facet) joints Contribute to stability
Ligamentum flavum	Maintains upright posture, preserves spinal curvature, and straightens the spine after flexion Yellow elastic ligament connecting lamina Always under tension Shingle pattern: anterior surface of the inferior border of the cephalad lamina to the posterior leading surface of the caudad superior lamina There are usually gaps at the midline to allow veins to exit Elasticity decreases with age and may be associated with hypertrophy and buckling, which contribute to nerve compression and stenosis
Interspinous ligament	Run between spinous processes and prevent hyperflexion
Supraspinous ligament	Acts as a tension band to limit hyperflexion and is a site of attachment for the fascial coverings of the medial spinal muscles Runs dorsal to while connecting the spinous processes Cervical portion is the ligamentum nuchae and extends from C7 spinous process to the external occipital protuberance; also attaches to the remaining cervical spinous processes and the posterior tubercle of the atlas
Apical ligament	Longitudinal ligament from tip of dens between alar ligaments to occiput
Alar ligament	Paired oblique ligaments connect the dens to the clivus of the occiput
Transverse ligament	Major stabilizer of the median atlantoaxial (C1-2) joint Sits transversely behind the dens Along with apical ligament, comprises the "cruciate" ligament
Iliolumbar ligament	Stout ligament connects L5 transverse process with ilium Avulsion fractures of L5 transverse process signals a vertical shear pelvic fracture
Denticulate ligament	Intradural ligaments that attach neural elements to the overlying membranes

TABLE 7.3 Musculature of the Spine

Muscles	Features	Innervation
Platysma	Anterior and superficial neck	CN VII
Stylohyoid and digastric	Anterior neck above hyoid	CN XII
Strap Sternohyoid Omohyoid	Superficial below hyoid	Ansa cervicalis
Strap Thyrohyoid Sternothyroid	Deep below hyoid	Ansa cervicalis
Sternocleidomastoid	Lateral and runs obliquely across the neck Rotates head to the contralateral side	CN X1 and ansa cervicalis
Trapezius	Superior back from spinous process of C7-T12 Insert on clavicle, scapula (AC, SP) Rotate scapula	CN XI
Latissimus dorsi	Inferior back from spinous process of T6-S5 and ilium Insert on humerus (ITG) Extend, adduct, internally rotate humerus	Thoracodorsal
Rhomboid major	Deep back Spinous process T2-5 Insert on medial scapula border Adduct scapula	Dorsal scapular
Rhomboid minor	Deep back Spinous process C7-T1 Insert on medial scapula spine Adduct scapula	Dorsal scapular
Levator scapulae	Deep back from spinous process C1-4 Insert on superior border of scapula Elevate and rotate scapula	C3, C4
Erector spinae group	Group of deep muscles (other group is transversospinalis) Runs from transverse and spinous processes of inferior vertebrae to spinous processes of superior vertebrae Stabilize and extends back	Dorsal primary rami of spinal nerves

CN, cranial nerve; AC, acromion; SP, spinous process; ITG, intertubercular groove

within the foramen. The S1 dorsal root ganglion more frequently lies intraspinally. The nerve becomes extradural as it approaches the foramen (dura becomes epineurium) at all levels above L1 but remains within the cauda equina below. In the cervical spine, the nerve root exits above the pedicle (example C5 exits at C4-5) but below the pedicle in the remainder of the spine. Spinal nerves exit the foramen and deliver dorsal primary rami which innervate the muscle and skin of the neck and back (Table 7.4). The ventral rami supply the anteromedial trunk and limbs. Ventral rami are grouped into plexuses before delivering sensorimotor functions with the exception of the thoracic nerves.

Pedicle and Nerves. The mean distance between the pedicle and dural sac is 1.5 mm. The mean distance between the pedicle and adjacent nerve root superiorly is 5.3 mm but 1.5 mm inferiorly in the lumbar spine.

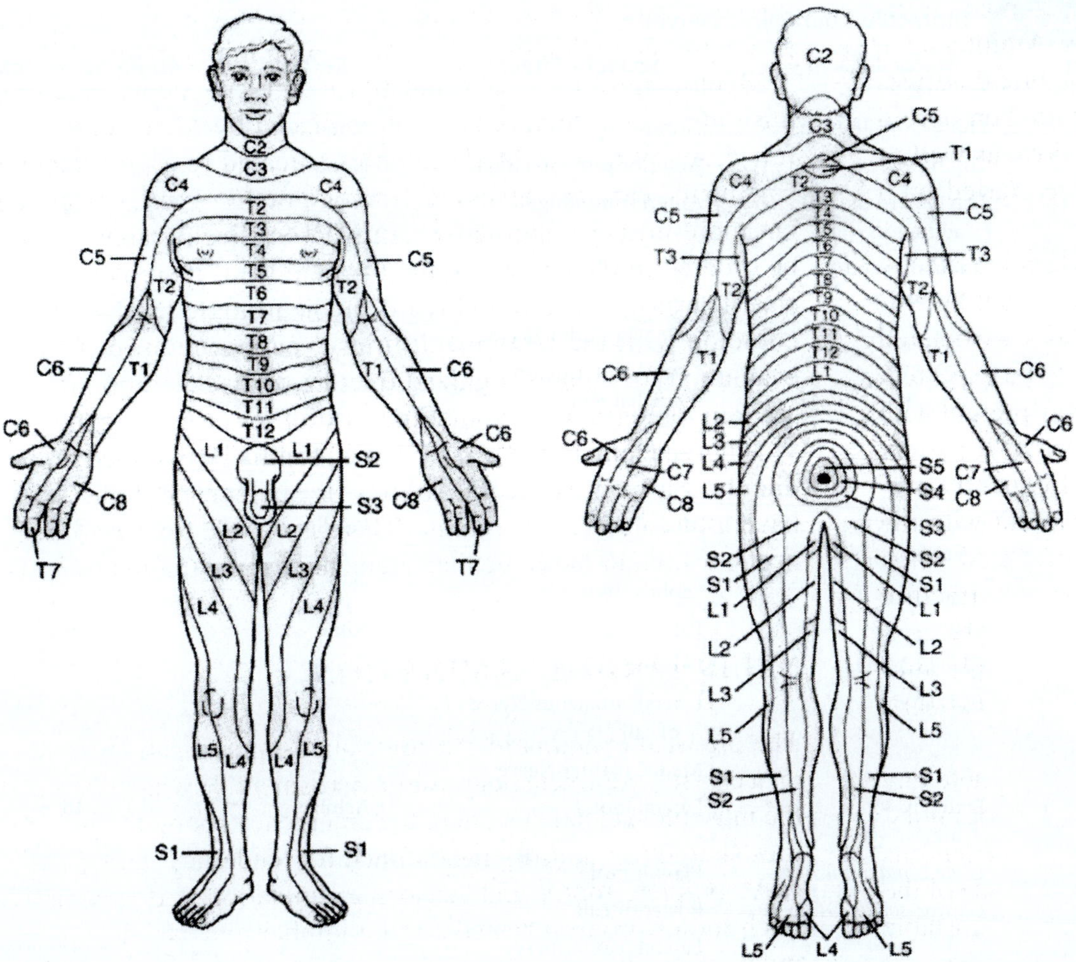

FIGURE 7.3 Dermatomes. (*Source*: Frymoyer JW, Wiesel SW, An HS, et al. (eds.), *The Adult and Pediatric Spine*, 3rd ed. Philadelphia: Lippincott Williams & Wilkins, 2004;826.)

TABLE 7.4 Cervicothoracic Nerves

Level	Nerve Root	Motor Effects	Sensory Effects	Reflex
C1-2	C2	Clavicular head of sternocleidomastoid	Head and neck	None
C2-3	C3	Trapezius, diaphragm	Head and neck	None
C3-4	C4	Scapula, diaphragm	Lateral neck/shoulder	None
C4-5	C5	Diaphragm, deltoid, biceps (elbow flexion)	Lateral arm (axillary nerve)	Biceps
C5-6	C6	Wrist extensors, biceps, triceps (supination)	Radial forearm, thumb, and index fingers (musculocutaneous nerve)	Brachioradialis
C6-7	C7	Triceps (elbow extension), wrist flexors, finger extensors Pronation	Middle finger	Triceps
C7-8	C8	Finger flexors, interossei	Ring and little fingers (ulnar hand), medial forearm (Medial antebrachial cutaneous nerve)	None
T1-2	T1	Finger abductors (interossei)	Medial arm (ulnar forearm) (medial brachial cutaneous nerve)	None

TABLE 7.5 Thoracolumbar Spinal Nerves

Root	Motor Effects	Sensory Effects	Reflex	Angle Nerve Takeoff
T12	Hip flexor (iliopsoas)	Groin	None	40
L1	Hip flexors	Anterior proximal thigh	None	32
L2	Hip flexors and adductors	Anterior midthigh	None	30
L3	Adductors and quadriceps	Distal thigh	Patellar (L2-L4)	27
		Lateral, anterior (L1-3)		
		Lateral, anterior, and medial femoral cutaneous nerves of the thigh and obturator nerve		
L4	Quadriceps and anterior tibialis	Medial leg	Patellar (L2-L4)	27
		Saphenous nerve		
L5	EHL	Lateral leg	None	27
	Gluteus Medius	Dorsum of foot		
	EDL/EDB	Lateral cutaneous Nerve of calf		
		Medial plantar Nerve		
S1	Peroneus longus and brevis	Lateral foot	Achilles	18
	Gluteus maximus	Plantar foot		
	Gastroc-soleus (S1/2)	Posterior calf		
		Lateral plantar nerve		
S1-4	Bowel/bladder	Perianal region	None	
	Foot intrinsics			
S4-5	Sphincter	Perianal	None	

Thus the nerve root is at greatest risk medially and inferiorly to the pedicle in the lumbar spine. In the thoracic spine, the mean distance from the pedicle to the superior nerve root ranges from 1.97 to 3.9 mm from T1 to T12, while the mean distance to the inferior root ranges from 1.7 mm to 3.7 mm (Table 7.5).

Sympathetic Chain. The cervical chain runs posterior to the carotid sheath and deep in association with the longus capitis and colli muscles. It runs anterior to the longus colli muscle and the transverse process and is *most vulnerable at C6.* There are three ganglia: superior, middle, and inferior (Table 7.6). Disruption of the inferior ganglia leads to Horner syndrome (meiosis, ptosis, and anhidrosis). Muscle strength and sensory and reflex grading are described in Tables 7.7 and 7.8.

Brachial Plexus. The brachial plexus gives off the peripheral nerve branches to the upper extremities and should be considered a potential site of pathology for patients with upper extremity complaints (Fig. 7.4; Table 7.9). It is formed from the ventral primary rami of C5-T1 and travels beneath the clavicle and between the scalenus medius and anterior to the axilla. The mnemonic **R**ob **T**aylor **D**rinks **C**old **B**eer describes the organization of the brachial plexus into five components: roots, trunks, divisions, cords, and branches. There are 5 roots (C5-T1 with occasional

TABLE 7.6 Ganglia

Ganglia	Location	Features
Superior	C2-3	Largest
Middle	C6	Variable
Inferior	C7-T1	"Stellate"

TABLE 7.7 Muscle Strength and Sensory Grading

Muscle Grade	Muscle Function	Clinical Findings	Sensory Grade
0	Absent	Paralysis	0–None
1	Trace	Palpable or visible contractions	1–Impaired
2	Poor	Active movement through full of motion with gravity eliminated	2–Normal
3	Fair	Active movement through full range of motion against gravity	
4	Good	Active movement through full range of motion against resistance	
5	Normal	Normal strength	

middle, lower), 6 divisions (two from each trunk), 3 cords (posterior, lateral, medial), and multiple branches. There are 4 preclavicular branches: dorsal scapular nerve, long thoracic nerve, suprascapular nerve, and nerve to subclavius. The plexus terminates into the musculocutaneous nerve (C5, C6, C7), axillary nerve (C5, C6), radial nerve (C5-T1), median nerve (C5-T1), and ulnar nerve (C7-T1). A prefixed brachial plexus has a large C4 contribution and T1 contribution, while a postfixed brachial plexus has T2 contribution but none from C5.

Lumbosacral Plexus. The lumbar plexus (consists of the ventral primary rami of T12-L4) travels on the surface of the quadratus lumborum and under and within the psoas major muscle (Fig. 7.5). It may have a prefixed (T11-L3) and postfixed (L1-5) variation. The sacral plexus usually involves the ventral primary rami of L4-S3. The sacral plexus is described further in Table 7.10. The genitofemoral nerve pierces the psoas and lies on the anteromedial surface. The femoral nerve lies between the iliacus and psoas. The lateral femoral cutaneous nerve (LFCN) lies on the iliacus and exits the pelvis under the lateral attachment of the inguinal ligament. The superior gluteal neurovascular bundle lies above the piriformis muscle, and the remaining neurovascular structures leave the pelvis below the muscle. The mnemonic 'POP'S IQ' describes the nerves from lateral to medial (pudendal, obturator internus, posterior femoral cutaneous, sciatic, inferior gluteal, and quadratus femoris). The pudendal and nerve to the obturator internus uniquely leave the greater sciatic foramen and reenter the pelvis via the lesser foramen.

TABLE 7.8 Reflex Grading

Reflex	Grade
Absence	0
Diminished	1
Normal	2
Hyperactive	3
Clonus	4

Femoral Nerve. The femoral nerve descends between the iliacus and psoas anteriorly into the thigh through the femoral triangle and under the inguinal ligament. An iliacus hematoma may irritate the nerve. The femoral triangle is bordered by the sartorius laterally, the pectineus medially, and the inguinal ligament superiorly. From lateral to medial, the floor is made of the iliacus, psoas, pectineus, and the adductor longus. From lateral to medial, the femoral triangle contains the femoral nerve, artery, vein, and lymphatic vessels (NAVL).

Sciatic Nerve. The sciatic nerve consists of the peroneal and tibial nerves and emerges from the pelvis anterior to the piriformis muscle and travels posterior to the other short external rotators lying superficially on the quadratus. It travels posteriorly to the adductor magnus and between the long head of the biceps and the semimembranosus.

Spinal Cord. The spinal cord is shorter than the vertebral column, ending in the conus medullaris at around L1 or L2. Nerve roots continue distally in the cauda equine (horse tail) until the thecal sac terminates in the filum terminale. The cord is covered by the meninges. The pia mater is closely adherent to the cord and cannot be dissected away (gives off denticulate ligaments to anchor the cord to the arachnoid though to the dura), the arachnoid (intermediate layer), and dura (outermost layer): remember 'PAD'. The arachnoid is transparent and encases the subarachnoid space that is filled with cerebrospinal fluid. The space extends to S2 (lumbar cistern is from L1 to S2). Between the dura and the arachnoid is the subdural space, which also extends to S2. The epidural space is outside the dura and contains the internal venous plexus and epidural fat (Fig. 7.6).

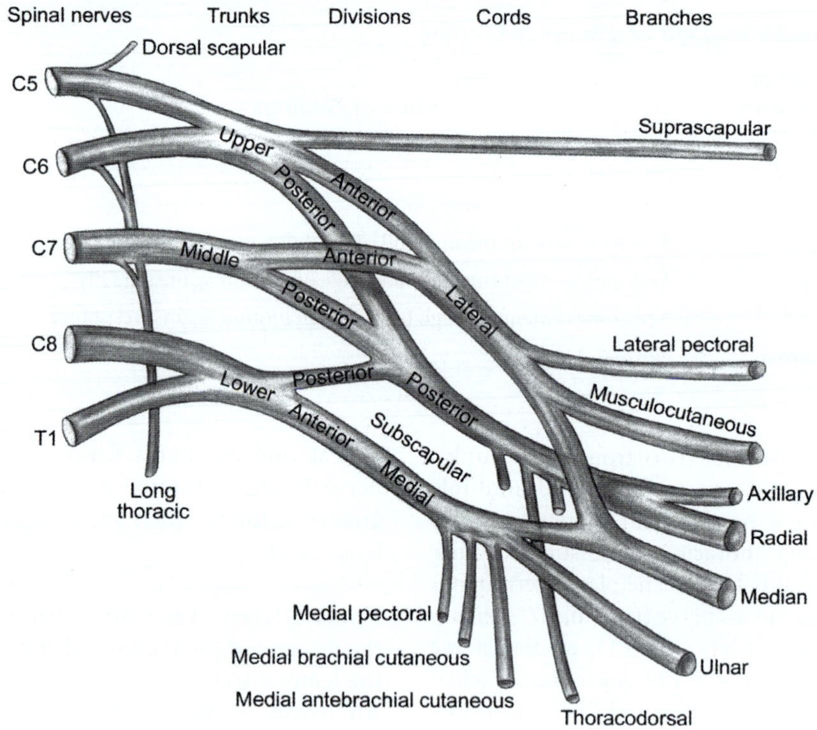

FIGURE 7.4 **Brachial plexus. (*Source*: Berger RA, Weiss AC. *Hand Surgery*, Vol 2 . Philadelphia: Lippincott Williams & Wilkins, 2004;980.)**

Cervical Spine. Tables 7.11, 7.12, and 7.13 describe the tracts, triangles, and topographical landmarks of the cervical spine.

Physical Examination and Special Tests. Diagnosing spine pathology starts with a careful history and physical examination. A history of localized pain may suggest tumor, infection, or trauma (such as pathologic compression fractures), while mechanical pain suggests instability or discogenic pain. Radicular pain suggests nerve compression such as a herniated disk, while claudication suggest spinal stenosis. Some special tests are listed in Table 7.14. Upper motor neuron (UMN) lesions caused by central nervous system pathology

TABLE 7.9 **Brachial Plexus Contributions**

Subdivision	*Roots*	*Terminal Branches*	*Muscles*
Roots	Dorsal scapular nerve	C5	Rhomboid major, minor
	Branch to phrenic nerve	C4, 5	Diaphragm
	Long thoracic nerve	C5, 6, 7	Serratus anterior
	First intercostals nerve	—	
Trunk	Suprascapular nerve	C5, 6	Supraspinatus
	Nerve to subclavius	C5, 6	Subclavius
Cord	Lateral pectoral nerve	C5, 6, 7	Pectoralis major
	Upper subscapular nerve	C5, 6	Subscapularis
	Thoracodorsal nerve	C7, 8–6	Latissimus dorsi
	Lower subscapular nerve	C5, 6	Subscapularis
	Medial pectoral nerve	C8, T1	Pectoralis minor
	Medial brachial cutaneous nerve	T1	Sensory
	Medial antebrachial cutaneous nerve	C8, T1	Sensory

Adapted from Monaghan BA. Anatomy. In: Beredjiklian PK, Bozentka DJ (eds.), *Review of Hand Surgery*. Philadelphia: Saunders, 2004;25.

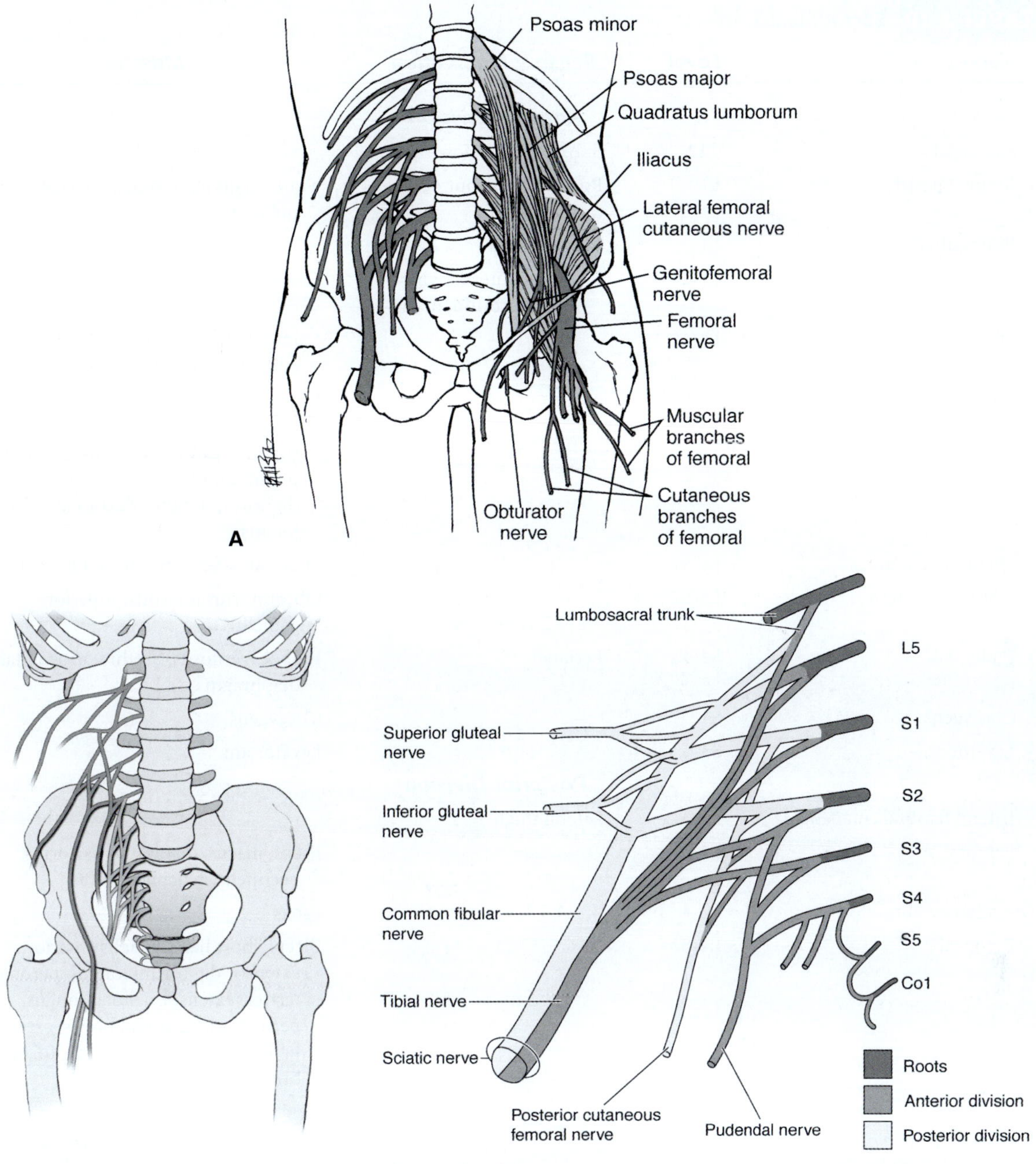

FIGURE 7.5 **Sacral plexus. (*Source*: *A from* Premkumar K. *The Massage Connection: Anatomy and Physiology*. Baltimore: Lippincott Williams & Wilkins 2004. *B from* Hendrickson T. *Massage for Orthopedic Conditions*. Chapter 16, Philadelphia: Lippincott Williams & Wilkins, 2002.)**

produce signs such as spasticity, hyperreflexia, clonus, and positive Hoffman and Babinski signs. Lower motor neuron (LMN) lesions are caused by peripheral nerve lesions and produce signs such as flaccid paralysis, areflexia, atrophy, and fasciculations. Herpes zoster is a rare cause of thoracic or lumbar radicularlike symptoms with pain preceding the skin eruptions. Night pain and weight loss in patients older than 50 years suggest tumor, and fevers and pain suggest infection. Back pain is a common complaint and accounts for the second most common reason to visit the physician after upper respiratory complaints, with a lifetime prevalence of 60% to 80%. It is difficult to separate patients with treatable causes from those malingering for secondary gains. Be aware that back pain can be referred from other sources, such as cholecystitis, nephrolithiasis, peptic ulcers, pancreatitis, a dissecting aortic aneurysm, and pelvic inflammatory disease. A history of back pain

TABLE 7.10 Sacral Plexus

Nerves	Level	Sensory Innervation	Muscles
		Anterior Division	
Subcostal	T12	Subxiphoid region	
Iliohypogastric	L1	Posterolateral buttock, above pubis	Transversus abdominis, internal oblique
Ilioinguinal	L1	Inguinal area	
Genitofemoral	L1-2	Proximal anteromedial thigh, scrotum, mons	Cremasteric
Obturator	L2-4		External oblique, adductor longus, adductor magnus (anterior), gracilis
Tibial	L4-S3		Semimembranosus, semitendinosus, long head biceps, adductor magnus, superior gamellus, soleus, plantaris, popliteus, tibialis posterior, flexor digitorum longus, flexor hallucis longus
Quadratus femoris	L4-S1		Quadratus femoris, inferior gamellus
Obturator internus	L5-S2		Obturatorius internus, superior gamellus
Pudendal	S2-4	Perianal	Bulbocavernosus, urethra, urogenital diaphragm
Coccygeus	S4		Coccygeus
Levator ani	S3-4		Levator ani
		Posterior Division	
Lateral femoral cutaneous	L2-3	Lateral thigh	
Femoral	L2-4		Psoas, iliacus, quadratus, sartorius, pectineus, articularis genu
Accessory obturator	L2-4		Psoas
Peroneal	L4-S2		Biceps short head, tibialis anterior, extensor digitorum longus, peroneus tertius, extensor hallucis longus, peroneus longus and brevis, extensor hallucis brevis, extensor digitorum brevis

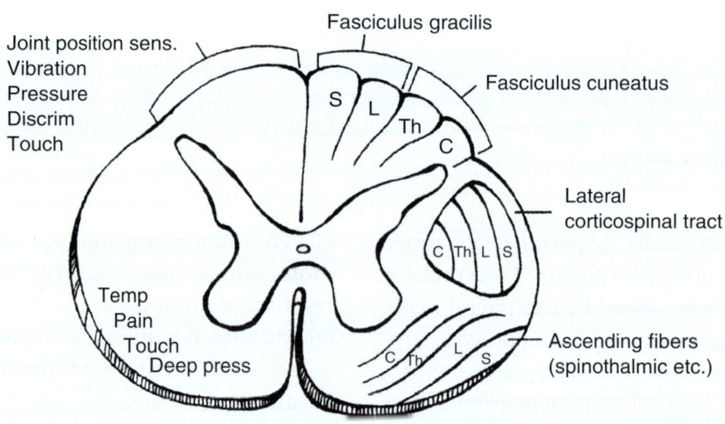

FIGURE 7.6 Spinal cord. (*Source*: Frymoyer JW, Wiesel SW, An HS, et al., (eds.), *The Adult and Pediatric Spine*, 3rd ed. Philadelphia: Lippincott Williams & Wilkins, 2004;620.)

TABLE 7.11 Tracts of the Cervical Spine

Tract	Features	Decussation
Lateral corticospinal tract	Motor: UE medial, LE lateral	Craniocervical
Posterior column	Proprioception, deep pressure, vibration	Craniocervical
Lateral spinothalamic tract	Pain and temperature (UE medial, LE lateral)	Spinal cord

is a risk factor for future complaints, especially with short intervals between complaints. Other risk factors include age over 30 but less than 60 years, smoking, heavy lifting, prolonged sitting, repetitive lifting, and repetitive vibrations (such as operating a jack hammer). Intradiskal pressure is reduced when lying supine and is the highest when sitting flexed forward with hand weights. Table 7.15 discusses nonorganic pathology, and Table 7.16 lists cervical spine radiographic parameters.

TABLE 7.12 Triangles of the Cervical Spine

Triangle	Borders
Anterior	Sternocleidomastoid
	Midline of the neck
	Lower border of the mandible
	Largest area
Submandibular	
Carotid	Posterior aspect of digastric
	Posterior aspect of omohyoid
Posterior	Trapezius
	Sternocleidomastoid
	Clavicle
Suboccipital	Superior and inferior heads of obliquus capitis and rectus capitis posterior major
	Contains vertebral artery, first cervical nerve, and greater occipital (C2) nerve superficially

TABLE 7.13 Topographical Landmarks

Hard palate	Arch of Atlas
Mandible	C2-3
Hyoid cartilage	C3
Thyroid cartilage	C4-5
First cricoid ring	C6
Carotid (Chassaignac tubercle)	C6 (anterior tubercle of the transverse process of C6)
Vertebra prominens	C7
Scapula spine	T3
Scapula tip	T7
Umbilicus	L3-4 disk space
Top of iliac crest	L4-5 interspace
PSIS	S2 spinous process

II. SPINAL CORD INJURIES

Approximately 12,000 to 14,000 acute spinal cord injuries occur annually in North America, with most affecting adolescent males secondary to motor vehicle collisions.

Manifestations of Spinal Shock. After a spinal cord injury, spinal shock occurs, manifested by flaccid paralysis, hypotonia, areflexia, and an absent bulbocavernosus reflex (BCR). At this time, the neurologic level cannot be determined. The BCR typically returns during the first 24 to 48 hours after the injury and can be tested by squeezing the glans penis, pubis, or pulling on a Foley and eliciting contraction of the anal sphincter.

Complete Spinal Cord Injury (SCI). Indicates no function below a given levels after spinal shock is over, where an incomplete injury has some distal neurologic function present especially sacral sparing. Approximately 80% of patients with a complete injury can anticipate improvement of one nerve root level around the injured level, and about 20% regain function at two levels (Fig. 7.7).

Incomplete SCI Syndromes. Incomplete are described in Table 7.17.

Foix-Alajouanine Syndrome. Rapid loss of spinal cord function caused by venous engorgement and ischemic infarction of the spinal cord due to obstruction of venous outflow typically from an arteriovenous malformation characterize Foix-Alajouanine syndrome. It

TABLE 7.14 Special Tests to Determine Spine Pathology

Sign	Pathology
Long Tract Signs	
Babinski: first toe dorsiflexion with fanning out of other toes when sharp instrument is rubbed on lateral border of foot from calcaneus to head of first metatarsal	Upper motor neuron lesion; corticospinal tract.
Hoffman: flick distal phalanx away from palm; look for pincer effect between thumb and index finger; look for asymmetry.	Cord compression; CNS dysfunction; brisk muscle stretch reflex
Trömner reflex: Elevate middle finger above other fingers and flick distal phalanx toward palm; look for pincer effect between thumb and index finger; look for asymmetry.	Cord compression; CNS dysfunction; brisk muscle stretch reflex
Inverted radial reflex: finger flexion upon testing brachioradialis reflex	Cervical myelopathy
Finger escape: abduction of fifth finger because of weak hand intrinsics	Cervical myelopathy
Lhermitte: neck flexion causing lightning-like sensation radiating down back	Cervical stenosis; disk herniation; multiple sclerosis with posterior column dysfunction (original description)
Cross adductor: stimulate patellar reflex and note contralateral thigh adductor contraction	UMN lesion
Chaddock: laterally abduct the little toe briskly and let it slap back against the other toes or flick the third or fourth toe down rapidly; note dorsiflexion of the great toe.	UMN lesion
Jaw jerk reflex: gently tap on patient's jaw with patient's mouth slightly open; a positive reflex is when the jaw closes	In a patient with UMN signs, a positive jaw jerk test suggests that the etiology is not in the cervical spine but that the pathology is located above the level of the pons
Nerve Root Compression	
Spurling: extend and bend the neck laterally and apply axial load to the top of the head; patient will report radicular pain.	Cervical nerve root compression
Straight-leg raise (SLR): with patient supine or sitting perform, SLR and patient will report pain in the distribution of the nerve root irritated; for sciatic involvement, the pain must extend distal to the knee	Nerve root compression
Contralateral SLR (Frajerstajn): raising asymptomatic side causes pain down symptomatic side	Indicates either a central disk herniation or an axillary herniation on the symptomatic side
Lasègue: perform SLR and then dorsiflex the ankle; should exacerbate SLR radiculopathy; less than 70 degrees of hip flexion is a positive Lasègue sign	Nerve root compression
Bowstring: with patient supine, raise leg, flex knee, then apply pressure to popliteal fossa to elicit radicular pain	Nerve root compression
Cram test: similar to Lasègue sign; extend hip then straighten leg to elicit pain	Nerve root compression
Milgram: patient raises both legs off examining table and holds for 30 seconds; note radiculopathy	Nerve root compression

TABLE 7.14 (continued)

Sign	Pathology
Naffziger: compress neck veins for 10 seconds with patient supine; coughing produces radiculopathy	Nerve root compression
Hoover: examiner places hands under patient's heel while the supine patient tries to perform SLR with the contralateral leg	If the patient is malingering or not trying, then there will be a lack of downward pressure on the hand under the heel (opposite foot not performing the SLR)
Femoral stretch: with patient prone or lying on side, the hip is held in extension and the knee is flexed	Femoral neuritis or L3 or L4 radiculopathy
Other Signs	
Wartenberg: unopposed abduction of the little finger	Ulnar nerve paresis
Beevor: have patient perform a quarter abdominal sit-up with arms crossed behind head; note any up, down, or sideways movement of the umbilicus	Lower abdominal muscles (controlled by spinal cord below T9) are weaker than upper abdominal muscles
Cremasteric reflex (males): stroke the inner thigh (genitofemoral nerve) and note ascent of the ipsilateral testicle	
Bulbocavernosus reflex: compress glans penis or pull on a Foley catheter; note contraction of the anal sphincter	When present, signals end of spinal cord shock after cord injury
Anal wink: apply sharp stimulus and note contraction of the external anal sphincter	When present, signals end of spinal cord shock after cord injury
Patrick (FABER) test: the hip is placed in a flexed, abducted, and externally rotated position, and ipsilateral foot is placed on opposite knee; pressure is put on ipsilateral knee and opposite ASIS	Sacroiliac pain
Localizing dermatomes	C6: thumb C7: middle finger C8: small finger T4: nipple T10: umbilicus L1: inguinal ligament

TABLE 7.15 Waddell Signs for Nonorganic Pathology

Signs	Outcome
Observations: Pain out of proportion to stimulus (example, light touch) Pain in a nonanatomic distribution Exaggerated pain response Four tests (none should be positive): 1. Skin roll test: roll skin between index and thumb and note radicular symptoms 2. Head compression: apply 5 pounds of load and note 3. Twist test: patient standing with feet planted, examiner rotates torso left and right and notes pain 4. Flip test: Perform sitting and supine SLR and note any difference in pain	Poor outcome after operative or nonoperative treatment if 3 or more positive signs

TABLE 7.16 Cervical Radiographic Parameters

Name	Findings
Atlantodens interval (ADI)	Anterior subluxation of 0–3 mm is normal in adults (0–5 mm in children), 3–6 mm suggests C1-2 instability (disruption of the transverse ligament), 5–7 mm suggests disruption of the alar ligaments, and 9 mm or more suggest disruption of the entire periodontoid-ligamentous and capsular structures, with gross instability
Pavlov/Torg ratio	Canal width, vertebral body width: normal approximately 1.0; stenosis less than 0.8; increased risk of transient quadriparesis but not predictive of permanent quadriplegia
McGregor line	Distance from the tip of odontoid to a line between hand palate and base of occiput on a lateral view; the tip should not project more than 4.5 mm above this line
McCrae line	A line across base of occiput from the anterior to posterior rim of the foramen magnum; the tip of the dens should not cross this line
Ranawat index	The distance along the odontoid is measured from the C2 pedicle to the transverse axis of the ring of C1; this technique prevents problems with changes in odontoid anatomy and identifying the bony landmarks at the base of the skull and hard palate; cranial settling is positive if the distance is less than 15 mm in males and 13 mm in females
Cervicomedullary angle	Normal angle is 135–175 degrees; applicable primarily in rheumatoids to diagnose basilar invagination if less than 135 degrees; this angle measures the intersection of vertical lines drawn along the anterior surface of the brainstem and the cord on a sagittal MRI
Power ratio	The distance from the anterior base of the occiput (basion) to the posterior arch of C1 divided by the distance from the anterior arch of C1 to the posterior base of the occiput (opisthion); should be 1.0 or less

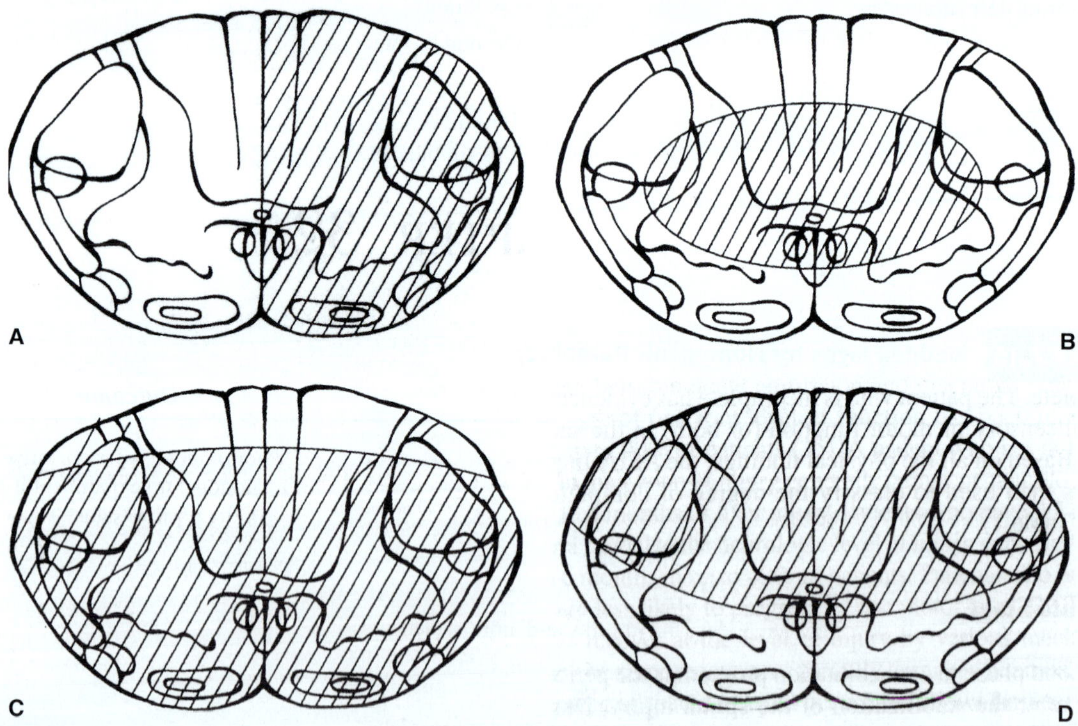

FIGURE 7.7 Complete spinal cord injury syndrome. (*Source*: Frymoyer JW, Wiesel SW, An HS, et al. (eds.), *The Adult and Pediatric Spine*, 3rd ed. Philadelphia: Lippincott Williams & Wilkins, 2004;620–621.)

TABLE 7.17 Incomplete Spinal Cord Injury Syndromes

Syndrome	*Mechanism*	*Injury (At or Below Level)*	*Prognosis*
Brown-Séquard syndrome: hemisection of spinal cord	Penetrating trauma; flexion-compression; vertebral artery	Ipsilateral loss of motor (UMN signs) Ipsilateral loss of proprioception and vibration Contralateral loss of pain and temperature	Best
Central cord syndrome: typically occurs in elderly patients with preexisting cervical stenosis	Extension injury	Most common Loss of motor and sensory upper ext > lower ext	Fair
Anterior cord syndrome: damage to anterior two thirds of spinal cord	Flexion-compression; spinal artery	Proprioception and vibration preserved Loss of motor at the level: LMN signs Loss of motor below the level: UMN signs Loss of pain and temperature	Poor
Posterior cord syndrome: very rare	Isolated injury to the posterior column with sparing of the anterior two thirds of the cord	Loss of deep pressure, joint position, and vibration No motor loss, but ambulation requires visual feedback	Good

is commonly seen in the lower thoracic and lumbar levels. Gray matter structures are more severely affected, and masses of enlarged, tortuous, and thick-walled subarachnoid veins can be seen overlying the cord mostly on the posterior aspect. Increasing unilateral and/or bilateral extremity weakness and numbness or tingling in the lower extremity may be asymmetric. Neurogenic claudication is common with brief exertion, and symptoms gradually worsen over months, eventually leading to fecal and urinary incontinence. Lumbosacral and coccygeal pan may be common. The upper extremities may become numb and weak with time.

Acute Management for SCI. Initial management of an SCI includes spine immobilization with or without traction, full trauma work-up, and methylprednisolone within the first 8 hours after injury. It is imperative during the trauma evaluation that the C7-T1 is seen because up to 10% of cervical spine fractures occur in this region. If C7-T1 is not clearly visualized, then a CT scan imaging is necessary.

Steroid Protocol for SCI. The steroid protocol for giving methylprednisolone after SCI is controversial as to whether any benefits outweigh the potentially significant side effects. Steroid treatment, if given, is dependent on time from injury to treatment:

- 0 to 3 hours: 30 mg/kg loading dose, then 5.4 mg/kg for 23 hours
- 3 to 8 hours: 30 mg/kg loading dose, then 5.4 mg/kg for 48 hours
- 8 hours: no methylprednisolone

This steroid protocol may improve spinal nerve root function at or near the level of injury, but not all neurologic function, as initially thought. In the NASCIS studies, significant complications included wound infection, pulmonary embolus, severe pneumonia, sepsis, and death, especially in the group receiving steroids longer than 48 hours. There was no statistical significance between groups.

Determination of Spinal Functional Level. On the basis of the American Spinal Injury Association's classification for determining a patient's functional level, the key muscles at the functional level must be at least at three-fifths motor strength (Table 7.18).

Baclofen Pumps in the Treatment of SCI. Intrathecal baclofen pumps have been shown to diminish spasticity

TABLE 7.18 American Spinal Injury Association Scale According to Level of Impairment

Grade	Motor Score Caudal to Injury level	Motor Function	Sensory Deficit Caudal to Injury Level
A	0:5	None	Complete
B	0:5	None	Incomplete
C	3:5	More than $\frac{1}{2}$ of key muscles below injury have less than grade-3 strength	Incomplete
D	> 3:5	More than $\frac{1}{2}$ of key muscles below injury have greater than grade-3 strength	Incomplete
E	5:5	Normal or radicular loss	None

Source: International Standards for Neurological and Functional Classification of Spinal Cord Injury. Chicago: American Spinal Injury Association Publication, 1996.

and improve function and quality of life in patients with severe spasticity related to an SPI.

Cauda Equina Syndrome (CES). CES is a surgical emergency and presents with bilateral buttock and leg pain, saddle back anesthesia, loss of lower extremity motor function, and bowel and bladder dysfunction (most commonly urinary retention). The nerve roots that control bowel and bladder function are S2, S3, and S4. Diminished reflexes and decreased rectal tone are also present. It is important to test perianal sensation and perform a digital rectal examination if CES suspected. If left untreated, patients with CES have a poor functional recovery. After surgical decompression, most patients will have return of normal motor function; however, nearly one third of patients will have some degree of voiding difficulties or sexual dysfunction.

Conus Medullaris Syndrome. This syndrome manifests as isolated loss of bowel and bladder function. Usually, it is the result of a neurologic injury at T12-L1, but it can be from T11 to L2.

Transient Quadriparesis. Typically seen with axial load injury or forced hyperextension or hyperflexion, transient quadriparesis presents with immediate motor weakness or paralysis and loss of sensation or paresthesia. It is often associated with cervical stenosis. Also, it has been associated with congenital fusions, HNP, and cervical instability. However, the decision whether to resume sports participation remains controversial. Loss of cerebrospinal fluid (CSF) space around the spinal cord may pose an unacceptable risk of future SCI if the patient resumes sports activity. On the other hand, multiple studies have shown no increased risk of SCI in athletes with narrowed spinal canal, even in high-contact sports such as football. The decision whether the athlete should resume participation in high-energy or contact sports should be left up to the athlete after he or she is informed accurately of the risks involved. In any case, the athlete should not be allowed to return until symptoms have resolved and the physical examination findings have returned to normal. If initial symptoms persist longer than 36 hours, then sports return should not be allowed.

Manifestations of Neurogenic Shock Versus Hypovolemic Shock. Neurogenic shock is the result of a traumatic sympathectomy with subsequent loss of the autonomic nervous systems control of vasoconstriction. It is associated with high thoracic and cervical spine injuries and manifests as hypotension and bradycardia. On the other hand, hypovolemic shock manifests as hypotension with resultant tachycardia.

Autonomic Dysreflexia. This condition is seen in patients who are paralyzed and have sympathetic nervous system overstimulation. Gastrointestinal and genitourinary obstructions, with resultant overdistension of visceral structures, are the most common reasons for autonomic dysreflexia to occur. It manifests with severe headaches, elevated blood pressure, blurred vision, diaphoresis, and anxiety. Initial treatment should include Foley catheterization or fecal disimpaction, as well as pharmacologic interventions for decreased blood pressure. Other causes have been described, such as fractures of the sacrum and femur and hip dislocations.

Treatment of Gunshots to the Spine. If a low-energy bullet is in the vertebral body, not causing any neurologic deficits, then the treatment should be to leave the bullet. Attempts at retrieval had worse complications then leaving it in place. However, if the bullet is lodged in the spinal canal causing neurologic deficits secondarily to compression, then the bullet should be removed via laminectomy. If the bullet is lodged in the vertebral body after it has penetrated a viscus (such as the colon), then the treatment is broad spectrum IV antibiotics administered for 7 days without surgical retrieval of the fragment.

III. CERVICAL SPINE

Fractures and Associated Injuries

Atlanto-occiput Dislocations. The tectorial membrane and the alar ligaments provide stability to the atlanto-occipital joint. Injuries to these structures results in gross joint instability. An atlanto-occiput dislocation is a rare injury with a very high mortality rate. Rare survivors have neurologic deficits with CN VII to CN X. High-resolution CT scan for diagnosis. There are 3 types:

- *I*—Anterior displacement of occiput on the C1; power's ratio greater than 1.0
- *II*—Longitudinal distraction
- *III*—Posterior subluxation or displacement

Initial treatment is placement of a halo vest. Since these are unstable fractures, an occiput cervical stabilization and fusion to C2 procedure is often necessary (Fig. 7.8).

Occipital Condyle Fractures. Occipital condyle fractures are rare, but 33% occur in conjunction with atlanto-occipital dislocations. They usually require CT scan for diagnosis. Patients may complain of headaches but may be neurologically intact. CN IX to CN XII are sometimes affected. Unstable fractures require posterior occipitocervical fusion. The classification is provided in Table 7.19.

Atlas Fractures. Atlas fractures are caused by axial loading and occur as an isolated injury less than 50% of the time. Neurologic injury is rare because of the wide canal diameter at this level. Fracture stability is determined by the diastasis of the lateral masses as determined by open-mouth odontoid view, but CT scan is the modality of choice. If there is spreading of the lateral masses greater than 6.9 mm, then there is transverse ligament insufficiency and instability is indicated. There are three types of Atlas fractures: posterior, anterior, and combined (Jefferson fracture).

Recommended treatment by fracture type is as follows.

- *Posterior Ring Fractures (Stable Fracture)*—Soft cervical orthosis. Injury pattern is an axial load with head in hyperextension.

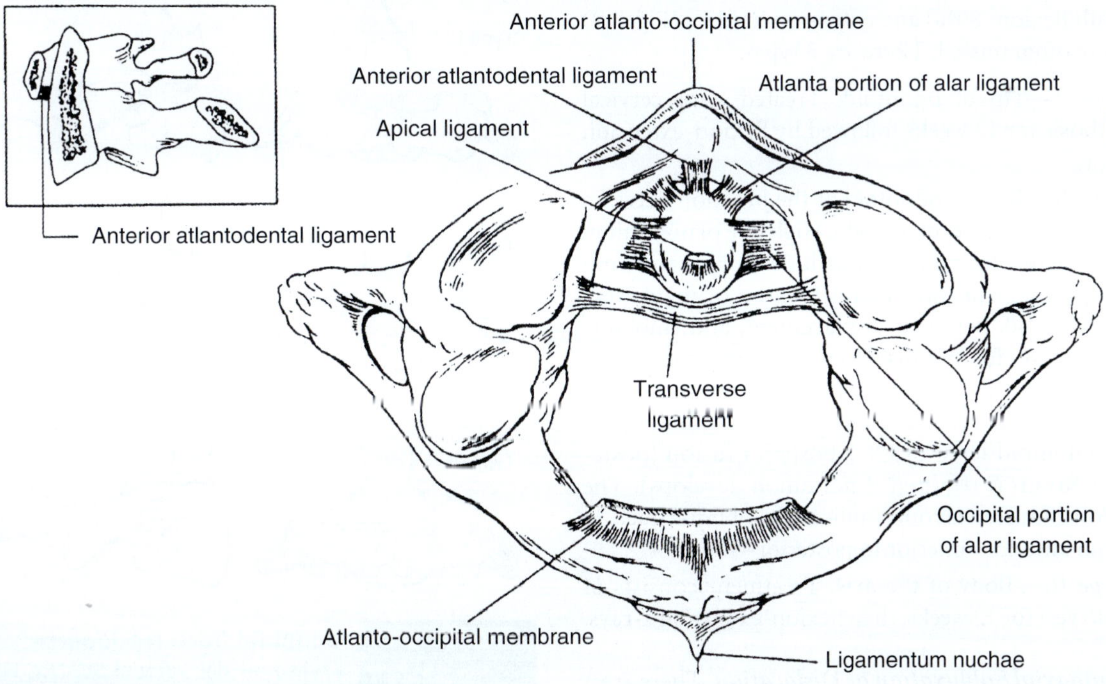

FIGURE 7.8 **Top view of the C1-2 joint. (*Source*: Herkowitz HN (ed.), *The Cervical Spine Surgery Atlas*, 2nd ed. Philadelphia: Lippincott Williams & Wilkins, 2004;342.)**

TABLE 7.19 Anderson and Montesano Classification of Occipital Condyle Fractures

Fracture Type	Stability	Fracture Description	Treatment
I	Stable	Axial impaction against lateral mass; comminuted but undisplaced	Cervical collar
II	Stable	A linear fracture associated with basilar skull fracture	Collar
III	Unstable	Avulsion fracture of the attachment site for the alar ligament	Halo or posterior fusion

Source: Anderson PA, Montesano PX. Morphology and treatment of occipital condyle fracture. *Spine* 1988; 13(7):731–736.

- *Fractures with less than 6.9 mm Lateral Mass Spreading*—Halo vest for 3 months, then test for C1-2 stability with flexion-extension lateral radiographs.
- *Fractures with more than 6.9 mm Lateral Mass Spreading*—Treatment is controversial: either halo vest for 3 months or traction for 6 to 8weeks then halo vest for 6 weeks followed by flexion-extension x-rays.

Surgery is necessary when there is a nonunion, malunion, or 5 mm or more of C1-2 instability present on the flexion-extension x-rays after removal of the halo vest. If the posterior arch is intact, then a posterior C1-2 fusion is performed. If the posterior ring is not intact, then fusion from the occiput to C2 is carried out.

Odontoid Fractures. Odontoid fractures are caused by both flexion (80%) and extension injuries (Fig. 7.9) and are often missed. There are 3 types:

- *Type I*—Tip of odontoid. Treated with cervical orthosis for 12 weeks followed by flexion-extension x-rays.
- *Type II*—Base of odontoid at the junction between the dens and C2 central body. High rate of nonunion. Risk factors for nonunion include more than 5 mm of displacement, more than 10 degrees of angulation, age over 40, posterior displacement, and smoking. Treatment for nondisplaced fractures consists of halo vest for 12 weeks, then flexion-extension x-rays. If there are 2 or more risk factors for nonunion, use an odontoid screw or C1-2 posterior fusion (posterior fusion is required if nonunion develops). The odontoid screw is contraindicated if oblique fracture from anterior–inferior to posterior–superior.
- *Type III*—Body of the axis. Treatment consists of halo vest for 12 weeks, then flexion-extension x-rays.

Atlantoaxial Subluxation or Dislocation. There are 3 types.

- *Anterior Subluxation with or without Fracture*—Transverse ligament disruption; treatment entails traction for reduction, then halo vest.
- *Posterior Subluxation with or without Fracture*—Rupture of alar and apical ligaments, high rate of recurrence if treated nonoperatively; treatment entails C1-2 posterior fusion.
- *Rotatory Subluxation (Grisel Syndrome)*—Rupture of transverse ligament; treatment entails initial trial of traction for reduction up to 3 weeks, then halo vest, or if traction fails, open reduction and C1-2 fusion

If patients are treated nonoperatively and follow up flexion-extension lateral radiographs reveal an atlantodens interval (ADI) greater than 5 mm, a C1-2 fusion is warranted.

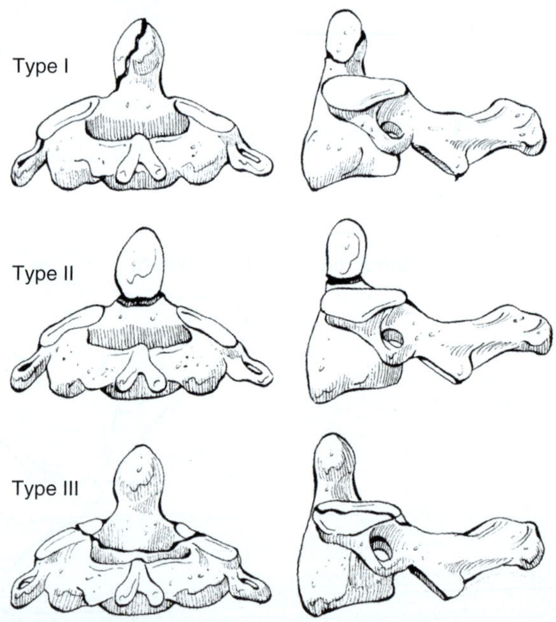

FIGURE 7.9 Odontoid fractures. (*Source:* Frymoyer JW, Wiesel SW, An HS, et al. (eds.), *The Adult and Pediatric Spine*, 3rd ed. Philadelphia: Lippincott Williams & Wilkins, 2004: Fig. 13, p. 649.)

Hangman Fracture (Traumatic Spondylolisthesis of the Axis). This type of fracture occurs through the neural arch of C2 (Fig. 7.10). A modified Effendi classification is as follows:

- *Type I*—Vertical fracture with less than 3 mm displacement and no angulation is treated with a rigid cervical collar or halo for 12 weeks.
- *Type II*—A fracture with more than 3 mm displacement, more than 11 degrees of angulation, and usually inferior body of C2 wedge compression and C3 anterior–superior endplate compression is treated with traction or halo vest 3 months
- *Type IIA*—For fractures with minimal translation, significant angulation, C2-3 disk and PLL disruption but ALL intact, treatment includes reduction in extension but *no traction*, followed by halo. Posterior fusion.
- *Type III*—For type III, unstable (increased likelihood of neurologic damage), vertical fractures with unilateral or bilateral C2-3 facet dislocations, treatment may include closed reduction followed by open stabilization with halo immobilization. Surgical stabilization and posterior C2-3 fusion is recommended.

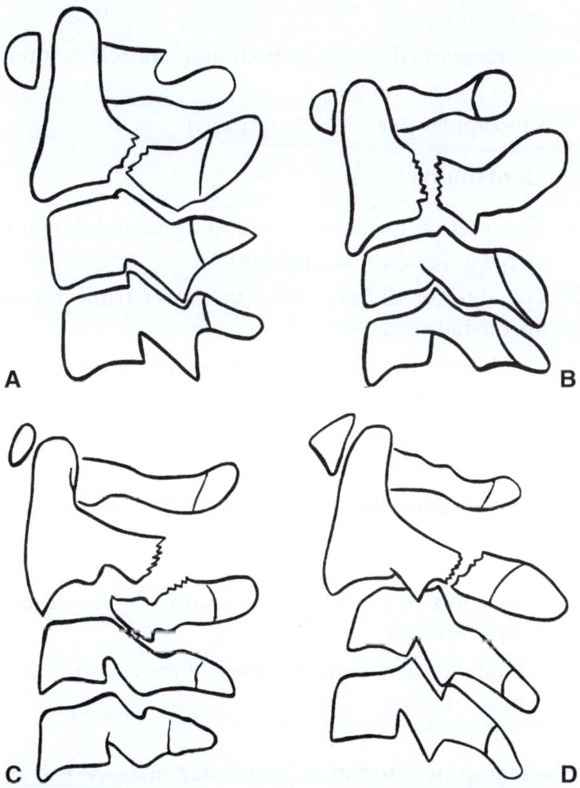

FIGURE 7.10 **Hangman fractures. (*Source*: Frymoyer JW, Wiesel SW, An HS, et al. (eds.), *The Adult and Pediatric Spine*, 3rd ed. Philadelphia: Lippincott Williams & Wilkins, 2004;652.)**

Facet Joint Dislocation. Facet joint dislocation is characterized by unilateral translation of less than 50% and bilateral translation of more than 50% (increased risk for nerve root injury or SCI). Treatment for bilateral jumped facets in an awake and alert patient includes closed reduction in Gardner-Wells tongs, serial traction, and serial examinations. MRI is indicated when there is progression of a neurologic deficit in an awake reduction, if the patient cannot give a reliable examination (e.g., is unconscious), or an open reduction is necessary, since open reduction may worsen the deficit if an HNP exists. If the MRI demonstrates an HNP, then an anterior decompression and fusion is warranted. After anatomic reduction, prevention of flexion is necessary to adequately treat this injury. Various posterior instrumentation systems have been biomechanically tested and proven to be equally efficacious in neutralizing the deforming force of flexion. However, if interspinous wiring is used, immobilization of the cervical spine is necessary with either a halo or rigid orthosis, since wiring does not immediately stabilize the cervical spine.

Cervical Burst Fracture. Burst fractures of the cervical spine result from a significant axial load and have a high association with complete or incomplete SCI. Treatment includes anterior cervical corpectomy and fusion with strut graft and instrumentation. Additional posterior instrumentation is necessary when there is severe posterior element disruption. Even performed late, anterior decompression has been shown to give improvement of an additional nerve root level.

Anterior Cervical Wedge Fractures. These fractures are caused by axial loading in flexion and typically occur at C4-5 and C5-6. Stable fractures are treated with 12 weeks in a rigid cervical orthosis. Unstable fractures, either more than 3.5 mm translation or more than 11 degrees angulation, are treated with posterior fusion, and fusion may be considered to prevent kyphosis if there is a loss of greater than 25% body height.

Subaxial Cervical Fractures. The Allen-Ferguson classification categorizes subaxial cervical fractures into 6 major classes based on mechanism: compression-flexion, compression-extension, vertical-compression, distractive-extension, distractive-flexion, and lateral-flexion. Compression fractures without posterior ligamentous injury will heal after 8 to 12 weeks in a rigid collar. A wedge compression fracture is suggested when the posterior vertebral body height is greater than the anterior by 3 mm or more. Posterior ligamentous injury is likely with loss of greater than 25% of the anterior vertebral height or when there is greater than 11 degrees of angulation between adjacent vertebrae. Surgery is recommended to prevent posttraumatic kyphosis.

Vertebrobasilar Artery Insufficiency Syndrome. This syndrome is seen in patients with cervical spine injury; the greatest risk is with flexion injuries. The brain stem, cerebellum, and occipital lobe are supplied by the vertebrobasilar (posterior) circulation. It can manifest with *vertigo*, visual disturbances (diplopia), facial numbness or paresthesias, dysphagia, dysarthria, and hoarseness. Physical examination may reveal nystagmus, limb ataxia, truncal ataxia (falling to the side of the lesion), contralateral deficit in pain and temperature perception, ipsilateral limb and trunk numbness, ipsilateral loss of taste, and visual field defects.

Brachial Plexus Injuries

Brachial plexus injuries may mimic cervical spine pathology. Patients with brachial plexus injury have a poor prognosis if they present with a history of persistent pain lasting more than 6 months. The differential diagnosis includes:

- Breast cancer (lower plexus and painful)
- Radiation therapy (upper plexus and painless)
- Parsonage-Turner syndrome (may first affect suprascapular)
- Pancoast tumor

Examination. Examination should include assessment for an axillary artery avulsion (may be as high as 20%). Consider an arteriogram in these patients. Perform a neurologic examination to determine the potential location of the lesion. Preganglionic and postganglionic lesions have different characteristics:

- Preganglionic injuries have limited spontaneous or potential for recovery
- Preganglionic lesions represent root avulsions from the spinal cord

These root avulsions can be divided into 2 categories:

- *Central avulsions*—The nerves are avulsed directly from the spinal cord
- *Intradural ruptures*—The rootlets are ruptured proximal to the dorsal root ganglion

Injuries in which roots of the upper plexus are avulsed from the spinal cord should be recognized, since surgical repair is not possible. The differential diagnosis includes a C6 root lesion, which may mimic a brachial plexus lesion. Examination will reveal weak elbow flexion and inability to supinate against resistance with the elbow held in extension. Patients will have anesthesia above the clavicle and may have a Horner syndrome caused by avulsion of the T1 root resulting in interruption of the T1 sympathetic ganglion, which interrupts the sympathetic nerve supply to the eye (miosis, or pupil constriction) ptosis (drooping of the upper eyelid), enophthalmos (sinking of the orbit), and anhydrosis (dry eyes).

Supraclavicular deficits involve the following structures:

- Suprascapular nerve (supraspinatus muscle)
- Dorsal scapular nerve (rhomboids)
- Long thoracic nerve (serratus)

Therefore, winging of the scapula may indicate preganglionic injury.

Infraclavicular deficits involve the following structures:

- Medial and lateral pectoral nerves (pectoralis major and minor)
- Thoracodorsal nerve (latissimus): muscle is fired when patient coughs
- Subscapular nerve (subscapularis)

Cord injury:

- The anterior divisions of the upper and middle trunk merge to form the lateral cord
- The anterior division from the lower trunk forms the medial cord
- The posterior divisions merge to become the posterior cord
  - Shoulder abduction determines function of the axillary nerve
  - Wrist extension determines low radial nerve function, and elbow extension determines high radial nerve function; median and ulnar nerve function are determined by examining finger and wrist motion
  - Elbow flexion evaluates musculocutaneous function

Radiographic Studies. Chest x-ray may reveal an elevated hemidiaphragm, while a cervical spine x-ray may show cervical spine fractures

- Arteriogram for a vascular lesion
- CT myelogram (rarely necessary):
  - May be used to help diagnose a preganglionic lesion

   - Should be delayed 6 to 12 weeks because a clot of blood may occlude the opening of a pseudomeningocele
   - The finding of a large diverticula or meningocele is diagnostic for a preganglionic root avulsion (as opposed to a postganglionic extraforaminal rupture)
- EMG should be considered after 7 to 10 days. Look for denervating potentials in the segmental paraspinal muscles innervated by the posterior primary rami. A normal sensory-evoked potential obtained from an anesthetic finger indicates that the lesion is preganglionic (otherwise, there is a more distal nerve injury). Early EMG may be limited because preganglionic injuries may occur along with dorsal root ganglion injuries, which will falsely indicate a postganglionic injury. An early EMG cannot distinguish between axonotmesis and neurotmesis. Usually, EMG is performed at 3 to 4 weeks to look for F wave. With a preganglionic lesion, one may see denervating potentials in segmental paraspinal muscles innervated by the posterior primary rami. Nerve conduction studies may show absent motor conduction with intact sensory conduction. Afferent sensory fibers will not undergo Wallerian degeneration following nerve root avulsion because cell bodies of afferent sensory fibers are located in the root ganglion, which resides distally. If nerve conduction velocity demonstrates absence of both sensory and motor, then the lesion is postganglionic.

Histamine Test. A histamine test may differentiate preganglionic and postganglionic lesions. If the nerve is interrupted proximal to the ganglion, there is anesthesia along its cutaneous course, but the normal axon response remains intact and can be demonstrated by placing a drop of histamine on the skin. The skin is then scratched through the histamine. There may be seen a triple response (cutaneous vasodilatation, wheel formation, and flare). A normal response implies a preganglionic lesion and portends a poor prognosis. If the flare response is negative, then the lesion may be at a site where recovery may be possible after repair.

Treatment. Refrain from using a sling because of the propensity to acquire a fixed internally rotated and flexed shoulder and elbow stiffness. Keep the patient in a cervical collar until a cervical spine fracture is ruled out. In children and adults, if biceps function has not returned after 3 months, surgery should be considered. Techniques include Steindler flexorplasty. With a severe injury, AEA is an option if the shoulder muscles are functioning.

Fixation of the Cervical Spine

Cervical Immobilization. The multiple types of rigid immobilization for the cervical spine include the following:

- *Cervical orthosis (like Philadelphia collar)*— Provides rigid immobilization in the midcervical spine
- *Cervicothoracic orthosis*— Restricts motion in the lower cervical/thoracic region, C7 and T1
- *Halo vest*— Provides rotational control and restricts motion in the extremes of the cervical spine: C1-2, C7, and T1. A halo vest provides the most rigid immobilization at these levels.

A soft collar provides minimal immobilization of the cervical spine and is used mainly for patient comfort. Mastication in a rigid collar can cause motion at the occipitocervical junction.

Application of a Halo. In adults, 4 pins should be placed and tightened to 8 pounds per inch in adults; 6 to 8 pins should be used and tightened to 4 pounds per inch in children. The pins should be retightened once at 24 to 48 hours. The location of the pins is as follows: 2 anterior pins are placed over the lateral 1/2 of the eyebrow, medial to the temporal fossa, and just superior to the eyebrow (below the greater circumference of the skull; Fig. 7.11). The pins are placed laterally because the supraorbital and supratrochlear nerves are located over the medial 1/2 of the eyebrow. The temporal fossa contains the muscles of mastication and is thin, making pin penetration possible. The 2 posterior pins should be placed about 1/4 inch above the ears. The most common halo complication is loosening of the pins. If there is no sign of obvious infection, then the pins should be retightened rather than replaced. If the cervical spine is immobilized in excessive extension, then patients may have difficulty swallowing.

Application of Cervical Traction. Start with Gardner-Wells tongs in the skull and the bed inclined slightly (Fig. 7.12). Place the pins a finger breadth above the ear. Apply 5 to 10 pounds initially, then add 5 to 7 pounds at a time with serial plain radiographs between applications. With steel tongs, traction up to 140 pounds was safe and efficacious, while graphite tongs can accommodate up to 60 pounds.

Cervical Stenosis

Parameters for Assessment. The diameter of the cervical spinal cord is approximately 10 mm. The SAC (space available for the cord) is normally over 17 mm. Stenosis is defined by a SAC of 13 mm or less, and absolute cord compression occurs with a SAC of

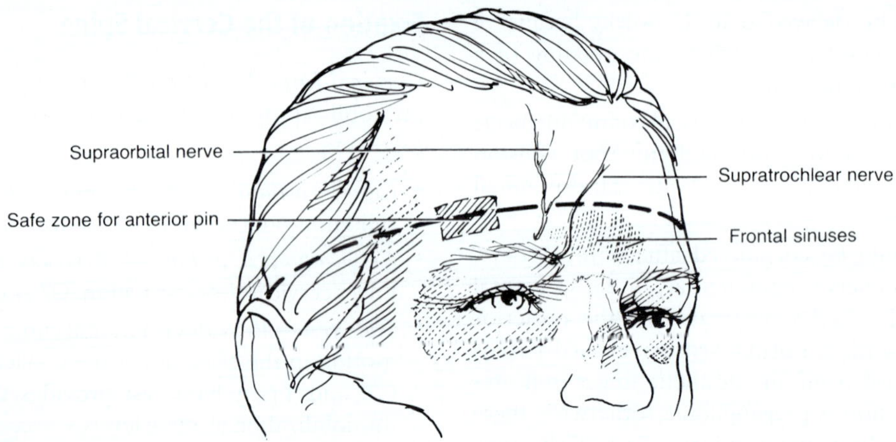

FIGURE 7.11 **Diagram of location for halo pins. (*Source*: Herkowitz HN, (ed.). *The Cervical Spine Surgery Atlas*, 2nd ed. Philadelphia: Lippincott Williams & Wilkins, 2004;8.)**

less than 10 mm. The Torg ratio is the ratio of canal width to vertebral body width. Normal is at least 1.0, and stenosis is less than 0.8. The compressive ratio is the anterior–posterior diameter of cord/transverse diameter of the cord on MRI. Normal is over 0.4; the anterior–posterior diameter should be at least 40% of the transverse diameter. Stenosis is defined by a ratio of under 0.4.

Cervical Spondylosis

Pathology and Risk Factors. Degenerative disk disease (DDD) of the cervical spine is part of the normal aging process. C5-6 is the most common level of involvement, followed by C6-7 and C4-5. The pathology behind cervical DDD is disk desiccation, loss of disk height, disk bulging, loss of intersegmental lordosis, uncinate osteophyte formation, facet joint arthritis, and disk herniation. Risk factors include a history of lifting, tobacco, or prolonged driving.

Signs and Symptoms. Cervical DDD can manifest in three different ways or in combination.

- *Discogenic Neck Pain*—Axial neck pain with or without trapezius radiation.
- *Cervical Radiculopathy*—Root compression (HNP, foraminal stenosis): neck pain, pain radiating to

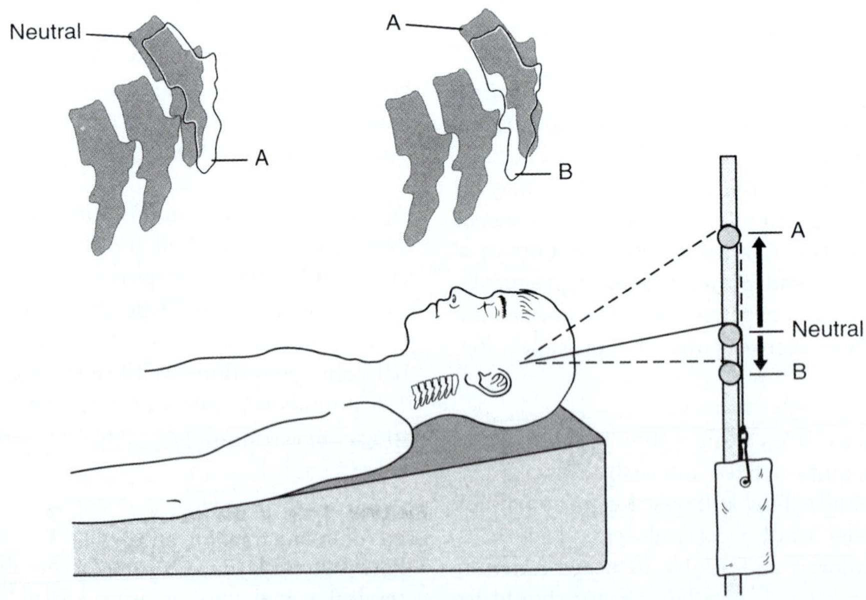

FIGURE 7.12 **Diagram of traction with bed elevated. (*Source*: Herkowitz HN (ed.). *The Cervical Spine Surgery Atlas*, 2nd ed. Philadelphia: Lippincott Williams & Wilkins, 2004;12.)**

upper extremities in a dermatomal pattern, and weakness in upper extremities. The signs are lower motor neuron signs, diminished reflexes, atrophy, and decreased sensation in a dermatomal distribution. The lower numbered nerve root is always involved, cervical DDD: C4-5, the C5 nerve root is involved.

- *Myelopathy*—Discussed later in chapter.

Nonoperative Treatment. Typical conservative treatment includes NSAIDs, heat, physical therapy, and epidural or selective nerve root injections. Some clinicians advocate the use of a cervical collar or consider cervical traction to alleviate symptoms.

Operative Procedures. Indications for operative intervention in the face of radiologic evidence of neural compression include more than 6 weeks of persistent radicular pain, progressive significant weakness, and cervical myelopathy. The most common operation is anterior cervical discectomy and fusion (ACDF) with or without a plate and bone graft (Fig. 7.13). For a 1-level fusion, the outcome is similar for allograft and autograft bone with or without plate fixation. Plates improve fusion rates for 2 or more levels. Other procedures are ACD without fusion and a keyhole foraminotomy for posterior decompression of the exiting nerve root. The posterior muscle-splitting approach for a keyhole foraminotomy may allow an athlete to return sooner than would a fusion secondarily to shorter recovery time and no need to wait for fusion of the graft.

Arthritis in the Atlantoaxial Joints. This disease process typically manifests with pain at the base of the occiput and the most superior portion of the posterior neck, severe headaches, and pain worse with rotation (and not usually flexion and extension). Atlantoaxial lateral mass arthritis is a frequently overlooked reason for significant pain in the occipitocervical region. Consider an open-mouth radiographic view and/or a CT scan. If the typical nonoperative treatments fail, then a posterior atlantoaxial fusion is the surgical treatment of choice to alleviate the symptoms.

Cervical Myelopathy

Pathology. Cervical myelopathy is a result of compression of the cervical spinal cord. It is seen with cervical stenosis (congenital and degenerative), cervical degenerative disk disease, and ossification of the posterior longitudinal ligament (OPLL; typically seen in the Asian population). The natural history of cervical myelopathy is that the disease will most likely progress.

Signs and Symptoms. The diagnosis of cervical myelopathy is based on history and physical examination (Table 7.20). X-rays may reveal cervical stenosis and/or spondylosis. MRI will reveal cord compression, stenosis, and possibly increase cord signal on T2-weighted MRI.

Nonoperative Treatment. Treatment is similar to that for cervical DDD without traction. Earlier surgical intervention has a better prognosis compared to waiting more than 6 months after symptom onset. Indications for operative intervention in cervical myelopathy include gait deterioration, progressive involvement, and significant hand involvement.

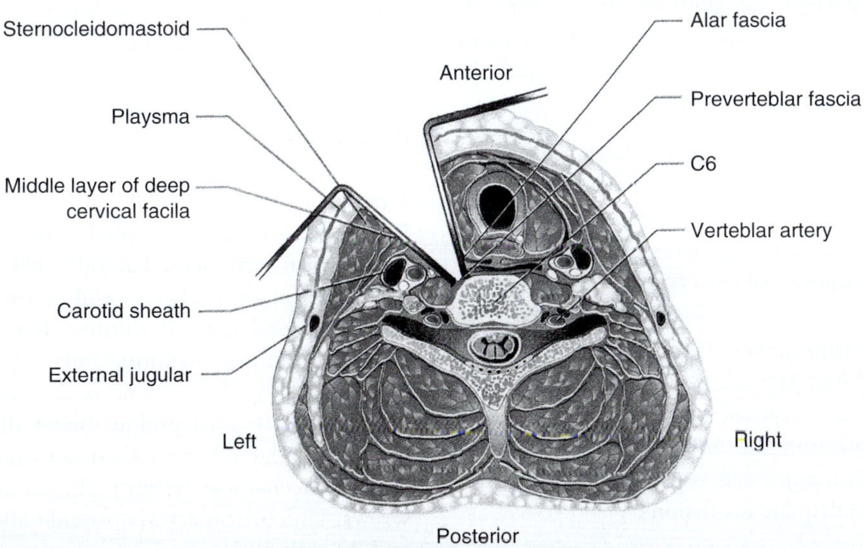

FIGURE 7.13 **Anterior approach to cervical spine. (*Source*: Herkowitz HN, (ed.). *The Cervical Spine Surgery Atlas*, 2nd ed. Philadelphia: Lippincott Williams & Wilkins, 2004;91.)**

TABLE 7.20 Symptoms and Signs of Cervical Myelopathy

Symptoms	Signs
• Gait disturbances: broad-base, shuffling gait (earliest and most important indicator) • Hand dysfunction (clumsiness) • Bowel and bladder problems (rare)	• UMN signs • Hoffman • Finger escape sign • Inverted radia reflex

Operative Treatment. Surgical intervention of cervical myelopathy can be approached anteriorly or posteriorly. The anterior approach is seen most commonly in orthopedics because most pathology is located anteriorly. Options include ACDF with or without plating, or corpectomy with strut graft with or without plating. This treatment is good for multilevel disease, and multilevel fusion decreases the risk of repeated surgery for adjacent level disease. It has been reported that adjacent level disease is present in up to 25% of patients within 10 years of their initial fusion at a rate of 2.9% per year per level. Operations performed posteriorly include:

- *Laminaplasty*—Used in multilevel disease; prevents postsurgery kyphosis and preserves motion.
- *Laminectomy*—Not a good option unless accompanied by fusion because patients may develop cervical kyphosis; laminectomy is therefore contraindicated in patients who have loss of their cervical lordosis.
- *Laminectomy and Instrumented Fusion*—Used when patient has straight or kyphotic spine, but on extension, radiographs move into lordosis. Perform laminectomy and instrument the cervical spine in lordosis.

The most important factor in determining the success of an operation is the degree of myelopathy. Patients with more severe myelopathy do worse than those with less severe disease progression. Other factors involved are the amount of cord compression and age.

Other Cervical Approaches. The transoral or mandibular split subglottal approach may provide anterior access to the upper cervical spine but is associated with increased infection rates and limited visualization. The lateral cervical approach is good for performing biopsies but not adequate for fusions.

Posterior Cervical Instrumentation Techniques. Instrumentation is increasingly used to stabilize the posterior cervical spine. Lateral mass screws and pedicle screws are commonly used today, and interspinous wire fixation plays a supplemental role.

Wire Techniques

Gallie Wiring Technique Plus Bone Graft. Described in 1939 for fracture fixation in the cervical spine, sublaminar wire fixation is obtained on the C1 ring and around the C2 spinous process.

Brooks Modification of the Gallie Technique. This technique utilizes bilateral sublaminar wires beneath C1 and C2. A laminotomy may be done between C2 and C3 to facilitate wire passage, and a 20-gauge wire is looped and the looped end threaded beneath the lamina of C2 and C1 on either side of midline. Near full-thickness corticocancellous iliac crest bone grafts are harvested and placed on the lamina of C1 and C2. Alternatively, a full bone block may be used with a space in the caudad end to fit around the C2 spinous process. The wires are then tightened down in a longitudinal fashion over the bone block on either side. This fixation may provide more rotational stability than does the Gallie technique because of fixation on both sides of midline.

Bohlman Triple-Wire Technique. An improvement on the Brooks-Gallie technique. The first 20-gauge wire is woven in a figure-of-8 fashion through holes burred into the base of the spinous processes of the involved vertebrae. This is the midline tethering wire. The wire is typically looped to itself after passing through the spinous process to help distribute stress. Twenty-two-gauge wires can then individually pass through the same holes to loop around the spinous processes at the ends of the segments to be fused. The ends of these wires are passed through drill holes in the rectangular corticocancellous iliac crest autografts. The wires are tightened down on the graft to force the graft against the laminas.

Lateral Mass and Pedicle Screws. The lateral mass is situated between the cephalad and caudad facets of the cervical vertebrae. Lateral mass screws provide excellent fixation at C1 and C3-6 (Table 7.21). The C7 lateral mass is thinner than the others and can be used for fixation, but a pedicle screw is preferred. A pedicle screw is also preferred at C2. Pedicle screws resist pullout better than lateral mass screws, but lateral mass C5-6 and pedicle screw C7 had biomechanical stability similar to C5-7 pedicle screws. Unicortical screws provide adequate fixation, and 14-mm unicortical lateral mass screws without laminectomy are equivalent to bicortical screws. Lateral mass screws at C1 risks injury to the C2 ganglion just caudad, the vertebral artery lateral and cephalad,

TABLE 7.21 Lateral Mass Screw Techniques

Method	Cephalad	Lateral	Start Point
Roy-Camille	0 degree	10 degrees	Center of lateral mass
Magerl	40–60 degrees	25 degrees	1–3 mm medial to midpoint of lateral mass
An	15 degrees	30 degrees	1 mm medial to midpoint of lateral mass

and the internal carotid and hypoglossal nerve just anterior with bicortical screws. The hypoglossal nerve is approximately 2 to 3 mm anterolateral to the middle of the C1 lateral mass. The internal carotid artery lies within 1 mm of the ideal exit point of bicortical C1-2 transarticular screw or C1 lateral mass screw. For lateral mass screws, the spinous processes can be used as an approximate guide for the lateral and cephalad angles according to the An technique. Using the starting point of 1 mm medial to the middle of the lateral mass, angling the drill halfway between the C3 and C4 spinous processes will approximate the C3 lateral mass screw trajectory. Angling the drill from halfway between the C4 and C5 spinous processes will approximate the C4 lateral mass screw angle. Resting the drill against the cephalad lateral border of the C6 and C7 spinous processes will approximate the angles for the C5 and C6 lateral mass screws respectively.

Transarticular Screw Fixation. Transarticular screw fixation provides the most rigid fixation for C1-2 atlantoaxial fusion and can be used in conjunction with wire techniques to provide 3-point fixation. Preoperative CT scan is necessary to adequately define the vertebral artery anatomy and to ensure that the C2 isthmus is wide enough to accept at least a 3.5-mm screw and that the lateral mass of C1 is reduced and aligned with the superior facet of C2. Other considerations that may preclude the use of this technique include significant cranial settling with collapsed lateral masses, irreducible subluxations, substantial osteoporosis and osteopenia, comminuted fractures of the atlas and axis vertebrae, and an anomalous vertebral artery.

Occipital Fixation. Occipital fixation is used for occipitocervical stabilization. Placing occipital screws risks injury to the confluence of sinuses and transverse sinuses located immediately beneath the thickest portions of the occiput; therefore, safer screw placement is suggested at least 2 cm below the superior nuchal line. The external occipital protuberance (EOP) has the thickest bone from 11.5 to 15.1 mm in males and 9.7 to 12.0 mm in females. The thickness decreases below 8 mm greater than 2 cm lateral to the EOP.

Complications of Anterior Cervical Decompression and Fusion

Recurrent Laryngeal Nerve (RLN) Injury. RLN has an approximately 1% incidence rate. During the Smith-Robinson anterior approach to the cervical spine, the RLN and superior laryngeal nerve are at risk for injury. The RLN (a medial branch of the vagus nerve CN X) supplies the main innervation to the larynx. Damage to the RLN results in a partial paralysis of the vocal cords, manifested by hoarseness, persistent dry cough, and possibly aspiration secondary to vocal cord laxity. On the left side of the neck, the RLN descends into the thoracic cavity within the carotid sheath, then curves under the aortic arch and ascends the neck between the trachea and esophagus (tracheoesophageal grove). On the right side of the neck, the RLN has a more unpredictable course. In 50% of cases, the right recurrent laryngeal nerve reaches the tracheoesophageal grove at C5–6. It exits the carotid sheath at variable levels, loops around the subclavian artery, and then ascends into the neck at a higher level then on the left, crossing the operative field around C6-7. The superior laryngeal nerve originates from the vagus nerve in the carotid sheath an average 20 mm (range 5 to 32 mm) proximal to the bifurcation of the carotid artery and, after traveling approximately 15 mm (range, 3 to 20 mm), bifurcates into internal (sensory) and external (motor) branches. Distally, the internal branch is located around C3-4 and courses close to the superior laryngeal artery and inserts within 1 cm superior to the artery into the thyrohyoid membrane. It innervates the mucosa of the larynx and has an important sensory reflex that protects the lungs from aspiration.

Thus, upon approaching the anterior cervical spine from the right side, there is an increased risk of directly injuring the RLN. However, the RLN may suffer a stretch injury when approached from the left with overzealous retraction. If the RLN is injured, typically symptoms will spontaneously resolve. However, if symptoms persist more than 6 weeks, then a direct laryngoscopy by an ENT physician is warranted. It is expected that patients will have throat pain and difficulty swallowing after surgery.

Respiratory Distress. After a corpectomy has been performed, patients may develop retropharyngeal edema or hematoma that may compress upon the larynx. Patient symptoms may include difficulty lying flat, changes in voice, difficulty swallowing, and diaphoresis. Patients should be promptly evaluated for possible intubation. Fiberoptic intubation may be necessary to find the airway because of the edema. In a hyperacute airway, intubation may provoke laryngospasm, and a cricothyroidotomy may be necessary.

Superior Laryngeal Nerve (SLN) Injury. The SLN is vital to professional singers because it is responsible for high-note phonation. During common vertical anterior approaches (extension of the traditional Smith-Robinson anterior approach) to the upper cervical spine, the SLN may be damaged secondarily to retraction. However, reports of a modified submandibular approach as an anterior retropharyngeal approach with a vertical extension (modification of the superior extension of Smith-Robinson) have shown that good visualization of the SLN can be obtained with prevention of injury to the SLN.

Vertebral Artery Injury. Vertebral artery injury can occur while an anterior corpectomy is being performed. It has been associated with use of a high-speed burr, loss of orientation of midline, and soft bone. Injury to the left vertebral artery can be catastrophic because the left vertebral artery is often dominant. Initial treatment is as follows:

- Neutral rotation of the head helps to prevent kinking of the contralateral vertebral artery and maintain cerebral blood flow.
- Tamponade the bleeding with the use of cottonoids with thrombostatic agents, and suction.
- Arteriography of the vertebral artery to determine location of injury and patency of vessel.
- Blind suturing is not recommended.
- After arteriography, microvascular repair can be performed after the damaged vertebral artery has been exposed.

Neurologic Injury. Neurologic injury is a rare but devastating complication.

Pseudoarthrosis. Single-level 10% to 12%, 3-level up to 44%. The patient is not always symptomatic. If asymptomatic, then just follow patient. If the patient is symptomatic and has documented motion on radiographs, then consider a posterior spinal fusion with or without foraminotomy with autograft or a repeat anterior spinal fusion. Both have been shown to have good results, but posterior spinal fusion with foraminotomy has better results, with significantly less risk of dysphagia than a revision anterior surgery.

Vocal Cord Paralysis (Not from Extrinsic RLN Palsy). Vocal cord paralysis may occur when the retractors are placed under the longus colli muscles can compress the laryngeal-tracheal branches within the larynx against the tented endotracheal tube. Deflating the endotracheal tube's cuff after the retractors are placed, allowing the tube to recenter itself, and then reinflating the cuff may decrease the risk of this occurrence.

Horner Syndrome. Horner syndrome can be caused by injury to the sympathetic chain. Manifestations include unilateral miosis (pupil constriction), ptosis, and anhydrosis (lack of sweat). The sympathetic chain is more susceptible to injury during the anterior approach to the cervical spine as it courses near the lateral border of the longus colli at C6. Protection of the sympathetic chain can be done with subperiosteal dissection on the midline.

Cervical Spine Abnormalities in Rheumatoid Arthritis (RA)

The cervical spine is commonly affected by RA. Most patients are symptomatic, but cervical involvement should be suspected and proactively evaluated in patients with peripheral involvement. Symptoms may include:

- Neck pain
- Headaches
- Crepitus in the cervical spine with a palpable clunk on movement; symptoms of cord and nerve root compression
- Basilar invagination causing vertebrobasilar insufficiency (tinnitus, vertigo, loss of equilibrium, visual disturbances, nystagmus, diplopia, and dysphagia)
- Urinary dysfunction
- Trigeminal nerve tract and facial sensory impairment
- Frozen shoulder secondary to myelopathy

Patients with progressive disease are at risk of sudden death in about 10% of cases, and 50% will die within 1 year of onset of myelopathy.

Atlantoaxial Subluxation. Up to 90% of patients with RA have pathologic changes in their cervical spine, thus flexion–extension x-rays of the cervical spine should be taken before elective surgery in these patients. Subluxation of the cervical spine is the most common manifestation and occurs at C1-2 about 65% of the time. Approximately one half of these atlantoaxial subluxations occur anteriorly, and the other half occur lateral and posterior. A greater than 3.5-mm difference of the ADI in flexion and extension lateral cervical spine x-rays is indicative of instability but not an absolute indication for surgery. Subluxation occurs from pannus destruction of facet joints, spinous ligaments, intervertebral disks, and bony architecture. A cervicomedullary angle less than 135 degrees on MRI suggests significant compression and basilar invagination and is an indication for C1-2 fusion. The pannus will resorb after stabilization and reduce the compression. The posterior atlantodens interval (PADI) is not the same as space available for the cord (SAC) since the retro-odontoid pannus may occupy as much as 3 mm of space not visible on plain radiographs. The PADI is an important predictor of recovery of function, more so than the anterior atlantodens interval (AADI). PADI of less than 14 mm is an indication for surgery and has a 97% sensitivity to predict paralysis. The PADI of 14 mm has a negative predictive value of 94% and means that a PADI of 14 mm or more has a 94% chance that the patient will not have paralysis. PADI of less than 10 mm has a poor prognosis for recovery of function. These observations can also be explained by the anatomy of the spinal cord at the C1 level because the dura occupies an average space of 1 mm on the anterior and posterior sides, the cerebrospinal fluid occupies 2 mm, and the cord 10 mm, for a total space of 14 mm. The open-mouth view is useful to identify lateral subluxation, defined as more than 2 mm of lateral displacement of C1-2 lateral masses, which occurs more commonly in patients with spinal cord compression than those without.

Basilar Invagination. Basilar invagination occurs in approximately 40% of patients with RA. The dens migrates cranially through the foramen magnum, violating the McRae line. Progressive cranial settling is secondary to bone loss between the atlas and occiput condyles and C1 and C2. Neurologic deterioration may be due to direct bony and soft tissue compression of the cervical medullary junction and/or ischemia from compression of the blood supply to this region. Occipitocervical stabilization is indicated with a patient with symptomatic basilar invagination.

Subaxial Spine Involvement. Subaxial spine involvement occurs in approximately 20% of cases with destruction of the intervertebral disks, uncovertebral joints of Luschka, and the facets. However, within 5 years of serologic diagnosis, 30% to 50% develop subluxation and 2% to 3% of these will develop myelopathy 10 years later. Lateral radiographs may reveal a "staircase" pattern to the vertebral bodies because of subluxations. Risk factors include male gender with steroid use, seropositive RA, presence of rheumatoid nodules, and severe RA. Vertebral subluxations of more than 4 mm or 20% of the vertebral bodies suggest cord compression. A cervical height index (cervical body height/width) of less than 2.0 is approximately 100% sensitive and specific in predicting neurologic compromise. Posterior stabilization and fusion is the treatment of choice.

Classification of Rheumatoid Myelopathy. Neurologic progression of rheumatoid myelopathy has been categorized by the Ranawat classification (Table 7.22). Surgery is less successful in patients with grade IIIB neurologic deficits.

Surgical Indications of Rheumatoid Cervical Spine. Indications for surgical stabilization of the cervical spine in RA patients with or without neurologic involvement is recommended in patients with:

- Atlantoaxial subluxation and PADI of 14 mm or less
- Atlantoaxial subluxation and basilar invagination of 5 mm or more
- Subaxial subluxation and SAC of 14 mm or less
- Cervicomedullary angle less than 135 degrees

The results of surgical stabilization with or without decompression are worse in patients with myelopathy. However, of patients with myelopathy who do not have a surgical intervention, about three quarters have a poor outcome with disease progression. Early intervention before significant neurologic compromise is important to hopefully improve the poor prognosis of patients with this disorder. The best predictor of any neurologic recovery after surgery in a patient with RA, C1-2 instability, and paralysis is the preoperative posterior atlanto-odontoid interval of 10 mm or more.

Increased Risk for Cervical Spine Injury. The cervical spine has an increased risk of injury during contact sports from axial loading when the neck is flexed at a minimum of 30 degrees. The paraspinal muscles, the intervertebral disks, and normal lordotic curvature of the cervical spine help absorb energy from an axial load. Beginning around 30 degrees, the cervical spine flattens out putting the cervical spine at increase risk.

Effect of Neck Flexion and Extension. Neck flexion causes the spinal cord to unfold and undergo elastic

TABLE 7.22 Ranawat Classification of Rheumatoid Myelopathy

Grade	Features
I	Subjective paresthesias
II	Subjective weakness; UMN findings
III	Objective weakness; UMN findings
IIIA	Ambulatory
IIIB	Nonambulatory

deformation, and the spinal canal lengthens. During the neck extension, the spinal canal shortens and the cord relaxes (folds similar to an accordion). Neck flexion will increase the canal dimensions but may cause worsening anterior compression if there is a herniated disk. Neck extension decreases the canal diameter (pincer effect) because of infolding of the ligamentum flavum posteriorly and compression from degenerative hypertrophic facets and anterior disk herniation if present. OPLL (common in Asians but also affects non-Asians) also causes narrowing of the canal and myelopathy.

Treatment of Whiplash. Whiplash is a hyperextension soft tissue injury to the neck. Treatment should include early mobilization and return to normal activities. Subjective decrease in symptoms and better functional outcomes 6 months after the injury have resulted from this treatment approach.

Athletes with Acute Cervical Disk Herniations. An athlete who suffers an acute cervical disk herniation should not be allow to return to play until symptoms have resolved and his or her physical examination returns to normal, unless there is a large disk herniation needing surgical decompression.

Cervical Spine MRI. Positive cervical spine MRI in asymptomatic patients (false-positives) is approximately 14% under age 40 and approximately 28% over age 40.

Vertebral Artery in the Cervical Spine. The vertebral artery transverses the cervical spine in the vertebral foramen; it ascends cephalad laterally to medial. It begins at C6, located directly anterior to the lateral mass of C6 and medial to the lateral masses at C3 to C5.

Preoperative Assessment of the Vertebral Artery in the Cervical Spine. Thin-cut CT scans are the best for assessing anomalous vertebral artery pathways in the upper cervical spine when planning to use posterior transarticular screw fixation. It has been reported that there is a greater than 10% incidence of vertebral artery anomalies at the C1-2 junction. MRI is helpful when looking at soft tissue and spinal cord pathology but is not as good as CT scan for evaluating the vertebral artery foramina.

Assessment Tools for Cervical Pathology. These tools fall into 2 categories: tools for assessing general status and disease-specific tools. General status instruments measure the whole person's functional status. The SF-36 health questionnaire is the best example and is considered the standard. It assesses a patient's physical, social, role function, emotional, and mental health; energy/fatigue; pain; health perception; health change; and overall daily function, general health, and well being. Attempts have been made to shorten the SF-36 to 12 items, but the shortened form may limit its accuracy and usefulness. Nurick criteria is an evaluation of physical function with gradations for ambulation and daily function. Oswestry neck disability index evaluates the effect of neck pain on daily living. The Odom criteria is the surgeon's evaluations of the impact of the patient's neck pain/radiculopathy on activities of daily living.

IV. THORACOLUMBAR SPINE

Thoracolumbar Fractures

Compression Fractures of the Thoracolumbar Spine. Compression fracture of the thoracolumbar spine is failure of the anterior spinal column with an intact middle column. Treatment of choice is typically nonoperatively with a thoracolumbosacral orthosis (TLSO) brace. Surgical indications include 50% loss on anterior body vertebral height and initial kyphosis of 20 to 30 degrees.

Factors Increasing the Risk of Compression Fracture in Postmenopausal Women. The biggest risk factor for a compression fracture is a history of 2 or more prior osteoporotic compression fractures (12-fold increased risk). In postmenopausal women, osteoporosis (a decrease in bone mineral density greater than 2 standard deviations) present a 4- to 6-fold increased risk; a positive family history of compression factors, a 2.7-fold increased risk; premature menopause, a 1.7-fold increased risk; and tobacco smoking history, a 1.2-fold increased risk. Prolonged steroid use also places an individual at an increased risk of a compression fracture even with minor trauma.

Thoracolumbar Burst Fracture. Burst fractures are typically a result of an axial compressive force with or without a flexion/distraction component. This mechanism of injury leads to failure of the anterior and middle column of the vertebrae, retropulsion of the posterior vertebral body into the spinal canal, and lateral spreading of the pedicles. In addition, posterior spinal column disruption can also occur. Neurologic injury may accompany these injuries and can occur approximately 40% to 50% of the time. Nonoperative treatment can be considered in patients with stable thoracolumbar burst fractures (no significant posterior column disruption). Patients can be treated with isometric exercises and early mobilization in an extension brace (TLSO), which has shown to provide good results of returning patients to full function. Nonoperative therapy is used when there is no neurologic deficit, kyphosis is less than 20 to 30 degrees, less than 50% of the canal is compromised. Operative indications include the following:

- Neurologic deficit with signs of spinal instability or canal compromise by osseous or soft tissue structures
- Evidence of posterior column disruption (indicative of unstable spine) without neurologic deficits:
  - Local kyphosis of more than 20 to 30 degrees
  - Loss of more than 50% anterior body height
  - Increase in interspinous process distance
  - Posterior facet subluxation

Thoracolumbar Bracing

TLSO Versus Jewett Brace. TLSO braces are used to immobilized stable thoracolumbar burst or compression fractures. *Rotational* control is the major advantage of a TLSO over a 3-point fixation brace (Jewett). Flexion or extension forces can be exerted with these Jewett-like braces but provide inadequate rotational stability. It is necessary to add a thigh extension to a TLSO when trying to immobilized the L5-S1 region.

Thoracolumbar Disk Disease

Thoracic Disk Disease (TDD)

Clinically significant TDD is rare (less than 1%), but there is a high rate of false-positive MRI scans, so clinical correlation is necessary. Most TDD occurs from T8 to T12. Patients may present with axial thoracic back pain, radiculopathy with pain radiating around into the chest or abdominal wall, or myelopathy with UMN signs in the lower extremities. Physical examination is important to detect signs of myelopathy and to determine the sensory level by pinprick testing.

Surgical Indications and Operative Approaches. Surgery is indicated in cases of myelopathy or persistent pain despite nonoperative therapies in patients with clinically correlated MRI findings. Central HNP is approached transthoracically or endoscopically. A costotransversectomy or a transpedicular approach can be utilized for a lateral HNP. A far lateral HNP can be approached transpedicularly. Laminectomies and posterior approach to the thoracic spine are associated with a high rate of neurologic complications, such as paraplegia, because the spinal cord must be retracted to gain access to the intervertebral disk.

Herpes Zoster and Disk Disease. Herpes zoster can present with a painful radiculopathy, but the key to diagnosis is the presence or history of a painful vesicular lesions in a dermatomal pattern.

Lumbar Herniated Disk

The most common location of a lumbar HNP is L4-5. The 3 types are as follows:

- *Posterior Lateral*—Most common; gets lowered nerve root (L4-5 involves L5 nerve root).
- *Foraminal/Far Lateral*—Gets upper nerve root as it passes out of foramina (L4-5 involves the L4 nerve root). Occurs more frequently in the older population, average age 65.
- *Central*—Rare.

Signs and Symptoms. Patients with a lumbar HNP complain of back pain, pain radiating down the leg typically below knee in a dermatomal pattern (sciatic), paresthesias, and possibly weakness. Physical examination findings include positive straight leg sign, which is the most predicative finding if it reproduces leg pain for HNP with L5 or S1 radiculopathy. If the patient has L3 or L4 nerve root involvement, then femoral nerve stretch is the important physical examination finding. Lateral bending may differentiate axillary disk herniations from those above the shoulder of the nerve root. Bending away from the disk herniation increases pain in axillary HNP as the nerve is pulled over the HNP. Lateral bending toward the side of the HNP increases symptoms in patients with HNP above the nerve root sleeve.

Natural History. Symptomatic lumbar HNP has a lifetime incidence of 2% of the general population. Risk factors include male gender, age 30 to 50 years, heavy lifting with twisting, poor job satisfaction or low income, cigarette smoking, and prolonged exposure to vibration. Ninety to ninety-five percent are observed at L4-5 or L5-S1 levels. Most HNP (more than 90%) of patients with symptomatic HNP will improve within 4 to 6 weeks. At 4 years, the results from operative and nonoperative treatment are approximately equal because of residual back pain. Operative treatment outstanding from eliminating radiculopathy, however, typically does not improve back pain.

Nonoperative Treatment. Initial treatment should last for at least 4 to 6 weeks (if an acute disk) and include rest, heat, antiinflammatory medications, and possibly physical therapy and injections.

Operative Indications, Treatment, and Results. Surgical indications include progressive weakness, persistent significant pain lasting more than 4 to 6 weeks, and cauda equina syndrome. The surgical treatment of an HNP is discectomy. The surgical results are as follows: leg pain is relieved in 90% of patients if surgery is performed within 3 months from the onset of

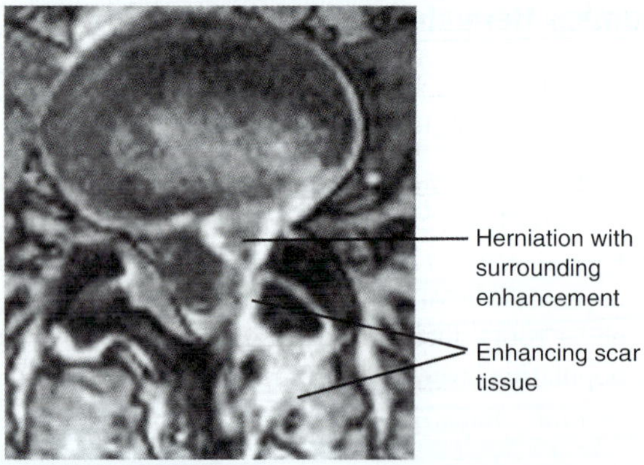

FIGURE 7.14 Enhancing ring due to HNP. (*Source*: Herkowitz H, Dvorak J, Bell GR, Nordin M, Grob D (eds.). *The Lumbar Spine*, 3rd ed. Philadelphia: Lippincott Williams & Wilkins, 2004.)

pain (result is worrisome if surgery is performed more than a year from the onset of symptoms); 15% to 30% of patients will have residual back pain; approximately 50% will regain motor and sensory deficit, but only 25% will regain normal reflexes,

Recurrent Disk Herniation. Recurrent disk herniation occurs on average in 5% to 10% of cases. An MRI with gadolinium will differentiate scar from a recurrent HNP (Fig. 7.14). Scar will have a consistent high signal, while an HNP may have a ring-enhancing appearance.

Lumbar Spinal Stenosis (LSS)

Types. There are five types of LSS.

- *Congenital/Developmental*—Short pedicles and a medially placed facet joint with a "trefoil" (triangular shaped) canal (seen in achondroplastic dwarfs)
- *Acquired*—Degenerative changes with facet joint enlargement, thickening of the facet capsule, hypertrophy of the ligamentum flavum, herniated or bulging disk, loss of disk height, osteophyte formation, and uncinate spurring (Fig. 7.15)
- *Combined*—Spondylotic changes with underlying congenital stenosis
- *Postsurgical*
- *Spondylolisthesis (Fig. 7.16)*

Classification. Classification of LSS is based on location.

- *Central Stenosis*—Compression of the thecal sac producing nonspecific nerve root involvement. Etiology may include enlargement of inferior articular facet and ligamentum flavum.

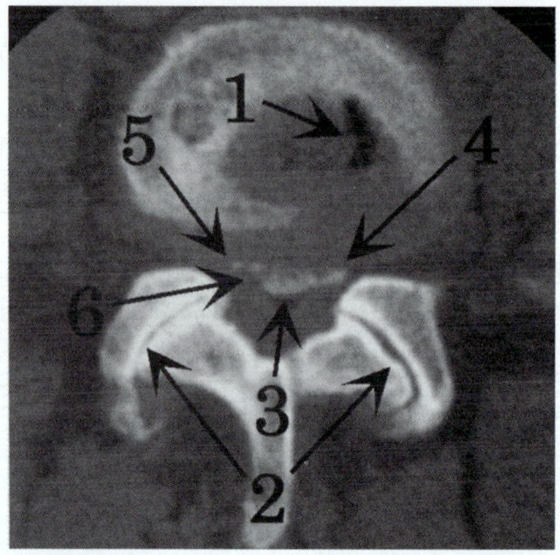

FIGURE 7.15 Stenosis. (*Source*: Herkowitz H, Dvorak J, Bell GR, Nordin M, Grob D (eds.). *The Lumbar Spine*, 3rd ed. Philadelphia: Lippincott Williams & Wilkins, 2004;473.)

- *Lateral Recess Stenosis*—Thecal sac to medial wall of the pedicle. Produces compression of the traversing nerve root from impingement. Etiology may include superior facet enlargement and facet capsular thickening with or without disk bulging.

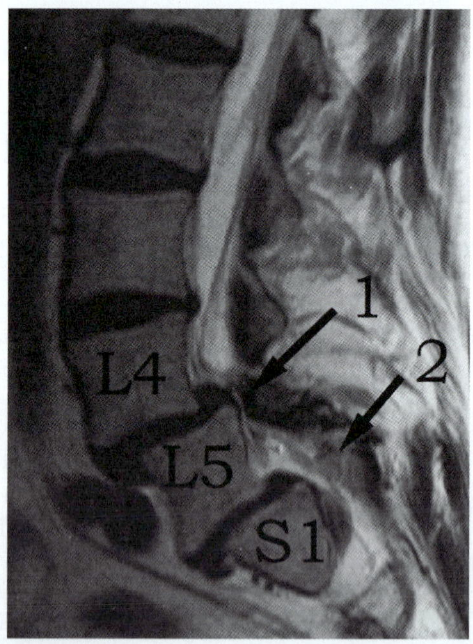

FIGURE 7.16 Spondylolisthesis deg and lytic. (*Source*: Herkowitz H, Dvorak J, Bell GR, Nordin M, Grob D (eds.). *The Lumbar Spine*, 3rd ed. Philadelphia: Lippincott Williams & Wilkins, 2004;485.)

- *Foraminal Stenosis*—Lateral to medial wall of pedicle. Produces exiting nerve root impingement. Etiology may include enlarged medial border of the superior facet, uncinate spur, and a far lateral disk herniation.

Signs and Symptoms. Patients with LSS typically complain of back pain and stiffness. Occasionally, radiculopathy is seen. Patients with subarticular stenosis have pain due to the traversing nerve, while foraminal stenosis affects the exiting nerve root at that level. Buttock pain is a very common compliant. Neurogenic claudication is seen in only about 50% of cases (Table 7.23). It is described as pain radiating proximally and extending distally into legs, typically worse with walking and better with forward flexion. Physical examination findings are limited extension and loss of lordosis. Typically, there is no neurologic deficit and a negative SLR. Bowel and bladder symptoms are rare. MRI/CT scans are confirmatory studies based on history. X-rays may reveal degenerative changes; MRI/CT scan will reveal stenosis of the spinal canal, and it is important to access the lateral recess and foraminal region for stenosis. The natural history of LSS is that one third of patients worsen, one third plateau, and one third improve with treatment.

Nonoperative Treatment. Conservative treatment of LSS includes physical therapy, NSAIDs, bracing, and either epidural or transforaminal steroid injections.

Operative Indications and Treatment. Indications for surgical treatment of LSS are persistent significant pain after nonoperative treatment or progressive weakness (very uncommon). There are 2 operations that can be performed.

- Laminectomy and decompression of all involved nerve roots
- Laminectomy with fusion (with or without instrumentation), performed in cases with degenerative spondylolisthesis or scoliosis or spinal instability

Lumbar Spondylolysis/Spondylolithesis

Background. Spondylolysis is a defect in the pars interarticularis, which occurs most commonly at L5-S1 (Fig. 7.17). It occurs in approximately 5% of the population, with a 27% to 69% familial predisposition. The defect develops in 75% of the cases by 5 to 6 years of age. Of these, 75% present with spondylolisthesis. However, in adults, progression of spondylolysis to spondylolisthesis is very unlikely.

Manifestations in Children. Spondylolysis is one of the more common causes of low back pain in children, adolescents, and young adults, and it is typically seen in gymnasts, wrestlers, and football down linemen. It is thought to be a fatigue fracture in the pars interarticularis due to shear stress on the pars from the repetitive hyperextension. Physical examination reveals limited extension and pain with extension. Initial treatment is activity restriction and bracing.

Radiographic Evaluation. Eighty percent of the pars defect will be picked up on the lateral radiograph, and oblique views will pick up an additional 15% of the cases. The defect shows up as "the Scottie dog" with a collar (Fig. 7.18). Bone scan allows for early detection. MRI will demonstrate nerve root compression if spondylolisthesis is present.

Classes. Classes of spondylolisthesis are listed in Table 7.24.

Meyerding Classification. The severity of the slip has been classified by Meyerding on the basis of the degree of anterior translation (relative to the S1 width):

- I. 0% to 25%
- II. 26% to 50%
- III. 51% to 75%
- IV. 76% to 99%
- greater than 99% (spondyloptosis)

Other Radiographic Measurements. These measurements are useful in evaluating spondylolisthesis.

TABLE 7.23 Neurogenic Versus Vascular Claudication

Activity	Vascular (Pseudo) Claudication	Neurogenic Claudication
Walking	Distal to proximal leg and calf pain; relieved with standing still; weak pulses	Proximal to distal thigh pain; relieved with sitting or flexion
Walking distance	Constant	Variable
Uphill walking	Symptoms develop sooner	Symptoms develop later
Bicycling	Symptoms develop	Symptoms do not develop
Lying flat	Relief	May exacerbate symptoms

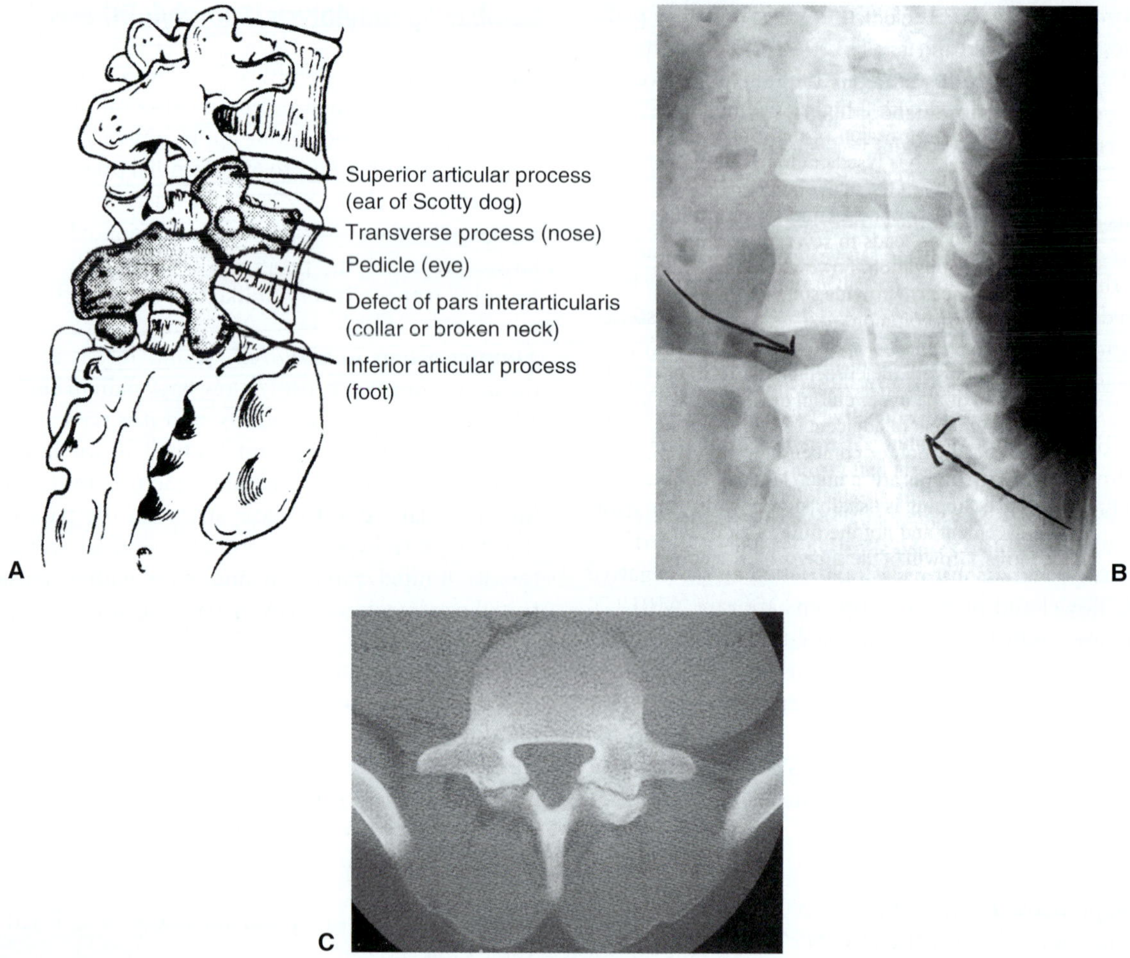

FIGURE 7.17 Pars defect. (*Source*: Frymoyer JW, Wiesel SW, An HS, et al. (eds.). *The Adult and Pediatric Spine*, 3rd ed. Philadelphia: Lippincott Williams & Wilkins, 2004;406.)

- *Sacral Inclination*—Sacral inclination is the measurement of the verticalization of the sacrum, which is normally 30 degrees. With increased slippage, the sacrum becomes more vertically orientated, while the L5 vertebra becomes more kyphotic.
- *Slip Angle*—The slip angle is determined from a line parallel to the superior endplate of L5 and a line perpendicular to the posterior S1-2. A low angle is normal, but an increased angle represents increasing kyphosis on L5 on S1.

Isthmic Spondylolisthesis. This condition is secondary to spondylolysis and is seen more commonly in young white males. It is very common in the Eskimo population (50%). Patients typically present with back pain and associated tightness of the hamstrings. With slip progression, there is increased narrowing of the neural foramen impinging on the outgoing nerve root (L5). The foraminal stenosis occurs from impingement of the pars stump, disk material, pedicle, and stress fracture fibrous tissue. Initial treatment is typically nonoperative: physical therapy with flexion exercises, NSAIDs, possible bracing, and activity modification.

Surgical Indications and Treatment for Isthmic Spondylolisthesis. Reasons for operative treatment are significant pain after failure of conservative treatment and/or slip progression. For grade I or II slips, treatment is an in situ L5-S1 posterior fusion. With more severe slips, grade III or IV, surgery is typically a posterior fusion from L4 to S1. Decompression is considered if leg pain is a major component of symptoms. Instrumentation should be used in patients with a history of smoking. Slip reduction remains controversial and is associated with injury to the L5 nerve root (20% to 30%).

Adult Scoliosis (Patients Older than 20 Years)

Etiology, Signs, and Symptoms. The etiology of adult scoliosis is neuromuscular, degenerative (spondylosis or osteoporosis), and/or posttraumatic or postsurgical.

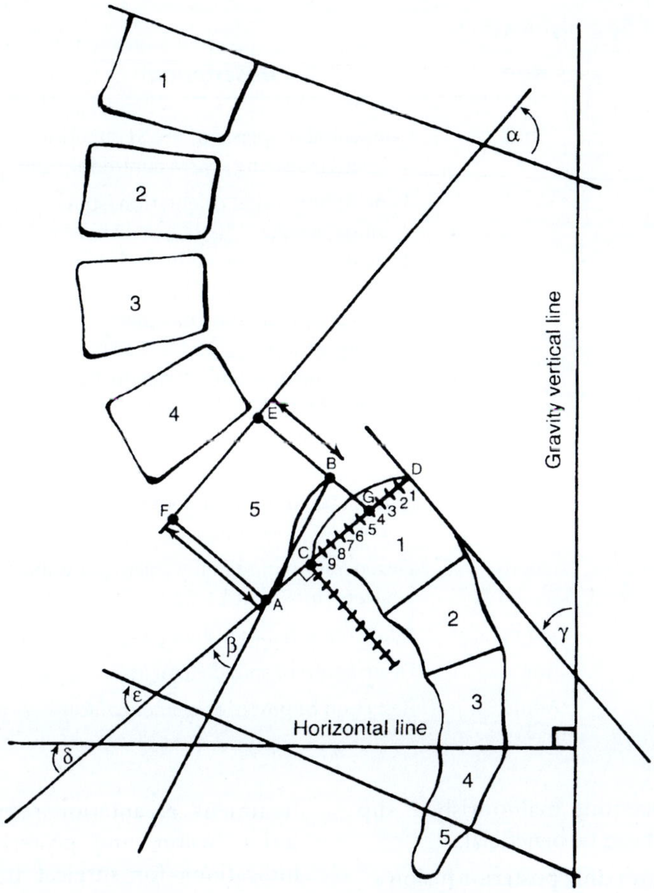

FIGURE 7.18 **Slip angles. (*Source*: Frymoyer JW, Wiesel SW, An HS, et al. (eds.). *The Adult and Pediatric Spine*, 3rd ed. Philadelphia: Lippincott Williams & Wilkins, 2004; 407.)**

Patients typically complain of back pain, which usually starts with pain at the convexity of the curve and progresses to the concavity, and concerns of the cosmetic deformity. Some people may have radicular pain if stenosis develops. With curve progression, the patient may develop cardiopulmonary compromise. Alterations in pulmonary function tests (PFT) may be seen with thoracic curves greater than 60 to 65 degrees.

Curve Progression. Curves less than 30 degrees are unlikely to progress, whereas curves greater than 60 to 80 degrees are likely to progress. The highest risk curve for progression is right thoracic (more than 50 degrees). The rate of progression is usually 1 degree a year, and pregnancy does not increase risk of curve progression.

Surgical Indications and Treatment. Operative indications for adult scoliosis include symptomatic curves greater than 60 degrees, progressive curves, cardiopulmonary problems, and refractory stenosis. Surgery is typically a posterior instrumented fusion with anterior release for rigid curves and curves greater than 70 degrees. Anterior fusion is included with long scoliosis curves in ambulatory adults. The goal is to maintain normal lumbar lordosis and thoracic kyphosis.

Complications in Surgical Treatment. The complications of surgery are much higher in older patients (thus cosmetic and radiographic deformities are not indications for surgery).

- *Malnourishment*—Adult patients undergoing combined anterior/posterior procedures for scoliosis

TABLE 7.24 Classes of Spondylolisthesis

Class	Type	Age	Description	Level
I	Congenital	Child	Congenital dysplasia of the S1 superior facet; hamstring spasm commonly seen **Type A:** horizontal orientation, spina bifida occulta **Type B:** asymmetric sagittal malorientation with intact neural arch, cauda equina syndrome, nerve compression **Type C:** failed vertebral body formation, lumbosacral angle deformities, congenital kyphosis	L5-S1
II	Isthmic	5–50	Most common; fracture or elongation of L5 pars; common in football linemen; gymnasts; ballet dancers	L5-S1
III	Degenerative	Elderly	Degeneration of sagitally oriented lumbar facets (mostly at L4-5)	L4-5 (90%); L3-4 or L5-S1 (10%)
IV	Traumatic	Young	Acute fracture other than pars	L5-S1
V	Pathologic	Any	Destruction of spinal elements	Any
VI	Postsurgical	Adult	Resection of posterior elements/facets	Any

have a high risk of becoming malnourished; supplemental nourishment can be beneficial.

- *Pseudoarthrosis* (15% with only posterior fusion)
- *Instrumentation Failure*
- *Infection* (up to 5%)
- *Neurologic Deficits*—Neural monitoring with the Stagnara wake-up test is the best for preserving function in both lower extremities.

Scheuermann Kyphosis

Diagnosis. Scheuermann kyphosis is usually seen in skeletally immature adolescents. It has a strong hereditary component, with an unknown etiology. Diagnosis is made from standing lateral radiographs.

The criteria for diagnosis are as follows:

- Thoracic kyphosis greater than 45 degrees
- Thoracolumbar kyphosis greater than 30 degrees (thoracolumbar spine normally straight)
- Wedging greater than 5 degrees of 3 adjacent vertebrae

Associated features include vertebral endplate irregularities, Schmorl node (erosion of endplates), and scoliosis (in one third of patients); the apex is usually located at T7 and T8.

Treatment. Nonoperative treatment is bracing and hamstring stretching. Curves less than 50 degrees do not progress after skeletal maturity. The operative treatment is anterior release, interbody and posterior fusion, and posterior instrumentation. The indications for surgical interventions are kyphosis greater than 75 degrees, persistent pain after nonoperative treatment, and rigid kyphosis greater than 55 degrees.

Miscellaneous Thoracolumbar Spine Pathology

Low Back Pain (LBP). Up to 60% to 90% of the adult population will experience an episode of low back pain in their lifetime. It is the leading cause of disability in patients younger than 45 years and the third leading cause in those older than 45 years. Fortunately, 50% will respond to conservative treatment and improve within 1 week, and 90% within 1 to 3 months. In comparison, 50% of patients with sciatica will improve in 1 month. Risk factors are overweight, tobacco, male gender, prolonged sitting, significant lifting or vibration, and job dissatisfaction. In acute low back pain (less than 4 weeks), radiographs are warranted if there is radiculopathy, weakness, trauma, or suspicion of malignancy, infection, fracture, or cauda equine syndrome. Initial treatment of acute low back pain is a maximum of 1 to 2 days of bed rest if symptoms are severe, activity modification, and NSAIDs. Physical therapy can be used as an adjuvant treatment. Education and aerobic exercises are the most important factors in avoiding missed work days and returning patients to work.

Diagnosis of Discogenic Low Back Pain. Patients will complain of primarily low back pain that is worse with flexion and activities. Radiographic signs may be nonspecific, but often there is loss of disk height and/or retrolisthesis on plain radiographs. Schmorl nodes may be seen in the endplates, but this is not considered a sign for low back pain. Schmorl nodes represent disk invaginating into the endplates, and histologic studies suggest collapse of the endplate due to osteonecrosis as a potential precursor. MRI may reveal a dark signal in the disk on T2-weighted images due to loss of water content. There may be a high-intensity zone (HIZ) on T2-weighted images suggesting a torn annulus. HIZ is predictive of a positive diskogram but is also seen in patients without low back pain and is therefore nonspecific. There may be endplate changes as described by Modic. Modic I changes show low signal on T1-weighted MRI but high signal on T2-weighted MRI because of fibrous changes in the endplate. Modic II changes show high signal on T1- and T2-weighted images and is due to fatty degeneration of the endplate. Modic III changes show dark signal on T1- and T2-weighted images and is due to sclerosis of the endplates. Diskography (Fig. 7.19) is a useful adjunct to MRI but can be positive in patients with or without back pain.

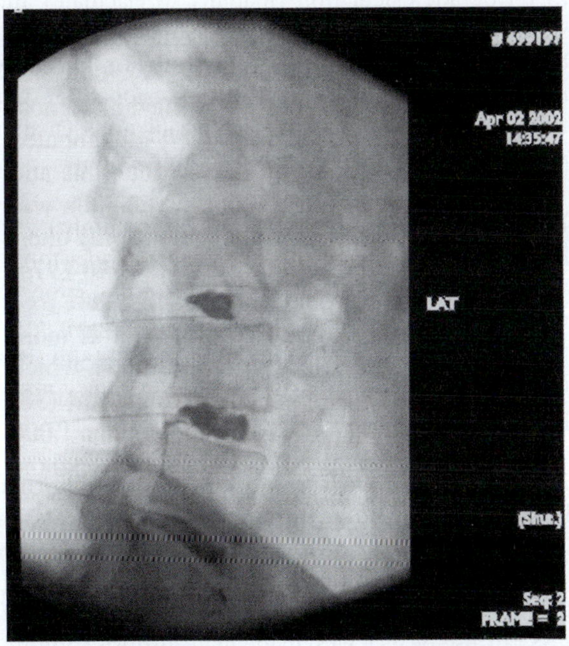

FIGURE 7.19 **Diskogram showing posterior annular defect at L4-5 and disk degeneration at L5-S1. (*Source:* Frymoyer JW, Wiesel SW, An HS, et al., (eds.). *The Adult and Pediatric Spine*, 3rd ed. Philadelphia: Lippincott Williams & Wilkins, 2004;97.)**

Procedurally, a needle is placed in the disk and the disk is hydrodynamically pressurized with contrast dye. The patient is asked to report whether there is pain (concordant if the same as preoperative pain or discordant if not the same). The pain level is graded on the visual analog scale of 10. Low-pressure pain is considered chemical, while high-pressure pain is considered mechanical pain. The best result of a diskography is a negative diskography and suggests a nonpainful disk. A positive diskogram result is controversial, especially in multilevel disease. The ideal candidate is a patient with 1 concordant, painful black disk and nonpainful disk above and below. The person performing the diskogram can affect the results both from a technique perspective and by interpreting the pain response.

Facet-Mediated Low Back Pain. Facet pain is responsible for 15% to 40% of chronic low back pain. The facets are innervated by the medial branches of the dorsal rami of the vertebrae above it and at the same level. The facets contain high-threshold mechanosensitive afferent nerve fibers that serve as nociceptors and low-threshold afferent fibers that modulate proprioceptive feedback. Pain is provoked with compression of the facets when the patient extends or bends laterally. Microfractures can result in posttraumatic lumbozygapophyseal pain.

Chiropractic Care Versus Physiotherapy in the Treatment of Low Back Pain. The cost benefit and effectiveness of chiropractic care and physiotherapy are essentially equal. Chiropractic care is slightly more beneficial in acute conditions, and physiotherapy showed slight benefit in chronic conditions.

Work-Related Injuries and Return to Work. Employee dissatisfaction, particularly after a poor performance evaluation, is the best predicator of a patient's potential of returning to work after sustaining a job-related back injury.

MRIs of the Lumbar Spine. An MRI, as a rule, should be considered a preoperative test. Criteria for positive lumbar spine in asymptomatic patients is shown in Table 7.25.

TABLE 7.25 **Positive Lumbar Spine MRI in Asymptomatic Patients**

Age	*HNP*	*Disk Bulge, Degeneration*	*Stenosis*
20–39	21%	34%–56%	
40–59	22%	50%–59%	
60–79	36%	79%–93%	21%

Diffuse Idiopathic Skeletal Hyperostosis (DISH). Also called Forestier disease, DISH is characterized by ossifications of unknown ligaments (ALL most often affected) and presents radiographically as non-marginal syndesmophytes at 3 adjacent levels (that is, the osteophytes bulge laterally beyond the outer margins of the vertebra). In contrast, ankylosing spondylitis has marginal syndesmophytes. Any location of the spine can be affected, but DISH is most common in the thoracic spine and on the right side. The incidence has been reported to be 28% in autopsy specimens. In males older than 50 years, the prevalence is 25%, and in females older than 50 years, it is 15%. Patients with diabetes and gout have a high prevalence, and it is less common in African Americans and Native Americans. Patients may have low back pain, but there is no relationship. Patients are at increased risk of spinal cord injury due to fractures from hyperextension injuries with minimal trauma. Unstable fractures do not respond to bracing and should be surgically stabilized. There may be associated extraspinal ossification at several joints. Heterotopic bone formation is common at extraspinal sites, such as after hip arthroplasty.

Destructive Spondyloarthropathy. This condition is typically seen in patients on hemodialysis with chronic renal failure. Three adjacent vertebra are usually involved with two intervening disks. Radiographic changes include subluxation, degeneration, and narrowed disk heights, and the changes resemble infection. The underlying pathology may be due to amyloid or crystal deposition.

Complications with Lumbar Spine Surgery

Injuries from Iliac Crest Bone Graft (ICBG) Harvesting. Damage to multiple structures can occur when harvesting ICBG, and symptoms may be seen in approximately 30% of patients, depending on the approach used. The lateral cutaneous branch of the T12 subcostal nerve may lie as close as 6 cm from the ASIS. The ilioinguinal and iliohypogastric nerves can be injured with retraction of the iliacus during dissection on the inner wall of the ilium.

- Anterior Crest Harvest
  - *Lateral Femoral Cutaneous Nerve*—Supplies skin sensation to the anterolateral thigh, injured directly as it courses near the ASIS (may deviate up to 2 cm away from ASIS) or indirectly from retraction after iliacus elevation
  - *Ilioinguinal Nerve*—Supplies skin sensation to the medial thigh and groin region; injury is due to excessive retraction of the iliacus when approaching the inner anterior ileum
- Posterior Crest Harvest
  - *Superior Gluteal Artery*—Injured with retractors placed into sciatic notch
  - *Superior Cluneal Nerve*—Supplies skin sensation in the gluteal region and can be damage with a horizontal skin incision extending more than 8 cm anterolateral of the PSIS

Retrograde Ejaculation. This condition is a complication of anterior approaches to the lower lumbar spine. The incidence of retrograde ejaculation in men after anterior lumbosacral spinal surgery has been reported to range from 0.42% to 5.9%. A transperitoneal approach to the lumbar spine at L4-5 and L5-S1 has a 10-fold greater chance of causing retrograde ejaculation in men than does a retroperitoneal approach. The parasympathetic nervous system is responsible for penile erection, and ejaculation is a function of the sympathetic nervous system. The superior hypogastric sympathetic plexus courses anteriorly over the L5-S1 disk space and can be damaged with anterior and transperitoneal approaches to this region. To limit risk of injury, dissect from left to right to avoid injury to the superior hypogastric plexus as it crosses the L5-S1 disk and refrain from using monopolar electrocautery. Damage to the sympathetic plexus leads to retrograde ejaculation (inability to ejaculate) and sterility. Erectile function and orgasm are not affected by sympathetic injury. Erectile dysfunction is usually related to nonorganic causes but occasionally results from a parasympathetic injury, typically not seen after an anterior approach to the lower lumbar spine.

Damage to the Iliolumbar Vein. The iliolumbar vein is encountered during the left-sided retroperitoneal approach to the lumbar spine as it crosses the L5 vertebral body. It originates from the left paraspinous region and feeds into the inferior vena cava, and once it is encountered, further mobilization of the aorta is prevented by this tether.

Flat Back Syndrome (FBS). FBS is the loss of normal lumbar lordosis, and patients may have difficulty standing erect. It is most often seen after scoliosis surgery with Harrington distraction instrumentation, which lengthens the posterior column of the lumbar spine. FBS can also be seen with inadequate lordosis contouring with segmental spinal instrumentation, anterior spinal column shortening, ankylosing spondylitis, and osteoporosis.

Discectomy/Laminectomy Complications

Dural Tear. 1% incidence, should repair tear primarily. If the tear is too large or dura substance of poor quality, then the defect should be covered with Gelfoam or fibrin glue with a fascial graft. The use of fibrin glue supplementation has been shown to promote a greater inflammatory reaction than does a suture alone. A subarachnoid drain should be used in large irreparable defects; studies have shown that it can decompress the dural tear, leading to spontaneous healing in 4 to 10 days. The drains should not be left more than 4 days because of increased risk of infection. The patient is kept on bed rest, and the lumbar drain is kept at 200 to 300 cc per 24 hour for 72 to 96 hours. During the initial healing phase of these dural tears, pia and arachnoid from the surrounding nerve roots fill the defect and create a pia–arachnoid plug.

Discitis. With less than a 1% incidence rate, diskitis manifests with increasing and severe back pain, elevated ESR, and often a normal peripheral WBC. An MRI with gadolinium should be performed to confirm the diagnosis, then a percutaneous biopsy performed to determine the offending organisms. Treatment should include IV antibiotics, bed rest, and spinal immobilization. Surgery is indicated when the biopsy fails to provide the diagnosis, nonoperative treatment does not provide relief, or the patient is septic.

Vascular Injury from Penetrating the Disk. The development of an arteriovenous fistula is more likely than an acute life-threatening bleed when a vascular insult occurs from penetrating the disk. The formation of an arteriovenous fistula may not be discovered until months after the injury and most commonly manifest with cardiomegaly and high out cardiac failure.

Incomplete Decompression. Lateral recess stenosis is the most common means of failure in percutaneous lumbar discectomy with a 6.9 mm cannula.

Reflexive Sympathetic Dystrophy (RSD). RSD can occur after lumbar spine surgery and manifests with hyperesthesia, hypersensitivity, and burning in the involved extremity. Early recognition is important in treating this entity. Treatment should include aggressive physical therapy, NSAIDs, and possibly a sympathetic block. Rest and analgesics are not effective in treatment of symptoms.

V. SACRUM AND COCCYX

Background. The sacrum provides strength and stability to the pelvis and transmits the body's weight from the spine to the pelvic girdle through the sacroiliac joints. Fractures through the sacrum can therefore propagate from the pelvis to the vertebral column.

Sacral Fractures. Fractures about the sacrum are described by the Denis classification.

- *Type I*—Fracture in sacral ala, lateral to neuroforamina
- *Type II*—Through neuroforamina
- *Type III*—Medial to neuroforamina; highest rate of neurologic injury (56%)

If there are no other pelvic ring fractures, minimal displacement, and no neurologic deficit, then treatment is nonoperative, with gradual mobilization with limited weight bearing. Treatment of a sacral fracture dislocation with neurologic deficit is decompression, realignment, and internal fixation. Sacral fractures with other pelvic ring injuries need to be assessed in terms of pelvis stability.

Sacral Insufficiency Fractures. These fractures are seen in the elderly osteopenic population, typically with a history of no or minor trauma, and can be associated with fractures of the pubic ramus. Patients present with back or groin pain. Bone scans or CT scans are the imaging modalities of choice for the diagnosis. A Technetium bone scan may show an H-type uptake pattern that is diagnostic. Treatment is supportive with activity modification, use of nonnarcotic analgesic, and ambulatory assistive devices (walker, cane, or crutches) until symptoms have resolved.

Coccygodynia. Coccygodynia is pain in the coccyx region that typically occurs while a person is sitting. It is 5 times more likely to occur in women than in man. The mean age of onset of symptoms is around 40. Many of the causes of coccygodynia are posttraumatic, occurring after fracture or contusion, as well as after a traumatic vaginal birth. In most cases, there is hypermobility of the coccyx seen on dynamic radiographs with increased flexion, posterior subluxation, and coccygeal spicule formation. If there is no increased mobility, then the patient has idiopathic coccygodynia, often associated with bursitis at the coccygeal tip. Initial treatment of coccygodynia includes rest, avoidance of sitting position, sitting on donut pillow, NSAIDS, and stool softeners. If this treatment does not relieve symptoms, then dynamic imaging studies should be done to look for the presence of hypermobility. MRI or bone scan will demonstrate inflammation and edema in this region. Steroid/anesthetic injections at the site of radiographic abnormality and massage/stretching of the levator ani muscle. However, if the patient continues to have severe coccygodynia despite nonoperative treatment, then a coccygectomy is considered.

Sacroiliac Pain. The sacroiliac joints may cause low back pain in 5% to 10% of patients. Palpation over the ilium and sacrum may elicit pain. The FABER test may elicit pain, but no test is considered sensitive or specific for sacroiliac dysfunction. Multiple pathologies may affect the sacroiliac joint and include spondyloarthropathy, crystal and pyogenic arthropathy, fractures causing late arthrosis, and diastasis secondary to pregnancy or childbirth.

VI. SPONDYLOARTHOPATHIES

Characteristics of Ankylosing Spondylitis (AS). AS is an inflammatory spondylitis that primarily affects the axial skeleton, starting with sacroiliitis (Fig. 7.20). It is more common in men, associated with HLA-B27, and characterized by an insidious onset of chronic low back pain (morning pain and stiffness, getting better throughout the day), typically beginning in the third or fourth decade of life. Radiographic features of progressive AS are symmetric sacroiliac erosion, squaring of the vertebrae, formation of marginal syndesmophytes (bamboo spine), and eventual ankylosis with kyphosis of the spine. Nonspinal manifestations of AS include arthritis of the peripheral joints, acute anterior uveitis, enthesopathy, hip flexion contractures, aortitis, renal amyloidosis, colitis, and arachnoiditis.

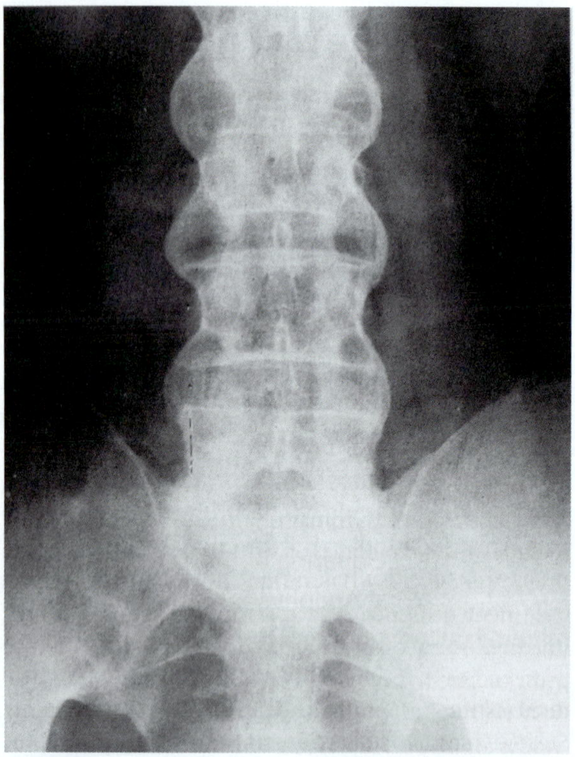

FIGURE 7.20 **Ankylosing spondylitis. (*Source*: Frymoyer JW, Wiesel SW, An HS, et al., (eds.). *The Adult and Pediatric Spine*, 3rd ed. Philadelphia: Lippincott Williams & Wilkins, 2004;146.)**

Management of AS. Initial management of AS is physical therapy and NSAIDs. With progressive spinal involvement in the cervical spine, worsening kyphosis leads to the development of "chin to chest" deformity, which can limit the patient's visual field and impair eating and swallowing ability. A cervical extension osteotomy can be performed to alleviate this situation.

Cervical Spine Fractures with AS. Minor trauma in a patient with AS can cause occult fractures about the cervical spine. Prompt evaluation is necessary. Fractures can extend through the disk space or vertebral body and involve the facet joint, leading to subluxation. Injury to the spinal cord can occur with direct spinal cord injury or from the formation of an epidural hematoma. The treatment of an ankylosing spondylitic cervical spine fracture should be reduction and decompression (if necessary) followed by rigid immobilization.

Reiter Syndrome (Reactive Arthritis). Reiter syndrome is a seronegative spondyloarthropathy, which manifests with arthritis, redness of the eyes (uveitis), and nonpurulent urethral discharge (urethritis). It usually presents with an acute onset of back pain, buttock pain, and a mixed small-joint polyarthritis after a nongonococcal urethritis discharge. It is associated with a positive HLA-B27 (90% of the time) and an elevated ESR (72% of the time). Other symptoms can include sacroiliitis, spondylitis, enthesopathy (pain at tendon and ligament insertion sites), and skin lesions, typically pustular lesions on the soles of the feet.

VII. BIOLOGY, BIOMECHANICS, AND BIOMATERIALS

Determination of Sagittal Plane Balance. Sagittal plane balance is determine by taking a standing, long-cassette, lateral radiograph, then dropping a plumb from C2 or C7 and determining the relationship of the plumb to the L5-1 disk:

- *Positive*—Plumb anterior to L5-1 disk
- *Neutral*—Plumb through L5-1 disk
- *Negative*—Plumb posterior to L5-1 disk

Thoracic Pedicle Diameter. Pedicle screws are now being used more often in the thoracic spine. The diameter of the pedicle in the transverse plane is the main limitation to their use. Anatomic studies have revealed that the thoracic pedicle diameter in the transverse plane, on average, is less than 5 mm and even smaller in deformed spines, such as in scoliosis or kyphosis. On average, anatomic studies have revealed that T5 has the narrowest pedicle diameter (if there is not significant spinal deformity). A study showed the T7 on the concave side of a scoliotic spine was narrower than T5.

Posterior Lumbar Facet Load Sharing. Approximately 20% of the vertical load, in an upright position, is borne by the posterior lumbar facets and 80% by the anterior column of the spine.

Biologic Breakdown of Intervertebral Disks. With DDD, there is a reduction in the disk's water and glycosaminoglycan content as well as an increase in noncollagen glycoprotein.

Effect of Tobacco on Spinal Fusions. Tobacco (and nicotine patches/gum) have been shown to have a negative impact on spinal fusion and wound healing. Smoking negatively affects the spinal artery supply through vasoconstriction or arterial atheromatous changes or both. Cessation of smoking just prior to surgery and until fusion has occurred has resulted in significant improvement in outcomes in patients who smoke and are undergoing spinal fusion. It is recommended that patients do not smoke up to 6 months after fusion.

Effect of Ketorolac (Toradol) on Spinal Fusions. Toradol is contraindicated in lumbar spinal fusion because it has been specifically associated with an increased risk of pseudoarthrosis. It also has been associated with epidural hematomas and other bleeding difficulties, especially in the gastrointestinal tract. Other NSAIDs have been shown to affect bone formation in animal and clinical studies and should not be used for postoperative analgesia.

Bone Morphogenic Protein and Spinal Fusion. The dose of bone morphogenic protein (BMP) is the most critical factor in successful fusion in experimental lumbar intertransverse fusions in rabbits and rhesus monkeys.

Titanium Implants. Titanium implants are being used more often than they previously were in spinal surgery. When compared to cobalt-chromium and stainless steel implants, titanium has a lower modulus of elasticity, which allows for less stress shielding. Also, titanium implants are MRI compatible.

Cross-Linking. The effect of cross-links in rigid pedicle screw systems increases torsional stability. There are recent emerging concerns that cross-link sites are predisposed to pseudoarthrosis.

Factors Affecting Pedicle Screw Fixation. The presence of osteopenia or low bone density has the greatest effect on the pullout strength of lumbar transpedicular screws fixation. Other factors that effect pullout strength are the depth of vertebral body penetration, screw diameter, the percentage of the pedicle filled by the screw, and tapping of the pedicle.

VIII. SPINAL TUMORS

The spine is a common site of tumors. Patients may complain of back pain mostly at night and may notice weight loss. Radiographic findings include absent pedicle on anteroposterior radiographs (owl wink sign), cortical erosion or expansion, and vertebral destruction. Bone scan can be useful in localizing the tumor and assessing for extraspinal involvement. MRI is also useful and with the addition of gadolinium can increase the sensitivity of identifying malignant tumors. A decreased T1 and increased T2 signal suggest malignancy. Malignant tumors most commonly affect the lower lumbar, then the thoracic, then the cervical spine. Locations of spinal tumors are described in Table 7.26.

Lesions Primarily of the Spine

Osteoid Osteoma. Osteoid osteoma is common in the posterior elements of the spine and occurs most often in adolescents. Scoliosis is commonly seen with this lesion but typically does not need surgical correction. Bone scan is helpful in localizing the lesion, and a fine CT scan can help direct treatment options. Initially, NSAIDs may alleviate the pain. However, if pain persists, then surgical resection may be required with or without fusion. Excellent results have been achieved with resection as well as percutaneous CT-guided thermocoagulation.

TABLE 7.26 Location of Spinal Tumors

Vertebral Body	Posterior Elements
Metastatic (most common)	Osteoid osteoma
Histiocytosis X	Aneurysmal bone cysts (ABC)
Giant cell tumor	Osteoblastoma
Chordoma	
Osteosarcoma	
Marrow cell tumors (lymphoma, myeloma)	
Hemangiomas	

Osteoblastoma. Up to 40% of osteoblastomas occur in the spine. They typically are located in the posterior elements in older patients. They can become large and locally aggressive, resulting in neurologic involvement in more than 50% of the spine cases. Treatment of choice is en bloc excision with or without fusion.

Aneurysmal Bone Cyst. In the spine, aneurysmal bone cysts typically occur in the posterior elements but may occur in the anterior elements as well. Excision and/or radiation is the treatment.

Histiocytosis X. This condition often presents in the thoracic spine of children under 10 years old, with progressive back pain. Classic lateral radiographic finding is vertebral flattening (vertebra plana). Biopsy is necessary for diagnosis. If the disease is present systemically, then treatment is chemotherapy. To prevent the development of significant kyphosis, bracing may be needed. If neurologic symptoms are present, then low-dose radiation may be used. The symptoms are usually self-limited.

Giant Cell Tumor. Seen in the fourth or fifth decades of life, giant cell tumor presents in the anterior elements of the spine as a destructive, expansible lesion. Treatment is typically surgical resection and fusion. Malignant transformation may occur with radiation therapy.

Chordoma. Chordomas are rare, slow-growing tumors arising from remnants of the notochord in axial skeleton of middle-aged adults. They present as lytic lesions in the base of the skull or more commonly in the sacrum. Patients will have intraabdominal complaints and a presacral mass. Chordomas are not chemo or radiation sensitive. Treatment for a chordoma is "en bloc" resection if possible with subsequent reconstruction fusion to adjacent levels. Bowel and bladder function can be maintained with excision of up to half of the sacral roots. Chordoma has a high recurrence rate, but patients typically survive 10 to 15 years after initial presentation.

Osteosarcoma. Osteosarcomas and other malignant primary skeletal lesions, such as Ewing or chondrosarcoma, rarely present in the spine. The overall prognosis is poor; initial treatment is chemotherapy and XRT. Surgical excision may also be necessary.

Hemangioma. Often asymptomatic, hemangioma lesions are found upon radiographic imaging of the spine. They are typically well-defined lesions that are hyperintense on both T1 and T2 MRI images. Vertical striations (jailhouse striations) may be seen on plain radiographs if the hemangioma is large enough. CT scan often shows a speckled pattern. Patients may present with a pathologic fracture through these lesions. Treatment, most of the time, is observation; however, if a patient has continued pain, then XRT may alleviate symptoms.

Lymphoma. Often associated with systemic disease, lymphoma presents with 'ivory' vertebrae. Once histologic diagnosis is confirmed, treatment is with XRT and chemotherapy.

Multiple Myeloma. Multiple myeloma is common in the spine, presenting with pain and lytic lesions. Laboratory findings include elevated calcium, decreased hematocrit, and abnormal protein studies, SPEP, and UPEP. XRT is the treatment; surgical intervention is reserved for cases of instability and persistent neurologic involvement. Bone scan is helpful but can be negative.

Intradural Extramedullary Lesions. Intradural extramedullary lesions usually are neurofibroma or meningioma (Table 7.27).

Dural Ectasia. Dural ectasia is a protrusion of the meninges outside the confines of the normal thecal sac, which causes lateral meningoceles or posterior scalloping of the vertebral bodies. It is seen in about 60% of patients with Marfan syndrome and is seen commonly in patients with neurofibromatous.

Sacral Tumors. Tumors commonly associated with the sacrum are the chordoma and giant cell tumor.

Winking Owl Sign. The winking owl sign is when the pedicle is missing on an anterior–posterior radiograph and is characteristic of tumor invasion of the cortical bone of the pedicle.

TABLE 7.27 Intradural Extramedullary Lesions by Type

	Spine Predilection	T1-Weighted MRI	T2-Weighted MRI
Neurofibroma	Evenly between cervical, thoracic, lumbar	Isointense	Increased signal
Meningioma (80% female)	Thoracic most often	Isointense	Isointense

Metastatic Lesions of the Spine

Spinal Metastasis. Metastatic disease in the spine is the most common tumor in the spine. The most common metastates to the spine are breast, lung, and prostate. These are typically osteolytic lesions except prostate, which is usually osteoblastic. The tumor usually spreads to the vertebral body first, then invades the pedicle. Plain radiograph evidence of an osteolytic process does not occur until greater than 30% invasion has occurred. Signs and symptoms (red flags) of possible metastatic lesion in the spine are cancer history, pain at night, recent weight loss, and age over 50 years. Diagnosis can be made by CT-guided biopsy or surgical biopsy, if necessary. Initial treatment is XRT and chemotherapy. Radiosensitive lesions are lymphoid tumors and prostate; radioresistant lesions are renal cell and gastrointestinal. Most (70%) breast metastases are radiosensitive.

Treatment of Metastatic Renal Cell Carcinoma to the Spine. Renal cell carcinoma is not chemo or radiation sensitive. Surgery is usually necessary, but since these lesions are extremely vascular, preoperative embolization is warranted.

Treatment of Spinal Metastasis with Compressive Neuropathy. The treatment most likely to restore or maintain function in a patient with progressive paraparesis from spinal cord compression secondary to a metastatic lesion is surgical decompression and stabilization. The decompression is performed on the compressive side, either anteriorly or posteriorly. Other surgical indications include persistent pain despite XRT, need for biopsy, and the development of spinal instability.

IX. SPINAL INFECTIONS

Vertebral Osteomyelitis. The diagnosis of vertebral osteomyelitis is often delayed (weeks). Patients present with unrelenting back pain, fevers, a history of prior infection, and sometimes neurologic involvement. Elderly patients, patients with systemic diseases (diabetes), IV drug abusers, and immunocompromised hosts are at increased risk for infection. Hematogenous spread is the most common route of invasion. Tissue diagnosis or positive blood cultures are imperative for treatment. CT guided needle biopsy can be helpful in early infection but can yield false-negatives.

Treatment of Vertebral Osteomyelitis. Initial therapy includes symptomatic pain relief and long-term organism-specific IV antibiotics (6 to 12 weeks). Indications for surgery include:

- Progressive spinal destruction despite antibiotic therapy
- Neurologic involvement
- Focal abscess
- Need for a diagnosis
- Instability of the spine

Débridement of the infection is performed to viable bone; decompression of the canal may be warranted. Strut grafts are used to replace destroyed anterior spinal elements. Posterior augmentation may be necessary depending on the amount of bony destruction.

Epidural Abscess. An epidural abscess needs surgical débridement. If there is no anterior pathology, such as discitis or vertebral body osteomyelitis, then a posterior approach is sufficient. If a patient presents with an epidural abscess and neurologic deficit, then it is a medical and surgical emergency. Epidural abscesses may develop (rarely) after an epidural injection.

Arachnoiditis. Arachnoiditis is visualized with MRI or myelography with abnormal clumping of the nerve roots.

Tuberculosis (TB). The spine is the most common skeletal location of TB, with the thoracic spine most commonly involved. There is hematogenesis spread to the anterior vertebral body with bone destruction and sequestrum formation. The vertebral disk is spared until late in the disease process. Multiple levels are usually involved with skip lesions. Paraspinal abscesses are common. With progressive bone destruction, the anterior vertebral body can collapse, resulting in kyphosis. Pott paraplegia develops from cord compression as a result of progressive kyphosis. Treatment is with chemotherapy with or without bracing and with or without radical anterior débridement with strut autografting (Hong Kong procedure).

Postoperative Infection in Instrumented Fusions. The treatment of postoperative infection in an instrumented fusion depends on the time course after surgery. An early, deep infection occurring prior to fusion should be treated with aggressive irrigation and débridement with retention of the hardware followed by a prolonged course of IV antibiotics. A late, deep infection or persistent infection after fusion has occurred should be treated with I&D, removal of the hardware, and IV antibiotics.

References

1. Abumi K, Panjabi MM, Kramer KM, et al. Biomechanical evaluation of lumbar spinal stability after graded facetectomies. *Spine* 1990;15:1142–1147.

2. Admas MA, Hutton WC. The effect of posture on the role of the apophyseal joints in resisting intervertebral compressive forces. *J Bone Joint Surg Br* 1980;62:358–362.
3. Ahn NU, Sponseller PD, Ahn UM, Nallamshetty L, Kuszyk BS, Zinreich SJ. Dural ectasia is associated with back pain in Marfan' syndrome. *Spine* 2000;25:1562–1568.
4. Anderson PA. Nonsurgical treatment of patients with thoracolumbar fractures. In: Jackson DW (ed.), *Instructional Course Lectures 44*. Rosemont, IL: American Academy of Orthopaedic Surgeons, 1995;57–65.
5. Anderson PA, Steinmann JC. Internal fixation of the cervical spine, In: Frymoyer JW (ed.), *The Adult Spine, Principles and Practice*, 2nd ed. Philadelphia: Lippincott Raven, 1997;1119–1147.
6. Apfelbaum RI, Kriskovich MD, Haller JR. On the incidence, cause, and prevention of recurrent laryngeal nerve palsy during anterior cervical spine surgery. *Spine* 2000;25:2906–2912.
7. Apple DF Jr. Spinal cord injury rehabilitation. In: Rothman RH, Simeone FA (eds.), *The Spine*, 3rd ed. Philadelphia: WB Saunders, 1992, Chap. 31.
8. Azouvi P, Mane M, Thiebaut J, et al. Intrathecal baclofen administration for control of severe spinal spasticity: Functional improvement and long-term follow-up. *Arch Phys Med Rehabil* 1996;77:35–39.
9. Beaty JH (ed.). *Orthopaedic Knowledge Update 6*. Rosemont, IL: American Academy of Orthopaedic Surgeons, 1999;673–698.
10. Benz R, Abitbol JJ, Ozanne S, Garfin SR. Cervical burst fractures. In: Levine AM, Eismont FJ, Garfin SR, Zigler JE (ed.), *Spine Trauma*. Philadelphia: WB Saunders, 1998;300–330.
11. Bernhardt M, Bridwell KH. Segmental analysis of the sagittal plane alignment of the normal thoracic and lumbar spines and thoracolumbar junction. *Spine* 1989;14:717–721.
12. Bigos S, Boyer O, Braen GR, et al. Acute low back pain problems in adults: Clinical practice guideline No 14. AHCPR Publication No 95–0642. Rockville, MD: Agency for Health Care Policy and Research, Public Health Service, US Department of Health and Human Services, December 1994.
13. Bigos SJ, Spengler DM, Martin NA, et al. Back injuries in industry: A retrospective study. III: Employee-related factors. *Spine* 1986;11:252–256.
14. Boden SD, Dodge LD, Bohlman HH et al. Rheumatoid arthritis of the cervical spine. *J Bone Joint Surg* 1993;75A:1282–1297.
15. Boden SD, Schimandle JH, Hutton WC. The use of an osteoinductive growth factor for lumbar spinal fusion: Part II. Study of dose, carrier, and species. *Spine* 1995;20:2633–2644.
16. Bohlman HH. Acute fractures and dislocations of the cervical spine: An analysis of three hundred hospitalized patients and review of the literature. *J Bone Joint Surg* 1979;61A:1119–1142.
17. Bohlman HH, Emery SE, Goodfellow DB, et al. Robinson anterior cervical discectomy and arthrodesis for cervical radiculopathy. *J Bone Joint Surg* 1993;75A:1298–1306.
18. Bonney G, Gilliatt RW. Sensory nerve conduction after traction injuries of the brachial plexus. *Proc R Soc Med* 1958;51:365–367.
19. Borchgrevink GE, Kaasa A, McDonagh D, Stiles TC, Haraldseth O, Lereim I. Acute treatment of whiplash neck injuries: A randomized trial during the first 14 days after a car accident. *Spine* 1998;23:25–31.
20. Botte MJ, Byrne TP, Abrams RA, et al. The halo skeletal fixator: Techniques of application and prevention of complications. *J Am Acad Orthop Surg* 1996;4:44–53.
21. Botte MJ, Garfin SR, Byrne TP, et al. The halo skeletal fixator: Principles of application and maintenance. *Clin Orthop* 1989;239:12–18.
22. Boxall D, Bradford DS, Winter RB, et al. Management of severe spondylolisthesis in children and adolescents. *J Bone Joint Surg* 1979;61A:479–495.
23. Bozkus H, Ames CP, Chamberlain RH, et al. Biomechanical analysis of rigid stabilization techniques for three-column injury in the lower cervical spine. *Spine* 2005 Apr 15;30(8):915–922.
24. Bracken MB, Shepard MJ, Holford TR, et al. Administration of methylprednisolone for 24 or 48 hours or tirilazad mesylate for 48 hours in the treatment of acute spinal cord injury: Results of the Third National Acute Spinal Cord Injury Randomized Controlled Trial. National Acute Spinal Cord Injury Study. *JAMA* 1997;277:1597–1604.
25. Bridwell KH, Ogilvie JW. Primary tumors of the spine. In: Bridwell KH, DeWald RL (eds.), *The Textbook of Spinal Surgery*. Philadelphia: JB Lippincott, 1991;1143–1185.
26. Brigham CD. Ankylosing spondylitis and seronegative spondyloarthropathies. In: Clark CR (ed.). *The Cervical Spine*, 3rd ed. Philadelphia: Lippincott-Raven, 1998;724–727.
27. Brodsky AE, Khalil MA, Sassard WR, et al. Repair of symptomatic pseudoarthrosis of anterior cervical fusion: Posterior versus anterior repair. *Spine* 1992;17:1137–1143.
28. Broom MJ, Raycroft JF. Complications of fractures of the cervical spine in ankylosing spondylitis. *Spine* 1988;13:763–766.
29. Buckwalker JA, Einhorn TA, Simon SR (ed.). *Orthopedics Basic Science: Biology and Biomechanics of the Musculoskeletal System*, 2nd ed. Rosemont, IL: American Academy of Orthopedic Surgeons, 1999;182–215.
30. Buirski G, Silberstein M. The symptomatic lumbar disk in patients with low-back pain: Magnetic resonance imaging appearances in both the symptomatic and controlled population. *Spine* 1993;18:1808–1811.
31. Cain JE Jr, Dryer RF, Barton BR. Evaluation of dural closure techniques: Suture methods, fibrin adhesive sealant, and cyanoacrylate polymer. *Spine* 1988;13:720–725.

32. Cain JE Jr, Lauerman WC, Rosenthal HG, Broom MJ, Jacobs RR. The histomorphologic sequence of dural repair: Observations in the canine model. *Spine* 1991;16:S319–S323.

33. Calin A. Ankylosing spondylitis. *Clin Rheum Dis* 1985; 11:41–60.

34. Campanacci M, Boriani S, Giunti A. Giant cell tumors of the spine. In: Sundaresan N, Schmidek HH, Schiller AL, et al (eds.), *Tumors of the Spine*. Philadelphia: WB Saunders, 1990;163–180.

35. Carragee EJ. Single level posterolateral arthrodesis, with or without posterior decompression, for the treatment of isthmic spondylolisthesis in adults: A prospective, randomized study. *J Bone Joint Surg* 1997;79A: 1175–1180.

36. Chen BH, Natarajan RN, An H, Anderson GB. Comparison of biomechanical response to surgical procedures used for cervical radiculopathy: Posterior keyhole foraminotomy versus anterior foraminotomy and discectomy versus anterior discectomy with fusion. *J Spinal Disord* 2001;14;17–20.

37. Chin KR, Auerbach JD, Adams SB, Sodl JF, Riew KD. Mastication causing segmental spinal motion in common cervical orthoses. *Spine* 2006 Feb 15;31(4):430–434.

38. Chin KR, Eiszner JR, Roh J, Bohlman HH. Use of spinous processes to determine drill trajectory during placement of lateral mass screws: A cadaveric analysis. *J Spinal Disord Tech* 2006 Feb;19(1):18–21.

39. Coe JD, Warden KE, Sutterlin CE III, et al. Biomechanical evaluation of cervical spinal stabilization methods in a human cadaveric model. *Spine* 1989;14:1122–1131.

40. Cove JA, Taminiau AH, Obermann WR, Vanderschueren GM. Osteoid osteoma of the spine treated with percutaneous computed tomography–guided thermocoagulation. *Spine* 2000;25:1283–1286.

41. Currier BL, Eismont FJ. Infections of the spine. In: Rothman RH, Simeone FA (eds.), *The Spine*, 3rd ed. Philadelphia: WB Saunders, 1992;1319–1380.

42. Denis F. The three column spine and its significance in the classification of acute thoracolumbar spinal injuries. *Spine* 1983;8:817–831.

43. Denis F, Davis S, Comfort T. Sacral fractures: An important problem. Retrospective analysis of 236 cases. *Clin Orthop* 1988;227:67–81.

44. DeWald RL. Revision surgery for spinal deformity. In: Eilert RE, (ed.), *Instructional Course Lectures XLI*. Park Ridge, IL: American Academy of Orthopaedic Surgeons, 1992;235–250.

45. Dick J, Boachie-Adjei O, Wilson M. One stage versus two-stage anterior and posterior spinal reconstruction in adults: Comparison of outcomes including nutritional status, complications rates, hospital costs, and other factors. *Spine* 1992;17:S310–S316.

46. Dick JC, Zdeblick TA, Bartel BD. Mechanical evaluation of cross-link designs in rigid pedicle screw systems. *Spine* 1997;22:370–375.

47. Dimar JR II, Ante WA, Zhang YP, et al. The effects of nonsteroidal antiinflammatory drugs on posterior spinal fusions in the rat. *Spine* 1996;21:1870–1876.

48. Dommisse GF. The blood supply of the spinal cord. A critical vascular zone in spinal surgery. *J Bone Joint Surg* 1974;56B:225–235.

49. Donaldson WF III, Star MJ, Thorne RP. Surgical treatment for the far lateral herniated lumbar disk. *Spine* 1993;18:1263–1267.

50. Ebraheim NA, Hoeflinger MJ, Salpietro B, et al. Anatomic consideration in posterior plating of the cervical spine. *J Orthop Trauma* 1991;5:196–199.

51. Ebraheim NA, Jabaly G, Xu R, Yeasting RA. Anatomic relations of the thoracic pedicle to the adjacent neural structures. *Spine* 1997;22:1553–1557.

52. Ebraheim NA, Lu J, Brown, et al. Vulnerability of vertebral artery in anterolateral decompression for cervical spondylosis. *Clin Orthop Rel Res* 1996;322:146–151.

53. Ebraheim NA, Lu J, Yang H, Heck BE, Yeasting RA. Vulnerability of the sympathetic trunk during the anterior approach to the cervical spine. *Spine* 2000;25:1603–1606.

54. Ebraheim NA, Xu R, Ahmad M, Heck B. The quantitative anatomy of the vertebral artery groove of the atlas and its relation to the posterior atlantoaxial approach. *Spine* 1998;23:320–323.

55. Ebraheim NA, Xu R, Darwich M, Yeasting RA. Anatomic relations between the lumbar pedicle and the adjacent neural structures. *Spine* 1997;22:2338–2341.

56. Ebraheim NA, Xu R, Yeasting RA. The location of the vertebral artery foramen and its relation to posterior lateral mass screw fixation. *Spine* 1996;21:1291–1295.

57. Eismont FJ, Arena MJ, Green BA. Extrusion of an intervertebral disk associated with traumatic subluxation or dislocation of cervical facets: Case report. *J Bone Joint Surg* 1991;73A:1555–1560.

58. Emery SE, Chan DP, Woodward HR. Treatment of hematogenous pyogenic vertebral osteomyelitis with anterior débridement and primary bone grafting. *Spine* 1989;14:284–291.

59. Emery SE, Smith MD, Bohlman HH. Upper-airway obstruction after multilevel cervical corpectomy for myelopathy. *J Bone Joint Surg Am* 1991;73:544–551.

60. Fardon DF, Garfin SR (eds.). *Orthopaedic Knowledge Update: Spine 2*. Rosemont, IL: American Academy of Orthopaedic Surgeons, 2002;254–261, 393–396.

61. Fidler MW, Plasmans CM. The effect of four types of support on the segmental mobility of the lumbosacral spine. *J Bone Joint Surg* 1983; 65A:943–947.

62. Flynn JC, Price CT. Sexual complications of anterior fusions of the lumbar spine. *Spine* 1984;9:480–492.

63. Fogel GR, Cunningham PY III, Esses SI. Coccygodynia: Evaluation and management. *J Am Aced Orthop Surg* 2004;12:49–54.

64. Fowler BL, Dall BE, Rowe DE. Complications associated with harvesting autogenous iliac bone graft. *Am J Orthop* 1995;24:895–903.

65. Fredrickson BE, Baker D, McHolick WJ, et al. The natural history of spondylolysis and spondylolisthesis. *J Bone Joint Surg* 1984;66A:699–707.

66. Fredrickson BE, Yuan HA, Bagley JC. The nonsurgical treatment of thoracolumbar injuries. *Semin Spine Surg* 1990;2:70–78.

67. Garfin SR, Botte MJ, Waters RL, et al. Complications in the use of the halo fixation device. *J Bone Joint Surg* 1986;68A:320–325.

68. Garfin SR, Vaccaro AR (eds.). *Orthopaedic Knowledge Update: Spine*. Rosemont, IL: American Academy of Orthopedic Surgeons, 1997.

69. Ghanayem AJ, Leventhal M, Bohlman HH. Osteoarthritis of the atlanto-axial joints: Long-term follow-up after treatment with arthrodesis. *J Bone Joint Surg Am* 1996;78:1300–1307.

70. Ghanayem AJ, Zdeblick TA, Panjabi MM. Biomechanics of nonacute cervical spine trauma. In: Clark CR (ed.), *The Cervical Spine*, 3rd ed.. Philadelphia: Lippincott Raven, 1998;103–105.

71. Giacobetti FB, Vaccaro AR, Deeley DM, et al. Vertebral artery occlusion associated with cervical spine trauma: A prospective analysis. *Spine* 1997;22:188–192.

72. Ginsburg HH, Shetter AG, Raudzens PA. Postoperative paraplegia with preserved intraoperative somatosensory evoked potentials: Case report. *J Neurosurg* 1985;63:296–300.

73. Givre S, Freed HA. Autonomic dysreflexia: A potentially fatal complication of somatic stress in quadriplegics. *J Emerg Med* 1989;7:461–463.

74. Glassman SD, Anagnost SC, Parker A, Burke D, Johnson JR, Dimar JR. The effect of cigarette smoking and smoking cessation on spinal fusion. *Spine* 2000;25:2608–2615.

75. Glassman SD, Rose SM, Dimar JR, Puno RM, Campbell MJ, Johnson JR. The effect of postoperative nonsteroidal antiinflammatory drug administration on spinal fusion. *Spine* 1998;23:834–838.

76. Hadler NM, Curtis P, Gilling DB, et al. A benefit of spinal manipulation as adjunctive therapy for acute low back pain: A stratified control trial. *Spine* 1987;12:702–706.

77. Hakelius A. Prognosis in sciatica: A clinical follow-up of surgical and nonsurgical treatment. *Acta Ortho Scand Suppl* 1970;129:1–76.

78. Hansraj KK, O'Leary PF, Cammisa FP Jr, et al. Decompression, fusion and instrumentation for complex lumbar spinal stenosis. *Clin Orthop* 2001;384:18–25.

79. Harrington KD. Metastatic tumors of the spine: Diagnosis and treatment. *J Am Acad Orthop Surg* 1993;1:76–86.

80. Heary RF, Albert TJ, Ludwig SC, et al. Surgical anatomy of the vertebral arteries. *Spine* 1996;21:2074–2080.

81. Heller JG, Levine MJ. Postoperative infections of the spine. *Semin Spine Surg* 1996;8:105–114.

82. Henderson CM, Hennessy RG, Shuey HM Jr, Schackelford EG. Posterior-lateral foraminotomy as an exclusive operative technique for cervical radiculopathy: A review of 846 consecutively operated cases. *Neurosurgery* 1983;13:504–512.

83. Hensinger RN. Spondylolysis and spondylolisthesis in children and adolescents. *J Bone Joint Surg* 1989;71A:1098–1107.

84. Herkowitz HN, Garfin SR. Decompressive surgery for spinal stenosis. *Semin Spine Surg* 1989;1:163–167.

85. Hilibrand AS, Carlson GD, Palumbo MA, Jones PK, Bohlman HH. Radiculopathy and myelopathy at segments adjacent to the site of previous anterior cervical arthrodesis. *J Bone Surg Am* 1999;81:519–528.

86. Hollingshead WH (ed.). *Anatomy for Surgeons, The Head and Neck*, 3rd ed. Philadelphia: Harper-Rowe, 1982;1:430–436.

87. Hoppenfeld S. *Physical Examination of the Spine & Extremities*. Norwalk, CT: Appleton & Lange, 1976.

88. *International Standards for Neurological and Functional Classification of Spinal Cord Injury*. Chicago, IL: American Spinal Injury Association Publication, 1996.

89. Jarret PJ, Whitesides TE Jr. Injuries of the cervicocranium, In: Browner BD, Jupiter JB, Levine AM, Trafton PG (eds.), *Skeletal Trauma*. Philadelphia: WB Saunders, 1992;665–697.

90. Johnson RM, Hart DL, Simmons EF, et al. Cervical orthoses: A study comparing their effectiveness in restricting cervical motion in normal subjects. *J Bone Joint Surg* 1977;59A:332–339.

91. Johnson RM, Owen JR, Hart DL, et al. Cervical orthoses: A guide to their selection and use. *Clin Orthop* 1981;154:34–45.

92. Johnsson KE, Rosen I, Uden A. The natural course of lumbar spinal stenosis. *Clin Orthop* 1992;279:82–86.

93. Kambin P, O'Brien E, Zhou L, et al. Arthroscopic microdiskectomy and selective fragmentectomy. *Clin Orthop* 1998;347:150–167.

94. Kellam JP. Sacral fractures. In: Tile M (ed.), *Fractures of the Pelvis and Acetabulum*, 2nd.ed. Media, PA: Williams & Wilkins, 1995;200–209.

95. Kibins NP, Noonan KJ, Weinstein WJN. Chordoma of the lumbar spine: Surgical approach and rationale. *Contemp Orthop* 1991;22:163.

96. Miller MD, Brinker MR (eds.), *Review of Orthopaedics*, 3rd ed. Philadelphia: WB Saunders, 2000;372–373.

97. King GJ, Kostuik JP, McBroom RJ, et al. Surgical management of metastatic renal carcinoma of the spine. *Spine* 1991;16:265–271.

98. Kitchel SH, Eismont FJ, Green BA. Closed subarachnoid drainage for management of cerebrospinal fluid leakage after an operation on the spine. *J Bone Joint Surg* 1989;71A:984–987.

99. Klippel J (ed.), *Primer on the Rheumatoid Diseases*, 11th ed. Atlanta: Arthritis Foundation, 1997;184–187.

100. Knight JW, Cordingley JJ, Palazzo MG. Epidural abscess following epidural steroid and local anaesthetic injection. *Anaesthesia* 1997;52:576–578.

101. Kostuik JP. Adult scoliosis: The lumbar spine. In: Bridwell KH, DeWald RL (eds.), *The Textbook of*

Spinal Surgery, 2nd ed. Philadelphia: Lippincott-Raven, 1997;733–775.

102. Kostuik JP, Harrington I, Alexander D, Rand W, Evans D. Cauda Equina Syndrome and Lumber Disc Herniation. *J Bone Joint Surg Am* 1986;68:386–391.
103. Kurz LT, Garfin SR, Booth RE. Harvesting autogenous iliac bone grafts: A review of complications and techniques. *Spine* 1989;14:1324–1331.
104. LaGrone MO, Bradford DS, Moe JH, et al. Treatment of symptomatic flat back after spinal fusion. *J Bone Joint Surg* 1988;70A:569–580.
105. Landells CD, Van Peteghem PK. Fractures of the atlas: Classification, treatment and morbidity. *Spine* 1988;13:450–452.
106. Landi A, Copeland SA, Parry CB, Jones SJ. The role of somatosensory evoked potentials and nerve conduction studies in the surgical management of brachial plexus injuries. *J Bone Joint Surg* 1980;62B:492–496.
107. Lane JM, Bostrom MP. Bone grafting and new composite biosynthetic graft materials. In: Cannon WD Jr (ed.), *Instructional Course Lectures 47*. Rosemont, IL: American Academy of Orthopaedic Surgeons, 1998;525–534.
108. Lauerman WC, Cain JE. Isthmic spondylolisthesis in the adult. *J Am Acad Orthop Surg* 1996;4:201–208.
109. Lees F, Aldren-Turner JW. Natural history and prognosis of cervical spondylosis. *Br Med J* 1963;2:1607–1610.
110. Lijenquist UR, Halm HF, Link TM. Pedicle screw instrumentation of the thoracic spine in idiopathic scoliosis. *Spine* 1997;22:2239–2245.
111. Louw JA, Mafoyane NA, Small B, et al. Occlusion of the vertebral artery in cervical spine dislocations. *J Bone Joint Surg* 1990;72B:679–681.
112. Lowe TG. Scheuermann's disease. In: Bridwell KH, DeWald RL (eds.), *The Textbook of Spinal Surgery*, 2nd ed. Philadelphia: Lippincott-Raven, 1997;1173–1198.
113. Lu J, Ebraheim NA, Biyani JA, Yeasting RA, Vulnerability of great medullary artery. *Spine* 1996;21:1852–1855.
114. Ludwig SC, Albert TJ. Measuring outcomes in cervical myelopathy and radiculopathy. *Instr Course Lect* 1999;48:417–421.
115. Malmivaara A, Hakkinen U, Ro T, et al. The treatment of low back pain: Bed rest, exercise, therapy, or ordinary activity? *N Engl J Med* 1995;332:351–355.
116. Malone DG, Benzyl EC. Laminotomy and laminectomy for spinal stenosis causing radiculopathy or myelopathy. In: Clark CR (ed.), *The Cervical Spine*, 3rd ed. Philadelphia: Lippincott Raven 1998; 817–825.
117. Matthew WB. Neuropathies. In: *Handbook of Clinical Neurology*, Vol. 51, Chap. 11 (Revised Series 7). New York: Elsevier Science.
118. McAfee PC, Bohlman HH, Riley LH Jr, et al. The anterior retropharyngeal approach to the upper part of the cervical spine. *J Bone Joint Surg* 1987;69A:1371–1383.
119. Mclain R, Weinstein J. Tumors of the spine. In: Herkowitz HH (ed.), *The Spine*, 4th ed. Philadelphia: WB Saunders, 1992;1173.
120. Mealy K, Brennan H, Fenelson GC. Early mobilization of acute whiplash injuries. *Br Med J* 1986;292:656–657.
121. Melton LJ III. Epidemiology of spinal osteoporosis. *Spine* 1997;22:2S–11S.
122. Montgomery DM, Aronson DD, Lee CL, et al. Posterior spinal fusion: Allograft versus autograft bone. *J Spinal Disord* 1990;3:370–375.
123. Montgomery DM, Brower RS. Cervical spondylotic myelopathy: Clinical syndrome and natural history. *Orthop Clin North AM* 1992;23:487–493.
124. Morganti C, Sweeney CA, Albanese SA, Burak C, Hosea T, Connolly PJ. Return to play after cervical spine injury. *Spine* 2001;26:1131–1136.
125. Muffolleto AJ, et al. Cervical stability with lateral mass plating: Unicortical versus bicortical screw purchase. *Spine* 2003 Apr 15;28(8):778–781.
126. Naylor A, Shentall R. Biomechanical aspects of intervertebral discs in aging and disease. In: Jayson M (ed.), *The Lumbar Spine and Back Pain*. New York: Grune & Stratton, 1976;317–326.
127. Newhouse KE, el-Khoury GY, Buckwalter JA. Occult sacral fractures in osteopenic patients. *J Bone Joint Surg Am* 1992;74(10):1472–1477.
128. Oda T, Fujiwara K, Yonenobu K, et al. Natural history of cervical spine lesions in rheumatoid arthritis. *Spine* 1995;20:1128–1135.
129. Paramore CG, Dickman CA, Sonntag VK. The anatomic suitability of the C1-2 complex for transarticular screw fixation. *J Neurosurg* 1996;85:221–224.
130. Penn R. Intrathecal baclofen for spasticity of spinal origin: Seven years of experience. *J Neurosurg* 1992;77: 236–240.
131. Petraco DM, Spivak JM, Cappadona JG, et al. An anatomic evaluation of L5 nerve stretch in spondylolisthesis reduction. *Spine* 1996;21:1133–1138.
132. Pettine KA, Klassen RA. Osteoid-osteoma and osteoblastoma of the spine. *J Bone Joint Surg Am* 1986;68:354–361.
133. Poussa M, Schlenzka D, Seitsalo S, et al. Surgical treatment of severe isthmic spondylolisthesis in adolescents: Reduction or fusion in situ. *Spine* 1993;18:894–901.
134. Roffi RP, Waters RL, Adkins RH. Gunshots wounds to the spine associated with a perforated viscus. *Spine* 1989;14:808–811.
135. Ross PD, Davis JW, Epstein RS, Wasnich RD. Pre-existing fractures and bone mass predict vertebral fracture incidence in women. *Ann Intern Med* 1991;114:919–923.
136. Rothman RH, Simeone FA. *The Spine*. Philadelphia: WB Saunders, 1982;33–36.
137. Saal JA, Saal JS, Herzog RJ. The natural history of lumbar intervertebral disk extrusions treated nonoperatively. *Spine* 1990;15:683–686.
138. Saal JS, Saal JA, Yurth EF. Non-operative management of herniated cervical intervertebral disc with radiculopathy. *Spine* 1996;21:1877–1883.
139. Sachs BL. Differential diagnosis of neck pain, arm pain, and myelopathy. In: Clark CR (ed.), *The cervical*

Spine, 3rd ed. Philadelphia: Lippincott Raven, 1998; 741–742.

140. Sachs BL, Zindrick MR, Beasley RD. Reflex sympathetic dystrophy after operative procedures on the lumbar spine. *J Bone Joint Surg* 1993;75A:721–725.
141. Saer EH III, Winter RB, Lonstein JE. Long scoliosis fusion to the sacrum in adults with nonparalytic scoliosis: An improved method. *Spine* 1990;15:650–653.
142. Sasso RC, Burkus KJ, LeHuec JC. Retrograde ejaculation after anterior lumbar interbody fusion: Transperitoneal versus retroperitoneal exposure. *Spine* 2003 May 15;28(10):1023–1026.
143. Schaffer JL, Kambin P. Percutaneous posterolateral lumbar diskectomy and decompression with a 6.9-mm cannula: Analysis of operative failures and complications. *J Bone Joint Surg* 1991;73A:822–831.
144. Seitsalo S, Osterman K, Hyvarinen H, et al. Progression of spondylolisthesis in children and adolescents: A long-term follow-up of 272 patients. *Spine* 1991;16:417–421.
145. Shapiro SA, Scully T. Closed continuous drainage of cerebrospinal fluid via a lumbar subarachnoid catheter for treatment or prevention of cranial/spinal cerebrospinal fluid fistula. *Neurosurgery* 1992;30:241–245.
146. Silcox DH III, Dafarti T, Boden SD, Schimandle JH, Hutton WC, Whitesides TE Jr. The effect of nicotine on spinal fusion. *Spine* 1995; 20:1549–1553.
147. Skargren EI, Oberg BE, Carlsson PG, et al. Cost and effectiveness analysis of chiropractic and physiotherapy treatment for low back and neck pain: Six-month follow-up. *Spine* 1997;22:2167–2177.
148. Smith MD, Emery SE, Dudley A, et al. Vertebral artery injury during anterior decompression of the cervical spine: A retrospective review of ten patients. *J Bone Joint Surg* 1993;75B:410–415.
149. Spivak JM, Vaccaro AR, Cotler JM. Thoracolumbar spine trauma: Principles of management. *J Am Acad Orthop Surg* 1995;3:345–360.
150. Stambough JL, Simeone FA. Vascular complications in spine surgery. In: Garfin SR (ed.), *Complications of Spine Surgery*. Baltimore: Williams & Wilkins, 1989;323–341.
151. Stauffer ES, Wood RW, Kelly EG. Gunshot wounds of the spine: The effects of laminectomy. *J Bone Joint Surg Am* 1979;61:389–392.
152. Sunahara N, Matsunaga S, Mori T. Clinical course of conservatively managed rheumatoid arthritis patients with myelopathy. *Spine* 1997;22:2603–2608.
153. Sutterlin CE III, McAfee PC, Warden KE, et al. A biomechanical evaluation of cervical spinal stabilization methods in a bovine model: Static and cyclical loading. *Spine* 1988;13:795–802.
154. Thomas BE, McCullen GM, Yuan HA. Cervical spine injuries in football players. *J Am Aced Orthop Surg* 1999;7:338–347.
155. Torg JS. Cervical spinal stenosis with cord neuropraxia and transient quadriplegia. *Clin Sports Med* 1990;9:279–296.
156. Torg JS, Naranja RJ, Pavlov H, et al. The relationship of developmental narrowing of the cervical spinal canal to reversible and irreversible injury of the cervical spinal cord in football players. *J Bone Joint Surg* 1996;78A:1308–1314.
157. Ulrich C, Woersdoerfer O, Kalff R, et al. Biomechanics of fixation systems to the cervical spine. *Spine* 1991;16:S4–S9.
158. Vaccaro AR, Rizzolo SJ, Barderston RA, et al. Placement of pedicle screws in the thoracic spine, Part II: An anatomical and radiographic assessment. *J Bone Joint Surg* 1995;77A:1193–1199, 1200–1206.
159. Vollmer DG. Intradural extramedullary spinal tumors. In: Bridwell KH, DeWald RL (eds.), *The Textbook of Spinal Surgery*, 2nd ed. Philadelphia: Lippincott-Raven, 1997;2:2103–2116.
160. Wang JC, Bohlman HH, Riew KD. Dural tears secondary to operations on the lumbar spine. Management and results after a two-year-minimum follow-up of eighty-eight patients. *J Bone Joint Surg Am.* 1998 Dec;80(12):1728–32.
161. Waters RL, Adkins RH. The effects of removal of bullet fragments retained in the spinal canal: A collaborative study by the National Spinal Cord Injury model systems. *Spine* 1991;16:934–939.
162. Watkins RG. Cervical, thoracic, and lumbar complications: Anterior approach. In: Garfin SR (ed.), *Complications of Spine Surgery*. Baltimore: Williams & Wilkins, 1989;211–224.
163. Watkins RG. History, physical examination, and diagnostic tests for lower extremity problems, In: Watkins RG (ed.), *The Spine in Sports*. St. Louis: Mosby, 1996;7.
164. Watkins RG. *Surgical Approaches to the Spine*. New York: Springer-Verlag, 1983.
165. Weber H. Lumbar disk herniation: A controlled, prospective study with ten years of observation. *Spine* 1983;8:131–140.
166. Weinstein SL, Ponseti IV. Curve progression in idiopathic scoliosis. *J Bone Joint Surg* 1983;65A:447–455.
167. Whiffen JR, Neuwirth MG. Spinal stenosis. In: Bridwell KH, DeWald RL (eds.), *The Textbook of Spinal Surgery*, 2nd ed. Philadelphia: Lippincott-Raven, 1997;2:1561–1580.
168. Wiltse LL, Jackson DN. Treatment of spondylolisthesis and spondylolysis in children. *Clin Orthop* 1976;117:92–100.
169. Wiltse LL, Rothman SL. Spondylolisthesis. Classification, diagnosis, and natural history. *Sem Spine Surg* 1993;5:264–280.
170. Wittenberg RH, Shea M, Swartz DE, Lee KS, White AA III, Hayes WC. Importance of bone mineral density in instrumented spine fusions. *Spine* 1991;16:647–652.
171. Woodall B, Hayes GJ. The well-leg raising test of Fajerszajn in the diagnosis of ruptured lumbar intervertebral disk. *J Bone Joint Surg* 1980;32A:786–792.
172. Zeidman SM, Ellenbogen RG, Ducker TB. Intradural tumors. *Semin Spine Surg* 1995;7:323–338.
173. Zindrick MR, Wiltse LL, Widell EH, et al. A biomechanical study of intrapeduncular screw fixation in the lumbosacral spine. *Clin Orthop* 1986;203:99–112.

Key References

Aprill C, Bogduk N. High intensity zone: A diagnostic sign of painful lumbar disk on magnetic resonance imaging. *Br J Radiol* 1992; 65(773):361–369.

This article was the original description of the HIZ on MRI in LBP patients undergoing discography. This study was done without knowledge of how frequently HIZ was found in asymptomatic or minimally symptomatic patients.

Carragee EJ, Paragioudakis SJ, Khurana S, et al. Lumbar high-intensity zone and discography in subjects without low back problems (2000 Volvo Award winner in clinical studies). *Spine* 2000; 25(23):2987–2992.

Twenty-five percent of asymptomatic patients were found to have HIZ lesions. Subjects were closely matched by age and risk of lumbar disk degeneration to patients with chronic LBP. Disks with HIZ were more likely than not to elicit pain on disk injection even in asymptomatic patients.

Fritzell P, Hagg O, Nordwall A. Complications in lumbar fusion surgery for chronic low back pain: Comparison of three surgical techniques used in a prospective randomized study. A report from the Swedish Lumbar Spine Study Group. *Eur Spine J* 2003; 12(2):178–89.

In a previous paper, the Swedish Lumbar Spine Study Group reported on the clinical outcome of lumbar spine fusion for chronic low back pain in a comparably homogeneous patient population. In this report, they compared the complication rates of the surgical procedures used in that study and analyzed the association between complications and baseline variables, and between outcome results and complications. A multicenter randomized study was conducted in which 211 patients aged 25 to 65 were treated with lumbar fusion according to three different surgical techniques: noninstrumented posterolateral fusion (PLF, n = 71), instrumented posterolateral fusion (VSP, n = 68), and interbody fusion with solid autogenous bone grafts ("360", n = 72). Complications were categorized as: early/late, major/minor. The association between complications and sociodemographic characteristics (age, gender, comorbidity, previous surgery, smoking), and technical variables (surgical technique, levels fused, hospital category) was analyzed. The association between outcome variables (patient global assessment, pain, disability, depressive symptoms) and complications was analyzed. A literature review was conducted. There was no mortality. There was no significant difference in clinical outcome between the surgical groups after 2 years, although the power to detect such a difference was low. The total complication rate after 2 years in the PLF group was 12%, compared with 22% in the VSP group, and 40% in the "360" group (P = 0.0003).

Fritzell P, Hagg O, Wessberg P, Nordwall A. 2001 Volvo Award Winner in Clinical Studies: Lumbar fusion versus nonsurgical treatment for chronic low back pain: A multicenter randomized controlled trial from the Swedish Lumbar Spine Study Group. *Spine* 2001; Dec 1;26(23):2521-2532–; discussion 2532-2534.

This is a randomized controlled multicenter study with a 2-year follow-up by an independent observer to compare fusion of the lower lumbar spine with nonsurgical treatment in patients with severe chronic low back pain (CLBP). A total of 294 patients were randomized blindly into 4 treatment groups. Patients aged 25 to 65 years with CLBP for at least 2 years and with radiologic evidence of disk degeneration at L4-L5, L5-S1, or both were eligible to participate in the study. The surgical group (n = 222) included 3 different fusion techniques. Patients in the nonsurgical group (n = 72) were treated with different kinds of physical therapy. The Visual Analogue Scale (VAS) was used to measure pain. The Oswestry Low Back Pain Questionnaire, the Million Score, and the General Function Score (GFS) were used to measure disability. The Zung Depression Scale was used to measure depressive symptoms. At the 2-year follow-up, 289 of 294 (98%) patients, including 25 who had changed groups, were examined. The study concluded that lumbar fusion in a well-informed and selected group of patients with severe CLBP can diminish pain and decrease disability more efficiently than commonly used nonsurgical treatment.

Carette S, Leclaire R, Marcoux S, et al. Epidural corticosteroid injections for sciatica due to herniated nucleus pulposus. *N Eng J Med* 1997;336:1634–1640.

This is a randomized, double-blind trial assessing 3 non-fluoroscopically guided interlaminar epidural injections of methylprednisolone acetate to patients with sciatica due to a herniated nucleus pulposus. Injections only had significant benefits in the first 6 weeks. After 3 months, the groups had no significant differences. At 12 months, there was a cumulative probability of back surgery in the placebo group of 25.8%.

Riew KD, Yin Y, Gilula L, et al. The effect of nerve-root injections on the need for operative treatment of lumbar radicular pan: A prospective, randomized, controlled, double-blind study. *J Bone Joint Surg Am* 2000;82:1589–1593.

This is the only well-designed study of fluoroscopically guided transforaminal ESI. Fifty-five patients with nerve root compression confirmed radiographically who requested surgery were randomized to receive selective root injection with bupivicaine or bupivicaine with betamethasone. Patients were given 3 injections each. Thirty-three point three percent of the control group versus 75% of the group receiving corticosteroids elected not to undergo surgery due to improved pain at follow-ups between 13 to 26 months.

Ahn UM, Ahn NU, Buchowski JM, et al. Cauda equina syndrome secondary to lumbar disk herniation: A metaanalysis of surgical outcomes. *Spine* 25:1515–1522.

The authors performed a metaanalysis of studies covering a total of 322 patients and found significant advantage to treating patients with cauda equine syndrome within 48 hours versus more than 48 hours after onset. Older age and preexisting bowel or bladder dysfunction were associated with worse outcomes.

Refresher Questions

1. The most common cervical spine abnormality in patients with Down syndrome (trisomy 21) and rheumatoid arthritis is:
   a) subaxial instability
   b) os odontoideum

c) cranial settling (superior migration of the odontoid)
d) atlantoaxial subluxation
e) congenital fusion

2. During posterior C1 lateral mass fixation, bicortical screws risk injury to:
a) vertebral artery
b) greater occipital nerve
c) spinal accessory nerve
d) hypoglossal nerve and internal carotid artery
e) common carotid artery

3. Physical examination of a patient with spinal cord injury revealed deltoid 5/5, biceps 5/5, wrist extension 4/5 bilaterally, finger extension 3/5 bilaterally, triceps 3/5 bilaterally, and finger flexion 2/5 bilaterally. Pinprick sensation is intact in the C6 distribution bilaterally. According to the ASIA standards, the patient's functional spinal cord level is:
a) C4
b) C5
c) C6
d) C7
e) C8

4. A 30-year-old male sustained a gunshot to the thorax and complained of ipsilateral loss of motor (UMN signs), ipsilateral loss of proprioception and vibration, and contralateral loss of pain and temperature. He most likely has:
a) posterior cord syndrome
b) anterior cord syndrome
c) Brown-Séquard syndrome
d) central cord syndrome
e) cauda equina

5. A 60-year-old Japanese female complains of insidious onset of gait imbalance, clumsiness of the hands, and urinary incontinence. Radiographs show 4 levels of ossification of the posterior longitudinal ligament and cervical lordosis. The best treatment should be:
a) epidural steroids
b) multilevel discectomies and fusion
c) multilevel corpectomies and fusion
d) multilevel laminoplasty
e) multilevel laminectomy

6. Which of the following is not a major risk factor for nonunion of a type II odontoid fracture?
a) posterior displacement more than 5 mm
b) anterior displacement more than 5 mm
c) angulation more than 10 degrees
d) age over 40 years
e) smoking

7. A type II Anderson and Montesano fracture of the occipitocondyle is best described as:
a) an occipital condyle avulsion fracture from the alar ligament
b) an impacted comminuted fracture of the occipital condyle
c) an occipital condyle fracture associated with a basilar skull fracture
d) an occipital condyle-C1 dislocation
e) an occipital condyle fracture and odontoid fracture

8. The major predictor of outcome in patients with rheumatoid arthritis is
a) AADI more than 3.5 mm
b) PADI less than 14 mm
c) cervicomedullary angle greater than 135 degrees
d) basilar invagination
e) retroodontoid pannus

9. A patient with a right positive femoral stretch test and anterior thigh pain will most likely have a herniated disk located:
a) right paracentral at L3-4
b) right paracentral at L4-5
c) right far lateral at L3-4
d) right far lateral at L4-5
e) central at L4-5

10. A patient with a right paracentral herniated disk causing foraminal stenosis at C6-7 will most likely have:
a) numbness and weakness over the deltoid
b) numbness around the thumb and weakness of the biceps and wrist extensor
c) numbness and weakness of the thumb, index, and middle finger
d) numbness over the volar tip of the middle finger and triceps and pronator weakness
e) numbness of the small finger and medial forearm and intrinsic weakness

Chapter 8

Musculoskeletal Tumors

HARISH S. HOSALKAR, JESSE T. TORBERT, GREGORY CAROLAN, and RICHARD D. LACKMAN

I. DIFFERENTIAL DIAGNOSIS

History and Examination. History, physical examination, and imaging can all impact the differential diagnosis in cases of bone tumors. Biopsy is usually the gold standard for diagnosis. The history mainly defines the clinical context of the lesion. Age, sex, duration of symptoms, presence and quality of pain, history of trauma, weight loss, smoking history, and history of prior malignancy are all-important historical factors. Early symptoms associated with skeletal neoplasms mimic all types of ordinary musculoskeletal disorders. Any pain that extends beyond the expected duration associated with a tentative diagnosis should raise the suspicion of an underlying tumor. Night pain is another red flag, again suspicious for an occult lesion, although many nonneoplastic conditions may also cause pain at night.

The 3 Lists for Common Tumor Differentials. A simple way to assemble a comprehensive differential diagnosis is to have a reasonable list of common lesions to review while approaching the tumor (Table 8.1). These 3 lists can be separated into bone-forming, cartilage-forming, and additional lesions. By going through the mental checklist of these differentials, one can systematically approach a tumor case and review the radiographs to arrive at a diagnosis.

Relevance of Age. The age of the patient is an important factor in establishing a differential diagnosis, because

TABLE 8.1 Lists for radiographic differential diagnosis

Radiographic Differential Diagnosis		
Bone-Forming Tumors	**Cartilage-Forming Tumors**	**Third List**
• Osteoid osteoma • Osteoblastoma • Osteochondroma • Osteosarcoma • Blastic metastases • Paget disease	• Osteochondroma • Chondromyxoid fibroma • Chondroblastoma • Enchondroma • Chondrosarcoma	• Infection • Metastasis • Round cell tumors • Ewing • Lymphoma • Myeloma • Neuroblastoma • Fibrous dysplasia • Nonossifying fibroma • Simple bone cyst • Aneurysmal bone cyst • Eosinophilic granuloma (histiocytosis) • Giant cell tumor • Stress fracture • Metabolic condition • Hemangioma

Lackman RD. Orthopaedic tumors. In: Vaccaro AR (ed.), *Orthopaedic Knowledge Update 8*. Rosemont, IL: American Academy of Orthopaedic Surgeons, 2005.

certain tumors tend to occur in certain age groups (Fig. 8.1).

Tissue of Origin. Primary bone and soft tissue tumors can be classified on the basis of their origin (Table 8.2).

Sex Predilection. Most musculoskeletal tumors tend to occur more commonly in males than females. Demographic features of osteosarcoma, Ewing sarcoma, and rhabdomyosarcoma are presented in Table 8.3.

Anatomic Location. The anatomic location of the tumor may be epiphyseal, metaphyseal, or diaphyseal, and central or eccentric (Table 8.4; Figs. 8.2, 8.3, and 8.4).

Etiology and Molecular Genetics. Cancer is now recognized as a genetic disease. Specific genetic tools, including molecular biology and cytogenetics, may help characterize malignancies and prognosis. The biology of sarcomas is being better understood and will undoubtedly change the evaluation, treatment, and outcome of patients with musculoskeletal cancer. Somatic cell mutations can activate an oncogene or inactivate a tumor suppressor gene, thus inducing neoplasia. A germline mutation can also occur, creating a heritable susceptibility to cancer (Table 8.5). Some common cytogenetic associations of musculoskeletal tumors are outlined in Table 8.6.

Staging. Staging of a patient with a suspected malignant tumor is mandatory prior to any biopsy. It is important to learn as much about a lesion and its differential diagnosis before the biopsy so as to avoid wrong decisions that may alter the eventual outcome of management. Staging includes a total body scan, a CT scan of the chest, and an MRI of the primary lesion. MRI should include the involved portion of the extremity, including the joint above and below. The Musculoskeletal Tumor Society (MSTS) adopted the Enneking surgical staging system for bone sarcomas. The Enneking staging system is based on the GTM classification: grade (G), tumor site (T), and metastases (M) (Table 8.7). In addition to the Enneking staging, various other staging systems also exist for staging the soft tissue sarcomas including the AJCC (American Joint Committee on Cancer) system staging, the Hajdu system and the Intergroup rhabdomyosarcoma study system. Each of these systems for soft tissue sarcomas directly or indirectly incorporates the important prognostic variables of grade, location, size, depth, and lymph node or distant metastasis. Enneking also proposed a classification system for benign tumors:

- *Stage 1*: Inactive lesions, asymptomatic with little or no growth
- *Stage 2*: Active lesions that are growing and symptomatic

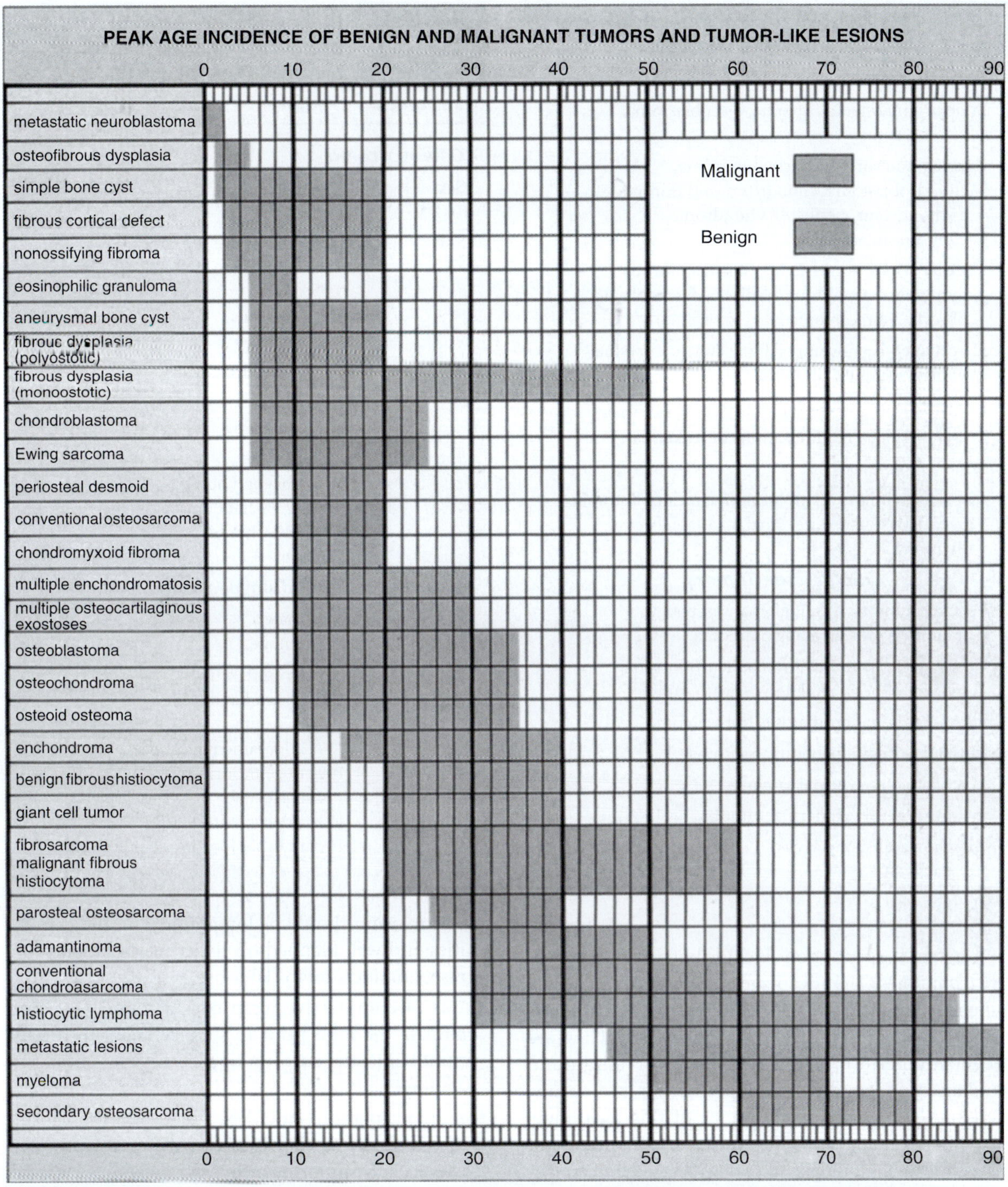

FIGURE 8.1 **Peak age incidence of benign and malignant tumors and malignantlike conditions. (*Source:* Greenspan A, Remagen W. *Differential Diagnosis of Tumors and Tumor-like Lesions of Bones and Joints*. Philadelphia: Lippincott-Raven, 1998;5.)**

- *Stage 3*: Lesions are aggressive, growing rapidly, and invading adjacent tissues

Biopsy. Not all lesions require a biopsy because many benign and inactive lesions may be diagnosed via imaging studies alone. The ideal biopsy is one that provides all tissue needed to establish a histologic diagnosis without affecting subsequent treatment options. Intrinsic in this decision to biopsy a particular lesion is the idea that the treating surgeon should be very familiar with the guidelines concerning type of biopsy performed and biopsy techniques.

TABLE 8.2 Classification of musculoskeletal tumors based on origin

Bone Tumors
Bone origin: osteoid osteoma, osteoblastoma, osteosarcoma
Cartilaginous origin: osteochondroma, chondroblastoma, chondromyxoid fibroma, enchondroma, periosteal chondroma, chondrosarcoma
Fibrous origin: nonossifying fibroma, fibrous dysplasia, osteofibrous dysplasia, desmoplastic fibroma, fibrosarcoma.
Miscellaneous: unicameral bone cyst, aneurysmal bone cyst, giant cell tumor
Langerhans cell histiocytosis, Ewing sarcoma
Musculoskeletal manifestations of leukemia
Bone lymphomas
Metastatic tumors: neuroblastoma, retinoblastoma, hepatoblastoma, lung, renal, prostate, breast, thyroid
Soft Tissue Tumors
Vascular tumors: hemangioma, vascular malformations, hemangiosarcoma
Nerve origin: neurolemmoma, neurofibroma, malignant peripheral nerve sheath tumor
Fibrous origin: fibromatosis, fibrosarcoma
Muscular origin: rhabdomyosarcoma
Miscellaneous: synovial sarcoma
Primitive neuroectodermal tumors
Ganglion and synovial cyst

TABLE 8.3 Demographic features of osteosarcoma, Ewing sarcoma, and rhabdomyosarcoma

Variables	*Features*
Osteosarcoma	
Sex	60% male 40% female
Site	50% arise above the knee 42% femur 18% tibia 10% humerus 8% pelvis
Ewing Sarcoma	
Sex	62% male 38% female
Site	25% femur 15% tibia and fibula 20%–25% flat bones of the pelvic girdle 5%–10% shoulder girdle 10% ribs
Rhabdomyosarcoma	
Sex	60% male 40% female
Site	20% in extremities 10% in head and neck 10% in orbit 15% at parameningeal sites 10% in genitourinary tract, bladder, and prostate 15% in pelvic sites 20% in other locations

Current biopsy options include both open and needle techniques. The advantage of percutaneous needle biopsies is that they cause little soft tissue contamination and require little or no anesthesia. They are frequently performed under CT scan or ultrasound guidance and can direct a biopsy needle into an underlying lesion. The disadvantage of this technique, however, is that it provides only a small amount of tissue for the pathologist to review. As such, it can frequently be nondiagnostic. More importantly, it must be remembered that primary bone tumors are notoriously heterogeneous, thereby creating a great potential for sampling error with closed techniques. Needle biopsies are optimal for initial sampling of lesions in anatomically inaccessible areas such as the spine or pelvis. In most locations, however, the carefully performed open biopsy is still the gold standard. The following principles for open biopsy are as follows:

- As small an incision as possible should be placed over the lesion
- The incision should be longitudinal on the extremities and well planned on the trunk to be part of a resection incision for later use.
- Use of compressive wrap over a tumor to exsanguinate the limb prior to surgery may rupture the tumor into the surrounding tissues and should be avoided.
- A small incision should be made into the capsule of the tumor so that it can be closed readily. This is especially important when no tourniquet is used, because bleeding may be appreciable and difficult to control with a large incision.
- The neurovascular bundle should be avoided to prevent contamination and dissemination.
- Major flap structures (e.g., gluteus maximus) or functionally important structures (e.g., rectus femoris) should be avoided.
- Minimal retraction should be utilized to limit soft tissue contamination.
- When approaching a tumor, a single large muscle belly can be violated as opposed to developing a plane

TABLE 8.4 Common locations of bone tumors

Epiphysis

Chondroblastoma
Brodie abscess of the epiphyses
Giant cell tumor
Fibrous dysplasia

Metaphysis

Any tumor

Diaphysis

Fibrous dysplasia
Osteofibrous dysplasia, adamantinoma
Langerhans cell histiocytosis
Ewing sarcoma
Leukemia, lymphoma
Occasional diaphyseal
  Osteoid osteoma
  Unicameral bone cyst

Multiple

Leukemia (metastasis)
Multiple hereditary exostoses
Langerhans cell histiocytosis
Polyostotic fibrous dysplasia
Enchondromatosis

Pelvis

Ewing sarcoma
Osteosarcoma
Osteochondroma
Metastasis
Fibrous dysplasia

Anterior Elements of Spine

Langerhans cell histiocytosis
Leukemia
Metastasis
Giant cell tumor

Posterior Elements of Spine

Aneurysmal bone cyst
Osteoblastoma
Osteoid osteoma

Rib

Fibrous dysplasia
Langerhans cell histiocytosis
Ewing sarcoma
Metastasis

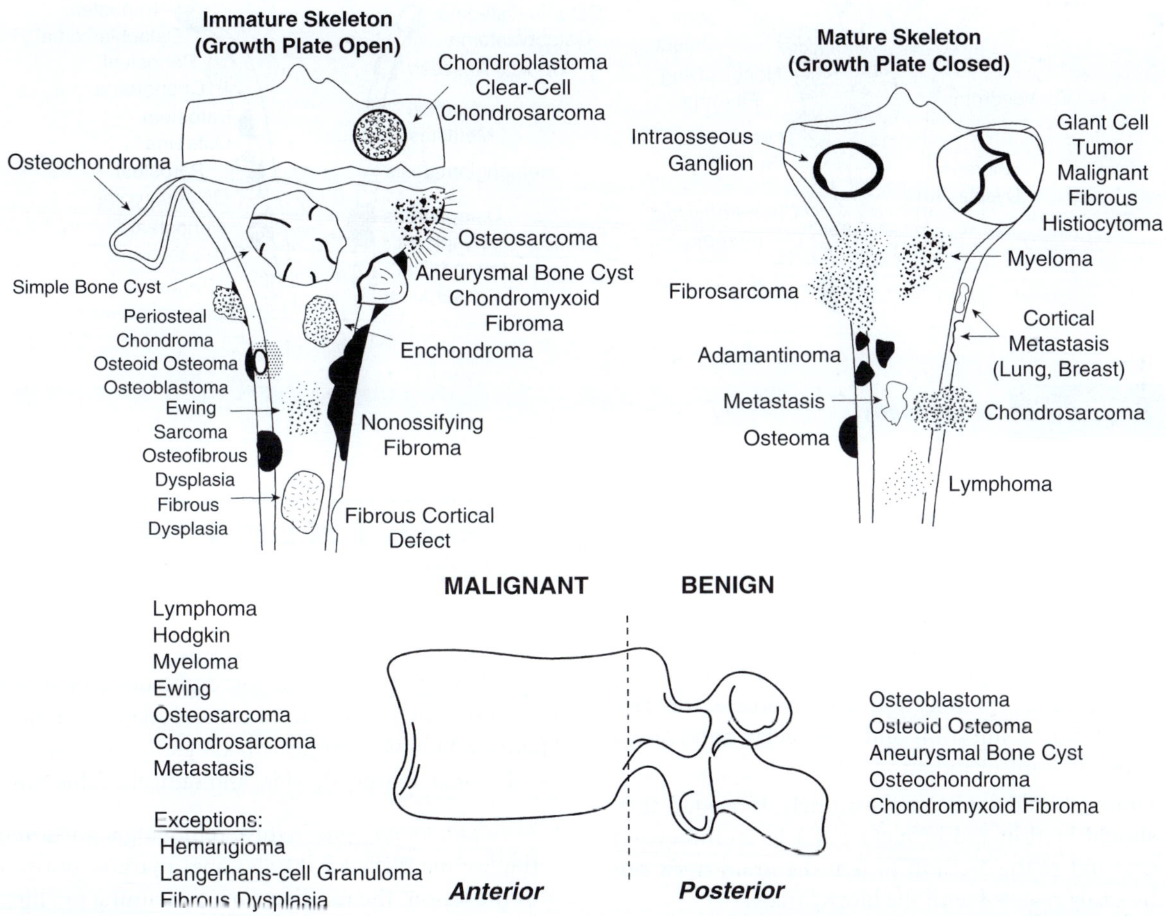

FIGURE 8.2 **(A, B) Distribution of various tumors. (*Source:* Greenspan A, Remagen W. *Differential Diagnosis of Tumors and Tumor-like Lesions of Bones and Joints*. Philadelphia: Lippincott-Raven, 1998;7,9.)**

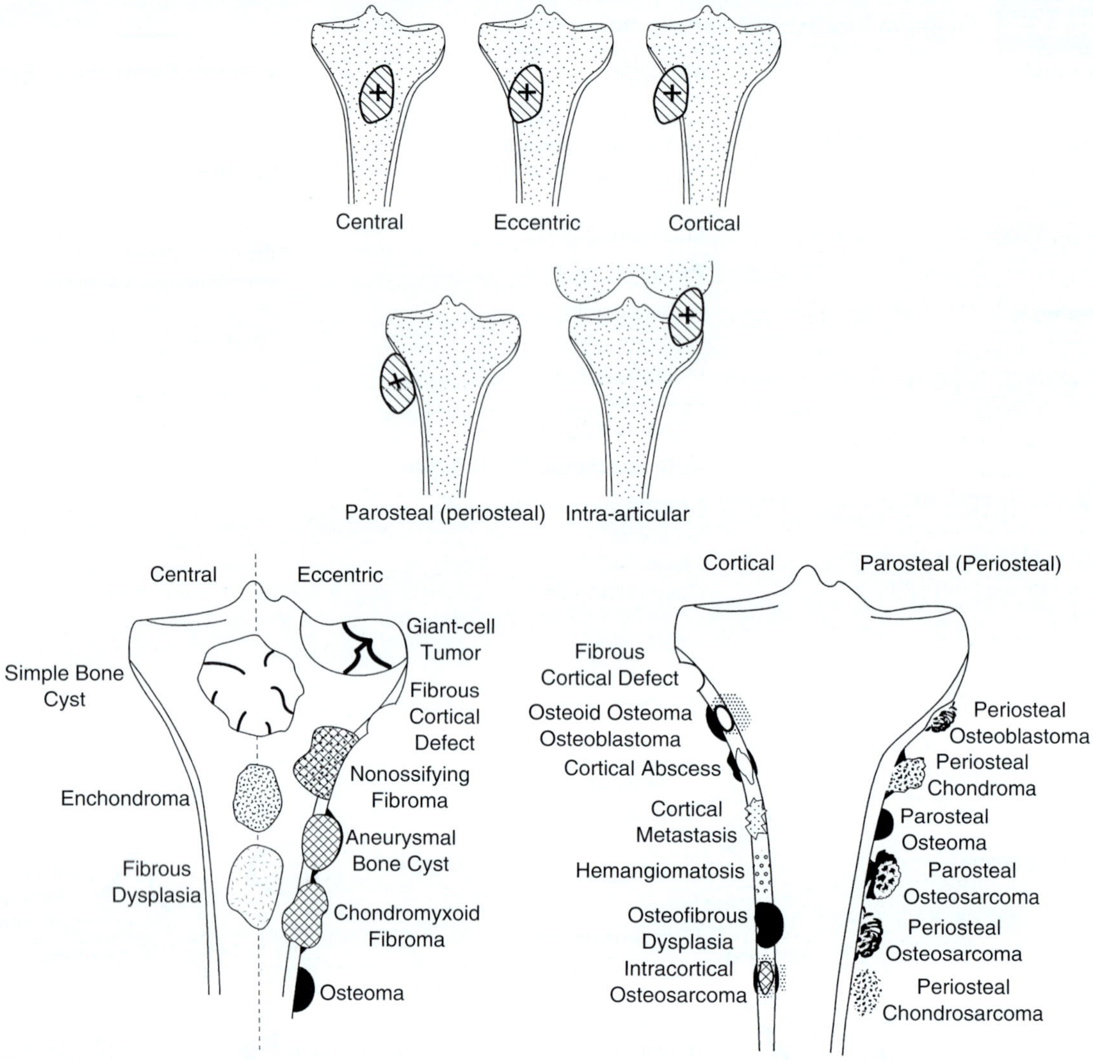

FIGURE 8.2 *(continued).*

between two muscle groups and contaminating both compartments.

- Hemostasis through a meticulous, multilayered, water-tight closure is essential. Many large tumors put the closure under pressure, and the vascularity commonly seen predisposes to subsequent drainage. Any wound complication will increase the risk of secondary infection and may delay subsequent chemotherapy or radiation.
- Drains should not be used routinely. If needed, they should be thin and brought out 1 to 2 cm beyond one end of the incision so that the drain track can be easily resected with the biopsy track.
- A frozen section should be obtained, when feasible, to insure that diagnostic material has been obtained. Tumors can often be very necrotic, and it may take a large volume of tissue before diagnostic material is encountered.

II. SURGERY FOR LOCAL TUMOR CONTROL

Margins. A precise definition and classification of surgical margins is useful for evaluation, planning, and treatment in the care of musculoskeletal tumors. There are 4 kinds of surgical oncologic wound margins: intralesional, marginal, wide, and radical (Table 8.8).

- *Intralesional margins* involve removing a portion of the lesion. With an intralesional margin, portions of the lesion, the reactive zone containing satellites, and skip lesions in the surrounding normal tissues are all left behind.
- *Marginal margins* involve removing the lesion en bloc with an extracapsular plane of dissection through the reactive zone of inflammation. Satellite

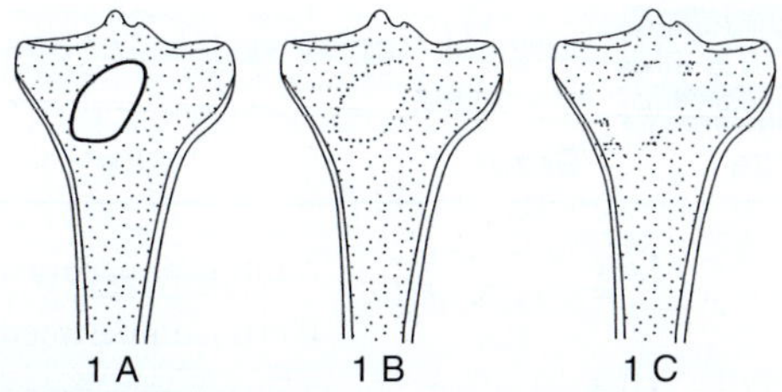

FIGURE 8.3 **Various border types of tumors. (*Source:* Greenspan A, Remagen W. *Differential Diagnosis of Tumors and Tumor-like Lesions of Bones and Joints*. Philadelphia: Lippincott-Raven, 1998;10; *modified from* Madewell JE, Ragsdale BD, Sweet DE. Radiologic and pathologic analysis of solitary bone lesions. Part I. Internal margins. *Radiol Clin North Am* 1981;19:715–748.)**

and skip lesions are left behind in the normal surrounding tissue.

- *Wide margins* require en block excision of the lesion in a plane of dissection that is peripheral to the reactive zone through normal tissue. The distance away from the tumor required to achieve this margin has not been strictly established and depends on factors such as tissue involved, type of tumor, and response to chemotherapy. With better imaging and the development and progress of limb salvage surgery, decreasing distances from the tumor while still maintaining a cuff of normal tissue around the tumor are being accepted.
- *Radical margins* involve removing the entire compartment(s) in which the tumor has extended.

An important principle in musculoskeletal tumor surgery is that the tumor itself should not be visualized or encountered at the time of surgery. If the surgeon does visualize or enter the substance of the tumor, he or she will no longer have a wide margin, and contamination of the tumor bed occurs; microscopic or gross residual tumor is left behind; and the likelihood of local recurrence increases.

Surgical Procedures. The margin of the wound is the criteria by which the procedures are defined. Margin may be obtained by either a local or an ablative procedure. Since there are 4 possible margins, there are 8 distinct oncologic surgical procedures possible (see Table 8.8).

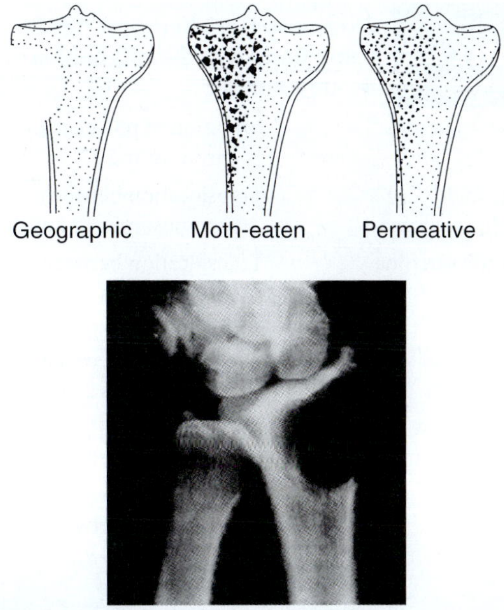

FIGURE 8.4 **Patterns of bone destruction. (*Source:* Greenspan A, Remagen W. *Differential Diagnosis of Tumors and Tumor-like Lesions of Bones and Joints*. Philadelphia: Lippincott-Raven, 1998;10; *modified from* Madewell JE, Ragsdale BD, Sweet DE. Radiologic and pathologic analysis of solitary bone lesions. Part I. Internal margins. *Radiol Clin North Am* 1981;19: 715–748.)**

Surgical Intentions. There are 4 different reasons for doing oncosurgical procedures: diagnostic, palliative, adjunctive, and definitive.

- *Diagnostic procedure*—May be performed open or closed by incision or needle. It could also be accomplished by marginal excision.
- *Palliative procedure*—Undertaken to relieve pain or to improve function temporarily. There is no intent to cure, and recurrence is accepted as inevitable. The benefits of a palliative procedure are accepted as temporary and are generally performed when no alternative surgical methods are desirable.
- *Adjunctive procedure*—Done with the intent of local control and usually followed by a definitive modality of treatment.
- *Definitive procedure*—Done with the intent of local control by the procedure itself. Nonsurgical modalities may be used as adjuncts in these cases.

TABLE 8.5 Chromosomal abnormalities in some benign and malignant soft tissue tumors

Osteosarcoma	Mutation of p53 gene on chromosome 17
Myxoid liposarcoma	Translocation between chromosomes 12 and 16
Ewing sarcoma	Translocation between chromosomes 11 and 22 in 90%–95%.
	Translocation between chromosomes 21 and 22 in 5%–10%.
Synovial sarcoma	Translocation between chromosomes X and 18
Myxoid chondrosarcoma	Translocation between chromosomes 9 and 22

TABLE 8.7 Surgical staging system for bone sarcomas

Stage	*Grade*	*Site**
I	Low	A intracompartmental
		B extracompartmental
II	High	A intracompartmental
		B extracompartmental
III	Any grade with regional or distant metastasis	Any

*A compartment is an anatomic structure or space bounded by natural barriers to tumor extension. A whole bone, a joint, or a functional muscle group are each considered compartments in this staging system.

Source: Enneking WF. A system of staging musculoskeletal neoplasms. *Clin Orthop Relat Res* 1986 Mar;(204):9–24.

TABLE 8.6 Common cytogenetic associations of sarcomas

Musculoskeletal Tumor	*Associations*
Osteosarcoma	RB gene locus on chromosome 13q (60%–75%) Mutation of p53 gene on chromosome 17 (30%–50%) Increased risk in individuals with inherited abnormality of p53 (Li-Fraumeni familial cancer syndrome) Increased risk in individuals with inherited abnormality of RB (heritable RB)
Ewing sarcoma	Reciprocal t(11;22) translocation (90%–95%) Reciprocal t(21;22) translocation (5%–10%) Poor prognosis associated with ○ p53 alterations ○ Deletions of INK4A (cell cycle regulator gene) ○ Gain of 1q chromosomal aberration is associated with adverse outcome, and loss of 16q is associated with disseminated disease at diagnosis
Rhabdomyosarcoma	Diagnostic markers ○ Myogenin mRNA ○ MyoD1 ○ Gamma subunit of fetal type acetylcholine receptor (AChR) Autosomal dominant NF1 have increased incidence of rhabdomyosarcoma Rhabdomyosarcoma is the most frequently diagnosed soft tissue sarcoma in the Li-Fraumeni cancer syndrome Alveolar rhabdomyosarcoma: t(2;13); t(1;13)
Other soft tissue sarcomas	Familial syndromes with increased risk: ○ Neurofibromatosis 1 ○ Li-Fraumeni cancer syndrome ○ Familial pleuropulmonary blastomas Synovial sarcoma: t(X;18) Myxoid liposarcoma: t(12;16)

TABLE 8.8 Surgical margins

Surgical Margins	*Limb Salvage*	*Amputation*	*Histology*
Intralesional	Curettage, piecemeal resection within lesion	Through tumor	Tumor at margin
Marginal	Marginal excision through reactive tissue	Along reactive tissue	Reactive tissue with or without satellites
Wide	Wide excision through normal surrounding tissue	Through normal tissue in compartment	Normal tissue with or without skip lesions
Radical	Radical resection with entire compartment	Extracompartmental amputation or disarticulation	Normal tissue

Source: Enneking WF, Spanier SS, Goodman MA. A system for the surgical staging of musculoskeletal sarcoma. *Clin Orthop Relat Res* 1980 Nov-Dec;(153):106–120.

III. CLASSIFICATION OF BONE AND SOFT TISSUE TUMORS

The following is a summary of the radiographic and clinical features associated with each of the common lesions and imaging studies showing a prototype or typical lesion. WHO classification of bone and soft tissue tumors is presented in Tables 8.9 and 8.10.

Primary Benign Lesion

Bone Forming

Osteoid Osteoma. A common benign bone tumor that affects mostly children and young adults, osteoid osteomas are associated with a classic pattern of constant pain that is relieved well for short periods with prostaglandin-inhibiting drugs such as NSAIDs. Night pain is common. Femur, tibia, and posterior spine are the most common sites. In the spine, these lesions may result in a secondary scoliosis due to pain. The nidus may be small and difficult to find on x-ray. MRI scans will show extensive edema, which may be confused with a marrow-replacing neoplasm and is therefore not recommended if osteoid osteoma is the suspected lesion. CT scans with fine cuts (i.e., 1 mm) are the study of choice for finding the lesion. The nidus and its sclerotic rim are best identified with CT imaging. Bone scintigraphy shows focal intense uptake. It appears as a small lytic nidus (less than 2 cm in diameter) surrounded by significant sclerosis. Histogram is shown in Figure 8.5.

Treatment of these lesions is based on symptoms, because they eventually become asymptomatic. If NSAID use is not tolerated or significant pain persists, surgical treatment may be considered. Procedures include mechanical evacuation via curettage and burring. Radiofrequency ablation has also been used with promising results (symptomatic improvement, rapid recovery, rare recurrence).

Osteoblastoma. Osteoblastoma is a rare neoplasm most often seen in the posterior elements of the spine or in the metadiaphyseal region of long bones. It has a very variable appearance and may be blastic or lytic. The classic appearance is that of a calcified lesion in the posterior elements of the spine (Fig. 8.6). Radiographically, osteoblastoma appears more lytic and destructive than osteoid osteoma. The nidus, greater than 1 to 2 cm, has less sclerotic surrounding bone and may take on the appearance of an aneurysmal bone cyst. Histologically, the nidus of osteoblastoma is nearly identical to that of osteoid osteoma, showing excessive osteoblastic activity and osteoid formation with numerous giant cells in a vascular fibrous stroma (Fig. 8.7). Marginal resection is usually the best surgical option. When complete excision of the osteoblastoma is not feasible, curettage and bone grafting may provide an acceptable long-term result. Aggressive osteoblastomas can recur at a rate of 50% if positive margins are obtained.

Osteochondroma (Exostosis). This tumor occurs on the outer edge of the growth plate causing radial growth of bone during childhood. The lesion grows out away from the bone at an angle from the adjacent growth plate (Figs. 8.8 and 8.9). The cortex of the bone is continuous with the cortex of the lesion, and the medullary canal is also continuous. A tumor that is sitting on an intact cortex is never an osteochondroma. Osteochondroma presents most commonly in the second decade, and the most common locations are the femur, humerus, and tibia. The most common symptom is a mass, with or without pain. Osteochondromas can be sessile (broad base) or pedunculated (narrow base). Many that grow out of the flat bones or the proximal femur can be very large and take on a "cauliflower" appearance. Secondary chondrosarcomatous degeneration (Fig. 8.10) should be suspected in any osteochondroma in an adult, which grows, causes pain, or has a cartilage cap of greater than 2 cm. Multiple hereditary exostoses (MHE) is an autosomal dominant disorder that is rare. Malignant degeneration is more common in MHE (due to a mutation in EXT1 and EXT2); there is a 2.8% rate of conversion, more often in the larger, more proximal lesions. Patients with MHE often have angular deformities with bone shortening. Treatment in most cases of osteochondroma is observation. Surgery may be indicated for pain, deformity, or malignant degeneration.

Chondroid Forming

Osteochondroma. Osteochondromas and enchondromas are the most common benign tumors of the

TABLE 8.9 The world health organization classification of primary bone tumors and tumorlike conditions

I. Bone-forming tumors
  A. Benign
    1. Osteoma
    2. Osteoid osteoma and osteoblastoma (i.e., benign osteoblastoma)
  B. Malignant
    1. Osteosarcoma (i.e., osteogenic sarcoma)
    2. Juxtacortical osteosarcoma (i.e., parosteal osteosarcoma)

II. Cartilage-forming tumors
  A. Benign
    1. Chondroma
    2. Osteochondroma (i.e., osteocartilaginous exostosis)
    3. Chondroblastoma (i.e., benign chondroblastoma, epiphyseal chondroblastoma)
    4. Chondromyxoid fibroma
  B. Malignant
    1. Chondrosarcoma
    2. Juxtacortical chondrosarcoma
    3. Mesenchymal chondrosarcoma

III. Giant cell tumors (i.e., osteoclastoma)

IV. Marrow tumors
  A. Ewing sarcoma
  B. Reticulosarcoma of bone
  C. Lymphosarcoma of bone
  D. Myeloma

V. Vascular tumors
  A. Benign
    1. Hemangioma
    2. Lymphangioma
    3. Glomus tumor (i.e., glomangioma)
  B. Intermediate or indeterminate
    1. Hemangioendothelioma
    2. Hemangiopericytoma
  C. Malignant
    1. Angiosarcoma

VI. Other connective tissue tumors
  A. Benign
    1. Desmoplastic fibroma
    2. Lipoma
  B. Malignant
    1. Fibrosarcoma
    2. Liposarcoma
    3. Malignant mesenchymoma
    4. Undifferentiated sarcoma

VII. Other tumors
  A. Chordoma
  B. Adamantinoma of long bones
  C. Neurilemoma (i.e., schwannoma, neurinoma)
  D. Neurofibroma

VIII. Unclassified tumors

IX. Tumor-like lesions
  A. Solitary bone cyst (i.e., simple or unicameral bone cyst)
  B. Aneurysmal bone cyst
  C. Juxtaarticular bone cyst (i.e., intraosseous ganglion)
  D. Metaphyseal fibrous defect (i.e., nonossifying fibroma)
  E. Eosinophilic granuloma
  F. Fibrous dysplasia
  G. Myositis ossificans
  H. Brown tumor of hyperparathyroidism

Osteoid osteoma: 2, 3
Unicameral bone cyst: 1, 2
Aneurysmal bone cyst: 2, 3
Source: Greenfield GB, Arrington JA. *Imaging of Bone Tumors: A Multimodality Approach.* Philadelphia. Lippincott, 1995;47.

TABLE 8.10 Classification of soft-tissue tumors

I. Tumors and tumor-like lesions of fibrous tissue
   A. Benign
      1. Fibroma
      2. Nodular fasciitis, including intravascular and cranial types
      3. Proliferative fasciitis
      4. Proliferative myositis
      5. Fibroma of tendon sheath
      6. Elastofibroma
      7. Nuchal fibroma
      8. Nasopharyngeal fibroma
      9. Keloid
   B. Fibrous tumors of infancy and childhood
      1. Fibrous hamartoma of infancy
      2. Myofibromatosis (solitary, multicentric)
      3. Fibromatosis colli
      4. Infantile digital fibromatosis
      5. Infantile fibromatosis, desmoid type
      6. Giant cell fibroblastoma
      7. Gingival fibromatosis
      8. Calcifying aponeurotic fibroma
      9. Hyalin fibromatosis
   C. Fibromatoses
      1. Superficial fibromatoses
         a. Palmar and plantar fibromatosis
         b. Penile (i.e., Peyronie) fibromatosis
         c. Knuckle pads
      2. Deep fibromatoses
         a. Abdominal fibromatosis
         b. Extraabdominal fibromatosis
         c. Intraabdominal fibromatosis
         d. Mesenteric fibromatosis (i.e., Gardner syndrome)
         e. Postradiation fibromatosis
         f. Cicatricial fibromatosis
   D. Malignant
      1. Adult fibrosarcoma
      2. Congenital and infantile fibrosarcoma
      3. Inflammatory fibrosarcoma
      4. Postradiation fibrosarcoma
      5. Cicatricial fibrosarcoma

II. Fibrohistiocytic tumors
   A. Benign
      1. Fibrous histiocytoma
         a. Cutaneous (i.e., dermatofibroma)
         b. Deep
      2. Atypical fibroxanthoma
      3. Juvenile xanthogranuloma
      4. Reticulohistiocytoma
      5. Xanthoma
   B. Intermediate
      1. Dermatofibrosarcoma protuberans
      2. Bednar tumor
   C. Malignant
      1. Malignant fibrous histiocytoma
         a. Storiform-pleomorphic
         b. Myxoid (i.e., myxofibrosarcoma)
         c. Giant cell (i.e., malignant giant cell tumor of soft parts)
         d. Inflammatory (i.e., malignant xanthogranuloma, xanthosarcoma)
         e. Angiomatoid

III. Tumors and tumor-like lesions of adipose tissue
   A. Benign
      1. Lipoma (cutaneous, deep, and multiple)
      2. Angiolipoma
      3. Spindle cell and pleomorphic lipoma
      4. Lipoblastoma and lipoblastomatosis
      5. Angiomyolipoma
      6. Myelolipoma
      7. Intramuscular and intermuscular lipoma
      8. Lipoma of tendon sheath
      9. Lumbosacral lipoma
      10. Interneural and perineural fibrolipoma
      11. Diffuse lipomatosis
      12. Cervical symmetrical lipomatosis (i.e., Madelung disease)
      13. Pelvic lipomatosis
      14. Hibernoma
   B. Malignant
      1. Liposarcoma, predominantly
         a. Well-differentiated
            (1) Lipoma-like
            (2) Sclerosing
            (3) Inflammatory
         b. Myxoid
         c. Round cell (i.e., poorly differentiated myxoid)
         d. Pleomorphic
         e. Dedifferentiated

(*continued*)

TABLE 8.10 *(continued)*

IV. Tumors of muscle tissue
- A. Smooth muscle
  - 1. Benign
    - a. Leiomyoma (cutaneous and deep)
    - b. Angiomyoma (i.e., vascular leiomyoma)
    - c. Epitheliod leiomyoma (i.e., benign leiomyoblastoma)
    - d. Intravenous leiomyomatosis
    - e. Leiomyomatosis peritonealis disseminata
  - 2. Malignant
    - a. Leiomyosarcoma
    - b. Epitheliod leiomyosarcoma (i.e., malignant leiomyoblastoma)
- B. Striated muscle
  - 1. Benign
    - a. Adult rhabdomyoma
    - b. Genital rhabdomyoma
    - c. Fetal rhabdomyoma
  - 2. Malignant
    - a. Rhabdomyosarcoma, predominantly
      - (1) Embryonal, including botryoid
      - (2) Alveolar
      - (3) Pleomorphic
      - (4) Mixed
    - b. Ectomesenchymoma (i.e., rhabdomyosarcoma with ganglion cell differentiation)

V. Tumors and tumor-like lesions of blood vessels
- A. Benign
  - 1. Hemangioma
    - a. Capillary, including juvenile
    - b. Cavernous
    - c. Arteriovenous
    - d. Venous
    - e. Epitheliod (i.e., angiolymphoid hyperplasia, Kimura disease)
    - f. Granulation tissue type (i.e., pyogenic, granuloma)
  - 2. Deep hemangioma (intramuscular, synovial, perineural)
  - 3. Hemangiomatosis
  - 4. Glomus tumor
  - 5. Hemangiopericytoma
  - 6. Papillary endothelial hyperplasia (i.e., intravascular vegetant hemangioendothelioma of Masson)
- B. Intermediate
  - 1. Hemangioendothelioma
    - a. Epitheliod
    - b. Spindle cell
    - c. Malignant endovascular papillary angioendothelioma
- C. Malignant
  - 1. Angiosarcoma
  - 2. Kaposi sarcoma
  - 3. Malignant glomus tumor
  - 4. Malignant hemangiopericytoma

VI. Tumors of lymph vessels
- A. Benign
  - 1. Lymphangioma
    - a. Cavernous
    - b. Cystic (i.e., cystic hygroma)
  - 2. Lymphangiomatosis
  - 3. Lymphangiomyoma and lymphangiomyomatosis
- B. Malignant
  - 1. Angiosarcoma

VII. Tumors and tumor-like lesions of synovial tissue
- A. Benign
  - 1. Giant cell tumor of tendon sheath
    - a. Localized (i.e., nodular tenosynovitis)
    - b. Diffuse (i.e., florid synovitis)
- B. Malignant
  - 1. Synovial sarcoma (i.e., malignant synovioma), predominantly
    - a. Biphasic (fibrous and epithelial)
    - b. Monophasic (fibrous or epithelial)
  - 2. Malignant giant cell tumor of tendon sheath

VIII. Tumors of mesothelial tissue
- A. Benign
  - 1. Localized fibrous mesothelioma (i.e., subserosal fibroma)
  - 2. Multicystic peritoneal mesothelioma
  - 3. Mesothelioma of the genital tract (i.e., adenomatoid tumor)
- B. Malignant
  - 1. Diffuse and localized mesothelioma, predominantly
    - a. Epithelial
    - b. Fibrous
    - c. Biphasic

TABLE 8.10 *(continued)*

IX. Tumors and tumor-like lesions of peripheral nerves
- A. Benign
  1. Traumatic neuroma
  2. Morton neuroma
  3. Neuromuscular hamartoma
  4. Nerve sheath ganglion
  5. Neurilemonma (i.e., benign schwannoma)
  6. Neurofibroma, solitary
     - a. Localized
     - b. Diffuse
     - c. Pacinian
     - d. Pigmented
  7. Granular cell tumor
  8. Neurofibromatosis (i.e., von Recklinghausen disease)
     - a. Localized
     - b. Plexiform
     - c. Diffuse
  9. Pigmented neuroectodermal tumor of infancy (i.e., retinal anlage tumor)
  10. Ectopic meningioma
  11. Nasal glioma
  12. Neurothekeoma
- B. Malignant
  1. Malignant schwannoma, including malignant schwannoma with rhabdomyoblastic differentiation (i.e., malignant Triton tumor), glandular malignant schwannoma, and epithelioid malignant schwannoma
  2. Peripheral tumors of primitive neuroectodermal tissues (i.e., neuroepithelioma)
  3. Malignant pigmented neuroectodermal tumor of infancy (i.e., retinal anlage tumor)
  4. Malignant granular cell tumor

X. Tumors of autonomic ganglia
- A. Benign
  1. Ganglioneuroma
  2. Melanocytic schwannoma
- B. Malignant
  1. Neuroblastoma
  2. Ganglioneuroblastoma
  3. Malignant melanocytic schwannoma

XI. Tumors of paraganglionic structures
- A. Benign
  1. Paraganglioma (solitary, multiple, familial)
- B. Malignant
  1. Malignant paraganglioma

XII. Tumors and tumor-like lesions of cartilage and boneforming tissues
- A. Benign
  1. Panniculitis ossificans
  2. Myositis ossificans
  3. Fibrodysplasia (i.e., myositis) ossificans progressiva
  4. Extraskeletal chondroma or osteochondroma
  5. Extraskeletal osteoma
- B. Malignant
  1. Extraskeletal chondrosarcoma
     - a. Well-differentiated
     - b. Myxoid (i.e., chordoid sarcoma)
     - c. Mesenchymal
  2. Extraskeletal osteosracoma

XIII. Tumors and tumor-like lesions of pluripotential mesenchyme
- A. Benign
  1. Mesenchymoma
- B. Malignant
  1. Malignant mesenchymoma

XIV. Tumors and tumor-like lesions of disputed or uncertain histogenesis
- A. Benign
  1. Congenital granular cell tumor
  2. Tumoral calcinosis
  3. Myxoma (cutaneous and intramuscular)
  4. Aggressive angiomyxoma
  5. Amyloid tumor
  6. Parachordoma
- B. Malignant
  1. Alveolar soft part sarcoma
  2. Epithelioid sarcoma
  3. Clear cell sarcoma of tendons and aponeuroses (i.e., malignant melanoma, soft parts)
  4. Extraskeletal Ewing sarcoma

XV. Unclassified soft-tissue tumors and tumor-like lesions

Source: Greenfield GB, Arrington JA. *Imaging of Bone Tumors: A Multimodality Approach.* Philadelphia: JB Lippincott, 1995;269–271.

skeleton. The risk of developing a sarcoma (most likely chondrosarcoma) within either is extremely low. The incidence is far below 1%. However, one must keep in mind that malignant degeneration of osteochondromas is more common in multiple hereditary exostoses; there is a 2.8% rate of conversion. Similarly, enchondromas present in Maffucci syndrome (multiple enchondromas associated with systemic hemangiomas) and Ollier disease (multiple enchondromas, typically on one side of the body) have a higher rate of malignant degeneration to chondrosarcoma than do solitary enchondromas.

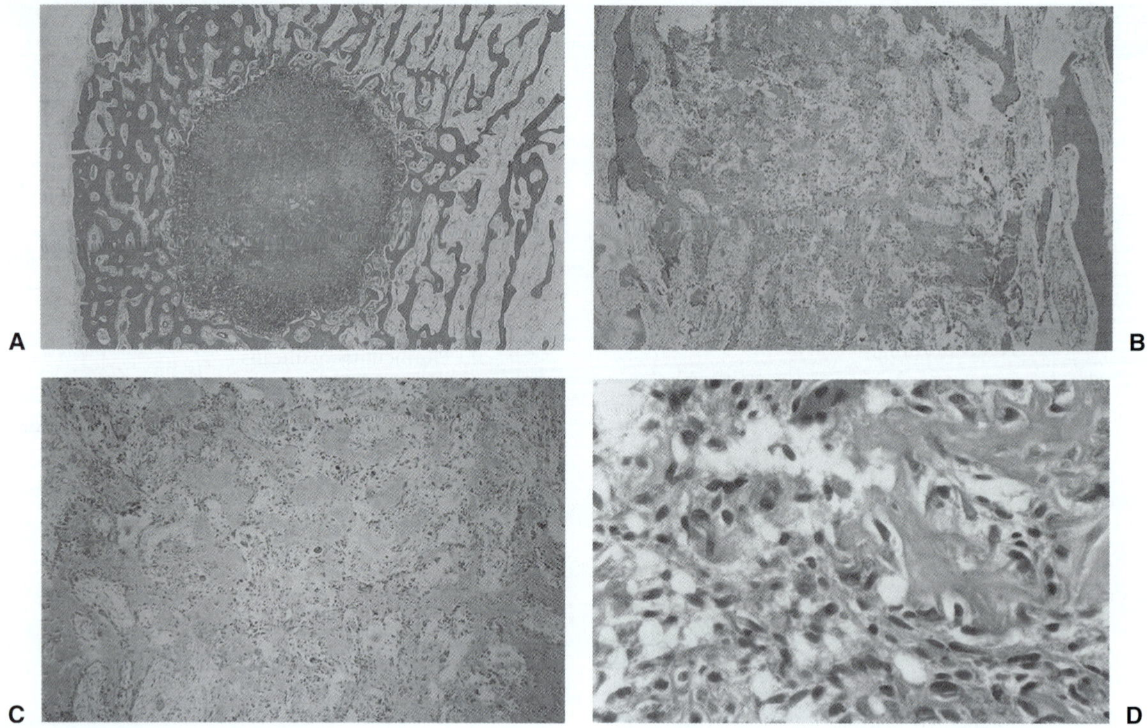

FIGURE 8.5 (A–D) Histopathology of osteoid osteoma. (*Source:* Greenspan A, Remagen W. *Differential Diagnosis of Tumors and Tumor-like Lesions of Bones and Joints.* Philadelphia: Lippincott-Raven, 1998;43; *D, courtesy of* Dr. KK Unni, Rochester, MN.)

Enchondroma. Enchondroma is a nest of cartilage tissue typically in a metaphyseal region that is usually encountered as an incidental finding in adulthood (Figs. 8.11 through 8.14). Multiple enchondromas are rare but exist in Maffucci syndrome and Ollier disease. Patients with these diseases have a higher rate of malignant degeneration to chondrosarcoma than do those with solitary enchondromas. Enchondromas are most common in the short tubular bones of the hands and in the femur and humerus. They are commonly discovered incidentally when an x-ray of the adjacent joint is obtained for reasons unrelated to the enchondroma itself. These lesions tend to be noncalcified or minimally calcified in young adults

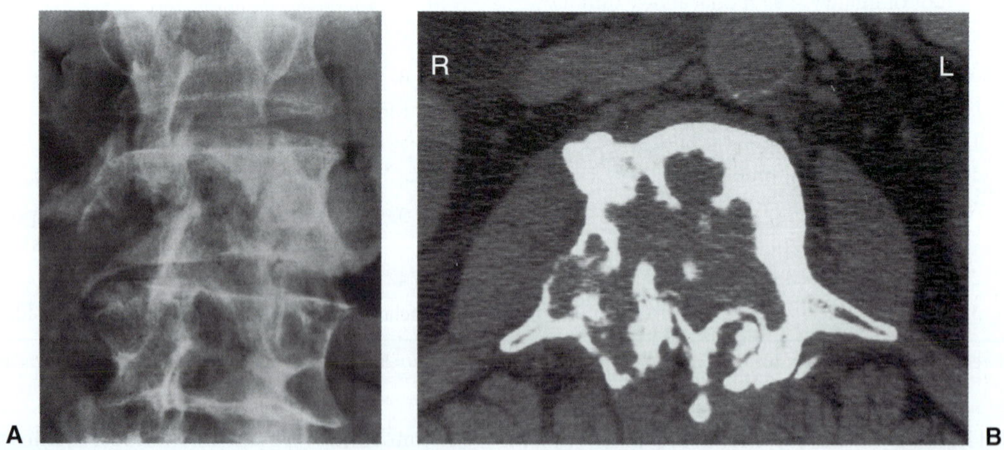

FIGURE 8.6 Aggressive osteoblastoma. (A) Destructive lytic lesion in the right half of the vertebral body of L3. (B) CT shows focal areas of bone formation within the lesion and invasion of cortex. (*Courtesy of* Ibrahim F. Abdelwahab, MD, New York, NY; *from* Greenspan A. Benign bone-forming lesions. *Skeletal Radiol* 1993;22:494.)

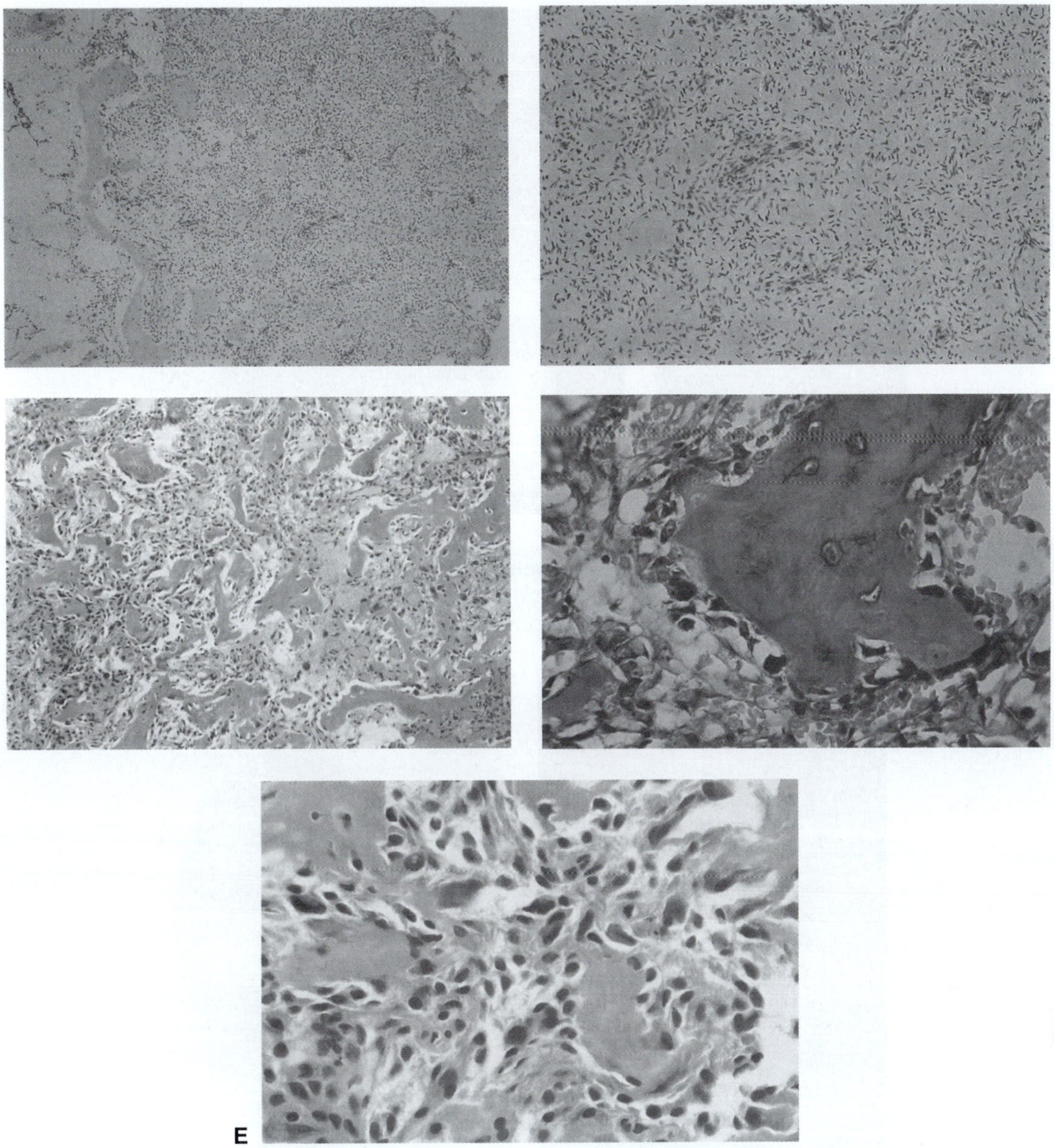

FIGURE 8.7 **(A–E) Histopathology of osteoblastoma.** *(A, B, D from* Greenspan A, Remagen W. *Differential Diagnosis of Tumors and Tumor-like Lesions of Bones and Joints.* Philadelphia: Lippincott-Raven, 1998;57. *C, E courtesy of* Ibrahim F. Abdelwahab, MD, New York, NY; *from* Greenspan A. Benign bone-forming lesions. *Skeletal Radiol* 1993;22;496.)

and usually show an increase in calcification but not an increase in size with follow-up over many years. The calcification has a typical stippled or "popcorn" pattern. They usually do not cause pain, but they are typically hot on technetium bone scan. Unlike chondrosarcomas, enchondromas do not cause damage to the host bone because they typically do not cause cortical thinning or expansion. They may cause some slight scalloping, with scallops usually less than 1 cm each. Some expansion may be seen in thin or small bones such as the fibular head or scapula.

Chondroblastoma. Chondroblastoma typically appears as a painful lytic lesion in the epiphysis of a child with significant edema seen on MRI scan. In older adolescents, it can occasionally grow across an old epiphyseal line to involve the adjacent metaphysis. The most common locations are the distal femur, proximal tibia, and proximal humerus (Figs. 8.15 and 8.16). The look of this painful epiphyseal lytic lesion with abundant edema may cause it to be confused with infection and even osteochondritis desiccans. Malignant degeneration is rare. Even though chondroblastoma is

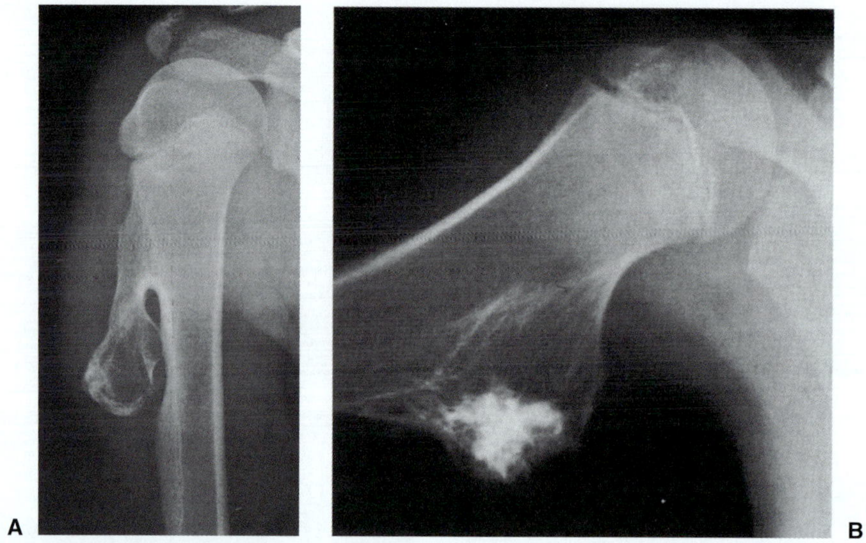

FIGURE 8.8 Osteochondroma ilium, preoperatively. (A) Pedunculated. (B) Sessile. (*Source:* Greenspan A, Remagen W. *Differential Diagnosis of Tumors and Tumor-like Lesions of Bones and Joints*. Philadelphia: Lippincott-Raven, 1998;148.)

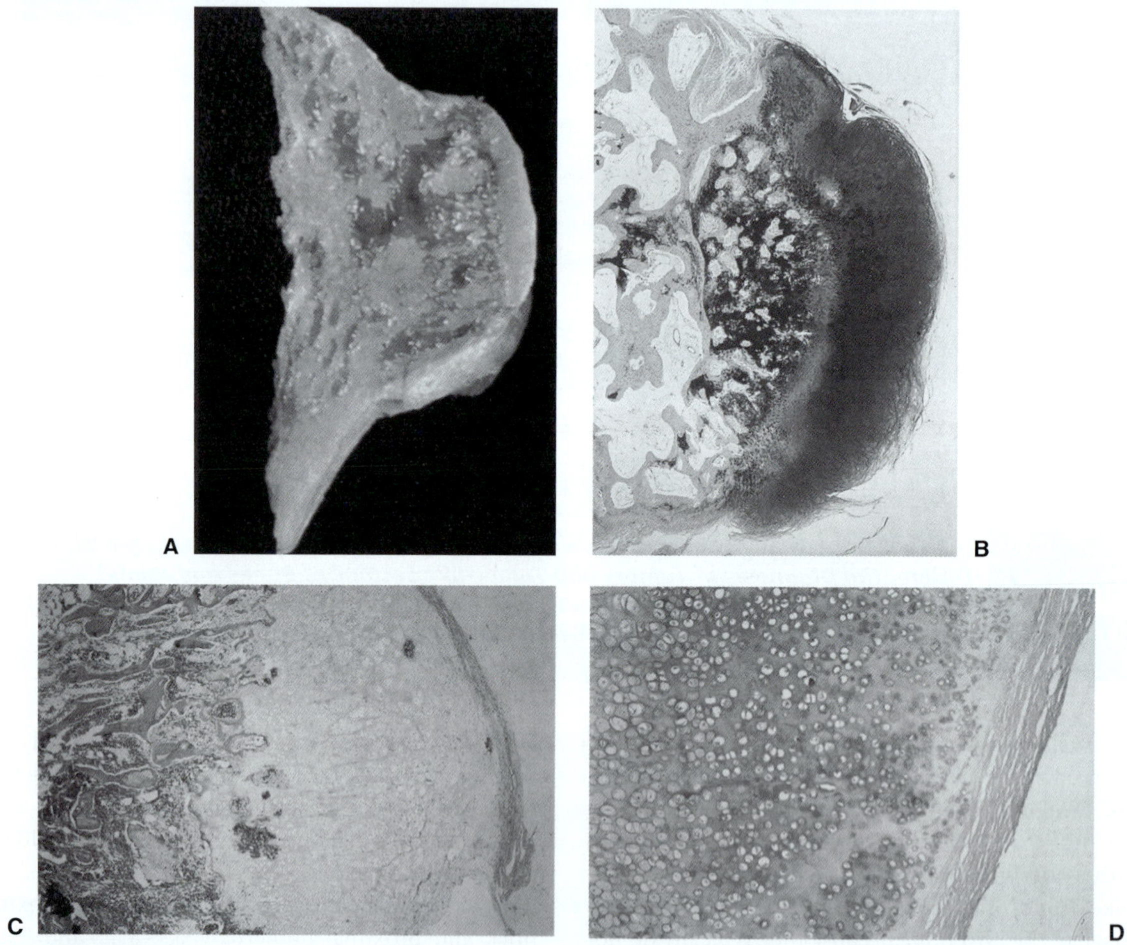

FIGURE 8.9 Osteochondroma ilium. (A) Gross specimen. (B, C, D) Histopathology. (*Source:* Greenspan A, Remagen W. *Differential Diagnosis of Tumors and Tumor-like Lesions of Bones and Joints*. Philadelphia: Lippincott-Raven, 1998;151.)

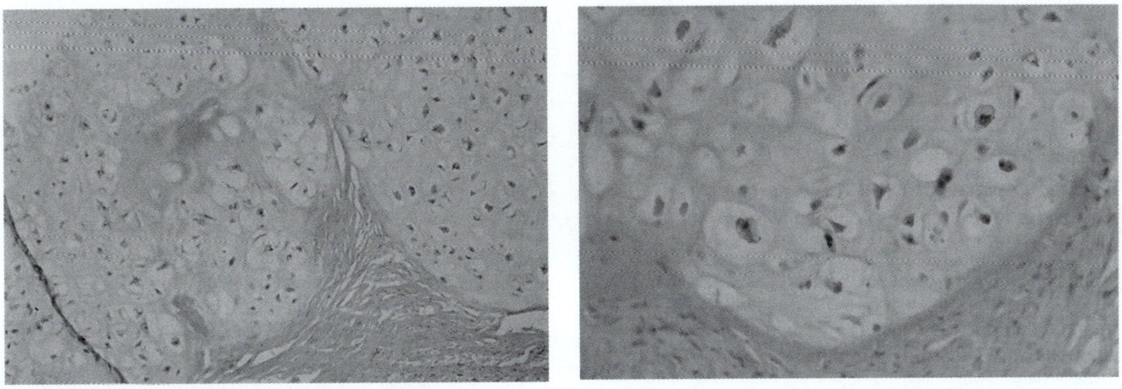

A B

FIGURE 8.10 (A, B) Histopathology of secondary chondrosarcomatous degeneration. (*Source:* Greenspan A, Remagen W. *Differential Diagnosis of Tumors and Tumor-like Lesions of Bones and Joints*. Philadelphia: Lippincott-Raven, 1998;158.)

benign, it has been reported to metastasize to the lung. Prognosis for chondroblastoma is good, and treatment consists of intralesional curettage and bone grafting or cementation.

Chondromyxoid Fibroma. A chondromyxoid fibroma contains variable amounts of chondroid, fibromatoid, and myxoid elements. It affects mostly males in their second and third decade and is commonly found in the proximal tibia, distal femur, and foot. The tumor is usually slow growing and mildly painful. Radiographically, the lesion is typically metaphyseal, lytic, destructive, and sharply demarcated from the adjacent bone with cortical thinning but no periosteal reaction (Figs. 8.17 and 8.18). It frequently has the appearance of a very large, nonossifying fibroma. Because the recurrence rate can reach up to 25% with simple curettage and bone grafting, a more aggressive margin is justified.

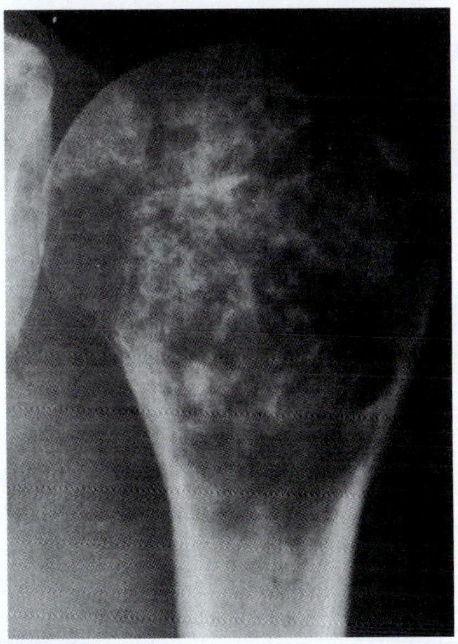

FIGURE 8.11 Radiologic characteristics of enchondroma. (*Source:* Greenspan A, Remagen W. *Differential Diagnosis of Tumors and Tumor-like Lesions of Bones and Joints*. Philadelphia: Lippincott-Raven, 1998;124.)

Nonosseus, Nonchondroid

Fibrous Dysplasia. Fibrous dysplasia is a dysplastic anomaly of bone-forming tissue that lacks the ability to produce mature lamellar bone with the bone being arrested in the woven state (Figs 8.19 8.20 and

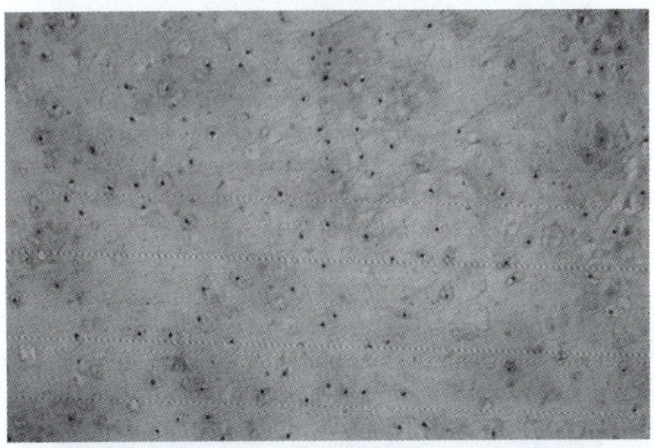

FIGURE 8.12 Histopathology of a benign cartilage tumor. (*Courtesy of* Dr. M. J. Klein, New York, NY. *From* Greenspan A, Remagen W. *Differential Diagnosis of Tumors and Tumor-like Lesions of Bones and Joints*. Philadelphia: Lippincott-Raven, 1998;124.)

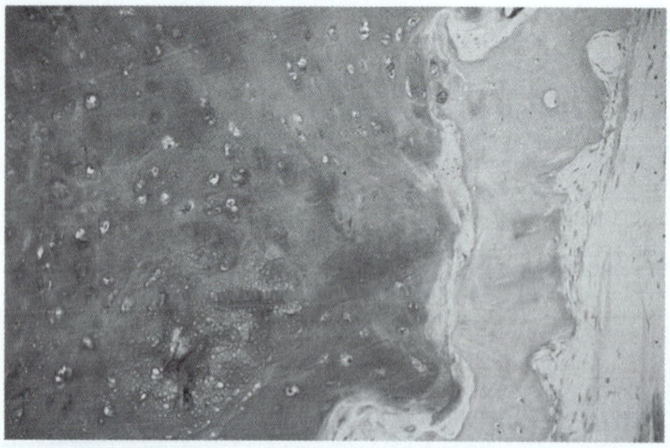

FIGURE 8.13 Histopathology of an enchondroma eroding the cortex but with no evidence of invasion. (*Source:* Greenspan A, Remagen W. *Differential Diagnosis of Tumors and Tumor-like Lesions of Bones and Joints*. Philadelphia: Lippincott-Raven, 1998;124.)

8.21). It most commonly diagnosed in the second or third decade. Three clinical forms of fibrous dysplasia exist: monostotic, polyostotic (Fig. 8.22), and McCune-Albright syndrome (multiple bone lesions, brown skin patches [café-au-lait spots], and endocrine abnormalities including precocious puberty). Solitary

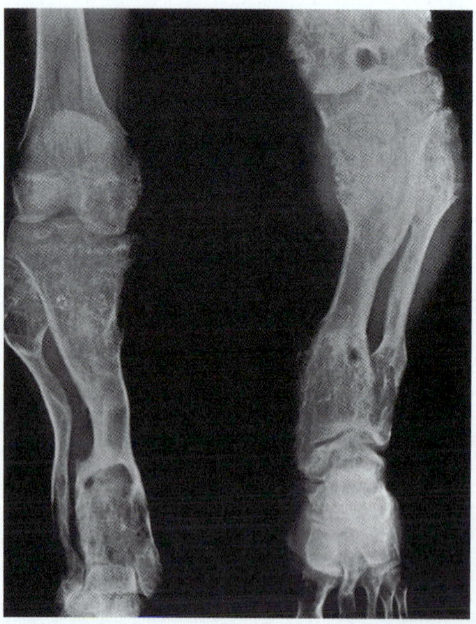

FIGURE 8.14 Enchondromatosis (Ollier disease). (*Source:* Greenspan A, Remagen W. *Differential Diagnosis of Tumors and Tumor-like Lesions of Bones and Joints*. Philadelphia: Lippincott-Raven, 1998;137.)

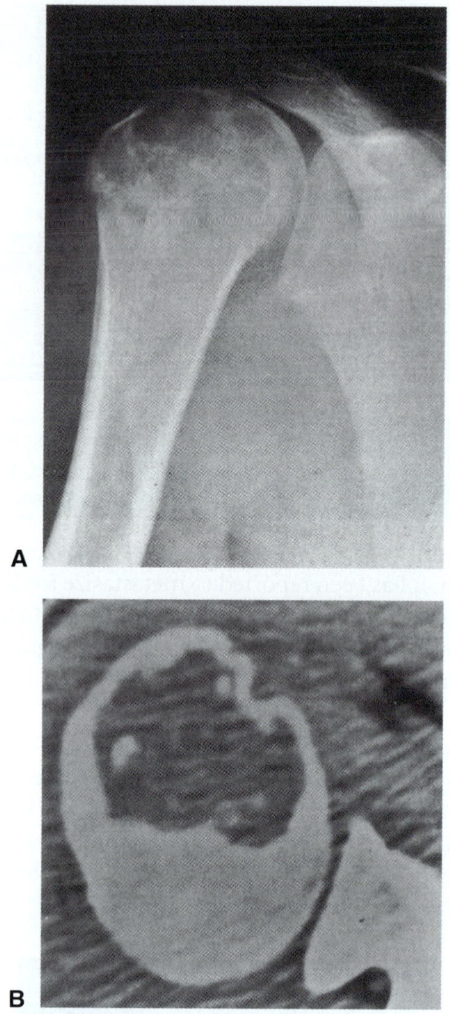

FIGURE 8.15 Chondroblastoma. (A) Radiograph of lesion in proximal humeral epiphysis. (B) CT shows the calcifications clearly. (*Source:* Greenspan A, Remagen W. *Differential Diagnosis of Tumors and Tumor-like Lesions of Bones and Joints*. Philadelphia: Lippincott-Raven, 1998;161.)

lesions are quite common, while polyostotic disease is rare. Virtually any bone may be involved, but the proximal femur is most common. Other areas frequently involved include the tibia, pelvis, humerus, radius, and ribs. Polyostotic disease tends to remain unilateral. Monostotic disease is typically an incidental radiographic finding in an asymptomatic patient. Occasionally, patients will present with localized pain from pathologic fracture or bone deformity, such as a shepard's crook deformity of the proximal femur. The classic fibrous dysplasia lesion occurs as a long

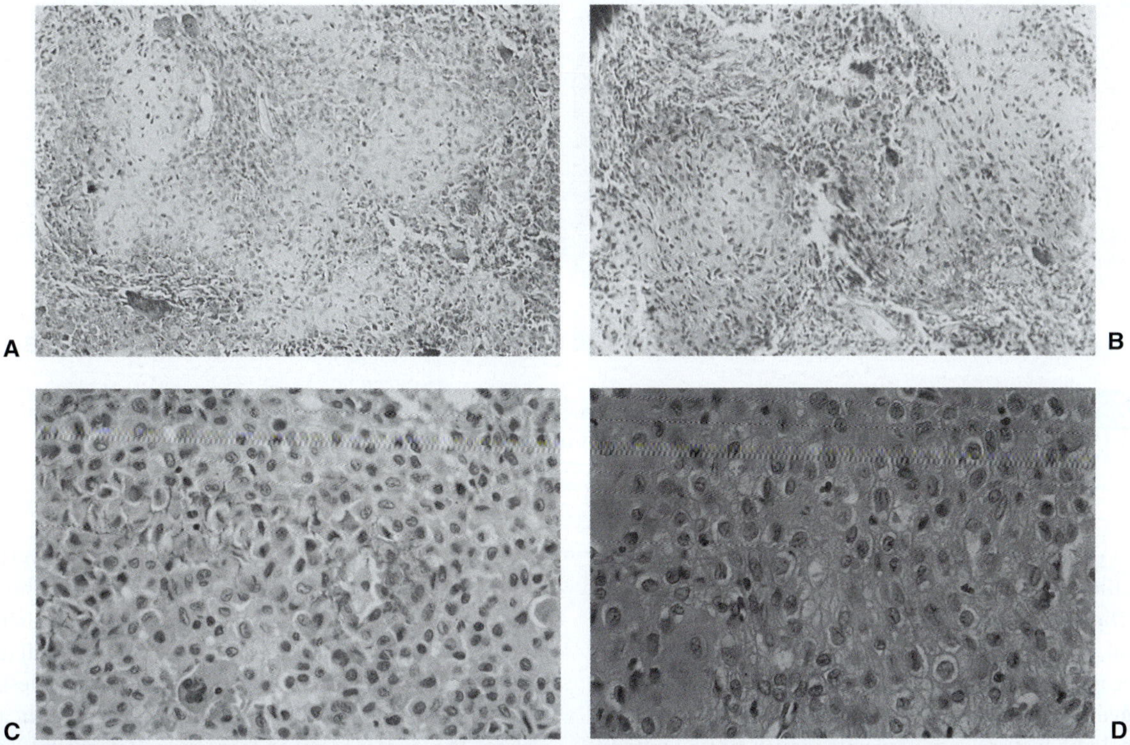

FIGURE 8.16 (A–D) Histopathology of chondroblastoma. (*Source:* Greenspan A, Remagen W. *Differential Diagnosis of Tumors and Tumor-like Lesions of Bones and Joints*. Philadelphia: Lippincott-Raven, 1998;163.)

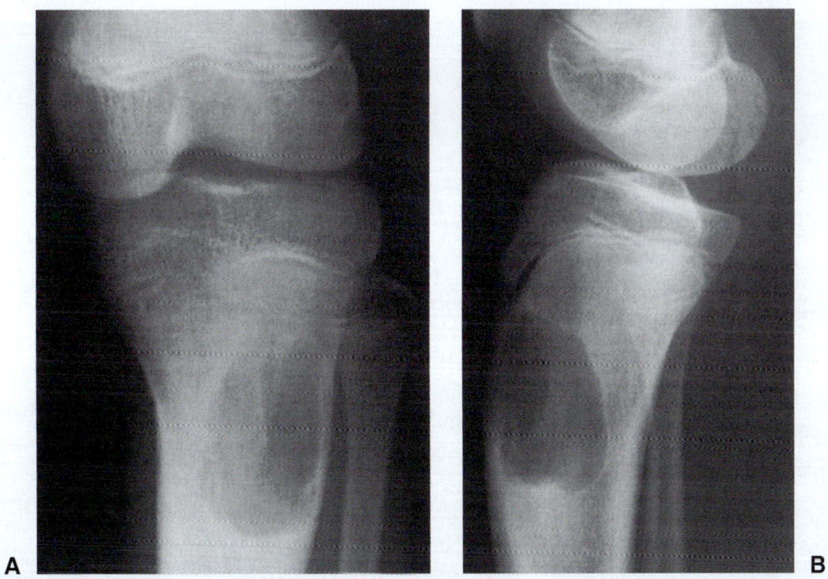

FIGURE 8.17 Chondromyxoid fibroma. (A) Anteroposterior radiograph. (B) Lateral radiograph. (*Source:* Greenspan A, Remagen W. *Differential Diagnosis of Tumors and Tumor-like Lesions of Bones and Joints*. Philadelphia: Lippincott-Raven, 1998;167.)

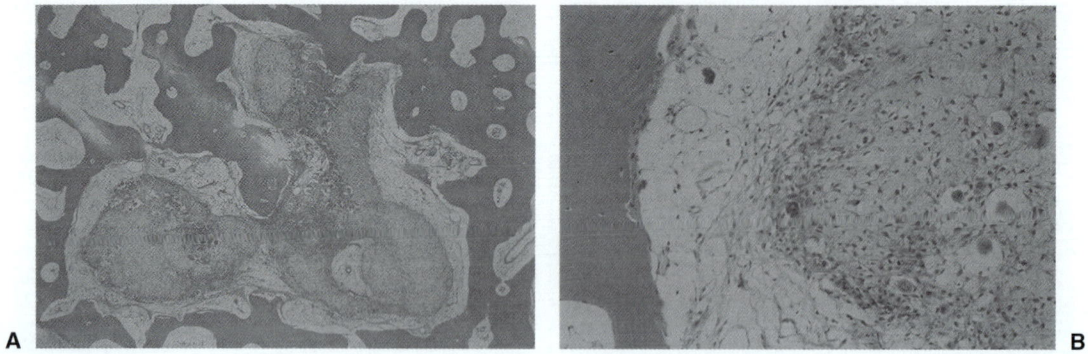

FIGURE 8.18 **(A, B) Histopathology of chondromyxoid fibroma. (*Source:* Greenspan A, Remagen W. *Differential Diagnosis of Tumors and Tumor-like Lesions of Bones and Joints.* Philadelphia: Lippincott-Raven, 1998;169.)**

lesion in a long bone with ground glass, medullary calcification, and cortical thinning but no periosteal reaction. It is commonly located centrally within the canal. Fibrous dysplasia can have a very variable appearance and should be included in the differential of every benign-appearing lesion in bone. The major histologic feature is metaplastic woven bone scattered through a benign fibrous tissue stroma. Often, the woven trabeculae are disorganized and have been described as having a "Chinese letter" appearance. Areas of cartilage formation are commonly present. Fibrous dysplasia tends to be active during the growing years and then becomes quiescent in the skeletally mature. Fibrous dysplasia can convert to malignancy, most commonly osteosarcoma, although the conversion rate is less than 1%. Irradiation is contraindicated because of the risk of radiation induced sarcoma later in life. Asymptomatic lesions can be observed for progression. Surgery is indicated when the patient has progressive deformity, large lesions with pain, nonunion, failure of nonsurgical therapy, or malignancy. Pain and deformity are signs that microfractures are developing in a lesion and should be addressed. Treatment typically consists of curettage, bone grafting or cementation, and internal fixation if necessary.

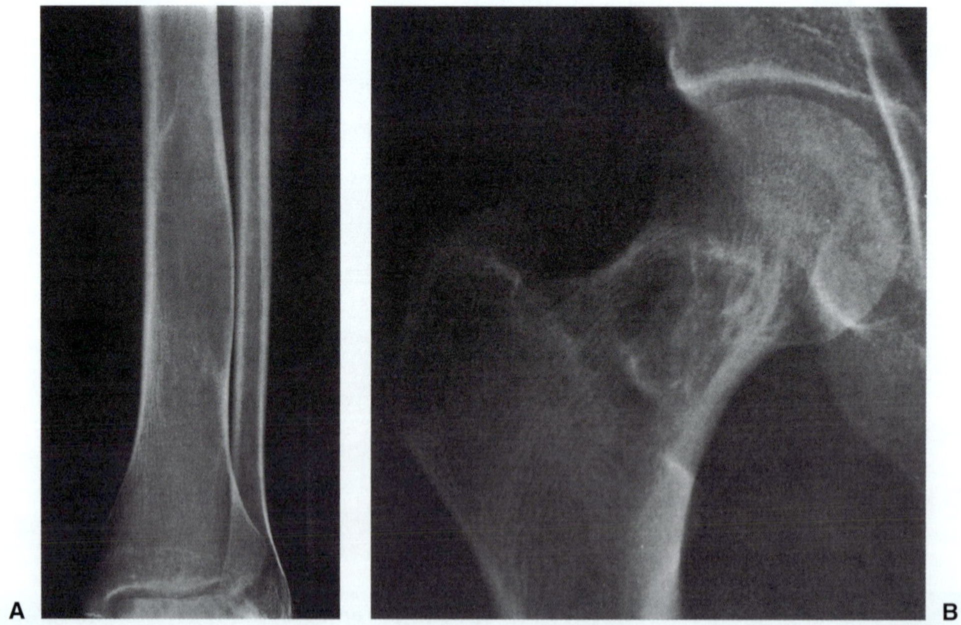

FIGURE 8.19 **Monostotic fibrous dysplasia. (A) Focus in the diaphysis of the tibia. (B) More sclerotic-appearing lesion in the femoral neck. (*Source:* Greenspan A, Remagen W. *Differential Diagnosis of Tumors and Tumor-like Lesions of Bones and Joints.* Philadelphia: Lippincott-Raven, 1998;217.)**

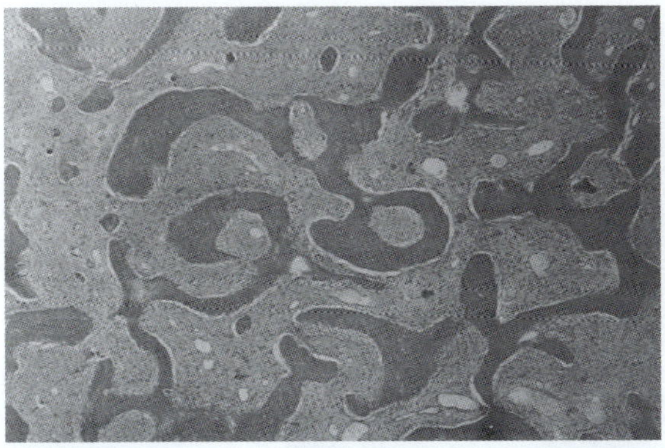

FIGURE 8.20 Classic histopathology of fibrous dysplasia. (*Source:* Greenspan A, Remagen W. *Differential Diagnosis of Tumors and Tumor-like Lesions of Bones and Joints*. Philadelphia: Lippincott-Raven, 1998;219.)

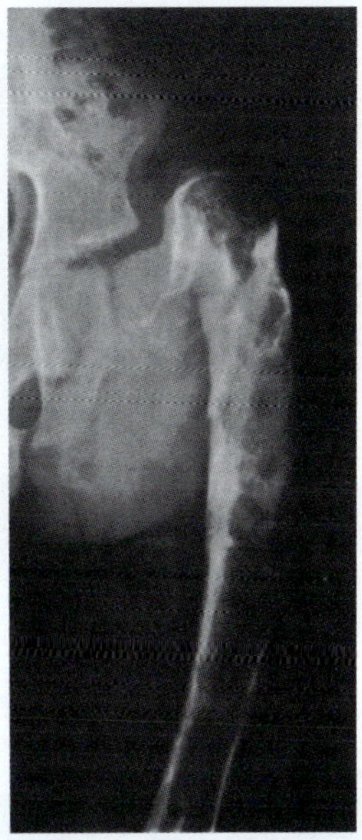

FIGURE 8.22 Polyostotic fibrous dysplasia. (*Source:* Greenspan A, Remagen W. *Differential Diagnosis of Tumors and Tumor-like Lesions of Bones and Joints*. Philadelphia: Lippincott-Raven, 1998;221.)

Aneurysmal Bone Cyst (ABC). This lesion is a nonneoplastic reactive condition found in the first 3 decades of life. ABCs occur in bone primarily or in association with other tumors, such as giant cell tumor, chondroblastoma, and osteosarcoma. They usually occur in the metaphyses of long bones, especially in the femur and tibia, but are also seen in the posterior spine. Patients often present with pain and swelling lasting months to years. The classic radiographic finding is an eccentric, lytic, ballooning expansion within the metaphysis (Fig. 8.23). Lesions frequently have a delicate rim of expanded cortical bone which may be best seen on CT scan. Fluid-filled levels are frequently seen (Fig. 8.24). Typical histologic features are blood-filled spaces without endothelial lining (Fig. 8.25). Not all lesions require treatment because they sometimes reach an inactive state.

Treatment is curettage and bone grafting with local recurrence as high as 25%. Hemorrhage from these lesions can be significant, and embolization should be considered when treating lesions of the spine and pelvis.

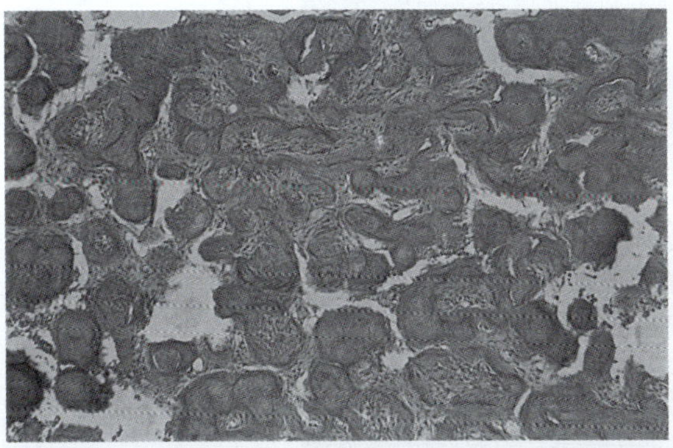

FIGURE 8.21 Variant of histologic appearance of fibrous dysplasia. (*Source:* Greenspan A, Remagen W. *Differential Diagnosis of Tumors and Tumor-like Lesions of Bones and Joints*. Philadelphia: Lippincott-Raven, 1998;219.)

Simple Bone Cyst. Simple bone cyst, or unicameral bone cyst, is an extremely common lesion that presents in the first 2 decades of life. Simple bone cysts are the most frequent cause of pathologic fracture in children. They are typically asymptomatic until fracture and occur almost exclusively in the metaphyses of long bones, especially in the proximal humerus, proximal femur, and proximal tibia. Radiographically, they appear as a central lytic area with symmetric cortical thinning. The bone is often expanded. Unlike the ABCs, they are rarely greater than the width of the adjacent physeal plate. The "fallen leaf" or "fallen fragment" sign, signifying a piece of cortical bone that fell into the intramedullary cyst as a result of fracture, is often seen (Fig. 8.26). Histopathology is shown in Figure 8.27. Simple bone cysts usually heal on their own by skeletal maturity, allowing for observation in most cases. In a weight-bearing location, such as the proximal femur,

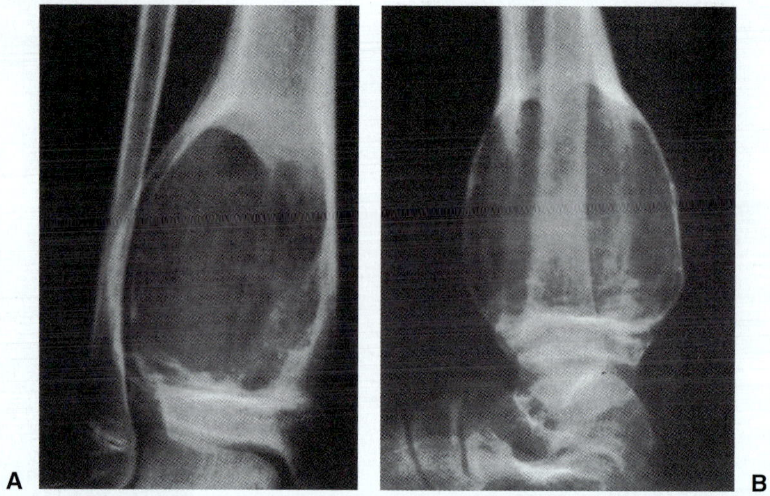

FIGURE 8.23 Aneurysmal bone cyst. (A) Anteroposterior radiograph. (B) Lateral radiograph. (*Source:* Greenspan A, Remagen W. *Differential Diagnosis of Tumors and Tumor-like Lesions of Bones and Joints.* Philadelphia: Lippincott-Raven, 1998;331.)

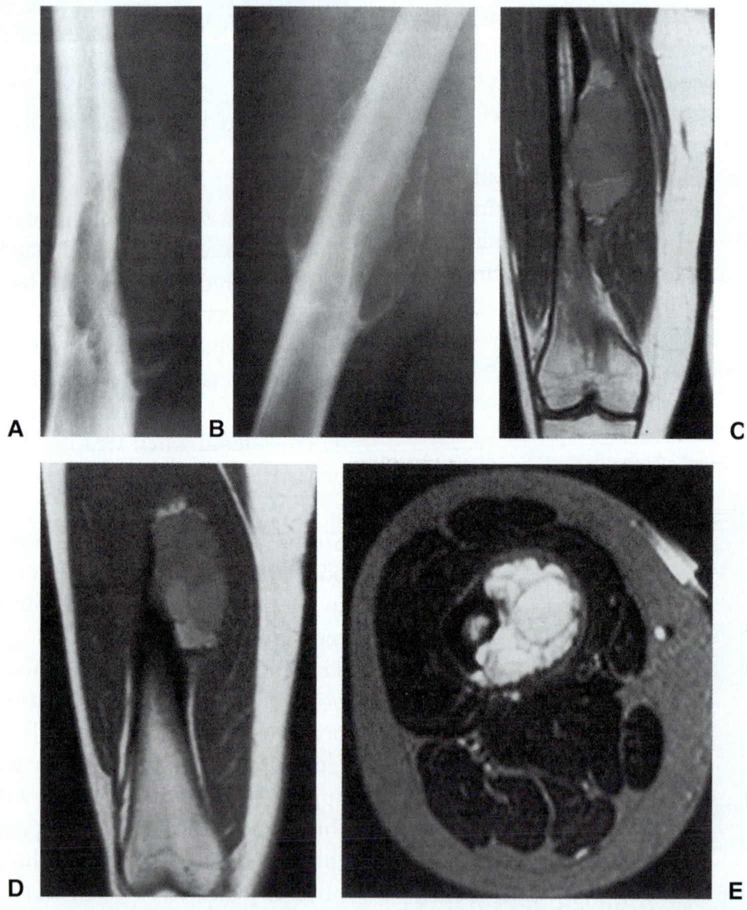

FIGURE 8.24 Aneurysmal bone cyst. (A) Anteroposterior and (B) lateral radiographs. (C, D) Coronal T1-weighted MRI shows inhomogeneity of the lesion and internal septations. (E) Axial T2-weighted MRI shows high-signal intensity lesion with a fluid-filled level. (*Source:* Greenspan A, Remagen W. *Differential Diagnosis of Tumors and Tumor-like Lesions of Bones and Joints.* Philadelphia: Lippincott-Raven, 1998;336.)

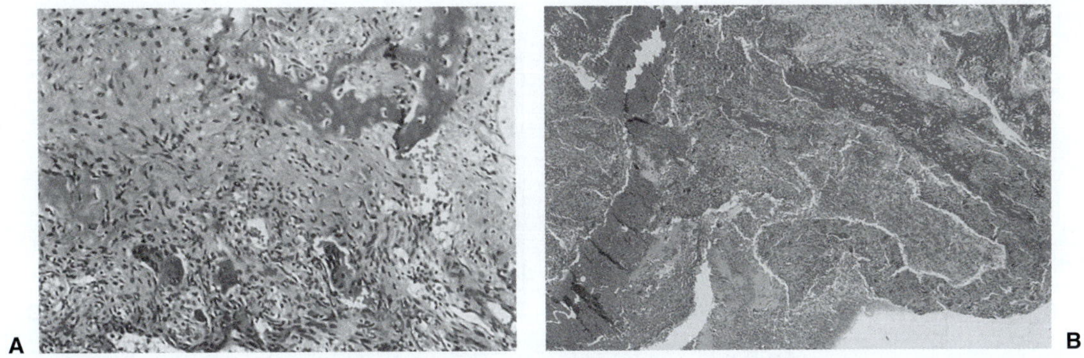

FIGURE 8.25 (A, B) Histopathology of aneurysmal bone cyst. (*Source:* Greenspan A, Remagen W. *Differential Diagnosis of Tumors and Tumor-like Lesions of Bones and Joints.* Philadelphia: Lippincott-Raven, 1998;337.)

lesions should be treated more aggressively. These lesions can be treated with repeated aspiration and injection with methylprednisolone, bone marrow and bone substitute, or with curettage and bone graft.

Eosinophilic Granuloma (Langerhans Cell Histiocytosis). Also known as solitary Langerhans cell histiocytosis (LCH), eosinophilic granuloma is the most benign member of a group of disorders of the reticuloendothelial system, including Hand-Schüller-Christian disease and disseminated LCH. Eosinophilic granuloma is a self-limiting process that can lead to focal destruction of bone. It is most prevalent in the first and second decade, with half of patients under the age of 10 years. It is more common in males. The etiology is unknown. The lesion is composed of lipid-containing histiocytes from the reticuloendothelial system and eosinophils. Lesions are most common in the skull, although virtually any bone may be affected, with vertebral involvement occurring in approximately 10% to 15% of cases. The most common appearance is a well-circumscribed, punched-out lesion with no periosteal reaction. Less common is the moth-eaten pattern with periosteal reaction (Figs. 8.28 through 8.34). Complete collapse of the vertebral body without spine deformity can occur and is classically referred to as *vertebra plana.* Treatment of symptomatic lesions includes curettage and bone grafting. Local steroid injections have also been used. Chemotherapy is recommended in cases of disseminated LCH.

Fibrous Cortical Defect. These lesions can occur in as many as 40% of children. They are small cortical defects found almost exclusively in the metaphyseal areas of

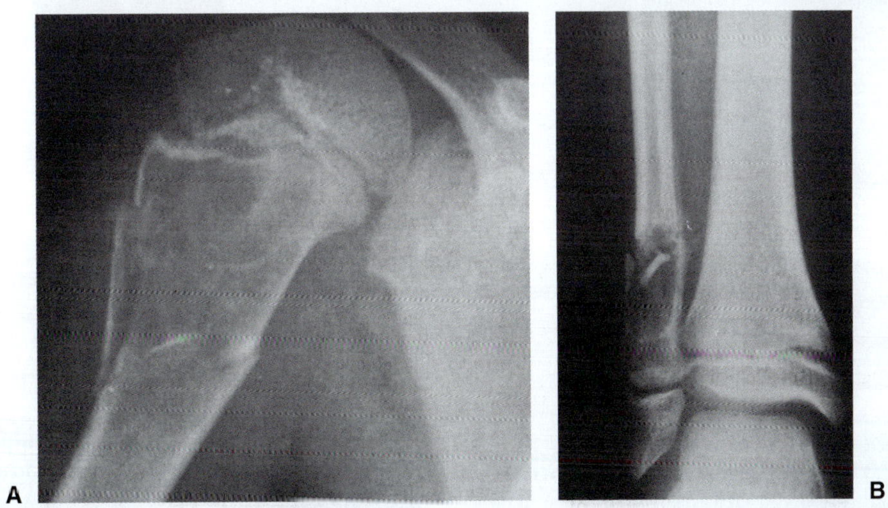

FIGURE 8.26 Simple bone cyst: "fallen fragment" sign. (A) Pathologic fracture of proximal humeral diaphysis. (B) Radiolucent lesion in the distal diaphysis of the fibula. (*Source:* Greenspan A, Remagen W. *Differential Diagnosis of Tumors and Tumor-like Lesions of Bones and Joints.* Philadelphia: Lippincott-Raven, 1998;325.)

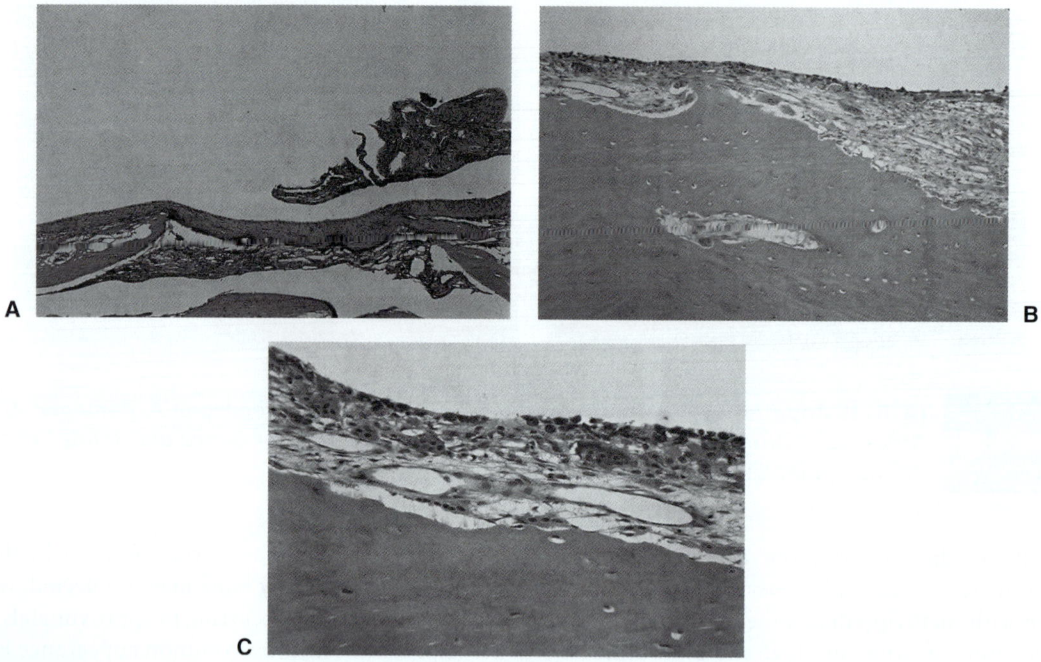

FIGURE 8.27 Histopathology of simple bone cyst. (A) Flattened fibrous lining contains a few bone trabeculae. (B, C) Several giant cells present within a fibrous lining. (*Source:* Greenspan A, Remagen W. *Differential Diagnosis of Tumors and Tumor-like Lesions of Bones and Joints*. Philadelphia: Lippincott-Raven, 1998;3327.)

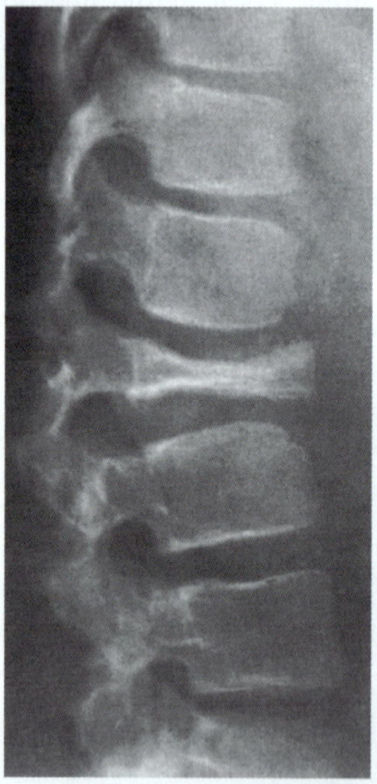

FIGURE 8.28 Eosinophilic granuloma (Langerhans cell histiocytosis). (*Source:* Greenspan A, Remagen W. *Differential Diagnosis of Tumors and Tumor-like Lesions of Bones and Joints*. Philadelphia: Lippincott-Raven, 1998;249.)

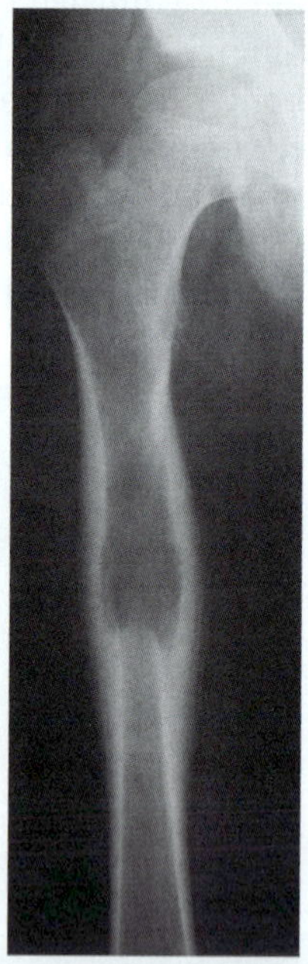

FIGURE 8.29 Eosinophilic granuloma: anteroposterior radiograph. (*Source:* Greenspan A, Remagen W. *Differential Diagnosis of Tumors and Tumor-like Lesions of Bones and Joints*. Philadelphia: Lippincott-Raven, 1998;251.)

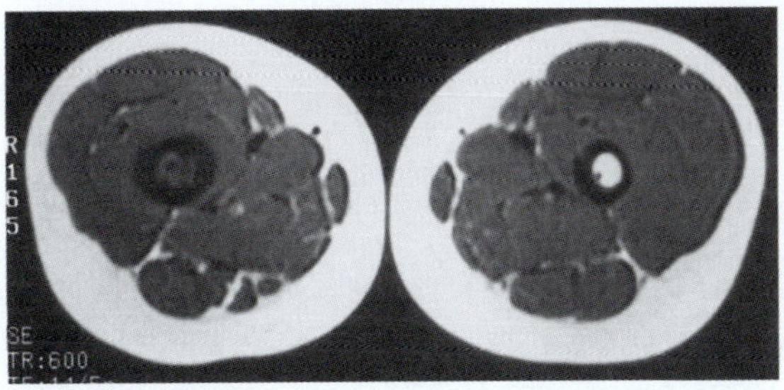

FIGURE 8.30 **Eosinophilic granuloma: axial T1-weighted MRI. (*Source:* Greenspan A, Remagen W. *Differential Diagnosis of Tumors and Tumor-like Lesions of Bones and Joints.* Philadelphia: Lippincott-Raven, 1998;251.)**

the lower extremities, most commonly about the knee. Lesions typically disappear as the bone remodels, but they can cause pain. The radiographic appearance of this eccentric metaphyseal radiolucency surrounded by a rim of sclerotic bone is usually enough to diagnose these lesions, which can generally be observed (Fig. 8.35).

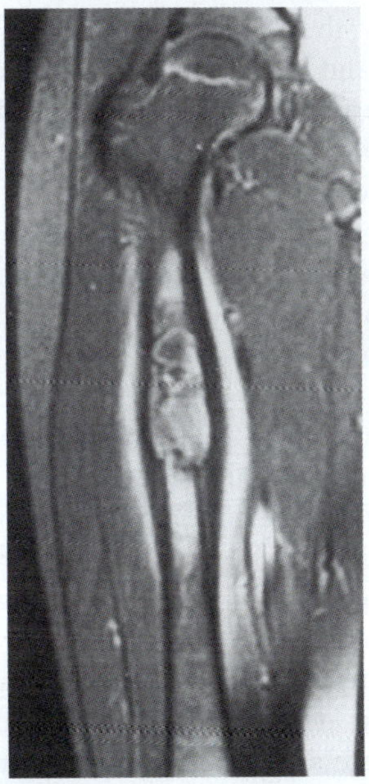

FIGURE 8.31 **Eosinophilic granuloma: coronal T1-weighted MRI with gadolinium. The healing stage mimics chronic osteomyelitis. (*Source:* Greenspan A, Remagen W. *Differential Diagnosis of Tumors and Tumor-like Lesions of Bones and Joints.* Philadelphia: Lippincott-Raven, 1998;251.)**

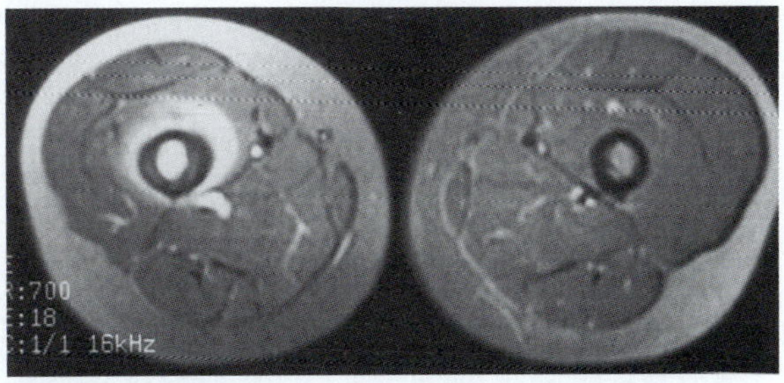

FIGURE 8.32 **Eosinophilic granuloma: axial T1-weighted MRI with gadolinium. (*Source:* Greenspan A, Remagen W. *Differential Diagnosis of Tumors and Tumor-like Lesions of Bones and Joints.* Philadelphia: Lippincott-Raven, 1998;251.)**

Nonossifying Fibroma (Metaphyseal Fibrous Defect). Nonossifying fibroma is likely a larger, more active form of the fibrous cortical defect (Fig. 8.36). It is typically seen in the lower extremity of children and, because of its size, may persist into adult life. They are usually eccentric metaphyseal lesions in children. As growth of the patient continues and external remodeling occurs, lesions that were previously intramedullary in the metaphysis become intracortical in the metadiaphysis. This cortical disruption creates a mechanical insufficiency and causes the bone to replace the lesion with new bone formation as the lesion heals in. This is a common lesion, which only rarely requires surgical intervention. Most of these lesions are incidental findings and require no specific treatment other than occasional x-rays to document stability and healing. On occasion, however, they may be large enough to cause mechanical pain and limit the ability of the child or adolescent to participate in desired activities. In these cases, or when the specific diagnosis remains elusive, open biopsy with curettage and some form of bone grafting is reasonable. Following surgical excision and grafting, these lesions will typically heal completely in about 8 weeks, whereas healing would commonly take 2 years or more with no intervention. Histologically, these lesions have a characteristic appearance showing benign spindle cells with a good number of benign giant cells mixed in. Surgical intervention is indicated for pathologic fracture and impending fracture.

Giant Cell Tumor. These benign but locally aggressive tumors occur in the juxtaarticular regions of skeletally mature individuals, usually in the third decade of life,

A 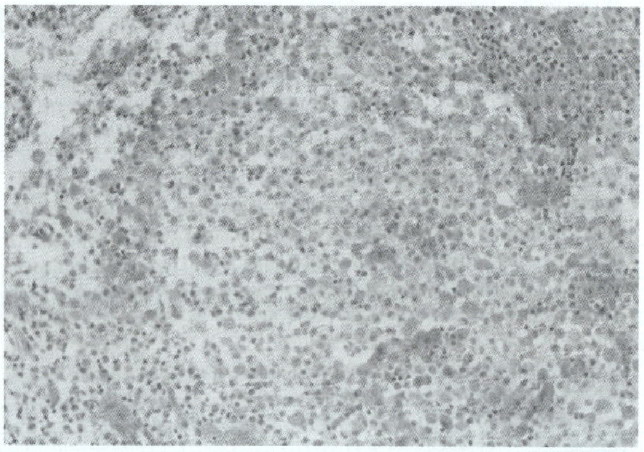 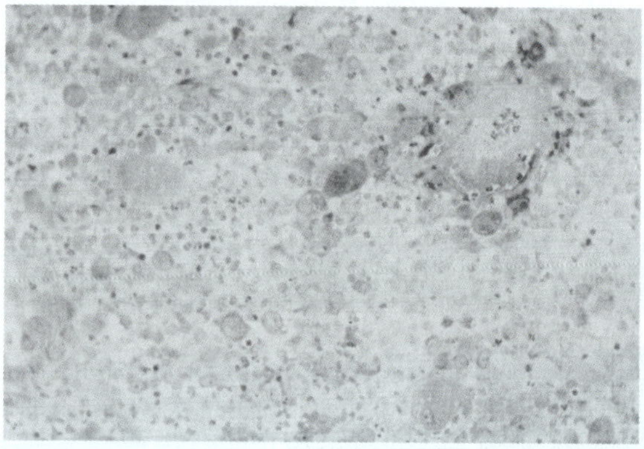 B

FIGURE 8.33 **(A, B) Histopathology of eosinophilic granuloma. (*Source:* Greenspan A, Remagen W. *Differential Diagnosis of Tumors and Tumor-like Lesions of Bones and Joints.* Philadelphia: Lippincott-Raven, 1998;253.)**

rarely after the age of 50 years. Most common locations are about the knee: the distal femur and proximal tibia account for about 50% of all cases. The distal radius, pelvis, and sacrum can also be involved. There is a slight female predominance. Pain is common and can be due to an effusion in the joint because of the proximity to the articular surface. Pathologic fractures often occur. Even though the tumor is classified as benign, it metastasizes to the lungs in approximately 2% of the cases. Therefore, a chest radiograph or CT should be part of the work-up for this lesion. The diagnosis of benign giant cell tumor is usually fairly simple when the histologic findings are coupled with typical radiographic changes. Located at the metaphyseal–epiphyseal junction, these lesions appear lytic on radiographs, frequently with a moth-eaten margin, cortical thinning or erosion and expansion, possible soft tissue extension, but usually no periosteal reaction. They tend to grow toward the joint surface and, rarely, they can break through (Fig. 8.37). Histologically, the lesion is composed of multinucleate giant cells and mononuclear stromal cells. The characteristic finding is that the nuclei of the giant cells look identical to the nuclei of the stromal cells. Mitotic figures may be found in all of these lesions and may be prominent in some. Small areas of woven bone may also be seen along with areas of spindle cells with spindled nuclei (Fig. 8.38). Some giant cell–rich osteosarcomas are indistinguishable from benign giant cell tumor. In these lesions, there is often only a malignant pattern of subsequent growth and metastasis that elucidates the true nature of the neoplasm. Giant cell tumors are most prone to recur locally. Studies have shown local failure rates as high as 50% following just curettage and grafting. Local failure rates as high as 25% have been reported with curettage and local adjuvant therapy (phenol, liquid nitrogen, and hydrogen peroxide). Currently, most surgeons treat with aggressive curettage, adjuvant therapy, and subsequent packing with bone cement. This approach has been shown to produce recurrence rates of 6% to 25%. One recent study showed this treatment was equally effective for lesions with extraosseous extension when the extraosseous component was carefully resected. Close follow-up for recurrent disease and pulmonary involvement is important. A chest radiograph or CT should be obtained every 6 to 12 months for the first 3 years.

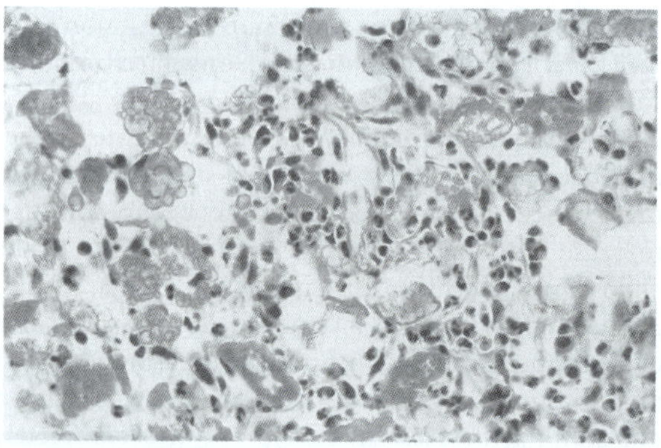

FIGURE 8.34 **Eosinophilic granuloma showing mulberry-like foam cells, eosinophilic granulocytes, and hyaline bodies. (*Source:* Greenspan A, Remagen W. *Differential Diagnosis of Tumors and Tumor-like Lesions of Bones and Joints.* Philadelphia: Lippincott-Raven, 1998;253.)**

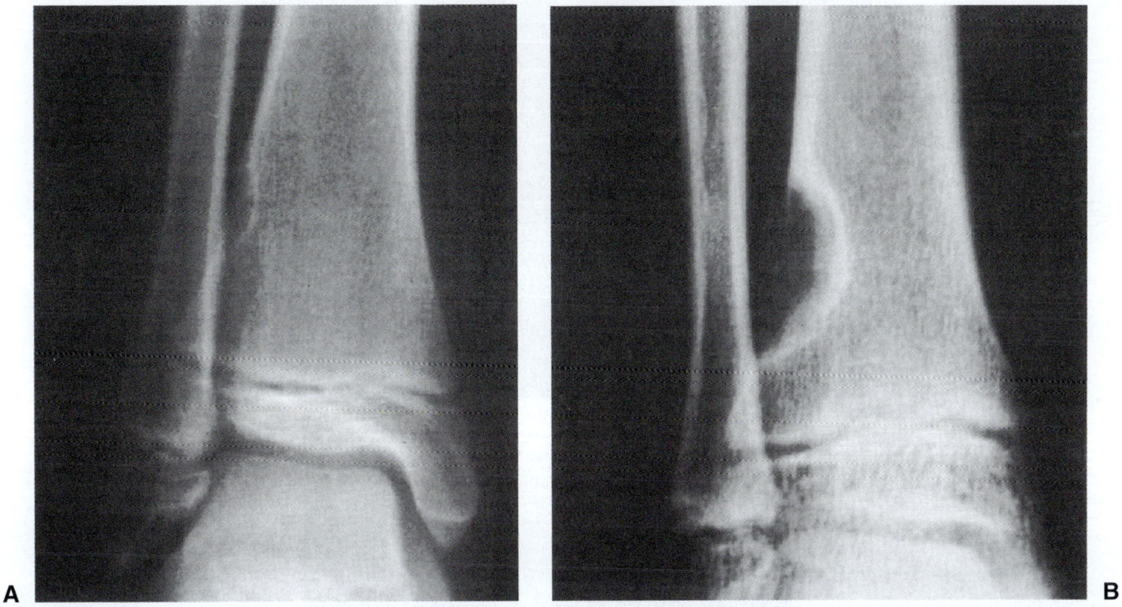

FIGURE 8.35 (A) Fibrous cortical defect. (B) When a fibrous cortical defect encroaches on the medullary cavity, it is called a nonossifying fibroma. (*Source:* Greenspan A, Remagen W. *Differential Diagnosis of Tumors and Tumor-like Lesions of Bones and Joints*. Philadelphia: Lippincott-Raven, 1998;207.)

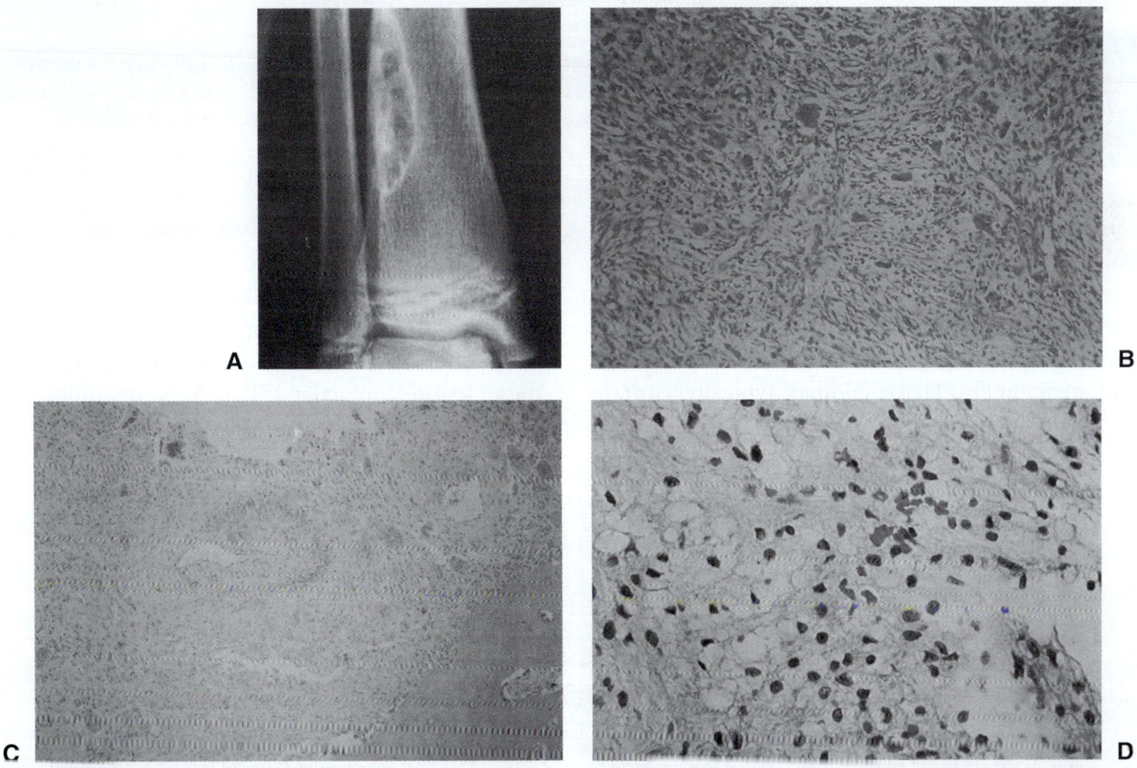

FIGURE 8.36 (A) Nonossifying fibroma. (B, C, D) Histopathology of nonossifying fibroma. (*Source:* Greenspan A, Remagen W. *Differential Diagnosis of Tumors and Tumor-like Lesions of Bones and Joints*. Philadelphia: Lippincott-Raven, 1998;207, 208.)

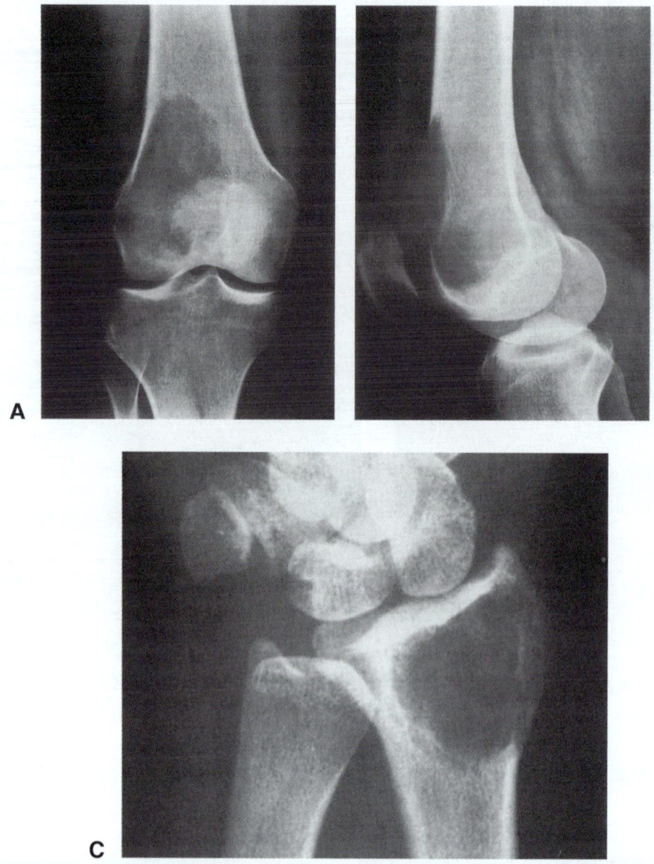

FIGURE 8.37 Giant cell tumor. (A) Anteroposterior and (B) lateral radiographs of a purely osteolytic lesion. (C) An eccentric osteolytic lesion. (*Source:* Greenspan A, Remagen W. *Differential Diagnosis of Tumors and Tumor-like Lesions of Bones and Joints*. Philadelphia: Lippincott-Raven, 1998;313.)

Hemangioma. When found in bone, these benign vascular tumors are often found in the vertebral bodies. Hemangiomas of the spine are common, occurring in approximately 10% of all adults. These lesions are rarely symptomatic and are typically found incidentally. Hemangiomas typically contain trabecular condensations surrounded by abnormal vascular channels, which are more lucent on plain films and CT, giving the vertebral body vertical striations on plain films, which are popularly referred to as the "jailhouse" vertebra (Fig. 8.39). The appearance of these lesions on axial CT images resembles polka

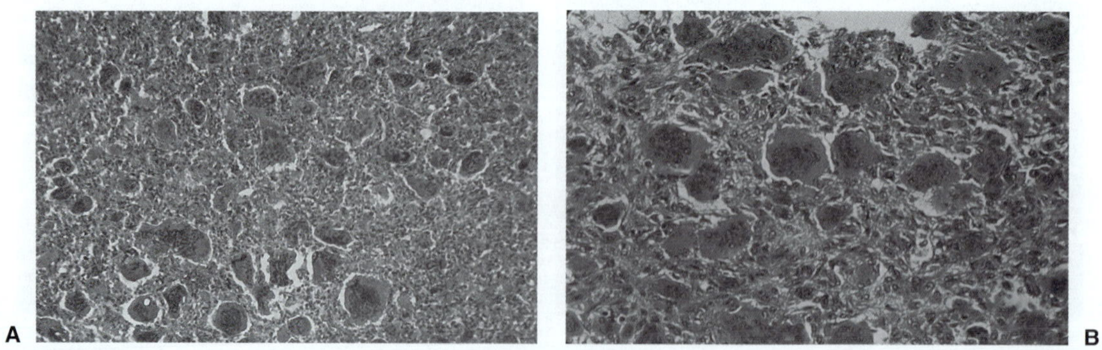

FIGURE 8.38 (A, B) Histopathology of a giant cell tumor. (*Source:* Greenspan A, Remagen W. *Differential Diagnosis of Tumors and Tumor-like Lesions of Bones and Joints*. Philadelphia: Lippincott-Raven, 1998;318.)

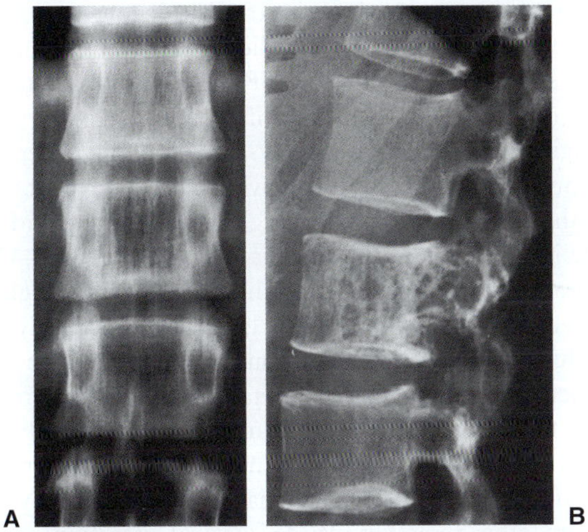

FIGURE 8.39 Vertebral hemangioma. (A) "Corduroy cloth" pattern. (B) "Honeycomb" pattern. (*Source:* Greenspan A, Remagen W. *Differential Diagnosis of Tumors and Tumor-like Lesions of Bones and Joints*. Philadelphia: Lippincott-Raven, 1998;291.)

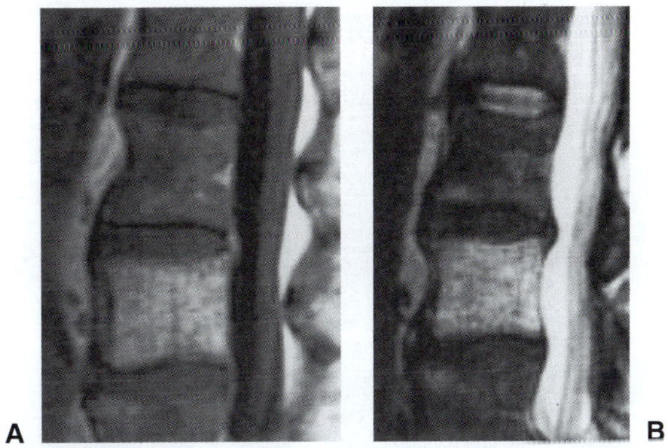

FIGURE 8.40 Vertebral hemangioma. (A) Sagittal T1-weighted and (B) T2-weighted MRI show high signal intensity lesion. (*Source:* Greenspan A, Remagen W. *Differential Diagnosis of Tumors and Tumor-like Lesions of Bones and Joints*. Philadelphia: Lippincott-Raven, 1998;292.)

dots. MRI images are provided in Figure 8.40 and histopathology in Figure 8.41. Asymptomatic hemangiomas rarely develop into symptomatic lesions. Symptomatic hemangiomas usually respond well to conservative surgical procedures. Selective arterial embolization may be a safer and more effective treatment than radiation. Anterior resection and fusion are reserved for pathologic collapse and neural compromise or refractory cases.

Osteofibrous Dysplasia (Kempson-Campanacci Lesion; Ossifying Fibroma). This rare condition is seen in the tibia of children younger than 10 years and is most often found in boys. The anterior diaphysis of the tibia is most commonly affected, often resulting in anterior cortical bowing. The lytic lesion with surrounding sclerosis creates a soap bubble appearance on radiographs, similar to that of fibrous dysplasia or adamantinoma (Fig. 8.42). Histologically, it is similar to fibrous dysplasia with a benign trabecular pattern within a fibrous stroma (Fig. 8.43). Osteofibrous dysplasia tends to involute spontaneously with skeletal maturity and recur if surgical intervention is performed before skeletal maturity. Therefore, surgical intervention should be limited to those with pain, impending fracture, or progressing deformity.

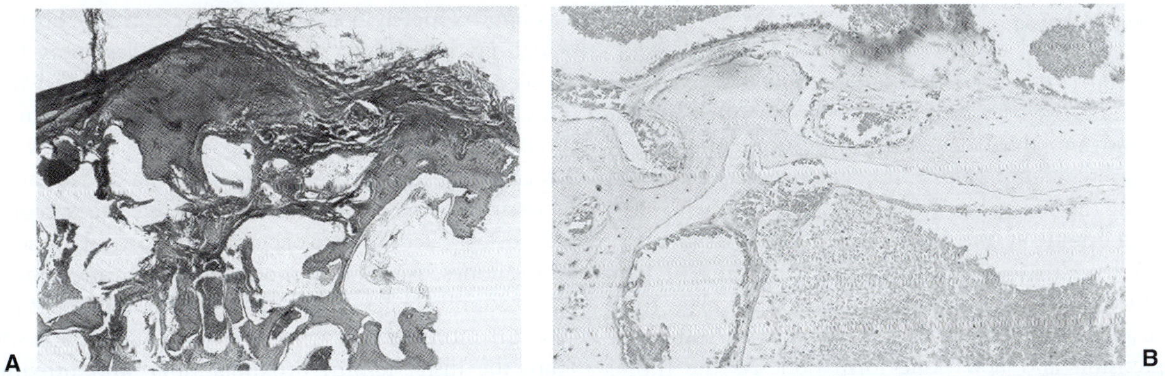

FIGURE 8.41 (A, B) Histopathology of cavernous intraosseous hemangioma. (*Source:* Greenspan A, Remagen W. *Differential Diagnosis of Tumors and Tumor-like Lesions of Bones and Joints*. Philadelphia: Lippincott-Raven, 1998;293.)

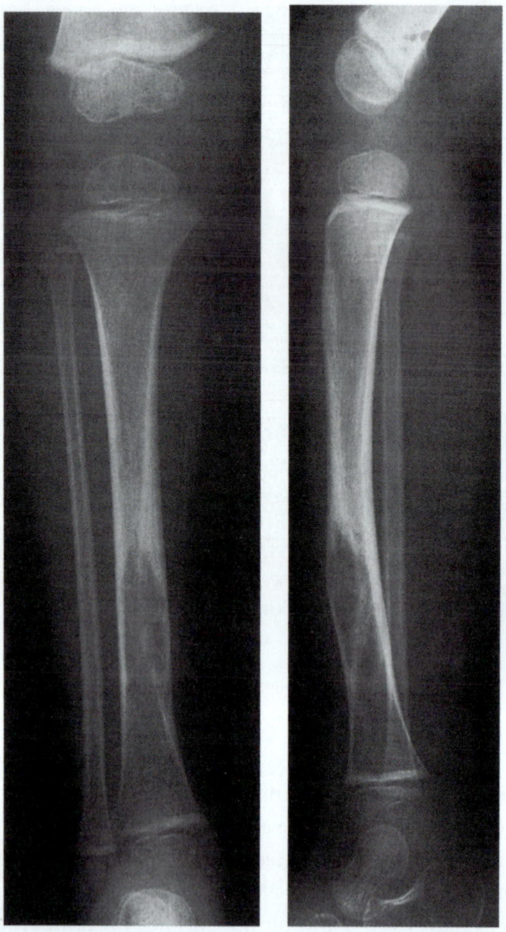

FIGURE 8.42 (A, B) Osteofibrous dysplasia. (*Source:* Greenspan A, Remagen W. *Differential Diagnosis of Tumors and Tumor-like Lesions of Bones and Joints.* Philadelphia: Lippincott-Raven, 1998;228.)

Primary Malignant

Bone Forming

Osteosarcoma (Osteogenic Sarcoma). The classic form of osteosarcoma is seen most often in the second and third decades, mostly occurring during the growth spurt (Fig. 8.44). The majority of lesions are in the metaphyses of the long bones, with 50% being found at the knee. Males are at higher risk (1.5 to 2). Most patients have symptoms of pain before a mass is noticed. Radiographically, these are permeative, metaphyseal lesions with soft tissue extension and new bone formation. As the tumor breaks through the cortex into the subperiosteal space, it forms a Codman triangle. Periosteal reaction is common, and frequently the new neoplastic bone takes on a sunburst or "hair on-end" appearance as the tumor continues to expand into the soft tissue (Fig. 8.45). Chest radiographs or CT studies are essential for evaluation of pulmonary metastasis. MRI provides anatomical information necessary in staging and planning surgery. Histologically, there is a presence of neoplastic woven bone (woven bone with no osteoblastic rimming) in association with a malignant spindle cell stroma (Figs. 8.46 and 8.47). Treatment consists of chemotherapy and wide surgical resection. Chemotherapy is given preoperatively to reduce tumor burden and kill malignant cells in the reactive zone and in micrometastases. Tumor necrosis due to chemotherapy is a prognostic indicator, with the survival rate of patients with more than 90% necrosis approaching 85%. Maintenance chemotherapy is given after resection. Wide surgical resection most often involves resection with reconstruction using replacement endoprostheses or allografts. Currently, with the use of adjuvant chemotherapy, limb salvage surgeries result in survival rates similar to those who receive radical amputations.

Hemorrhagic Osteosarcoma (Telangiectatic). Hemorrhagic osteosarcoma is a high-grade variant that is extremely lytic and destructive. On radiographs, it resembles an aneurysmal bone cyst (Fig. 8.48). Histologically, it is hemorrhagic with malignant stromal cells and giant cells (Fig. 8.49). The incidence of pathologic fracture is high because of the amount of destruction. When nearby neurovascular structures are contaminated, the possibility of limb salvage can be eliminated. Therefore, in patients at risk for pathologic fracture, earlier surgery or immobilization can reduce this risk. Treatment is otherwise similar to classic osteosarcoma with similar outcomes.

Parosteal Osteosarcoma. Parosteal osteosarcoma is a low-grade form of osteosarcoma. The tumor is well differentiated (Fig. 8.50), and when local control of the lesion is achieved, the risk of pulmonary metastases is approximately 5%. If the tumor contains areas of high-grade sarcoma (Fig. 8.51), the lesion is then called a dedifferentiated parosteal osteosarcoma, which has a higher rate of metastases. The approximate risk of pulmonary metastasis is 25% for low- to medium-grade parosteal osteosarcoma and 85% for classic, pagetoid, and radiation-induced osteosarcoma. Parosteal osteosarcoma occurs on the cortical surface of long bones, usually near the location of the metaphysis. It accounts for less than 5% of all osteosarcomas and occurs more often in females. The most common sites are the distal femur, proximal tibia, and proximal humerus. Treatment is wide surgical resection, which is often curative. Approximately 15% possess a high-grade component on histological analysis, which carries a worse prognosis and requires chemotherapy.

TABLE 8.11 Histologic grading of chondrosarcoma

Grade	Histologic Features
0.5 (borderline)	Histologic features similar to enchondroma, but radiographic features more aggressive.
1 (low-grade)	Cellularity: slightly increased. Cytologic atypia: slight increase in size and variation in shape of the nuclei; slightly increased hyperchromasia of the nuclei. Binucleation: few binucleate cells are present. Stromal myxoid change: may or may not present.
2 (intermediate)	Cellularity: moderately increased. Cytologic atypia: moderate increase in size and variation in shape of the nuclei; moderately increased hyperchromasia of the nuclei. Binucleation: large number of double- and tri-nucleated cells. Stromal myxoid change: focally present.
3 (high-grade)	Cellularity: markedly increased. Cytologic atypia: marked enlargement and irregularity of the nuclei; markedly increased hyperchromasia of the nuclei. Binucleation: large number of double- and multi-nucleated cells. Stromal myxoid change: commonly present. Other: small foci of spindling at the periphery of the lobules of chondrocytes.

Modified from Dahlin and Unni, 1988.

Source: Greenspan A, Remagen W. *Differential Diagnosis of Tumors and Tumor-like Lesions of Bones and Joints.* Philadelphia: Lippincott-Raven, 1998;173.

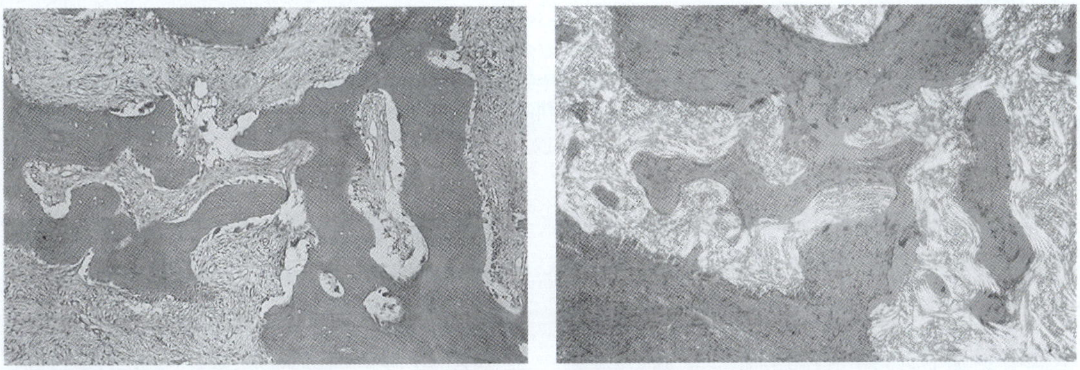

FIGURE 8.43 (A, B) Histopathology of osteofibrous dysplasia. (*Source:* Greenspan A, Remagen W. *Differential Diagnosis of Tumors and Tumor-like Lesions of Bones and Joints.* Philadelphia: Lippincott-Raven, 1998;228.)

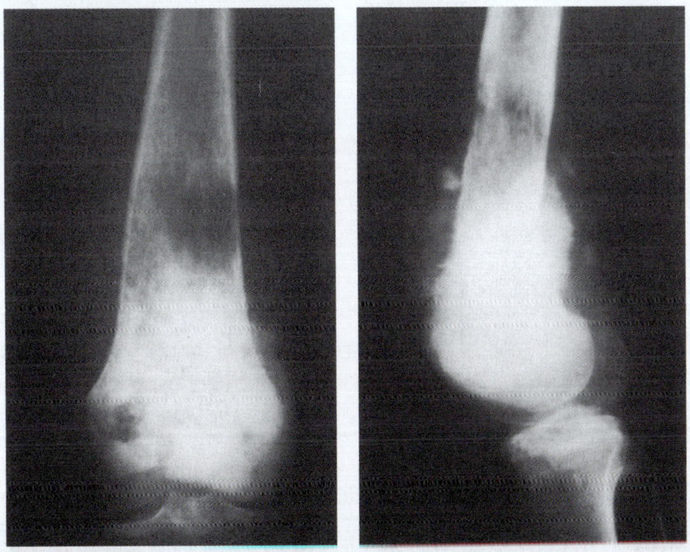

FIGURE 8.44 Conventional osteosarcoma. (A) Anteroposterior. (B) Lateral. (*Source:* Greenspan A, Remagen W. *Differential Diagnosis of Tumors and Tumor-like Lesions of Bones and Joints*. Philadelphia: Lippincott-Raven, 1998;65.)

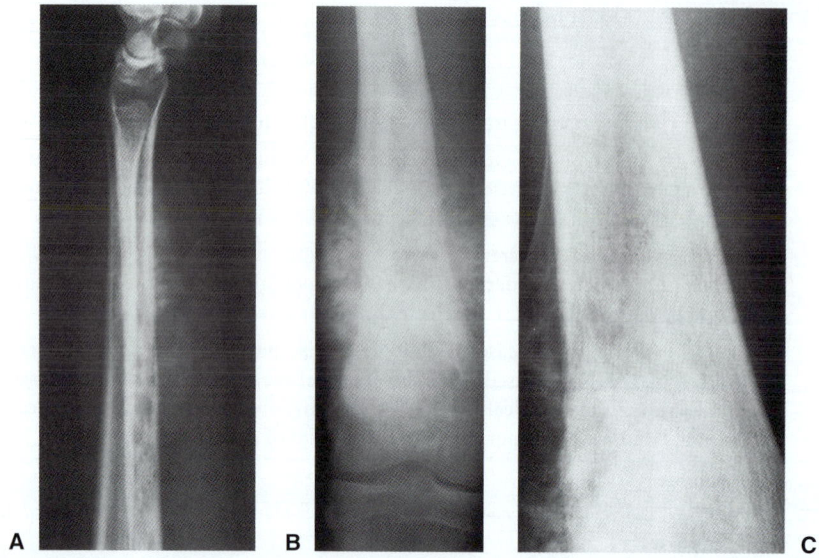

FIGURE 8.45 Types of periosteal reaction in osteosarcoma. (A, B) Sunburst type is the most common. (C) Typical Codman triangle in the distal femur. (*Source:* Greenspan A, Remagen W. *Differential Diagnosis of Tumors and Tumor-like Lesions of Bones and Joints*. Philadelphia: Lippincott-Raven, 1998;67.)

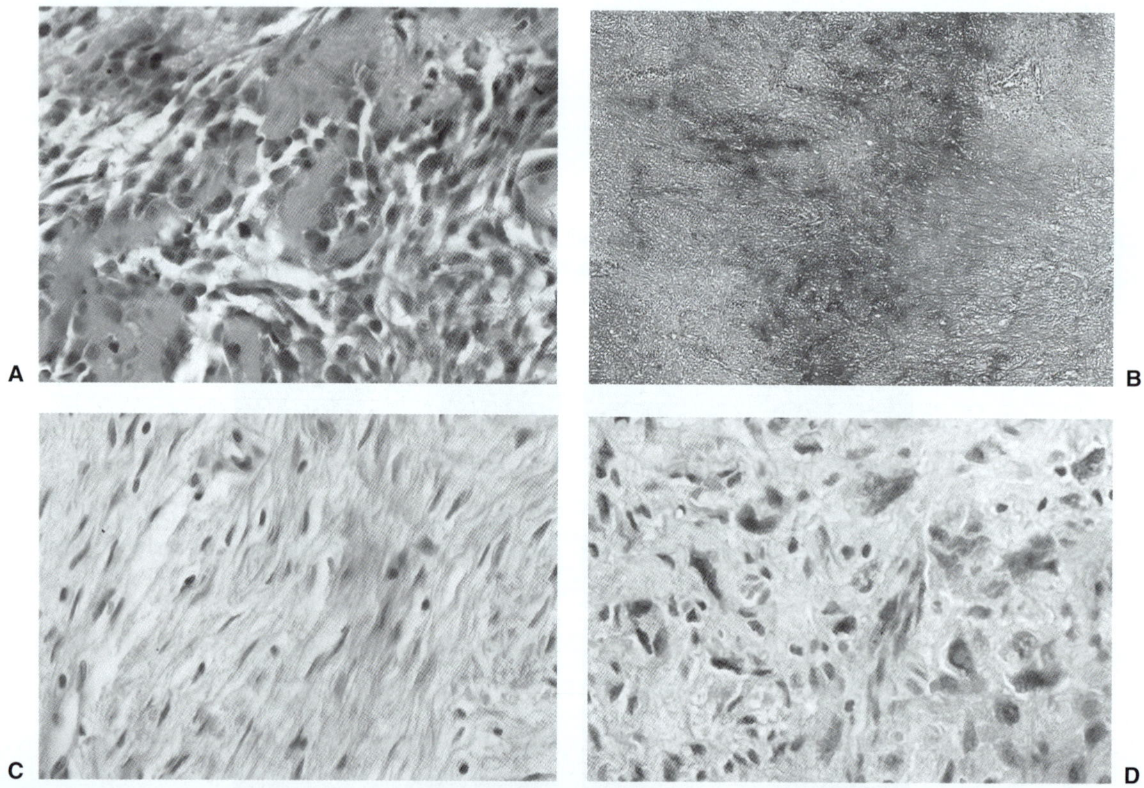

FIGURE 8.46 Histologic subtypes of osteosarcoma. (A) Osteoblastic. (B) Chondroblastic. (C) Fibroblastic. (D) Fibroblastic with malignant cells producing osteoid. (*Source:* Greenspan A, Remagen W. *Differential Diagnosis of Tumors and Tumor-like Lesions of Bones and Joints*. Philadelphia: Lippincott-Raven, 1998;74; *D. Courtesy of* Dr. L. Wold, Rochester, MN.)

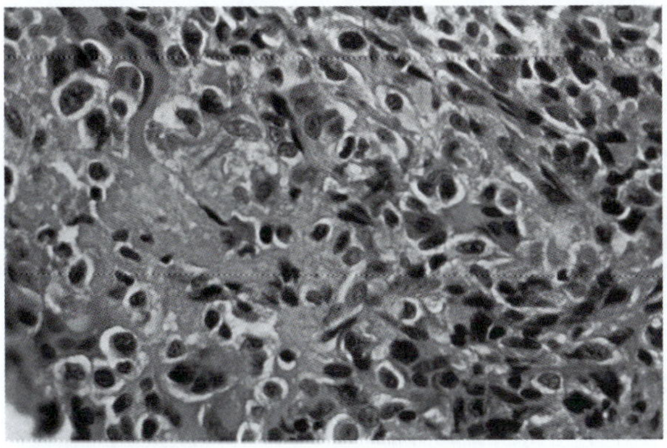

FIGURE 8.47 **Histopathology of conventional osteosarcoma. (*Source:* Greenspan A, Remagen W. *Differential Diagnosis of Tumors and Tumor-like Lesions of Bones and Joints.* Philadelphia: Lippincott-Raven, 1998;75.)**

Periosteal Osteosarcoma. A surface-based osteosarcoma arising in long bones, periosteal osteosarcoma occurs typically in the diaphyses and is low to intermediate in grade. It accounts for less than 2% of all osteosarcoma. The most common sites are the distal femur, proximal tibia, and proximal humerus. It arises under the periosteum, giving rise to the typical radiographic appearance of a sunburst-type lesion over a depressed cortical base (Figs. 8.52 and 8.53). Treatment is wide surgical resection, with adjuvant chemotherapy in more advanced, higher grade lesions.

Secondary Osteosarcoma. Secondary osteosarcoma may arise from many benign conditions including fibrous dysplasia, giant cell tumor, osteoblastoma, osteochondroma, Paget disease, and chronic osteomyelitis. The classic example of secondary osteosarcoma is that due to Paget, most commonly found in the humerus (Figs. 8.54 and 8.55). The prognosis in pagetoid osteosarcoma is very poor, with less than 10% surviving 5 years. Chemotherapeutic and surgical options may be limited by the old age and fragility of these patients. Radiation-induced osteosarcoma (Fig. 8.56) can result after any significant radiation exposure, typically greater than 30 Gy. The average delay in onset is approximately 15 years but can vary widely. These osteosarcomas carry a poor prognosis and have a high rate of metastasis.

Chondroid Forming

Chondrosarcoma. These common malignant cartilage tumors are primarily tumors of adulthood and old age. They also cause pain. About 85% of chondrosarcomas are low-grade and slow-growing. Chondrosarcomas are active lesions that grow and alter the host bone over time. Changes associated with chondrosarcoma include intralesional lysis, endosteal scalloping, cortical thinning, and expansion (Fig. 8.57). Most will show chondroid calcification, but high-grade lesions may take on a purely lytic appearance. Histological grading of chondrosarcoma is presented in Table 8.11 and Figure 8.58. Chondrosarcomas are relatively resistant to radiation and chemotherapy. Chondrosarcomas tend to recur locally and require complete surgical resection with a wide margin of uninvolved tissue to achieve cure. The treatment of low-grade

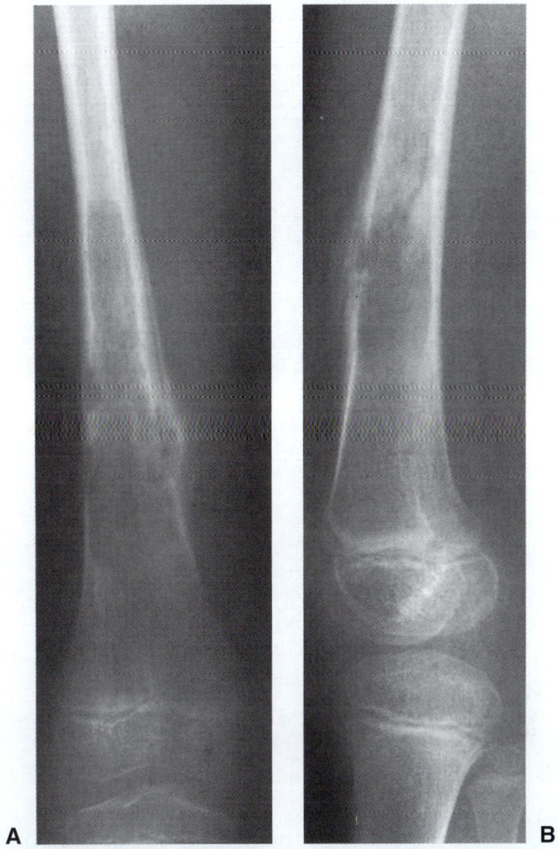

FIGURE 8.48 **Hemorrhagic (telangiectatic) osteosarcoma. (A) Predominantly lytic tumor associated with periosteal reaction. (B) Lateral view reveals an oblique pathologic fracture. (*Source:* Greenspan A, Remagen W. *Differential Diagnosis of Tumors and Tumor-like Lesions of Bones and Joints.* Philadelphia: Lippincott-Raven, 1998;79. *Courtesy of* Dr. K.K. Unni, Rochester, MN.)**

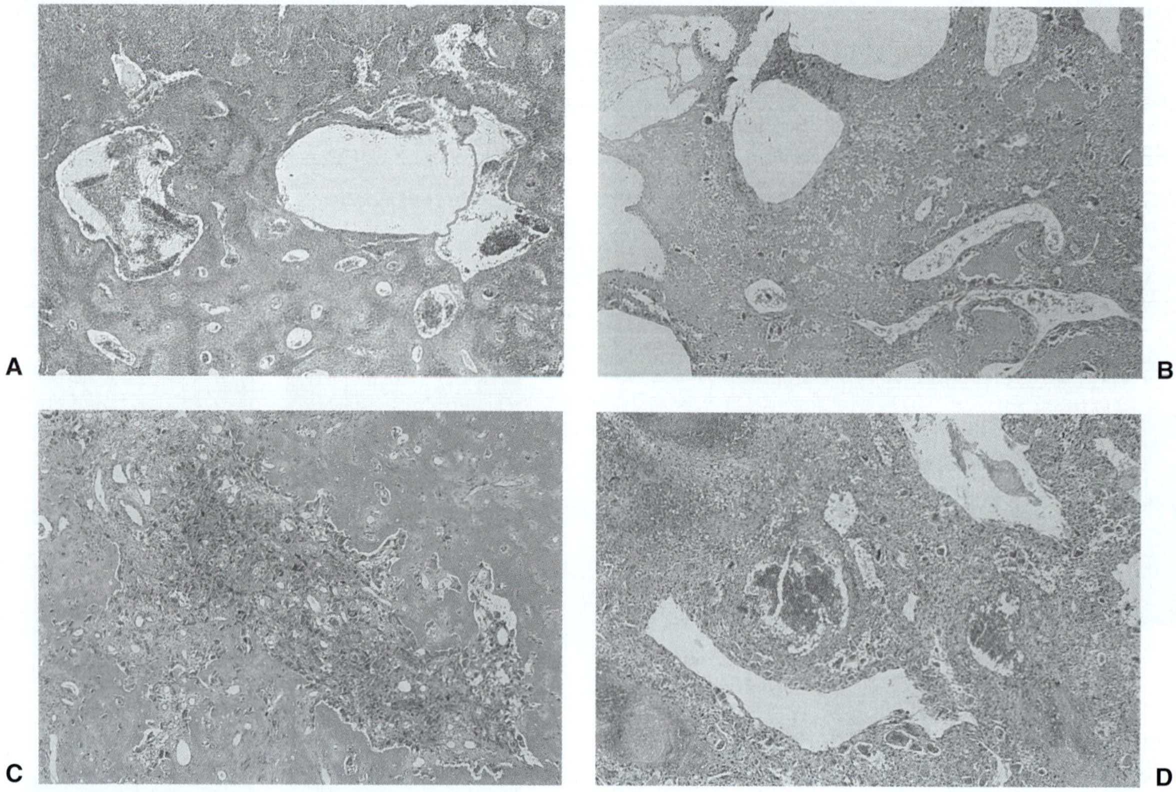

FIGURE 8.49 **(A–D) Histopathology of hemorrhagic osteosarcoma. (*Source:* Greenspan A, Remagen W. *Differential Diagnosis of Tumors and Tumor-like Lesions of Bones and Joints*. Philadelphia: Lippincott-Raven, 1998;80.)**

chondrosarcomas is somewhat controversial: some clinicians prefer aggressive intralesional curettage and adjuvant therapy with phenol or liquid nitrogen; others prefer wide excision. For intermediate and high-grade chondrosarcoma, wide margins are required.

Enchondromas and chondrosarcomas are both intramedullary cartilage lesions. In the adult patient, enchondromas do not grow. When an intramedullary cartilage lesion grows and destroys the bone, the lesion is very likely a chondrosarcoma. The hallmark feature of almost all chondrosarcomas is involvement of the cortical bone. Erosion of the cortex (more than 50% of cortex), cortical thickening, and destruction of the cortex are worrisome for chondrosarcoma.

Nonosseus, Nonchondroid

Ewing Sarcoma. Ewing sarcoma is an undifferentiated tumor in the family of neural tumors. It is characterized by the t(11;22) translocation in 90% of cases. It occurs primarily in patients between 5 and 25 years of age. Males are affected more frequently. Twenty percent of patients will have associated systemic symptoms such as fever, chills, and a high erythrocyte sedimentation rate and white blood cell count, which may cause the lesion to mimic osteomyelitis. Ewing classically presents as a diaphyseal, permeative lesion with "onion skin" periosteal reaction and a large, associated soft tissue mass. Other times it may be more metaphyseal and destructive. The most common locations are the femur, pelvis, tibia, and humerus (Fig. 8.59). Histologically, Ewing consists of small, round cells arranged in sheets (Fig. 8.60). Ewing is an aggressive disease with approximately 20% having metastases on presentation. Those with locally resectable disease fare well, but those with advanced metastatic disease have a 30% survival rate at 5 years. Excision of lung metastases, if possible, can improve survival. Treatment is typically preoperative chemotherapy, wide surgical excision, and maintenance chemotherapy. Ewing is a radiosensitive tumor, and studies have not clearly demonstrated that surgery improves survival without radiation. Therefore, in contaminated margins, postoperative radiation is needed. Radiation may replace surgical resection in areas where wide surgical excision is either impossible or associated with poor outcome.

Solitary Lymphoma. Lymphoma and myeloma are the two most common malignant hematopoietic tumors found in bone. Lymphoma may present as an isolated

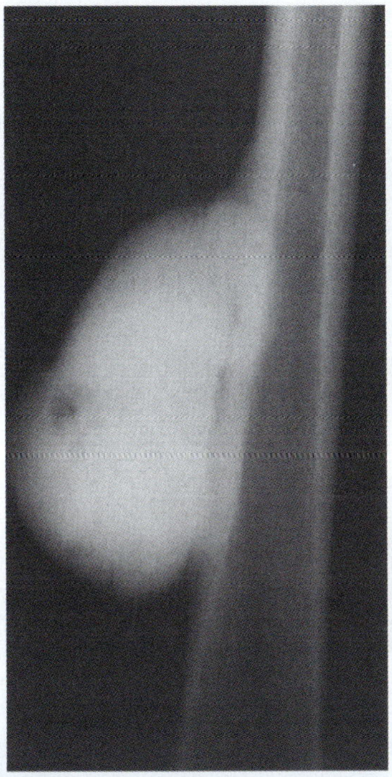

FIGURE 8.50 **Parosteal osteosarcoma. (*Source:* Greenspan A, Remagen W. *Differential Diagnosis of Tumors and Tumor-like Lesions of Bones and Joints*. Philadelphia: Lippincott-Raven, 1998;89.)**

tumor within bone, referred to in the past as reticulum cell sarcoma, or as a systemic disease. Primary lymphomas of the bone account for 3% of all malignant bone tumors. These patients typically have none of the general constitutional complaints so commonly associated with systemic lymphoma, even when lesions are extensive. However, those lesions that involve the spine frequently have neurologic symptoms. Lymphoma is typically a very permeative but minimally destructive lesion. The usual progression is that lymphomas fill up the medullary canal and then grow into the surrounding soft tissues while causing little destruction of the bone itself. X-rays may be remarkably normal, while MRI scans show marrow replacement and often an associated soft tissue mass (Figs. 8.61 and 8.62). Histopathology is shown in Figures 8.63 and 8.64. Surgical intervention is typically reserved for select cases to achieve local control, but treatment centers around radiation and multiagent chemotherapy.

Solitary Myeloma (Plasma Cell Tumor). Solitary myeloma is one of many B-cell lymphoproliferative diseases, which include multiple myeloma. True solitary myeloma is relatively rare, constituting only 3% of all plasma cell neoplasms. Monoclonal proteins are more often absent or undetectable in solitary myeloma compared to multiple myeloma. Diagnostic criteria for solitary myeloma includes solitary lesion on skeletal survey, histologic confirmation, and bone marrow plasmacytosis of less than 10%. Solitary myeloma is an isolated lesion, and treatment may result in cure. Treatment of choice in solitary plasmacytoma and multiple myeloma is radiation. The prognosis for patients with solitary plasmacytoma is much better than that for multiple myeloma. Surgical intervention is typically reserved for decompression of neural structures in the case of spinal involvement and stabilization in cases of severe destruction. Postoperative adjuvant radiation is recommended. Surgery is the treatment of choice for recurrent lesions or those that do not respond to radiotherapy in which en bloc resection and prophylactic reconstruction with repeat radiotherapy may provide extended disease-free survival. Dissemination of myeloma can occur

A 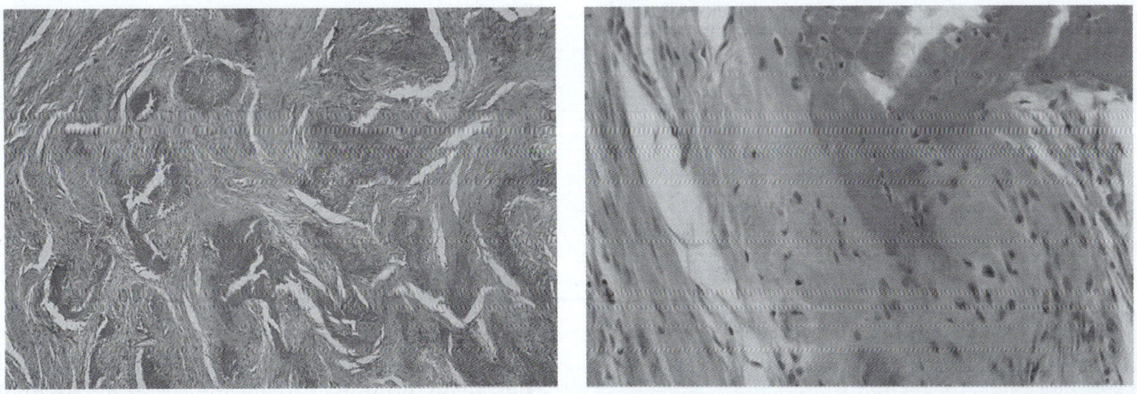 B

FIGURE 8.51 **(A, B) Histopathology of parosteal osteosarcoma. (*Source:* Greenspan A, Remagen W. *Differential Diagnosis of Tumors and Tumor-like Lesions of Bones and Joints*. Philadelphia: Lippincott-Raven, 1998;90.)**

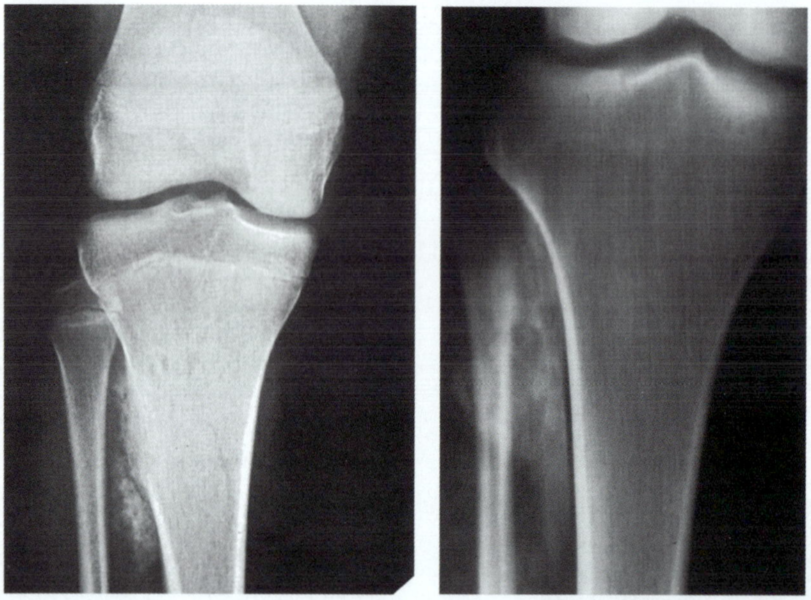

FIGURE 8.52 (A, B) Periosteal osteosarcoma. (*Source:* Greenspan A, Remagen W. *Differential Diagnosis of Tumors and Tumor-like Lesions of Bones and Joints*. Philadelphia: Lippincott-Raven, 1998;91.)

after years of disease-free survival, and patients should undergo regularly scheduled follow-up. MRI provides the earliest indication of local recurrence, and serum protein electrophoresis (SPEP) has proven to be the best indicator of dissemination. The treatment for disseminated myeloma is systemic chemotherapy.

Multiple Myeloma. Radiographic appearance of multiple myeloma is shown in Figures 8.65 and 8.66.

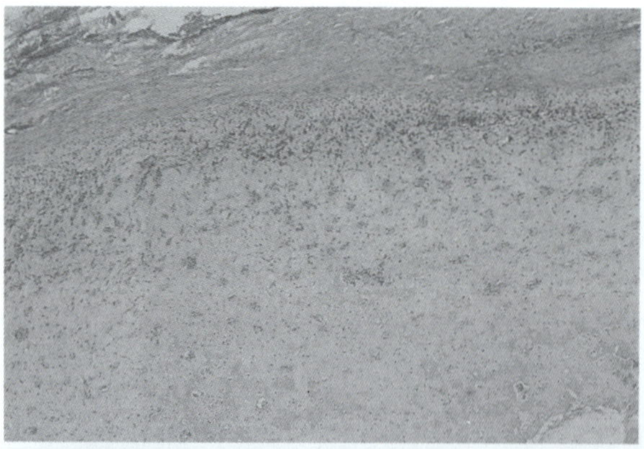

FIGURE 8.53 Histopathology of periosteal osteosarcoma. (*Source:* Greenspan A, Remagen W. *Differential Diagnosis of Tumors and Tumor-like Lesions of Bones and Joints*. Philadelphia: Lippincott-Raven, 1998;93.)

Brown tumors appear in Figure 8.67 and Gaucher disease in Figure 8.68.

Malignant Fibrous Histiocytoma (MFH). MFH is an aggressive tumor found in bone and in soft tissue. When in bone, it is most commonly found in the femur, tibia, innominate, and humerus. A painful, fixed mass adjacent to a major joint is a common presentation. Pain, tenderness, and localized swelling are also common. Radiographically, these lesions are variable in size and located centrally within the bone (Fig. 8.69). Cortical destruction with soft tissue extension is very common. Osseous expansion is unusual but may occur in flat and irregular bones. Histological diagnosis is often made by exclusion. The tumor is composed of fibroblasts in a storiform pattern with giant and inflammatory cells (Fig. 8.70). MFH is characterized by a high rate of local recurrence and metastasis. The mainstay of treatment of low-grade nonmetastatic MFH is wide surgical excision, while high-grade lesions are treated with preoperative chemotherapy similar to that of osteosarcoma.

Adamantinoma. A rare tumor of long bones, adamantinoma is predominately found in the anterior cortex of the midtibia. Patients typically present with pain, months to years in duration. Radiographically, adamantinoma usually appears as a soap bubble sclerotic lesion and can mimic cortical fibrous dysplasia (Fig. 8.71). Cortical fibrous dysplasia occurs predominately in males in the first two decades, while adamantinoma occurs in both sexes and all ages,

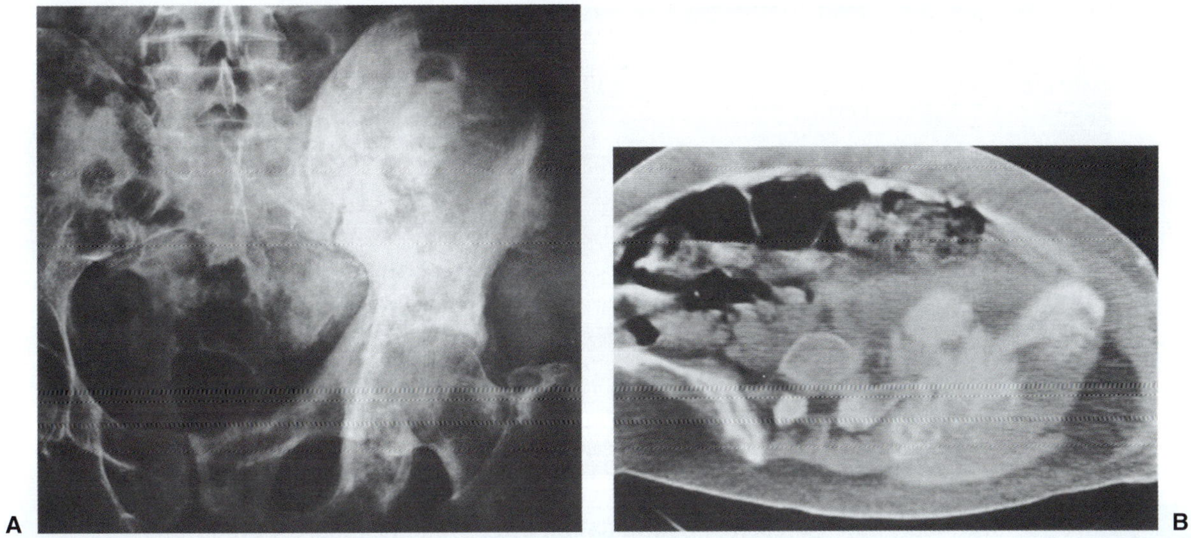

FIGURE 8.54 Secondary osteosarcoma: Paget sarcoma. (A) Anteroposterior radiograph of the pelvis. (B) CT scan demonstrates bone formation in soft tissue more clearly. (*Source:* Greenspan A, Remagen W. *Differential Diagnosis of Tumors and Tumor-like Lesions of Bones and Joints*. Philadelphia: Lippincott-Raven, 1998;97.)

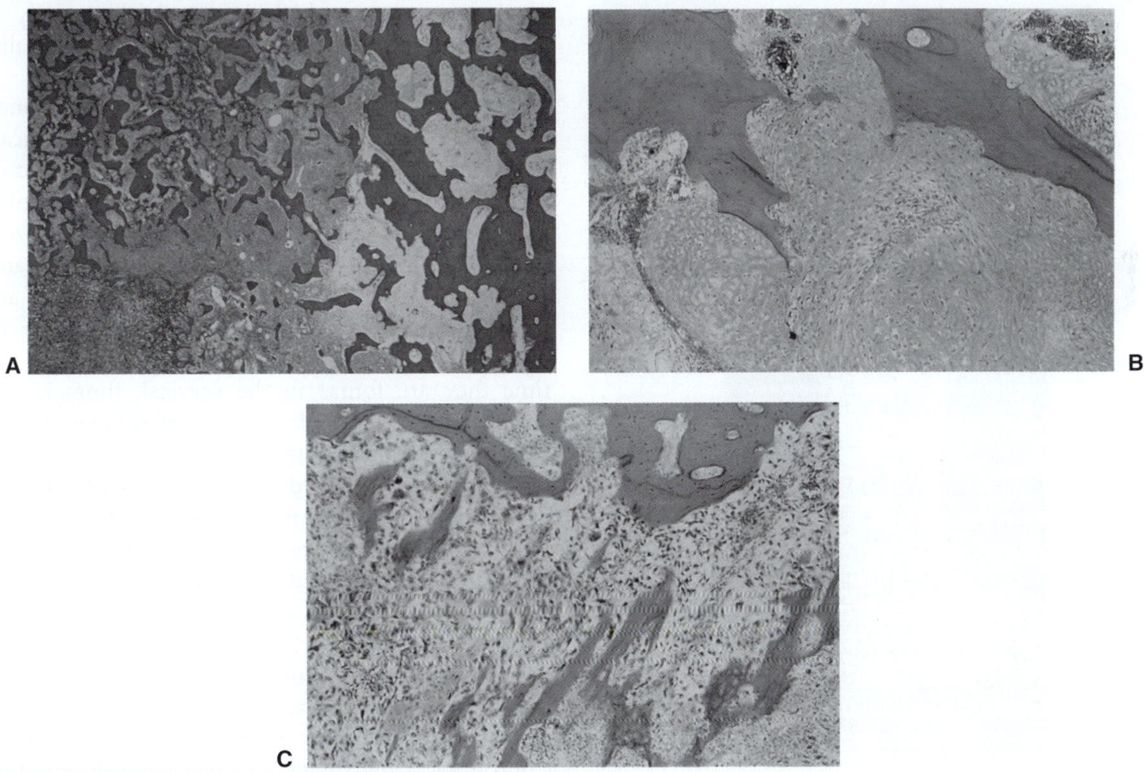

FIGURE 8.55 (A, B, C) Histopathology of Paget sarcoma. (*Source:* Greenspan A, Remagen W. *Differential Diagnosis of Tumors and Tumor-like Lesions of Bones and Joints*. Philadelphia: Lippincott-Raven, 1998;98.)

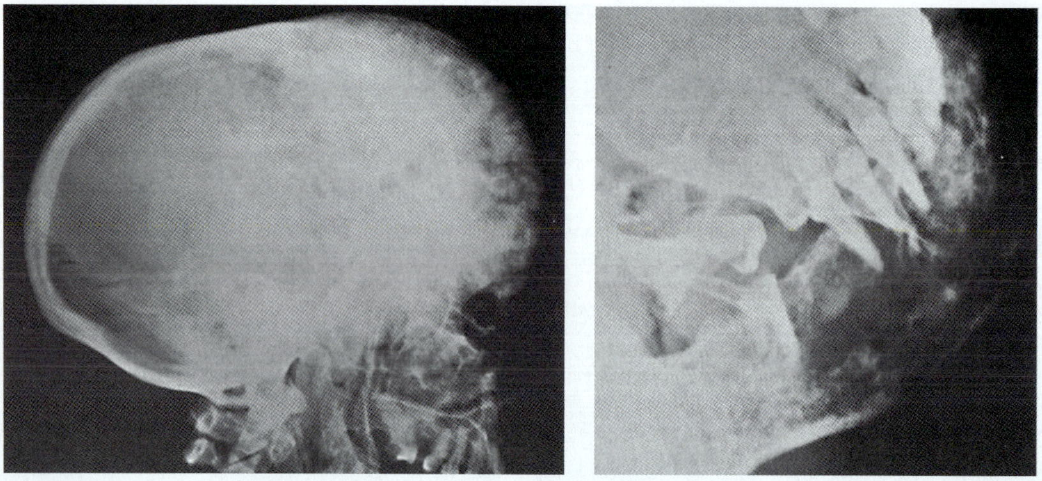

FIGURE 8.56 Secondary osteosarcoma: Postirradiation osteosarcoma. (*Source:* Greenspan A, Remagen W. *Differential Diagnosis of Tumors and Tumor-like Lesions of Bones and Joints*. Philadelphia: Lippincott-Raven, 1998;98.)

though typically during the first four decades. Histologically, adamantinoma is a low-grade spindle cell sarcoma with islands of epithelial cells that may resemble cutaneous basal cells (Fig. 8.72). A second pattern consists of islands of neoplastic cells surrounded by columnar cells in a palisading fashion. These findings are usually fairly diagnostic when seen with the usual presentation via imaging studies. Treatment is wide surgical resection, which is often followed by an allograft reconstruction over an intramedullary nail.

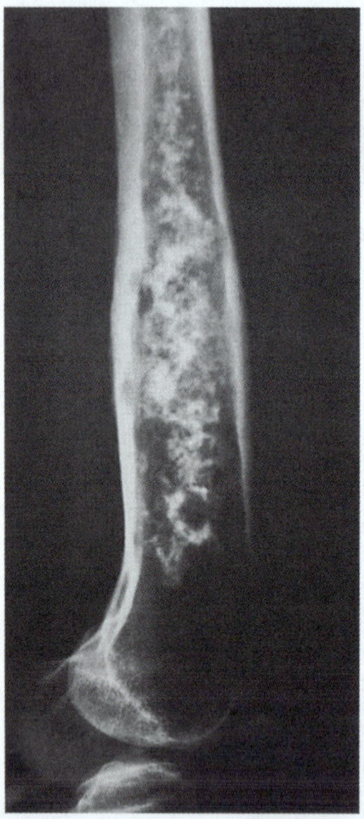

FIGURE 8.57 Conventional chondrosarcoma. (*Source:* Greenspan A, Remagen W. *Differential Diagnosis of Tumors and Tumor-like Lesions of Bones and Joints*. Philadelphia: Lippincott-Raven, 1998;176.)

Chordoma. Chordoma is a low-grade sarcoma and a relatively common malignancy of the spine typically found in patients in their fourth to sixth decade. It accounts for approximately 6% of all primary malignant bone tumors. Chordomas always localize to the midline, arise from primitive notochord remnants, and are primarily found in the sacrococcygeal area (47%) and spheno-occipital region (38%) in the base of the skull (Fig. 8.73). The rest of the time they are found in the cervical, thoracic, and lumbar areas. Approximately 5% of patients develop metastases. Clinically, these lesions present with low back pain of varying duration and frequently with a history of referred pain or numbness involving the rectum and perineum. It is essential for the clinician to recognize that normal sciatica does not cause pain in a perineal distribution and that pain or numbness referred to this area is indicative of a pelvis tumor compromising the sacral plexus until proven otherwise. Initial symptoms are typically mild in nature and progress as the tumor slowly enlarges. Chordomas grow slowly and progressively, reaching considerable size before metastasizing, sometimes causing nerve root compression, constipation, and urinary frequency. Occasionally, an advanced, very large chordoma can be palpated posteriorly on rectal examination. Histologically, chordoma has a typical presentation showing a myxoid or loose appearing mucinous lesion with strands or chords of syncytial

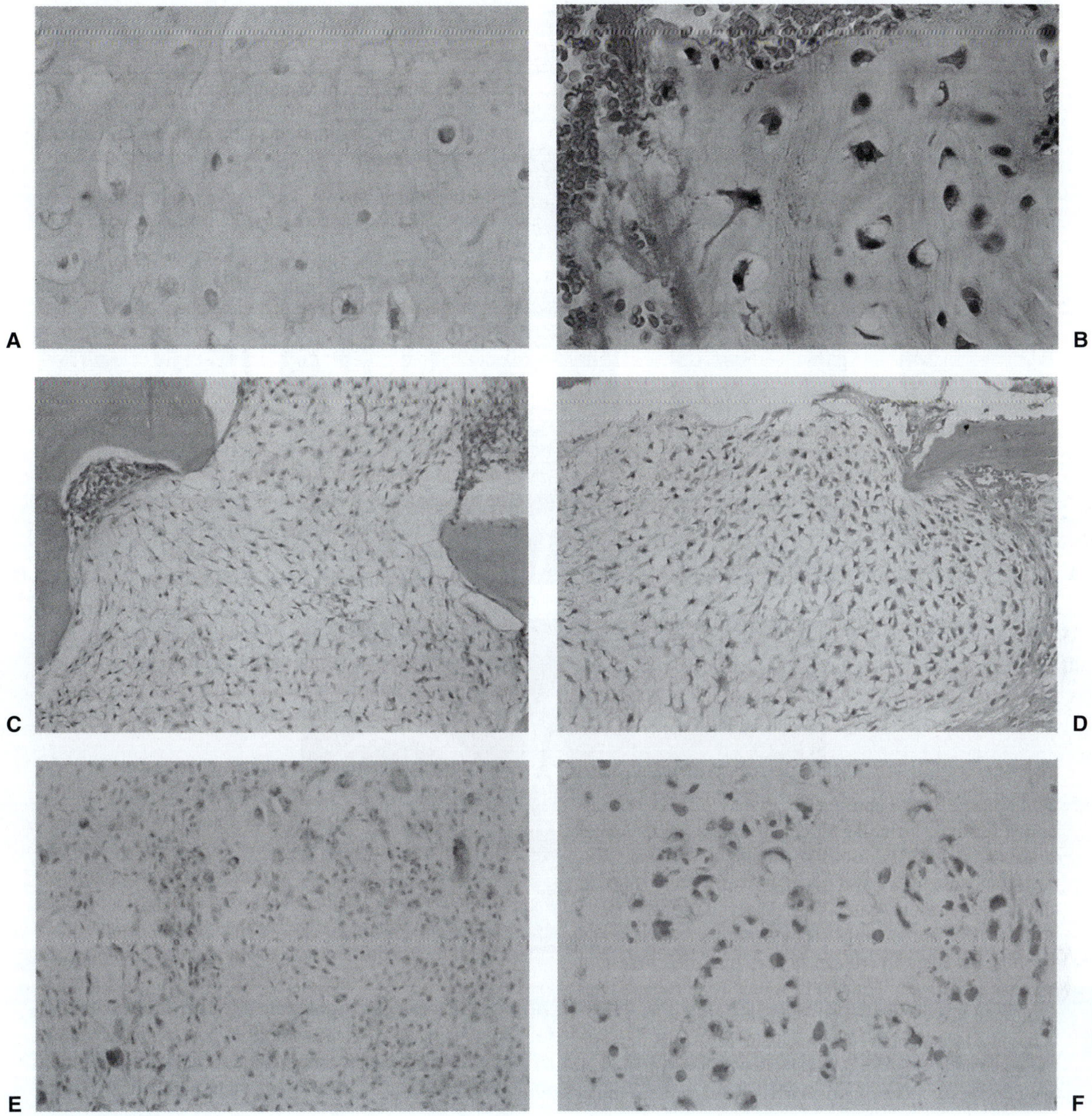

FIGURE 8.58 **Histologic grades of chondrosarcoma. (A, B) Grade 1. (C, D) Grade 2. (E, F) Grade 3. (*Source:* Greenspan A, Remagen W. *Differential Diagnosis of Tumors and Tumor-like Lesions of Bones and Joints.* Philadelphia: Lippincott-Raven, 1998;174.)**

cells where the cell margins are indistinct and the cells flow together (Fig. 8.74). Also, physaliferous ("foam") cells, which are large multivacuolated cells that take on a foamy appearance, can be seen. All of these cells float in a mucinous matrix that gives the tissue a very runny texture. While this lesion is usually characteristic, the histologic pattern may occasionally mimic chondrosarcoma. Surgical resection with wide margins is the only curative procedure.

Metastatic. The most common primary malignancies that metastasize to the bone are breast, lung, kidney, prostate, and thyroid carcinomas, which account for approximately 700,000 new cases annually. On autopsy, patients with cancer of the breast, lungs, prostate, and kidney have metastases to bone approximately 50% of the time. Skeletal metastases are most common in the elderly. However, certain metastatic tumors to bone are more likely to occur in children: Ewing sarcoma and osteosarcoma (from other skeletal sites), neuroblastoma, and rhabdomyosarcoma. The origins of osteolytic and osteoblastic metastases are shown in Figs. 8.75 and 8.76, and examples of appearance are shown in Figure 8.77.

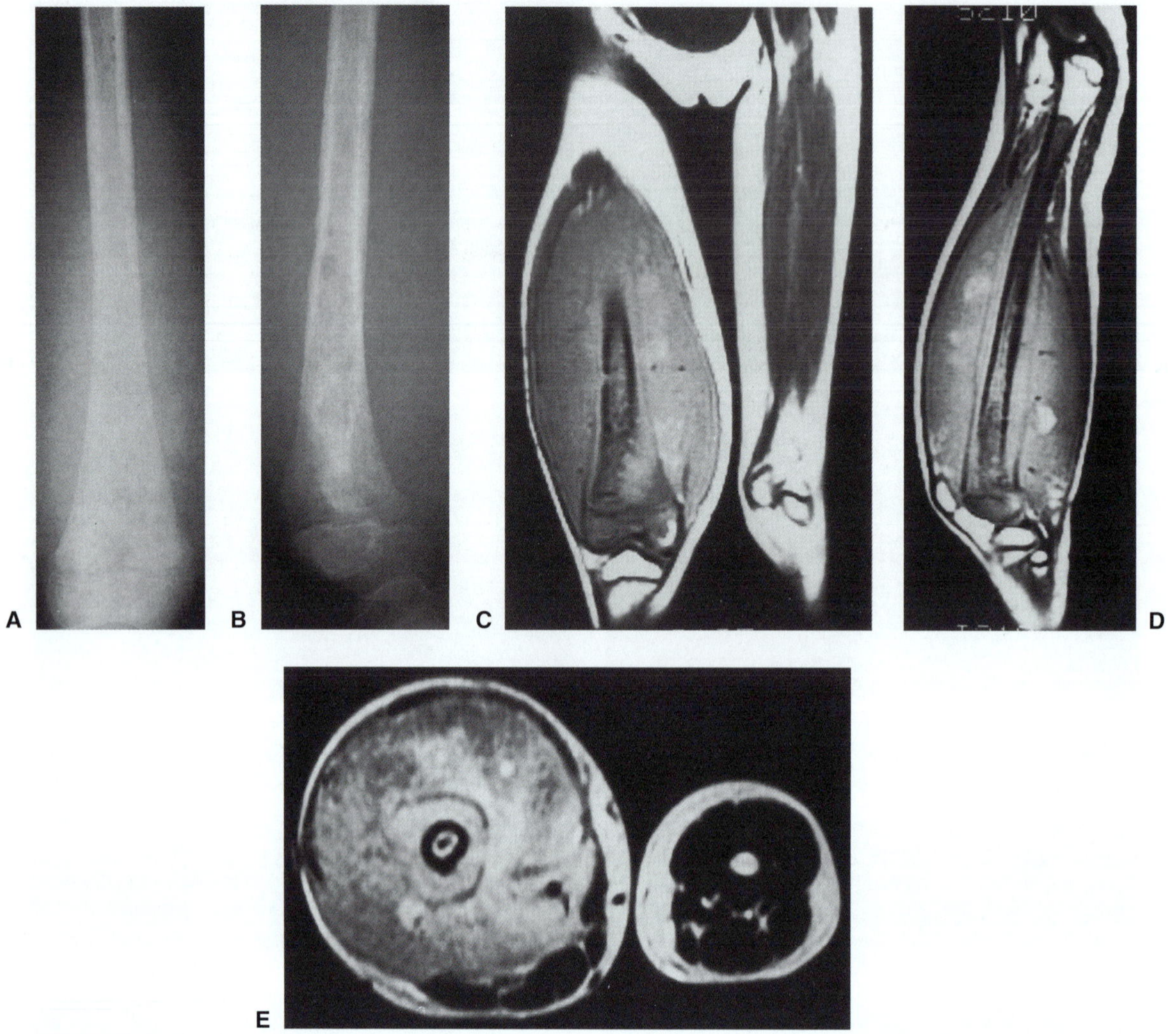

FIGURE 8.59 **Ewing sarcoma. (A) Anteroposterior and (B) lateral radiographs. (C) Coronal and (D) sagittal T1-weighted MRI. (E) Axial T2-weighted MRI. (*Source:* Greenspan A, Remagen W. *Differential Diagnosis of Tumors and Tumor-like Lesions of Bones and Joints*. Philadelphia: Lippincott-Raven, 1998;260.)**

IV. IMAGING

Subsequent to a careful history and physical examination, assessment of the imaging studies becomes the next step in evaluation. Plain radiographs offer detailed information for skeletal lesions. It is necessary to take good-quality plain radiographs, at least two views (anteroposterior and lateral), showing the entire involved bone including the joint above and below. It is estimated that about 30% to 40% of the bone must be destroyed before the changes can be seen in plain radiographs. It is useful to ask some questions when evaluating plain radiographs of bony lesions:

- Where is the lesion located in the bone?
- What is the lesion doing to the bone?
- What is the bone doing to the lesion?
- What is the periosteal response?

Bone metastases are typically seen in one of three patterns: predominantly lytic, mixed lytic-blastic, and purely blastic (Table 8.12). The type of bone destruction (geographic, moth-eaten, or permeative) may suggest a benign or a malignant process. The cortex and periosteum adjacent to the tumor are involved in the response of the bone to the neoplastic process. The lesion may be contained by the cortex or walled off by dense, sclerotic bone, implying a very slow-growing or static lesion, or it may destroy the cortex and form a soft tissue mass, indicating an aggressive neoplastic process. The pattern of periosteal reaction is also an indicator of

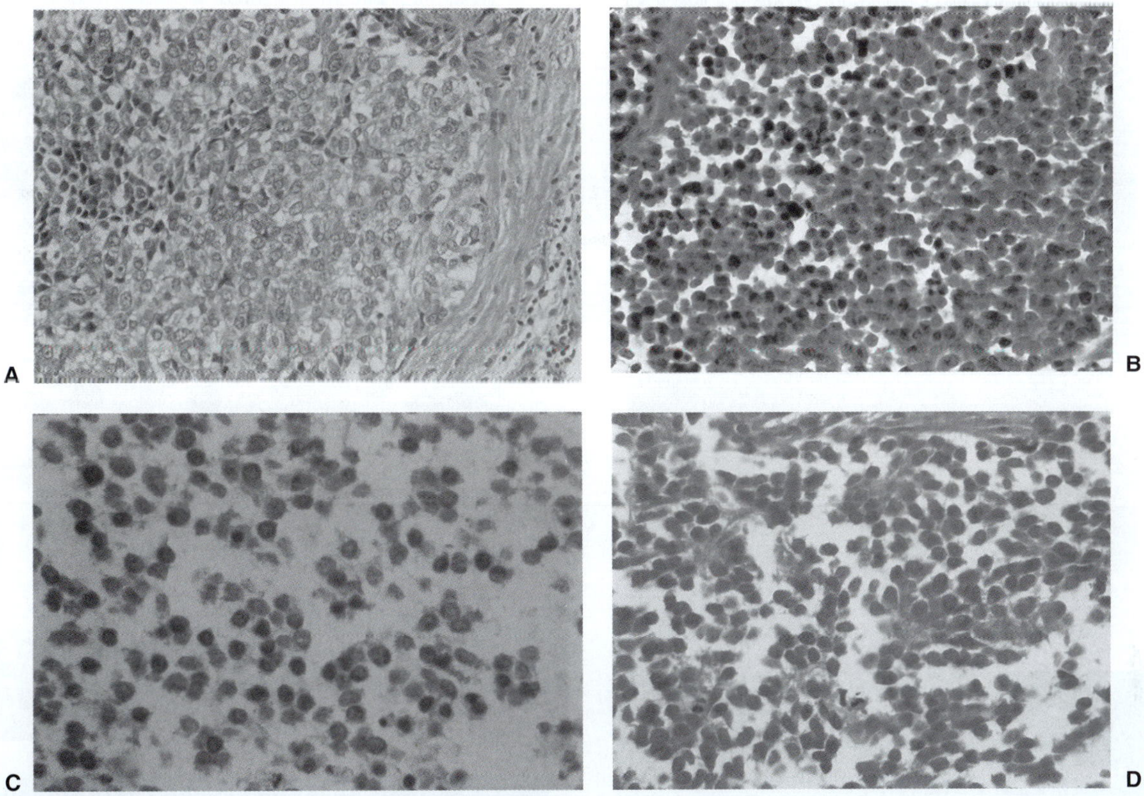

FIGURE 8.60 (A–D) Histopathology of Ewing sarcoma. (*Source:* Greenspan A, Remagen W. *Differential Diagnosis of Tumors and Tumor-like Lesions of Bones and Joints*. Philadelphia: Lippincott-Raven, 1998;261.)

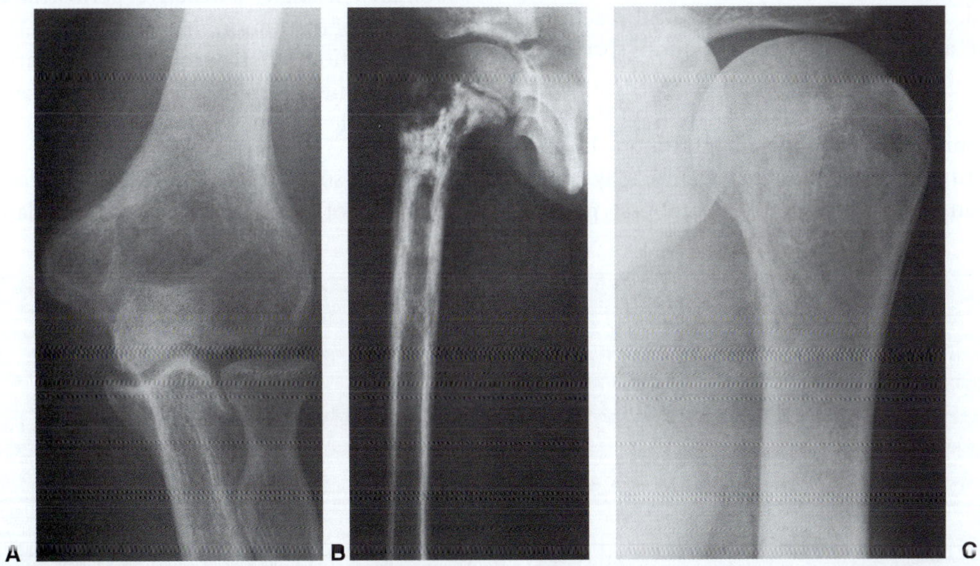

FIGURE 8.61 (A, B, C) Solitary malignant lymphoma. (*Source:* Greenspan A, Remagen W. *Differential Diagnosis of Tumors and Tumor-like Lesions of Bones and Joints*. Philadelphia: Lippincott-Raven, 1998;268.)

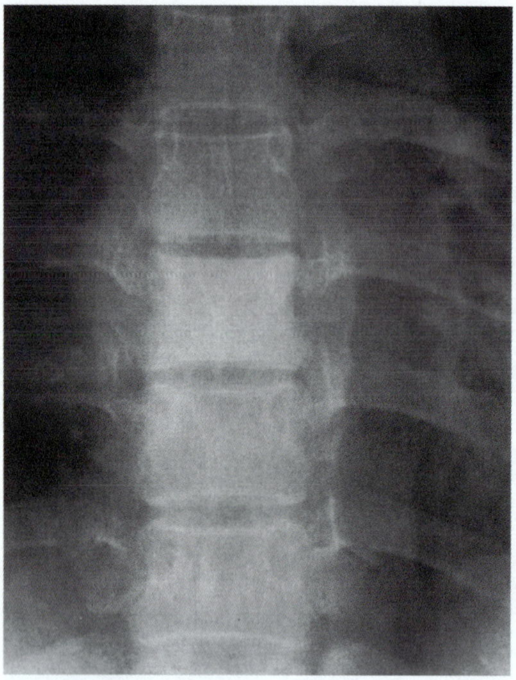

FIGURE 8.62 Solitary malignant lymphoma. (*Source:* Greenspan A, Remagen W. *Differential Diagnosis of Tumors and Tumor-like Lesions of Bones and Joints.* Philadelphia: Lippincott-Raven, 1998;269.)

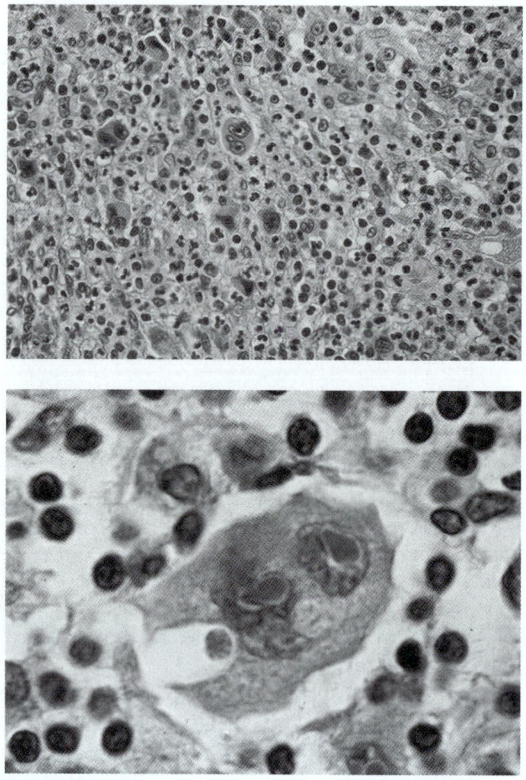

FIGURE 8.64 (A, B) Histopathology of solitary Hodgkin lymphoma. (*Source:* Bullough PG. *Atlas of Orthopedic Pathology*, 2nd ed. New York: Gower, 1992;17.16.)

biologic activity of a lesion. Periosteal reactions elicited by tumors can be categorized as continuous or interrupted. Although no single periosteal reaction is unique for a given tumor, a continuous periosteal reaction indicates a long-standing (slow-growing) benign process. An interrupted reaction, on the other hand, is commonly seen in malignant tumors. In these malignant tumors, the periosteal response may appear in an onion-skin (lamellated) or sunburst pattern. Codman's triangle, a reactive periosteal cuff at the periphery of the tumor, may also be seen.

In addition, there are specific differentials that should come to mind in the presence of certain radiographic findings.

- Sclerotic soap bubble lesion in the anterior cortex of the shaft of the tibia is likely either an adamantinoma

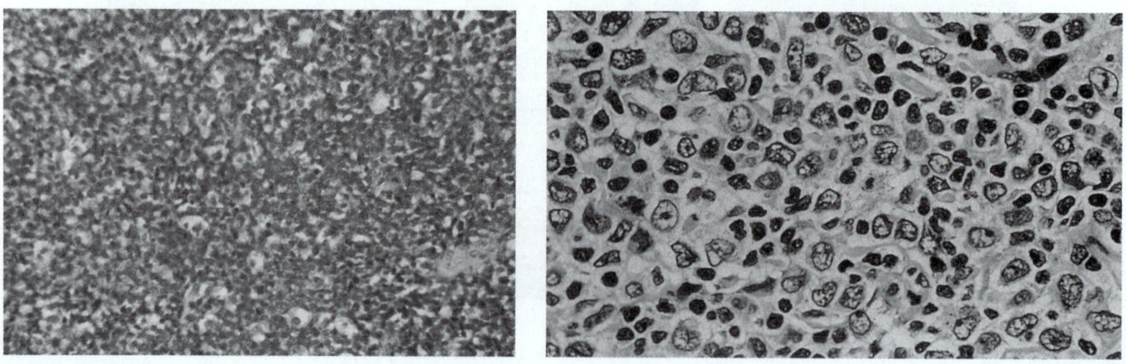

FIGURE 8.65 (A, B) Histopathology of solitary malignant lymphoma. (*Source:* Bullough PG. *Atlas of Orthopedic Pathology*, 2nd ed. New York: Gower, 1992;17.15.)

or a cortical fibrous dysplasia (the patient's age will likely assist in diagnosis).

- The differential for a sclerotic lesion with a central lytic nidus is osteoid osteoma, stress fracture, or infection. Since many stress fractures or stress reactions involve intramedullary edema, they can mimic lymphomas, which also cause intramedullary MRI changes, and so lymphoma should always be considered in the differential diagnosis of a stress reaction. Sequential MRI scans will demonstrate healing of a stress reaction but no healing of a lymphoma, which may appear stable or progressive.
- Cauliflower exophytic lesions on radiographs are indicative of either cauliflower osteochondroma or secondary chondrosarcoma arising in an osteochondroma. The thickness of the cartilage cap will assist in diagnosis.
- Multiple lesions in a single bone could be metastases, myeloma, enchondromas, histiocytosis, fibrous dysplasia, or nonossifying fibromas.
- Lytic lesion in the humeral shaft in a child with no periosteal reaction is likely a simple bone cyst.
- Lytic lesions in the sacrum may be a chordoma, chondrosarcoma, giant cell tumor, metastasis, or myeloma.

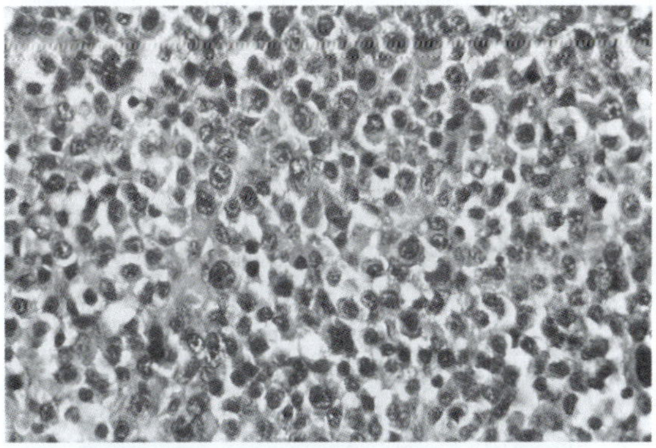

FIGURE 8.65 **Histopathology of multiple myeloma. (*Source:* Greenspan A, Remagen W. *Differential Diagnosis of Tumors and Tumor-like Lesions of Bones and Joints.* Philadelphia: Lippincott-Raven, 1998;280.)**

- A calcified lesion on the surface of a bone includes a differential of osteochondroma, periosteal osteosarcoma, parosteal osteosarcoma, myositis ossificans, periosteal chondroma, or periosteal chondrosarcoma.

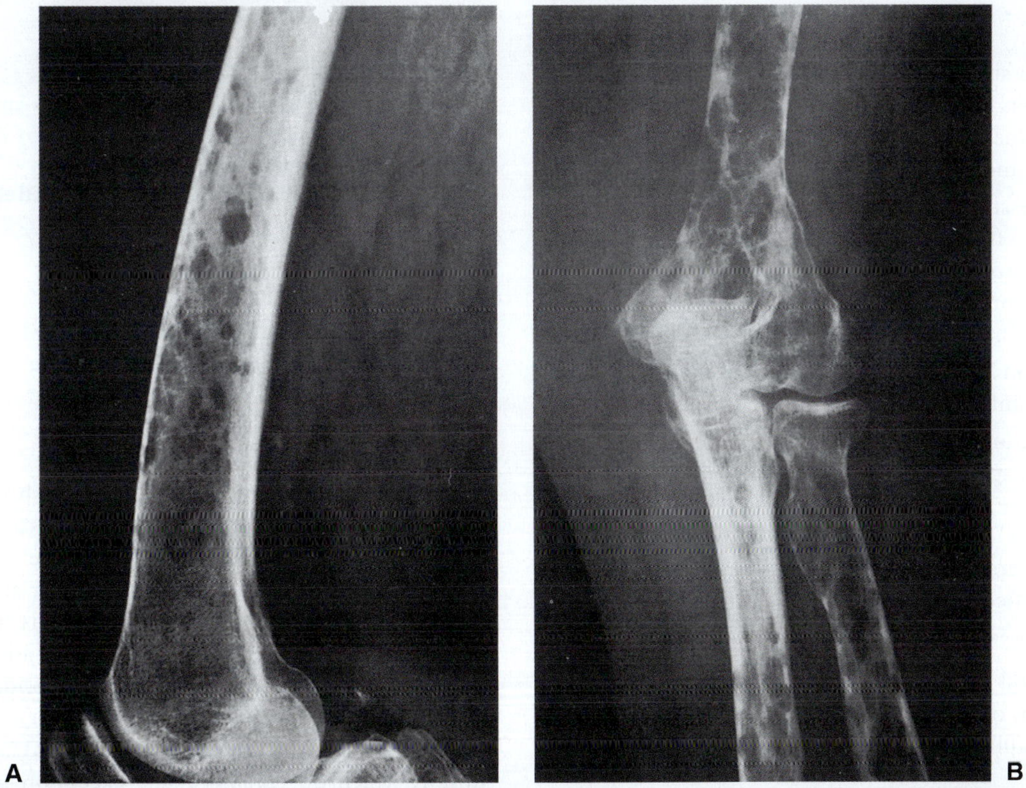

FIGURE 8.66 **(A, B) Multiple myeloma. (*Source:* Greenspan A, Remagen W. *Differential Diagnosis of Tumors and Tumor-like Lesions of Bones and Joints.* Philadelphia: Lippincott-Raven, 1998;279.)**

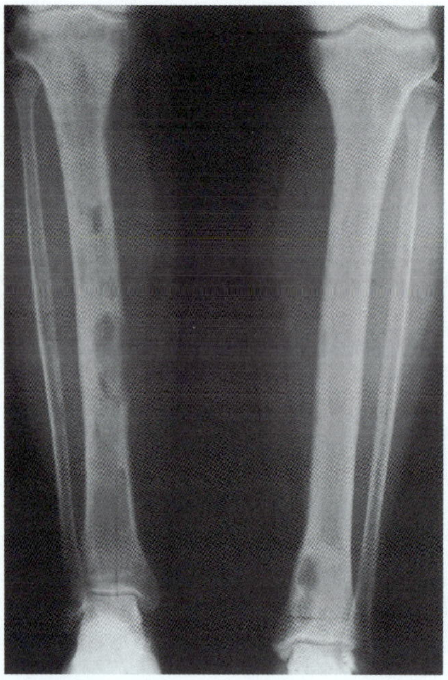

FIGURE 8.67 Brown tumors. (*Source:* Greenspan A, Remagen W. *Differential Diagnosis of Tumors and Tumor-like Lesions of Bones and Joints.* Philadelphia: Lippincott-Raven, 1998;281.)

- Aggressive metaepiphyseal lesion in young patients (under 30 years) could be osteosarcoma, Ewing sarcoma, infection, aneurysmal bone cyst, or giant cell tumor.
- Aggressive metaepiphyseal lesion in older patients (over 30 years) is likely osteosarcoma, chondrosarcoma, metastasis, adult round cell tumors, or giant cell tumor.
- Lytic lesion in the epiphysis of a child with edema seen on MRI may be likely either a chondroblastoma or an infection.
- Additional imaging studies should be requested only if the specific diagnosis cannot be made or when they are necessary for treatment. Radioisotope bone scan, CT, and MRI can show early bone lesions when conventional radiographs appear normal. CT is particularly helpful in difficult imaging areas like pelvis, sacrum, and vertebrae.

Several factors should be considered when evaluating or ordering imaging studies other than plain radiographs.

CT Scans. The major value of a CT scan is to show bone detail, including bone formation as well as bone destruction. CT scans are the best study to see how much bone is destroyed and whether or not soft tissue calcification is present. It is not optimal for looking for the extent of a permeative lesion in bone, soft tissue extension from a bone lesion, or the extent of a lesion in soft tissue.

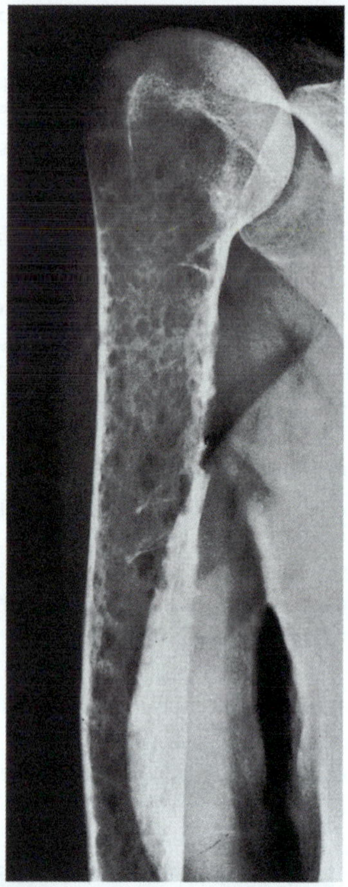

FIGURE 8.68 Gaucher disease. (*Source:* Greenspan A, Remagen W. *Differential Diagnosis of Tumors and Tumor-like Lesions of Bones and Joints.* Philadelphia: Lippincott-Raven, 1998;282.)

MRI Scans. MRI scans are excellent for showing the extent of a lesion in bone (i.e., where it starts and stops). It is also excellent for showing the presence and extent of edema within bone and the presence or absence of an associated soft tissue extension. MRI is the study of choice for any soft tissue lesion. The addition of contrast to an MRI scan can also help elucidate areas of cyst formation, which do not contrast enhance (but may show rim enhancement), from areas of solid tumor, which do enhance. One exception to this is chondroid lesions such as low-grade chondrosarcoma, which may also show rim enhancement with little internal enhancement and thus mimic a cyst. One must always be careful in differentiating between edema

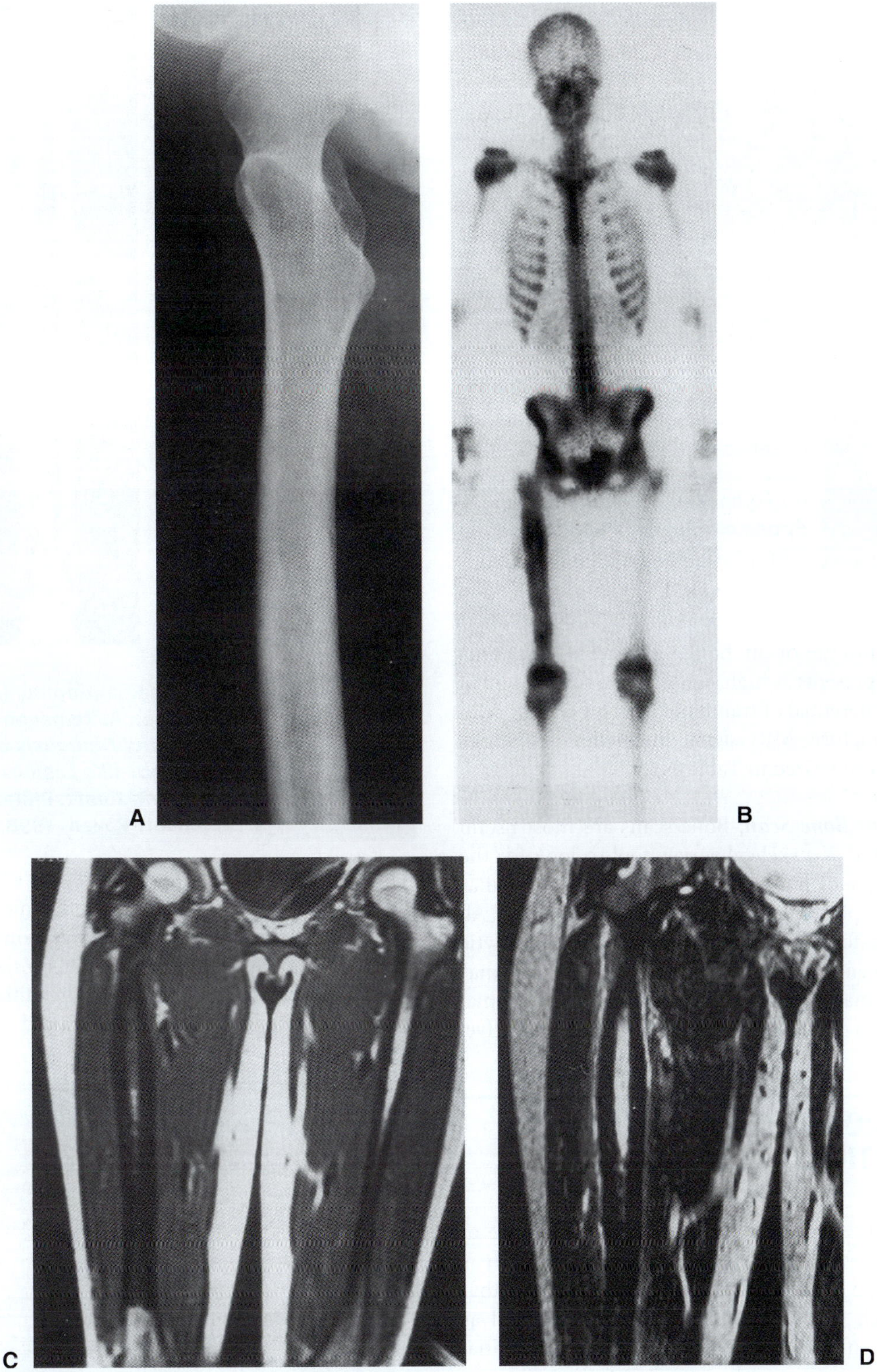

FIGURE 0.69 Malignant fibrous histiocytoma. (A) Oblique radiograph. (B) Radionuclide bone scan. (C) Coronal T1-weighted MRI. (D) Coronal T2-weighted MRI. (*Source:* Greenspan A, Remagen W. *Differential Diagnosis of Tumors and Tumor-like Lesions of Bones and Joints*. Philadelphia: Lippincott-Raven, 1998;237.)

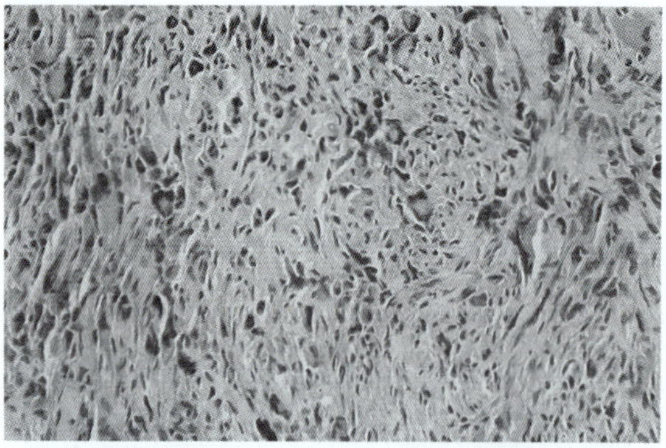

FIGURE 8.70 **Malignant fibrous histiocytoma: starry night pattern. (*Source:* Greenspan A, Remagen W. *Differential Diagnosis of Tumors and Tumor-like Lesions of Bones and Joints.* Philadelphia: Lippincott-Raven, 1998;239.)**

in bone and tumor in bone. As such, lymphoma frequently presents as high signal in marrow and must be in the differential of traumatic marrow lesions such as stress fracture. MRI signal intensities of various tissues is summarized in Table 8.13.

Technetium Bone Scan. Bone scans are most useful when utilized as a skeletal survey tool to look for the total number of lesions present or when a singular lesion is suspected but not seen on initial x-ray. All active bone-forming lesions are hot, while some lytic lesions that engender no bone reaction (e.g., myeloma) may be normal or cold. Sclerotic lesions appear normal on bone scan because they are usually old and inactive.

V. APPROACH TO HISTOLOGIC EVALUATION

A systematic approach to histologic diagnoses of musculoskeletal tumors is extremely important. It is important to focus on the trends and patterns that run through groups of histologic lesions as well as the relationship of histologic findings to a differential diagnosis based on available imaging studies.

Bone-Forming Tumors. There are several lesions to be considered, including fracture callus, myositis ossificans, osteoid osteoma, osteoblastoma, fibrous dysplasia, parosteal osteosarcoma, and osteosarcoma. These lesions typically contain woven bone and a spindle cell stroma, each of which need to be scrutinized to understand the nature of the lesion. It should be understood that in looking at bone-forming lesions, it is the bone that differentiates reactive from neoplastic lesions and the stromal cells that differentiate between benign and malignant neoplasms. The initial approach should be to look at the bone produced by a specific

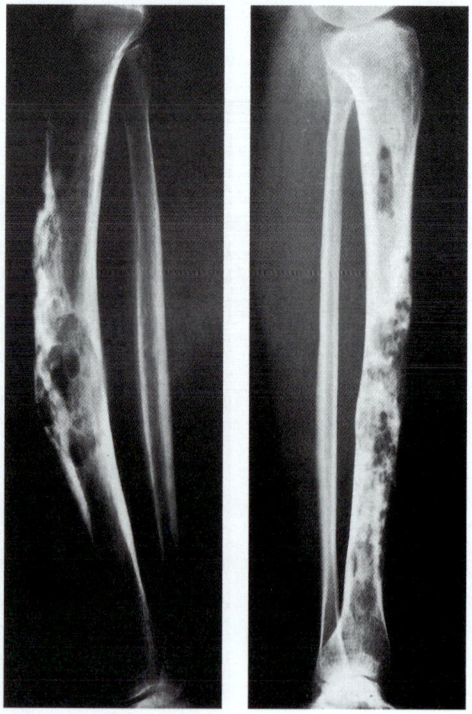

FIGURE 8.71 **(A, B) Adamantinoma. (*Source:* Greenspan A, Remagen W. *Differential Diagnosis of Tumors and Tumor-like Lesions of Bones and Joints.* Philadelphia: Lippincott-Raven, 1998;349.)**

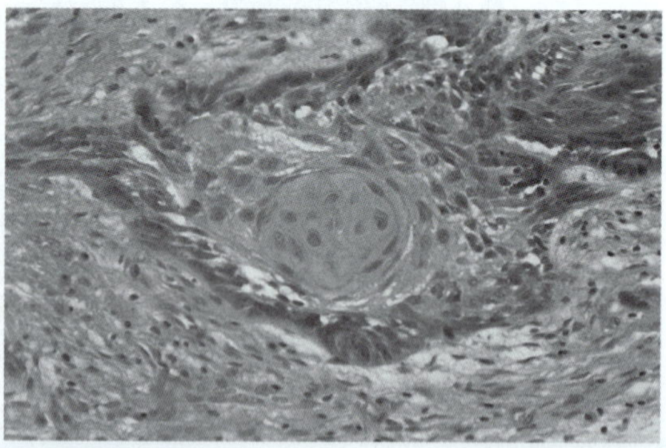

FIGURE 8.72 **Histopathology of adamantinoma. (*Source:* Greenspan A, Remagen W. *Differential Diagnosis of Tumors and Tumor-like Lesions of Bones and Joints.* Philadelphia: Lippincott-Raven, 1998;351.)**

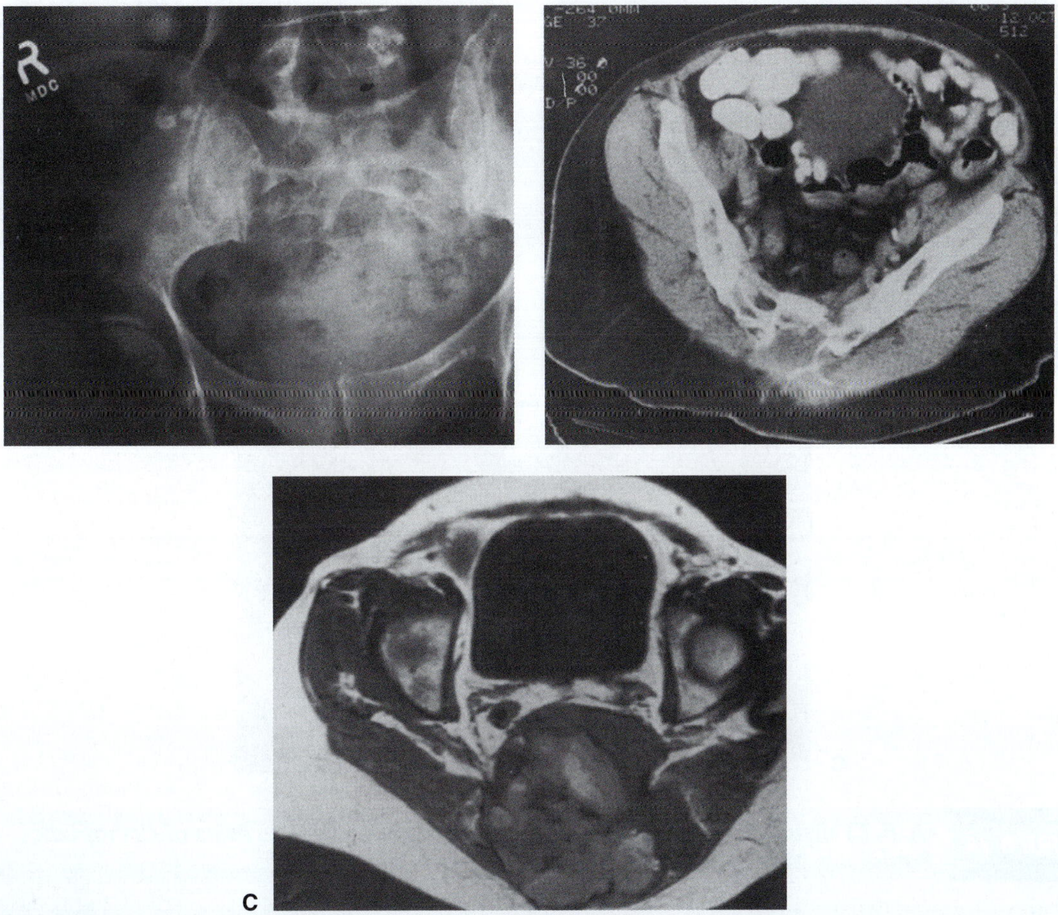

A
B
C

FIGURE 8.73 **Chordoma. (A) Anteroposterior radiograph. (B) CT section. (C) Axial T1-weighted MRI. (*Source:* Greenspan A, Remagen W. *Differential Diagnosis of Tumors and Tumor-like Lesions of Bones and Joints.* Philadelphia: Lippincott-Raven, 1998;355.)**

lesion. Lamellar bone is rarely produced by tumors and is usually native host bone part of a mature bone reaction. On the other hand, woven bone can be either neoplastic or reactive, and woven bone discloses this by the presence or absence of osteoblastic rimming. Typically, woven bone with significant osteoblastic rimming is reactive and indicative of fracture callus, periosteal reaction, or myositis ossificans. In all of these lesions, spindled stromal cells may also be present and may have some mild atypia (especially in early myositis or early fracture callus). On the contrary, woven bone that shows no osteoblastic rimming is usually neoplastic in origin and can be seen with both benign and malignant bone-forming neoplasms. Neoplastic woven bone (i.e., with no osteoblastic rimming) seen in association with a benign spindle cell stroma is indicative of a benign bone-forming neoplasm. These include osteoid osteoma, osteoblastoma, and fibrous dysplasia. Also included in this histologic differential is parosteal osteosarcoma, which is a grade-1 malignant tumor and as such presents with a stroma that shows little overt atypia. Thus, the histologic differential diagnosis for lesions showing neoplastic woven bone and a bland spindle cell stroma include osteoid osteoma, osteoblastoma, fibrous dysplasia, and parosteal osteosarcoma. The final pattern seen in bone-forming lesions is the presence of neoplastic woven bone (again, woven bone with no osteoblastic rimming) in association with a malignant spindle cell stroma, which constitutes osteosarcoma. The findings that make a spindle cell stroma appear malignant include increased cellularity, spontaneous necrosis, the presence of significant atypia or pleomorphism, and a high mitotic rate with many abnormal mitoses.

The patterns to be understood in bone-forming lesions are:

- *Reactive lesion*—Woven bone with osteoblastic rimming and a benign spindle cell stroma (fracture callus, periosteal reaction, myositis ossificans)
- *Benign or low-grade bone-forming neoplasm*—Woven bone with no osteoblastic rimming and a bland-appearing spindle cell stroma (osteoid osteoma,

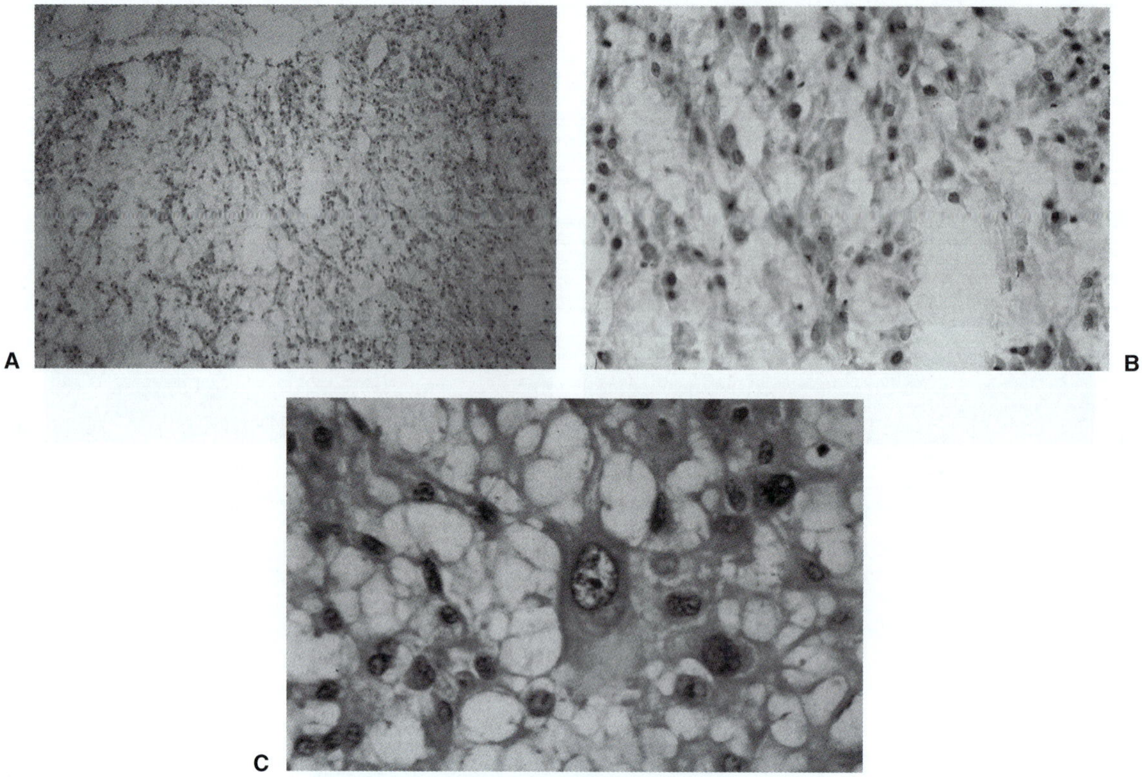

FIGURE 8.74 (A, B, C) Histopathology of chordoma. (*Source:* Bullough PG. *Atlas of Orthopedic Pathology*, 2nd ed. New York: Gower, 1992;16.28.)

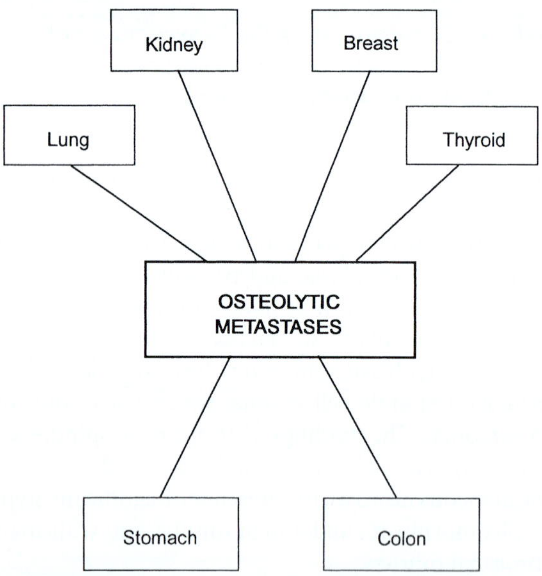

FIGURE 8.75 Origin of osteolytic metastases. (*Source:* Greenspan A, Remagen W. *Differential Diagnosis of Tumors and Tumor-like Lesions of Bones and Joints*. Philadelphia: Lippincott-Raven, 1998;369.)

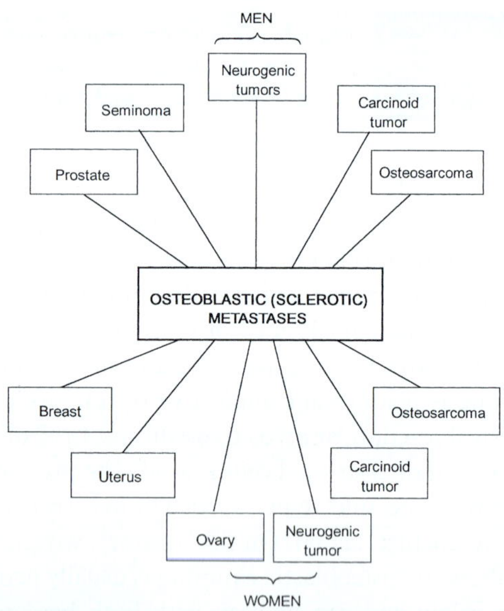

FIGURE 8.76 Origin of osteoblastic metastases. (*Source:* Greenspan A, Remagen W. *Differential Diagnosis of Tumors and Tumor-like Lesions of Bones and Joints*. Philadelphia: Lippincott-Raven, 1998;371.)

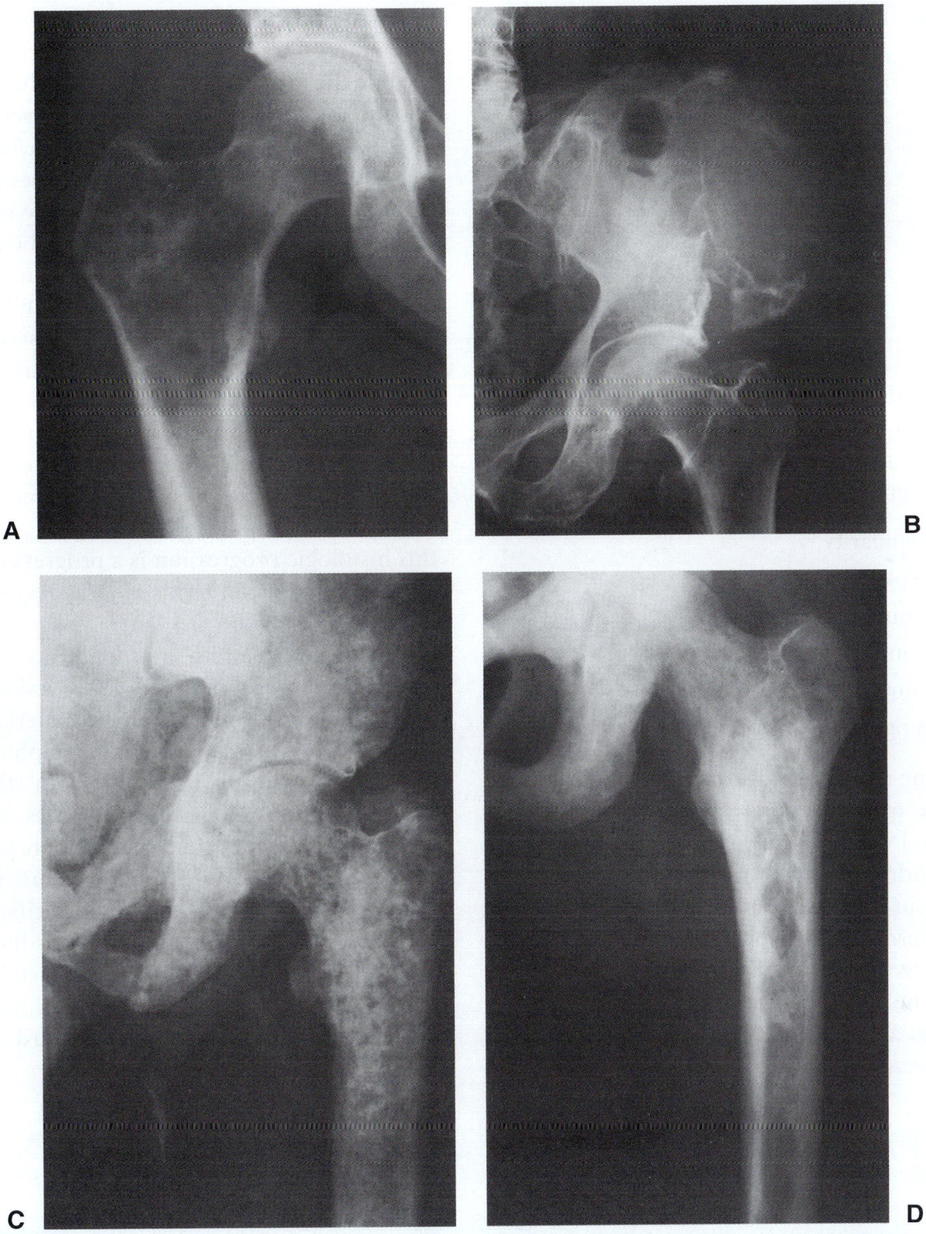

FIGURE 8.77 **(A, B) Osteolytic metastases. (C, D) Sclerotic metastases. (*Source:* Greenspan A, Remagen W. *Differential Diagnosis of Tumors and Tumor-like Lesions of Bones and Joints.* Philadelphia: Lippincott-Raven, 1998;370.)**

osteoblastoma, fibrous dysplasia, parosteal osteosarcoma)

- *Malignant bone tumor*—Woven bone with no osteoblastic rimming associated with a malignant spindle cell stroma (osteosarcoma)

Cartilage-Forming Tumors. There are 3 patterns of cartilage tumors:

- Benign cartilage (enchondroma) merging into low-grade cartilage that merges into intermediate and high-grade chondrosarcoma
- Chondroblastoma: cobblestone chondroblasts and intervening chicken-wire calcification with immature cartilage
- Chondromyxoid fibroma: a benign spindle cell lesion with some areas of immature cartilage

Normal cartilage has two components, cells and matrix. Both are important in evaluating cartilage histologically. Normal cartilage is sparsely cellular. The cells have small, oval (pinocytotic) nuclei and only one nucleus per cell. There is only one cell per lacuna, and there are rare cells outside of lacunae. The matrix is

TABLE 8.12 Common patterns of bone metastases

Purely Lytic	*Mixed Lytic and Blastic*	*Purely Blastic*
Kidney	Breast	Prostate
Lung		Breast
Thyroid		

well formed and regular with no areas that are loose or falling apart (myxoid change).

The changes that occur in cartilage as one goes from benign to low grade are:

- Increased cellularity
- Presence of plump nuclei
- Occasional binucleate cells
- More than one cell in some lacunae
- Some cells outside lacunae
- Myxoid change in the matrix

This finding of "low-grade cartilage" basically puts one in the spectrum of lesions ranging from cellular or active enchondroma to what some authors have called "grade I chondrosarcoma." It is critical to appreciate that tumors in this range have a variable biologic potential in terms of their propensity to continue to grow. The key for the treating physician is to look carefully at the clinical history and imaging studies and to assess what would constitute a reasonable course of treatment. Options for treatment may range from careful observation to curettage to resection, depending on a whole host of factors. These factors include the presence or absence of pain, the age of the patient, the bone involved, and the presence or absence of radiographic changes typical of *chondrosarcoma*, as were listed previously. As one goes further away from normal and closer to high-grade malignant, the chondrocytes look less normal and behave in a less normal fashion. They develop dark, plump nuclei. The cellularity increases appreciably and mitoses become more common. The cells make less or no matrix, or they start making abnormal matrix, which may look nothing like recognizable chondroid. At the end of this progression of dedifferentiation is high-grade sarcoma, not otherwise specified, which is no longer recognizable as chondrosarcoma because it no longer has any chondroid phenotype. Associated with this histologic progression is a progressive increase in biologic potential in terms of local aggressiveness and metastatic behavior.

The second pattern in chondroid lesions is that seen in chondroblastoma. This lesion is usually suspected even before histologic material is available because of its characteristic radiographic and clinical features: a painful lytic lesion in the epiphysis of a child. Histologically, one sees a pattern of "cobblestone" chondroblasts, which are polygonal cells with well-defined cell borders. In association with these cells, a branching pattern of calcification labeled "chicken wire" is also common, as is the presence of immature chondroid matrix. These histologic findings in association with an epiphyseal lytic lesion in a child yield a fairly straightforward diagnosis of chondroblastoma.

TABLE 8.13 MRI signal intensities of various tissues

Tissue	*Image*	
	T1-weighted	*T2-weighted*
Hematoma	High	High
Fat, fatty marrow	High	Intermediate
Muscle, nerves, hyaline cartilage	Intermediate	Intermediate
Cortical bone, tendons, ligaments, fibrocartilage, scar tissue, air	Low	Low
Hyaline cartilage	Intermediate	Intermediate
Red (hematopoietic) marrow	Low	Intermediate
Fluid	Intermediate	High
Tumors (generally)	Intermediate-to-low	High
Lipoma	High	Intermediate
Hemangioma	Intermediate (slightly higher than muscle)	High

Source: Greenspan A, Remagen W. *Differential Diagnosis of Tumors and Tumor-like Lesions of Bones and Joints.* Philadelphia: Lippincott-Raven, 1998;3.

The final pattern seen in cartilage tumors is that seen in chondromyxoid fibroma. This is a rare lesion that is composed of benign spindle cells in a collagenous matrix. In association with this is a varying amount of immature chondroid. This histologic pattern seen in association with the typical radiographic findings helps to suggest this diagnosis.

Round Cell Tumors. These tumors include Ewing sarcoma and neuroblastoma in children as well as myeloma; lymphoma; and small, round-cell metastatic carcinomas in adults. Also included in the differential diagnosis of this group are nonmalignant lesions such as eosinophilic granuloma and infection. All of these lesions are composed in part or in whole of small, round cells. A round cell infiltrate in a histologic slide from a bone lesion points toward the following classes of disorders:

- Infection (i.e., osteomyelitis)
- Eosinophilic granuloma (Langerhans cell histiocytosis)
- Primary round cell tumors
- Small round cell metastatic carcinomas

The histology of bone infection includes the presence of acute and chronic inflammatory cells. While lymphocytes that tend to be associated with chronic inflammatory conditions may resemble lymphoid cells seen in lymphoma, polymorphonuclear leucocytes (polys) are usually easy to visualize and, when present in large numbers, lead to a diagnosis of infection. Thus, when a round cell infiltrate is seen and most of the cells can be shown to be polys, then infection is the likely diagnosis. Confirmation of course requires culture of an appropriate pathogenic bacterium.

- Langerhans' cell histiocytosis is also a type of inflammatory condition in bone. It is composed of foci of proliferating histiocytes but also demonstrates varying numbers of small, round cells, including lymphocytes, neutrophils, and most notably, eosinophils. Histiocytes are large cells with ill-defined cytoplasmic borders and an oval or indented nucleus, while eosinophils are small, round cells with bilobed nuclei and red cytoplasm.
- Pediatric round cell tumors occurring in bone include Ewing sarcoma and metastatic neuroblastoma.
  - Ewing sarcoma is a malignant tumor of unknown histogenesis composed of uniform sheets of small, round, blue cells. These cells show round or oval nuclei of uniform size with poor delineation of cytoplasm. Stains for intracellular glycogen are typically positive.
  - Neuroblastoma occurring in bone is usually a metastasis from a primary tumor in the midline of the body (e.g., spine, brain). The cells of neuroblastoma look similar to those of Ewing sarcoma. The presence of pseudorosettes, circles of round cells surrounding a pink ground substance, on the histologic specimen from a neuroblastoma lesion differentiates these from Ewing.
- Adult round cell tumors include myeloma; lymphoma and small, round-cell metastatic carcinomas. Myeloma is, for the most part, easily recognizable (when well differentiated) because it is composed of sheets of plasma cells. Plasma cells have a single, round or oval nucleus with eccentric cytoplasm. The cell outlines are distinct, and the nuclei often show prominent clumping of chromatin, which produces a "clock face" or "wheel spoke" appearance. Thus, sheets of recognizable plasma cells define myeloma. Lymphoma and small, round-cell carcinoma metastases are much more difficult to differentiate by routine light microscopy and may require immunohistochemical stains for final verification. As such, metastases usually stain positive for cytokeratin, while lymphomas stain for lymphoid markers such as leukocyte common antigen or B or T cell markers.

Bone Cysts. The final group of lesions that can be considered categorically are bone cysts. These include unicameral (simple) and aneurysmal bone cysts. Histologically, unicameral bone cysts appear as a thin layer of fibrous tissue lining large, empty spaces. Benign giant cells, hemosiderin pigment, and a few chronic inflammatory cells may also be present. ABCs have a different histologic appearance and feature the presence of blood-filled cavernous spaces, the walls of which lack the normal features of blood vessels. There is some overlap between these two lesions, and some cysts have characteristics of both. This overlap is most evident in the case of cysts directly abutting the growth plate in skeletally immature individuals, especially in young children. In these instances, the cyst is often central as opposed to eccentric and often not very expansile. Still, these lesions can have a very aggressive course. They tend not to respond to percutaneous treatments and often require open treatments associated with ABCs, such as curettage, bone grafting, and embolization. In these cases, great care needs to be directed toward preservation of the adjacent growth plate.

Immunohistochemistry. One of the major advances in diagnostic pathology that has occurred over the past 2 decades has been the development of sophisticated immunohistochemical techniques. These stains have greatly improved the diagnostic acumen of tissues seen via light microscopy and have added a new area of classification based on specific cell proteins. While it is beyond most orthopaedic surgeons to have a detailed knowledge of this field, these stains are commonly referred to in pathology reports of musculoskeletal lesions and so should be familiar at a basic level to all orthopaedic surgeons. Immunohistochemical stains bind to intermediate filament proteins (IFPs) that are basic structural components of all human cells. These proteins include 6 distinct moieties, which are separated biochemically and include vimentin, desmin, keratins, neurofilament proteins (NFPs), glial fibrillary proteins (GFAPs), and lamins (nuclear envelope proteins). In terms of cell function, the IFPs serve a nucleic acid–binding function and may also act as modulators of nuclear function at a translational or transcriptional level. It should be emphasized that while certain tumors have typical immunohistochemical profiles, the profile can vary from tumor to tumor because individual tumors exhibit specific genotypes and phenotypes. Small, round-cell tumors of bone and their typical immunohistochemistry results are outlined in Table 8.14.

Keratins. Keratins are commonly seen in epithelial tissues and epithelial cells. From a bone tumor standpoint, keratins are the classic marker of metastatic carcinomas. They may be seen, however, in almost any form of sarcoma in rare instances. Keratins are also commonly seen in those sarcomas that show some epithelial differentiation, including synovial sarcoma, adamantinoma, and epithelioid sarcoma, where they can be seen to label cells in the epithelial component of these lesions.

Vimentin. Vimentin is the typical stain of all tumors of mesothelial origin. It thus stains almost all *sarcomas*, but it is usually negative in carcinomas. Its presence is widespread among sarcomas, so it is not very useful in distinguishing between specific sarcoma types.

Desmin. Desmin is typically found in muscle cells and in tumors with myodifferentiation. These tumors most commonly present in soft tissue and include rhabdomyomas, rhabdomyosarcomas, leiomyomas, and leiomyosarcomas. They are also occasionally seen to be present in desmoid tumors and in primitive neuroectodermal tumors.

Actins. As with desmins, actins are indicative of myodifferentiation and are seen in tumors showing these changes, which parallel desmin in muscle-restricted immunoreactivity.

TABLE 8.14 Small, round-cell tumors of bone and typical immunocytochemistry results

Tumor	Keratin	Vimentin	Desmin	Neurofilament	HBA-71B (Mic 2)	Leu7 (CD 57)	NSE	LCA (CD 45)	κ or λ light chains
Ewing sarcoma	+/[a]	+	−	−/*	+	(+)	−	−	−
Primitive neuroectodermal tumor of bone	−	+	−	(+)	+	(+)	+	−	−
Askin tumor	−	+	−	(+)	+	(+)	+	−	−
Malignant lymphoma	−	+	−	−	−	(+)	−	+	+/−
Myeloma	−	−/+	−	−	−	−	−	−/+	+
Small cell osteosarcoma	−	+	−	−	−	−	−	−	−
Mesenchymal chondrosarcoma	−	+	−	−	−	−	−	−	−
Metastatic neuroblastoma	−	−	−	+	−	(+)	+	−	−
Rhabdomyosarcoma	−	(+)	+	−	−	−	(+)	−	−
Synovial sarcoma	+	+	−	−	−	−	−	−	−

[a] Positive in single cases.
(+) Weak reaction.

Source: Greenspan A, Remagen W. *Differential Diagnosis of Tumors and Tumor-like Lesions of Bones and Joints.* Philadelphia: Lippincott-Raven, 1998;263; modified from Triche T, Cavazzana A. Round cell tumors of bone. In: Unni KK (ed.), *Bone Tumors.* New York: Churchill Livingstone, 1998;199–223.

S 100. This protein derives its name from the fact that it is soluble in 100% solution of ammonium sulfate. It has a wide distribution in human tissues. The stains are most commonly associated with *neural, chondroid,* or *melanocytic* differentiation.

Factor VIII-Related Antigen. Also called von Willebrand factor, factor VIII stains in lesions with *vascular* differentiation. It is typically seen in benign and low-grade vascular lesions such as hemangiomas and hemangioendotheliomas but is not commonly present in high-grade angiosarcomas.

Soft Tissue Tumors

A systematic approach to the diagnosis of these lesions reveals a limited number of clinical presentations. Histologically, however, they do form a large and diverse group with fewer trends in the histology than shown in bone tumors.

Clinical Presentations. Most soft tissue tumors present with pain and/or a mass. As noted previously, there may be a history of trauma, as patients tend to relate mass lesions with trauma to that site. It is also remarkable that even very large soft tissue masses, including sarcomas, can reach tremendous size and yet cause minimal, if no, symptoms. Many patients falsely assume that because the lesion is painless it must also be harmless. This is obviously not the case but is often responsible for long delays in diagnosis on the part of the patient or, less frequently, the physician. Ironically, the lesions in soft tissue that are most commonly painful are the benign soft tissue tumors, including desmoid tumors, hemangiomas, benign nerve sheath tumors, and soft tissue infections. Desmoid tumors are very prone to local recurrence. Despite adequate surgery, these lesions may recur in up to 50% of patients. This lesion has an infiltrative growth pattern with prominent invasion of surrounding muscle. Local recurrences may be treated with repeat excision, external beam irradiation, or low-dose chemotherapy. If the lesion does not display active and progressive growth, then the local recurrence can be observed. Many benign lesions can be treated with simple excision with a very low risk of local recurrence. Examples of these include nodular fasciitis, lipoma, angiolipoma, and schwannoma.

Imaging Studies

Plain Radiographs. Most soft tissue masses are seen poorly or not at all on plain x-rays. Those that show calcification will be more apparent, however. While the most common lesion to present with soft tissue calcification is myositis ossificans, synovial sarcoma can present this way also. The calcification seen in synovial sarcomas can vary considerably from minute, almost imperceptible calcifications to very dense calcification that may mimic a benign lesion.

MRI. MRI is the gold standard for the evaluation of lesions in soft tissue. MRI scans are very useful in showing the location of the lesion but not in delineating the nature of the lesion. The classic MRI finding in most soft tissue tumors is a lesion that is well circumscribed and dark on T1, high signal on T2, or Short T1 Inversion Recovery (STIR). Such a lesion would include benign tumor, malignant tumor, abscess, cyst, and hematoma in the differential diagnosis. Most soft tissue sarcomas are very distinct, while often showing a bit of edema in the compartment in which they occur. On the contrary, many benign lesions are poorly marginated on MRI scans, and these include desmoid tumors, hemangiomas, inflammation, injury, and infection. It is often wrongly thought that soft tissue sarcomas are grossly invasive while benign lesions are radiographically distinct and encapsulated.

Fatty Lipoma. Lipoma is one of the few histologic diagnoses that can be made confidently on the basis of MRI and clinical findings alone. Benign lipomas appear as masses of uniform fat density and so parallel the appearance of normal subcutaneous fat on all sequences. Thus, they are bright on T1 and T2 views but suppress as does the normal fat on fat-suppressed T2 and STIR views. Therefore, a mass seen on MRI as a uniform fat density with no interstitial markings is diagnostic of benign lipoma. Without symptoms, these lesions can be monitored. If excision is warranted, marginal resection has a low recurrence rate.

Atypical Lipoma. This benign tumor has also been labeled well-differentiated liposarcoma and lipomalike well-differentiated liposarcoma. It is a fat-containing lesion characterized by lobules of fat signal on MRI with surrounding layers of fibrous tissue, which show as thin layers of high signal. The critical difference between this lesion and higher grade liposarcoma is that the lobules in this lesion look fatty on MRI. Ordinary liposarcoma looks like the typical nonlipomatous lesion, which shows dark on T1 and bright on T2, fat-suppressed T2, and STIR views. While atypical lipomas do not metastasize, they do carry a 10% risk of malignant transformation, usually to high-grade liposarcoma.

Fibrous Nodular Fasciitis. This benign proliferation of fibroblasts is a common lesion most often found in the upper extremity. It is typically less than 2 cm, and there is a low risk of recurrence with local excision.

Malignant Fibrous Histiocytoma. Also found in bone, malignant fibrous histiocytoma is the most common soft tissue sarcoma. These tumors usually occur in adults and are slightly more common in men. They are typically found subfascially in the lower extremities. Because it is believed that this class of tumor actually represents a diverse group of unrelated sarcomas that appear similar on histology, this name may not remain in favor. However, regardless of subtype, this diagnosis is worrisome with high recurrence rates and poor survival rates.

Neural

Schwannoma (Neurilemoma). Schwannoma is a benign round tumor found in peripheral nerves, most commonly in the spinal roots and superficial nerves on the flexor surfaces of the extremities. Histologically, the lesion is described as having Antoni A (compact spindle cells, often in a whorl-like pattern) and Antoni B (less cellular and orderly) areas. Malignant degeneration is rare. When symptoms require treatment, excision is performed.

Neurofibroma. Solitary neurofibroma is a benign, fibrotic, fusiform tumor arising from a peripheral nerve. It occurs most commonly in the third to sixth decades. The lesion is usually asymptomatic except for the presence of a mass. Treatment is excision. In neurofibromatosis or von Recklinghausen disease, small café-au-lait spots appear in the first few years of life with multiple neurofibromas developing later. The neurofibromas appear as soft, pedunculated nodules. Malignant degeneration of these neurofibromas is much more common (3% to 5% of patients) than in the solitary disease. Definitive treatment is excision; however unlike the schwannoma, which is easily excised, excision typically requires sacrifice of the involved nerve.

Vascular

Hemangioma. When found in soft tissue, these benign tumors are typically diffuse, heterogeneous lesions with serpiginous borders. The classic findings of a hemangioma include the presence of a painful lesion in soft tissue which presents with a soft tissue mass seen on MRI scan but with no mass effect. Atrophy from the underlying pain and smooth soft tissue calcifications (phleboliths) are common. Lesions may spontaneously regress. Curative treatment for persistent, symptomatic lesions is surgical excision although it may be difficult due to infiltrative nature of this tumor, and recurrence is common.

Other

Synovial Sarcoma. Despite the name, synovial sarcoma (Figs. 8.78 and 8.79) does not arise from synovium. It comprises 8% to 10% of soft tissue sarcomas and typically occurs before the age of 50. The most common sites are around the knee and foot. Most of these tumors occur in extraarticular locations and in exceptional cases may be intraarticular. The radiologic features of synovial sarcoma include a soft tissue mass, often close to a joint. Soft tissue calcifications are present in about 30% of cases.

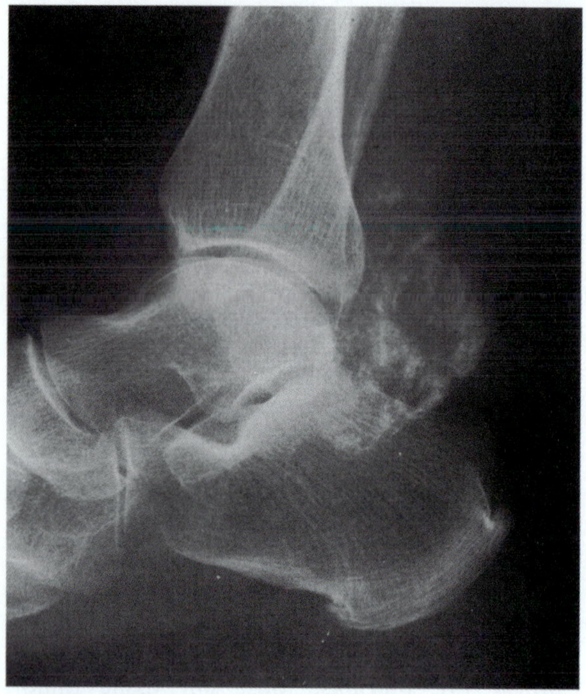

FIGURE 8.78 Synovial sarcoma. (*Source:* Greenspan A, Remagen W. *Differential Diagnosis of Tumors and Tumor-like Lesions of Bones and Joints.* Philadelphia: Lippincott-Raven, 1998;410.)

Synovial Chondromatosis. Synovial chondromatosis is a benign, uncommon disorder characterized by metaplastic proliferation of cartilaginous nodules in the synovial membrane of joints, bursae, and tendon sheaths. Typically diagnosed in the third to fifth decade, it is most often found in the knee followed by hip, shoulder, and elbow. Pain and swelling are the most common complaints, but joint effusion, tenderness, and limited range of motion occur. The radiographic findings range from mere joint effusion to multiple radiopaque joint bodies, depending on the degree of calcification in the cartilaginous nodules. MRI may show the calcifications as signal void on T2-weighted images with a high-signal intensity background of inflamed, hyperplastic synovium.

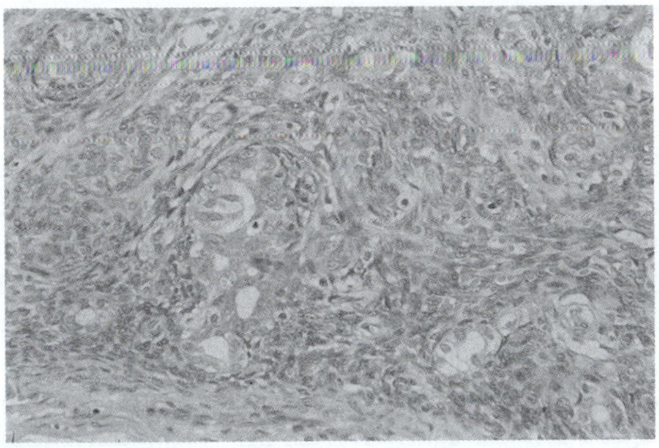

FIGURE 8.79 Histopathology of synovial sarcoma. (*Source:* Greenspan A, Remagen W. *Differential Diagnosis of Tumors and Tumor-like Lesions of Bones and Joints*. Philadelphia: Lippincott-Raven, 1998;413.)

PVNS (Pigmented Villonodular Synovitis). PVNS (Fig. 8.80) is a locally destructive fibrohistiocytic proliferation that affects joints, bursae, and tendon sheaths. There is the diffuse (proliferative) and the nodular (localized) form. Clinically, PVNS is a slowly progressing process that causes pain and joint swelling, often with limited range of motion. The knee is the most common location. More than half of patients present with a bloody joint effusion. Thus, a patient with bloody effusion of the knee without trauma is suggestive of this diagnosis. On radiographs, a soft tissue density is often present in the affected joint, which is sometimes interpreted as a joint effusion but is more dense, because it is hemorrhagic fluid and lobulated synovial tissue. Calcifications are rare.

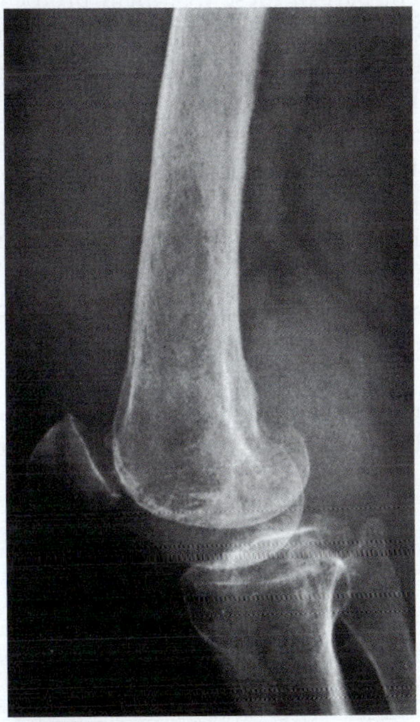

FIGURE 8.80 Pigmented villonodular synovitis. (*Source:* Greenspan A, Remagen W. *Differential Diagnosis of Tumors and Tumor-like Lesions of Bones and Joints*. Philadelphia: Lippincott-Raven, 1998;397.)

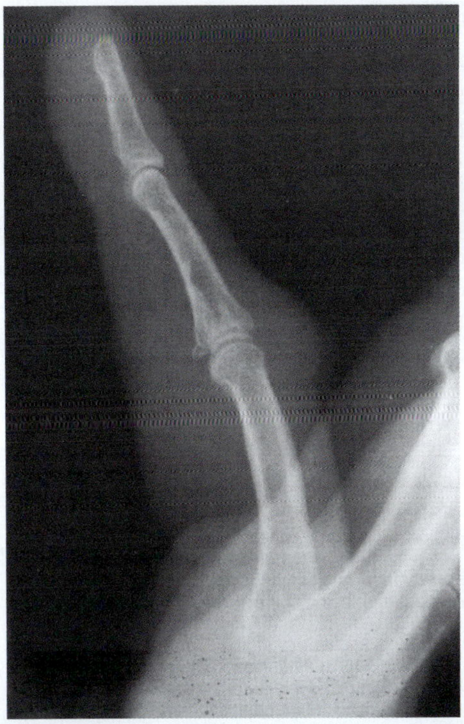

FIGURE 8.81 Localized pigmented nodular tenosynovitis. (*Source:* Bullough PG. *Atlas of Orthopedic Pathology*, 2nd ed. New York: Gower, 1992;17.25.)

Giant Cell Tumor of Tendon Sheath. Giant cell tumor of the tendon sheath occurs mainly on the palmar aspect of the phalanges and occasionally in the articular synovium. It is a well-circumscribed lesion that affects a small area of the synovium or tendon sheath. The most common symptom is pain, but it can be asymptomatic. Radiologically, it is seen as a well-circumscribed, dense soft tissue mass, often accompanied by a bony erosion. Because of the iron stored in the histiocytes, the nonenhanced MRI appearance is characteristic. On T1- and T2-weighted images, lesions are of low signal intensity, similar to muscle. On enhanced T1-weighted images, strong homogenous enhancement due to the numerous proliferative capillaries in the collagenous stroma is seen.

TABLE 8.15	Surgical steps for effective intralesional surgery

1. Extensive soft tissue exposure
2. Large bone window to completely expose all surfaces of the underlying cavity
3. Wide resection of any area of soft tissue extension
4. Complete curettage of all gross tumor in the cavity
5. Burring the perimeter of the boney cavity to extend the curettage beyond all visible areas of tumor extension
6. Pulsatile lavage to expose clean surfaces of adjacent bone
7. Cauterization of the boney surface of the cavity (90% phenol or liquid nitrogen)
8. Reconstruction with bone cement or bone graft with or without internal fixation as needed for boney stability and joint surface support

Myositis Ossificans. The hallmark of late lesions radiographically is the presence of well-formed and benign-appearing calcification in soft tissue, which often is more prominent peripherally and is termed *eggshell calcification.* Early lesions show little or no calcification but do show tremendous inflammation and edema in the adjacent soft tissues. In these cases, the edema greatly exceeds in volume the area of the lesion itself.

Metastasis. Bone metastases are most commonly found in the spine. Metastases are approximately five times more common in the vertebral body when compared to the posterior elements. The common distribution of bone metastases is to the spine, ribs, pelvis, skull, and proximal long bones. Lesions in the hands and feet are uncommon.

Treatment of Musculoskeletal Tumors

Treatment Options. There are several potential treatment options for musculoskeletal tumors. For those lesions in bone, these range from simple curettage to aggressive intralesional excision to wide and radical resection. Simple curettage is sufficient for lesions that tend to be self-limited, such as nonossifying fibroma and eosinophilic granuloma. Aggressive benign lesions such as giant cell tumor, ABC, chondromyxoid fibroma, and osteoblastoma require a more aggressive surgical technique, which usually entails several steps that together allow the surgeon to control the tumor bed and result in a high likelihood of local control. These steps for aggressive intralesional excision are shown in Table 8.15. It is only through the meticulous and methodic application of these steps that eradication of the underlying lesion can be attained with high frequency.

Sarcomas. The treatment of sarcomas of bone and soft tissue are summarized in Table 8.16. Low-grade bone sarcomas such as chondrosarcoma, chordoma, and adamantinoma respond only to surgery, so that is the only modality utilized in their treatment. High-grade bone sarcomas such as osteosarcoma and Ewing sarcoma respond well to chemotherapy, so it is therefore a consistent part of these treatment protocols. Other high-grade bone sarcomas, such as malignant fibrous histiocytoma in bone, high-grade chondrosarcoma, and dedifferentiated chondrosarcoma, present a challenge because of their significant metastatic rate. While there is less data than is present for osteosarcoma, chemotherapy is commonly utilized in an attempt to both increase resectability and decrease the appearance or progression of systemic spread. Radiation is still a possible local treatment for Ewing sarcoma but has been largely replaced by surgery because of the potential for postradiation morbidity and malignant transformation. Despite the risk, radiation is still utilized and reasonable in cases where resection carries

TABLE 8.16 Sarcoma treatment modalities

	Radio-Resistant	*Radio-Sensitive*
LOW GRADE	**Surgery** Chondrosarcoma Chordoma Adamantinoma	**Surgery and Radiation** Low-grade soft tissue sarcomas
HIGH GRADE	**Surgery and Chemotherapy** Osteosarcoma Ewing sarcoma Other high-grade bone sarcomas	**Surgery, Radiation, and Chemotherapy** High-grade soft tissue sarcomas

unacceptable morbidity or when surgical margins are closer than desired. This reasoning also applies to other high-grade bone sarcomas: a treatment plan for each sarcoma should be individualized to each patient in light of the potential benefits of each treatment option. Low-grade soft tissue sarcomas respond well to a combination of wide resection surgery and local radiation. The radiation can be given either preoperatively or postoperatively. In either case, there is no difference in local control as long as the treatments are well planned. The major advantage to preoperative radiation is that the presence of the lesion in situallows the radiation oncologist to concentrate the radiation field on the lesion, and therefore, the oncologist can use a smaller field size than can be use if the lesion was removed previously. Radiation also has many beneficial effects on the local tumor, which commonly will decrease in size and vascularity as well as increase in firmness, thereby greatly facilitating resection. The disadvantage of preoperative treatment is that it necessitates operating through tissues that have been damaged by receiving usually 50 centigray (5000 rads) of radiation. This damaged tissue carries a 20% risk of major wound complications in most series. High-grade soft tissue sarcomas still present a major challenge to the oncology team. Local control can be accomplished with radiation and wide resection, as with the low-grade malignant lesions. Ideally, high-grade lesions should also receive systemic treatment in the form of chemotherapy in light of the higher rate of metastasis associated with high-grade histology. While patients with high-grade lesions are commonly treated with protocols that include multidrug chemotherapy, the results of this treatment in terms of improved survival are not as dramatic as hoped. Chemotherapy for high-grade soft tissue sarcomas continues to be a controversial topic to which much research has been directed. New findings regarding the molecular and genetic bases of these diseases will spawn new drug treatments for all types of sarcomas and further improve the survival of these patients.

References

1. Bataille R, Sany J. Solitary myeloma: Clinical and prognostic features of a review of 114 cases. *Cancer* 1981;483: 845–851.
2. Chin KR, Barr SJ, Winalski C, Zurakowski, Brick GW. Treatment of advanced primary and recurrent diffuse pigmented villonodular synovitis of the knee. *J Bone Joint Surg Am* 2002 Dec;84A(12): 2192–2202.
3. Chin KR, Brick GW. Extraarticular pigmented villonodular synovitis: A cause for failed knee arthroscopy. *Clin Orthop Relat Res* 2002 Nov;(404): 330–338.
4. Chin KR, Kharrazi FD, Miller BS, Mankin HJ, Gephardt MC. Osteochondromas of the distal aspect of the tibia or fibula. Natural history and treatment. *J Bone Joint Surg Am* 2000 Sep;82(9): 1269–1278.
5. Corwin JLR. Solitary plasmacytoma of bone vs. extramedullary plasmacytoma and their relationship to multiple myeloma. *Cancer* 1979;43: 1007–1013.
6. Eckardt JJ, Eilber FR, Dorey FJ, Mirra JM. The UCLA experience in limb: Salvage surgery for malignant tumors. *Orthopaedics* 1985;8: 612–621.
7. Enneking WF. A system of staging musculoskeletal neoplasms. *Clin Orthop Relat Res* 1986 Mar;(204): 9–24.
8. Enneking WF, Spanier SS, Goodman MA. A system for the surgical staging of musculoskeletal sarcoma. *Clin Orthop Relat Res* 1980 Nov-Dec;(153): 106–120.
9. Gebhardt MC, Goorin A, Traina J. Long term results of limb salvage and amputation in extremity osteosarcoma. In: Yamamuro T (ed.), *New Developments for Limb Salvage in Musculoskeletal Tumors*. New York: Springer, 1989; 99–109.
10. Hosalkar HS, Garg S, Moroz L. Diagnostic accuracy of MRI vs. CT imaging for osteoid osteoma in children. *Clin Orthop Rel Res* 2005;436: 286.
11. Lackman RD. Orthopaedic tumors. In: Vaccaro AR (ed.), *Orthopaedic Knowledge Update 8*. Rosemont, IL: American Academy of Orthopaedic Surgeons, 2005.
12. Lackman RD, Hosalkar HS, Ogilvie CM, Torbert JT, Fox EJ. Intralesional curettage for grades II and III giant cell tumors of bone. *Clin Orthop Relat Res* 2005;(438): 123–127.
13. Lin PP, Thenappan A, Deavers MT, Lewis VO, Yasko AW. Treatment and prognosis of chondroblastoma. *Clin Orthop Relat Res* 2005 Sep;(438): 103–109.
14. Mankin HJ, Mankin CJ, Simon MA. The hazards of the biopsy, revisited. Members of the musculoskeletal tumor society. *J Bone Joint Surg Am* 1996 May;78(5): 656–663.
15. Martinez V, Sissons HA. Aneurysmal bone cyst: A review of 123 cases including primary lesions and those secondary to other bone pathology. *Cancer* 1988 Jun 1;61(11): 2291–2304.
16. National Cancer Institute. Estimated new cancer cases and deaths for 2004;September 14, 2004. Online: www.seer.cancer.gov.
17. Papagelopoulos PJ, Galanis EC, Sim FH, Unni KK. Clinicopathologic features, diagnosis, and treatment of malignant fibrous histiocytoma of bone. *Orthopedics* 2000 Jan;23(1): 59–65.
18. Parekh SG, Donthineni-Rao R, Ricchetti E, Lackman RD. Fibrous Dysplasia. *J Am Acad Orthop Surg* 2004;12(5): 305–313.
19. Rosenthal DI, Springfield DS, Gebhardt MC, Rosenberg AE, Mankin HJ. Osteoid osteoma: Percutaneous radio-frequency ablation. *Radiology* 1995 Nov;197(2): 451–454.
20. Rougraff B, Kling TJ. Treatment of active unicameral bone cysts with percutaneous injection of demineralized bone matrix and autogenous bone marrow. *J Bone Joint Surg Am* 2002;84: 921–929.
21. Scaglietti O, Marchetti PG, Bartolozzi P. The effects of methylprednisolone acetate in the treatment of bone

cysts. Results of three years follow-up. *J Bone Joint Surg Br* 1979;61: 200–2004.

22. Unni KK. In: Dahlin DC (ed.), *Dahlin's Bone Tumors*. Philadelphia: Lippincott, 1996.
23. Wicklund CL, Pauli RM, Johnston D, Hecht JT. Natural history study of hereditary multiple exostoses. *Am J Med Genet* 1995 Jan 2;55(1): 43–46.

Key References

Lackman RD. Orthopaedic tumors. In: Vaccaro AR (ed.), *Orthopaedic Knowledge Update 8*. Rosemont, IL: American Academy of Orthopaedic Surgeons, 2005.

Published by the AAOS, this text is intended to keep both resident and experienced surgeons up to date with the most current orthopaedic principles and data.

Lackman RD, Torbert JT, Hosalkar HS, Fox EJ, Ogilvie CM. Treatment of metastases to the extremities and pelvis. *Oper Techn Orthop* 2005; 14: 288–295.

This article offers information on the presentation and management of metastases to both the extremities and the pelvis. One section is devoted to imaging modalities and their efficacy. Both surgical and nonsurgical management strategies are included, as well as a concise table demonstrating the most commonly used surgical interventions for bone metastases in the extremities.

Hahn WC, Weinberg RA. Rules making human tumor cells. *New Engl J Med* 2000;347 (20): 1593–1603.

This paper presents a review of 121 articles on the pathogenesis of cancer. The authors conclude that a cell must demonstrate specific acquired capabilities to transform into a malignant cell.

Sanjay BKS, Sim FH, Ummi KK, et al. Giant cell tumors of the spine. *J Bone Joint Surg Br* 1993;75B: 148–154.

The authors studied 24 patients with giant cell tumors of the spine. They recommend surgical excision with wide margins because of high recurrence rates and that radiotherapy should not be used because of the 10% rate of sarcomatous change.

Lackman RD, Khoury LD, Esmail A, Donthinini-Rao R. The treatment of sacral giant-cell tumours by serial arterial embolisation. *J Bone Joint Surg Br* 2002 Aug;84(6): 873–877.

Because radiation is only effective in some patients but has a risk of malignant change, the authors evaluated the effectiveness of serial arterial embolization as an alternative to surgery. Five patients with giant cell tumors of the sacrum, which had been primarily treated by serial embolization, were retrospectively reviewed for changes in the size of the tumor. In 4, the symptoms resolved with full return of function and arrest in the growth of the tumor. They remained free from growth, recurrence, or metastases at follow-up (4 to 17 years). One patient died from metastatic disease within 18 months of the initial diagnosis.

Grubb MR, Currier BL, Pritchard DJ, et al. Primary Ewing's sarcoma of the spine. *Spine* 19(3): 309–313.

This report describes a retrospective study of 36 patients with primary Ewing sarcoma of the spine. There was a 5-year survival rate of 33%, and there was no correlation between prognosis and location of the tumor.

Refresher Questions

1. Which of the following tumors has the best prognosis (least risk of pulmonary metastases)?
   a) classic osteosarcoma
   b) parosteal osteosarcoma
   c) periosteal osteosarcoma
   d) osteosarcoma secondary to Paget disease
   e) osteosarcoma secondary to irradiation
2. What is the most common site of bone metastases?
   a) proximal humerus
   b) hands/feet
   c) spine
   d) pelvis
   e) proximal femur
3. Which of the following benign bone lesions is the most likely to recur following curettage?
   a) chondroblastoma
   b) nonossifying fibroma
   c) osteoid osteoma
   d) giant cell tumor
   e) enchondroma
4. The risk of developing a sarcoma in an enchondroma or an osteochondroma is approximately:
   a) less than 1%
   b) 3% to 5%
   c) 5% to 10%
   d) 10% to 20%
   e) 20% to 30%
5. In which of the following bone tumors is CT scanning superior to MRI?
   a) osteoid osteoma
   b) Ewing tumor
   c) giant cell tumor of bone
   d) intramedullary osteosarcoma
   e) malignant fibrous histiocytoma
6. Which of the following benign soft tissue tumors is very prone to local recurrence after surgical removal?
   a) nodular fasciitis
   b) lipoma
   c) angiolipoma
   d) schwannoma
   e) desmoid tumor

7. Which of the following radiographic features helps in differentiating a chondrosarcoma from an enchondroma?
   a) expansion of the cortex in a small bone
   b) small endosteal erosions
   c) cortical perforation
   d) absence of matrix calcifications
   e) stippled calcification

8. Ewing sarcoma has which of the following cytogenetic abnormalities?
   a) mutation on chromosome 17
   b) reciprocal translocation between chromosomes 12 and 16
   c) translocation between chromosomes 11 and 22
   d) reciprocal translocation of chromosomes X and 18
   e) translocation between chromosomes 9 and 22

9. A 15-year-old boy has a destructive lesion in his proximal tibia. The MRI shows soft tissue extension, and a CT scan of the chest shows no evidence of pulmonary metastases. A technetium bone scan shows a solitary lesion, and a needle biopsy shows a high-grade osteosarcoma. Which of the following is the correct surgical stage?
   a) stage IA
   b) stage IB
   c) stage IIA
   d) stage IIB
   e) stage III

10. Which of the following carcinomas typically produces purely lytic bone metastases?
    a) lung and breast
    b) lung and prostate
    c) kidney and lung
    d) kidney and breast
    e) breast and prostate

Chapter 9

Rehabilitation

RICHARD SCARLETT, SAMIR MEHTA, and MARY ANN KEENAN

I. AMBULATION

The Gait Cycle. The gait cycle (Fig. 9.1) refers to the complete sequence of all of the functions of a single limb during walking. Walking is the process by which the body moves forward while maintaining stance stability. Normal walking is a cyclical, energy-efficient process. The gait cycle is divided into 2 periods, stance and swing. Stance refers to the period while the foot is in contact with the ground. At any point during walking, 1 foot is always in contact with the ground, which is termed single limb stance. When both feet are in contact with the ground, it is referred to as double-limb stance. Swing refers to the period when the foot is in the air, enabling limb advancement. The stance period constitutes approximately 60% of the gait cycle, while the swing period constitutes the remaining 40%. As the body moves forward, 1 limb serves as a mobile source of support while the other limb advances the body to a new support site. Each leg alternates its role during walking. When the period of double stance is absent, the person is termed to be running.

Step vs. Stride. The gait cycle can also be described in terms of step and stride. Step is the distance between the initial contact of alternating feet. Stride is the distance between consecutive initial contact points of the same foot (Fig. 9.2).

Periods of the Gait Cycle. Stance is divided into 5 periods: initial contact, loading response, midstance, terminal stance, and preswing. Swing is divided into 3 periods: initial swing, midswing, and terminal swing. The sequential combinations of the 8 periods of gait can be divided into 3 basic tasks: weight acceptance, single-limb support, and limb advancement (Table 9.1; Fig. 9.3).

- *Initial Contact*—In normal gait, the heel is the first part of the foot to touch the ground. The hip is flexed,

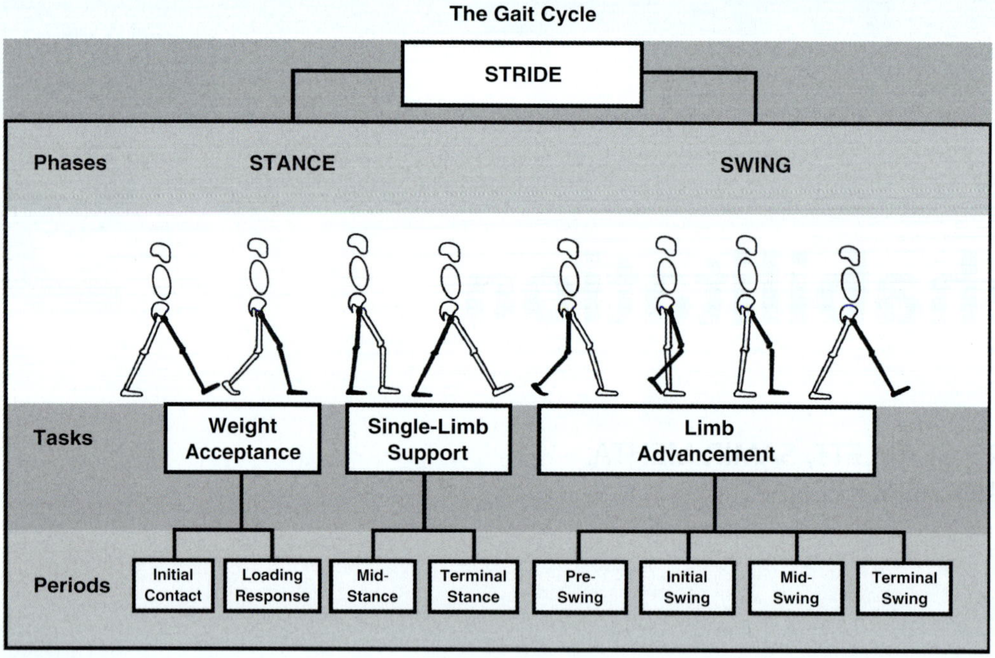

FIGURE 9.1 The two phases of the gait cycle: stance phase when the foot is on the floor and swing phase when the foot is in the air. The gait cycle is further subdivided into tasks as well as periods. (*Source:* Rose J, Gamble JG. *Human Walking*. Philadelphia: Lippincott Williams & Wilkins, 2006;224.)

the knee is extended, and the ankle is dorsiflexed to neutral.

- *Loading Response*—Marks the beginning of double-stance period when the foot contacts the floor and continues until the opposite foot is lifted for swing. Body weight is transferred onto a supporting leg. The opposite leg is in the preswing phase.

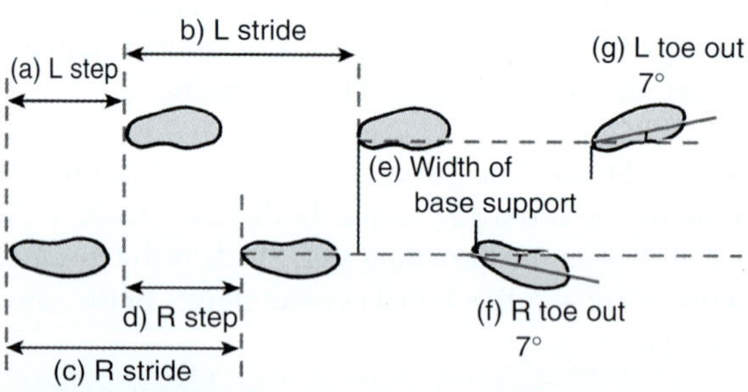

FIGURE 9.2 Distance variables of gait. (a) Left step length. (b) Left stride length. (c) Right stride length. (d) Right step length. (e) Width of base of support. (f) Right toe-out. (g) Left toe-out. (*Source:* Seymour R. *Prosthetics and Orthotics, Lower Limb and Spinal*. Philadelphia: Lippincott Williams & Wilkins, 2002;98.)

- *Midstance*—The first half of the single-limb support interval. It begins with the lifting of the opposite foot and continues until body weight is aligned over the supporting foot. The supporting leg advances over the supporting foot by ankle dorsiflexion while the hip and knee extend. The opposite leg is advancing in its midswing phase.
- *Terminal Stance*—Begins when the supporting heel rises and continues until the heel of the opposite foot hits the ground. Body weight progresses beyond the supporting foot as increased hip extension puts the leg in a more trailing position.
- *Preswing*—Marks the second double-stance interval in the gait cycle. It begins with the initial contact of the previous swing limb and ends with toe-off of the previously supporting leg. Ground contact by the leg making initial contact causes the soon-to-be swing leg to increase ankle plantarflexion, increase knee flexion, and decrease hip extension. Transfer of body weight from ipsilateral to opposite limb takes place.
- *Initial Swing*—Begins when the foot is lifted from the floor and ends when the swinging foot is opposite the stance foot. The swing leg is advanced by increased hip flexion and increased knee flexion. The ankle only partially dorsiflexes to ensure ground clearance. The supporting leg is in midstance.
- *Midswing*—Continues from the endpoint of the initial swing and continues until the swinging limb is in

TABLE 9.1 Summary of gait phases

R	0%–10% (10%)	10%–30% (20%)	30%–50% (20%)		50%–60% (10%)	60%–73% (13%)	73%–87% (14%)	87%–100% (13%)
R	Initial & loading	Midstance	Terminal stance		Preswing	Initial swing	Midswing	Terminal swing
L	Preswing	Initial swing	Midswing	Terminal swing	Initial & loading	Midstance	Terminal stance	
L	0%–10% (10%)	10%–23% (13%)	23%–37% (14%)	37%–50% (13%)	50%–60% (10%)	60%–80% (20%)	80%–100% (20%)	

Key: Swing (shaded) *Stance* (unshaded)

front of the body and the tibia is vertical. Advancement of the swing leg is accomplished by further hip flexion. The knee is allowed to extend in response to gravity while the ankle continues dorsiflexion to neutral. The supporting leg is in late midstance.

- *Terminal Swing*—Begins when the tibia is vertical and ends when the foot touches the floor. Limb advancement is completed by knee extension. The hip maintains its flexion, and the ankle remains dorsiflexed to neutral.

Center of Mass. A human center of mass (COM) is located just anterior to the second sacral vertebra (S2), midway between both hip joints. The least amount of energy is required when a body moves along a straight line, with the COM deviating neither up nor down nor side to side. The COM deviates from the straight line in vertical and lateral sinusoidal displacements (Fig. 9.4). With respect to vertical displacement, the COM goes through rhythmic upward and downward motion as it moves forward. The highest point occurs at midstance, the lowest point occurs at time of double support. The average amount of vertical displacement in the average adult male is approximately 5 cm. With respect to lateral displacements, as weight is transferred from one leg to the other, there is shift of the pelvis to the weight-bearing side. The oscillation of the COM amounts to side-to-side displacement of approximately 5 cm. The lateral limits are reached at midstance.

Muscle Activity. During the normal gait cycle, agonist and antagonist muscle groups work in concert to advance the limb. Most muscle groups undergo eccentric contractions (lengthening with contraction), such as the quadriceps during initial contact, enabling the muscles to serve as shock absorbers during walking. However, the quadriceps undergo concentric contracture (muscle shortening) during midstance. Alternatively, some muscle groups undergo isocentric contracture (muscle length stays constant); an example of this is the hip abductors during midstance. For muscle activity during the gait cycle, see Figure 9.5A to E.

Pathologic Gait. Pathologic gait patterns can be broadly divided into either neuromuscular or musculoskeletal etiologies. Gait deviations may be a result of structural abnormalities of the bone, joints, or soft tissue. Other general causes of pathologic gait include neuromuscular and myopathic conditions as well as pain. Generally, as the efficiency of the gait pattern is reduced, the energy expenditure is increased.

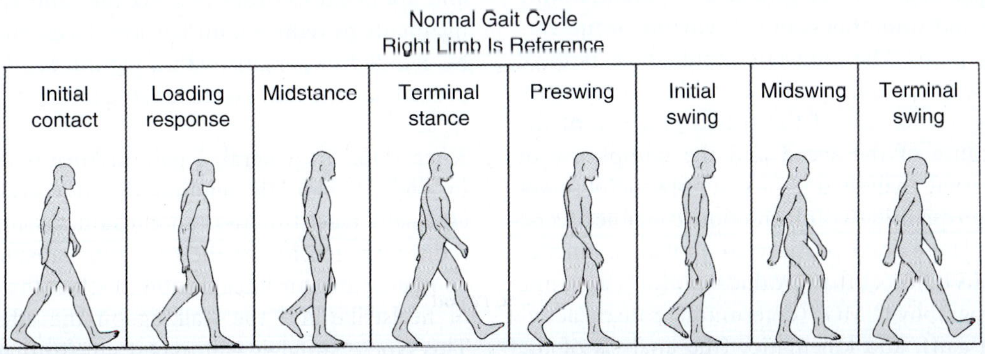

FIGURE 9.3 Phases of the gait cycle. (*Source:* Seymour R. *Prosthetics and Orthotics, Lower Limb and Spinal*. Philadelphia: Lippincott Williams & Wilkins, 2002;100.)

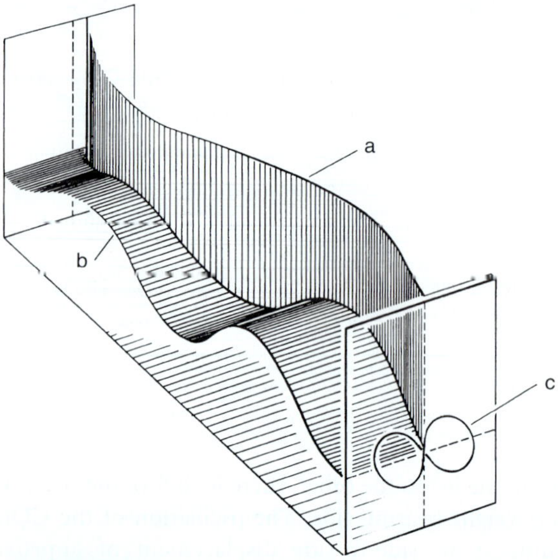

FIGURE 9.4 Displacements of center of mass in three planes of space during single stride (cycle). The actual displacements have been greatly exaggerated. (a) Lateral displacement in a horizontal plane. (b) Vertical displacement. Combined displacement of *a* and *b* as projected onto a plane perpendicular to the plane of progression are shown in c. (*Source:* Rose J, Gamble JG. *Human Walking*. Philadelphia: Lippincott Williams & Wilkins, 2006;3.)

Gait Analysis. Gait analysis is a method of diagnosing the way people walk. Analysis may be done through visual observation or with quantitative measurements. Since the entire gait cycle ends in approximately 1 second, a systematic and disciplined approach must be used to clinically evaluate a patient's gait. The observation of gait begins with a general assessment, noting symmetry and smoothness of movements of the various body parts. The clinician should take note of the cadence (steps/minute), base width, stride length, arm swing, movement of the trunk, and rise of the body. Because of the speed and the complexity of walking, visual analysis does not supply the observer with enough quantitative information to enable precise diagnosis. There are 3 primary components: kinetics (the analysis of forces that produce motion), dynamic electromyography (EMG) (determining muscle activity during gait), and kinematics (the analysis of the motion produced during the gait cycle).

Three instruments that are commonly used in quantitative gait analysis are dynamic EMG, force plate studies, and motion analysis. Dynamic EMG measures and records the electrical activity in the multiple muscle groups working during functional activity (Fig. 9.6). Force plate studies measure ground reactive forces and changes in the center of pressure as a patient walks. This allows quantification of balance disturbances and other gait problems. Motion analysis uses multiple cameras that detect sensors on a patient. The data from the cameras can be used to recreate a 3-dimensional model of the patient's gait pattern. Quantitative gait analysis is essential in determining treatment options (e.g., orthoses, prosthetic positioning, and surgical intervention) that will be most beneficial to the patient.

Musculoskeletal Causes of Pathologic Gait

Hip Pain. Osteoarthritis is the most common abnormality of the hip, resulting in gait abnormalities. The first changes noted are diminished hip range of motion, especially in internal rotation and flexion. This often results in exaggerated compensatory motion in the lumbar spine and the opposite unaffected hip. In severely restricted hip joints, there will be a reduction in hip flexion in the swing phase and in hip extension during the stance phase. These restrictions will be somewhat compensated by other joints (e.g., hip hiking on the unaffected side or 'tiptoeing' on the affected side) (Fig. 9.7A).

The term *antalgic gait* refers to any gait abnormality that results from pain. Hip pain may create an antalgic gait that is characterized by limiting of weight bearing on the affected side and a decrease in the stance phase on that limb in an attempt to unload the mechanical stresses on the painful hip joint. In addition, a trunk lurch toward the painful hip of the stance leg brings the COM over the joint and decreases the mechanical stress across the joint. This is done by dipping the shoulder on the affected side, elevating the opposite shoulder, and shifting the pelvis over the stance leg during the stance phase of the gait cycle (Fig. 9.7B). During the swing phase, the hip is slightly flexed, externally rotated, and abducted in order to relax the joint capsule and ligaments to reduce joint tension. Heelstrike tends to be avoided in persons with a painful hip in order to prevent jarring and excess loading of the joint.

Knee Pain. In general, a painful knee is maintained in slight flexion throughout the gait cycle. This is especially true if there is an effusion, as slight flexion reduces the tension on the knee joint capsule. Another compensation for knee flexion involves the avoidance of heelstrike and toe walking on the affected side. This type of antalgic gait may result from any painful condition of the knee joint, including a meniscal tear, loose body, fracture, infection, or inflammatory synovitis.

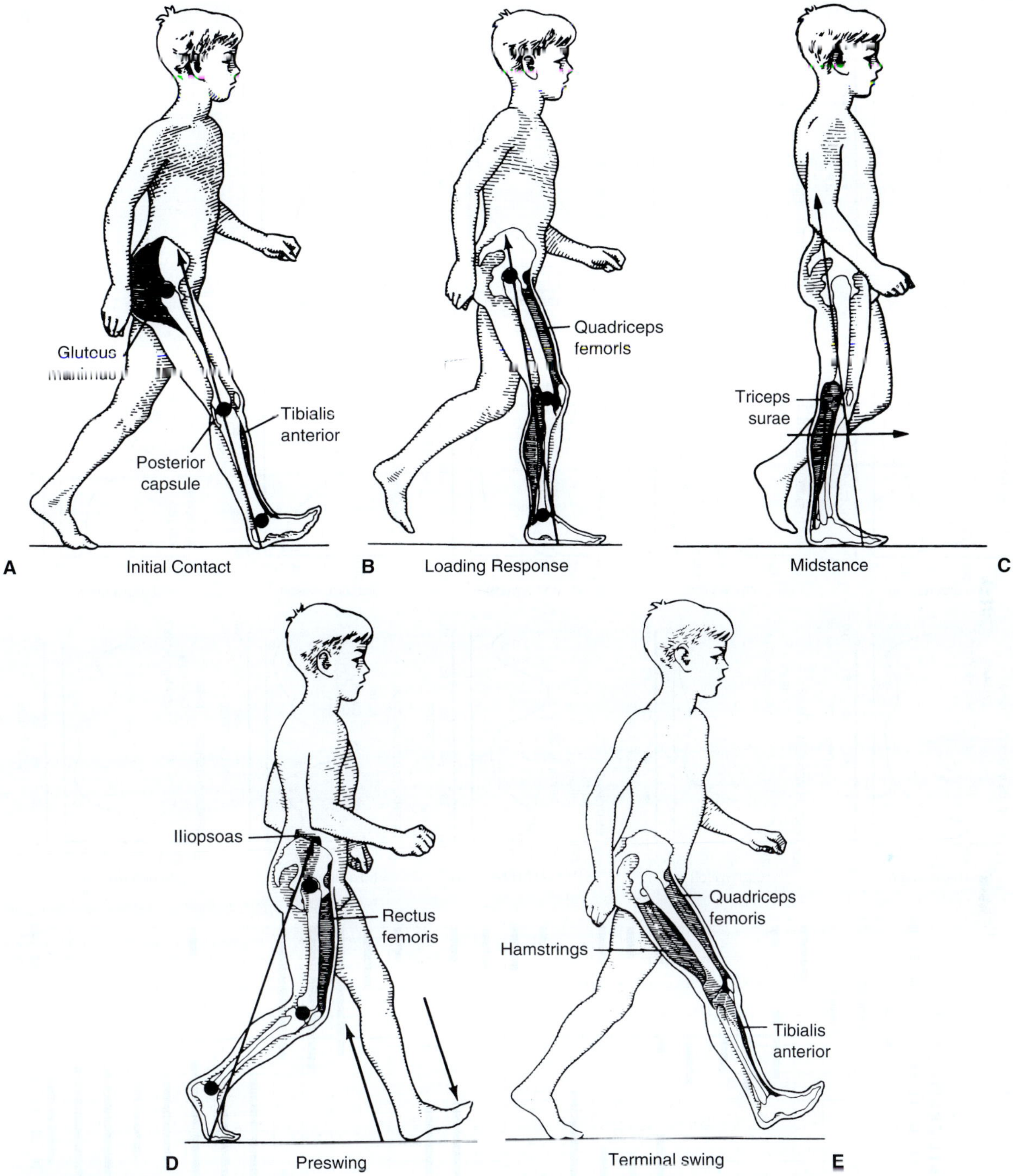

FIGURE 9.5 **(A) Muscle activity and line of floor reaction force at initial foot contact. (B) Muscle activity and line of floor reaction force during loading response. (C) Muscle activity and line of floor reaction force at midstance. (D) Muscle activity and line of floor reaction force at preswing. (E) Muscle activity and line of floor reaction force during terminal swing. (*Source:* Gage Jr. An overview of normal walking. *Instr Course Lect* 1990;39:297–300.)**

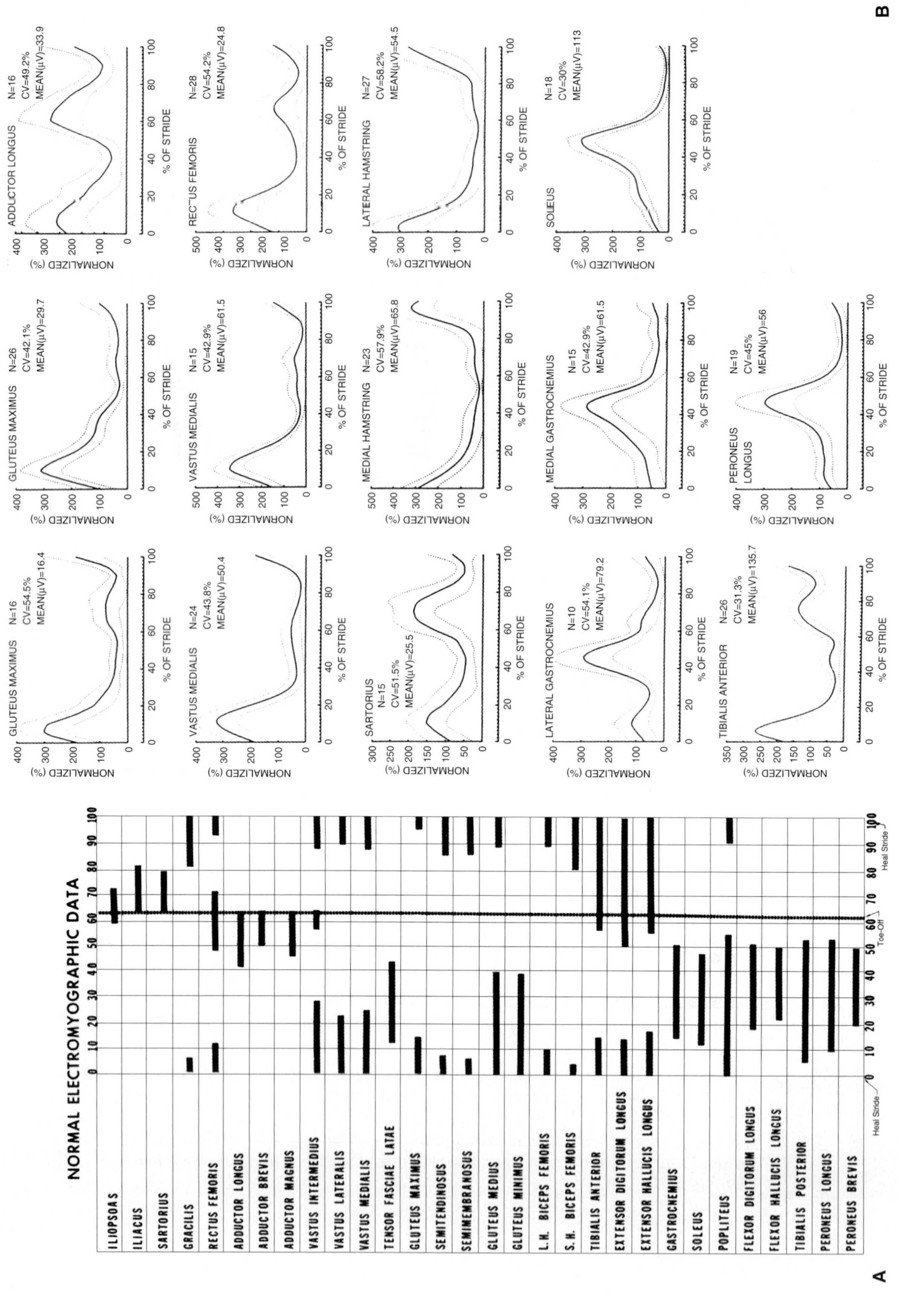
NORMAL ELECTROMYOGRAPHIC DATA
ILIOPSOAS
ILIACUS
SARTORIUS
GRACILIS
RECTUS FEMORIS
ADDUCTOR LONGUS
ADDUCTOR BREVIS
ADDUCTOR MAGNUS
VASTUS INTERMEDIUS
VASTUS LATERALIS
VASTUS MEDIALIS
TENSOR FASCIAE LATAE
GLUTEUS MAXIMUS
SEMITENDINOSUS
SEMIMEMBRANOSUS
GLUTEUS MEDIUS
GLUTEUS MINIMUS
L.H. BICEPS FEMORIS
S.H. BICEPS FEMORIS
TIBIALIS ANTERIOR
EXTENSOR DIGITORUM LONGUS
EXTENSOR HALLUCIS LONGUS
GASTROCNEMIUS
SOLEUS
POPLITEUS
FLEXOR DIGITORUM LONGUS
FLEXOR HALLUCIS LONGUS
TIBIALIS POSTERIOR
PERONEUS LONGUS
PERONEUS BREVIS
Heal Stride
Toe-Off
A
GLUTEUS MAXIMUS N=16 CV=54.5% MEAN(μV)=16.4
VASTUS MEDIALIS N=24 CV=43.8% MEAN(μV)=50.4
SARTORIUS N=15 CV=51.5% MEAN(μV)=25.5
LATERAL GASTROCNEMIUS N=10 CV=54.1% MEAN(μV)=79.2
TIBIALIS ANTERIOR N=26 CV=31.3% MEAN(μV)=135.7
GLUTEUS MAXIMUS N=26 CV=42.1% MEAN(μV)=29.7
VASTUS MEDIALIS N=15 CV=42.9% MEAN(μV)=61.5
MEDIAL HAMSTRING N=23 CV=57.9% MEAN(μV)=65.8
MEDIAL GASTROCNEMIUS N=15 CV=42.9% MEAN(μV)=61.5
PERONEUS LONGUS N=19 CV=45% MEAN(μV)=56
ADDUCTOR LONGUS N=16 CV=49.2% MEAN(μV)=33.9
RECTUS FEMORIS N=28 CV=54.2% MEAN(μV)=24.8
LATERAL HAMSTRING N=27 CV=58.2% MEAN(μV)=54.5
SOLEUS N=18 CV=30% MEAN(μV)=113
NORMALIZED (%)
% OF STRIDE
B

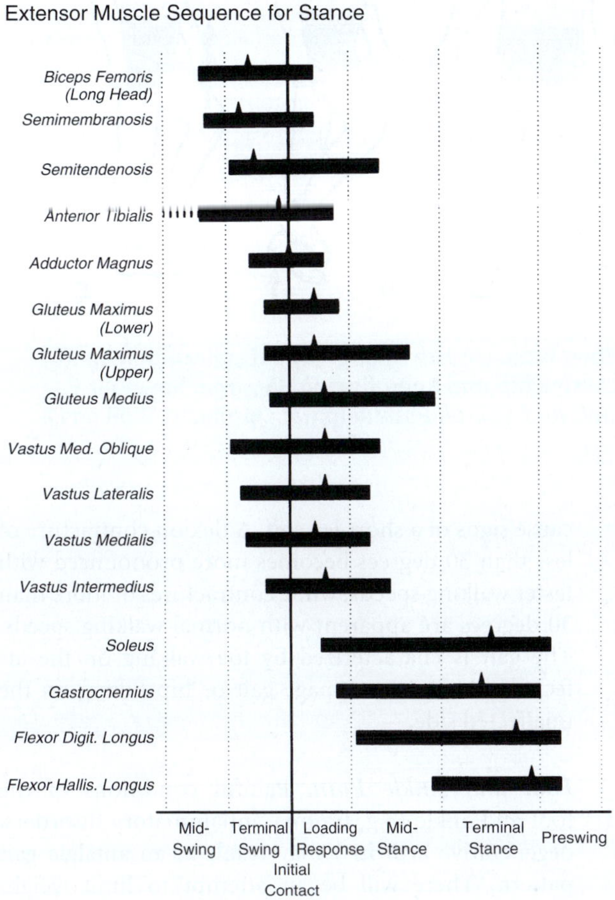

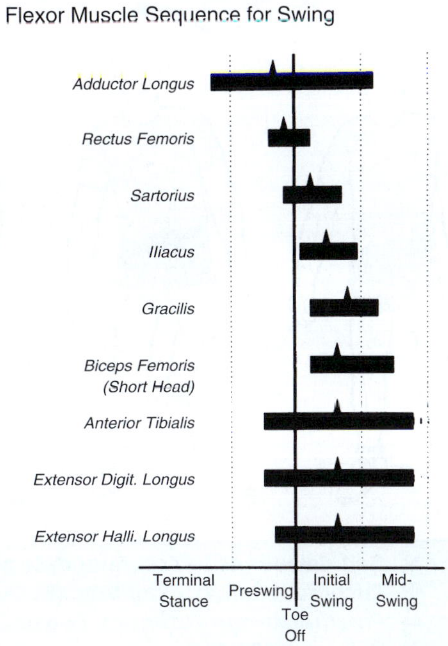

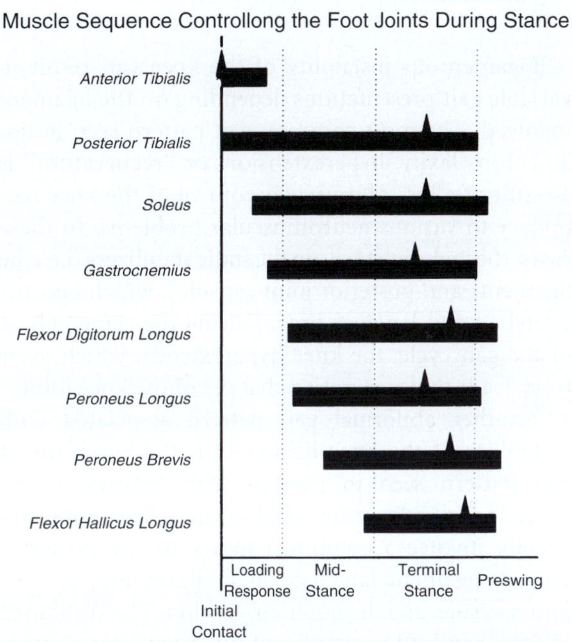

C

FIGURE 9.6 **Examples of normal EMG activity during gait (A) "On-Off" diagrams of activity from the University of California, San Francisco, based on fine-wire EMG. (*Modified from* Lieber RL. *Skeletal Muscle Structure and Function*. Williams & Wilkins, 1992; 122.) (B) *Curves* are normalized EMG envelopes (data from University of Waterloo). (*Modified from* Stulen FB, DeLuca CJ. Frequency parameters of the myoelectric signal as a measure of muscle conduction velocity. *IEEE Trans Biomed Eng* 1981;28:515–523.) (C) Timing of functional muscle activity with peak activity noted (data from Rancho Los Amigos Hospital). (*Modified from* Perry J. *Gait Analysis–Normal and Pathological Function*. Thorofare, NJ: Slack, 1992.) Differences between these types of data reflect the measure variability in phasic activity that has been observed during human walking. (A, B, and C from Rose J, Gamble JG. *Human Walking*. Philadelphia: Lippincott Williams & Wilkins, 2006:111–115.)**

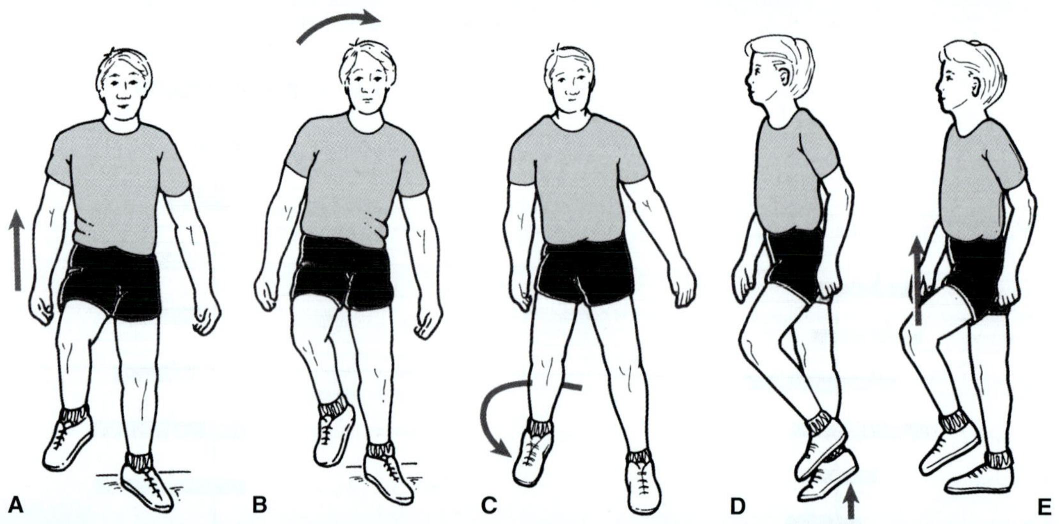

FIGURE 9.7 **Gait deviations to accommodate a long limb. (A) Hip hiking. (B) Lateral trunk lean. (C) Circumduction. (D) Vaulting. (E) Excessive hip and knee flexion. (*Source:* Seymour R. *Prosthetics and Orthotics, Lower Limb and Spinal*. Philadelphia: Lippincott Williams & Wilkins, 2002;109.)**

Ligamentous instability of the knee can result in variable gait presentations depending on the ligament involved. The most common gait pattern seen in ligamentous laxity, hyperextension, or "recurvatum" is a result of a loss of muscular control of the knee secondary to various neuromuscular problems. In these cases, the knee must rely on the static stabilizers (i.e., the ligaments and posterior joint capsule), which become stretched and lax over time. During the stance phase of the gait cycle, the knee hyperextends, which, over time, leads to degenerative changes of the knee joint.

Another abnormal gait pattern associated with instability of the knee ligaments is the varus thrust gait pattern seen in persons with injuries of the posterior-lateral corner of the knee. These injuries usually involve a combined injury to the posterior cruciate ligament, lateral collateral ligament, posterior joint capsule, and the popliteus tendon. The combined injuries can lead to significant functional impairment requiring reconstructive surgery. The gait pattern seen in these people is characterized by varus thrust, which occurs at the knee during the stance phase of gait.

The quadriceps avoidance gait occurs in those who have suffered an injury to their anterior cruciate ligament (ACL). The quadriceps muscle provides an anterior force to the tibia, which becomes a problem in someone with an ACL deficiency because the tibia is prone to anterior subluxation. The person will attempt to decrease the load response phase on the affected limb by decreasing the stride length and avoiding knee flexion during the midportion of stance.

Knee joint contractures will also lead to abnormal gait patterns. A flexion contraction of the knee will cause signs of a short leg gait. A flexion contracture of less than 30 degrees becomes more pronounced with faster walking speeds, while contractures of more than 30 degrees are apparent with normal walking speeds. The gait is characterized by toe walking on the affected side and a steppage gait or hip hiking on the unaffected side.

Foot and Ankle Pain. Painful conditions of the foot and ankle (e.g, trauma, inflammatory disorders, degenerative arthritis) may result in an antalgic gait pattern. There will be an attempt to limit weight bearing through the affected area. The stride length will be greatly shortened, and normal heel-to-toe motion will be lost. If the problem involves the forefoot, the person will tend to avoid plantarflexion and toe-off. If the problem involves the ankle or hindfoot, then the person will avoid heelstrike at initial contact and will ambulate with a tiptoeing gait on the affected side with compensations on the unaffected side (Fig. 9.7D).

People with ankle instability will have great difficulty with supporting body weight during initial contact on the stance leg. At initial contact, the unstable ankle will often buckle with a resultant antalgic gait limiting the load response phase on the affected side.

Joint contractures of the ankle are often seen after trauma, immobilization, and neurologic problems affecting the muscles of the ankle and foot. The most common contracture seen in clinical practice is contracture of the gastrocsoleus complex or "heel cord." A tight or contracted heel cord will result in a steppage type gait pattern (Fig. 9.7E). There will be a loss of normal heel contact and heel-to-toe motion, along with exaggerated hip and knee flexion during the swing phase in order to clear the toe. In long-standing contracture, hyperextension of the ipsilateral knee may occur as plantarflexion at the ankle causes an extension moment at the knee.

Problems of the hindfoot, particularly of the calcaneus, will produce a similar gait pattern (e.g., elimination of heelstrike and a promotion of toe contact during stance). These problems include calcaneal fractures, plantar fasciitis, stress fractures of the ankle or calcaneus, and so forth. An antalgic or avoidance gait with a decrease in the loading of the heel is the typical pattern. In contrast, problems of the forefoot (sprain, fracture, arthritis, metatarsalgia, etc.) will result in an antalgic gait, which minimizes loading on the forefoot by decreasing plantarflexion during the stance phase and push off. People with these problems tend to increase loading to the heel and hindfoot and shorten the time of forefoot loading.

Leg Length Discrepancy. Leg length discrepancy can be the result of various factors affecting any segment of the kinetic chain, including scoliosis and contracture of the hip, knee, and ankle, and is termed a *relative leg length discrepancy*. A true leg length discrepancy is the result of asymmetry in length of the pelvis, femur, or tibia. In either case, a leg length discrepancy can result in pelvic obliquity with a drop of the pelvis, decreased hip and knee flexion, ankle plantarflexion, and/or hyperpronation, which all occur ipsilateral to the shortened side. It is important to determine the etiology of the leg length discrepancy and to properly treat the underlying cause rather than treating all leg length discrepancy with a heel lift. In leg length discrepancy of less than 1.27 cm during the entire stance phase, one sees dipping of the shoulder on the affected side and a compensatory pelvic drop. There is an apparent elevation of the shoulder on the opposite (swing side) and an exaggerated flexion of the hip, knee, and ankle on the ipsilateral side. For shortening more than 3.81 cm, he or she will walk on tiptoes on the shortened limb during the stance phase with full knee extension.

Neurologic Causes of Abnormal Gait

Any dysfunction of the central nervous system, spinal cord, peripheral nerves, or muscles can result in an abnormal gait. It is important to know the segmental innervation of the trunk and lower limbs to evaluate for abnormal gait patterns, particularly the peripheral nerve innervation of each muscle and region. In addition, neurologic injury may result in changes in motor tone and control. The more common disease problems leading to pathologic gait will be reviewed.

Hemiplegic Gait. Cerebrovascular and traumatic brain injuries commonly result in various gait abnormalities, the most common of which is the hemiplegic gait. It is characterized by abnormal arm swing with the arm carried in adduction with flexion at the shoulder, elbow, wrist, and fingers. Also, in many individuals, there is an extensor synergy of the affected lower limb, consisting of extension, adduction, and internal rotation at the hip, extension at the knee, and plantarflexion and inversion of the ankle and foot. This synergy pattern is often initiated by weight bearing over the involved limb and can be useful in supporting the subject. The hemiplegic gait tends to be quite slow with a decrease in step length and an increase in the stance phase with circumduction to allow toe clearance (see Fig. 9.7C). Compensatory changes include hip hiking from lack of knee flexion of the stance leg, a decreased lateral shift over the affected side, a lack of heelstrike secondary to the plantarflexion of the ankle, and recurvatum of the affected knee. The extension moment at the knee is created by the plantar flexion moment occurring at the ankle. Swing phase is characterized by an absent or markedly reduced knee flexion (stiff-knee gait) due to quadriceps spasticity. The flexor synergy gait occurs less commonly and consists of hip flexion, abduction and external rotation, knee flexion, and ankle dorsiflexion. This synergy pattern does not allow the person to stand, thereby eliminating ambulation potential.

Spastic Gait. A spastic gait can develop from an insult to the central nervous system that affects motor tone, particularly of the lower limbs. This can result in "scissoring" of the lower limbs from overactivity of the hip adductors and a narrow, crossing base. There is associated tiptoeing to maintain balance, and great effort is exerted to swing the legs forward, all of which create an unsteady, fatiguing gait. In addition, isolated muscles or muscle groups may develop increased tone and spasticity. For example, spasticity of the tibialis posterior, a powerful plantarflexor and inverter of the foot, causes significant changes in gait during both the stance and swing phases of gait. During stance phase, the initial contact will occur on the lateral aspect of the foot and plantarflexion at the ankle results in an extension moment at the knee. Plantarflexion will also result in a relative lengthening of the limb, often causing dragging of the toes and requiring increased hip and knee flexion.

Parkinsonian Gait. Parkinson disease results from lesions of the basal ganglia affecting motor control and function bilaterally. It is characterized by a paucity of movement of the facial, trunk, and upper and lower limb muscles, resulting in a gait that is slow and shuffling with short, rapid steps, described as being festinating. The trunk is flexed forward, and the person may have difficulties with stops and turns, appearing to chase after his or her COM. Joint motion is reduced because of rigidity, and there is usually little or no arm swing to help in balancing the individual, with falls being a common result.

Ataxic Gait. Injury to the cerebellum or its pathways may disrupt the normal coordination and precision of motor function. The gait of these individuals will be unsteady and associated with a broad-standing base and a lurching or staggering of the trunk and lower limbs. Movements are uncoordinated and appear exaggerated. Leg placement will be variable, and reproducibility is lost. An ataxic gait may also be seen in persons with sensory deficits of the lower limb. In these people, the base is wide, and there may be slapping of their feet as they hit the ground. In addition, these individuals tend to look at their feet because of the lack of proprioceptive feedback and therefore have more problems at night or in the dark.

Isolated Motor Weakness Gait Problems

Gluteus Maximus (Lurch) Gait. The gluteus maximus, a major hip extensor and stabilizer of the trunk, prevents the trunk from falling forward as the COM moves forward at heelstrike. In weakness of the gluteus maximus, the hip is supported by the ligament of Bigelow, which becomes taut in hyperextension. The individual will throw the hip backward with a "lurch" using abdominal and paraspinal muscle activation just after heelstrike on the affected side. The backward trunk lurch persists throughout stance to maintain the gravitational force line behind the hip axis, locking the hip in extension. There is an apparent forward protrusion of the affected hip due to the exaggerated trunk motion, and the person may also hold the shoulders backward to keep the center of gravity behind the hip joint. The hamstring muscles will often compensate for isolated gluteus maximus weakness, resulting in a near normal gait pattern; however, these muscles are often affected together (e.g., in S1 radiculopathy).

Gluteus Medius (Trendelenburg) Gait (Uncompensated and Compensated). In uncompensated gluteus medius weakness, there is a drop of the pelvis more than the usual 5 degrees on the unaffected side, beginning with heelstrike on the affected side and continuing until heelstrike on the unaffected side. There is also a lateral protrusion of the affected hip. In compensated gluteus medius gait due to severe or total paralysis of the hip abductors, the pelvic drop appears to be less as the subject laterally bends the trunk over the hip and drops the shoulder on the affected side. This serves to keep the center of gravity over the hip, which decreases the muscle force required to stabilize the pelvis. With both compensated and uncompensated gait, because the affected leg becomes functionally longer, there is an increase in hip and knee flexion and ankle dorsiflexion. This steppage gait allows for toe clearance.

Hip Flexor Weakness. Hip flexors are the major accelerators in the swing phase of gait. Weakness of the hip flexors results in a limp starting during the stance phase of gait at push-off, persisting throughout the swing phase of the affected side. The subject will demonstrate a trunk lurch backward and toward the unaffected side from push off to midswing, which results in locking of the hip joint on its ligaments, with further extension of the trunk as a unit from push-off to midswing carrying the affected leg forward. The inertia generated from trunk and hip activity carries the limb into flexion. The stride thus becomes shortened on the affected side.

Quadriceps Weakness. Weakness of the quadriceps is most apparent during heelstrike through the stance phase of gait. However, the limp affects all phases of the gait cycle. The affected knee must be locked in hyperextension at or preceding heelstrike by compensatory activity of the gluteus maximus extending the femur and the soleus, which extends the tibia. Extension at the femur results in flexion of the trunk and an extension moment at the knee. Some people place their hand on their thigh at heelstrike and stance to assist the knee into this extended position. With rapid walking, the affected leg lags during swing phase, resulting in excessive heel rise. Repetitive hyperextension of the knee results in stretching of the ligaments and capsule of the knee and resultant recurvatum of the knee during the stance phase.

Ankle Dorsiflexor Weakness (Drop Foot, Slap Foot, or Steppage Gait). With mild weakness, the gait abnormality will be noted at heelstrike and results in loss of plantarflexion control. Heelstrike to foot-flat phase occurs rapidly, and the foot may slap at heelstrike, as eccentric control of the dorsiflexors is decreased. In severe weakness or paralysis, the foot will fall into plantarflexion during swing phase, presenting as a footdrop. Heelstrike is absent, and the person comes down with the toes first or with the entire foot, causing a relative lengthening of the limb, compensated for by exaggerated hip and knee flexion to allow for toe clearance (steppage gait).

Gastrocsoleus Weakness. Gastrocsoleus weakness results in loss of ankle dorsiflexion control. Heel-off will

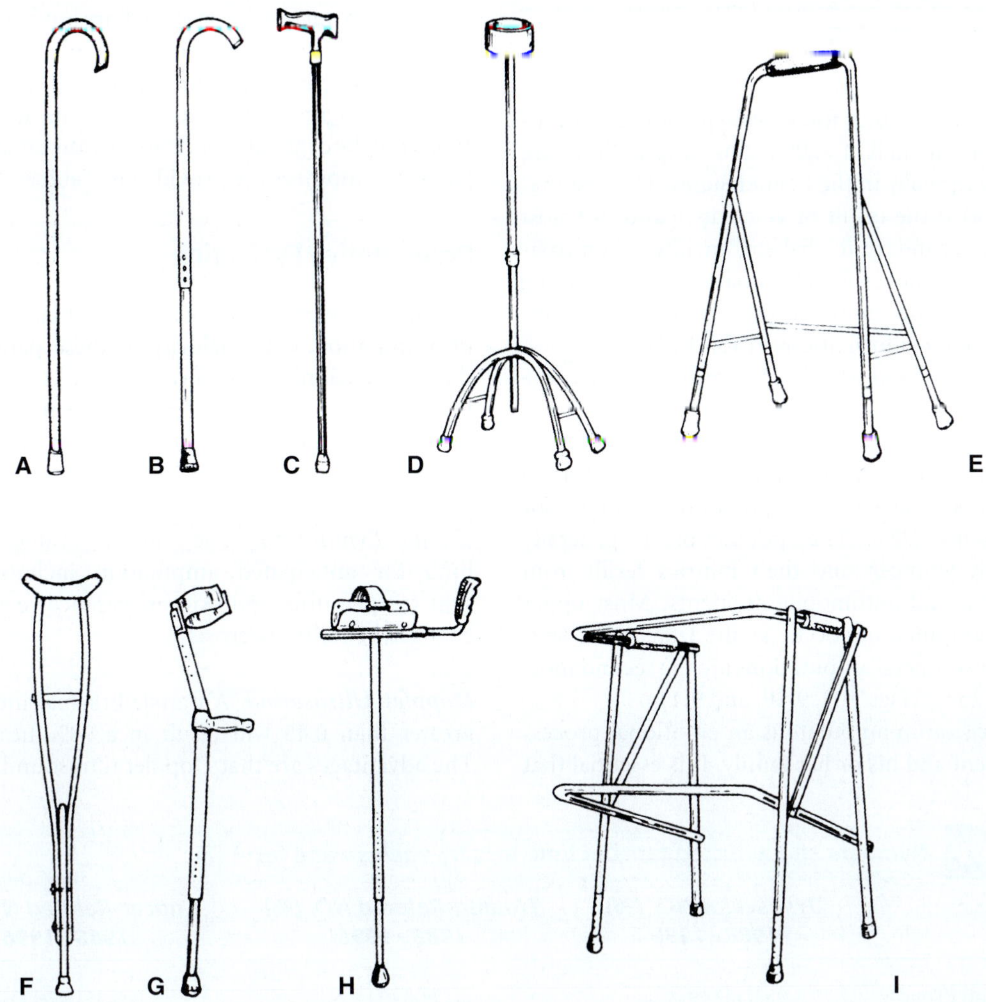

FIGURE 9.8 Canes, crutches and walkers. (A) C-handle or crook-top cane. (B) Adjustable aluminum cane. (C) Functional grip cane. (D) Adjustable wide-base quad cane. (E) Hemiwalker. (F) Adjustable wooden axillary crutch. (G) Adjustable aluminum Lofstrand crutch. (H) Forearm support or platform crutch. (I) Walker or walkerette. (*Source:* DeLisa JA, Gans BM, Walsh NE, et al. *Physical Medicine and Rehabilitation, Principles and Practice*, 4th ed., Vol. 2. Lippincott Williams & Wilkins, 2005;1390.)

be delayed, and the push-off phase will be decreased, resulting in a lag of forward movement of the pelvis on the unaffected side at the time of heelstrike and on the affected side during push off. There will be a shortening of the stride on the unaffected side due to the delay of forward movement of the ipsilateral hip. Altered ground reactive forces lead to a flexion moment behind the knee, which can result in knee buckling.

Assistive Devices. Ambulatory aids (e.g., canes, crutches, walkers) are used to provide an extension of the upper extremities to help transmit body weight and provide support for the patient (Fig. 9.8). The type of ambulatory aid needed depends on how much balance and weight-bearing assistance are needed. Generally, the more disabled the individual, the more complex a walking device is required. The walker supplies the most support, and the standard cane provides the least. Uses of assistive devices include the following:

- Redistribute and unload a weight-bearing lower limb
- Improve balance
- Reduce lower limb pain
- Provide sensory feedback

A cane should be used on the contralateral side to maximize the reduction of stress on the affected limb. Adequate upper limb strength, coordination, and hand function are required for the proper use of ambulation aids.

II. AMPUTATIONS

Amputations are done for several pathologic conditions. Approximately 130,000 new amputations are performed annually in the United States. The vast majority (80%) is the result of vascular disorders (most commonly secondary to diabetes mellitus), approximately 15% are the result of trauma, and the remaining 5% result from the combination of tumors, infections, and congenital malformations (Table 9.2).

The majority (80%) of amputations involve the lower extremities, with approximately 50% involving the toes and foot and the remaining half being evenly distributed between transtibial (25%) and transfemoral (25%). Upper extremity amputation accounts for the remaining 20%. This population is generally significantly younger, and their injuries result from work-related and automobile accidents. Most upper extremity amputations occur at the transradial level (57%); transhumeral amputations are the second most common (23%) (Figs. 9.9, 9.10, and 9.11).

The decision to amputate is an emotional process to the patient and his or her family. It is essential that amputation not be viewed as a failure but as a necessary step in recovery. The residual limb must be surgically constructed to maintain muscle balance, appropriately transfer weight loads, and assume its new role of replacing the original limb. Postoperative management goals for amputees are provided in Table 9.3.

Preoperative Evaluation

Peripheral vascular disease is the most common cause of amputation. The majority of these patients have diabetes mellitus. The preoperative assessment of these patients includes a physical examination and evaluation of perfusion, nutrition, and immunologic status.

Tissue Evaluation. The clinical evaluation of a limb for anticipated amputation includes pulses, skin temperature, and skin appearance (e.g., trophic changes, cellulitis, necrosis).

Doppler Ultrasound. An ankle/brachial index (ABI) greater than 0.45 will result in a 90% healing rate. The advantages are that Doppler ultrasound is readily

TABLE 9.2 Numbers and adjusted rates of limb loss by etiology and level (7)

Level	Dyvascular NO. (%) 1988–1996	Trauma-Related NO. (%) 1988–1996	Cancer-Related NO. (%) 1988–1996
Lower limb (Total)	953,367 (97)	61,605 (31)	8,351 (76.1)
Toe	309,589 (31.5)	27,233 (13.9)	1,466 (13.4)
Foot	102,872 (10.5)	4,483 (2.3)	482 (4.4)
Ankle	7,478 (0.8)	823 (0.4)	164 (1.5)
Transtibial	271,550 (27.6)	14,244 (7.3)	1,501 (13.7)
Through-knee	4,237 (0.4)	921 (0.5)	133 (1.2)
Transfemoral	253,145 (25.8)	10,821 (5.5)	2,499 (22.8)
Hip disarticulation	3,554 (0.4)	418 (0.2)	726 (6.6)
Pelvic	469 (0.1)	52 (0.03)	1,369 (12.5)
Bilateral	0 (0)	1,504 (0.8)	0 (0)
Upper limb (Total)	29,426 (3)	134,421 (68.6)	2,617 (23.9)
Thumb	2,344 (0.2)	24,325 (12.4)	352 (3.2)
Finger(s)	21,427 (2.2)	100,316 (51.2)	529 (4.8)
Hand	1,255 (0.1)	983 (0.5)	92 (0.8)
Wrist	514 (0.1)	415 (0.2)	21 (0.2)
Transradial	1,626 (0.2)	4,001 (2.0)	212 (1.9)
Through-elbow	385 (0.04)	346 (0.2)	123 (1.1)
Transhumeral	1,511 (0.2)	3,008 (1.5)	488 (4.4)
Shoulder	236 (0.02)	154 (0.1)	365 (3.3)
Bilateral	0 (0)	462 (0.2)	0 (0)
Forequarter	132 (0.01)	15 (0.01)	439 (4)

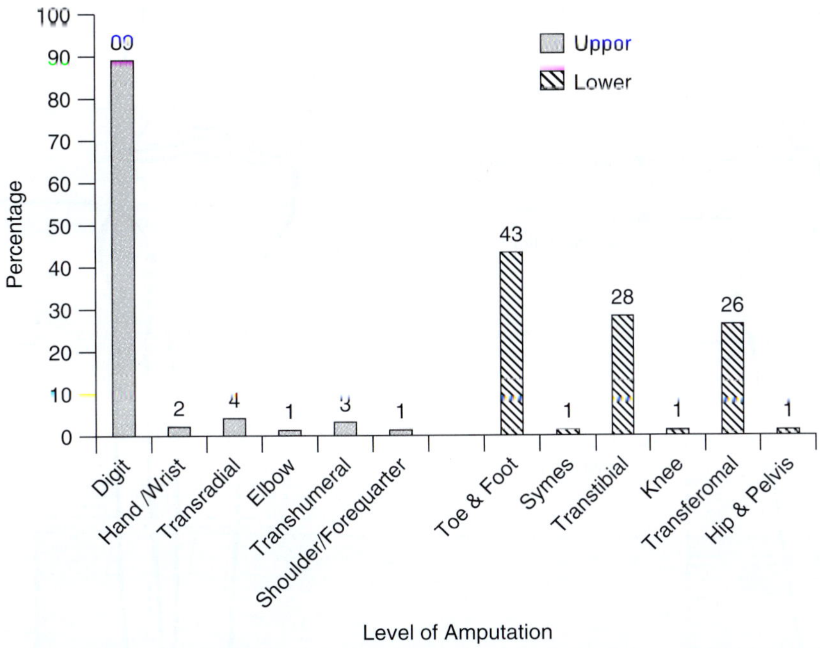

FIGURE 9.9 **Numbers and adjusted rates of limb loss by level. (*Source:* Glennon TP, Smith BS. Amputations. In: Garrison SJ, (ed.), *Handbook of Physical Medicine and Rehabilitation Basics*. Philadelphia: Lippincott-Raven, 1995;34–60.)**

available and noninvasive. However, the disadvantages are that arterial wall calcifications can give misleadingly elevated readings.

Toe Systolic Blood Pressure. A minimum of 55 mmHg is required for distal healing. The advantages of using toe systolic pressure are that it is noninvasive, readily available, and inexpensive, despite that it is inaccurate.

Transcutaneous Oxygen Tension. PO_2 higher than 35 is necessary for wound healing.

- *Advantages*—Noninvasive, highly accurate in determining wound healing
- *Disadvantages*—Results may be altered by skin disorders (e.g., edema or cellulitis)

Other Studies. Other means of evaluation that may prove useful include the following:

- *Skin blood flow (Xenon-133 clearance)*—Expensive, time consuming
- *Fluorescence studies*—Unreliable results
- *Arteriogram to visualize patency of vessels*—Invasive, not reliable in determining successful wound healing

Nutritional and Immune Competence. The following are in addition to general requirements for surgery.

- Serum albumin at least 3g/dL
- Total lymphocyte count of more than 1500/mL

Psychological Factors. It is important that patients view amputation as a step in recovery, not a failure. An early plan for prosthetic fitting and return to function should be in place, and preoperative counseling of the patient and family should take place. Amputee support groups are rated to be very helpful by many amputees; the Amputee Coalition of America is one such group.

Additional Factors. Activity level, ambulatory potential, cognitive skills, and overall health status must be evaluated in the potential amputee. Generally, for potentially ambulatory patients, the goal of amputation is to achieve healing at the most distal level that can be fitted with a prosthesis and allow successful rehabilitation. For nonambulatory patients, the goal is to improve sitting balance, ease of transfers, and hygienic requirements.

Surgical Principles

Levels of Amputations. Careful surgical techniques, especially soft tissue handling, is critical to wound healing and functional outcome in amputation surgery. Muscle flaps should be kept thick, and skin and flaps should be avoided because of the increased risk of wound failure (see Figs. 9.10 and 9.11).

Bone. The distal bone should be smoothed and beveled to decrease the likelihood of bony prominences. In adults, the periosteum should not be stripped.

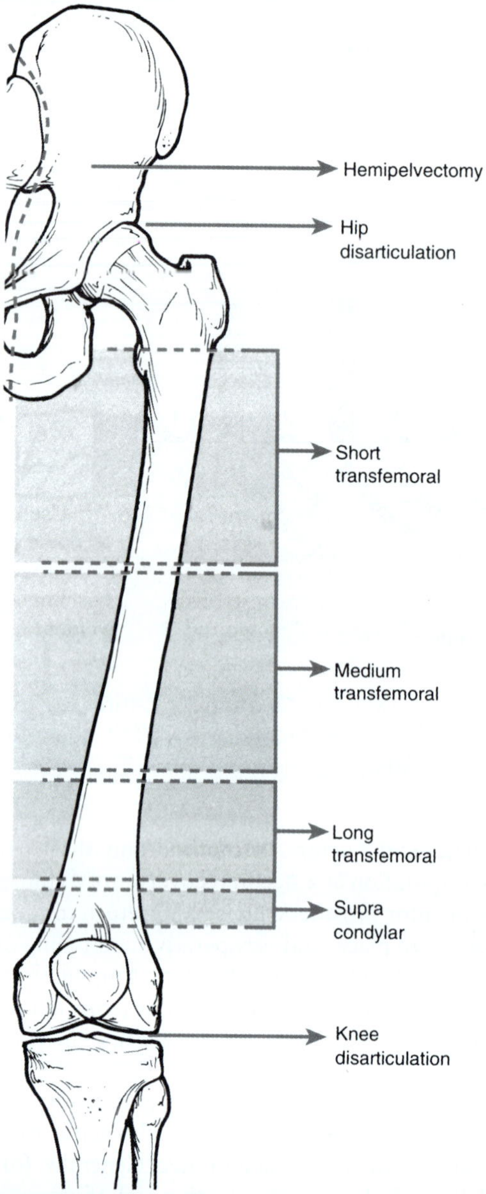

FIGURE 9.10 **Transfemoral amputation levels. (*Source:* Seymour R. *Prosthetics and Orthotics, Lower Limb and Spinal*. Lippincott Williams & Wilkins, 2002;22.)**

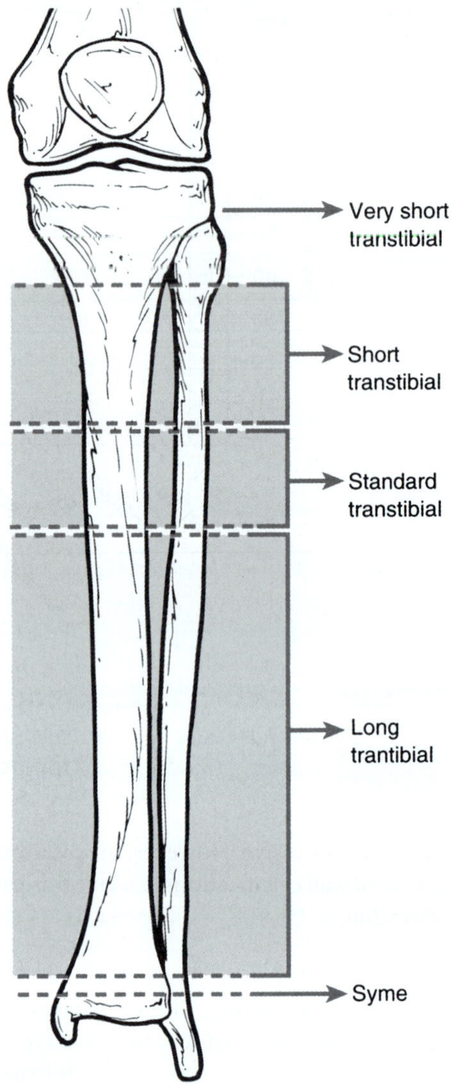

FIGURE 9.11 **Transtibial amputation levels. (*Source:* Seymour R. *Prosthetics and Orthotics, Lower Limb and Spinal*. Lippincott Williams & Wilkins, 2002;25.)**

However, in pediatric amputations it is advantageous to remove the distal 0.5 cm of the distal periosteum to prevent terminal overgrowth of the bone.

Muscle Attachment. Beveling or contouring may be required for good residual limb shape (Fig. 9.12A). Stabilization of the distal insertion of muscle can improve residual limb function by preventing muscle atrophy, providing counterbalance of the deforming forces resulting from amputation, and providing padding for the residual limb. Myodesis is the technique in which distal muscle is sutured directly to bone or tendon (Fig. 9.12B). Myodesis is most effective in securing large muscle groups (e.g., gastrocsoleus in a transtibial amputation). Myoplasty is the technique in which muscle is secured to periosteum or other muscle. In general, myodesis results in a more stable residual limb than myoplasty and decreases the likelihood of bursal formation in a poorly stabilized residual limb.

Nerve and Blood Vessel Management. The transection of nerves is inevitable during amputation surgery. Care must be taken to limit the incidence

TABLE 9.3 Goals of post operative management of the amputee

- Successful healing of the amputation
- Pain control
- Maintaining range of motion in the remaining proximal joints of the amputated extremity
- Strengthening of residual muscle groups needed for biomechanical compensation
- Preparation of the residual limb for prosthetic fitting
- Achieving independence in ADLs and mobility without a prosthetic limb
- Education about the process of prosthetic limb fitting and expected functional outcome.
- Psychosocial support for the adaptations resulting from the amputation.

of symptomatic neuroma formation. Meticulous isolation, application of gentle tension and sharp transaction allows the nerve to retract into the soft tissues where neuroma formation is less likely to be symptomatic. Larger nerves (e.g., sciatic) have well-vascularized perineurium that require ligation prior to transaction. Blood vessels, large arteries, and veins should be doubly ligated and hemostasis achieved prior to closure.

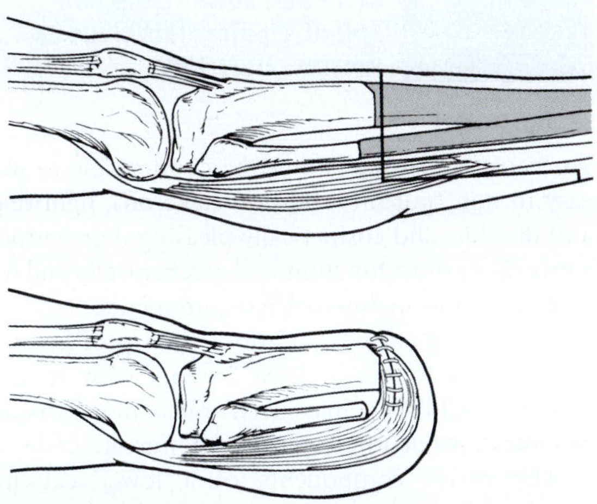

FIGURE 9.12 **Transtibial amputation procedure (A) Long posterior flap is used. (B) Fibula is cut higher than the tibia and the anterior surface of the tibia is beveled.** *(Adapted from Shea, JD. Surgical techniques for lower extremity amputation. Orthopedic Clinics of North America* 1972; 3:287–301; *from* Seymour R. *Prosthetics and Orthotics, Lower Limb and Spinal.* Lippincott Williams & Wilkins, 2002;25.)

Wound Closure. The wound may be closed primarily or wound closure may be delayed in the event of an ischemic limb. In either event, attention must be made to not close the wound with tension. Additionally, placement of a drain to decompress the underlying tissue is recommended.

Postoperative Management. Wound protection and edema control can be established with the use of a compressive dressing immediately postoperatively. Care should be taken to avoid too constrictive a dressing that could result in a tourniquet effect. A splint or cast may also be applied to help mold the residual limb and limit edema.

Complications of Amputation

Phantom Limb Sensation. Phantom limb sensation is the feeling that part or some of the amputated limb is still present. This sensation occurs in greater than 80% of transtibial and transfemoral amputates. This phenomenon usually decreases with time.

Phantom Limb Pain. Phantom limb pain is a painful condition that causes a burning sensation in the amputated limb. This is due to nerve irritation. It may be treated pharmacologically (e.g., with gabapentin) or with transdermal stimulation. Additionally, desensitization through physical therapy and prosthetic use helps to decrease phantom limb pain.

Hematoma. The result of insufficient hemostasis intraoperatively can result in hematoma formation. Use of a drain helps to evacuate the accumulating blood. Reexploration might be necessary if the hematoma is too large or compromising the overlying soft tissues.

Infection. Patients with poor circulation are at an increased risk for infection. If the amputation is performed as result of an infection or trauma, attention must be made to remove all of the devitalized tissue. Administration of perioperative antibiotics also decreases the risk of infection.

Wound Necrosis. Wound necrosis is another complication that may result. Careful closure of the wound, especially limited wound tension, is necessary to limit necrosis.

Contractures. Flexion contractures usually occur about the hip and knee. These can be avoided by careful balancing of distal muscle flaps intraoperatively, encouraging range of motion exercises, and careful positioning of the amputated limb in the early postoperative period.

Neuromas. Neuromas are inevitable once a nerve is transected. However, symptomatic neuromas are preventable. Injecting the nerve endings with lidocaine or bupivacaine prior to allowing sharply transected nerves to retract deep into the soft tissue limits the likelihood that they will develop into symptomatic neuromas.

Terminal Overgrowth of Bone. This phenomenon occurs most commonly in pediatric amputees. This condition commonly occurs as the result of diaphyseal amputation of patients with significant remaining growth. Attempts should be made to perform a disarticulation as opposed to a diaphyseal amputation in the pediatric population, if amputation is indicated. Overgrowth occurs most commonly at the humerus, followed by the fibula, tibia, and femur. Treatment consists of surgical revision of the residual limb. Alternatively, residual limb-capping procedures (with autologous bone) may be use to prevent this occurrence.

Limb Salvage. Limb salvage has become a viable alternative to amputation in some patients, particularly in tumor and trauma patients. However, recent data from multicenter studies have compared the results of limb salvage versus amputations in trauma patients. The results suggested that the outcomes of patients who underwent limb salvage measures were not significantly different from patients who underwent amputation. In fact, limb salvage patients had a higher rate of complications, additional surgeries, and rehospitalization. The absolute indication for amputation after trauma is an ischemic limb with a vascular injury that cannot be repaired (absence of neurologic function is not an absolute indication for amputation).

III. PROSTHETICS

A prosthesis is a device or an artificial substitute designed to replace, as much as possible, the function or appearance of a missing limb or body part. An orthosis is a device designed to supplement or augment the function of an existing limb or body part.

The level of motivation of the individual should be assessed. Ideally, discussions about prosthetic use should begin preoperatively and should involve the surgeon, physiatrist, prosthetist, and patient.

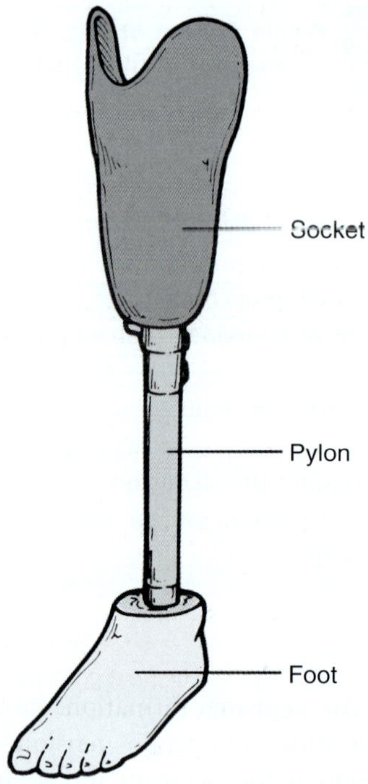

FIGURE 9.13 **Endoskeletal or modular design prosthetics depicting socket, pylon, and foot. (*Source:* Seymour R. *Prosthetics and Orthotics, Lower Limb and Spinal.* Lippincott Williams & Wilkins, 2002;177.)**

Foremost, a prosthesis must be comfortable to wear, easy to don (put on) and doff (take off), lightweight and durable, and cosmetically pleasing. Furthermore, a prosthesis must function well mechanically and have reasonably low maintenance requirements.

Minor cosmetic modifications aside, prostheses can be expected to last at least 2 years with standard daily use. Children may need much more frequent modifications or adjustments as they grow.

The major components of a lower extremity prosthesis are the socket, a sock or gel liner, a suspension system, an articulating joint (if needed), a pylon, and a terminal device (Fig. 9.13). The terminal device is typically a foot (Fig. 9.14) but may take other forms for water or sports activities.

The Socket. The socket is the connection between the residual limb and the prosthesis. It not only must protect the residual limb but also must transmit the forces associated with standing and ambulation. The preparatory socket (temporary) needs to be adjusted several times as the volume of the residual limb stabilizes. The preparatory socket can be created by using a plaster mold of the residual limb as a template. The transfemoral sockets allow for 10 degrees of

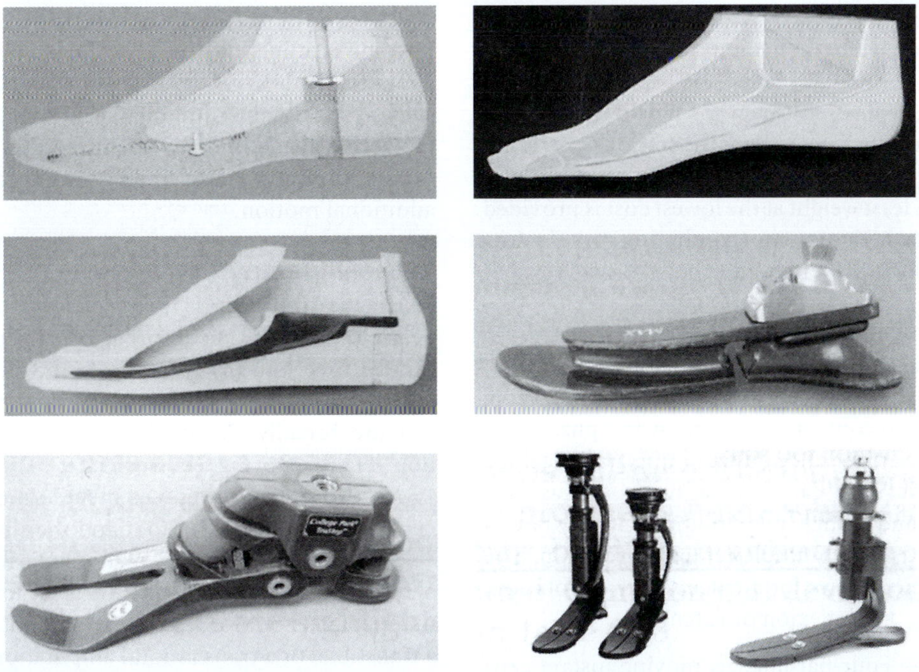

FIGURE 9.14 **Prosthetic feet from the single-axis cushion heel (SACH) and stationary-and-flexible endoskeletal (Safe II flexible keel) foot (top). The Carbon Copy II Lite Foot (dynamic response) and Luxon Max (dynamic response with multiaxis) (middle). The College Park TruStep (dynamic response, with some inversion, eversion, and transverse motion). The FlexFoot VSP (vertical shock pylon, dynamic response, multi-axis). The Ceterus (vertical shock pylon, dynamic response, multiaxis, and transverse motion) (bottom). The prosthetic manufacturers have numerous feet available for a wide range of patients, from homebound to paralympic. Courtesy of Kingsley, Ohio Willow Wood, Otto Block, CPI, and Ossur. See Web Site listings.) (*Source:* DeLisa JA, Gans BM, Walsh NE, et al. *Physical Medicine and Rehabilitation, Principles and Practice*, 4th ed., Vol. 2. Lippincott Williams & Wilkins, 2005;1332.)**

adduction of the femur (to stretch the gluteus medius, allowing adequate strength for midstance stability) and 5 degrees of flexion (to stretch the gluteus maximus and allow for greater hip extension). The most common socket used in a transtibial prosthesis is a patellar tendon-bearing design.

The Suspension Mechanism. The prosthesis can be attached to the residual limb by a variety of belts, wedges, straps, suction, or a combination of the above. Suction suspension is broken down into 2 categories: standard suction and silicon suspension suction. A standard suction is simply a form-fitting rigid or semirigid socket into which the residual limb is fitted. The silicon suction uses a silicon-based sock that slips onto the residual limb, which is then inserted into the socket. The silicon helps to form an airtight seal that stabilizes the prosthesis.

- *Transtibial suspension*—Gel liner suspension with a locking pin is most common; sleeve (made of silicone, urethane, or thermoplastic elastomer) rolls on to the stump and then is locked in with pin; liners use suction and friction to provide suspension; supracondylar suspension is used when the residual limb is less then 5 cm
- *Transfemoral suspension*—Vacuum suspension is frequently used; relies on surface tension, negative pressure, and muscle contraction; Silesian belts used to prevent socket rotation

Upper Limb. Limb salvage is more critical for the upper limb, where sensation is critical to function. An insensate prosthesis provides less function than a partially sensate, partially functional salvaged limb in the upper extremity. After amputation, prosthetic fitting should be done as soon as possible, even before complete wound healing has occurred. Outcomes of prosthetic limbs vary 75% to 85% when prosthetic fitting occurs within 30 days of amputation, for transradial amputation, in contrast with less than 30% when started late. With respect to the actual prosthetic device, the terminal device (particularly in heavy laborers) is activated by shoulder flexion and abduction. Elbow flexion and extension are controlled by shoulder extension and depression. Optimal mechanical efficiency of figure-8 harnesses requires the harness ring to be at the spinous process of C7 and slightly toward the nonamputated side. The best function with least weight at the lowest cost is provided by hybrid prosthetic systems (combining myoelectric, traditional body-powered and body-driven switch components).

Knee Joint. The prosthetic knee must fill 3 functions: provide support during the stance phase of ambulation, produce smooth control during the swing phase, and maintain unrestricted motion for sitting and kneeling. The prosthetic knee can have a single axis with a simple hinge and a single pivot point, or it may have a polycentric axis with multiple centers of rotation. The polycentric knee allows for a truer center of rotation, not sacrificing either flexion or extension.

- *Polycentric*—Four-bar linkage; moving instant center of rotation; different stability characteristics during gait cycle; increased flexion in sitting, recommended for transfemoral amputations, knee disarticulations, and bilateral amputees
- *Stance-phase control*—Weight-activated; constant-friction during swing phase; "freezes" during weight application; primarily for older patients, high-level amputees, or uneven terrain
- *Fluid control*—Hydraulic or pneumatic; cadence response by changing resistance to knee flexion; prevents excessive flexion; extended earlier in gait cycle
- *Constant friction*—General utility knee; uneven terrain; dampens knee swing; most common knee used in childhood prosthetics; allows only single-speed walking; relies solely on alignment for stance phase stability; not recommended for older or weaker patients
- *Variable friction*—Cadence control; resistance to knee flexion increases with extension; allows for different walking speeds; not durable; not available in endoskeleton systems
- *Manual locking*—Constant-friction knee hinge with a lock in extension; usually left locked in extension; used primarily in weak, unstable patients

The Pylon and Ankle. The pylon is a simple tube or shell that attaches the socket to the terminal device. Pylons have progressed from simple static shells to dynamic devices that allow axial rotation and absorb, store, and release energy. The pylon can be an exoskeleton (soft foam contoured to match the other limb with a hard laminated shell) or an endoskeleton (internal metal frame with cosmetic soft covering). The ankle function usually is incorporated into the terminal device. Separate ankle joints can be beneficial in heavy-duty industrial work or in sports such as mountain climbing, swimming, and rowing. However, the additional weight requires more energy expenditure and more limb strength to control the additional motion.

Terminal Devices. The 5 basic functions of the prosthetic foot are (1) to provide a stable, weight-bearing surface; (2) to absorb shock; (3) to replace lost muscle function; (4) to replicate the anatomic joint; and (5) to restore cosmetic appearance. Prosthetic feet are broadly classified as energy-storing feet or non–energy-storing feet (see Fig. 9.14).

Non–energy-storing feet include the solid-ankle/cushioned-heel (SACH) foot and the single-axis foot. The SACH foot mimics ankle plantarflexion, which allows for a smooth gait. It is a low-cost, low-maintenance foot for a sedentary patient who has had a transtibial or a transfemoral amputation. The single-axis foot adds passive plantarflexion and dorsiflexion, which increase stability during stance phase.

The energy-storing feet are the multiaxis foot and the dynamic-response foot. The multiaxis foot adds inversion, eversion, and rotation to plantar flexion and dorsiflexion. It handles uneven terrain well and is a good choice for the individual with a minimal-to-moderate activity level. The dynamic-response foot is the top-of-the-line foot and is commonly used by young, active individuals and athletic individuals with amputations.

Prosthetic Fitting and Testing. When the incision has completely healed, fitting for the prosthesis can begin. The prosthesis must be individually fitted to the patient. Prostheses are described at this stage as either preparatory or definitive. The preparatory prosthesis is fitted while the residual limb is still remodeling. This allows the patient to start the rehabilitation program of donning and doffing, transfer training, building wear tolerance, obtaining balance, and ambulating with the prosthesis several weeks earlier in the process. A preparatory prosthesis often allows a better fit in the definitive prosthesis as the preparatory socket can be used to mold the residual limb into the desired shape.

Sometimes, a preparatory prosthesis is not feasible because of financial considerations. In this case, the patient can only be fitted for the definitive prosthesis. If the patient is being fitted for a final prosthesis without ever having a preparatory prosthesis, delay fitting for the socket until the residual limb is fully mature (usually 3 to 4 months) or until general stabilization occurs in the patient's weight and residual limb circumference.

Initially, the patient is taught the basics of prosthetics care, including how to don and doff the prosthesis, how to inspect the residual limb for signs of skin breakdown (which should be checked daily), and how to perform safe transfers (moving from one position or surface to another). Then, shift emphasis to weight bearing with the prosthesis. Finally, address ambulation on level surfaces with a walker or other assistive device. Once the patient has mastered these skills, he or she can begin training on stairs, uneven surfaces, and ramps/inclines. The end goal is for the patient to safely ambulate on all usual surfaces without adaptive equipment.

Weight Bearing. An individual with a lower extremity amputation must bear full body weight on soft tissues not designed for that function. The socket must be designed such that these forces are distributed as much as possible and as evenly as possible over pressure-tolerant areas. These include the patellar tendon, the pretibial muscles, the residual posterior muscles, the medial flare of the tibia, and the lateral fibula. The presence of ongoing pain, skin breakdown, change in the ability to don and doff the prosthesis, and change in the number of sock plies indicates that the prosthesis needs to be modified. Erythema normally appears within a few minutes after removing the prosthesis and should fade quickly. Erythema that is present upon removing the prosthesis or that does not completely resolve within 20 minutes is particularly worrisome.

Choke Syndrome. When the proximal part of the socket has too snug a fit on the residual limb, venous outflow can be obstructed. When this is combined with an empty space more distally in the socket, swelling can occur until that empty space is filled. In an acute choke situation, the skin is red and indurated and may have an orange-peel appearance with prominent skin pores. If the constriction is not resolved, then chronic skin changes with hemosiderin deposits and venous stasis ulcers may develop.

Dermatologic Problems. Common skin management issues include contact dermatitis, sebaceous cysts, scar management, and excessive sweating. The liner, socks, and suspension mechanism are the usual culprits for contact dermatitis. The socket is a less likely cause. Treatment is identification and removal of the offending item and symptomatic treatment with topical Benadryl or cortisone creams. Cysts and sweating can be a sign of excessive shear forces and components that are improperly fitted. Scar management is focused on massaging and lubricating the scar to obtain a well-healed result without dog ears or adhesions.

TABLE 9.4 Increase in energy consumption by amputation level

Level	Percentage Above Normal
Below knee unilateral amputation	10%–20%
Below knee bilateral amputation	20%–40%
Above knee unilateral amputation	60%–70%
Above knee bilateral amputation	> 200%

Energy Expenditure of Amputees. The increase in energy requirements can be the limiting factor in ambulation. An individual who has a lower extremity amputation and requires a walker or crutches to ambulate uses 65% more energy than someone with a normal gait. Increased levels of energy consumption (percentage above normal) by amputation level are provided in Table 9.4. Energy consumption is actually less with a transtibial amputation prosthesis than ambulating with crutches. However, ambulating with a transfemoral amputation prosthesis requires more energy, which makes the cardiopulmonary status of these patients more significant.

IV. ORTHOTICS

A lower limb orthosis is an external device applied or attached to a lower body segment to improve function by controlling motion, providing support through stabilizing gait, reducing pain through transferring load to another area, correcting flexible deformities, and preventing progression of fixed deformities. Orthoses generally are named by the body regions that they involve, as demonstrated by the following abbreviations:

- *AFO*—Ankle-foot orthosis (Fig. 9.15)
- *KAFO*—Knee-ankle-foot orthosis (Fig. 9.16)
- *HKAFO*—Hip-knee-ankle-foot orthosis
- *THKAFO*—Trunk-hip-knee-ankle-foot orthosis

Lower Extremity Orthotics

An orthosis is classified as a static or dynamic device. A static orthosis is rigid and is used to support the weakened or paralyzed body parts in a particular position. A dynamic orthosis is used to facilitate body motion to allow optimal function. Most orthoses use

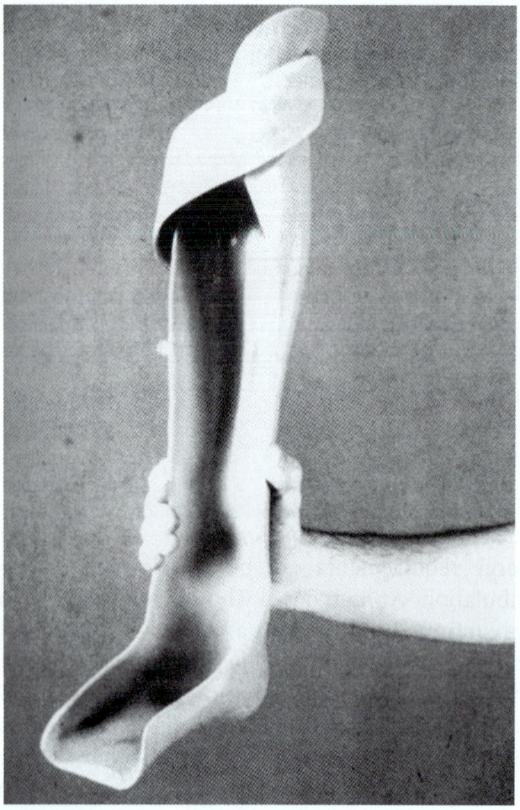

FIGURE 9.15 **Plastic solid ankle-foot orthosis. (*Source:* DeLisa JA, Gans BM, Walsh NE, et al. *Physical Medicine and Rehabilitation, Principles and Practice*, 4th ed., Vol. 2. Lippincott Williams & Wilkins, 2005;1385.)**

a 3-point system to ensure proper positioning of the lower limb inside the orthosis. A lower limb orthosis should be used only for specific management of a selected disorder. The orthotic joints should be aligned at the approximate anatomic joints.

The orthosis selected should be simple, lightweight, strong, durable, and cosmetically acceptable. Considerations for orthotic prescription should include the 3-point pressure control system, static or dynamic stabilization, flexible material, and tissue tolerance to compression and shear force.

An orthosis can be constructed from metal, plastic, leather, synthetic fabrics, or any combination. Plastic material, such as polypropylene, is the material most commonly used in the orthotic industry.

Shoes

Shoes are an important component of the lower limb orthosis. Shoes are used to protect and warm the feet, transfer body weight while walking, and reduce pressure or pain through redistributing weight. Shoes should be comfortable and properly fitted. They should be at least 1 cm longer than the longest toe and correspond to the shape of the feet.

Shoe Anatomy. The shoe can be divided into lower and upper parts. The lower parts consist of the sole, shank, ball, toe spring, and heel. The upper parts include the quarter, heel counter, vamp, toe box, tongue, and throat (Fig. 9.17).

Sole. Outer and inner soles are separated by compressible filler. Both of them are made preferably of leather for breathability. The ball is the widest part of the sole and corresponds to the area of the metatarsal heads. The shank area is from the anterior border of the heel to the ball. A steel piece may be used to reinforce the shank area. The toe spring is the space between the anterior sole and the floor.

The Heel. Leather with rubber on the plantar surface is commonly is used for the heel. The heel counter is the posterior portion of the upper part between the quarters. This structure is used to reinforce the quarters and support the calcaneus. The heel counter can increase the posterior stability of the shoe.

The Upper. The upper is the portion of the shoe above the sole. The vamp is the anterior section. The quarters are the posterior section. The throat is the base of the tongue. The tongue is the portion attached proximally to the vamp. The toe box is the reinforcement of the vamp to protect the shoe from trauma.

External Shoe Modifications

Heel Modifications. There are many types of heel modifications.

- *Cushioned heel*—A wedge of compressible rubber is inserted into the heel to absorb impact at heelstrike. This cushion often is used with a rigid ankle to reduce the knee flexion moment by allowing for more rapid ankle plantar flexion.
- *Heel flare*—A medial flare is used to resist inversion, and a lateral flare is used to resist eversion. Both flares are used to provide heel stability.
- *Heel wedge*—A medial wedge is used to promote inversion, and a lateral wedge is used to promote eversion. The heel counter should be strong enough to prevent the hindfoot from sliding down the incline created by the wedge.
- *Extended heel*—The Thomas heel projects anteriorly on the medial side to provide support to the medial longitudinal arch. The reverse Thomas heel projects anteriorly on the lateral side to provide stability to the lateral longitudinal arch.

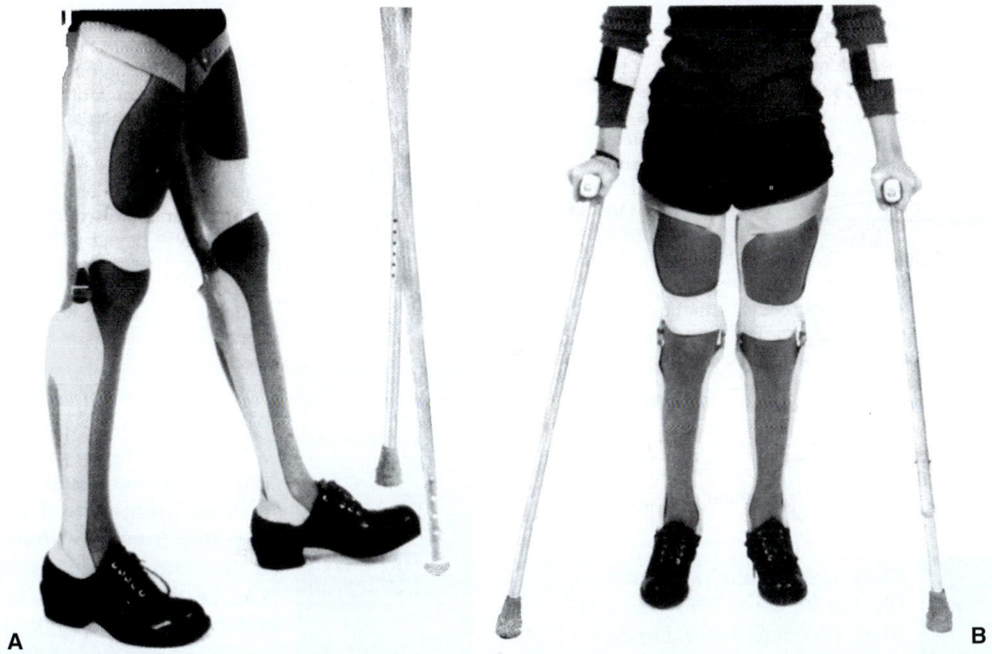

FIGURE 9.16 Plastic-laminated knee-ankle-foot orthoses viewed from side (A) and front (B). (*Source:* DeLisa JA, Gans BM, Walsh NE, et al. *Physical Medicine and Rehabilitation, Principles and Practice*, 4th ed., Vol. 2. Lippincott Williams & Wilkins, 2005;1387.)

- *Heel elevation*—A shoe lift is used to compensate for fixed equinus deformity or for any leg length discrepancy of more than one quarter of an inch.

Sole Modifications. Sole modifications are shown in Figure 9.18.

- *Rocker bar*—A convex structure placed posterior to the metatarsal head. The rocker bar is used to shift the rollover point from metatarsal head to metatarsal shaft to avoid irritation of ulcers along the metatarsal head in patients with diabetes mellitus.
- *Metatarsal bar*—A bar with a flat surface placed posterior to the metatarsal head. The metatarsal bar is used to relieve the pressure from the metatarsal heads.
- *Sole wedge*—A medial wedge is used to promote supination, and a lateral wedge is used to provide pronation.
- *Sole flare*—A medial flare is used to resist inversion, and a lateral flare is used to resist eversion. Both flares promote great stability.
- *Steel bar*—The steel bar is placed between the inner sole and outer sole. This bar is used to reduce forefoot motion to reduce the stress from phalanges and metatarsals.
- *Combination of sole and heel modifications*—If heel elevation is more than one half an inch, a sole elevation should be added to avoid equinus posture.

Internal Shoe Modifications

Heel modifications. Internal heel modification options include cushions and wedges.

- *Heel cushion relief*—This soft pad with excavation is placed under the painful point of the heel.
- *Heel wedges*—A medial heel wedge can rotate the hindfoot into inversion. A lateral heel wedge can evert the hindfoot to avoid pressure on the cuboid.

Sole Modifications. There are several options for internal sole modifications.

- *Metatarsal pad*—This domed pad is designed to reduce the stress from metatarsal heads by transferring the load to metatarsal shafts in metatarsalgia.
- *Inner sole excavation*—A soft pad filled with compressible material is placed under one or more metatarsal heads.
- *Scaphoid pad*—This type of pad extends from one half inch posterior to the first metatarsal head to the anterior tubercle of the calcaneus. The apex of the scaphoid pad is between the talonavicular joint and the navicular tuberosity. The scaphoid pad is used for medial arch support.
- *Toe crest*—A crescent-shaped pad is placed behind the second through fourth phalanges. The toe crest fills the void under the proximal phalanges and reduces the stress.

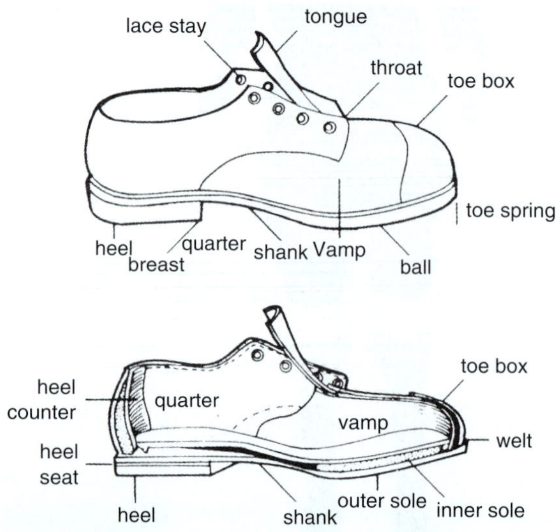

FIGURE 9.17 Shoe components. (*Source:* DeLisa JA, Gans BM, Walsh NE, et al. *Physical Medicine and Rehabilitation, Principles and Practice*, 4th ed., Vol. 2. Lippincott Williams & Wilkins, 2005;1379.)

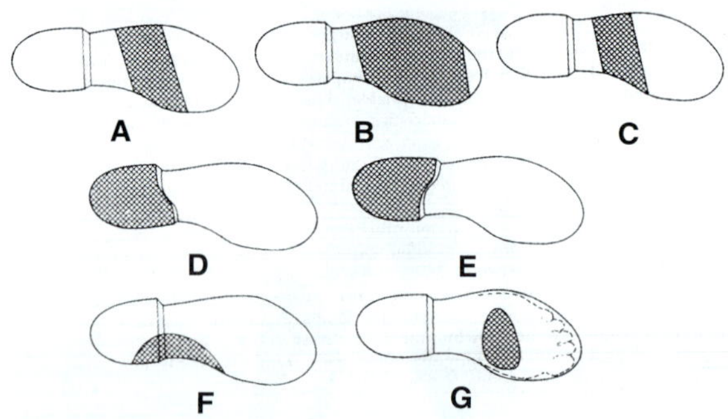

FIGURE 9.18 Common shoe modifications (plantar views). (A) Metatarsal bar. (B) Rocker bar. (C) Denver bar. (D) Thomas heel. (E) Reverse Thomas heel. (F) Scaphoid (navicular pad insert). (G) Metatarsal pad insert. (*Source:* DeLisa JA, Gans BM, Walsh NE, et al. *Physical Medicine and Rehabilitation, Principles and Practice*, 4th ed., Vol. 2. Lippincott Williams & Wilkins, 2005;1382.)

Foot Orthoses

The foot orthosis extends from the posterior border of the foot to a point just posterior to the metatarsal heads. This device is used to accommodate the abnormal foot to help restore more normalized lower limb biomechanics.

UCBL (University of California at Berkeley Laboratory) Insert. This insert is made of rigid plastic fabricated over a cast of the foot held in maximal manual correction. The UCBL encompasses the heel and midfoot, and it has rigid medial, lateral, and posterior walls.

Heel Cup. The heel cup is a rigid plastic insert that covers the plantar surface of the heel and extends posteriorly, medially, and laterally up the side of the heel. The heel cup is used to prevent lateral calcaneal shift in the flexible flat foot.

Sesamoid Insert. This addition to an orthosis is an insert amounting to three quarters of an inch with an extension under the hallux to transfer pressure off the short first metatarsal head and onto its shaft.

Ankle Foot Orthoses

An AFO is commonly is prescribed for weakness or paralysis of ankle dorsiflexion, plantarflexion, inversion, and eversion. AFOs are used to prevent or correct deformities and reduce weight bearing. The position of the ankle indirectly affects the stability of the knee with ankle plantarflexion providing a knee extension force and ankle dorsiflexion providing a knee flexion force. An AFO has been shown to reduce the energy cost of ambulation in a wide variety of conditions, such as spastic diplegia due to cerebral palsy, lower motor neuron weakness of poliomyelitis, and spastic hemiplegia in cerebral infarction.

Thermoplastic AFOs. These devices are plastic molded AFOs, consisting of a shoe insert, a calf shell, and a calf strap attached proximally (see Fig. 9.15). The rigidity depends on the thickness and composition of the plastic, as well as the trim line and shape. Thermoplastic AFOs are contraindicated in cases of fluctuating edema and insensation.

Posterior Leaf Spring (PLS). The PLS is the most common form of AFO with a narrow calf shell and a narrow ankle trim line behind the malleoli. The PLS is used for compensating for weak ankle dorsiflexors by resisting ankle plantarflexion at heelstrike and during swing phase with no mediolateral control.

Spiral AFO. This orthosis consists of a shoe insert, a spiral that starts medially, passes around the leg posteriorly, then passes anteriorly to terminate at the medial tibial flare where a calf band is attached. The spiral AFO allows for rotation in the transverse plane while controlling ankle dorsiflexion and plantarflexion, as well as eversion and inversion.

Hemispiral AFO. This orthosis consists of a shoe insert with a spiral starting on the lateral side of the shoe insert, passing up the posterior leg, and terminating at the medial tibial flare where the calf band is attached. This design is used for achieving better control of equinovarus than the spiral AFO can.

Hinged AFO. The adjustable ankle hinges can be set to the desired range of ankle dorsiflexion or plantarflexion.

Tone-Reducing AFO (TRAFO). The broad footplate is used to provide support around most of the foot, extending distally under the toes and up over the foot medially and laterally to maintain the subtalar joint in normal alignment. The TRAFO is indicated for patients with spastic hemiplegia.

Metal and Metal-Plastic AFO. This type of AFO consists of a shoe or foot attachment, ankle joint, 2 metal uprights (medial and lateral), with a calf band (application of force) connected proximally (Fig. 9.19). The stirrup anchors the uprights to the shoes between the sole and the heel. The caliper is a round tube placed in the heel of the shoe, which connects to the uprights and also allows for easy detachability of the uprights. A molded shoe insert is another alternative to fit the stirrup into the shoe, which also allows maximum control of the foot and aligns the anatomic and mechanical ankles.

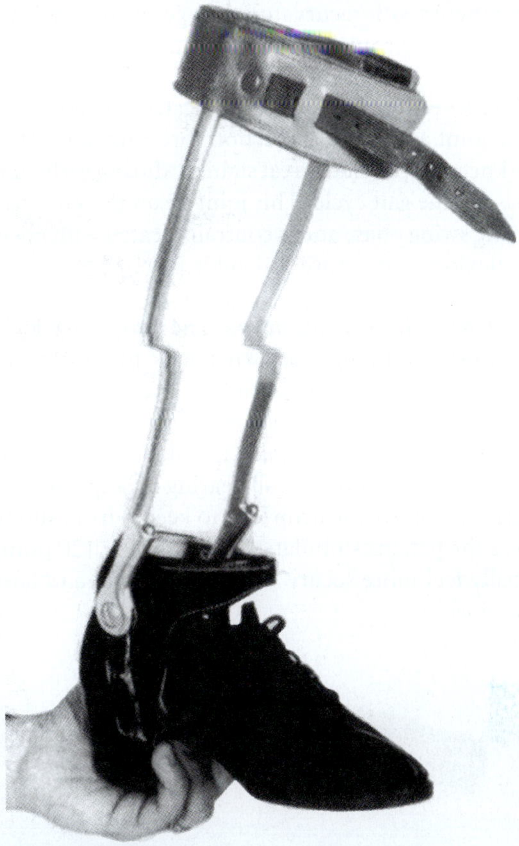

FIGURE 9.19 **Klenzak ankle-foot orthosis with a medial T-strap to control vagus. (*Source:* DeLisa JA, Gans BM, Walsh NE, et al. *Physical Medicine and Rehabilitation, Principles and Practice*, 4th ed., Vol. 2. Lippincott Williams & Wilkins, 2005;1378.)**

Ankle Joints

The mechanical ankle joints can control or assist ankle dorsiflexion or plantarflexion by means of stops (pins) or assists (springs). The mechanical ankle joint also controls mediolateral stability. Knee extension moment is promoted by ankle plantarflexion, and knee flexion moment is promoted by ankle dorsiflexion.

Knee-Ankle-Foot Orthoses. These orthoses consist of an AFO with metal uprights, a mechanical knee joint, and 2 thigh bands (see Fig. 9.16). KAFO can be used in quadriceps paralysis or weakness to maintain knee stability and control flexible genu valgum or varum. KAFO also is used to limit the weight bearing of the thigh, leg, and foot with quadrilateral or ischial containment brim. A KAFO is more difficult to don and doff than an AFO, so it is not recommended for patients who have moderate-to-severe cognitive dysfunction. KAFO orthosis can be made of metal-leather and metal-plastic or plastic and plastic-metal. The metal design includes double upright metal KAFO (most common), single upright metal KAFO (lateral upright only), and Scott-Craig metal KAFO (Fig. 9.20). The plastic designs are indicated for closer fit and maximum control of the foot, including supracondylar plastic KAFO, supracondylar plastic-metal KAFO, and plastic shells with metal uprights KAFO.

Knee Joints

The mechanical knee joint can be polycentric or single axis. Polycentric is used for significant knee motion, and a single axis is more common and is used for knee stabilization. Single axis knee joints include the following:

Free-Motion Knee Joint. This joint has unrestricted knee flexion and extension with a stop to prevent hyperextension. The free motion knee joint is used for patients with recurvatum but good strength of the quadriceps to control knee motion.

Offset Knee Joint. The hinge is located posterior to the knee joint and ground reaction force; thus, it extends the knee and provides great stability during early stance phase of the gait cycle. This joint flexes the knee freely during swing phase and is contraindicated with knee or hip flexion contracture and ankle plantarflexion stop.

Drop Ring Lock Knee Joint. The drop ring lock is the most commonly used knee lock to control knee flexion. The rings drop to unlock over the knee joint while the knee is in extension by gravity or manual assistance. This type of joint is stable, but gait is stiff without knee motion. A ball bearing on a spring can be added just above the drop lock to keep it from slipping up as the patient ambulates. Patients over 120 pounds usually feel more secure with both medial and lateral drop locks.

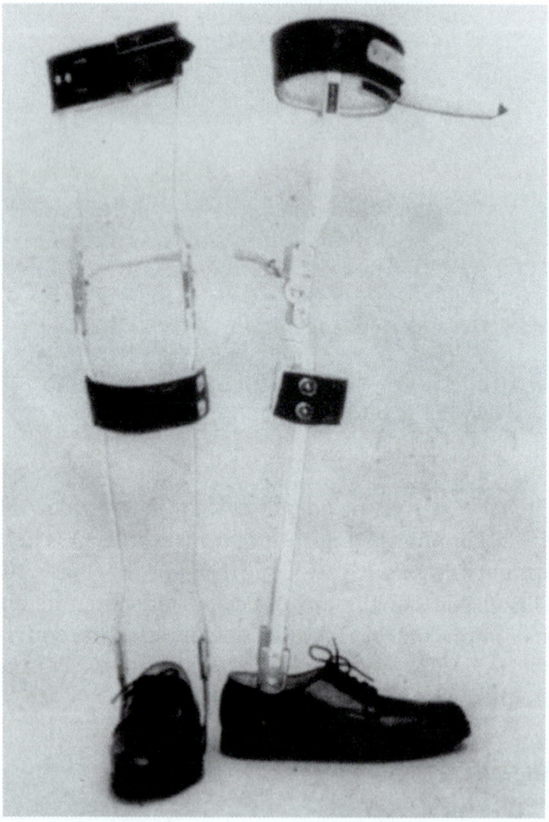

FIGURE 9.20 The Scott-Craig knee-ankle-foot orthosis. (*Source:* DeLisa JA, Gans BM, Walsh NE, et al. *Physical Medicine and Rehabilitation, Principles and Practice*, 4th ed., Vol. 2. Lippincott Williams & Wilkins, 2005;1387.)

Adjustable Knee Lock Joint (Dial Lock). The serrated adjustable knee joint allows knee locking at different degrees of flexion. This type of knee joint is used in patients with knee flexion contractures that are improving gradually with stretching. This type of orthosis is also used postoperatively for patients who are being temporarily partially immobilized (e.g., ACL reconstruction).

Knee Orthoses

A knee orthosis (KO) provides support or control only of the knee, not of the foot and ankle. The knee joint is centered over the medial femoral condyle. If the patient does not have adequate gastrocnemius delineation so that there is a shelf for the distal end of the orthosis to rest on, the brace may slide down the leg with wear. In that case, the brace needs to extend to the sole of the foot.

Knee Orthoses for Patellofemoral Disorder. These orthoses are used to supply mediolateral knee stability and to control tracking of the patella during knee flexion and extension. This type of orthosis includes an infrapatellar strap KO and Palumbo KO.

Knee Orthoses for Knee Control in the Sagittal Plane. These orthoses are used to control genu recurvatum with minimal mediolateral stability. This type of KO includes a Swedish knee cage and a 3-way knee stabilizer (Fig. 9.21).

Knee Orthoses for Knee Control in the Frontal Plane. These orthoses consist of thigh and calf cuffs joined by sidebars with mechanical knee joints. The knee joint usually is polycentric and closely mimics the anatomic joint motion. This type of KO includes traditional metal-leather KO, Miami KO, Canadian Arthritis and Rheumatism Society–University of British Columbia KO, and supracondylar KO.

Knee Orthoses for Axial Rotation Control. These orthoses can provide angular control of flexion–extension and mediolateral planes, in addition to controlling axial rotation. This orthosis is used mostly in management of sports injuries of the knee. This type of KO includes Lenox–Hill derotation orthosis and Lerman multiligamentous knee control orthosis.

Other Orthoses

Hip-Knee-Ankle-Foot Orthosis. The HKAFO consists of a hip joint and pelvic band in addition to a KAFO. The orthotic hip joint is positioned with the patient sitting upright at 90 degrees while the orthotic knee joint is centered over the medial femoral condyle. Pelvic bands complicate dressing after toileting unless the orthosis is worn under all clothing. Pelvic bands increase the energy demands for ambulation. The pelvic girdle is made of molded thermoplastic materials, providing a maximum degree of control in patients with bilateral involvement.

Trunk-Hip-Knee-Ankle-Foot Orthosis. The THKAFO consists of a spinal orthosis in addition to an HKAFO for control of trunk motion and spinal alignment. A THKAFO is indicated in patients with paraplegia and is very difficult to don and doff.

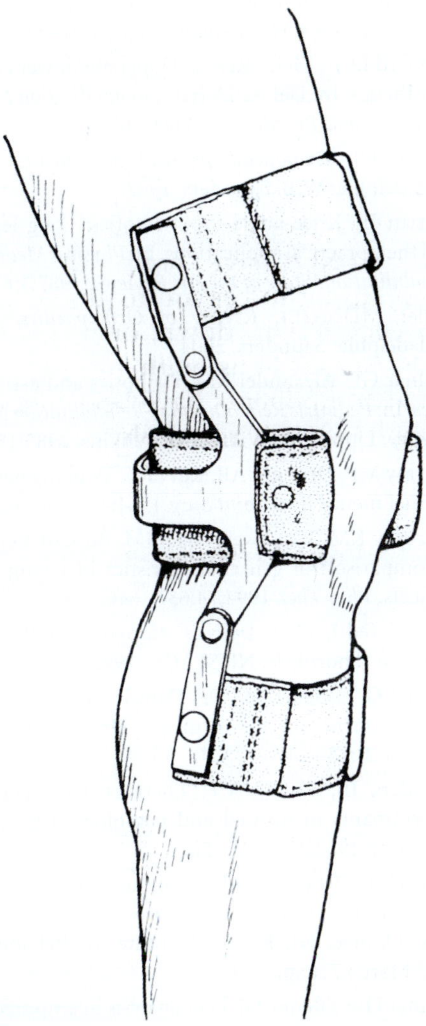

FIGURE 9.21 The Swedish knee cage is an example of a knee orthosis (KO). (*Source:* DeLisa JA, Gans BM, Walsh NE, et al. *Physical Medicine and Rehabilitation, Principles and Practice*, 4th ed., Vol. 2. Lippincott Williams & Wilkins, 2005;1388.)

Fracture Orthoses. These orthoses stabilize the fracture site and promote callus formation, while allowing weight bearing and joint movement after initial subsiding pain and edema. The bony motion at the fracture site is prevented through circumferential compression of the soft tissue. Fracture orthoses include the tibial fracture orthosis and femoral fracture orthosis.

Pediatric Hip Dislocation Orthoses. Congenital hip dislocation orthoses, such as Pavlik harness, Ilfeld splint, and Von Rosen splint are used to maintain the hip in flexion and abduction position to hold the femoral head within the acetabulum. The Scottish Rite, Toronto, and nonskeletal-bearing trilateral orthoses are used in Legg-Calvé-Perthes disease to maintain the hip in abduction and keep the femoral head in the acetabulum.

V. NEUROLOGIC CONDITIONS AFFECTING LIMBS

General Principles. Interventional modalities include orthotics, serial castings, and motor point nerve blocks with short-acting (bupivacaine) or long-standing (phenol or Botox) agents. Splinting a joint is often not sufficient to control deformity. Surgical intervention in the adult-acquired spasticity is delayed until the patient achieves maximum spontaneous motor recovery (6 months for stroke and 12 to 18 months for traumatic brain injury). When surgery is considered as a method of improving function, patients should be screened for cognitive deficits, motivation, and body-image awareness.

Lower Limb. Balance is the best predictor of a patient's ability to ambulate after acquired brain injury. The mainstay of treatment for the dynamic ankle equinus component of this gait deviation is to achieve ankle stability in neutral position during initial floor contact as well as floor clearance during swing phase. An adjustable AFO with ankle dorsiflexion and plantarflexion stop at neutral is often used during the recover period. When the dynamic equinus overpowers the holding power of the orthosis, the equinus deformity is treated by a percutaneous tendo-achilles lengthening. The dynamic varus deformity, resulting from an out-of-phase tibialis anterior muscle, is corrected by either split or complete lateral transfer of the anterior tibialis muscle.

Upper Limb. Surgical release of static contractures is generally performed to assist nursing care or hygiene when the fixed contracture and/or spastic component results in skin maceration or breakdown.

A functional use of static contracture release is to improve upper extremity tracking (e.g., arm swing) during walking. The goal of upper extremity surgery in this patient population is to improve prehensile hand function. Dynamic electromyography may be used when delineation of phasic motor activity is essential. Muscle unit lengthening, by fractional musculotendinous or step-cut methods, of the agonist-deforming muscle units is combined with motor-balancing tendon transfers of the antagonists to achieve muscle balance and improved prehensile hand function.

References

1. Andriacchi TP. Dynamics of pathological motion: Applied to the anterior cruciate deficient knee. *J Biomech* 1990;23 (Suppl 1):99–105.
2. Basmajiam JV. Crutch and cane exercises and use. In: Redford JB (ed.), *Orthotics Etcetera,* 2nd ed. Baltimore: Williams & Wilkins, 1980;125–138.
3. Berchuck M, Andriacchi TP, Bach BR, Reider B. Gait adaptations by patients who have a deficient anterior cruciate ligament. *J Bone Joint Surg Am* 1990;72A:871–877.
4. Braddom RL, Dumitru D, Johnson EW, et al (eds.). Lower limb orthoses. In: *Physical Medicine and Rehabilitation,* 1st ed. WB Saunders 1995;333–358.
5. Colwell MO, Spires MC. Lower extremity prosthesis and rehabilitation. In: Grabois M (ed.), *Physical Medicine and Rehabilitation: The Complete Approach*. 2000; 583–607.
6. Deathe AB, Hayes KC, Winter DA. The biomechanics of canes, crutches, and walkers. *Crit Rev Phys Rehab Med* 1993;5:15–29.
7. Glennon TP, Smith BS. Amputations. In: Garrison SJ (ed.), *Handbook of Physical Medicine and Rehabilitation Basics*. 1995;34–60.
8. Gyory AN, Chao EYS, Stauffer RN. Functional evaluation of normal and pathologic knees during gait. *Arch Phys Med Rehabil* 1976;57:571–577.
9. Hennessey WJ, Johnson EW. Lower limb orthoses. In: *Physical Medicine and Rehabilitation*, 2nd ed. Philadelphia: WB Saunders, 2000;326–352.
10. Iida H, Yamamuro T. Kinetic analysis of the center of gravity of the human body in normal and pathological gaits. *J Biomech* 1987;20:987–995.
11. Inman VT. Conservation of energy in ambulation. *Arch Phys Med Rehabil* 1967;47:484–488.
12. Inman VT. Human locomotion. *Can Med Assoc J* 1966;94:1047–1054.
13. Jacobs SR. Rehabilitation of the person with arthritis of the ankle and foot. *Clin Podiatry* 1984 Aug;1(2):373–99.
14. Kay RM, Dennis S, Rethlefsen S, Reynolds RA, Skaggs DL, Tolo VT. The effect of preoperative gait analysis on orthopaedic decision making. *Clin Orthop* 2000;372:217–222.
15. Kay RM, Dennis S, Rethlefsen S, Skaggs DL, Tolo VT. Impact of post-operative gait analysis on orthopaedic care. *Clin Orthop* 2000;374:259–264.
16. Keenan MA, Waters R. Rehabilitation. In: Skinner B (ed.), *Diagnosis and Treatment in Orthopaedics: A Lange Medical Book.* 1995;665–720.
17. Klopsteg PE, Wilson PD (eds.). *Human Limbs and Their Substitutes*. New York: McGraw-Hill, 1954.
18. Lehmann JF, de Lateur BJ, Price R. Biomechanics of normal gait. *Phys Med Rehabil Clin North Am* 1992;3:95–109.
19. Lehmann JF, de Lateur BJ, Price R. Biomechanics of abnormal gait. *Phys Med Rehabil Clin North Am* 1992;3:125–138.
20. Lehmann JF, Condon SM, de Lateur BJ, Smith JC. Gait abnormalities in tibial nerve paralysis: A biomechanical study. *Arch Phys Med Rehabil* 1985;66:80–85.
21. Leonard JA Jr, Meier RH III. Upper and lower extremity prosthetics. In: DeLisa JA (ed.), *Rehabilitation Medicine: Principles and Practice*. 1998;669–696.
22. Magee DJ. *Orthopedic physical assessment*, 2nd ed. Philadelphia: W.B. Saunders, 1992.
23. Merritt JL. Knee-ankle-foot orthotics: Long leg braces and their practical applications. In: *Physical Medicine and Rehabilitation: State of the Art Reviews*. 1987;1:67–82.
24. Miller MD (ed.). *Review of Orthopaedics,* 4th ed. Philadelphia: Saunders, 2004.
25. Molnar GE, Alexander MA. Orthotics and assistive devices. In: *Pediatric Rehabilitation, Rehabilitation Medicine Library*. Lippincott Williams & Wilkins, 1985:157–177.
26. Murray MP, Drought AB, Kory RC. Walking patterns of normal men. *J Bone Joint Surg* 1964;46:335–360.
27. Ostrosky KM, Van Swearingen JM, Burdett RG, Gee Z. A comparison of gait characteristics in young and old subjects. *Phys Ther* 1994;74:637–646.
28. Perry J (ed.), *Gait Analysis: Normal and Pathological Function*. Thorofare, NJ: SLACK, 1992.
29. Rubin G, Bonarrigo D, Danisi M. The shoe as a component of the orthosis. *Prosthet Orthot Int* 1976;30(2):13–25.
30. Saunders JB, Inman VT, Eberhart HD. The major determinants in normal and pathological gait. *J Bone Joint Surg* 1953;35A:543–58.
31. Schneck C. Normal and abnormal gait. *Ninth Annual Review Course in Physical Medicine and Rehabilitation*, West Orange, NJ: Kessler Institute for Rehabilitation; 1997 March 716; p. 4–9.
32. Skinner HB, Effeney DJ. Gait analysis in amputees. *Am J Phys Med* 1985;64:82–89.
33. Seymour R. *Prosthetics and Orthotics: Lower Limb and Spinal*. Lippincott Williams & Wilkins, 2002.
34. Sutherland DH. Gait analysis in neuromuscular disease. *Instr Course Lect* 1990;39:333–341.
35. Sutherland DH, Kaufman KR, Moitoza JR. Kinematics of normal human walking. In: Rose J, Gamble JG (eds.), *Human Walking*, 2nd ed. Baltimore: Williams & Wilkins, 1994;23–44.

36. Tan JC. Orthoses. In: *Practical Manual of Physical Medicine and Rehabilitation*, 1st ed. Mosby Year Book, 1998;178–228.

37. Tazawa E. Analysis of torso movement of transfemoral amputees during level walking. *Prosthet Orthot Int* 1997;21:129–140.

38. Torry MR, Decker MJ, Viola RW, O'Connor DD, Steadman JR. Intra-articular knee joint effusion induces quadriceps avoidance gait patterns. *Clin Biomech (Bristol, Avon)* 2000;15:147–159.

39. Vaccaro AR (ed.). *Orthopaedic Knowledge Update 8*. Rosemont, IL: AAOS, 2005.

40. Waters RL, Perry J, Antonelli D, Hislop H. Energy cost of walking of amputees: The influence of level of amputation. *J Bone Joint Surg Am* 1976;58:42–46.

41. Wyss C, Harrington, R, Burgess E, Matsen F. Transcutaneous oxygen tension as a predictor of success after an amputation. *J Bone Joint Surg Am* 1988;70:203.

42. Xing Y, Alexander M, Sarjoo M, Bhagia S, Cashen Y. Lower extremity orthotics. Available at: www.eMedicine.com. 2002.

Key References

Gyory AN, Choa EY, Stauffer RN. Functional evaluation of normal and pathologic knees during gait. *Arch Phys Med Rehab* 1976;57(12):571–577.

The functional performance of the knee joints in patients with degenerative joint disease and rheumatoid arthritis was studied according to clinical (historical, physical, and roentgenographic) and biomechanical gait parameters. Statistically significant correlations between various clinical and biomechanical gait parameters suggest that the techniques used are an objective measurement of knee joint function and may be employed as a means of evaluating various treatment modalities for the diseased knee.

Iida H, Yamamauro T. Kinetic analysis of the center of gravity of the human body in normal and pathological gaits. *J Biomech* 1987;20(10):987–995.

The kinetics of the body's center of gravity during level walking were analyzed in persons with normal and pathological gaits. Three-dimensional displacements of the center of gravity were computed by the integration of force plate data. The parameters obtained from the displacements and the energy variations of the center of gravity are considered useful in the evaluation of stability and efficiency for pathological gaits.

Kay RM, Dennis S, Rethlefsen S, Skaggs DL, Tolo VT. Impact of postoperative gait analysis on orthopaedic care. *Clin Orthop Rel Res* 2000;(374):259–264.

The impact of postoperative gait analysis on the ongoing orthopaedic care of patients with a static encephalopathy was evaluated. This study suggests that postoperative gait analysis serves not only as a measure of treatment outcome but also as a useful tool in planning ongoing care for these patients.

Waters RL, Perry J, Antonelli D, Hislop H. Energy cost of walking of amputees: The influence of level of amputation. *J Bone Joint Surg Am* 1976;58(1):42–46.

A comparison of selected gait parameters and the energy cost of prosthetic walking in patients with unilateral traumatic and vascular amputations above the knee, below the knee, and at the Syme level were compared. In both groups of amputees, performance was significantly better the lower the level of the amputation. When preservation of function is the chief concern, amputation should be performed at the lowest possible level.

Skinner HB, Effeney DJ. Gait analysis in amputees. *Am J Phys Med* 1985;64(2):82–89.

There are marked differences from normal in both AK and BK gait. This article examines differences in time–distance parameters of velocity, cadence, stride length, and gait cycle, and includes analysis of measurements of single-limb support times and motion analysis of the lower extremities as well as of the head, arms, and trunk. Asymmetry of motion increases the excursion of the center of mass during each cycle and thereby increases the energy cost of ambulation.

Refresher Questions

1. The adult human center of mass (COM) is slightly anterior to:
   a) L5
   b) S2
   c) S1
   d) L4
   e) L3

2. Which of the following muscles DOES NOT serve as decelerators of the leg during swing phase?
   a) gracilis
   b) semimembranosus
   c) semitendinosus
   d) adductor magnus
   e) biceps femoris

3. Which of the following conditions will most commonly result in a varus thrust gait pattern?
   a) spastic adductors
   b) ACL deficiency
   c) weak quadriceps
   d) posterior-lateral corner disruption
   e) weak hip abductors

4. Which of the following is NOT considered one of the functions of a cane?
   a) redistribute and unload a weight-bearing lower limb
   b) improve balance
   c) increase joint reactive forces across the contralateral leg
   d) reduce lower limb pain
   e) provide sensory feedback

5. Which of the following is NOT a preoperative indicator for successful wound healing after an amputation?
   a) complete lymphocyte count higher than 1500/mL
   b) ankle/brachial index (ABI) greater than 0.45
   c) serum albumen higher than 2g/dL
   d) toe systolic blood pressure greater than 55 mmHg
   e) transcutaneous oxygen tension: PO_2 greater than 35 mmHg

6. Approximately what percentage of amputees experience phantom limb sensation?
   a) 100
   b) 80
   c) 60
   d) 40
   e) 20

7. The increase in the level of energy consumption (percentage above normal) by a unilateral transfemoral amputee is approximately
   a) 60%
   b) 100%
   c) 200%
   d) 40%
   e) 25%

8. Which of the following is NOT a component of the upper portion of a shoe?
   a) shank
   b) throat
   c) vamp
   d) quarter
   e) counter

9. Which shoe modification is designed to unload the metatarsal heads while ambulating?
   a) lateral heel wedge
   b) rocker bar
   c) oxford heel
   d) scaphoid pad
   e) widened toe box

10. A patient with genu recurvatum might be best assisted with which of the following orthotics?
    a) HKAFO
    b) Palumbo strap
    c) infrapatellar strap
    d) Swedish knee cage
    e) Lenox-Hill derotational brace

Chapter 10

Trauma

SAMIR MEHTA

I. UPPER EXTREMITY

Fractures of the Scapula

Overview and Anatomy. Scapular function and motion is a composite of glenohumeral motion (120 degrees) and scapulothoracic motion (60 degrees). Eighteen muscles have their origins and insertions on the scapula, all of which contribute to the forces across the glenohumeral joint. Scapular fractures account for approximately 1% of all fractures and 3% to 5% of all injuries about the shoulder girdle. The most common age range for injury is 30 to 50 years old. Glenoid cavity fractures, including the rim and fossa, account for 10% of all scapular fractures, with 1% of these being significantly displaced. Glenoid neck fractures account for 25% of all scapular fractures, with 2% being significantly displaced.

Mechanism of Injury. The mechanism for scapular fractures can be divided into direct and indirect causes. Direct injury is usually a result of high energy and is associated with 80% to 95% of cases. Patients with this kind of mechanism should be evaluated for rib fractures, pneumo- or hemothorax, pulmonary contusion, brachial plexus injury, cervical spine fracture, skull fracture, or clavicular fracture. An indirect mechanism usually results from axial loading on an outstretched arm. The presentation of such injuries is often pain with passive or active shoulder motion; however, given the nature of this fracture, physical signs are difficult to assess, and therefore, diagnosis is ultimately based on imaging.

Imaging. Imaging in patients being evaluated for scapular fractures includes a chest radiograph and a lateral cervical spine film to assess the lungs and other potentially fatal injuries. If the patient is stable, anteroposterior, axillary, and scapular lateral views should be obtained, along with a Stryker view taken in 45 degrees of cephalic tilt to assess for coracoid fractures. In patients requiring a better understanding of their scapular fracture, a CT scan, including coronal, axial, and sagittal reconstruction views, to assess glenoid and glenoid neck fractures offers the highest yield in terms of preoperative planning and patient care (Fig. 10.1).

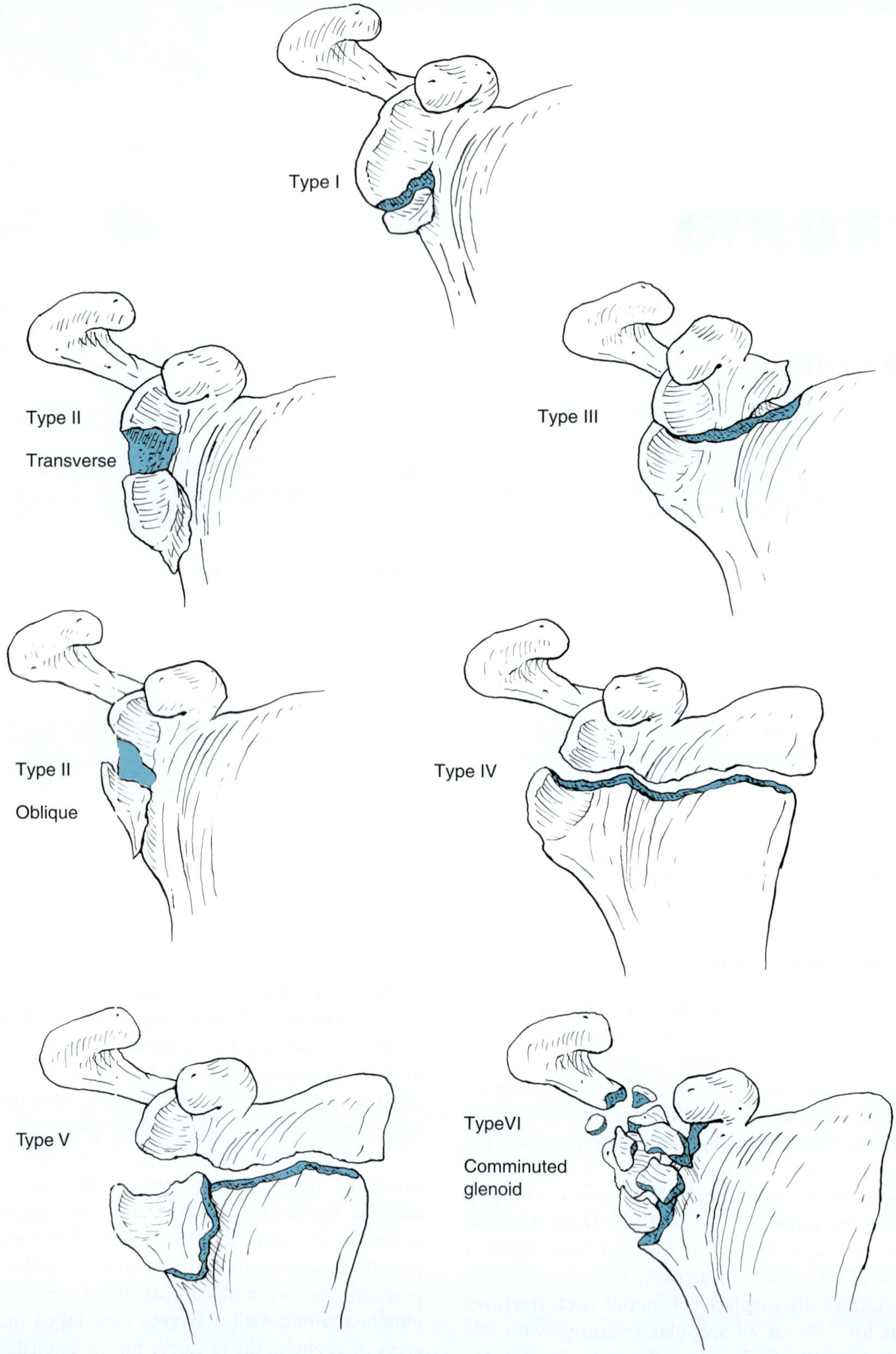

FIGURE 10.1 Ideberg classification of glenoid fractures into 5 types, with comminuted type VI of Goss added. (*Asset provided by* Anatomical Chart Co.)

Nonoperative Treatment. Nonoperative treatment of scapular fractures is often indicated because more than 90% are minimally displaced. Treatment for minimally displaced fractures includes a sling and swathe with a gradual increase in activity over 6 weeks. Radiographs are taken at 2-week intervals for 6 weeks to assess increasing displacement. If union is present on radiographs at 6 weeks, the sling and swathe are discontinued. However, despite union, it may take between 6 months and 1 year for full recovery.

Operative Treatment of Glenoid Fractures. Operative treatment of glenoid fractures is based on location and stability. Fractures of the glenoid cavity can be divided into those of the glenoid rim and those of the glenoid fossa. Fractures of the glenoid rim are considered unstable if there is greater than 10 mm of fracture displacement or if 25% to 33% of the posterior aspect of the glenoid rim is involved (resulting in the "inverted pear" shape). Anterior rim fractures can be approached anteriorly via a deltopectoral approach while posterior rim fractures can be fixed via a posterior Judet approach. Glenoid fossa fractures are considered operative if there is an articular step-off greater than 5 mm or if there is subluxation of the humeral head. These injuries are approached posteriorly. Type II fractures of the glenoid neck have a translational displacement greater than 10 mm and angulation greater than 40 degrees and therefore should be fixed operatively. This is different than type I fractures of the glenoid neck which have less than 10 mm of displacement and are considered nonoperative.

Treatment of Coracoid Fractures. Coracoid fractures are treated on the basis of their location and patient activity. Type I fractures occur at the tip of the coracoid and are treated nonoperatively except in athletes and manual laborers. This same exception holds true for type II fractures between the coracoacromial ligament and the coracoclavicular ligament. Fractures at the base of the coracoid (type III) are often minimally displaced and can be treated nonoperatively. Type IV (involving the superior body) and type V (fractures extending into the glenoid fossa) are treated operatively.

Scapula and Shoulder Girdle. There are several unique injury patterns involving the scapula and shoulder girdle. The "floating shoulder" (double disruption of the superior suspensory shoulder complex) is an injury to the ring that includes the glenoid fossa, coracoid process, coracoclavicular ligaments, distal clavicle, acromioclavicular joint, and acromial process. The superior strut is the middle third of the clavicle, and the inferior strut is the lateral scapular body and spine. Traumatic disruption of 2 or more components requires surgical treatment because the shoulder will collapse anteriorly, inferiorly, and medially. However, good results have been achieved with conservative care when each component of the injury has been evaluated for surgery, as the combination does not mandate operative intervention.

Often, treatment of the clavicular fracture component of the "floating shoulder" will address stability. Scapulothoracic dissociation is a closed, complete traumatic disruption of the scapula from the posterior chest wall. This injury often presents with a flail, pulseless, swollen extremity after high-energy trauma and is life-threatening. A lateral shift of the scapula is seen on chest radiographs, and associated injuries include avulsion of the subclavian, axillary, and brachial arteries (88%) and/or complete brachial plexopathy (81%). Treatment includes advanced trama life support (ATLS) protocol, angiography, vascular repair with brachial plexus exploration, stabilization of fractures, an EMG at 3 weeks, and a cervical myelogram at 6 weeks. Shoulder arthrodesis and/or an above elbow amputation (AEA) may be necessary. The prognosis in patients with a nerve avulsion of complete deficit is poor.

Clavicular, Acromioclavicular Joint, and Sternoclavicular Joint Injuries

Overview and Anatomy. The clavicle is the first bone to ossify via intramembranous ossification. An "S"-shaped bone, it is concave ventrally on the outer half and convex ventrally on the medial half. The medial extent is the sternoclavicular (SC) joint and the lateral extent is the acromioclavicular (AC) joint and coracoclavicular (CC) ligaments. Important muscles include the sternocleidomastoid medially and the trapezius and pectoralis major laterally. Essential ligaments about the clavicle include the AC and CC ligaments, which anchor the clavicle to the scapula and the SC and costoclavicular ligaments, which anchor the clavicle to the trunk. The acromioclavicular joint is a diarthrodial joint between the medial facet of the acromion and distal clavicle with an intraarticular disk. The AC ligaments control anteroposterior displacement with the superior portion being the most important. The coracoclavicular ligaments, composed of the trapezoid and conoid ligaments, are stronger than the AC ligament and provide vertical stability to the AC joint. The sternoclavicular joint is a poorly congruent, saddle-shaped diarthrodial joint with an intraarticular disk ligament dividing the SC joint into 2 separate spaces. The costoclavicular ligaments from the first rib to the clavicle resist rotation and medial and lateral displacement. The interclavicular ligament connects the superomedial aspects of the clavicle with the capsular ligaments and the upper sternum. Capsular ligaments cover the anterior and posterior aspects of the joint (the anterior portion is stronger). Of note, the epiphysis of the medial clavicle is the last ossification center to appear and the last epiphysis to close. It usually does not ossify until 20th year and does not unite with the clavicle until 24th year.

Imaging. Imaging of this region can be directed toward the specific area based on the clinical examination and suspected site of injury. Radiographs to evaluate the clavicle include an anteroposterior and 30-degree cephalic tilt view along with Quesana views taken at 45-degree angles superiorly and inferiorly, which provide a better assessment of the extent of displacement. A Zanca view to evaluate the AC joint is taken as an anteroposterior view centered over the AC joint with a 15-degree cephalic tilt. A serendipity view taken with a 40-degree cephalic tilt will evaluate SC joint pathology; however, CT imaging is the best modality to study displacement of this joint. Stress views taken with the patient holding a 10-pound weight in the injured extremity are rarely used, but they can demonstrate instability and allow the physician to differentiate grade III AC separations from grade I or grade II.

Classification. Classification of clavicle fractures is based on their anatomic location (Fig. 10.2). Group I fractures are those of the middle third of the clavicle and occur in 80% of patients. Group II fractures are of the distal third and occur in 15% of patients. Group II fractures are divided into 3 types. Type I are nondisplaced and usually occur between the CC ligaments (conoid and trapezoid), while the AC ligament is still intact. Type II fractures are medial to the CC ligaments and are therefore displaced superiorly. These fractures have the highest rates of nonunion. Group II type II fractures have two subtypes: subtype A fractures maintain attachment of the conoid and trapezoid to the distal fragment, while subtype B fractures maintain attachment of the trapezoid only. Group II type II fractures should be treated aggressively. Type III are articular fractures. Group III fractures are of the medial third of the clavicle and occur in 5% of cases. SC joint dislocations are classified by their anatomic position with anterior being more common than posterior. However, posterior dislocations can lead to mediastinal compression, pneumothorax, laceration of the SVC, or tracheal erosion. AC joint injuries are classified in Table 10.1 and Figure 10.3.

Treatment of Clavicle Injuries. Treatment of clavicle injuries is usually nonoperative because they unite rapidly. Even those that go to nonunion can be minimally symptomatic. Nonoperative interventions include a sling or figure of 8 treatment; outcomes are identical with less discomfort to the patient in a simple sling. Absolute operative indications include open fractures or associated neurovascular injury. Relative indications include fractures that are widely displaced, multitrauma, displaced distal-third fractures, floating shoulder, seizure disorder, cosmetic deformity, or an earlier return to work. Results of treatment reveal that less than 5 mm of shortening is acceptable at 5 years, while greater than 20 mm of shortening is associated with increased risk of nonunion and poor outcomes at 3 years. Increased risk of nonunions is seen in distal-third fractures, fractures with marked displacement, and those fractures undergoing primary open reduction. Treatment of nonunions includes restoration of clavicular length with rigid internal fixation and iliac crest bone graft.

Treatment of AC Joint Injuries. Type I and II AC joint injuries can be treated nonoperatively. Patients can return to activity as tolerated. Type II injuries recalcitrant to nonoperative treatment can be treated by resection of the distal clavicle and reconstruction of the CC ligament. Types III through VI are treated by an initial course of nonoperative treatment. However, operative repair should be considered in younger, active, dominant extremities, especially in athletes or heavy laborers, and in irreducible type IV, V, and VI injuries. The principles of fixation include primary AC joint and CC ligament fixation with excision of the distal clavicle and potentially performing dynamic muscle transfers. The Weaver-Dunn procedure can be utilized for late reconstruction by excising the distal clavicle, transferring the CA ligament to the remaining distal clavicle, and repairing or augmenting the CC ligaments with a CC screw or suture.

Anterior SC joint dislocations are usually treated nonoperatively, especially considering closed reduction is not usually successful. On the other hand, posterior dislocations are more concerning. A vascular evaluation is critical, along with a CT scan to rule out mediastinal compression. Closed reduction usually results in stable fixation and should be performed in the operating room. The reduction technique involves abduction with traction or adduction with traction, and a towel clip is used to apply an anterior force percutaneously. The chest and thorax should be prepped, and a thoracic or vascular surgeon should be available.

Proximal Humerus Fractures

Mechanism of Injury and Anatomy. Proximal humerus fractures often have a bimodal distribution with injuries in younger patients resulting from high-energy trauma and older patients resulting from low-energy falls. Forty-five percent of all humerus fractures occur proximally, with a female-to-male ratio of 4:1. The major blood supply to the articular

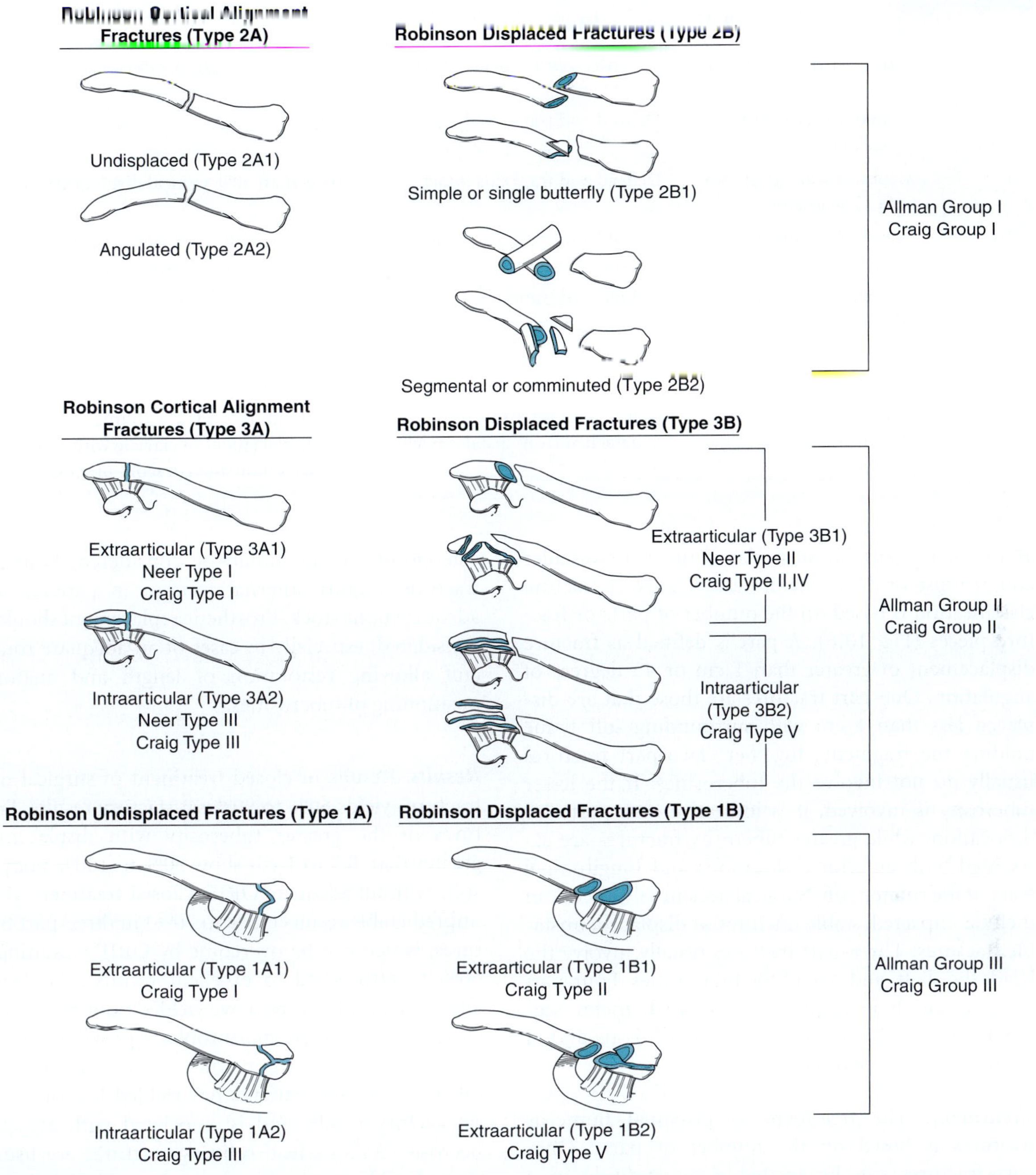

FIGURE 10.2 Clavicle fracture classification. (*Source:* Bucholz RW, Heckman JD. ***Rockwood & Green's Fractures in Adults***, 5th ed. Lippincott Williams & Wilkins, 2001.)

surface of the humeral head is the ascending branch of the anterior humeral circumflex artery with a smaller contribution from the posterior humeral circumflex artery. The ossification centers of the greater tuberosity appear at 3 years, the lesser tuberosity at 5 years, and the epiphysis at 4 months (Figs. 10.4 and 10.5).

Imaging. Imaging of the proximal humerus in patients with suspected fractures starts with radiographs including a true scapular anteroposterior view, an axillary view, and a Y view. A CT scan be used for further evaluation of articular fractures, including impaction injuries, head-splitting injuries, fractures of the glenoid, and tuberosity of fractures.

Classification. The classification of proximal humerus fractures can be based on the AO system or, more commonly, the Neer classification. The AO classification is divided into 3 types: A is a 2-part extracapsular fracture; B is a 3-part, partially intracapsular fracture;

TABLE 10.1 Classification of AC joint injuries

Type	Ligament Involvement	Muscle Involvement	Displacement
I	Sprain of AC (CC not involved)	Deltoid and trapezius intact	None
II	AC joint disrupted, sprain of CC ligaments	Deltoid and trapezius intact	Less than 50% vertical displacement
III	AC and CC ligaments disrupted	Deltoid and trapezius detached from clavicle	AC joint dislocated with clavicle 25% to 100% displaced from scapular
IV	AC and CC ligaments disrupted	Deltoid and trapezius detached from clavicle	
V	AC and CC ligaments disrupted	Deltoid and trapezius detached from distal half of clavicle	AC joint dislocated with 100% to 300% displacement of clavicle from scapula
VI	AC and CC ligaments disrupted	Deltoid and trapezius muscles detached from distal clavicle	AC joint dislocated with inferior displacement of clavicle with respect to acromion and coracoid process

and C is a 4-part intracapsular injury with vascular compromise of the humeral head. The Neer fracture classification is based on the number of parts or fracture pieces (Fig. 10.6). A part is defined as fracture displacement of greater than 1 cm or 45 degrees of angulation. One-part fractures are those that are displaced less than 1 cm with surrounding soft tissue holding the fragments together. Two-part fractures usually do not involve the tuberosities. If the lesser tuberosity is involved, it is indicative of a posterior dislocation, while greater tuberosity fractures are associated with anterior dislocations and longitudinal tears of the rotator cuff. Surgical neck involvement can include impacted, stable fractures or displaced, unstable fractures. Three-part fractures usually involve the head, the shaft, and one of the tuberosities. Four-part fractures result in displacement of each major segment, with the humeral head devoid of tissue and at an increased risk of osteonecrosis.

Treatment. The treatment of proximal humerus fractures is based on the number of parts. One-part fractures can be treated nonoperatively in a sling with early range of motion (ROM). Two-part fractures that are minimally displaced can be treated nonoperatively as well. However, the greater trochanter should have less than 5 mm of displacement to avoid impingement with abduction of the arm. Stable two-part neck fractures can be treated closed; however, unstable displaced fractures require open reduction with internal fixation (ORIF) or percutaneous pinning. Three-part fractures are difficult to manage closed because of the unopposed pull of the remaining tuberosity. ORIF with tension-band wiring and incorporation of the rotator cuff can provide improved fixation. Hemiarthroplasty in patients without secure fixation or with severely osteoporotic bone should be considered. Four-part fractures require internal fixation in patients with adequate bone stock. Prosthetic replacement should be considered, especially in cases of an adequate rotator cuff allowing restoration of length and anatomic positioning of tuberosities.

Results. Results of closed treatment of surgical neck fractures yields 60% to 90% satisfactory results. Fractures of the greater tuberosity with displacement greater than 0.5 to 1 cm show 50% to 100% poor results without adequate ORIF. Closed treatment yields unpredictable results (15% to 70%) in three-part fractures, which can be overcome by ORIF (resulting in 60% to 80% good to excellent results). Traditionally, four-part fractures have yielded poor results with closed treatment. Hemiarthroplasty provides satisfactory pain results but unpredictable functional results. ORIF in younger patients has yielded less than 50% satisfactory results and is associated with avascular necrosis (AVN). Head-splitting fractures are usually treated with hemiarthroplasty; however, if the CT shows a segment attached to the lesser tuberosity, then an ORIF is indicated.

Complications. Complications of proximal humerus fractures include decreased range of motion, loss of reduction, nonunion, HO, rotator cuff injuries, clavicular or scapular fractures, vascular disruption, and AVN. There is significant incidence of avascular necrosis (AVN) in 3-part and 4-part fractures and those fractures treated with an ORIF. Furthermore, palpable distal pulses do not eliminate the possibility of vascular injury because there is significant collateral flow about the proximal humerus.

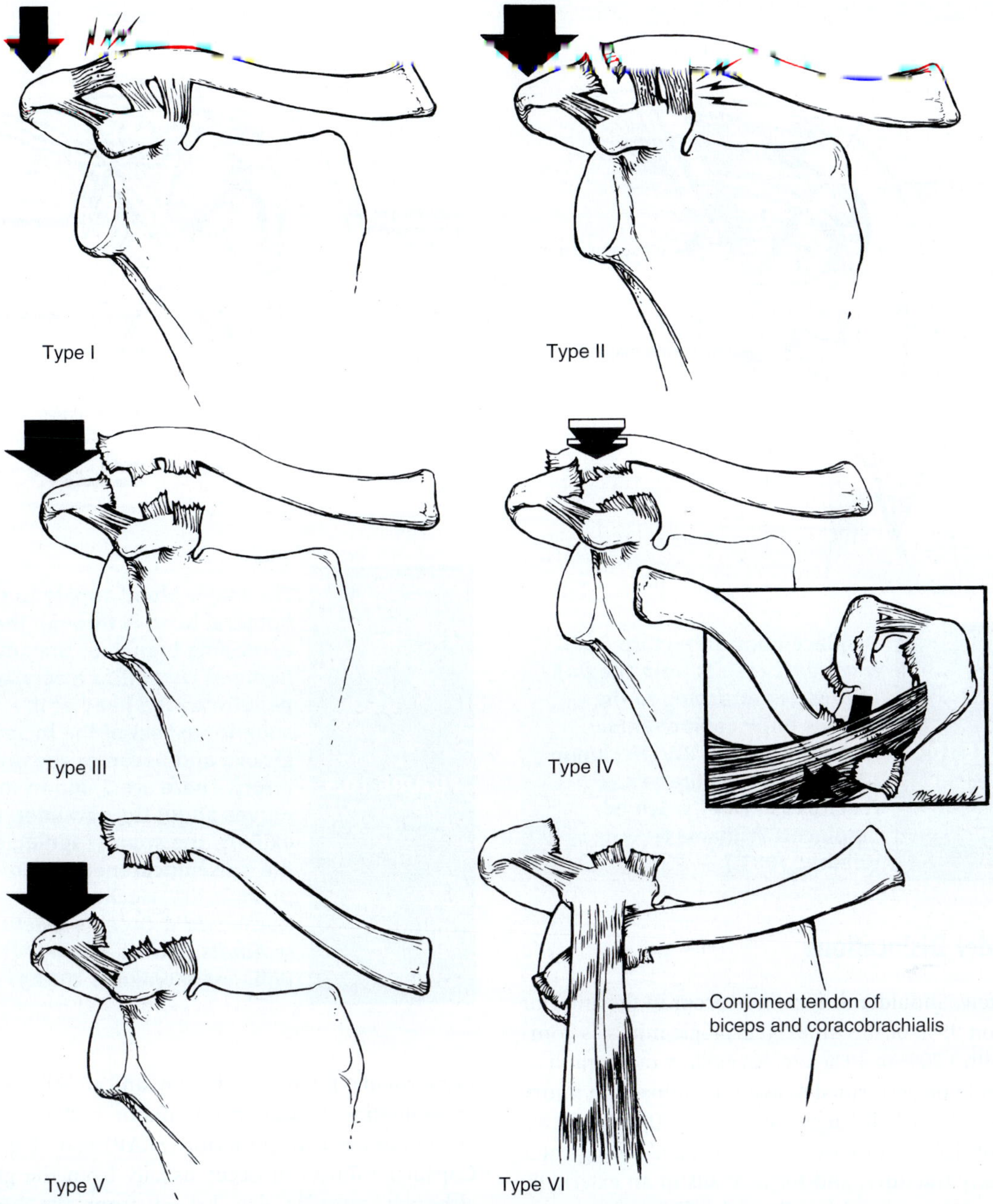

FIGURE 10.3 Classification of ligamentous injuries to the AC joint. **Top left:** Type I: mild force applied to the point of the shoulder does not disrupt either the AC or the CC ligaments. **Top right:** Type II: moderate to heavy force applied to the point of the shoulder will disrupt the AC ligaments, but the CC ligaments remain intact. **Center left:** Type III: when severe force is applied to the point of the shoulder, both the AC and the CC ligaments are disrupted. **Center right:** Type IV: Not only are the ligaments disrupted, but the distal end of the clavicle is also displaced posteriorly into or through the trapezius muscle. **Bottom left:** Type V: violent force applied to the point of the shoulder not only ruptures the AC and CC ligaments but also disrupts the muscle attachments and creates a major separation between the clavicle and the acromion. **Bottom right:** Type VI: an inferior dislocation of the distal clavicle in which the clavicle is inferior to the coracoid process and posterior to the biceps and coracobrachialis tendons. The AC and CC ligaments are also disrupted. AC, acromioclavicular; CC, coracoclavicular. (*Source:* Bucholz RW, Heckman JD. *Rockwood & Green's Fractures in Adults*, 5th ed. Lippincott Williams & Wilkins, 2001.)

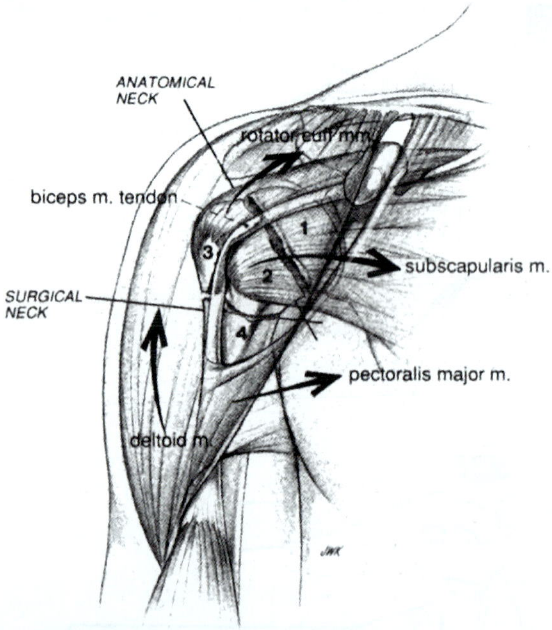

FIGURE 10.4 Displacement of fracture fragments results from the pull of muscles attaching to the various bony components. (*Source:* Bucholz RW, Heckman JD. *Rockwood & Green's Fractures in Adults*, 5th ed. Lippincott Williams & Wilkins, 2001.)

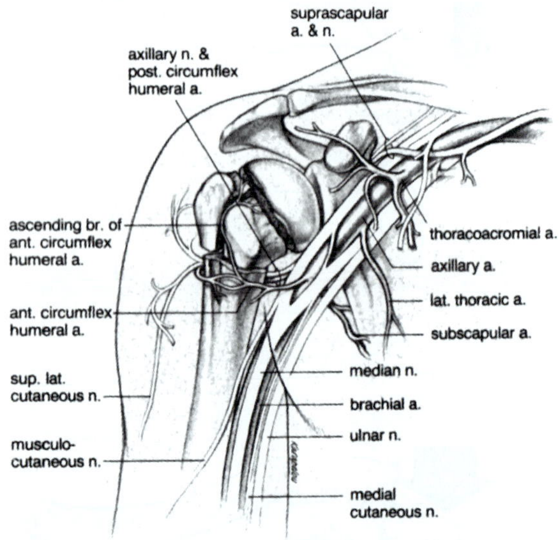

FIGURE 10.5 The major blood supply to the humeral head is through the ascending branch of the anterior humeral circumflex artery, which penetrates the head at the superior aspect of the bicipital groove and becomes the arcuate artery. There are 3 important nerves about the shoulder: the axillary, the suprascapular, and the musculocutaneous. (*Source:* Bucholz RW, Heckman JD. *Rockwood & Green's Fractures in Adults*, 5th ed. Lippincott Williams & Wilkins, 2001.)

Shoulder Dislocations

Overview. Shoulder dislocations occur in the anterior direction 95% of the time. Neurologic injury is common with a 20% to 40% rate. An axillary radiograph or CT should be performed to assess an impaction injury of the head or a Hill-Sachs lesion (Figs. 10.7 and 10.8). Anterior dislocations are often associated with greater tuberosity fractures, and the arm sits in an externally rotated, abducted position. Posterior dislocations comprise the remaining 5% of shoulder dislocations and are often associated with seizures or electric shock. Posterior dislocations can often be missed on radiographs, but the finding of a lesser tuberosity fracture should raise the examiner's suspicions. The arm sits in adducted, internally rotated position. Traumatic dislocations usually lead to a unidirectional instability pattern, while atraumatic dislocations are indicative of multidirectional injury complex.

Imaging. Imaging of the shoulder in suspected dislocation should include a standard shoulder series along with a Stryker notch view to better visualize a Hill-Sachs defect and a West Point view to assess the anteroinferior glenoid. A CT scan can be used to assess intraarticular fracture pathology, and an MRI can assist in evaluating a concurrent rotator cuff or superior labrum anterior to posterior (SLAP) tear (Fig. 10.9). Capsular injury can occur usually from the glenoid, although capsular detachment from the humerus (humeral avulsion of glenohumeral ligament [HAGL] lesion) is also a known entity. Labral damage including a Bankart lesion (avulsion of the anteroinferior labrum of the glenoid rim) or a bony Bankart (associated glenoid rim fracture) can lead to recurrent instability. A Hill-Sachs lesion results from the humeral head impacting on the glenoid and can result in a locked dislocation.

Treatment. Treatment of an acute dislocation necessitates immediate reduction and immobilization. Immobilization of the shoulder in external rotation provides the best reduction of the anterior labrum. Operative indications include an irreducible shoulder via closed techniques or patients with recurrent

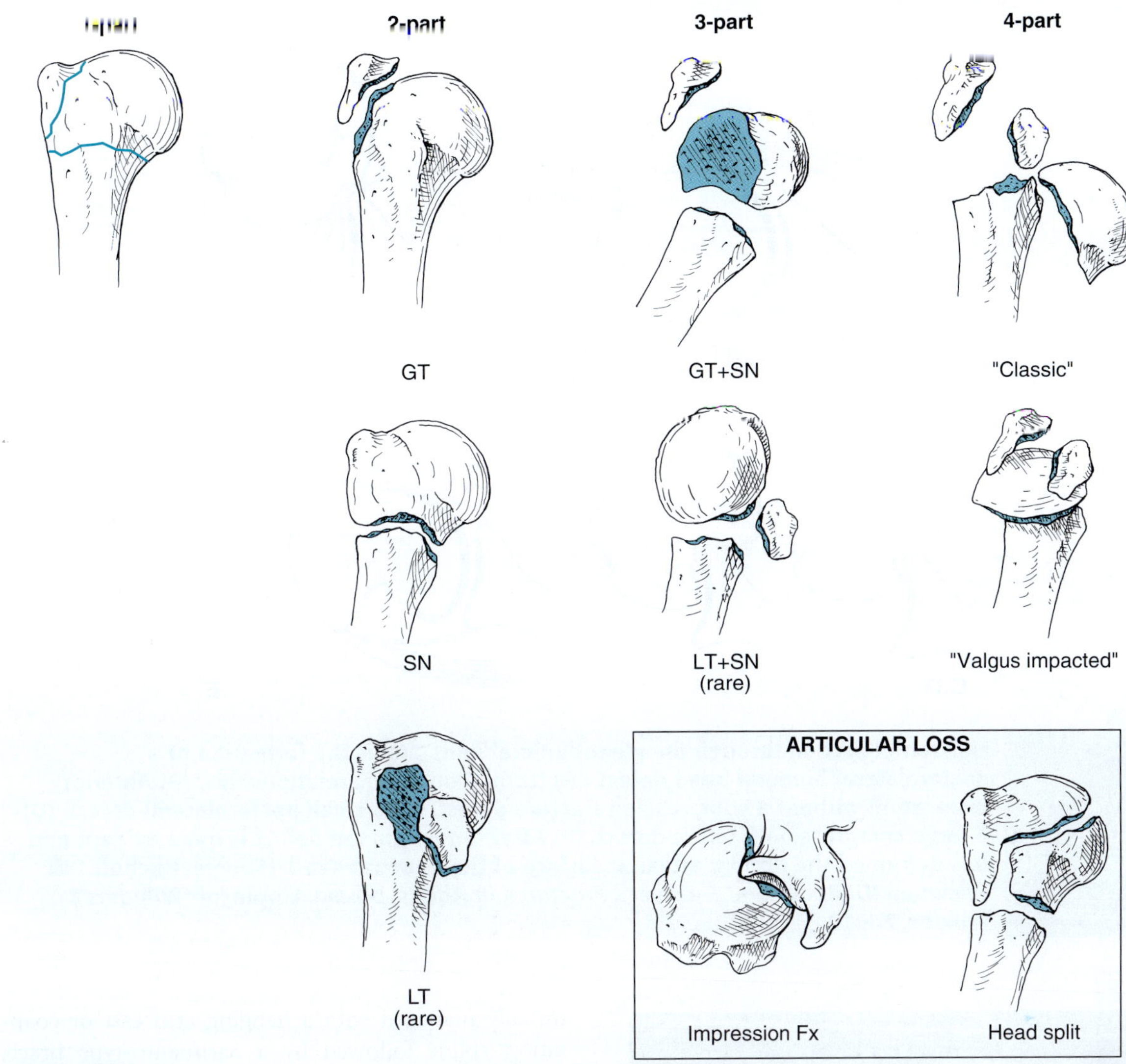

FIGURE 10.6 Simplified Neer classification with valgus-impacted 4-part fractures added. GT, greater tuberosity; LT, lesser tuberosity; SN, surgical neck. (*Source:* Bucholz RW, Heckman JD. *Rockwood & Green's Fractures in Adults*, 5th ed. Lippincott Williams & Wilkins, 2001.)

instability. In recurrent instability, open repair is the "gold standard," often requiring fixation of the Bankart lesion and a capsulorrhaphy. The outcomes after dislocation are often linked to age and the direction of dislocation. In patients under 20 years old, recurrence rates are near 100% after traumatic anterior dislocations, while patients over 45 have much less chance of recurrent dislocation.

Humeral Shaft Fractures

Overview and Anatomy. The diaphysis of the humeral shaft extends from the insertion of the pectoralis major to the supracondylar ridge. Fracture displacement is based on the muscular attachments. For example, if the fracture is distal to the pectoralis major and proximal to deltoid tuberosity, the proximal fragment is adducted. If the fracture is distal to the deltoid tuberosity, the proximal fragment is abducted and shortened because of the pull of the biceps and triceps. Because of the variable pattern of presentation, the classification is predominantly descriptive and based on location, pattern, amount of energy, and whether the injury is open or closed. Radiographic evaluation indicated for these injuries includes an anteroposterior and lateral view of the humerus. Imaging should also be performed of the shoulder and elbow joints to determine if there is associated pathology. CT and/or MRI are indicated if a pathologic fracture is suspected.

Closed Management. Treatment is often nonsurgical. Closed management of humeral shaft fractures is

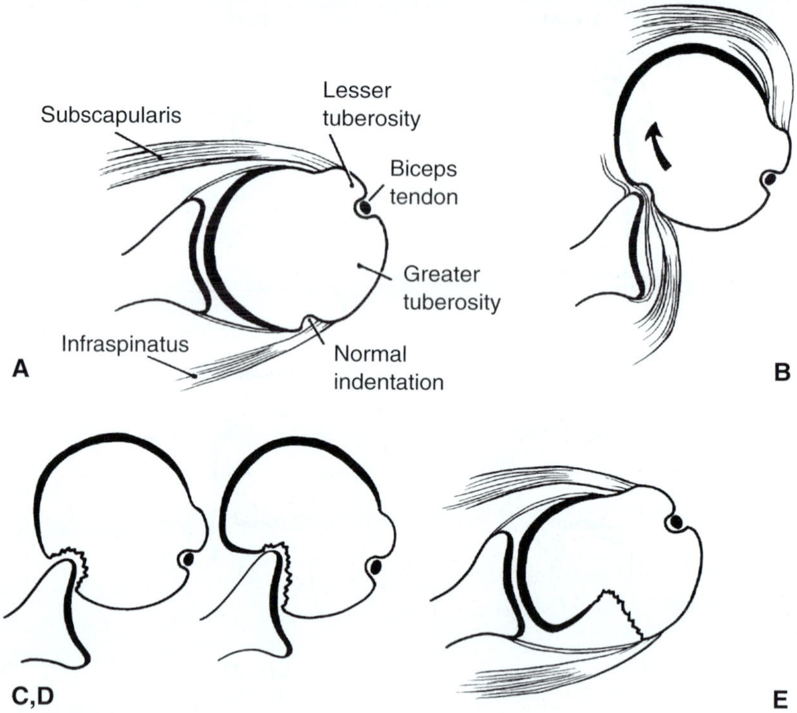

FIGURE 10.7 **Horizontal section through the glenohumeral joint shows the formation of a posterolateral humeral head defect. (A) Normal anatomic relationships. (B) Anterior dislocation without a compression fracture defect. (C) A small posterolateral defect. (D) A large compression fracture defect. (E) After reduction, the defect is quite evident and has deformed the normal articular surface of the humeral head. (*Source:* Bucholz RW, Heckman JD. *Rockwood & Green's Fractures in Adults*, 5th ed. Lippincott Williams & Wilkins, 2001.)**

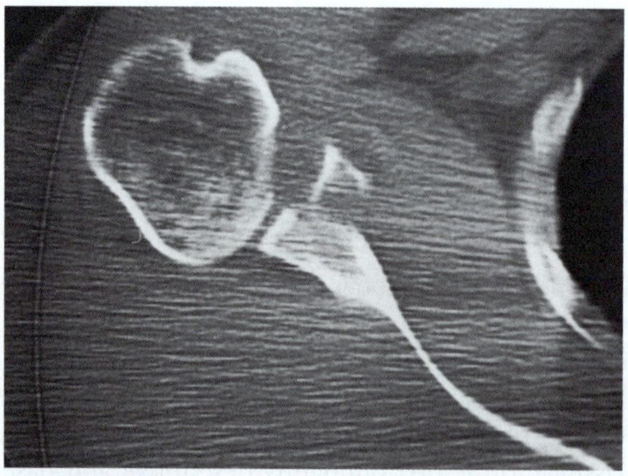

FIGURE 10.8 **CT scan shows a fracture of the anterior glenoid rim secondary to anterior glenohumeral dislocation. (*Source:* Matsen FA III, Thomas SC, Rockwood CA Jr. Glenohumeral instability. In: Rockwood CA, Matsen FA III (eds.), *The Shoulder.* Philadelphia: WB Saunders, 1990;611–689.)**

initially managed with a hanging arm cast or coaptation splint followed by a Sarmiento-type brace. Rigid immobilization and perfect alignment are not essential for adequate healing. Indications for continued closed treatment include less than 20 degrees of anterior or posterior angulation, less than 30 degrees of varus, and less than 3 cm of shortening. Closed management of these injuries has resulted in a 98% union rate with good functional restoration and minimal deformity; however, success depends on a compliant patient. Contraindications to closed management include massive soft tissue or bone loss, unreliable patient, inability to maintain acceptable fracture alignment, or presence of a fracture gap.

Operative Treatment. Surgical indications include failed closed treatment, open fractures, vascular or neurologic injury, segmental fractures, floating elbow, bilateral humeral shaft fractures, pathologic fractures, ipsilateral brachial plexus injuries, polytrauma patients, and Parkinson disease. Techniques for humeral shaft fracture fixation include plate osteosynthesis (Fig. 10.10), intramedullary fixation, and external

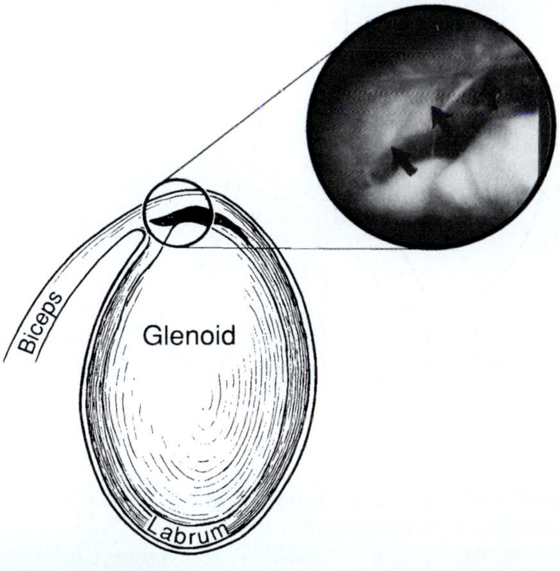

FIGURE 10.9 **(A, B, C) A so-called SLAP lesion of the long-head biceps tendon origin and superior glenoid labrum as seen on arthroscopic examinations. (*Source:* Bucholz RW, Heckman JD. *Rockwood & Green's Fractures in Adults*, 5th ed. Lippincott Williams & Wilkins, 2001.)**

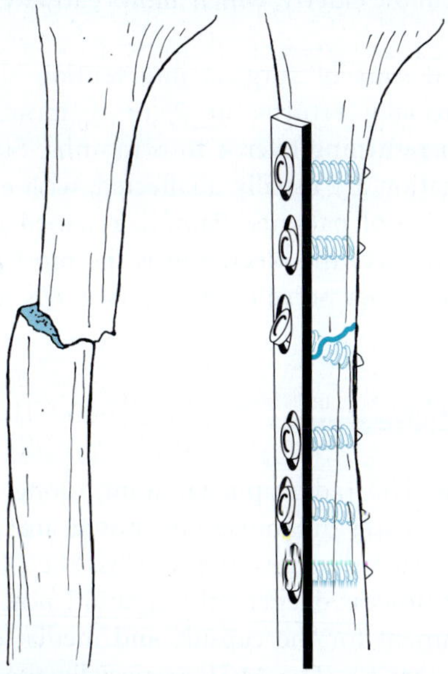

FIGURE 10.10 **Ideal configuration of compression plate and screws for fixation of a short oblique fracture. (*Source:* Bucholz RW, Heckman JD. *Rockwood & Green's Fractures in Adults*, 5th ed. Lippincott Williams & Wilkins, 2001.)**

fixation. External fixation is indicated for severe open fractures with soft tissue injury, burns or infected nonunions, and humeral shaft fracture with neurovascular injury. Plate fixation provides the best functional results and can be performed without violation of the rotator cuff. An anterolateral approach is preferred for proximal third fractures, while an anterolateral and posterior approach are appropriate for midshaft and distal third fractures.

Results. Operative intervention results in union rates of 96% with complications in 3% to 13% of patients. Intramedullary fixation minimizes soft tissue stripping, is less likely to fail because of fatigue since the implant is closer to the mechanical axis, is a load-sharing device if not statically locked, and has limited stress shielding. However, there is an extremely high incidence of shoulder pain due to violation of the rotator cuff during insertion. Indications for intramedullary fixation include segmental fractures requiring significant soft tissue stripping, osteopenic bone, pathologic fractures, and highly comminuted fractures with extension to the surgical neck. Complications associated with intramedullary fixation include potential injury to the radial nerve during reaming, avoiding anteroposterior proximal locking screws to prevent injury to the axillary nerve, and avoiding lateral-medial distal locking screws to prevent injury to the lateral antebrachial cutaneous nerve.

Complications. Complications include radial nerve injury, vascular injury, and nonunion. Radial nerve injury occurs in 1.8% to 24% of all shaft fracture. Primary injury occurs at time of injury, but secondary injury occurs during closed or open reduction. Transverse fractures of the middle third of the humerus are most commonly associated with neuropraxia. Holstein-Lewis fractures (spiral fractures of the distal third of the humerus) result in a higher risk of laceration or radial nerve entrapment. Spontaneous recovery is found in greater than 70% of patients, and secondary injuries often recover spontaneously (90% resolve in 3 to 4 months). Exploration for palsies associated with open fractures is the only indication that is not associated with conflicting data (unlike Holstein-Lewis fractures or secondary palsies). Vascular injury to the brachial artery is greatest with fractures in the proximal and distal third of arm. Nonunion occurs between 0% and 15% of the time, with the proximal and distal aspects of the humerus at greatest risk. Risk factors for nonunion include transverse fracture pattern, older age, poor nutritional status, osteoporosis, endocrine abnormalities, steroid use, anticoagulation, and previous radiation therapy. Compression plate fixation is the preferred treatment.

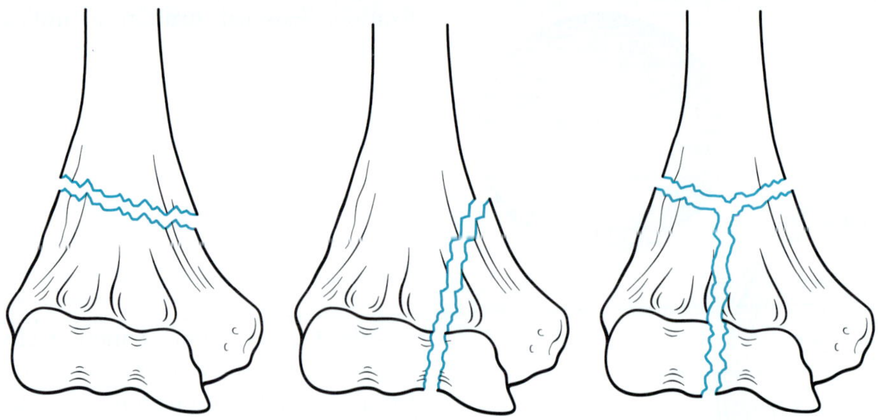

FIGURE 10.11 **Fractures of the distal humerus are divided into 3 types: A, nonarticular; B, partially articular; and C, no articular fracture fragments remain in continuity with the shaft fragment. (*Source:* Bucholz RW, Heckman JD. *Rockwood & Green's Fractures in Adults*, 5th ed. Lippincott Williams & Wilkins, 2001.)**

Distal Humerus Fractures

Overview and Anatomy. The elbow is a hinged joint with a single axis of rotation. The trochlea is the center of rotation with a medial and lateral column. The trochlear axis is 94 to 98 degrees in valgus relative to the longitudinal axis. The trochlear axis is 3 to 8 degrees externally rotated. The medial column diverges from the humeral shaft at a 45-degree angle, and the lateral column diverges at a 20-degree angle. The intramedullary canal ends 2 to 3 cm above the olecranon fossa. The functional ROM of the elbow is 30 to 130 degrees of extension and flexion and 50 to 50 degrees of pronation to supination. Fracture lines are related to the position of the elbow at the time of load application. The classification system (Fig. 10.11) is based on the location of the fracture line (Table 10.2).

Treatment. Treatment principles include anatomic articular reduction with stable internal fixation of the articular surface and restoration of articular axial alignment. Stable internal fixation of the articular segment to the metaphysis and diaphysis and early ROM is important for restoration of function. Comminution of the epicondyles is supported by small or mini-fragment buttress plates with bone graft as needed. Two-column plate fixation (which can be parallel or at 90 degrees to each other) provides greatest stability. Total elbow arthroplasty is indicated in severely comminuted fractures in the elderly, which allows early ROM.

Results. Results of surgical intervention show that flexion usually returns in 2 to 3 months, with extension returning over 4 to 6 months. Supination and pronation are usually unaffected, with exertional pain in 25% of patients. Painful, retained hardware medially or over the olecranon is the most common complaint. Ulnar nerve palsy occurs in 8% to 20% of patients.

TABLE 10.2 **Classification of elbow fracture**

Type	*Fracture Line Location*	*Subtype*
A	Extraarticular	Medial epicondyle Lateral epicondyle Distal metaphyseal humerus
B	Partial articular	Capitellum Trochlea
C	Complete articular	

Elbow Dislocations

Anatomy. The radiocapitellar joint, along with the coronoid process and the sigmoid notch, are secondary stabilizers against valgus forces across the elbow. The coronoid process deepens the sigmoid notch and is an attachment for the capsule and medial collateral ligament (MCL). The MCL (especially the anterior band) is the primary medial stabilizer of the elbow, which resists valgus forces, along with the lateral column (radial head and capitellum). In full extension, the MCL provides 30% of valgus stability, while at 90 degrees of flexion, it confers 50% of valgus stability. Resection of the anterior band causes gross instability except in extension. The three components of the MCL include the anterior oblique band (the primary stabilizer from 20 to 120 degrees flexion inserting near the coracoid process), the posterior oblique band, and the transverse band. The lateral ligaments prevent posterior subluxation and rotation of the ulna and protect against posterolateral rotatory instability.

Mechanisms of Injury. The elbow is the second most common joint dislocated, with over 90% being posterior and 50% including fracture with the dislocation. The mechanism of injury involves a sequential tear of the MCL, rupture of the capsule, tear of the lateral ligaments, and variable injury to the flexor-pronator mass as a result of a fall onto an extended elbow.

Evaluation. Neuropraxia is seen in up to 20% of cases (ulnar nerve or anterior interosseous nerve [AIN] injury). The wrist and distal radioulnar joint (DRUJ) should be evaluated along with radiographs of the elbow because associated fractures most commonly involved the radial head or coronoid process.

Classification. The classification system is predominantly descriptive and based on the direction of displacement of the ulna relative to the humerus.

Treatment. Treatment of acute elbow dislocations requires immediate closed reduction. After closed reduction, stability should be assessed by examining the anterior band of the MCL at 30 and 90 degrees of flexion with the forearm pronated. The elbow should be splinted for 5 to 10 days in 90 degrees of flexion and protected ROM should begin after 5 to 10 days. ROM should be advanced 3 to 6 weeks after injury. Currently, there is little advantage to acute ligament repair if the elbow is stable. Associated radial head or neck fractures require fixation if the joint is unstable. If the radial head is irreparable, radial head replacement should be considered along with ligamentous repair. Fractures of more than 50% of the coronoid process should be repaired if the elbow is unstable.

Olecranon Fractures

Mechanisms of Injury. The mechanisms of injury in olecranon fractures can be multifold. Acute tension overload when a tensile force is applied by the triceps with elbow flexion, chronic overload (e.g., stress fracture, pediatric injuries, osteopenia), or a direct blow can lead to fractures of the olecranon. The Mayo classification is shown in Table 10.3 and is subdivided with A and B modifiers for noncomminuted and comminuted respectively.

Treatment. Nonoperative treatment via a long-arm splint for 7 to 10 days followed by functional bracing for 4 to 6 weeks is indicated for nondisplaced fractures.

TABLE 10.3 Mayo classification of olecranon fractures

Type	Description	Rate of Occurrence
I	Nondisplaced	12%
II	Displaced, elbow stable	82%
III	Displaced, elbow unstable	6%

Operative indications for repair include disruption of extensor mechanism or articular incongruity. Excision of the olecranon and reattachment of the triceps anteriorly is indicated in elderly patients, osteoporosis, or involvement of less than 50% of joint. Open reduction and internal fixation can be performed with tension-band wires, plates, or an intramedullary screw. Tension-band wire with pins or an intramedullary screw is indicated for transverse fractures with an intact dorsal cortex (Fig. 10.12). Plate fixation can be

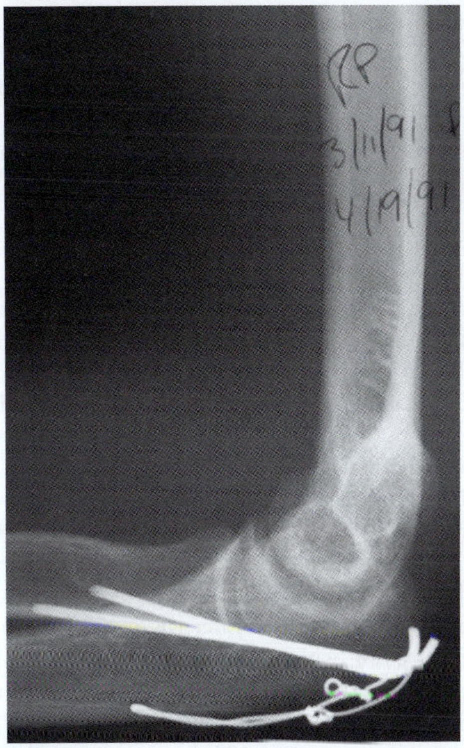

FIGURE 10.12 Displaced olecranon fracture union at 5 weeks, treated with transfixion wires and tensioned wire loop. (*Source:* Bucholz RW, Heckman JD. *Rockwood & Green's Fractures in Adults*, 5th ed. Lippincott Williams & Wilkins, 2001.)

useful in patients with oblique, complex fracture pattern and comminuted dorsal cortex. The plate is placed posteriorly or laterally (fewer problems with lateral placement). Intramedullary screw fixation can be utilized for an oblique fracture plane. However, a long screw may lead to medial shift of the tip of the olecranon. An additional tension-band wire may be needed to improve rigidity of the construct. These fractures, when treated appropriately, often go on to union.

Complications. Complications include painful retained hardware, often necessitating removal; pin migration; heterotopic ossification; and hardware failure.

Radial Head Fractures

Anatomy and Overview. The radial head acts as a secondary restraint to valgus force across the elbow and serves to shift the center of varus–valgus rotation laterally so that medial ligaments bear less force. The radial head acts to transfer load from wrist to radiocapitellar joint and also provides longitudinal stability (along with interosseous ligament). Radial head fractures often occur because of an axial load after a fall combined with a valgus force.

Imaging. Imaging of the radial head includes anteroposterior, lateral, and oblique radiographs. MRI and ultrasound are useful in diagnosing skeletally immature patients.

Classification. The modified Mason classification is used to describe these injuries (Table 10.4).

TABLE 10.4 Mason classification for radial head fractures

Type	Displacement	Description
I	Nondisplaced, less than 2 cm of articular step-off	No block to formation
II	Displaced more than 2 cm	Internal fixation possible
III	Displaced, severely comminuted	Usually irreparable; often requires excision to allow elbow movement

Treatment. Operative consideration for preserving the radial head versus replacing it requires assessing valgus instability associated with elbow dislocation and longitudinal instability with interosseous ligament injury. In isolated radial head or neck fracture, start with early ROM if minimally displaced or consider radial head excision if significantly displaced or comminuted. If there is an associated dislocation with fracture of the radial head, restoration of function is required. This can be done with either internal fixation of the radial head along with lateral ligament reconstruction (which is ideal) or prosthetic head replacement if the radial head is irreparable. The safe zone for radial head replacement is an arc of 100 degrees centered on the equator of the neutrally rotated forearm (Fig. 10.13). Complications of radial head fracture include hardware failure, loss of fixation, posterior interosseous nerve (PIN) injury, and elbow stiffness.

An Essex-Lopresti lesion is a longitudinal disruption of the interosseous ligament combined with radial head fracture and dislocation and disruption of the distal radioulnar joint. Treatment requires stabilizing both the elbow and DRUJ components of the injury. If the radial head is excised, it will lead to proximal migration of the radius.

Forearm Fractures

Anatomy. The 3 compartments of the forearm include the posterior (dorsal containing the extensors), the anterior (volar containing the flexors), and the mobile wad (brachioradialis, extensor carpi radialis longus [ECRL], and extensor carpi radialis brevis [ECRB]). The classification of forearm fracture is a descriptive one: isolated fractures of the radius or ulna (e.g., nightstick fracture of ulna), fractures of both bones (no ligament injury), and fractures of 1 bone with ligament rupture.

Fracture Types. Monteggia fractures involve fractures of the proximal third of the ulna with dislocation of the radial head and are described by the Bado Classification (Table 10.5). Plate fixation of the ulna often reduces the radial head (see Fig. 10.14).

Galeazzi fractures involve fractures of the distal one-third of the radius with disruption of the DRU (usually within seven centimeters). Signs of DRUJ injury include fracture at the base of the ulnar styloid, widening of the DRUJ on anteroposterior radiographs, subluxation of the ulna on lateral radiographs, or greater than 5 mm of radial shortening. Plate fixation of the radius with DRUJ stabilization is needed.

Classification. The AO/ASIF classification system is only for diaphyseal injuries and does not take into account intraarticular fractures. Type A fractures are simple with no comminution. Type B fractures are wedge fractures with a single butterfly fracture. Type C fractures are complex fractures that can be either segmental or comminuted.

Treatment. Treatment of forearm fractures requires maintaining anatomic reduction and normal

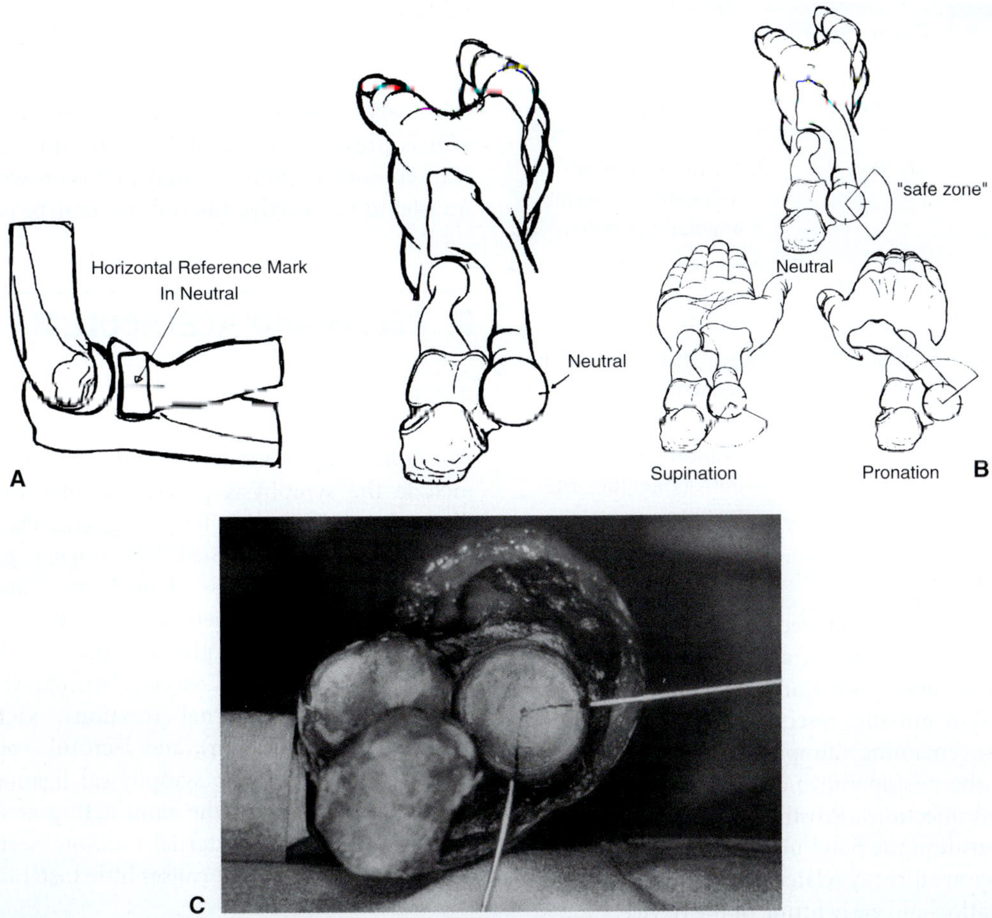

FIGURE 10.13 **Preserving the radial head after fracture. (A) A horizontal reference mark is made with the forearm in neutral position. (B) Two more horizontal marks are made in full pronation and full supination. By dividing each of these sectors in half, the safe zone is identified. (C) An anatomic specimen showing the safe zone with the forearm in full supination. (*Source:* Bucholz RW, Heckman JD. *Rockwood & Green's Fractures in Adults*, 5th ed. Lippincott Williams & Wilkins, 2001.)**

relationships. Closed reduction and casting have led to high rates of nonunion or malunion with poor functional results. Functional braces or casting of the ulna is possible if the fracture is in the stable distal one-third of the bone with less than 10 degrees of angulation. The radius can be treated nonoperatively if it is completely nondisplaced and the radial bow is maintained. Open reduction and internal fixation should be performed for all unstable or open fractures. Proper technique leads to high union rates (95%) with excellent function. The principles of fixation include anatomic reduction, restoration of ulnar and radial length, rotational alignment, and restoration of the radial bow. External fixation for Gustillo types IIIB and IIIC open fractures usually need to be revised to internal fixation when the soft tissues improve.

Complications. Complications of forearm injuries include compartment syndrome, especially in crush injury, high-energy trauma, and those with risk factors including coagulopathy, vascular injury, and limb compression. When performing a fasciotomy, all three compartments should be released. Neurovascular injuries occur to the PIN in proximal fractures, the superficial radial nerve during the anterior radius approach for distal fractures, and the AIN during reduction of radius fractures. Malunion with greater than 10 degrees of angulation leads to loss of motion and decreased grip strength (especially with loss of radial bow). In cases of nonunion, segmental bone loss should be replaced with an intercalary graft (vascularized fibula if more than 3.5 cm or iliac crest bone if less than 3.5 cm).

Amputations

General Indications. The indications for amputation of the upper extremity are severe open fractures with

TABLE 10.5 Bado classification

Type	Rate of Occurrence	Description
I	60%	Anterior radial head dislocation, anterior angulation of ulna
II	15%	Posterior radial head dislocation, posterior angulation of ulna
III	20%	Lateral dislocation of the radial head
IV	5%	Anterior radial head dislocation, proximal both-bones forearm fracture

extensive soft tissue and neurologic injury, tumors, peripheral vascular disease, and infection. The basic principles include maintaining length, maintaining all viable skin initially, resecting nerves sharply and burying the remaining stump to avoid neuromas, and managing the postoperative care as open wounds in trauma and infections. Prosthetic use in amputations serves to position the hand in space. Limb length and joint salvage are directly related to functional outcome, as are sensation and early fitting of the device.

Levels of Amputation. Forequarter amputations are primarily performed because of malignancy but result in difficult skin flaps and poor cosmesis. An above-elbow amputation is indicated in a flail arm with no scapulothoracic control (unloads the shoulder joint, reduces subluxation), but patients are still unlikely to be able to use a prosthesis. The proximal humeral amputations behave like shoulder disarticulations but have better cosmesis and prosthesis suspension. Similarly, distal humeral amputations (3.5 cm proximal to the elbow) have better function than elbow disarticulations. In performing below-elbow amputations, maintenance of forearm length to preserve strength and rotation is essential. If a flail arm is present but the ability exists to stabilize the scapulothoracic joint, a shoulder fusion with muscle transfer to allow active elbow flexion can be performed.

II. PELVIS AND ACETABULUM

Pelvic fractures

Anatomy. Important bony landmarks in the pelvis include the symphysis pubis, the anterior superior iliac spine (ASIS), the iliac wing, and the posterior superior iliac spine (PSIS). The normal gap in the pubic symphysis is less than 5 mm and the SI joint gap is usually between 2 and 4 mm. The ligamentous stabilizers give the pelvis stability and include the posterior iliosacral (strongest), anterior iliosacral (resists external rotation), sacrospinous (resists external rotation), and sacrotuberous (resists shear and flexion). The symphyseal ligament resists external rotation with the rami acting as a strut to resist compression in internal rotation. Sectioning of the symphyseal ligament causes little instability.

Associated Injuries. Associated injuries include neurologic damage, visceral injuries, and the Morel-Lavallière lesion (Fig. 10.15). Neurologic injury most commonly occurs at L5 and S1, but L2 to L4 are possible with the greatest risk occurring with sacral fractures (Table 10.6). Injuries to the bladder and urethra occur in 15% of cases. Clinical signs include blood at the meatus or a high-riding prostate or eventual swelling of scrotum and labia. A retrograde urethrogram is indicated in patients with pelvic injury to insure hemodynamic stability, with a Foley placed in the suprapubic

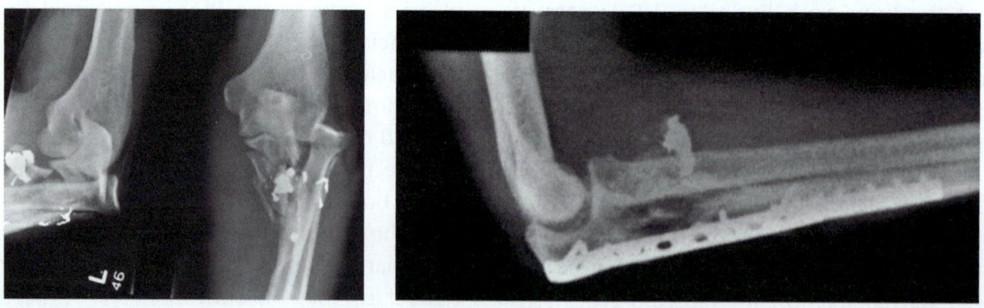

A B

FIGURE 10.14 (A) Bado type II Monteggia fracture secondary to a gunshot wound in a 35-year-old man. (B) Adequate fixation required use of overlapping plates because of extensive comminution. (*Source:* Bucholz RW, Heckman JD. *Rockwood & Green's Fractures in Adults*, 5th ed. Lippincott Williams & Wilkins, 2001.)

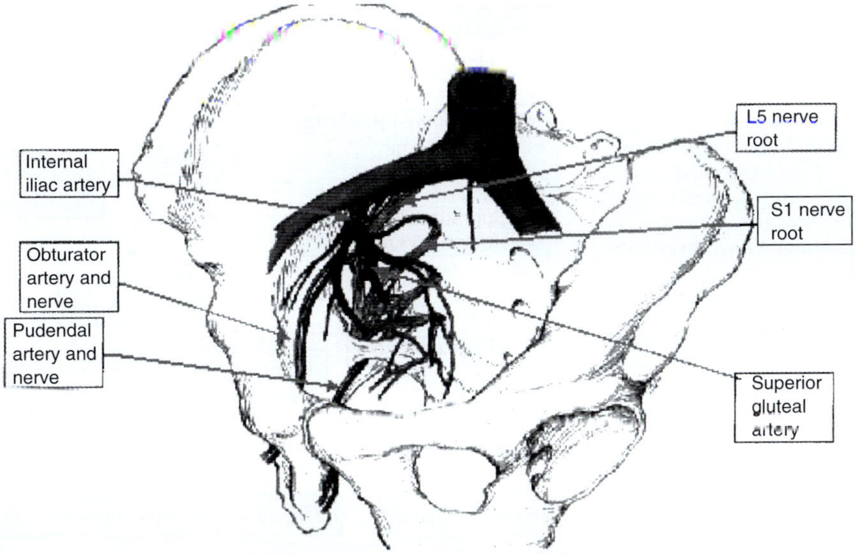

FIGURE 10.15 Vasculature and neurologic structures of the pelvis. (*Source:* Bucholz RW, Heckman JD. *Rockwood & Green's Fractures in Adults*, 5th ed. Lippincott Williams & Wilkins, 2001.)

region if needed. The Morel-Lavallière lesion is a skin degloving that occurs over the pelvic region. It becomes infected in one-third of cases and requires thorough débridement prior to definitive surgery.

Biomechanics of Deformity. The biomechanics of deformity are defined from an anatomically positioned pelvis in space and are a combination of rotational and translational deformities. The pelvis does not deform around a single point. Stability is determined by the integrity of posterior bone and ligamentous structures, injury to which leads to vertical instability and some rotational instability.

Acute Management. The acute management of patients with pelvic injuries involves a thorough primary survey, an anteroposterior radiograph of the pelvis, and assessment for bladder or urethral injury. An open-book injury with anterior displacement of the pubic symphysis greater than 2.5 cm should be stabilized to limit pelvic hemorrhage (Fig. 10.16) with either a posterior or anterior external fixator, a pelvic binder, embolization with unexplained blood loss after stabilization and aggressive resuscitation, or a sheet clamped around the pelvis.

TABLE 10.6 Risk of neurologic injury by Denis Type pelvic fracture

Denis Type	Location	Risk of Neurologic Injury
I	Lateral to foramen	6%
II	Through the foramen	28%
III	Medial to foramen	57%

Hypovolemic Shock. The etiology of hypovolemic shock may be intrathoracic bleeding, intraperitoneal bleeding (diagnosed by ultrasound, peritoneal tap, or CT), and/or retroperitoneal bleeding. The average blood loss in patients with a lateral compression injury is 3.6 units, in an anteroposterior compression injury is 14.8 units, and in vertical shear injuries is 9.2 units (Table 10.7). Bleeding is often due to venous disruption.

Imaging. Once a patient has been relatively stable, radiographs to review should include an anteroposterior view, and inlet view (taken with the beam 40 degrees caudad), and an outlet view (taken with the beam 40 degree cephalad). The inlet view provides information on horizontal plane rotation, posterior displacement, and the sacral ala. The outlet view assesses the sacrum, cephalad displacement, and the sacral foramina. CT scan provides much more detailed information than radiographs. The CT defines posterior injury, assesses displacement versus impaction, determines rotation and comminution, and completely visualizes the neural foramina. Radiographic signs of instability include SI displacement of 5 mm in any plane, posterior fracture gap, and or avulsions of the fifth lumbar transverse process.

Classification. There are 3 main classification systems.

- *Tile Classification*—This system focuses on stability and offers prognosis and treatment. Tile A fractures

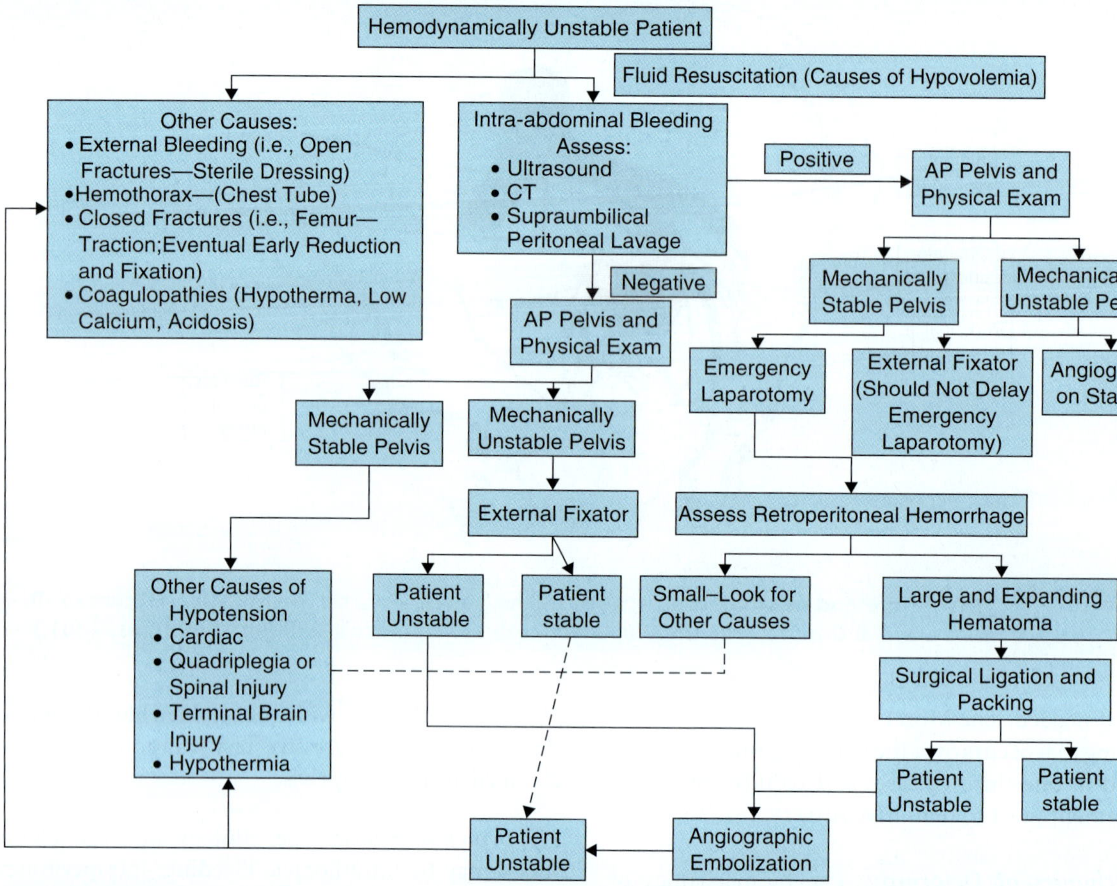

FIGURE 10.16 Algorithm for the acute management of hemodynamically unstable patients with pelvic injuries.

TABLE 10.7 Estimated fluid and blood losses* based on patient's initial presentation

	Class I	*Class II*	*Class III*	*Class IV*
Blood loss (mL)	Up to 750	750–1,500	1,500–2,000	> 2,000
Blood loss (% blood volume)	Up to 15%	15%–30%	30%–40%	> 40%
Pulse rate	< 00	> 100	> 120	> 140
Blood pressure	Normal	Normal	Decreased	Decreased
Pulse pressure (mm Hg)	Normal or increased	Decreased	Decreased	Decreased
Respiratory rate	14–20	20–30	30–40	> 35
Urine output (mL/hr)	> 30	20–30	5–15	Negligible
CNS/mental status	Slightly anxious	Mildly anxious	Anxious, confused	Confused, lethargic
Fluid replacement (3:1 rule)	Crystalloid	Crystalloid	Crystalloid and blood	Crystalloid and blood

*For a 70-kg man

TABLE 10.8 Tile B and C classification of pelvic fractures

Tile B		
Type	**Description**	**Notes**
B1	AP compression	Stage 1: less than 2.5 cm diastasis Stage 2: more than 2.5 cm diastasis, unilateral posterior injury Stage 3: more than 2.5 cm diastasis, bilateral posterior injury
B2	Lateral compression	Ipsilateral
B3	Lateral compression	Contralateral

Tile C	
Type	**Disruption**
C1	Ipsilateral anterior and posterior
C2	Bilateral hemipelvic
C3	Any pelvic fracture with an associated acetabular fracture

are considered stable fractures. Tile B fractures (Table 10.8) are rotationally unstable and vertically stable. Tile C fractures are rotationally and vertically unstable (see Table 10.8).

- *Young-Burgess Classification*—This system is based on the mechanism of injury and predicts resuscitation requirements and injury patterns (Table 10.9; Figs. 10.17 through 10.23). Head injury is a major cause of death in lateral compression injuries, while pelvic and visceral injuries result in death in patients with anteroposterior compression.
- *Buchholz Classification*—This system defines treatment options. Type I fractures have an anterior injury with minimal posterior involvement. Most injuries fall within the Buchholz type I description and are inherently stable. Type II fractures are rotationally unstable and vertically stable, and type III are rotationally and vertically unstable.

Treatment. Treatment is based on instability. Instability is determined through radiographic displacement or an inability to sustain loads required for mobilization. The sacrum is the keystone to the bony stability of the pelvis. Nonoperative treatment is indicated for Buchholz type I and type II fractures with less than 2.5 cm of anterior diastasis. Patients are followed with serial radiographs to assure fracture stability and are allowed to weight-bear with support. Operative fixation is indicated for Buchholz type II fractures with greater than 2.5 cm anterior diastasis via singe or double anterior plating of the pubic symphysis. Buchholz type III fractures require stabilization posteriorly and

TABLE 10.9 Young-Burgess classification of pelvic fracture

Mechanism	Subtype	Description	Figure
Lateral compression	LC I	Impaction of sacrum on side of injury	10.17
	LC II	Crescent fracture	10.18
	LC III	LC I & II with an open-book fracture on the opposite side ("windswept" pelvis)	10.19
Anteroposterior compression	APC I	Symphysis widened 1 to 2 cm	10.20
	APC II	Symphysis widened more than 2 cm and anterior SI ligaments disrupted	10.21
	APC III	Complete SI joint disruption	10.22
Vertical shear	Vertical displacement	Unstable	10.23

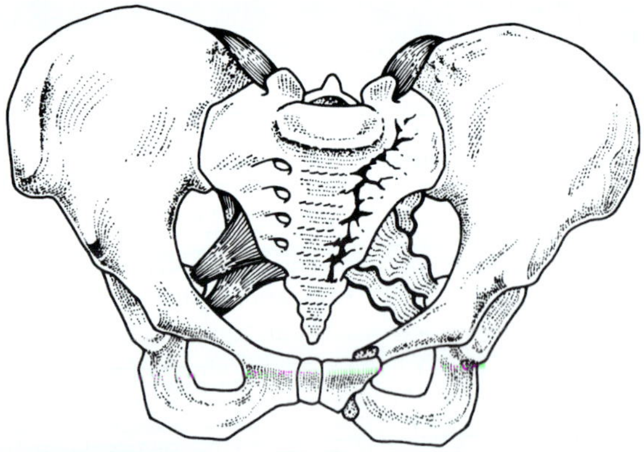

FIGURE 10.17 LC-I. Note impaction injury of the sacrum and the transverse nature of the anterior ring injury. (*Source:* Bucholz RW, Heckman JD. *Rockwood & Green's Fractures in Adults*, 5th ed. Lippincott Williams & Wilkins, 2001.)

may need additional treatment anteriorly. Timing has been shown to play an important role because early stabilization within 24 to 48 hours has been successful.

Acetabular Fractures

Anatomy. The acetabulum follows an inverted Y, 2-column concept. The anterior column extends from the anterior iliac crest to the symphysis pubis and consists of an iliac segment, acetabular segment, and pubic segment. The posterior (ilioischial) column extends from the greater sciatic notch to the inferior ischium.

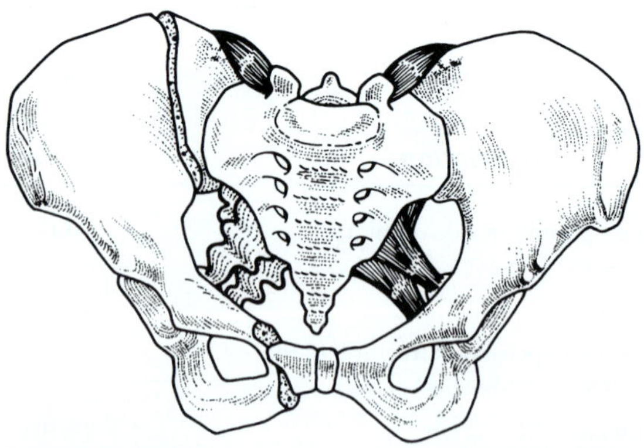

FIGURE 10.18 LC-II. Note the intact sacrospinous and sacrotuberous ligaments. (*Source:* Bucholz RW, Heckman JD. *Rockwood & Green's Fractures in Adults*, 5th ed. Lippincott Williams & Wilkins, 2001.)

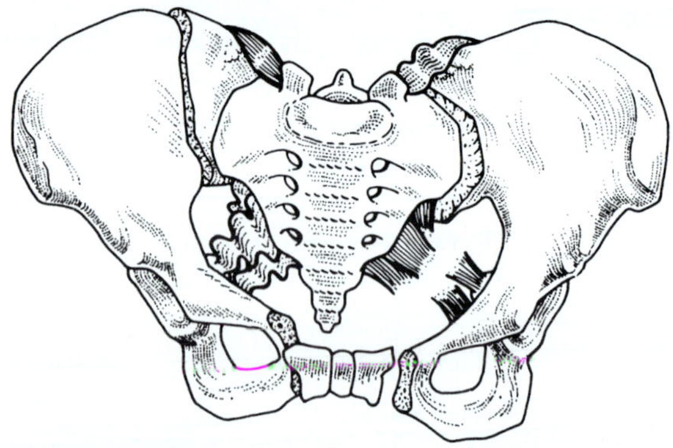

FIGURE 10.19 LC-III. Note ligamentous injury on the left side of the pelvis. (*Source:* Bucholz RW, Heckman JD. *Rockwood & Green's Fractures in Adults*, 5th ed. Lippincott Williams & Wilkins, 2001.)

The acetabular dome forms the keystone of the arch. The column concept leads to defining a classification system. The corona mortis is an anomalous branch of obturator artery, which occurs in 50% of patients and extends from the external iliac or inferior epigastric vessels. The ascending branch of medial circumflex is the main blood supply to the femoral head, which lies deep to the short external rotators and can be damaged with femoral head dislocation.

Imaging. Imaging of the acetabulum involves anteroposterior radiographs, Judet radiographs, and CT

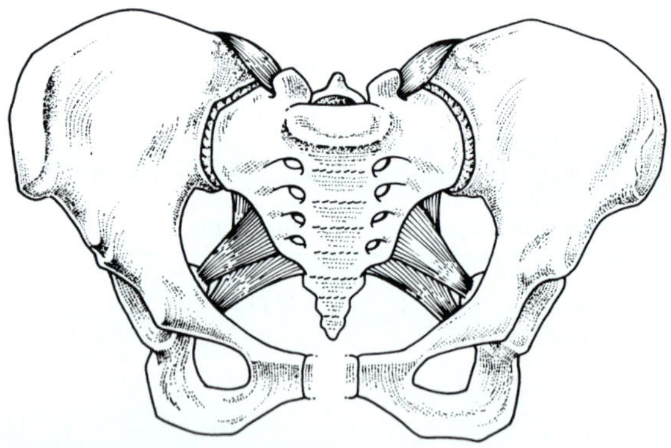

FIGURE 10.20 Anteroposterior compression type I (APC-I). Note the slight opening, yet ligamentous integrity, of the sacroiliac (SI) joints. (*Source:* Bucholz RW, Heckman JD. *Rockwood & Green's Fractures in Adults*, 5th ed. Lippincott Williams & Wilkins, 2001.)

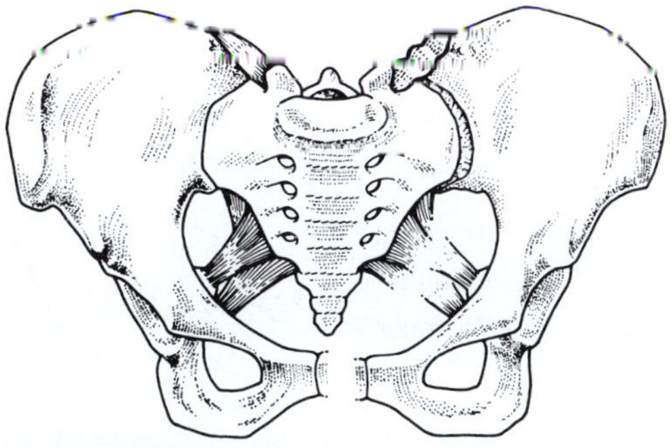

FIGURE 10.21 **APC-II. Note injury to the sacrotuberous and sacrospinous ligaments. (*Source:* Bucholz RW, Heckman JD. *Rockwood & Green's Fractures in Adults*, 5th ed. Lippincott Williams & Wilkins, 2001.)**

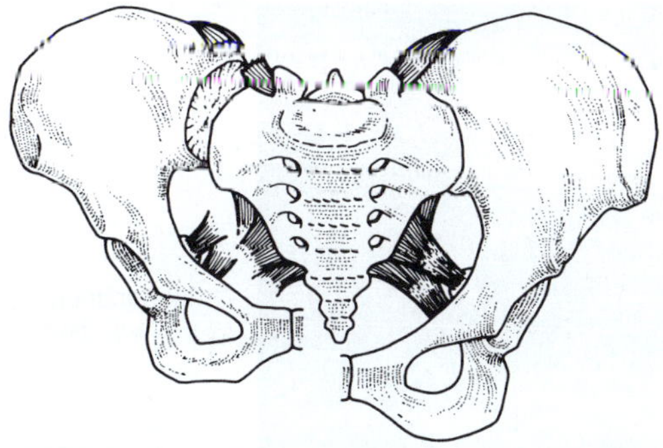

FIGURE 10.23 **Vertical shear (VS). Note vertical displacement of the hemipelvis. (*Source:* Bucholz RW, Heckman JD. *Rockwood & Green's Fractures in Adults*, 5th ed. Lippincott Williams & Wilkins, 2001.)**

scans. Anteroposterior radiographs provide information regarding associated pelvic ring injuries, bilateral acetabular fractures, femoral head fractures, fracture displacement, and congruency of the femoral head in the acetabulum. Important landmarks include the anterior wall, posterior wall, ilioischial line, iliopectineal line, teardrop, and acetabular roof (Fig. 10.24). The medial roof arc angle should be greater than 30 degrees. Judet radiographs are taken at 45-degree oblique angles to the pelvis with focus on the acetabular domes and the coccyx lying over the teardrop to ensure adequate rotation. The obturator oblique visualizes the anterior column and posterior wall with the obturator fossa on profile and the injured side up. Important lines include the iliopectineal, obturator foramen, and posterior wall (Fig. 10.25). The anterior roof arc angle is greater than 40 degrees. The iliac oblique visualizes the posterior column and anterior wall and is referenced with the image side down. Important radiographic lines include the iliac wing and crest, quadrilateral plate, and posterior border of the innominate bone (Fig. 10.26). The posterior roof arc angle is greater than 50 degrees. CT scans, imaged with 3-mm cuts through the pelvis, assess fracture comminution and associated injuries, intraarticular loose bodies, the vertical portion of T-type acetabular fracture, and sacral fractures.

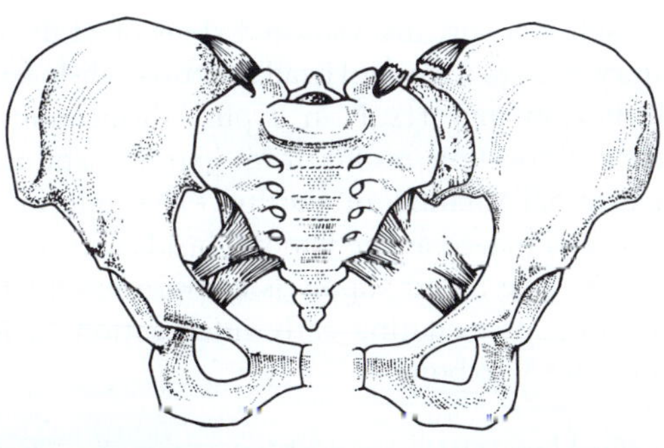

FIGURE 10.22 **APC-III. Note violation of all ligamentous structures on the left. (*Source:* Bucholz RW, Heckman JD. *Rockwood & Green's Fractures in Adults*, 5th ed. Lippincott Williams & Wilkins, 2001.)**

Classification. The classification system is descriptive and based on the location of fractures (see Fig. 10.27). Elementary fractures include those of the posterior wall (associated with posterior femoral head dislocation), posterior column (disruption of ischium and fracture of the ischiopubic ramus), anterior wall, anterior column (very low, low, intermediate, and high), and transverse through the anterior and posterior columns (can be transtectal, juxtatectal, and infratectal). Combined injuries include the following:

- Posterior wall/posterior column
- Transverse/posterior wall (highest incidence of preoperative sciatic nerve palsy)
- T-type
- Anterior wall or column/posterior hemitransverse fracture
- Both columns (where no articular surface remains intact)

Operative Treatment. Operative treatment of acetabular fractures rests on an anatomic reduction. Emergent indications for surgery include the rare open fracture and new-onset sciatic nerve palsy after closed

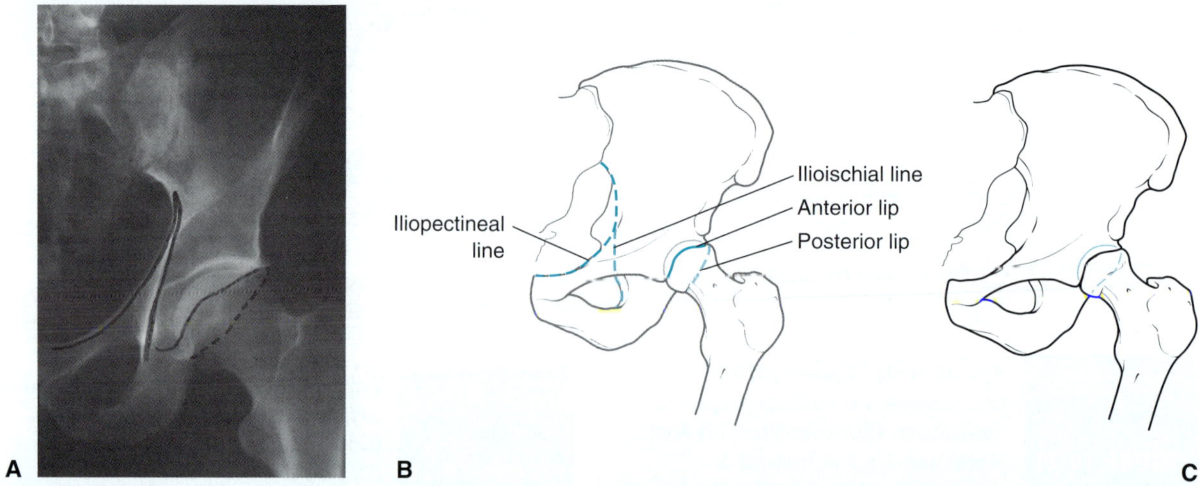

FIGURE 10.24 **(A) Anteroposterior x-ray of the left hemipelvis. (B) Major landmarks are the iliopectineal line (anterior column); the ilioischial line (posterior column); the anterior lip of the acetabulum; and the posterior lip of the acetabulum. (C) Anatomic landmarks as seen on the anteroposterior x-ray. (*Source:* Tile M. *Fractures of the Pelvis and Acetabulum.* Baltimore: Williams & Wilkins, 1984.)**

reduction. Urgent indications for surgery include an irreducible posterior hip dislocation and medial dislocation of the femoral head against the cancellous bone surface of the ilium. Factors that are predictive of outcome include injury to cartilage or bone of the femoral head, anatomic reduction, and age of patient. In treating pelvic fractures, a single surgical approach is preferred (Table 10.10). Of note, the surgical windows in the ilioinguinal approach are lateral, middle, and medial. The lateral window allows access to the internal iliac fossa, the SI joint, and the upper third of the pelvic brim. The middle window accesses the quadrilateral surface, the anterior rim, and the pelvic brim from the SI joint to the pectineal eminence. The medial window accesses the superior pubic ramus and the symphysis pubis.

III. LOWER EXTREMITY

Hip Dislocations

Overview and Anatomy. During the average ROM of the hip, 40% of the femoral head is in contact with articular cartilage and 10% of the femoral head is in contact with labrum. The labrum is a fibrous ring that increases femoral head coverage and contributes to joint stability. The capsule extends from the intertrochanteric ridge to the acetabulum. There are several fibrous bands of tissue, including the iliofemoral ligament (upside down Y), that block hip extension. The average anteversion of the femoral neck is 7 degrees (greater in females). The blood supply to the femoral head includes the artery of the ligamentum teres, which is most important in children. However, its contribution decreases with age, and it has a limited role in the elderly. The ascending cervical branches arise from the ring at the base of the neck. The ring is formed by the medial and lateral circumflex femoral arteries, which are susceptible to injury with hip dislocation.

Mechanism of Injury. The mechanism of injury usually involves high-energy trauma. A posterior dislocation occurs with an axial load applied to the femur while the hip is flexed. Most commonly, it is a result of a dashboard impact on the knee. The type of dislocation is based on the position of the hip at time of impact. If the leg is abducted, there will be a resultant fracture-dislocation; however, if the leg is adducted, it may result in a pure dislocation. Extension at the time of injury leads to a femoral head fracture—dislocation, while flexion may result in a pure dislocation. An anterior dislocation results from extreme abduction with external rotation of the hip. The anterior hip capsule is damaged as the femoral head is levered out anteriorly. The blood supply is compromised with a dislocation, necessitating early intervention to limit vascular insult to bone.

Classification. The classification system by Thomas and Epstein is shown in Table 10.11.

Examination. Physical findings in patients with posterior dislocation include a hip that is flexed, internally rotated, and adducted. On the other hand, an anterior dislocation results in an externally rotated, slightly abducted, and flexed hip.

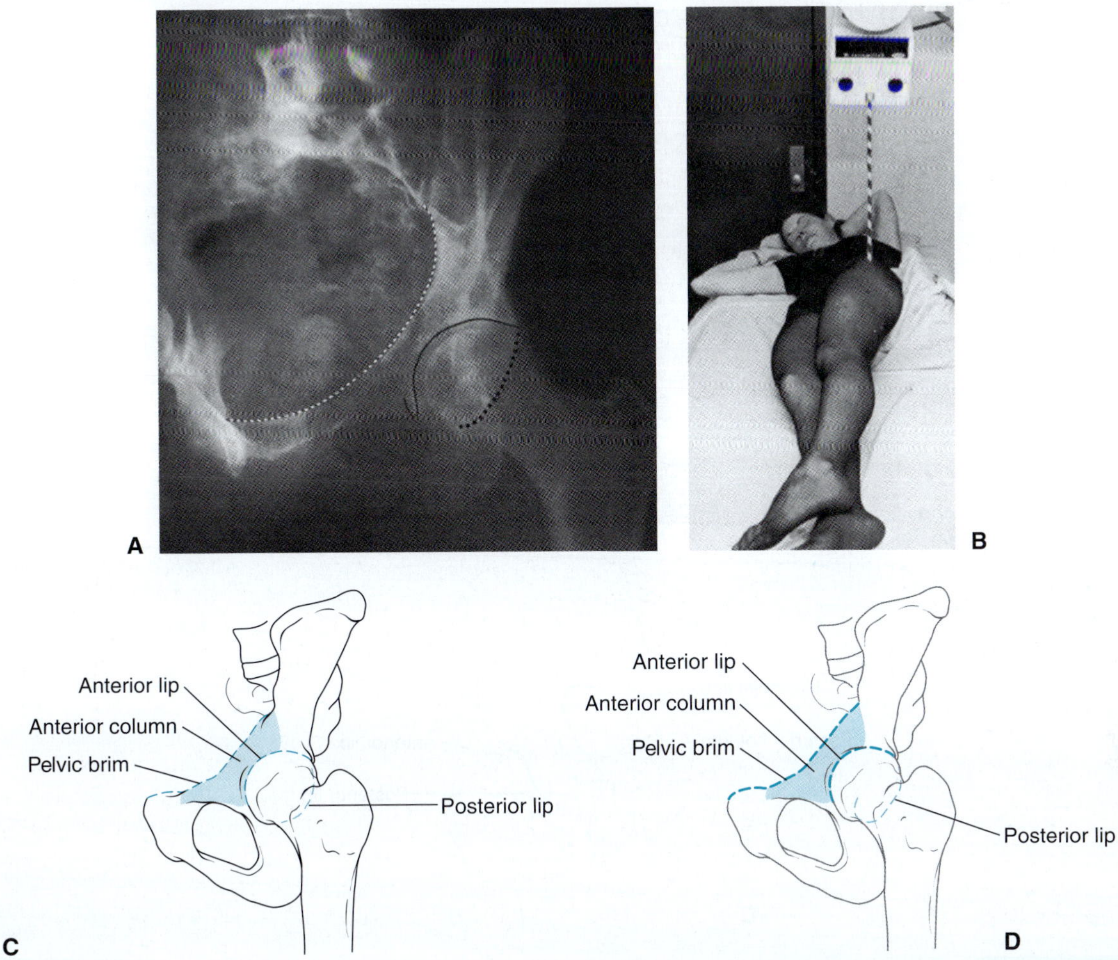

FIGURE 10.25 **(A) Obturator oblique x-ray of the left hemipelvis. (B) This view is taken by elevating the affected hip 45 degrees to the horizontal by means of a wedge and directing the beam through the hip joint with a 15-degrees upward tilt. (C) Diagram of the anatomy of the pelvis on the obturator oblique view. (D) Diagram of the important landmarks. Note particularly the pelvic brim indicating the border of the anterior column and the posterior lip of the acetabulum. (*Source:* Tile M. *Fractures of the Pelvis and Acetabulum.* Baltimore: Williams & Wilkins, 1984.)**

Imaging. Imaging should include an anteroposterior pelvis, which would reveal a femoral head not centered in acetabulum. If the head appears larger, then the dislocation is an anterior, but if it appears smaller, then the dislocation is posterior. The femoral neck should be thoroughly visualized to assess the femoral neck. Additional views or a CT scan may be necessary to assess the postreduction status of the hip, identify nondisplaced fractures, determine the congruity of reduction, and visualize and size intraarticular fragments.

Management. Acute management involves immediate reduction to minimize the risk of AVN and degenerative joint disease (DJD). The hip can be reduced through a variety of maneuvers. The Allis maneuver is performed with the patient in supine position with the pelvis stabilized. The hip is flexed to 90 degrees, and increased traction is placed with the hip adducted and extremity internally rotated. The Stimson maneuver is performed with the patient prone as the hip is flexed and the leg is placed off the stretcher, often an impractical maneuver in the trauma setting. Operative indications include an irreducible dislocation, which is approached anteriorly via the Smith-Peterson approach and posteriorly via the Kocher-Langenbeck approach; a dislocation with femoral neck fracture; an intraarticular fragment; an incongruent reduction; or an unstable hip after reduction.

Associated injuries include distal femoral contusions or fractures, patella fractures, foot and ankle injuries (especially when the knee is extended), and sciatic nerve injury in up to 10% of patients. AVN (1% to 20% of patients) is correlated with the duration of

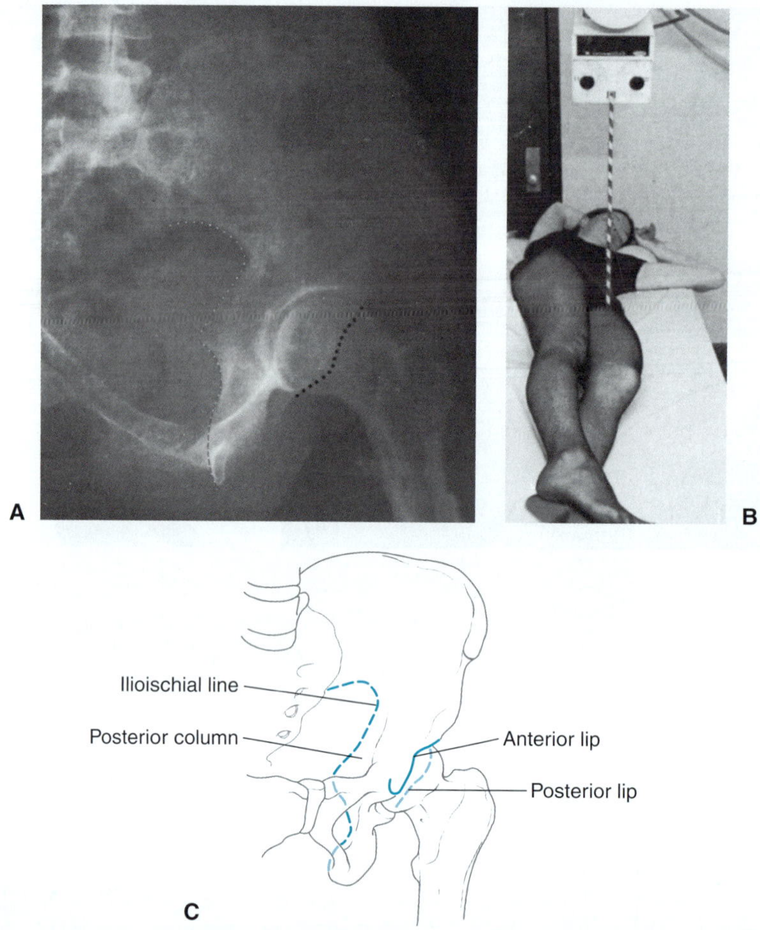

FIGURE 10.26 **(A) Iliac oblique radiographic view of the left hemipelvis. (B) This view is taken by rotating the patient into 45 degrees of external rotation by elevating the uninjured side on a wedge. (C) Anatomic landmarks of the left hemipelvis on the iliac oblique view are the posterior column of the acetabulum, outlined by the ilioischial line, the iliac crest, and the anterior lip of the acetabulum. (*Source:* Tile M. *Fractures of the Pelvis and Acetabulum*, 2nd ed. Baltimore: Williams & Wilkins, 1995.)**

dislocation, but the best results are if the hip is reduced within 6 hours. Posttraumatic osteoarthritis (OA) has increased incidence with concomitant femoral head or acetabular fractures, and anatomic reduction is key in preventing abrasive wear of cartilage. Sciatic nerve injury occurs in up to 20% of patients. With reduction, 40% see complete resolution and 25% to 35% have partial resolution. An EMG should be performed after 3 to 4 weeks if there is no improvement.

Femoral Head Fractures

Classification. The Pipkin classification stratifies femoral head fractures into 4 groups. Type I (Fig. 10.28A) fractures are inferior to the fovea, while type II (Fig. 10.28B) are superior to the fovea. Type III (Fig. 10.28C) fractures include a fracture of the acetabulum, and type IV (Fig. 10.28D) have an associated femoral neck fracture. Imaging of the femoral head includes anteroposterior, lateral, and Judet radiographs, followed by a postreduction CT scan if a reduction is performed.

Treatment. Nonoperative treatment can be considered in patients with infrafoveal fracture that is reduced. Operative treatment should be sought for displaced infrafoveal and suprafoveal fractures (through an anterior approach) for an ORIF. Elderly patients with a Pipkin IV may require a hemiarthroplasty or total hip arthroplasty.

Femoral Neck Fractures

Overview and Anatomy. The femoral neck physis closes at age 16. The average neck-shaft angle is 130 ± 7 degrees, and the average anteversion is

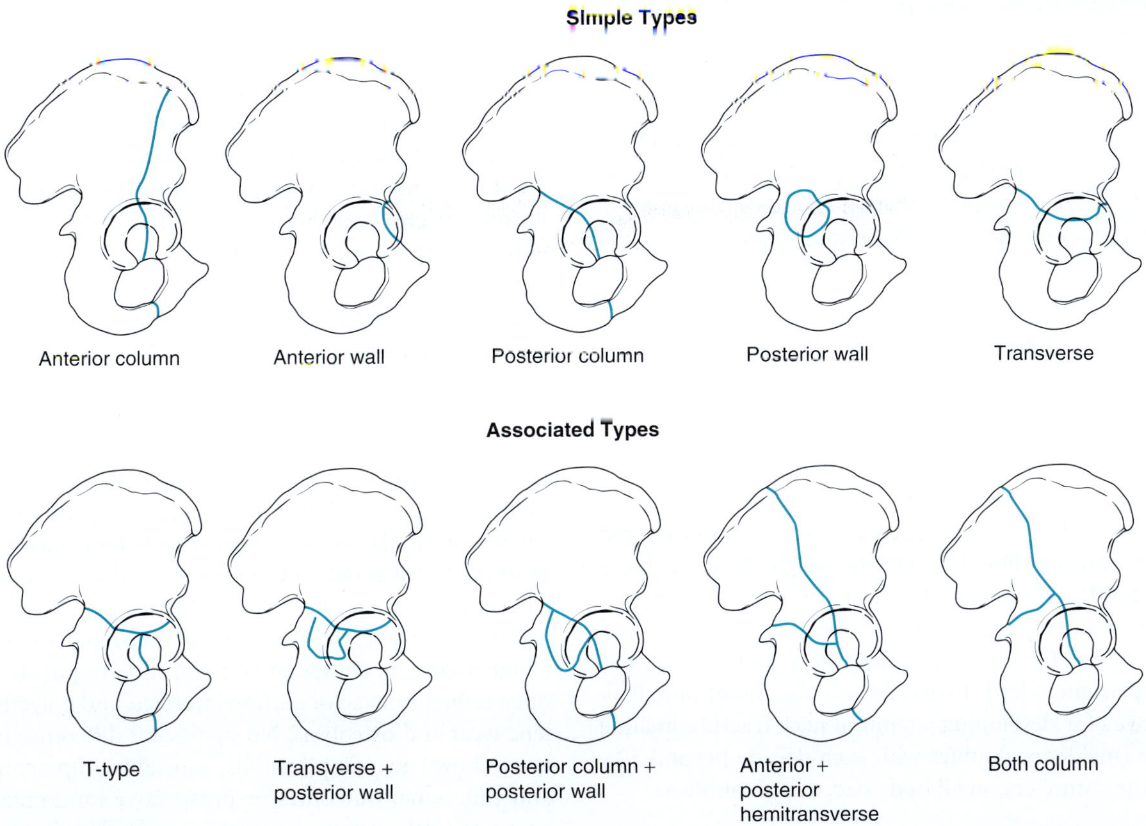

FIGURE 10.27 Letournel classification of acetabular fractures. (*Source:* Bucholz RW, Heckman JD. *Rockwood & Green's Fractures in Adults*, 5th ed. Lippincott Williams & Wilkins, 2001.)

TABLE 10.10 Surgical approaches for pelvic fractures

Surgical Approach	*General Indications*	*Fracture Patterns*	*Complications*
Kocher-Langenbeck	Posterior column and posterior articular surface	Posterior wall Posterior column Transverse Transverse with posterior wall Some T-shaped fractures	HO: 8%–25% Sciatic nerve palsy: 3%–5% Infection: 2%–5%
Ilioinguinal	Anterior column and anterior articular surface	Anterior wall Anterior column Transverse with anterior displacement Anterior column and posterior hemitransverse Associated both column	Lateral femoral cutaneous nerve dysesthesia (80%–90% returns by 1 year) HO: 2%–10% Femoral nerve palsy: 2% Infection: 2%–5%
Extended iliofemoral	Maximal simultaneous access to both columns	Transtectal transverse with posterior wall T-shaped fractures Greater than 21 days following injury Inability to reduce posterior column through ilioinguinal Associated SI joint disruption	Infection: 2%–5% Sciatic nerve palsy: 3%–5% HO: 20%–50%

TABLE 10.11 Thomas-Epstein classification of hip dislocation

Type	Description
I	Pure dislocation (may have a small posterior wall fragment)
II	Dislocation with large posterior wall fragment
III	Dislocation with comminuted posterior wall
IV	Dislocation with transverse and posterior wall acetabulum fracture
V	Dislocation with femoral head fracture

10 ± 7 degrees. The blood supply that surrounds the femoral neck includes the lateral epiphyseal artery (terminal branch of the medial femoral circumflex and predominant blood supply to weight-bearing dome of head), the artery of ligamentum teres (from the obturator supplying the anteroinferior head), and the lateral femoral circumflex artery. Greater fracture displacement leads to greater vascular disruption. Risk factors for developing a femoral neck fracture include age (incidence doubles with each decade beyond 50), whites, smokers, small body size, and alcoholism.

Classification. The Garden classification, which portends risk of AVN and nonunion, classifies femoral neck fractures on the basis of displacement. Type I are valgus impacted or incomplete; type II are complete, nondisplaced; Type III are complete with partial displacement; and type IV are complete fractures with full displacement. The fractures can also be classified from a functional standpoint as either stable or unstable. Stable fractures fall under Garden I or II type injuries. Unstable injures, such as Garden III and IV, require either hemiarthroplasty or ORIF.

Treatment Options. Hemiarthroplasty in the treatment of unstable femoral neck fractures has been shown to have a lower reoperation rate, improved functional scores, and less pain, and to be more cost effective, but to have slightly increased short-term mortality than open reduction internal fixation in the elderly patient population. Within hemiarthroplasty surgeries, the use of bipolar versus unipolar prosthesis has been examined. Advantages of a bipolar prosthesis include a lower dislocation rate, less acetabular wear, less pain, and more motion. Disadvantages of the bipolar include a higher cost, a postoperative dislocation requiring an open reduction, loss of motion interface, and polyethylene wear and osteolysis. No significant difference has been shown in complications, mortality, hip scores, and functional outcomes. A prospective randomized study of ORIF versus cemented bipolar hemiarthroplasty versus total hip arthroplasty (THA) showed that the THA group had best functional outcome.

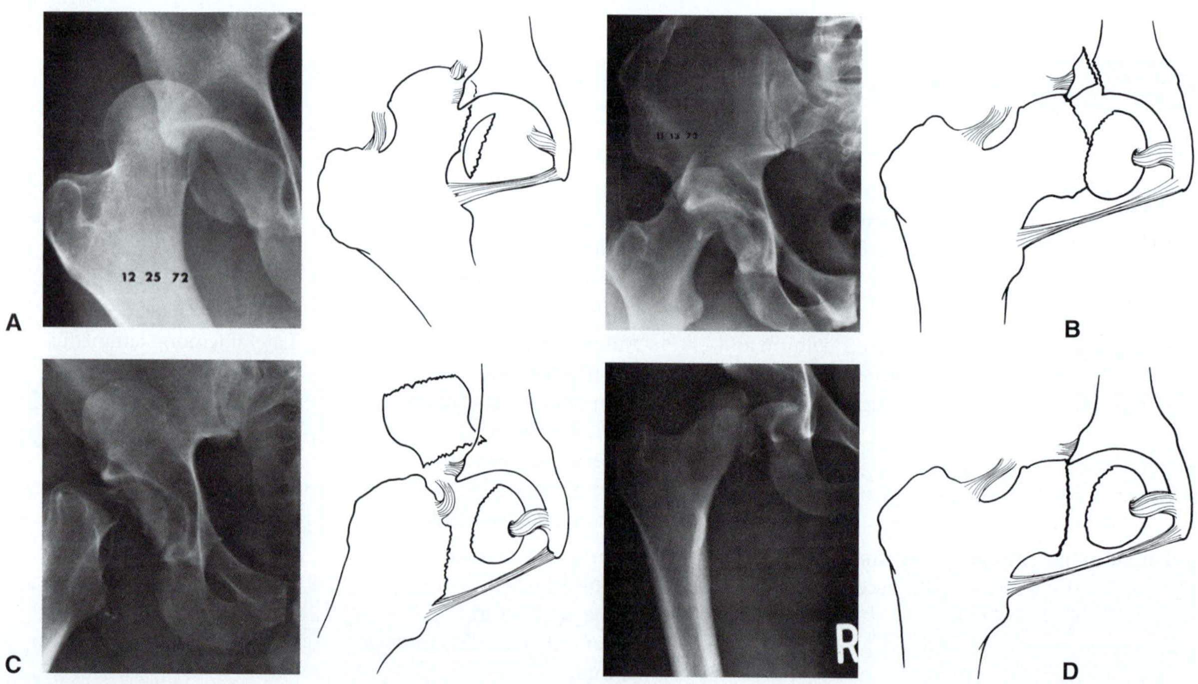

FIGURE 10.28 **The Pipkin classification of dislocations with femoral head fractures. (A) Type I. (B) Type II. (C) Type III. (D) Type IV. (*Source:* Bucholz RW, Heckman JD. *Rockwood & Green's Fractures in Adults,* 5th ed. Lippincott Williams & Wilkins, 2001.)**

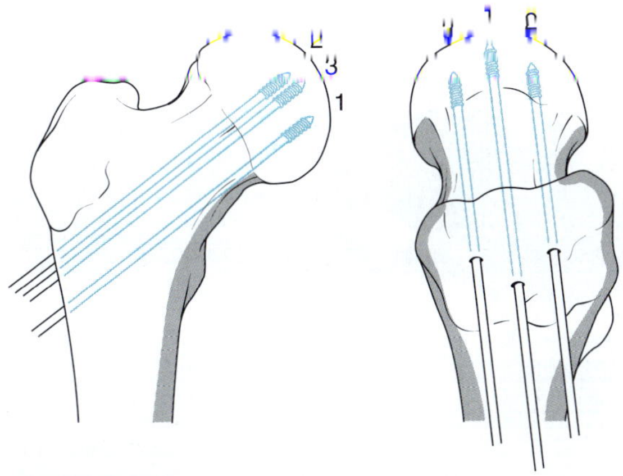

FIGURE 10.29 **Ideal placement for the 3 guide pins for cannulated screws. (*Source:* Bucholz RW, Heckman JD. *Rockwood & Green's Fractures in Adults,* 5th ed. Lippincott Williams & Wilkins, 2001.)**

Preoperative Interventions. Preoperative interventions show that skin traction is not beneficial because it does not have an effect on fracture reduction, and the traction position decreases capsular volume, thereby being detrimental on blood flow. Timing of surgical intervention can be delayed up to 72 hours for medical stabilization, which is warranted in unhealthy patients. However, surgical delay for medical clearance in healthy patients is not warranted. Nonoperative treatment has a limited role and can be offered along with activity modification and skeletal traction in those patients who have a significant medical risk for surgery.

Operative Techniques. Operative techniques include ORIF, hemiarthroplasty, and total hip replacement. ORIF is offered in an attempt to obtain an ideal reduction that is anatomic with less than 15 degrees of valgus and less than 10 degrees of anteroposterior angulation. No advantage has been shown in having more than 3 screws (Fig. 10.29). The inferior pin is placed first and must be buttressed by the intact cortex of the femoral neck. A parallel pin, placed proximally and posterior to the first, rests on the posterior cortex of the neck. A third pin is placed anteriorly. In situ pinning of impacted fractures is recommended because disimpaction increases the risk of AVN. The role of the intracapsular hematoma continues to remain unclear, but leg position (extension and internal rotation) can increase the pressure. The decision regarding type of operative intervention is based on patient characteristics (young versus elderly) and fracture characteristics (stable versus unstable). Young patients (physiologic age under 65) with nondisplaced fractures should undergo urgent ORIF because they are at risk for secondary displacement. Displaced fractures in this group should be treated with emergent ORIF because the native femoral head is the best and AVN is related to the duration and degree of displacement. In elderly patients with nondisplaced fractures, there is an unpredictable risk of secondary displacement, but the rate of AVN doubles. Displaced fractures in the elderly have unacceptable rates of mortality and morbidity and a very poor outcome is associated with nonoperative treatment. The standard of care is operative for all femoral neck fractures.

Complications. The complications from these fractures include nonunion of the femoral neck if there is no healing at 1 year. Nonhealing occurs in up to 5% of nondisplaced fractures and in 9% to 35% of displaced fractures. Risk factors include posterior comminution, initial displacement, inadequate reduction, and noncompressive fixation. The treatment of nonunions in the elderly is arthroplasty, with very limited indications for a Girdlestone. In younger patients, a valgus-producing osteotomy is an option in those with varus alignment or with limb shortening. In those with normal alignment, bone graft with repeat ORIF is suggested. The rate of AVN is 5% to 8% in nondisplaced fractures and 20% to 45% in displaced fractures (Fig. 10.30). The treatment of AVN includes arthroplasty, but results are not as good as with primary THA. The 1-year mortality is at 14% to 50%. Risk factors for death include medical comorbidities, surgical delay greater than 3 days, institutionalized or demented patients, arthroplasty (short term), and posterior approach to the hip.

Special Patient Groups. Stress fractures of the femoral neck are 4 to 10 times more common in women, due to amenorrhea, anorexia or bulimia, and decreased bone mineral density (10% less than control). Distance runners are also commonly involved because of their increase in athletic activity. The typical presentation is anterior groin pain that is directly activity related with limited ROM at extremes and an antalgic gait. Often, plain radiographs are negative (in 66% of cases), and therefore bone scan is recommended (sensitivity 93% to 100%, specificity 76% to 95%). MRI has been shown to be 100% sensitive and specific. Fractures on the compression side of the femoral neck (inferior aspect of femoral neck) are treated with activity and weight-bearing modification if they are stable and the fracture line does not extend more than halfway across the neck. If the fracture line does extend beyond half the neck width on the compression, ORIF should be considered. Any fracture lines on the tension side (superior aspect of femoral neck) or displaced fractures should be treated with emergent ORIF.

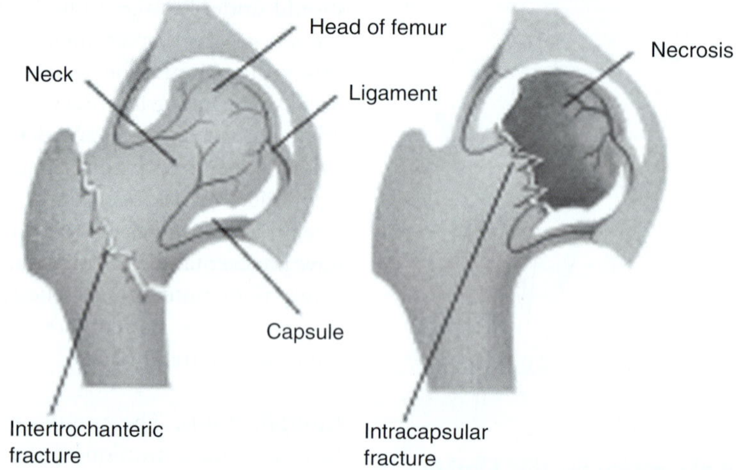

FIGURE 10.30 Sites of avascular necrosis in intertrochanteric versus intracapsular fracture.

Intertrochanteric Hip Fractures

Anatomy and Overview. The intertrochanteric region of the hip extends from the extracapsular portion of the femoral neck to the inferior border of the lesser trochanter. Ninety percent of intertrochanteric fractures occur in patients older than 65 years, with females at greatest risk. A peak incidence occurs at 80, and osteoporosis is thought to be a significant risk factor.

Imaging. Imaging of these injuries involves plain radiographs. CT scan has limited use in diagnosing intertrochanteric fractures. Bone scan can be useful for occult fractures (100% sensitivity) but will only provide a positive reading 72 hours after injury. An MRI can be utilized within 24 hours after injury if an occult fracture is suspected. Perioperative management includes optimizing medical problems, DVT prophylaxis, antibiotics, UTI treatment, and assessing and improving nutritional status. The fracture can be classified functional as stable (fractures resist medial and compressive loads with reduction and fixation) and unstable (collapse into varus or into shaft despite anatomic reduction). The OTA AO/ASIF also provides for a more part-based classification system (Table 10.12).

Treatment. Treatment goals include a stable reduction with internal fixation that permits immediate transfers. Treatment options include a compression hip screw and slide plate (that allow controlled impaction of fracture where higher angles allow for greater impaction), intramedullary sliding hip screw (that has decreased implant bending strength, a potential for percutaneous technique, reverse obliquity, pathologic shaft fracture), or a calcar-replacing prosthesis (for pathologic fracture, severe osteopenia, severe comminution, or rheumatoid arthritis). Implant positioning is essential, with the implant being centered in the femoral head on anteroposterior and lateral views. The tip–apex distance (TAD) is a predictor of cutout. If there is less than 25 mm between the end of the implant and the subchondral surface of the femoral head, failure approaches zero; if there is greater than 25 mm, chance of failure rapidly increases.

Femoral Shaft Fractures

Anatomy and Overview. The blood supply to the femoral shaft is through metaphyseal vessels, a single nutrient artery in the diaphysis that enters through the linea aspera, which communicates with medullary arteries in the intramedullary canal. Medullary arteries supply two-thirds of the endosteal blood supply. Of note, reaming destroys intramedullary endosteal

TABLE 10.12 OTA AO/ASIF classification of intertrochanteric hip fractures

Type	*Parts*	*Stability*	*Notes*
31-A1	Two	Stable	No comminution Fracture does not violate lateral cortex
31-A2	Two	Unstable	Comminution Fracture does not violate lateral cortex
31-A3	Two	Unstable	Comminution Enters lateral cortex Reverse obliquity

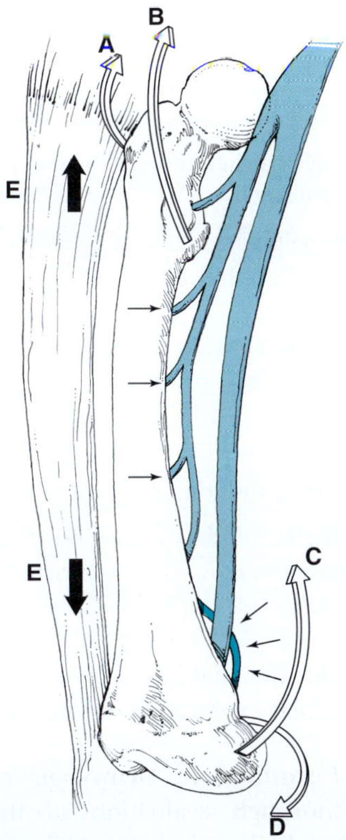

FIGURE 10.31 **Deforming muscle forces on the femur: Abductors (A), iliopsoas (B), adductors (C), and gastrocnemius origin (D). The medial angulating forces are resisted by the fascia lata (E). (*Source:* Bucholz RW, Heckman JD. *Rockwood & Green's Fractures in Adults*, 5th ed. Lippincott Williams & Wilkins, 2001.)**

blood supply, but periosteal blood flow increases and medullary blood supply is reestablished over 8 to 12 weeks. Muscle forces across the femoral shaft (especially important in fracture alignment) include the iliopsoas, leading to flexion of the proximal fragment; the adductors, leading to shortening of the femur; and the gluteal muscles, which abduct and extend the proximal piece (Fig. 10.31).

Classification. The Winquist classification system is used to describe these injuries. Type 0 have no comminution, type 1 have an insignificant butterfly fragment with a transverse or short oblique fracture line, type 2 have a larger butterfly of less than 50% bony width (more than 50% of the cortex is intact), type 3 have a yet larger butterfly leaving less than 50% of cortical contact, and type 4 is a femoral shaft with segmental comminution.

Treatment. Initial management includes traction with either a splint or transosseous pin. Timing of surgery is dependent on the level of patient resuscitation and additional injuries. Diaphyseal fractures are managed by intramedullary nailing through an antegrade or retrograde insertion. Proximal or distal one-third fractures may be managed with a plate depending on fracture morphology. Reaming allows for a decreased risk of nail incarceration, higher union rates, a more durable fracture–nail construct, earlier weight bearing, generation of fat emboli (unreamed nail insertion also generates fat emboli though), and no increased risk of ARDS. The risk of nonunion is 5 times greater without reaming.

Nailing Technique. Antegrade nailing is the gold standard, with highest union rates achieved with reamed nails. The starting point is extraarticular and can lead to varus alignment of proximal fractures with Trendelenburg gait. The starting point is the piriformis fossa. If the starting point is too posterior, loss of proximal fixation can occur, and a too anterior starting point can generate large forces that can lead to fracture of the proximal femur. Static locking is recommended in antegrade nailing. Retrograde nailing is easier to perform in obese patients because the piriformis fossa can be difficult to locate, and is better for combined fracture patterns, pregnancy, and floating knees. Retrograde nailing may require more dynamization than antegrade nails, but they yield equal union rates with reaming when compared to antegrade insertion. Retrograde nailing does require an intraarticular starting point. Open fractures show a high rate of healing when treated with a reamed, antegrade nail. Grade IIIB fractures may require débridement and skeletal traction prior to conversion to a nail. Subtrochanteric femur fractures extend from the base of the lesser trochanter to 5 cm distal. Proximal femoral nailing can lead to varus in these injuries. If the piriformis fossa is not involved and the lesser trochanter is fractured, a second-generation nail may be used. If a hypertrophic nonunion occurs, exchange nailing without dynamization is key because stability is essential.

Supracondylar Femur Fractures

Classification. The AO/OTA classification for supracondylar femur fractures divides the fractures into 3 groups. Type A are supracondylar with no articular extension, type B are unicondylar, and type C are supracondylar with intercondylar extension. The goals of treatment are to restore the articular surface and restore the mechanical axis.

Treatment. Intramedullary nailing for the treatment of supracondylar femur fractures is advantageous because it can be performed through smaller incisions and limited exposure, with percutaneous joint fixation, decreased blood loss, a load-sharing device with a longer lever arm, and maintenance of the soft tissues. The disadvantages of intramedullary nailing of this fracture pattern is lack of axial alignment control and insertion through cartilage. Indications for intramedullary nailing include type A or C1 fractures, long spirals, osteoporosis, or ipsilateral tibia or femoral neck fractures. Plating can be performed via direct visualization of the joint during fixation, which also allows for restoration of the mechanical axis (with a fixed device). Biologic fixation with indirect reduction and minimal soft tissue stripping is advocated, but this does not refer to that articular surface (needs accurate direct reduction). Indication for plating include type C2 or C3 fractures, shortening, good bone quality, low fractures, and biplanar fractures.

TABLE 10.13 Anatomic classification of knee dislocations

Type	Injury	Intact Structures
I	Single cruciate and collateral	Single cruciate and collateral
II	ACL and PCL	Collaterals
IIIM	ACL, PCL, and MCL	LCL and PLC
IIIL	ACL, PCL, MCL, and PLC	MCL
IV	ACL, PCL, MCL, LCL, and PCL	None
V	Fracture dislocation	Variable
C	Arterial injury	Variable
N	Nerve injury	Variable

Knee Dislocations

Overview and Mechanism of Injury. The true incidence of knee dislocations is underreported because usually 20% to 50% spontaneously reduce. The pathophysiology leading to a knee dislocation includes high-energy (MVA) and low-energy (sports) mechanisms, and knee position with respect to the direction of the applied force is essential. Hyperextension with varus or valgus force leads to anterior dislocation. The anterior cruciate ligament (ACL), posterior cruciate ligament (PCL), posterior capsule, and popliteal artery can all be involved. Flexion and a posterior force lead to posterior dislocation.

Classification. The classification of knee dislocations can be functional or anatomic. The functional method describes the position of the tibia with respect to the femur and is based on visual inspection and radiographs, but it does not define exact status of ligaments. The anatomic system takes into account the soft tissue and is seen in Table 10.13. Type III injuries are most common, with type IIIL having a poor outcome when compared to type IIIM. There is a high incidence of arterial injury (on average, 33%) including intimal tears rather than complete disruptions.

Vascular Examination. The vascular examination should assess the dorsalis pedis and posterior tibial arteries. If the pulses are absent or severely diminished, immediate closed reduction is recommended. If the pulses continue to be absent despite a reduction, the patient should consider going to the operating room for an exploration. However, if pulses return, consider an angiogram versus observation (in deference to a maximum 8-hour ischemic time). Finally, if pulses are present, an ankle brachial index (ABI) of less than 0.9 indicates a vascular exploration or angiogram.

Neurologic Examination. Neurologic examination includes a thorough evaluation of the peroneal nerve, including EHL and tibial anterior strength and sensation to the EHL and tibialis anterior strength. There is a 14% to 35% incidence of injury; the most common occurrence is type III L (varus) as a result of traction. The tibial nerve may be involved and can be assessed with FHL and gastrocnemius/soleus strength along with sensation over the lateral border and planter surface of the foot.

Imaging. Imaging should include plain radiographs as well as an MRI in all cases. Management consists of immediate closed reduction. A dimple sign (puckering of the anteromedial skin) is indicative of an irreducible (posterolateral) dislocation. A buttonhole of the medial femoral condyle through the medial retinaculum or capsule may also occur. Vascular exploration should be considered in all patients with decreased ABI. Acute management after reduction can include a knee immobilizer or external fixation. However, nonoperative treatment (immobilization for 6 weeks or external fixation) leads to poor results. Operative treatment with repair of affected structures is advocated by most surgeons where early ROM is essential after stable ligament fixation. Associated injuries (vascular, nerve, etc.) indicate limited surgical intervention acutely. Ligament avulsions portend early open surgery with reattachment. Complete PCL disruption is treated with early open repair (within 3 weeks) because repair later than that necessitates reconstruction. Furthermore, reconstruction of the PCL is important because it allows tibiofemoral positioning since the PCL is the central pivot point.

Patella Fractures

Anatomy and Overview. The patella is the largest sesamoid bone and has thick articular cartilage proximally. The articular surface is divided into medial and lateral facets by a longitudinal ridge. The distal pole is nonarticular. The retinaculum consists of longitudinal fibers and patellofemoral ligaments. The blood supply is primarily derived from the geniculate arteries. The patella translates approximately 7 cm from flexion to extension with 13% to 38% of the patellar surface in contact with the femur at any given time through the ROM. [The patella increases the moment arm about the knee (up to 30% during extension).] High compressive loads can be withstood by the patella with 2 times as much torque required to extend the knee from 15 degrees to full extension than to extend a fully flexed knee to 15 degrees.

Mechanism of Injury. The mechanism of injury to the extensor mechanism of the knee can be multifold. A direct blow (e.g., dashboard injury) can lead to comminution or articular damage. Rapid knee flexion with quadriceps resistance can result in a simple, transverse fracture. Depending on the type and mechanism of injury, a palpable defect or a soft tissue component may exist. The extensor mechanism can be evaluated by having the patient extend the knee against gravity or maintain knee extension against gravity.

Imaging. Imaging of the knee in suspected extensor mechanism injuries includes plain radiographs to assess for patella baja or patella alta, or to look for disruption in the normal contour of the patella fat pad, particularly on the lateral film. CT scan can be useful for occult fractures. The examiner should be aware of the bipartite patella, which is a normal variant that involves the superolateral corner of the patella because of an accessory ossification center. Radiographs of the other knee often reveal bilaterality. A descriptive classification system is used to describe these injuries as transverse (35% nondisplaced, likely because the retinaculum is intact), marginal, vertical (22% of all fractures resulting from compression of the patella with the knee flexed), and comminuted/stellate (65% displaced resulting from a direct blow leading to osteochondral injuries) (Fig. 10.32).

Nonoperative Treatment. Nonoperative treatment is indicated for nondisplaced fractures (less than 2 mm of articular step-off and less than 3 mm of diastasis with an intact extensor mechanism), for minimally displaced fractures in the elderly, and for patients with multiple medical problems. Nonoperative treatment includes a long-leg cylinder cast for 4 to 6 weeks (consider knee

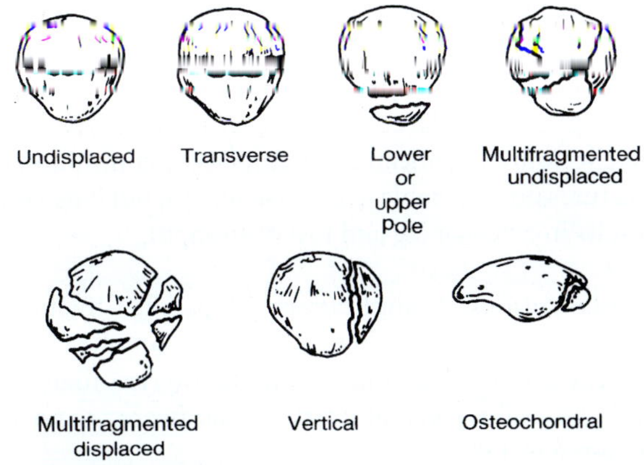

FIGURE 10.32 **Classification of patella fractures. (*Source:* Bucholz RW, Heckman JD. *Rockwood & Green's Fractures in Adults*, 5th ed. Lippincott Williams & Wilkins, 2001.)**

immobilizer for the elderly) with immediate weight bearing as tolerated after cast application.

Operative Treatment. A multitude of operative techniques exist, including modified tension-band wiring of fractures for transverse, noncomminuted fractures where the wire converts anterior distractive forces to compressive forces at the articular surface. Lag-screw fixation stabilizes comminuted fragments in conjunction with tension-band wiring but is contraindicated for extensive comminution and osteopenic bone. Cerclage wiring is an option for a stellate fracture pattern. The cannulated lag screw with tension bands is the most stable construct (Fig. 10.33). A partial patellectomy is

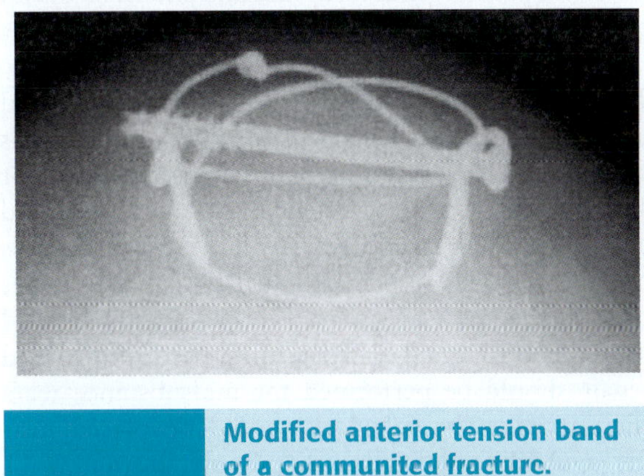

FIGURE 10.33 **Modified anterior tension band of a communited fracture. Anteroposterior axial view of internal fixation. (*Source:* Bucholz RW, Heckman JD. *Rockwood & Green's Fractures in Adults*, 5th ed. Lippincott Williams & Wilkins, 2001.)**

indicated for fractures involving extensive comminution not amenable to fixation. It usually involves the distal pole, and drill holes to reattach the patellar tendon should be placed near the articular surface. A patellectomy is indicated for displaced, comminuted fractures not amenable to reconstruction, but it usually results in extensor lag and loss of strength.

Complications. Complications of patellar fractures include knee stiffness (most common complication), infection, loss of fixation, OA, nonunion (less than 1% with surgical repair), and painful hardware (removal required in 15%).

Quadriceps Tendon Ruptures

Overview and Anatomy. Quadriceps tendon ruptures typically occur in patients older than 40 years. The ruptures often occur between 0 and 2 cm proximal to the superior pole of the patella. The level of injury is often associated with the age of the patient—ruptures occur at the bone–tendon junction in most patients older than 40, while patients under 40 often rupture within the midsubstance of the quadriceps. Risk factors for tendon rupture include chronic tendonitis, anabolic steroid use, local steroid injection, diabetes mellitus, inflammatory arthropathy, and chronic renal failure. Patients with quadriceps tendon rupture present with a sensation of a sudden pop while stressing the extensor mechanism. Tenderness at the upper pole of the patella with a palpable defect and loss of extension is often seen on physical examination. The lower pole of the patella should be at the level of a Blumensaat line projected anteriorly from the intercondylar as seen on a lateral radiograph of the knee with the knee in 30 degrees. Patella alta may be seen with patellar tendon rupture and patella baja with quadriceps tendon rupture.

Treatment. Nonoperative treatment can be utilized in incomplete tears in which active extension is preserved. The leg is immobilized in extension for 4 to 6 weeks. Operative repair of the tendon should be performed if active extension by the patient is not possible. The repair should be such that it lies close to the articular surface on the superior pole of the patella to avoid patellar tilting. An end-to-end repair should be performed for midsubstance tears (Fig. 10.34). The first lock should be placed near the avulsed tendon edge to prevent shortening or "accordionization" of the tendon repair. Chronic tears may require a V-Y advancement. Postoperative care includes a knee immobilizer or cylinder cast for 6 weeks with immediate versus delayed weight bearing.

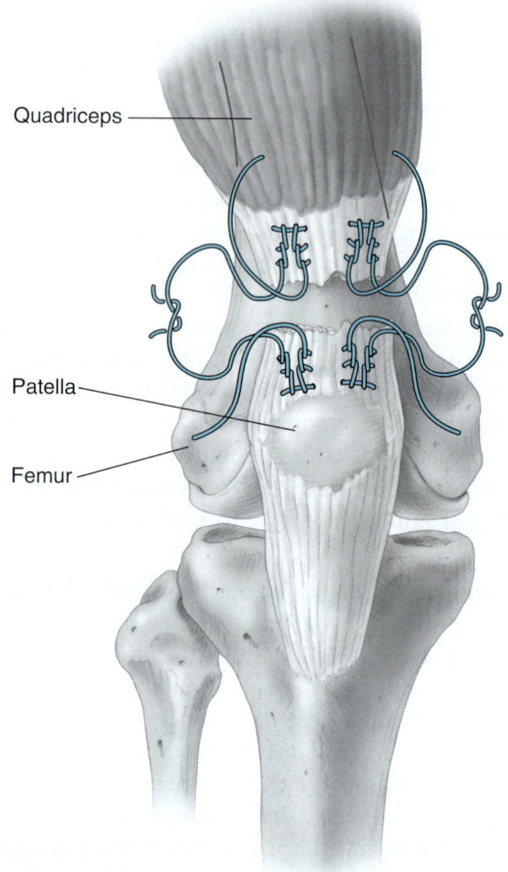

FIGURE 10.34 **Acute repair of a quadriceps tendon rupture using a Krackow suture technique and nonabsorbable heavy sutures. (*Source:* Bucholz RW, Heckman JD. *Rockwood & Green's Fractures in Adults*, 5th ed. Lippincott Williams & Wilkins, 2001.)**

Complications. Complications include rerupture of the quadriceps tendon, atrophy or weakness of the muscle, and loss of knee ROM.

Patellar Tendon Ruptures

Anatomy and Overview. Patellar tendon ruptures occur less commonly than quadriceps ruptures, often occurring in patients under 40 years old. The site of rupture is usually at the insertion site of the patellar tendon at the inferior pole of the patella. Risk factors for patellar tendon rupture include rheumatoid disease, Systemic lupus erythematosus (SLE), chronic renal failure, systemic or local steroid treatment, and chronic patellar tendinitis. The patellar tendon is approximately 4 mm thick at its midsubstance but widens to 5 to 6 mm at the tibial tubercle insertion. It is composed primarily of type I collagen (90%), receiving its blood supply from the fat pad posteriorly, which is supplied by the inferior medial and lateral geniculate arteries. The proximal and distal insertion sites are relatively avascular. The patellar tendon sees its greatest stress with the knee in 60 degrees of flexion. Force is distributed across the tendon such that 4 times greater strain is felt at the insertion site than within the midsubstance of the tendon. Patients often describe an audible "pop" after forceful quadriceps contraction against a flexed knee followed by an inability to bear weight. A palpable defect with painful passive knee flexion and inability to actively extend the knee may be their presentation. Patella alta can be seen on a lateral radiograph of the knee with ultrasound or MRI aiding in diagnosis (Fig. 10.35).

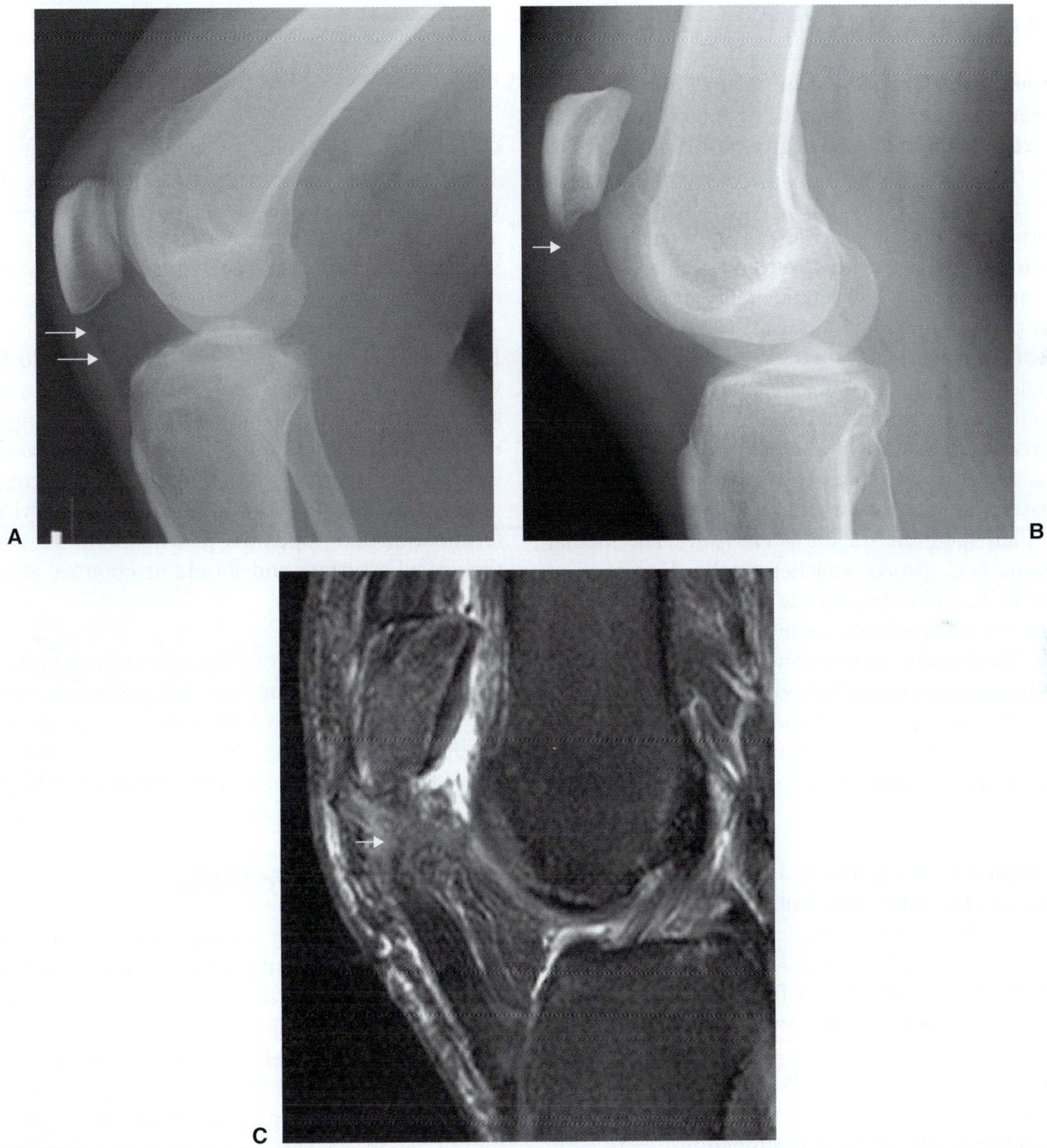

FIGURE 10.35 **(A) Lateral radiograph shows the normal contour of the patella fat pad (double arrows). (B) The fat pad contour is disrupted (single arrow), and there is patella alta. (C) MRI of the injured knee shows the ruptured tendon (single arrow).**

Treatment. Nonoperative treatment for partial tears with an intact extensor mechanism involves immobilization in full extension for 3 to 6 weeks. Results of operative involvement are based on timing between injury and surgery. Acute repairs, those occurring within 2 weeks of injury, can be performed via drill holes and sutures through the patella. This repair can be tested in the operating room with knee flexion. Delayed repair, occurring 6 weeks after injury, is associated with a poor outcome and often requires allograft or autograft augmentation.

Tibial Plateau Fractures

Anatomy and Overview. The medial tibial plateau is larger and more distal than the lateral plateau, is concave in shape with a 10-degree posterior slope, has 3 mm of articular cartilage, and sits more distal than the lateral side. The bone has a greater density because it bears 75% of the weight. The lateral plateau slopes posteriorly 7 degrees with 4 mm of articular cartilage covering the surface. The lateral meniscus lies atop the lateral plateau. It is more circular in shape and covers more of the articular surface than the medial meniscus. The lateral meniscus is attached to the PCL via the ligament of Humphrey (anterior) and the ligament of Wrisberg (posterior). There is no attachment of the meniscus to the lateral collateral ligament (LCL). The lateral meniscus bears more of the joint reactive force than the bone on the lateral side. The medial meniscus is C-shaped, attached to the deep portion of the MCL, and biomechanically bears load equal to that of bone with respect to joint reactive forces. Tibial plateau fractures occur in a bimodal distribution, with younger patients being injured secondary to high-energy injuries (e.g., MVA) and older patients due to low-energy injuries (e.g., fall from standing). The most common fracture pattern is a split-depression of the lateral tibia (80%).

Classification. If the injury is closed, the grading system of Tscherne and Gotzen is used, as seen in Table 10.14 and in Figure 10.36. Open fractures are classified by the Gustilo-Anderson system (Table 10.15). Tibial plateau fractures can be classified via the Schatzker classification on the basis of the location and type of fracture pattern (Table 10.16; Fig. 10.37).

Examination. The physical examination begins with an evaluation of the soft-tissue. C0, simple fracture configuration with little or no soft tissue injury; C1, superficial abrasion, mild to moderately severe fracture configuration; C2, deep contamination with local skin or muscle contusion; moderately severe fracture configuration; C3, extensive contusion or crushing of skin or destruction of muscle; severe fracture. The neurologic examination should include documentation of peroneal nerve activity. The popliteal artery is at risk with medial plateau injuries or fracture/dislocations of the knee. Therefore, the examination should also assess compartment and knee stability.

TABLE 10.14 Tscherne-Gotzen grading of closed tibial plateau fractures

Grade	Description
0	Minimal soft tissue damage, usually via indirect force
1	Superficial abrasion/contusion
2	Deep, contaminated abrasion with localized skin/muscle contusion Impending compartment syndrome
3	Extensive skin contusion/crush Subcutaneous avulsion Underlying muscle damage

Imaging. Imaging of the tibial plateau should begin with anteroposterior, lateral, and oblique views of the knee and the entire length of the tibia. Using ligamentotaxis, traction radiographs can provide valuable information regarding fracture patterns in complex plateau fractures. CT scan is essential to assist with determination of the operative plan in fractures involving the articular surface and should be obtained after the application of traction.

Treatment. Treatment is based on the type of fracture pattern, but the essential principles of fixation remain the same: restoration of the varus–valgus alignment of the proximal tibia, maintaining the meniscus, reconstruction of incompetent ligamentous structures, and addressing articular incongruity (5 mm or less).

Open Tibial Shaft Fractures

Overview. The acute management of tibial shaft fractures is a vital component to the overall success in the outcome of these injuries. An immediate assessment should be made of the associated injuries. Antibiotics (e.g., Ancef and tobramycin) along with tetanus should be administered in an urgent fashion. A circumferential inspection of soft tissue envelope should be made with grading of the open injury based on the Gustilo-Anderson system; however, true grading is performed at the time of surgical débridement (see Table 10.15). ABIs may be indicated on the basis of the soft tissue injury. All patients should obtain full-length tibia radiographs that include the knee and ankle because 30% of patients have multiple

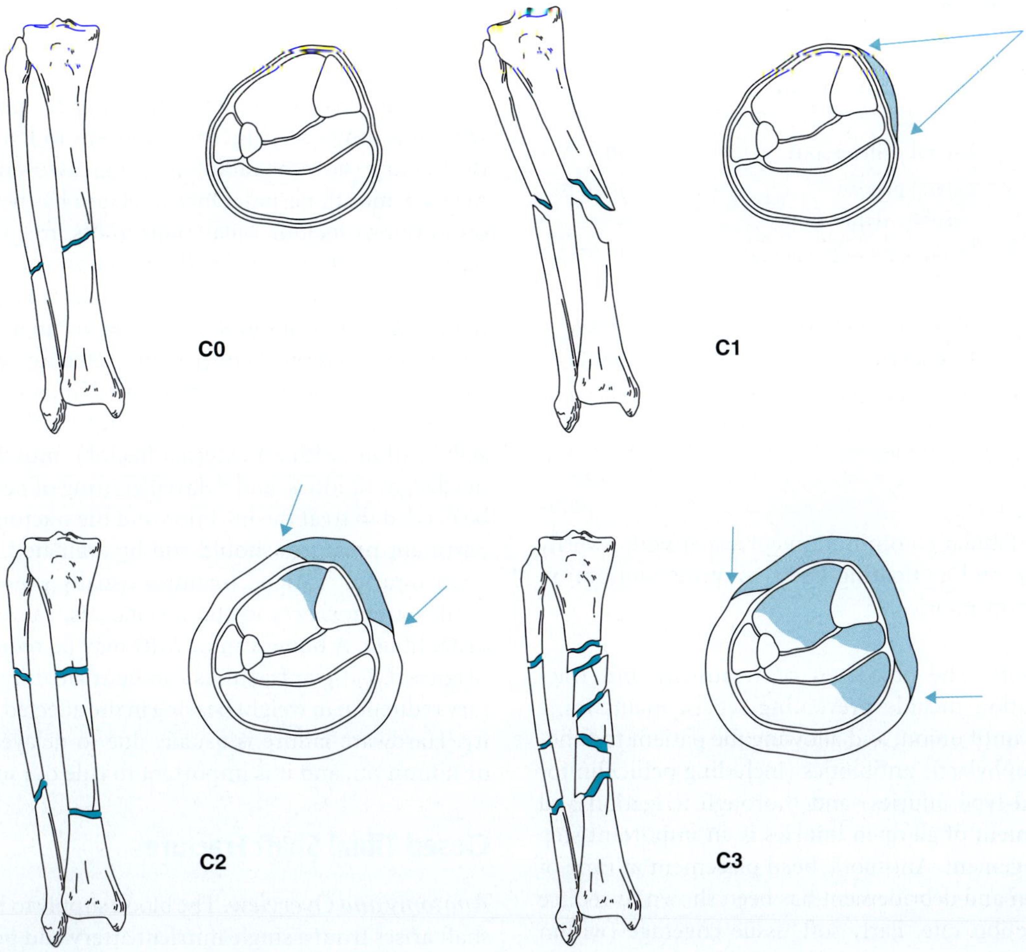

FIGURE 10.36 The Tscherne classification of closed fractures. (*Source:* Bucholz RW, Heckman JD. *Rockwood & Green's Fractures in Adults*, 5th ed. Lippincott Williams & Wilkins, 2001.)

TABLE 10.15 Gustilo-Anderson grading system of open tibial plateau fractures

Grade	Description	Suggested Fracture Fixation Method
1	Skin opening of less than 1 cm Minimal muscle contusion Usually inside-out mechanism	Reamed intramedullary nail (11% require secondary procedure)
2	Skin laceration 1 to 10 cm Extensive soft tissue damage	Reamed intramedullary nail Union time: 25 weeks Deep infection rate: 3.5%
3a	Extensive soft tissue injury (10 cm) Adequate bone coverage	Reamed intramedullary nail Union time: 25 weeks Deep infection rate: 3.5%
3b	Extensive soft tissue injury with periosteal stripping	Flap advancement or free flap Reamed intramedullary nail Union time: 50 weeks Infection rate: 23%
3c	Associated vascular injury	External fixation followed by vascular repair

TABLE 10.16 Schatzker classification of tibial plateau fractures

Type	Description	Figure
I	Lateral plateau split	10.37A
II	Lateral plateau split—depression	10.37B
III	Depression of the lateral plateau	10.37C
IV	Medial plateau fracture	10.37D
V	Bicondylar	10.37E
VI	Bicondylar fracture with metaphyseal dissociation	10.37F

injuries. Fibular comminution correlates with severity of injury, and a "floating knee" is more common in high-energy injuries.

Treatment. The objectives of treatment and fracture fixation include preventing sepsis, maintaining stability until union, and allowing the patient to function. Prophylactic antibiotics (including penicillin for barnyard-type injuries) and thorough irrigation and débridement of all open injuries is an important step in management. Antibiotic bead placement at time of irrigation and débridement has been shown to reduce the infection rate. Early soft tissue coverage (within 7 days) over the open wound is essential to limiting infection and maintaining fixation. If the wound occurs in the proximal third of the tibia, the gastrocnemius can be rotated; if the wound is in the middle third, the soleus can be rotated; and, if the wound is in the distal third, a free flap must be employed to cover the wound. External fixation has an increased rate of malunion and has a high risk of pin tract infection, which often necessitates a secondary procedure. Plate fixation offers minimally invasive techniques with less soft tissue stripping and locking capabilities.

Low-velocity gunshot wounds can be treated like closed injures, while high-velocity injuries (e.g., assault rifle, shot gun) should be treated as open injuries. Amputation can be considered in crush injury with a warm ischemia time greater than 6 hours with an anatomic division of the tibial nerve. The Mangled Extremity Severity Score (MESS) offers a guide to limb salvage versus amputation, where a score of 7 or higher is predicative of amputation. The NISSA score is a modification of MESS; it takes nerve injury into account along with ischemia, soft tissue injury, shock, and age. The LEAP study has shown that plantar sensation is not prognostic and that scoring systems do not work. Outcomes are affected by the severity of soft tissue and neurovascular injury with early soft tissue coverage important. Most studies show a major change in outcomes between type 3a and 3b/c fractures.

Complications. Complications include nonunion, with time limits varying from 6 months to 1 year when the fracture shows no radiologic progress toward union over a 3-month period. Once infection has been ruled out, options include onlay bone grafts, free vascularized bone grafts, reamed nailing, compression plating, or a ring fixator. Varus malunion is more of a problem than valgus, with surgical correction via an osteotomy an option in symptomatic patients. Infection should be suspected in patients who present with increasing pain, wound drainage, or sinus formation. Débridement, stabilization (with an external fixator), muscle flap if needed, antibiotics, and delayed grafting of defect may be needed to treat the infection and the fracture. Compartment pressures should still be evaluated, even in open injuries. Fatigue fractures usually present with localized tenderness in the metatarsals, calcaneus, or distal fibula. A bone scan or MRI may be required for diagnosis. Fatigue fractures can be treated by temporary reduction in weight bearing in the affected extremity. Hardware failure is usually due to delayed union or nonunion, and it is important to rule out infection.

Closed Tibial Shaft Fractures

Anatomy and Overview. The blood supply to the tibial shaft arises from a single nutrient artery and periosteal arteries. The 4 compartments with their contents and function are shown in Table 10.17. The tibial canal expands, and the cortex thins proximally and distally at the metaphyseal–diaphyseal junctions.

Associated Injuries. Associated injuries occur in up to 30% of patients; an ipsilateral fibula fracture is the most common additional injury. The ligamentous structures of the knee are at high risk in high-energy injuries.

Classification. There are multiple classification systems for closed tibial shaft fractures, but ultimately a descriptive system is most often employed. The Johner-Wruh classification (examines the extent of comminution and is prognostic for union time) divides fractures into 3 categories: A (simple), B (butterfly), and C (comminuted). Henly classification for tibial shaft fractures is an application of Winquist classification for the femur shown (Table 10.18). Finally, the soft tissue surrounding the tibia can be graded using the Tscherne-Gotzen classification (see Table 10.14) for closed injuries.

Compartment Syndrome. Compartment syndrome, in many instances, is predominantly a clinical

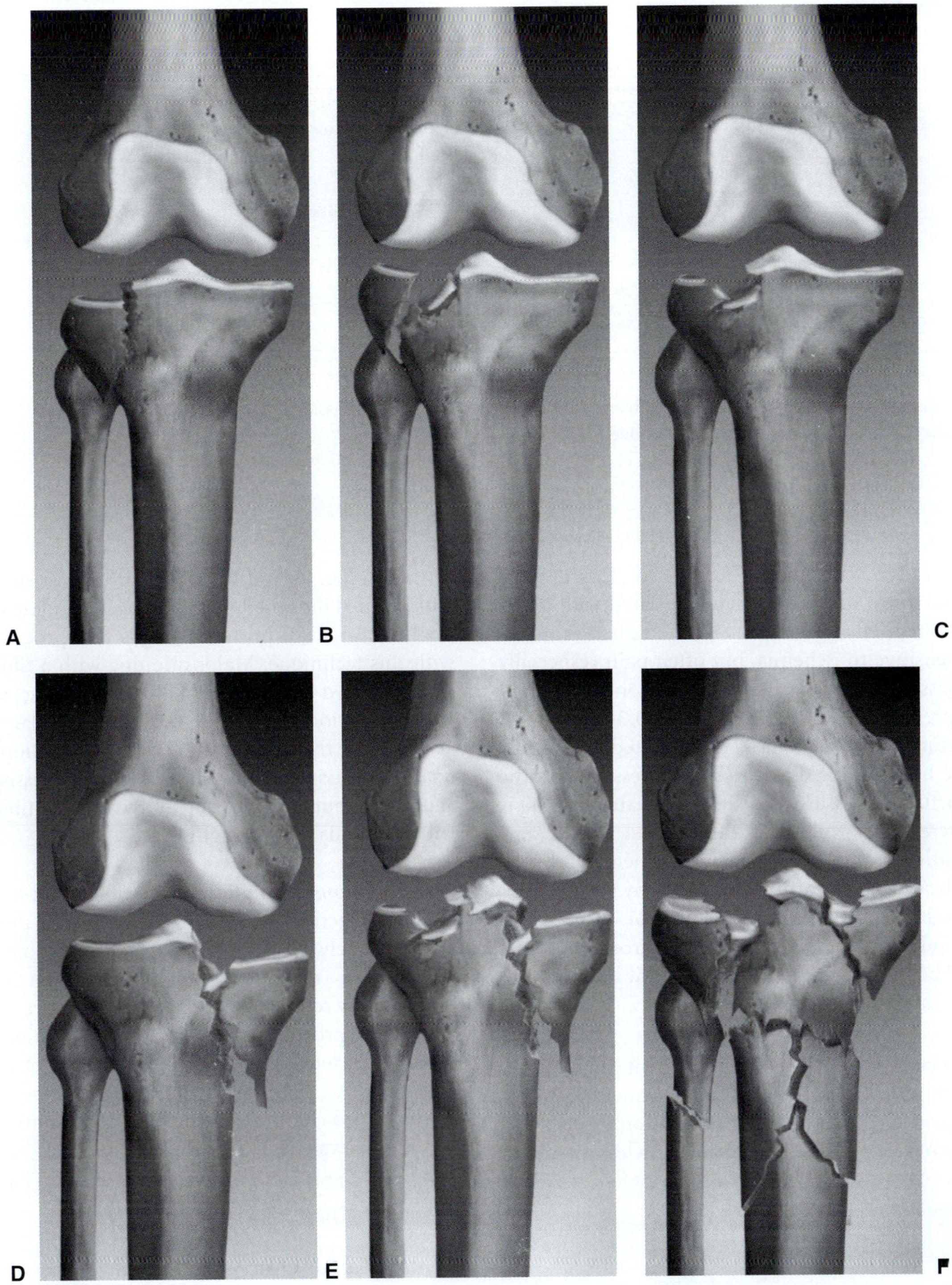

FIGURE 10.37 The Schatzker classification of tibial plateau fractures. (A) Type I. (B) Type II. (C) Type III. (D) Type IV. (E) Type V. (F) Type VI. (*Source:* Bucholz RW, Heckman JD. *Rockwood & Green's Fractures in Adults*, 5th ed. Lippincott Williams & Wilkins, 2001.)

TABLE 10.17 Tibial shaft compartments and functions

Compartment	Function	Muscles	Neurovascular Contents
Anterior	Ankle dorsiflexion	Tibialis anterior EDL EHL Peroneus tertius	Deep peroneal nerve Anterior tibial artery and vein
Lateral	Foot eversion Sensation to the dorsum of the foot (except the first web space)	Peroneus longus Peroneus brevis	Superficial peroneal nerve
Deep posterior	Plantar flexion and eversion of the foot	FDL FHL Tibialis posterior	Tibial nerve Posterior tibial vessels
Superficial posterior	Ankle plantar flexion Sensation to lateral heel	Gastrocnemius Soleus Popliteus Plantaris	Sural nerve Lesser saphenous veins

diagnosis. It occurs in 5% to 15% of closed tibial shaft fractures, which are often associated with a history of a high-energy or crush injury. The nerves are the most sensitive to ischemia, but often pain (especially with passive stretch) is the first symptom. Compartment pressure measurement (Figure 10.38) is highest at fracture site. The delta P is calculated as the difference between the diastolic blood pressure and the compartment pressure. A delta P of greater than 30 is considered safe, while a delta P less than 30 and clinical findings consistent with compartment syndrome are indicative to performing a fasciotomy (Fig. 10.39). An absolute pressure greater than 30 or 45 may also be an indication of compartment syndrome. Patients should be monitored closely with repeat examination and pressure measurements if needed.

Treatment. Nonoperative management is indicated for fractures with less than 50% displacement, less than 10 degrees of anteroposterior angulation, less than 5 degrees of varus–valgus angulation, and less than 2 cm of shortening. Operative treatment is most successful with reamed intramedullary nailing, noting that proximal fractures are prone to valgus and procurvatum with this technique. Malpositioning with a tibial nail can be limited with the use of blocking (Poller) screws, which functionally narrow the intramedullary canal and increase the strength and rigidity of fixation. Plate fixation of associated fibula fractures can assist with alignment, but it is difficult to dynamize a tibial nail with the fibula out to length.

TABLE 10.18 Henly classification for tibial shaft fractures

Type	Description
I	No comminution
II	Insignificant butterfly fragment with transverse or short oblique fracture
III	Large butterfly of less than 50% bony width (more than 50% of cortex intact)
IV	Larger butterfly leaving less than 50% of cortical contact
V	Segmental comminution

Complications. Complications of tibial shaft fractures include infection in 1% to 5% and non-union in approximately 10% of patients. Anterior knee pain is the most common complication, which may be improved by removal of the nail after fracture healing. Surgical approach through the patellar tendon or avoiding the tendon does not impact the rate of anterior knee pain. An epidural should be avoided because of the increased risk of neurologic complications and an inability to evaluate compartments.

Pilon Fractures

Anatomy and Overview. The incidence of pilon fractures has increased with the advent of air bags. Associated injuries occur in at least one-third of all patients. The average age range of patients is 35 to 40, with rare occurrence in children or the elderly. Males are 3 times more commonly involved. The soft tissue component predominantly drives injury management (particularly anteromedially) because of the thin skin, lack of adipose tissue, and lack of deep veins over the distal tibial. The biomechanics of fracture formation in the distal tibia involve a rapid axial load with a tremendous release of energy with a shift in the stress strain

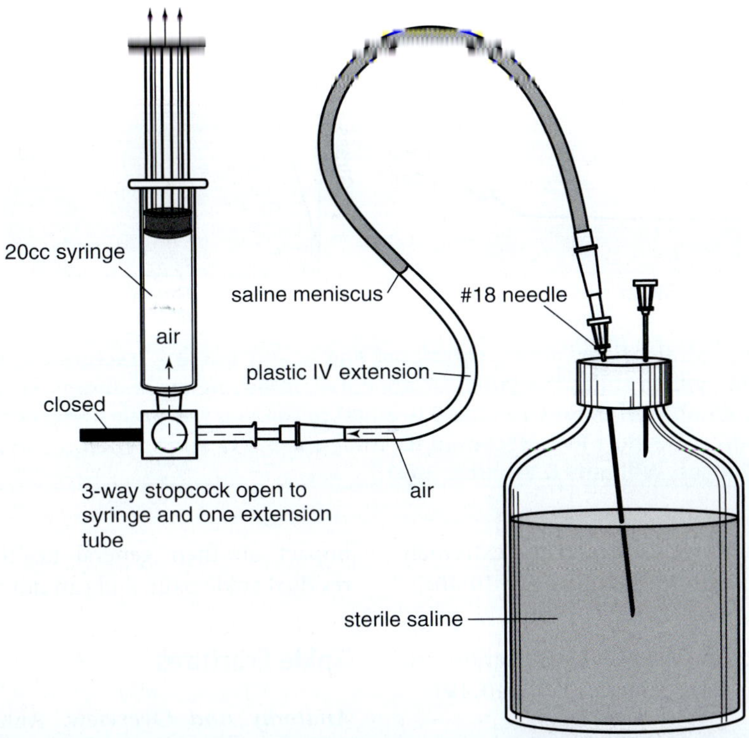

FIGURE 10.38 **System for measuring tissue pressures. (*Source:* Bucholz RW, Heckman JD. *Rockwood & Green's Fractures in Adults*, 5th ed. Lippincott Williams & Wilkins, 2001.)**

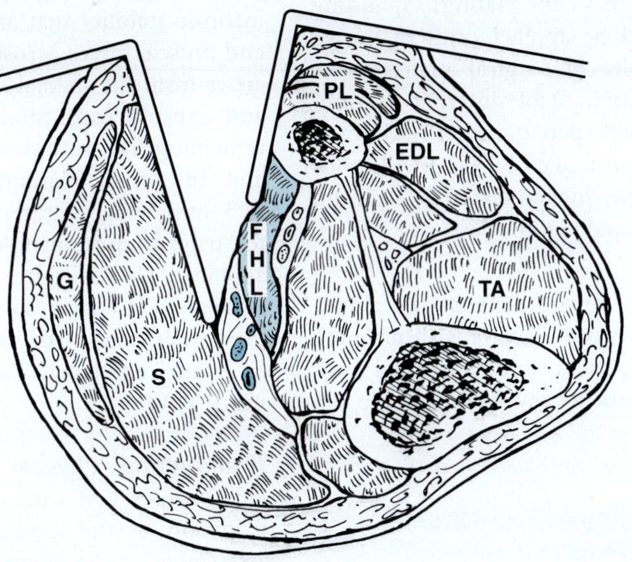

FIGURE 10.39 **Cross-section of perifibular approach to release posterior compartments. (*Source:* Bucholz RW, Heckman JD. *Rockwood & Green's Fractures in Adults*, 5th ed. Lippincott Williams & Wilkins, 2001.)**

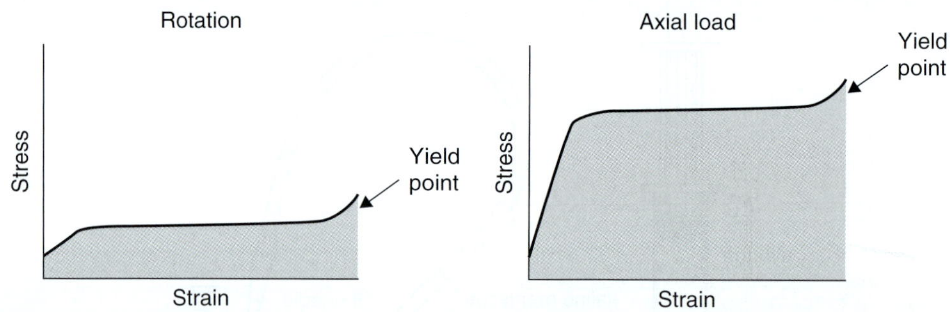

FIGURE 10.40 **Stress-strain diagrams for rotational and axially loading fractures. Axial loading is faster, which shifts the stress-strain curve, releasing more energy at the time of fracture. The amount of energy released is equal to the *shaded area* underneath the curves. (*Source*: Bucholz RW, Heckman JD. *Rockwood & Green's Fractures in Adults*, 5th ed. Lippincott Williams & Wilkins, 2001.)**

curve due to the viscoelastic nature of the extremely dense trabecular bone of the distal tibia (Fig. 10.40).

Classification. The Ruedi-Allgower classification system is used to describe these injuries (Table 10.19).

Management. Management of the soft tissue is the first priority in these injuries. Definitive surgical treatment should be delayed until the presence of a "wrinkle sign" (usually 10 to 28 days for plating). Spanning external fixation should be applied until definitive treatment. The principles of surgical management include anatomic reduction, stable internal fixation, atraumatic technique with percutaneous or limited approaches, and early pain-free mobilization. Options include external fixation, hinged external fixation, hybrid external fixation, and plating.

Results. Postoperative outcomes analysis shows arthrosis in 50% of patients at 2 years with ultimate arthrodesis in 5% of all patients initially treated for a plafond fracture. Most patients have a measurable impact on their general health status, have some residual ankle pain, and can not run or play sports.

TABLE 10.19 **Ruedi-Allgower classification of pilon fractures**

Type	*Description*
I	Articular fracture without significant displacement
II	Articular fracture with minimal articular incongruity
III	Articular fracture with significant comminution and central depression

Ankle Fractures

Anatomy and Overview. Ankle fractures are the most common weight-bearing skeletal injury, with the highest incidence in elderly women. Most commonly unimalleolar (68%), injuries can also be bimalleolar (25%), trimalleolar (7%), or open (2%). The ankle has intrinsic stability that arises from bony articulations and muscle forces across the joint. Extrinsic stability arises from the medial and lateral ligament complex and capsule with minimal contribution from the remaining thin soft tissue envelope. The talar dome and the tibial plafond are trapezoidal in shape (2.5 mm wider anteriorly). The ankle joint allows for triplane motion, tolerating 4 times body weight at stance. Normal range of motion is dorsiflexion to 20 degrees (10 degrees is needed for normal gait) and plantarflexion to 40 degrees. A lateral talar shift as little as 1 mm can change talotibial surface contact by as much as 40%.

Examination. Physical examination of an injured ankle begins first with inspection of the soft tissue, palpation of the medial and lateral malleoli, and assessment of the ligamentous stability. Pain during palpation of the entire course of the fibula or pain with side-to-side compression of the tibia and fibula at least 5 cm over the joint is indicative of a syndesmotic injury. Other associated injuries can include fifth metatarsal fractures or calcaneus fractures.

Imaging. Radiographs include anteroposterior, lateral, and mortise views. The anteroposterior radiograph will visualize tibiofibular overlap (greater than 10 mm is

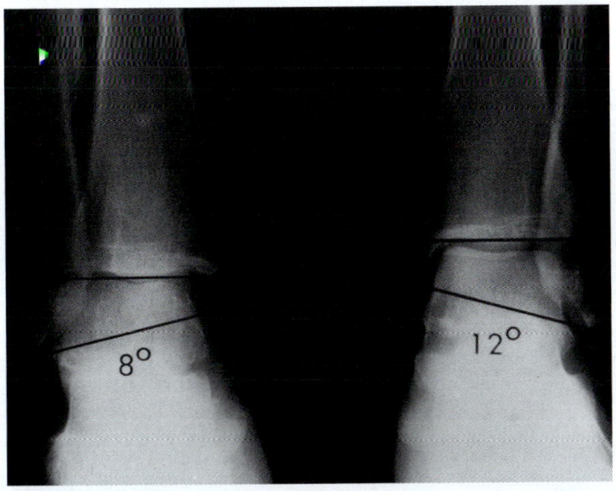

FIGURE 10.41 **Anteroposterior x-ray of both ankles shows a proximal fibula fracture that has healed with shortening and malrotation, resulting in malalignment of the ankle mortise and a loss of the normal talocrural angle compared to the opposite side. Persistent symptoms can be alleviated by corrective realignment of the fibula and ankle mortise. (*Source*: Bucholz RW, Heckman JD. *Rockwood & Green's Fractures in Adults*, 5th ed. Lippincott Williams & Wilkins, 2001.)**

normal, with less overlap indicative of syndesmotic injury), tibiofibular clear space (less than 5 mm is normal, with more indicative of a syndesmotic injury), and talar tilt (less than 2 mm is normal). Any medial joint-space widening on the mortise view is abnormal, as is a talocrural ankle of less than 8 degrees or greater than 15 degrees (Fig. 10.41). If there is less than 1 mm of tibiofibular overlap on the mortise view, syndesmotic injury should be considered. The lateral view allows assessment of posterior malleolar fractures, anteroposterior subluxation of the talus under the tibia, distal fibula translation, or a talus fracture. Stress views (external rotation) can evaluate the integrity of the syndesmosis.

Classification. There are multiple classification systems that categorize ankle fractures. The Lauge-Hansen system (Table 10.20) consists of 2 words, the first referring to the position of the foot at the time of injury and the second referring to the force applied to the foot relative to the tibia at the time of injury (Fig. 10.42 and 10.43). A supinated foot sustains either an external rotation or adduction force and creates the successive stages of injury. A pronated foot sustains either an external rotation or abduction force and creates the successive stages of injury. The injury starts on the tension side of the ankle (the lateral side is tight in supination and the medial side is tight in pronation). The Weber classification system is more simplified and is based on the location of fibula fracture with respect to the mortise (Fig. 10.44). Weber A is distal to the mortise (pronation–abduction), Weber B is at the level of the mortise (supination–external rotation), and Weber C is proximal to the mortise (pronation–external rotation).

Treatment. Nonoperative treatment is reserved for nondisplaced stable fractures with an intact syndesmosis or for medically unstable patients. Treatment involves casting for 4 to 6 weeks with serial x-rays and subsequent transition to a short-leg walking cast. Operative indications include talar subluxation, joint incongruity, or articular step-off. The posterior malleolus should be fixed if 25% of the joint surface is involved. This is associated with the pull of the posterior tibiofibular ligament (the fragment usually larger laterally than medially). The syndesmosis should be reduced anatomically, and dorsiflexion of the foot is recommended to prevent malreduction (to prevent overtightening), although the data is not conclusive.

Diabetic Patients. Ankle fractures in the diabetic patient population have a higher incidence because of neuropathy, nephropathy, retinopathy, and PVD. These patients are at a higher risk for amputations, with a 6% rate in closed injuries and 43% in open injuries. Diabetic patients are at increased risk for infection and malunion or nonunion. Furthermore, rehabilitation times are twice as long. Osteopenic ankle fractures occur in the older patient population and can be challenging to fix because of poor hardware fixation with increased risk of failure. Solutions can include maintaining the periosteum with fixation, using an antiglide plate on the fibula with posterior-to-anterior screws (better purchase), or using an intramedullary screw if there is inadequate distal bone.

Results. Poorer results can be expected in bimalleolar fractures, impaction injuries of the tibial plafond, large posterior malleolar fragments, talar dome injuries, talus fractures, associated foot and ankle injuries, delays in fixation, age greater than 50, and patients with diabetes.

TABLE 10.20 Lauge-Hansen classification of ankle fractures

Type	Mechanism	Injury
Supination, external rotation	Starts at mortise anteriorly and extends posteriorly and proximally	Short oblique fibula fracture Stage 2 (ATFL and fibula) can be managed closed Stage 4 (ATFL, fibula, posterior malleolus/posterior tibiofibular ligament, deltoid ligament/medial malleolus) are unstable
Supination, adduction	Marginal impaction at the medial edge of the plafond	Stage 1: transverse fibula fracture below mortise Stage 2: vertical medial malleolus fracture
Pronation, external rotation	Proximal spiral fibula fracture	Full-length leg films required to assess proximal fibula PER IV: syndesmosis usually disrupted (Maisonneuve fracture)
Pronation, abduction	Fibula fracture typically in distal of fibula	Medial malleolus may need to be tension-banded

Tarsal Fractures and Dislocations

Anatomy and Overview. The talus has no muscular insertions; 60% of the surface is covered by articular cartilage. The blood supply is predominantly via the artery of the tarsal canal with some contribution of the artery of the tarsal sinus and the deltoid artery through an anastomosis. Fractures of the talus compose 2% of all fractures and 6% to 8% of all foot fractures. These injuries have high complication rates, including AVN, posttraumatic arthritis, and malunion. The talar neck tolerates 1200 newtons of sheer force during active motion. Injury occurs when there is hyperdorsiflexion of the foot on the leg and the neck of the talus impinges against the anterior distal tibia, resulting in neck fracture. If there is continued force propagation, the talar body can dislocate posteromedially around the deltoid.

Imaging. Imaging includes multiple plain film views including a Canale view (ankle in plantarflexion with 15 degrees of pronation and the beam entering at 15 degrees from the vertical plane). CT scan can be useful to further delineate injury pattern, and MRI can be performed primarily to assess for complications (AVN). The Hawkins classification system, which is predictive of AVN, is used to describe these injuries (Table 10.21; Figs. 10.45 and 10.46).

Management. The goals of management include immediate reduction of dislocated joints and anatomic fracture reduction. Reduction can be achieved via a 1-incision technique or a 2-incision technique for the talus. The 1-incision technique allows for an anteromedial or anterolateral approach, resulting in less skin injury, but difficulty visualizing the talar neck and subtalar joint. The 2-incision technique allows for an anteromedial and direct lateral approach with 2 incisions leading to a tighter closure and with better fracture visualization. Stable fixation can be achieved with posterior-to-anterior fixation or anterior screw fixation. Posterior-to-anterior fixation is stronger than anteroposterior fixation with 2 screws perpendicular to the fracture site, which is able to withstand the shear forces of active motion. Anterior screw fixation is easier to perform with direct visualization and no cartilage damage.

Complications. Complications of treatment include AVN. Hawkins sign, the presence of subchondral lucency, implies revascularization and can be visualized on radiographs 6 to 8 weeks after injury. MRI is sensitive for diagnosis as well. Weight bearing should be modified prior to collapse. Malunion is common in 40% of cases where the hindfoot goes into varus. Greater than 3 degrees of malunion leads to decreased ROM, and greater than 2 mm of displacement alters subtalar contact forces. Treatment should consist of a calcaneal osteotomy and tendoachilles lengthening. While nonunion is uncommon, arthritis often occurs in the subtalar joint.

Classification and Mechanism of Injury with Dislocations. Subtalar dislocations are classified on the basis of direction of dislocation. Medial dislocations are often a result of low-energy injuries and make up 85% of all subtalar dislocations. Mechanical blocks to reduction include the capsule and the extensor digitorum brevis (EDB) tendon. Lateral dislocations are a result of higher energy injuries and comprise 15% of all subtalar dislocations. Reductions of lateral dislocations can be blocked by the posterior tibial tendon. Subtalar arthritis occurs in nearly 90% of patients.

Calcaneus Fractures

Anatomy and Overview. The calcaneus articulates with the talus and the cuboid. Bony landmarks medially are the sustentaculum tali and laterally are the sinus

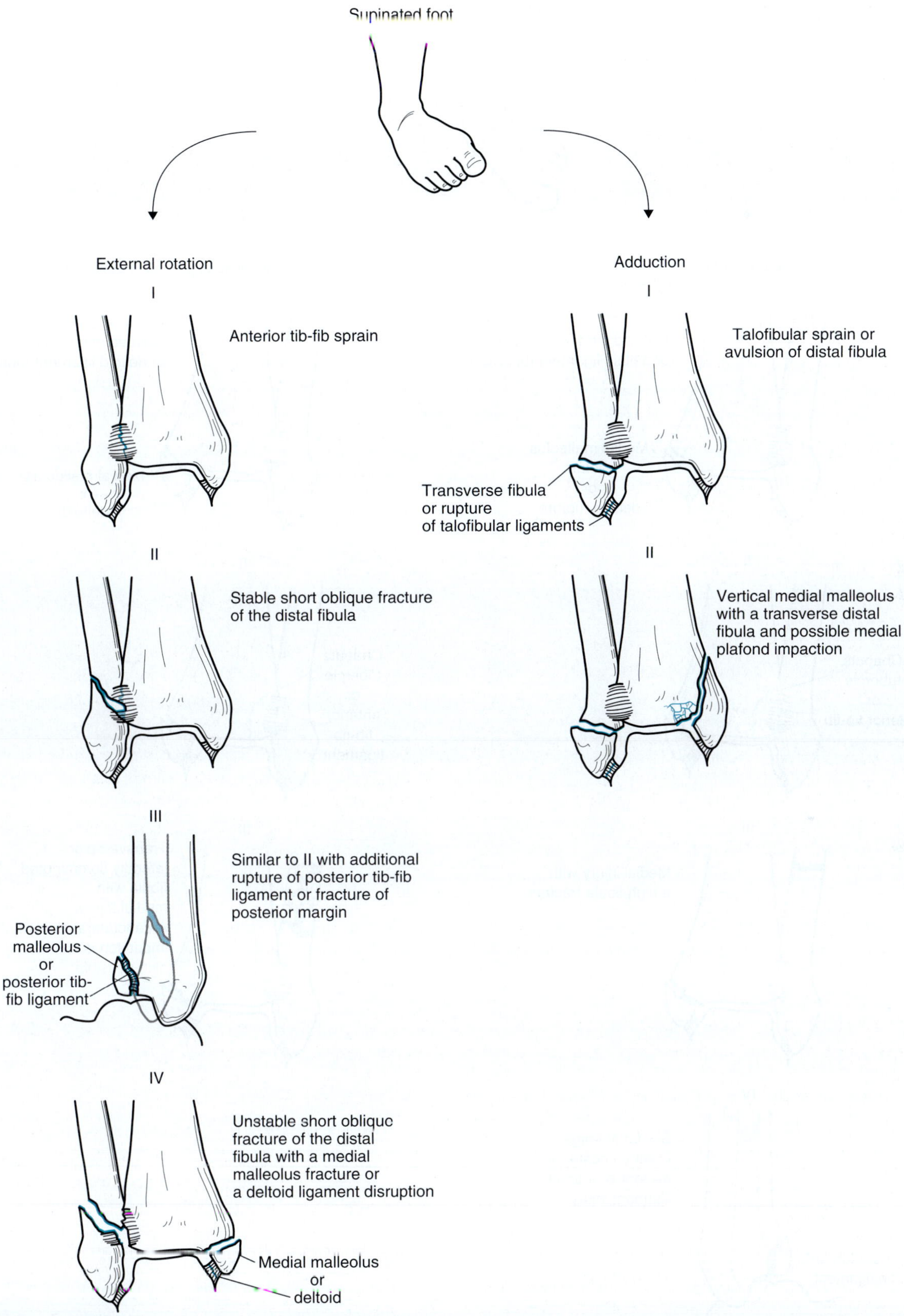

FIGURE 10.42 **Lauge-Hansen supination–external rotation and supination–adduction ankle fractures. (*Source:* Bucholz RW, Heckman JD. *Rockwood & Green's Fractures in Adults*, 5th ed. Lippincott Williams & Wilkins, 2001.)**

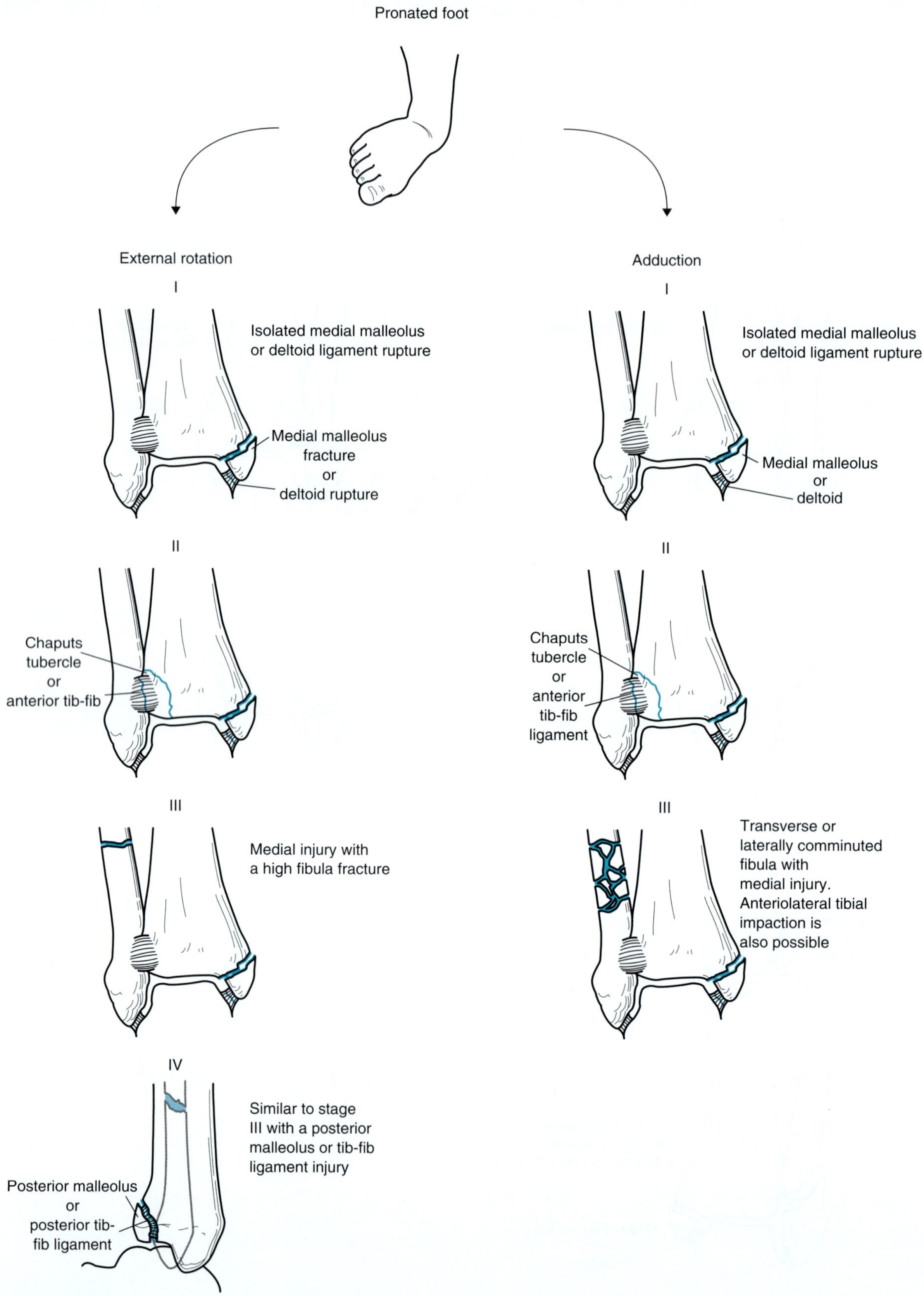

FIGURE 10.43 **Lauge-Hansen pronation–external rotation and pronation–abduction ankle fractures. (*Source:* Bucholz RW, Heckman JD. *Rockwood & Green's Fractures in Adults*, 5th ed. Lippincott Williams & Wilkins, 2001.)**

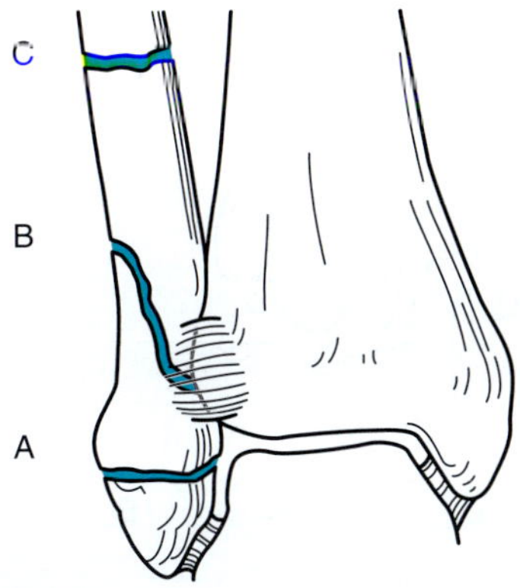

FIGURE 10.44 There are 3 types of ankle fractures in the AO/OTA classification: type A, type B, and type C. (*Source*: Bucholz RW, Heckman JD. *Rockwood & Green's Fractures in Adults*, 5th ed. Lippincott Williams & Wilkins, 2001.)

tarsi and anterior process. Facets of the subtalar joint include anterior, middle, and posterior. The calcaneus functions to support the lateral column of the foot with the subtalar joint inverting and everting the foot. The position of the hindfoot will lock and unlock the midfoot joint.

Associated Injuries. Extraarticular injuries of the calcaneus are common. Anterior process fractures result from an inversion injury and are often missed. Small pieces are treated like a sprain, but larger displaced fragments are reduced and fixed. A tuberosity fracture results from a fall from height or MVA and is usually managed nonoperatively. A calcaneal tuberosity avulsion is indicative of an Achilles avulsion with high risk for wound complications after surgical fixation of the avulsed piece with lag screws or tension band. Sustentacular fractures may alter subtalar joint mechanics. Small, nondisplaced injuries are treated conservatively, while large, displaced fragments are addressed with ORIF (through a medial approach) or buttress plate.

Mechanism of Injury. Intraarticular fractures are usually due to a high-energy mechanism (e.g., MVA, fall). The lateral process of the talus acts as a wedge leading to an impaction type injury. The primary fracture line is lateral to the sustentaculum tali, and the secondary fracture line extends posteriorly through the tuberosity, thus creating 3 parts of the calcaneus. The articular incongruity leads to the hindfoot being in varus. The shape of the foot is noted to be altered: it can be wider, shorter, and smaller in height. The heel pad can be crushed and the peroneals impinged.

Imaging. Lateral radiographs can reveal changes in the Bohler angle and the critical angle of Gissane. A Broden view examines the posterior facet and is taken with the foot positioned in 20 degrees of internal rotation with 10 to 40 degrees of plantar flexion. Axial radiographs assess varus–valgus angulation of the calcaneus with the image taken as a 45-degree axial of the heel with the second toe in line with the tibia (normal alignment is 10 degrees of valgus). The CT scan is a better tool for assessment of the posterior facet and extent of comminution and should be performed perpendicular to the posterior facet with sagittal cuts parallel to the plantar aspect of foot.

Classification. Prior to CT scanning, the classification of calcaneus fractures was based on the Essex-Lopresti system and was categorized in 3 broad categories: extraarticular, joint depression, and tongue. The Sanders classification is based on CT scans and is predictive of the results. The type of fracture is based on the number of joint fragments (II, III, or IV) present. The subtype (A, B, C) is dependent on the lateral to medial fracture lines present (Fig. 10.47).

Treatment. Nonoperative treatment has poor long-term outcomes with symptoms in nearly 60% of

TABLE 10.21 Hawkins classification of tarsal fracture and dislocation

Type	*Description*	*AVN*	*Notes*
I	Undisplaced	0%–13%	NWB cast for 4 to 6 weeks with motion in a brace after healing Percutaneous screw fixation and early motion
II	Displaced fracture with subtalar dislocation	20%–50%	Fracture line enters subtalar joint Subtalar joint intact
III	Subtalar and ankle joint dislocated	83%–100%	Talar body extrudes around deltoid ligament
IV	Type III with talonavicular subluxation	100%	Rare variant

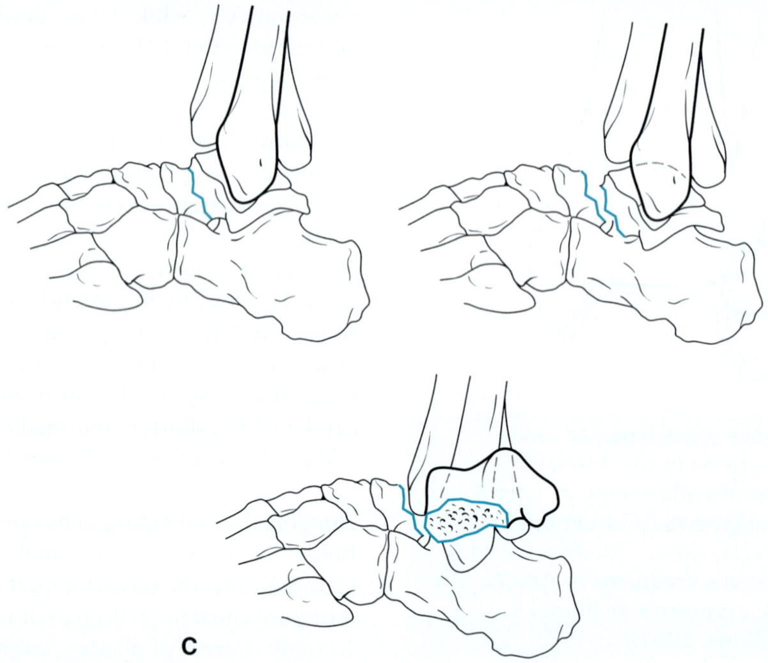

FIGURE 10.45 The 3 patterns of talar neck fractures as described by Hawkins. Note that type I fractures are nondisplaced. (A) Type I talar neck fracture with no displacement. (B) Type II talar neck fracture with displacement and subluxation of subtalar joint. (C) Type III talar neck fracture with displacement and dislocation of both ankle and subtalar joints. (*Source:* Bucholz RW, Heckman JD. *Rockwood & Green's Fractures in Adults,* 5th ed. Lippincott Williams & Wilkins, 2001.)

patients. Nonoperative management often leads to malunion with the varus hindfoot, resulting in locking of the midfoot and medialization of stance. This shortening of the foot leads to a shorter lever arm. Furthermore, fracture malunion can lead to peroneal tendon impingement or dislocation and problems with shoewear. Malunions can be treated with an orthosis or custom shoewear, a lateral wall exostectomy, peroneal tenodesis, or subtalar fusion or sliding wedge osteotomy. The goal of operative intervention is to restore shape and alignment of the hindfoot and articular congruency. Surgery should result in medial translation, restore height, and restore valgus.

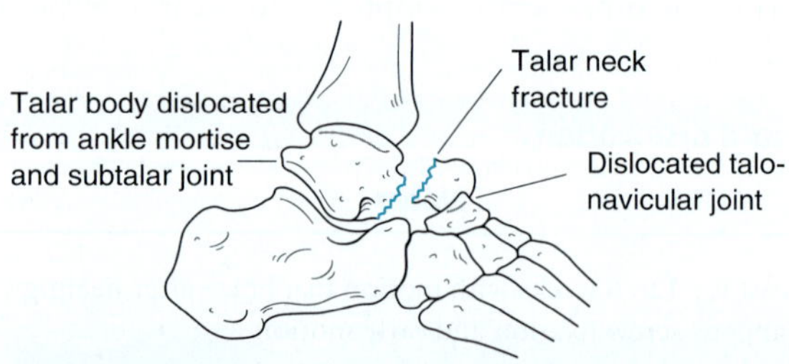

FIGURE 10.46 Type IV talar neck fracture. (*Source:* Bucholz RW, Heckman JD. *Rockwood & Green's Fractures in Adults,* 5th ed. Lippincott Williams & Wilkins, 2001.)

Contraindications to Surgery. Contraindications to surgery include diabetes, smoking, vascular insufficiency, severe swelling, open fractures, Sanders type IV, the elderly, the neuropathic joint, noncompliant patients, and an inexperienced surgeon. Skin wrinkling should be present prior to surgery, and a lateral approach to the fracture via removal of the lateral wall should be employed.

Complications. Complications include stiffness, loss of normal gait, shoewear problems, posttraumatic arthritis, peroneal pain, heel pad pain, and wound breakdown.

Lisfranc and Midfoot Injuries

Anatomy and Overview. The midfoot consists of an articulation between the 3 cuneiforms and cuboid and the bases of the 5 metatarsals. Osseus stability is provided by the Roman arch construct of the metatarsals and recessed keystone of the second metatarsal base. The Lisfranc ligament is a large, oblique ligament that extends from the plantar aspect of the medial cuneiform to the base of the second

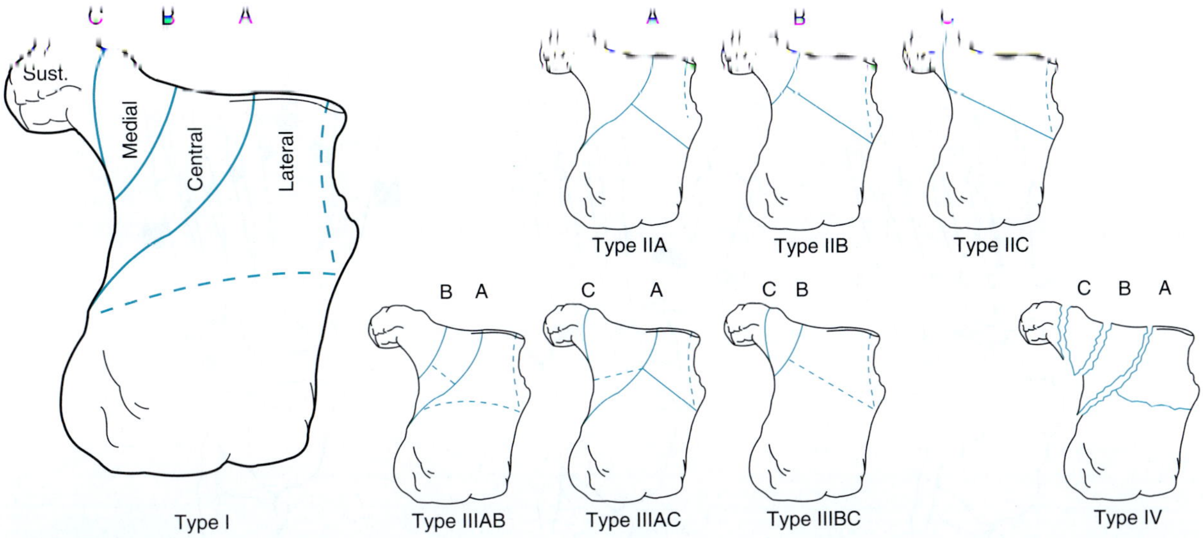

FIGURE 10.47 Sanders classification of intraarticular fractures of the calcaneus. Fracture lines *A*, *B*, and *C* describe the position of the primary fracture line in relation to the posterior facet and the subtalar joint. Types II and III have 2 or 3 fragments. Type IV represents severe comminution. (*Source:* Bucholz RW, Heckman JD. *Rockwood & Green's Fractures in Adults*, 5th ed. Lippincott Williams & Wilkins, 2001.)

metatarsal. The interosseus ligaments connect the second through fifth metatarsal bases on both the dorsal and plantar surfaces. The plantar ligaments are stronger and larger. The secondary stabilizers including plantar fascia, peroneus longus, and the intrinsics. The dorsalis pedis courses between the first and second metatarsal bases, and the deep peroneal nerve runs alongside the artery.

Mechanism of Injury. Lisfranc injuries are overlooked in 20% of patients (especially those in polytrauma situations). The mechanism of injury often includes MVC, crush injuries, and sports and results from either direct or indirect loading. In the direct loading scheme, force is applied directly to the dorsum of the Lisfranc joint. Plantar displacement is more common, and there is a greater risk of open fracture, compartment syndrome, and soft tissue injury. Indirect loading is more common than direct and results from axial loading and twisting leading to forceful abduction of the forefoot, a second metatarsal base fracture, and a possible compression fracture of the cuboid ("nutcracker"). The metatarsal bases dislocate dorsally more often than plantar, and dislocations are usually due to athletic injuries.

Types of Dislocations. The classification of these injuries is descriptive (Fig. 10.48). Homolateral dislocations are the most common, and all 5 metatarsals displace in a common direction (total). Often, there is a fracture at the base of the second metatarsal. Isolated dislocations are a displacement of one or more metatarsals away from the others (partial). Divergent dislocations are least common and result from a lateral displacement of the lesser metatarsals with medial displacement of the first metatarsal. The divergent dislocations may extend into the cuneiforms and talonavicular joint.

Diagnosis. The diagnosis of a Lisfranc injury is made with a high index of suspicion. Patients have midfoot pain with weight bearing and swelling across the dorsum of foot. Gentle stressing to plantarflexion and dorsiflexion and rotation will reveal instability and, along with assessment of compartments, will help lead to a diagnosis.

Imaging. An anteroposterior radiograph should show alignment of the medial margin of the second metatarsal base and medial margin of the medial cuneiform. An oblique radiograph should show alignment of the medial base of the fourth metatarsal and medial margin of the cuboid. The lateral radiograph should show the dorsal surface of the first and second metatarsals to be level to the corresponding cuneiforms. Standing stress films may demonstrate diastasis.

Treatment. Treatment necessitates anatomic reduction for best result, with a displacement of greater than 1 mm or gross instability unacceptable. Nonoperative treatment is reserved for nondisplaced injuries with normal stress radiographs and is performed by placing a patient in a short-leg cast for 4 to 6

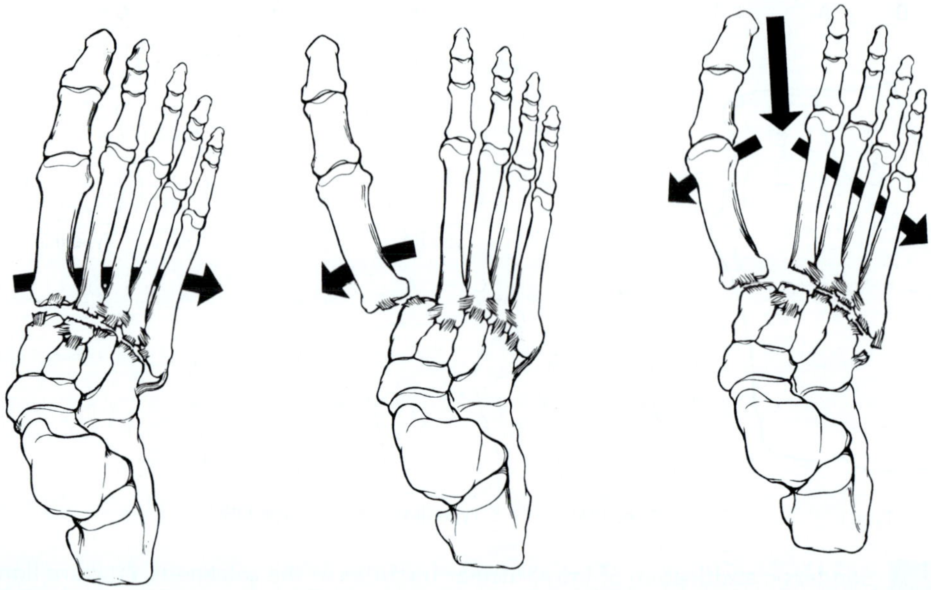

FIGURE 10.48 The common classification devised by Quenu and Kuss. Further subdivisions are used to identify the direction of dislocation in the homolateral pattern (medial or lateral) and the partial disruption (first or lesser). (*Source:* Bucholz RW, Heckman JD. *Rockwood & Green's Fractures in Adults,* 5th ed. Lippincott Williams & Wilkins, 2001.)

weeks with frequent radiographic evaluation. Operative treatment includes surgical emergencies (e.g., open, vascular compromise, compartment syndrome) and requires reduction and stabilization of the first and second tarsometatarsal (TMT) joints with screw fixation (not lag).

Associated Injuries. Numerous short ligaments attach dorsally, plantarly, and laterally to the navicular, with the deltoid attaching medially. Vessels enter dorsally, plantarly, and through the tuberosity. The central third is largely avascular; the number of vessels decreases with age. Avulsion fractures at the dorsal lip are treated with immobilization or excision of the fragment if painful. Tuberosity fractures can occur secondary to avulsion of the posterior tibial tendon or spring ligament and may be associated with calcaneocuboid impaction. ORIF is indicated if the fracture is displaced (more than 5 mm). Navicular body fractures are a result of high-energy trauma with axial loading of the foot. CT scans are recommended for operative planning with the goal to reduce these fractures anatomically. The classification system is described by Sangerozan. Type I fractures are in the coronal plane. Type II fractures have a primary fracture line from dorsolateral to plantar medial with medial displacement of the major fragment. Type III navicular body fractures are comminuted and have the worst prognosis because they often go on to have osteonecrosis. ORIF is indicated for displaced fractures.

Amputations

General Indications. Amputations of the lower extremity are a result of limb ischemia in 75% to 80% of cases (50% have diabetes). Trauma (10% to 15%), tumors (5%), and congenital deformity (5%) have a lower incidence as an indication for amputation. In patients with an acute traumatic amputation, immediate management includes control of hemorrhaging with a compression dressing and splinting to decrease pain, protect soft tissue, and help control bleeding. The amputated part should not be soaked in water but rather placed directly on ice.

Criteria. The MESS assesses skeletal and soft tissue injury, limb ischemia, shock, and age. A score greater than 7 indicates amputation, 6 or less indicates salvage. Absolute criteria for amputation include nonreconstructible vascular injury and severe bone and soft tissue loss. Tibial nerve disruption associated with soft tissue injury is an indication for amputation, while loss of plantar sensation alone is not. Relative criteria for amputations include shock in an elderly patient with a mangled limb, massive muscle loss associated with bone loss, and a MESS greater than 7, especially with no plantar sensation. Isolated tibial nerve disruption is not an indication for amputation.

Goals of Surgery. Surgical treatment involves preserving length, with the final bone cuts occurring at the

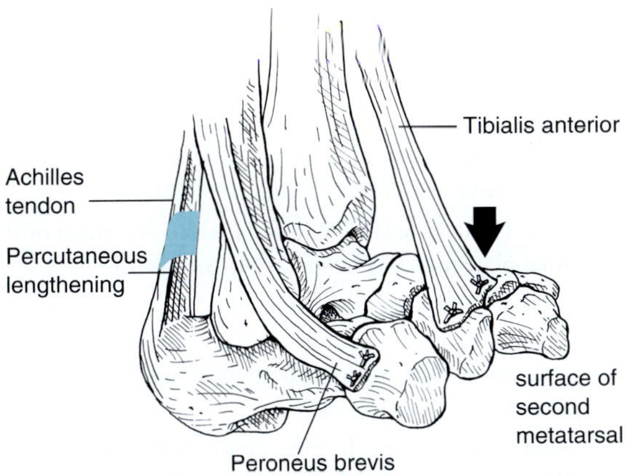

FIGURE 10.49 Tarsometatarsal (Lisfranc) amputation. Tibialis anterior is reattached to the midfoot, and the Achilles tendon is lengthened percutaneously. The peroneal tendons are reattached laterally. (*Source:* Bucholz RW, Heckman JD. *Rockwood & Green's Fractures in Adults*, 5th ed. Lippincott Williams & Wilkins, 2001.)

time of definitive treatment. Débridement of nonviable tissue is critical, but soft tissue coverage is essential. Obtaining full extension is more important than full knee flexion. Split-thickness skin grafts should be obtained from the contralateral limb.

Levels of Amputation. Levels of amputation are dependent on the extent of injury and the ability to provide soft tissue coverage.

- *Toes*—Amputation at the MTP is performed through the joint, leaving the cartilage intact (barrier to infection and better end bearing). There is a limited effect on gait with better biomechanics and good ankle motion and calf musculature compared with higher amputations. A ray amputation includes the toe with some or the entire corresponding metatarsal. The first ray bears one-third of the weight, and each additional ray bears one-sixth of the weight.
- *Midfoot*—A midfoot amputation, through the transmetatarsal or Lisfranc joint, needs a well padded flap and close monitoring to prevent postoperative equinus (Fig. 10.49).
- *Hindfoot*—Hindfoot amputations are divided into three types. A Chopart amputation saves the calcaneus and talus. A Boyd amputation is a talectomy with calcaneal–tibial fusion (translation of the calcaneus forward). A Pirogoff procedure is performed as a talectomy with calcaneal–tibial fusion (forward rotation of the calcaneus).
- *Ankle*—A Syme amputation is disarticulation of the ankle. Stabilization of the heel pad is critical and is performed by suturing the Achilles to the posterior tibia. It is difficult to walk on a Syme amputation without a prosthesis.
- *Transtibial*—During a transtibial amputation (BKA), it is important to maintain a posterior flap to obtain a cylindrical shape to the limb. Roughly, flap

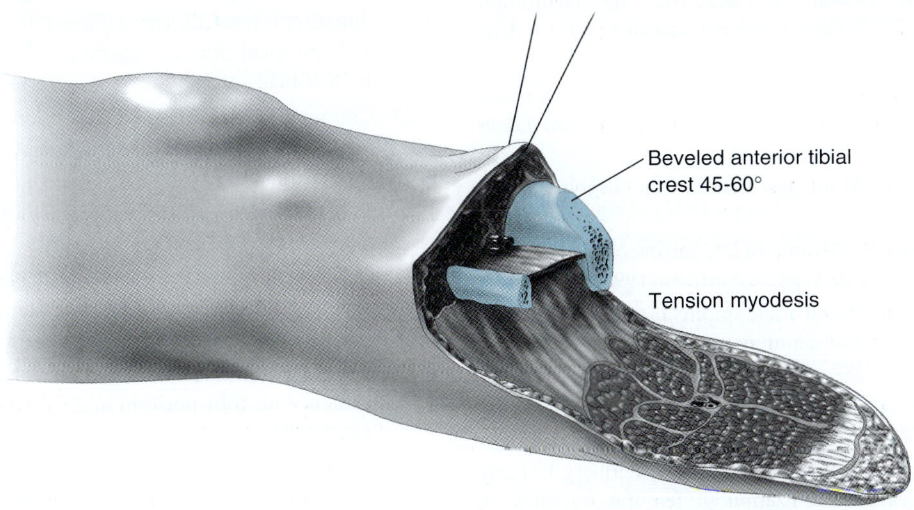

FIGURE 10.50 Transtibial amputation with a long posterior myocutaneous flap and a short anterior flap. The soleus has been removed and the tibia beveled 45 to 60 degrees. The fibula is 1 cm shorter than the tibia. Myodesis is performed to stabilize the soft tissues. (*Source:* Bucholz RW, Heckman JD. *Rockwood & Green's Fractures in Adults*, 5th ed. Lippincott Williams & Wilkins, 2001.)

length should be equivalent to the diameter plus 1 cm. The fibula should be cut 1 to 2 cm shorter than the tibia, and a myodesis of the musculature should be performed to the anterior tibia (Fig. 10.50). Limb length should be sufficient for a prosthesis (should not be done through the distal one-third of the tibia).

- *Knee*—Knee disarticulation is a consideration for ambulatory patients. There is some data to support that knee disarticulation is usually more functional than transfemoral amputation. It leaves the patient with a longer lever arm and balanced thigh muscles, allows for end bearing, and potentially improves sitting comfort.
- *Transfemoral*—Technical considerations during a transfemoral amputation (AKA) include muscle stabilization. The iliopsoas results in flexion, and the abductor muscle group forces abduction. Myodesis with the adductors is essential, and postoperative hip flexion contracture prophylaxis is essential.

Results. The LEAP review showed no difference in long-term outcomes between salvage, transtibial amputation, and transfemoral amputation; however, knee disarticulation scored the worst in the review.

References

1. Ackerman G, Jupiter JB. Nonunion of fractures of the distal end of the humerus. *J Bone Joint Surg* 1988;70A:75–83.
2. Ada JR, Miller ME. Scapular fractures: Analysis of 113 cases. *Clin Orthop* 1991;269:174–180.
3. Alpert SW, Koval KJ, Zuckerman JD. Neurologic arthropathy: Review of current knowledge. *J Am Acad Orthop Surg* 1996;4:100–108.
4. Arntz CT, Veith RG, Hansen ST Jr. Fractures and fracture-dislocations of the tarsometatarsal joint. *J Bone Joint Surg* 1983;65B:329–332.
5. Bado JL. The Monteggia Lesion. *Clin Orthop* 1967;50: 71–76.
6. Baumhauer JF, Alvarez RG. Controversies in treating talus fractures. *Orthop Clin North Am* 1995;17:164–169.
7. Bennett WF. Lateral ankle sprains I. Anatomy, biomechanics, diagnosis, and natural history. *Orthop Rev* 1994;23:381–387.
8. Bone LB. Fractures of the tibial plafond. *Orthop Clin North Am* 1987;18(1):95–104.
9. Bone LB, Johnson KD, Weiglet J, Scheinberg R. Early versus delayed stabilization of femoral fractures: A prospective, randomized study. *J Bone Joint Surg* 1989;71A (3):336–240.
10. Bostrom A. Fractures of the patella: A study of 422 patellar fractures. *Acta Orthop Scand* 1972;143:1–80.
11. Boyd HB, Griffin LL. Classification and treatment of trochanteric fractures. *Arch Surg* 1949;58:853–866.
12. Brumback RJ. Open tibial fractures: Current orthopaedic management. *Instr Course Lect* 1992;41: 101–117.
13. Burgess AR, Eastridge BJ, Young JWR, et al. Pelvic ring disruptions: Effective classification system and treatment protocols. *J Trauma* 1990;30:848–856.
14. Burri C, Bartzke G, Coldeway J, et al. Fractures of the tibial plateau. *Clin Orthop* 1979;138:84–93.
15. Cage DJ, Abrams RA, Callahan JJ, Botte MJ. Soft tissue attachments of the ulnar coronoid process: An anatomic study with radiographic correlation. *Clin Orthop* 1987;216:109–119.
16. Canale ST, Kelly FC Jr. Fractures of the neck and talus. *J Bone Joint Surg* 1978;60A:143–156.
17. Carpenter JE, Matthews LS. Fractures of the patella. *J Bone Joint Surg* 1993;75A(10):1550–1561.
18. Chapman MW, Gordon JE, Zissimos AG. Compression-plate fixation of acute fractures of the diaphyses of the radius and ulna. *J Bone Joint Surg* 1989;71A:159–169.
19. Chin KR, Sodl JF. Infrapatellar fat pad disruption: A radiographic sign of patellar tendon rupture. *Clin Orthop Relat Res* 2005 Nov;440:222–225.
20. Cofield RH. Comminuted fractures of the proximal humerus. *Clin Orthop* 1988;230:49–57.
21. Cohen MS, Hastings H II. Acute elbow dislocation: Evaluation and management. *J Am Acad Orthop Surg* 1998;6(1):15–23.
22. Cohen MS, Hastings H II. Rotary instability of the elbow: The anatomy and role of the lateral stabilizers. *J Bone Joint Surg* 1997;79A:225–233.
23. Colton CL. Fractures of the olecranon in adults: Classification and management. *Injury* 1973;5:121–129.
24. Court-Brown CM, Keating JF, McQueen MM. Infection after intramedullary nailing of the tibia: Incidence and protocol for management. *J Bone Joint Surg* 1958;40B:42–46.
25. Cramer KE, Moed BR. Patellar fractures: Contemporary approach to treatment. *J Am Acad Orthop Surg* 1997;5(6):323–331.
26. Dahl E. Mortality and life expectancy after hip fractures. *Acta Orthop Scan* 1980;51:163–170.
27. Dalal SA, Burgess AR, Siegel JH, et al. Pelvic fracture disruptions: Effective classification system and treatment protocols. *J Trauma* 1990;30(7):848–856.
28. Daniels T, Smith JW. Varus neck talar malunion: Its influence on foot position and subtalar motion. *Foot Ankle* 1993;14:302.
29. Ebraheim NA, An S, Jackson WT, et al. Scapulothoracic dissociation. *J Bone Joint Surg* 1988;70A:428–432.
30. Edwards GS, Jupiter JB. Radial head fractures with acute radioulnar dislocation: Essex-Lopresti revisited. *Clin Orthop* 1988;234:61–69.
31. Failinger MS, McGanity PLJ. Current concepts review: Unstable fractures of the pelvic ring. *J Bone Joint Surg* 1992;74A(5):781–791.

32. Flatow EL, Cuomo F, Mayday MG, et al. Open reduction and internal fixation of two-part displaced fractures of the greater tuberosity of the proximal part of the humerus. *J Bone Joint Surg* 1991;73A:1213–1218.
33. Garden RS. Low-angle fixation in fractures of the femoral neck. *J Bone Joint Surg* 1961;43B:647–663.
34. Goossens M, DeStoop N. Lisfranc's fracture-dislocation: Etiology, radiology, and results of treatment: A review of 20 cases. *Clin Orthop* 1983;176:154–162.
35. Green N, Allen B. Vascular injuries associated with dislocation of the knee. *J Bone Joint Surg* 1997;59A:236–239.
36. Gustilo RB, Mendoza RM, Williams DN. Problems in the management of type III (severe) open fractures: A new classification of type III open fractures. *J Trauma* 1984;24(8):742–746.
37. Gustilo RB, Merkow RL, Templeman D. Current concepts review: The management of open fractures. *J Bone Joint Surg* 1990;72A:299–303.
38. Hardegger FH, Simpson LA, Weber BG. The operative treatment of scapular fractures. *J Bone Joint Surg* 1984;66B:725–731.
39. Hawkins LG. Fractures of the neck and talus. *J Bone Joint Surg* 1970;52A:991–1002.
40. Healy WL, White GM, Mick CA, et al. Nonunion of the humeral shaft. *Clin Orthop* 1987;219:206–213.
41. Hidaka S, Gustilo RB. Refracture of bones of the forearm after plate removal. *J Bone Joint Surg* 1984;66A:1241–1243.
42. Helfet DL, Hotchkiss RN. Internal fixation of the distal humerus: A biomechanical comparison of methods. *J Orthop Trauma* 1990;4:260–264.
43. Helfet DL, Howey T, Sanders R, Johansen K. Limb salvage versus amputation—Preliminary results of the mangled extremity severity score. *Clin Orthop Relat Res* 1990;256:80–86.
44. Hill JM, McGuire MH, Crosby LA. Closed treatment of displaced middle-third fractures of the clavicle gives poor results. *J Bone Joint Surg* 1997;79B(4):537–539.
45. Hovelius L, Augustini BG, Fredin H, et al. Primary anterior dislocation of the shoulder in young patients: A ten year prospective study. *J Bone Joint Surg* 1996;78A:1677–1684.
46. Ingman AM, Waters DA. Locked intramedullary nailing of humeral shaft fractures: Implant design, surgical technique, and clinical results. *J Bone Joint Surg* 1994;76B:23–29.
47. Johansen K, Daines M, Howey T, Helfet D, Hansen ST Jr. Objective criteria accurately predict amputation following lower extremity trauma. *J Trauma* 1990;30(5):568–572.
48. Judet R, Judet J, Letournel E. Fractures of the acetabulum: Classification and surgical approaches for open reduction. *J Bone Joint Surg* 1964;46A:1615–1638.
49. Knight DJ, Rymaszewski AL, Amis AA, et al. Primary replacement of the fractured radial head with a metal prosthesis. *J Bone Joint Surg* 1993;75B:572–576.
50. Koval KJ, Zuckerman JD. Hip fractures I: Overview and evaluation and treatment of femoral neck fractures. *J Am Acad Orthop Surg* 1994;2(3):141–149.
51. Koval KJ, Zuckerman JD. Hip fractures II: Evaluation and treatment of intertrochanteric fractures. *J Am Acad Orthop Surg* 1994;2(3):150–156.
52. Lauge-Hansen N. Fractures of the ankle II: Combined experimental-surgical and experimental-roentgenologic investigations. *Arch Surg* 1950;60:957–985.
53. Littenberg B, Weinstein LP, McCarren M, et al. Closed fractures of the tibial shaft: A meta-analysis of three methods of treatment. *J Bone Joint Surg* 1998;80A:174–183.
54. Lowery RB, Calhoun JH. Fractures of the calcaneus I: Anatomy, injury, mechanism, and classification. *Foot Ankle* 1996;17:230–235.
55. Lowery RB, Calhoun JH. Fractures of the calcaneus II: Treatment. *Foot Ankle* 1996;17:360–366.
56. Lu J, Ebraheim NA, Skie M, et al. Radiographic and computer tomographic evaluation of Lisfranc dislocation: A cadaver study. *Foot Ankle* 1997;18:351–355.
57. Martin-Herrero T, Rodriguez-Merchan C, Munuera-Martinez L. Fractures of the coracoid process: Presentation of seven cases and review of the literature. *J Trauma* 1990;30(12):1597–1599.
58. Mast JW, Spiegel PG, Pappas JN. Fractures of the tibial pilon. *Clin Orthop Rel Res* 1988;230:68–82.
59. Matava MJ. Patellar tendon ruptures. *J Am Acad Orthop Surg* 1996;4(6):287–296.
60. Matta JM, Letournel E, Browner B. Surgical management of acetabular fractures. *Instr Course Lect* 1986;35:382–397.
61. Matta JM, Saucedo T. Internal fixation of pelvic ring fractures. *Clin Orthop* 1989;242:83–97.
62. Matta JM, Tornetta P III. Internal fixation of unstable pelvic ring injuries. *Clin Orthop* 1996;329:129–140.
63. McGahan JP, Rab GT, Dublin A. Fractures of the Scapula. *J Trauma* 1980;20:880–883.
64. McLaughlin HL, Francis KC. Operative repair of injuries to the quadriceps extensor mechanism. *Am J Surg* 1956;91:651–653.
65. McQueen MM, Christie J, Court-Brown CM. Compartment pressures after intramedullary nailing of the tibia. *J Bone Joint Surg* 1988;70A:900–911.
66. Morrey BF, An KN, Stormont TJ. Force transmission through the radial head. *J Bone Joint Surg* 1988;70A:250–256.
67. Myerson MS, Fisher RT, Burgess AR, et al. Fracture dislocations of the tarsometatarsal joints: End results correlated with pathology and treatment. *Foot Ankle* 1986;6:225–242.
68. Neer CS II. Displaced proximal humerus fractures. I. Classification & evaluation. *J Bone Joint Surg* 1970;52A:1077–1089.
69. Neer CS II. Treatment of three-part and four-part displacement. *J Bone Joint Surg* 1970;52A:1090–1103.

70. Nichter LS, Menendez LR. Reconstructive considerations for limb salvage surgery. *Orthop Clin North Am* 1993;24(3):511–521.
71. Phillips CS, Murphy MS. Vascular problems of the upper extremity: A primer for the orthopaedic surgeon. *J Amer Acad Orthop Surg* 2002;10:401–408.
72. Pipkin G. Treatment of grade IV fracture-dislocation of the hip: A review. *J Bone Joint Surg* 1957;39A:1027–1042.
73. Pisani G. Chronic laxity of the subtalar joint. *Orthopaedics* 1996;19:431–437.
74. Ring D, Chin K, Jupiter JB. Radial nerve palsy associated with high-energy humeral shaft fractures. *J Hand Surg Am* 2004 Jan;29(1):144–147.
75. Ring D, Gulotta L, Chin K, Jupiter JB. Olecranon osteotomy for exposure of fractures and nonunions of the distal humerus. *J Orthop Trauma.* 2004 Aug;18(7):446–449.
76. Ring D, Jupiter JB, Sanders RW, et al. Transolecranon fracture-dislocation of the elbow. *J Orthop Trauma* 1997;11:545–550.
77. Ring D, Jupiter JB. Current concepts review: Fracture-dislocation of the elbow. *J Bone Joint Surg* 1998;80A:566–580.
78. Ring D, Psychoyios VN, Chin KR, Jupiter JB. Nonunion of nonoperatively treated fractures of the radial head. *Clin Orthop Relat Res* 2002 May;(398):235–238.
79. Rizzo PF, Gould ES, Lyden JP, Asnis SE. Diagnosis of occult fractures about the hip: MRI compared with bone-scanning. *J Bone Joint Surg* 1995;75A:1551–1556.
80. Roberts CS, DeMaio M, Larkin JJ, Paine R. Eversion ankle sprains. *Orthopaedics* 1995;18:299–304.
81. Rockwood CA. Reconstruction of chronic and complete dislocations of the acromioclavicular joint. *Clin Orthop* 1998;347:138–149.
82. Rowe CR. Prognosis in the dislocations of the shoulder. *J Bone Joint Surg* 1956;38A:957–977.
83. Samardzic M, Grujicic D, Milinkovic ZB. Radial nerve lesions associated with fractures of the humeral shaft. *Injury* 1990;21:220–222.
84. Sanders R, Gregroy P. Operative treatment of intra-articular fractures of the calcaneus. *Orthop Clin North Am* 1995;26:203–214.
85. Sanders R, Regazzoni P, Reudi T. Treatment of supracondylar-intraarticular fractures of the femur using the dynamic condylar screw. *J Orthop Trauma* 1989;3:214–222.
86. Sanders R. Intra-articular fractures of the calcaneus: Present state of the art. *J Orthop Trauma* 1992;6:252–265.
87. Sangerozan BJ, Benirschke SK, Mosca V, et al. Displaced intra-articular fractures of the tarsal navicular. *J Bone Joint Surg* 1989;71A:1504–1510.
88. Sarmiento A, Kinman PB, Calvin EG, et al. Functional bracing of fractures of the humeral shaft. *J Bone Joint Surg* 1977;59A:596–601.
89. Schatzker J, McBroom R, Bruce D. The tibial plateau fracture: The Toronto experience, 1968–1976. *Clin Orthop* 1979;138:94–104.
90. Schenk R. The dislocated knee. *Inst Course Lect* 1994;43:127–136.
91. Shim SS. Circulatory and vascular changes in the hip following traumatic hip dislocation. *Clin Orthop* 1979;140:255–261.
92. Sisto D, Warren R. Complete knee dislocation: A follow-up study of operative treatment. *Clin Orthop* 1985;198:94–101.
93. Smith GR, Hotchkiss RN. Radial head and neck fractures: Anatomic guidelines for proper placement of internal fixation. *J Shoulder Elbow Surg* 1996;5:113–117.
94. Smith JJ, Agel J, Swiontkowski MF, Castillo R, Mackenzie E, Kellam JF. LEAP Study Group: Functional outcome of bilateral limb threatening: Lower extremity injuries at two years postinjury. *J Orthop Trauma* 2005;19(4):249–253.
95. Stewart MJ, Milford LW. Fracture-dislocation of the hip: An end-result study. *J Bone Joint Surg* 1954;36A:315–342.
96. Swiontkowski MF, Winquist RA, Hansen ST. Femoral neck fractures in patients aged 12–49. *J Bone Joint Surg* 1984;661:837–846.
97. Thompson DA, Flynn TC, Miller PW, et al. The significance of scapular fractures. *J Trauma* 1985;25:974–977.
98. Tile M. Acute pelvic fractures I: Causation and classification. *J Am Acad Orthop Surg* 1996;4(3):143–151.
99. Tile M. Acute pelvic fractures II: Principles of Management. *J Am Acad Orthop Surg* 1996;4(3):152–161.
100. Tornetta P III, Mustatari H. Hip dislocation: Current treatment regimens. *J Am Acad Orthop Surg* 1997;5:27–36.
101. Tscherne H, Lobenhoffer P. Tibial plateau fractures: Management and expected results. *Clin Orthop* 1993;292:87–100.
102. Tunturi T, Kemppainen K, Patiala H, et al. Importance of anatomical reduction for subjective recovery ankle fracturem. *Acta Orthop Scand* 1983;54:641–647.
103. Turkel Sj, Panio MW, Marshall JL, Girgis FG. Stabilizing mechanisms preventing anterior dislocations of the glenohumeral joint. *J Bone Joint Surg* 1981;63A:1208–1217.
104. Urist MR. Complete dislocation of the acromioclavicular joint. *J Bone Joint Surg* 1946;28A:813–837.
105. Wascher DC, Dvirnak PC, DeCoster TA. Knee dislocations: Initial assessment and complications for treatment. *J Orthop Trauma* 1997;11(7):525–529.
106. Winquist RA, Hansen ST. Segmental fractures of the femur treated by closed intramedullary nailing. *J Bone Joint Surg* 1978;60A(7):934–939.
107. Wirth MA, Rockwood CA. Acute and chronic traumatic injuries of the sternoclavicular joint. *J Am Acad Orthop Surg* 1996;4:268–278.
108. Zdravkovic D, Damholt VV. Comminuted and Severely Displaced Fractures of the Scapula. *Acta Orthop Scand* 1974;45:60–65.

Key References

Chapman MW, Gordon JE, Zissimos AG. Compression plate fixation of acute fractures of the diaphyses of the radius and ulna. *J Bone Joint Surg* 1989;71A:159–169.

This retrospective review of 129 diaphyseal forearm fractures in 87 patients plated using AO/ASIF techniques demonstrated union in 98% and an excellent or satisfactory functional result in 92%. Refracture occurred in only 2 patients, both fixed with 4.5-mm dynamic compression plates. Forty-nine fractures were open. The overall infection rate was less than 3%. Immediate fixation of open fractures had a low complication rate. Routine autogenous bone grafting was performed in all comminuted and open fractures.

Baumgaertner MR, Curtin SL, Lindskog DM, Keggi JM. The value of the tip–apex distance in predicting failure of fixation of peritrochanteric fractures of the hip. *J Bone Joint Surg* 1995;77A:1058–1064.

This study introduces the tip–apex distance as a way to summarize screw position. The authors demonstrate through multivariate logistic regression that although increasing patient age, unstable fracture pattens, and the use of high-angle devices are all independent predictors of increased risk for cutout failure, screw position as measured by the TAD is the strongest predictor. An odds ratio for failure by cutout based on the TAD is presented.

Carpenter JE, Kasman RA, Patel N, Lee ML, Goldstein SA. Biomechanical evaluation of current patella fracture fixation techniques. *J Orthop Trauma* 1997;11:351–356.

In this biomechanical study of cadaveric knees, the authors evaluated 3 forms of patellar fracture fixation: modified tension band, two 4.5-mm interfragmentary lag screws, and two 4.0-mm cannulated lag screws with a tension band wire through screws. The cannulated screws–tension band construct was found to be superior, with less displacement and a higher load to failure.

Schandelmaier P, Krettek MD, Rudolf J, Kohl A, Katz BE, Tscherne H. Superior results of tibial rodding versus external fixation in Grade IIIB fractures. *Clin Orthop* 1997;342:164–172.

Thirty-two grade IIIB open tibial fractures were followed for 2 years. Patients with intramedullary nailing had a shorter time to full weight bearing (11 versus 20 weeks), were less likely to need a bone graft, had better limb function scores, and had easier soft tissue coverage than patients with external fixators.

Hak DJ, Olson SA, Matta JM. Diagnosis and management of closed internal degloving injuries associated with pelvic and acetabular fractures: The Morel-Lavallière lesion. *J Trauma* 1997;42:1046–1051.

Twenty-four patients (6 lateral compression injuries, 6 sacroiliac joint dislocations and acetabular fractures, and 6 acetabular fractures alone) with closed internal degloving injury of the skin (Morel-Lavallière) were retrospectively reviewed. Forty-six percent of the cases had positive cultures, with staphylococcus and pseudomonas being the most common bacteria. Twenty-one percent of patients (3 out of 14) who received an open débridement and healing by secondary intention became secondarily infected, whereas no patient (0 out of 8) became secondarily infected after an open débridement and delayed primary closure. Recognition and thorough débridement either before or at the time of fracture fixation is recommended.

Refresher Questions

1. In the surgical management of comminuted talar neck fractures, what is the most common position of malreduction?
   a) varus
   b) valgus
   c) flexion
   d) internal rotation
   e) external rotation

2. Reconstruction or prosthetic replacement of the radial head is most important following an acute radial head fracture with associated distal radioulnar joint instability because the radial head is an important
   a) restraint to varus stress
   b) restraint to valgus stress
   c) restraint to proximal migration of the radius
   d) enabler of elbow flexion and extension
   e) enabler of forearm rotation

3. What is the best indication for intramedullary nailing of the humerus?
   a) impending pathologic fracture from metastatic disease
   b) open fracture
   c) closed fracture with associated femur fracture
   d) closed fracture with radial nerve palsy
   e) nonunion of a midshaft fracture

4. Nonsurgical management is most appropriate for which of the following transverse patellar fractures?
   a) nondisplaced fracture in an active 20-year-old laborer who can perform a straight leg raise
   b) minimally displaced fracture in a 40-year-old patient who cannot perform a straight leg raise
   c) displaced fracture in an 80-year-old retired farmer
   d) displaced fracture in a patient on renal dialysis
   e) displaced fracture in a patient with diabetes mellitus

5. Following surgical treatment of an intertrochanteric femur fracture with a fixed-angle dynamic hip screw, what factor has the greatest effect on the rate of implant cutout?
   a) length of the side plate
   b) length of the barrel

c) angle of the device
d) use of a compression screw
e) tip–apex distance

6. A young, healthy patient sustains a severe crush injury resulting in a comminuted midshaft tibia fracture and an 8 × 10-cm medial soft tissue defect with exposed bone. There is no associated vascular injury. Which of the following procedures will most predictably result in successful coverage?
   a) split-thickness skin graft
   b) fasciocutaneous flap
   c) soleus flap
   d) gastrocnemius flap
   e) free-tissue transfer

7. A 19-year-old man sustains an isolated, displaced transcervical femoral neck fracture in a motor vehicle accident. An urgent closed reduction attempt in the operating room results in residual varus angulation and 1 cm of displacement. Appropriate management should now consist of
   a) in situ fixation
   b) bipolar hemiarthroplasty
   c) total hip arthroplasty
   d) open reduction and internal fixation
   e) in situ fixation and bone grafting

8. In addition to the sinus tarsi artery, the arterial supply to the talar body comes from which of the following structures?
   a) lateral plantar artery and deltoid artery
   b) artery of the tarsal canal and recurrent plantar artery
   c) artery of the tarsal canal and lateral plantar artery
   d) artery of the tarsal canal and deltoid artery
   e) recurrent plantar artery and deltoid artery

9. What type of displaced unstable posterior pelvic ring injury will benefit most from open reduction and internal fixation?
   a) transforaminal sacral fracture
   b) sacral alar fracture
   c) iliac fracture
   d) sacroiliac fracture-dislocation
   e) sacroiliac dislocations

10. Which surgical approach to the acetabulum is associated with the highest rates of heterotopic ossification?
    a) Kocher-Langenbeck
    b) extended iliofemoral
    c) Watson-Jones
    d) Smith-Peterson
    e) ilioinguinal

Chapter 11

Biostatistics

G. RUSSELL HUFFMAN

I. INTRODUCTION

The systematic approach to accruing biomedical knowledge and accurately incorporating it into the practice of orthopaedic surgery involves the fields of epidemiology, biostatistics, and evidenced-based medicine. We apply methodologies from each of these areas of study into our everyday lives. It is therefore critical for the orthopaedic surgeon to be familiar with the tools of biostatistics in order to more accurately and critically assess the existing evidence justifying the assessment of at-risk populations, correctly diagnosing injury and illness, and treating musculoskeletal diseases. *Biostatistics* is the application of mathematical methods to the collection, organization, and interpretation of biological or medical data. *Inference* is the act of deriving logical conclusions from the existing knowledge regarding a condition. Biostatistical methods allow inferences to be made with a quantifiable degree of certainty. *Epidemiology* is the study of the distribution and determinants of disease frequency. Inferences are made regarding disease causes and associations, the success of treatments, and factors that may modify a condition by using biostatical methods in the framework of an epidemiologic study.

II. DATA

Data are factual information, especially information organized for analysis or used to reason or make decisions. This information may or may not be numerical. Biomedical data may be broadly characterized as one of 3 types: continuous, ordinal, or categorical. The type of data determines the appropriateness of given statistical methods to analyze a set of data.

Variables. Information acquired for a given characteristic is defined as a variable. For example, in a study assessing the incidence of low back pain, a researcher may obtain patient characteristics such as the estimated number of cigarettes smoked each day, an individual's body mass index, educational level in years, and type of work (sedentary or laborious). Each defined characteristic about which the researcher inquires and stores as data is a variable. Statistical methods may subsequently be used to find the likelihood of an association between the outcome of interest, in this case low back pain, and each variable or combination of variables.

- *Independent Variable*—One that determines the value of other variables according to its value. In an experimental trial, this variable would be controlled by the researcher (e.g., one treatment or another).
- *Dependent Variable*—The observed variable in an experiment or study the value of which is determined by the presence or degree of one or more independent variables. For example, a mathematical variable's value is determined by the value assumed by an independent variable. This is the outcome of interest.

Types of Data. Data are further categorized depending on whether they are numeric, ordered, or qualitative. The 3 categories of data are continuous, ordinal, and categorical.

- *Continuous Variable*—Describes numerical information that can be any given value within a range of values. Common examples of continuous variables used in medical research include age and body mass index. Common statistical methods for comparing continuous data values between 2 or more groups include means testing (student's t-test for comparison of the means of 2 groups and analysis of variance (ANOVA) for comparison of the means of 3 or more groups).
- *Ordinal Variable*—One in which the data is represented in an ordered fashion. For example, a researcher wishes to examine factors potentially associated with the severity of osteonecrosis of the femoral head. The researcher may employ a commonly used grading scale with a severity ranging from 1 to 4. Within the study, patients' hip radiographs are examined for the severity of osteonecrosis and assigned an integral number 1, 2, 3, or 4. For the purposes of statistical analysis, each number represents a discrete increase in the radiographic severity of the disease. In contrast, if a scale were continuous with a range of 1 to 4, then values could be any magnitude from 1 to 4 (e.g., 1.12, 2.35, 3.99).
- *Categorical (Nominal) Variable*—One in which the primary data is best described qualitatively rather than quantitatively. An example is an epidemiologic study designed to examine the risk of ulnar collateral injuries in baseball pitchers. Categorical variables a researcher might wish to consider might include type of pitcher: starting; middle reliever; closer; or the type of pitch that one typically throws most commonly: fastball; slider; change up; curve ball. Each variable is distinctly different from the other and may be assigned a numerical representation for the purposes of data analysis. However, there is no clear gradation between a curve ball, slider, or change up. In other words, there is no clear ordering of these variables. They simply are distinct qualitatively from one another.

Data Distribution. Continuous data may be parametric or nonparametric. Parametric data may be represented in a distribution explained by a single mathematical equation. The most widely recognized distribution of continuous, parametric data is Gaussian or normally distributed data (Fig. 11.1). The y-axis represents the probability (or percentage frequency) of observing a given value. The x-axis represents the range of possible continuous values. The area under the curve = 1.0, or the sum of probability of observing all given values. For a value to fall within "normal" limits, the value must fall within the mean ± 2 standard deviations. That is, with a normal distribution, 95% of the values will fall within ± 2 standard deviations of the mean. In a normal distribution, 69% of values will fall within ± 1 SD, 95% within ± 2 SD, and 99% within ± 3 SD of the mean. In a normal distribution, the mean, median, and mode are all equal. Each of these terms is a measurement of a data's central tendency, or the value that is most representative of the typical (or most predictable) value for an entire group.

- *Mean*—The sum of all observed measurements divided by the number of observations (i.e., the average value).

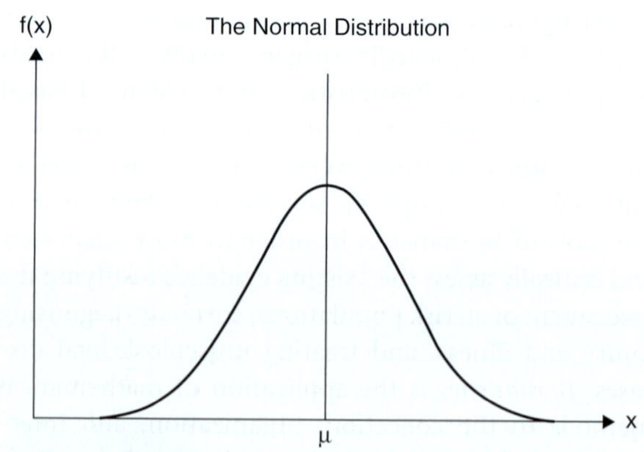

FIGURE 11.1 **Normal distribution.**

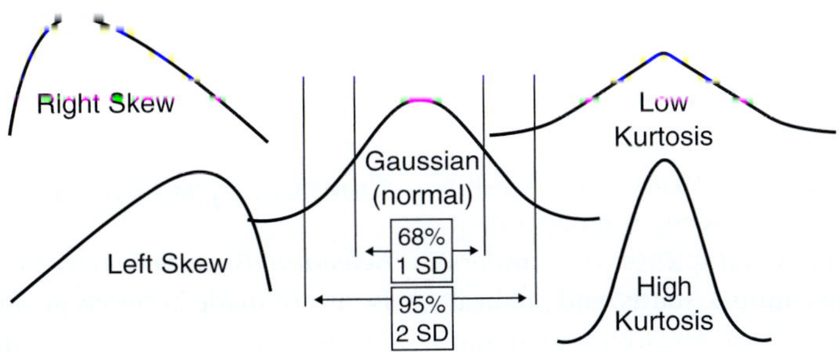

FIGURE 11.2 Types of data distribution and the effect on skew, kurtosis, and central tendency.

- *Median*—The 50th percentile, or the value below which half of the values fall. For nonparametric data, the median is a more robust measurement of the central tendency than the mean.
- *Mode*—The most frequently occurring observation.

Skewness. Continuous data may be skewed, or asymmetric about the mean (Fig. 11.2). Skewness is a statistical measure of the symmetry of the distribution of values about the mean for a given variable. For a normal distribution, the skewness = 0. In general, a right skew means that the median and mean have a smaller value than the mode. A left skew indicates that the mean and median have a greater value than the mode. Kurtosis is a measure of the peakedness of a unimodal distribution of data. Statistical tests for data skewness and kurtosis may be used to determine whether parametric means testing is appropriate.

- Normally distributed (Gaussian)
  - Area under curve = 1.0
  - 68.27% + / − 1 SD
  - 95.45% + / − 2 SD
  - 99.73% + / − 3 SD
- Mean, median, and mode are equal

Statistical Methods. Biostatistics applies mathematics to quantify the probability of occurrences and to analyze data.

III. INFERENCE

The purpose of a well-designed research study is to help us gain more knowledge that gives us insight into the truth about a clinical problem. This is the science of inference, a determination arrived at by reasoning using facts to derive a broader conclusion. In statistical assessment, we often draw conclusions about the population as a whole on the basis of information gathered from a sample, representative or not, of the whole. Our ability to accurately determine the truth from a limited sample of the whole is compromised by systematic error characterized by bias, confounding, and chance. The level of evidence, or weight to which we place our trust in a study's results, depends largely on the study's ability to minimize these errors in design.

Errors in Inference

There are 2 ways in which incorrect conclusions may be drawn about data. A study may have a systematic error or design flaw caused by bias or confounding, or chance may influence the interpretation of a study.

Bias. Bias is a nonrandom, systematic error in the design or conduct of a study that may result in mistaken inference about association or causation. In the orthopaedic literature, common types of bias include recall bias, or potential error introduced in a retrospective study in which patients or clinicians are asked to relay an exposure that previously occurred and about which imperfect records may exist. If a researcher is to examine an association between antibiotics and the risk of subsequent Achilles tendon rupture, he or she may wish to first identify patients with Achilles tendon ruptures. Once these patients are identified, the researcher then assesses exposure to antibiotics by asking these patients about history of antibiotic use prior to the tendon rupture. In a similar group of patients without tendon rupture, the exposure risk to antibiotics over the same time period is assessed in a similar fashion. The problem with this methodology is that patients may not remember perfectly their history of antibiotic exposure. Similarly, patients may be led by the manner in which a question is asked. This type of error is inherent in retrospective studies assessing exposure risk (antibiotics) to an outcome of interest (tendon rupture). A method to avoid recall bias is to enroll a cohort of persons without Achilles tendon rupture in a prospective study in which the use of antibiotics is carefully monitored. As each new case of tendon rupture is identified, the researchers are readily, and without bias, able to determine whether the person was exposed to antibiotics. The problem with this methodology is that it is extremely time consuming and costly, particularly for events that occur rarely.

Confounders. A confounder is a variable that has an association with both the independent and dependent variables of a study. Common examples of confounders include age, gender, socioeconomic status, and medical comorbidities. For example, if the researcher wishes to determine the longevity of implant A against implant B, then he or she should account for each patient's activity level and age. If it can be shown through preliminary data or historical data that young age is associated with accelerated implant wear, then it is vital that the researcher demonstrate that there is no statistical difference in the central tendency (mean or median) age of those treated with implant A compared to those treated with implant B. Each comparative study should have a clearly demarcated demographic table (Table 11.1) showing a value of central tendency (mean or median) for each variable that might possibly be related to both outcome (implant longevity) and exposure (implant A vs. B). Randomized clinical trials should eliminate potential confounders, making the probability distribution equal within each treatment arm unless differences occur by chance alone. In either event, if groups differ with respect to potential confounders, then these variables should be accounted for with appropriate statistical measures.

Chance. Chance is the probability that 2 unrelated events will appear associated by accident or through random occurrence. Studies that fail to adequately control for chance occurrences may make invalid conclusions based on the probability of type I error (concluding a true association exists between variables or risk factors and outcome when in reality there is none) and type II error (probability of failing to find a true association when one in fact does exist).

TABLE 11.1 Demographic table

Factor	*Implant A*	*Implant B*	*P-value*
Age (mean)	67	66	0.48
Gender (% male)	56	54	0.45
BMI	40	31	0.04

All comparative studies should display a demographic display of baseline characteristics in order to determine potential confounding variables. In this instance, body mass index (BMI) is statistically associated with the type of implant used. Even if this association occurs by chance, it should be accounted for statistically, either by stratification or in a multivariate analysis controlling for BMI, when one draws conclusions regarding the outcomes with implant A compared to implant B.

The methods to minimize bias, confounding, and chance are through study design and statistical analysis.

Common Types of Bias

Selection Bias. Selection bias occurs when comparisons are made between groups of patients who differ in important ways other than the main factor under consideration. This leads to confounding. An example the comparison of healing rates after lumbar spine fusion for 2 competing fixation devices. If 1 device is used exclusively in 1 geographical region and the other in a separate location, then factors such as education, smoking rates, median income, and surgeon experience may affect success and be different between the 2 locations.

Recall Bias. An individual's remembrance of an exposure may be influenced by having the outcome of interest. Means of controlling for this include randomization (bias equally likely in each treatment group) and prospective cohort (exposure recorded as it happens).

Measurement Bias. Measurement bias is possible when patients in one subgroup are more likely than another subgroup to have their outcome or exposure detected. This bias may be minimized by blinding researchers to each subgroup when determining exposure, establishing strict definitions of exposure or risk, and seeking to elucidate outcome events in all patient subgroups with equal vigor. In addition to blinding, prospective assessment of outcomes and having an independent assessment of outcome help minimize this type of bias.

Publication Bias. The tendency for published studies to differ systematically from all completed studies is called publication bias. The most common example is that more favorable (or statistically significant) results are more likely to reach formal publication (Fig. 11.3).

Sampling Bias. Sampling bias occurs when patients selected for a study are systematically different from the population to which the results are generalized. Sampling bias leads to a lack of external validity, or inability to extrapolate the study's findings to all populations equally.

Methods for Controlling Selection Bias

- Design phase of study
  - *Randomization*—Assign patients into treatment groups in a manner that affords an equal

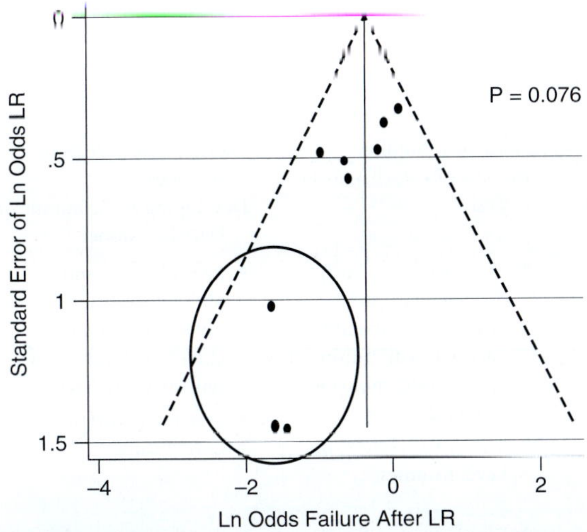

FIGURE 11.3 Funnel plot with pseudo 95% confidence limits for Ln failure after lateral release. Funnel plots are graphical means of assessing for publication bias. This plot shows the standard error compared to the effect, in this case the natural logarithm of the rate of recurrent instability following isolated lateral retinacular release for patellofemoral instability. As the SE increases, the sample size decreases. This plot shows a strong trend toward publication bias for isolated lateral release papers. Studies with a larger SE show a lower rate of instability (encircled studies) indicating publication bias, or better results in smaller studies. Publication bias may also be detected by assessing year of publication, journal type, and sample size.

probability of a given patient being given each treatment.

- *Restriction*—Limit the characteristics of patients studied; also called inclusion and exclusion criteria.
- *Matching*—Select control patients with characteristics similar to those of the group of interest with respect to potentially confounding characteristics save for the exposure or characteristic of interest to the study.

- Statistical analysis phase of study
    - *Stratification*—Compare rates within subgroups (strata) with otherwise similar probability of the outcome. An example is a comparison of outcomes after either surgical or nonsurgical treatment of a given fracture type. A logical stratification of outcomes would be according to fracture classification (severity).
    - *Simple Adjustment*—Mathematical adjustment of crude rates for a given characteristic so that equal weight is assigned to strata of similar risk.
    - *Multivariable Analysis*—Mathematical modeling that adjusts the risk assigned to a given factor based on the influence or association of this factor to other characteristics.

Other factors to consider when making inferences from a study include the characteristics deemed necessary for causality.

Causality

- *Temporality*—Cause precedes effect
- *Strength*—Large relative risk
- *Dose Response*—Larger exposures are associated with higher rates of disease or more severe disease
- *Reversibility*—Reduction in exposure is followed by lower rates of disease
- *Consistency*—Repeatedly observed by different researchers in different places and times
- *Biologic plausibility*—Reasonable based on current scientific understanding
- *Specificity*—One cause leads to one effect
- *Analogy*—Cause-and-effect relationship already established for a separate but similar exposure or disease

IV. STUDY DESIGN AND EVIDENCED-BASED MEDICINE

Overview. Evidenced-based medicine incorporates the conscientious, explicit, and judicious use of the current best evidence in making decisions about the care of individual patients. The best evidence is acquired through epidemiologic and scientific studies analyzed with biostatistical methods and from which inferences (conclusions) have been made. The more rigorously designed the study and the more carefully a study's authors have analyzed data to minimize error, the more confident one can be in the meaningfulness of a given study. An outline of the levels of evidence for clinical studies is demonstrated in Table 11.2.

Observational Versus Experimental Studies. One may more confidently draw inferences about a study that has adequately accounted for bias, confounding,

TABLE 11.2 Levels of evidence

	Types of Studies			
	Therapeutic Studies: Investigating the Results of Treatment	Prognostic Studies: Investigating the Effect of a Patient Characteristic on the Outcome of Disease	Diagnostic Studies: Investigating a Diagnostic Test	Economic and Decision Analyses: Developing an Economic or Decision Model
Level I	• High-quality randomized trial with statistically significant difference or no statistically significant difference but narrow confidence intervals[1] • Systematic review[2] of Level I RCTs (and study results were homogenous[3])	• High quality prospective study[4] (all patients were enrolled at the same point in their disease with ≥ 80% follow-up of enrolled patients) • Systematic review[2] of Level I studies	• Testing of previously developed diagnostic criteria on consecutive patients (with universally applied reference gold standard) • Systematic review[2] of Level I studies	• Sensible costs and alternatives; values obtained from many studies with multiway sensitivity analyses • Systematic review[2] of Level I studies
Level II	• Lesser quality RCT (e.g., < 80% follow-up, no blinding, or improper randomization) • Prospective[4] comparative study[5] • Systematic review[2] of Level II studies or Level I studies with inconsistent results	• Retrospective[6] study • Untreated controls from an RCT • Lesser quality prospective study (e.g., patients enrolled at different points in their disease or < 80% follow-up) • Systematic review[2] of Level II studies	• Development of diagnostic criteria on consecutive patients (with universally applied reference gold standard) • Systematic review[2] of Level II studies	• Sensible costs and alternatives; values obtained from limited studies with multiway sensitivity analyses • Systematic review[2] of Level II studies
Level III	• Case control study[7] • Retrospective[6] comparative study[5] • Systematic review[2] of Level III studies	• Case control study[7]	• Study of nonconsecutive patients; without consistently applied reference gold standard • Systematic review[2] of Level III studies	• Analyses based on limited alternatives and costs; and poor estimates • Systematic review[2] of Level III studies
Level IV	Case series[8]	Case series	• Case-control study • Poor reference standard	• Analyses with no sensitivity analyses
Level V	Expert opinion	Expert opinion	Expert opinion	Expert opinion

[1]A complete assessment of quality of individual studies requires critical appraisal of all aspects of the study design.
[2]A combination of results from two or more prior studies.
[3]Studies provided consistent results.
[4]Study was started before the first patient enrolled.
[5]Patients treated one way (e.g., cemented hip arthroplasty) compared with a group of patients treated in another way (e.g., uncemented hip arthroplasty) at the same institution.
[6]The study was started after the first patient enrolled.
[7]Patients identified for the study based on their outcome, called cases (e.g., failed total arthroplasty) are compared with patients who did not have outcome, called controls (e.g., successful total hip arthroplasty).
[8]Patients treated one way with no comparison group of patients treated in another way.
Source: Clinical Orthopaedics and Related Research, Information for Authors.

and chance. Clinical research studies may be broadly categorized as either observational or experimental in design. The majority of the orthopaedic surgery literature is observational (Figure 11.4).

- *Observational Studies*
  - Descriptive
    - Case reports
    - Case series
    - Cross-sectional studies
      - — Often unable to demonstrate causality but informative and useful for obtaining background information laying the groundwork for more sophisticated studies
  - Analytic
    - Case-control trials
    - Cohort studies
    - Meta-analyses
      - — No allocation of treatment groups
      - — Prospective or retrospective
      - — Useful in determining causality or the association between risk factors and an outcome of interest

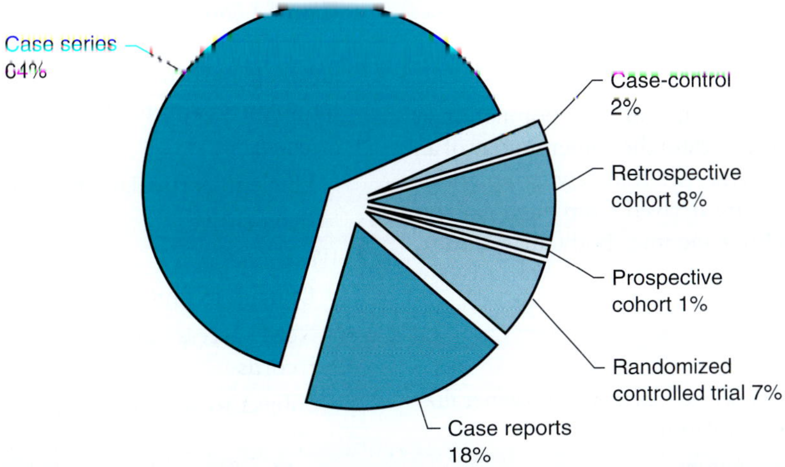

FIGURE 11.4 **Distribution of study types published in *JBJS* and *CORR*. (*Source*: Freedman KB, Bernstein J. *JBJS Br* 2001; 397.)**

- — Provide background information for designing experimental or further observational studies (e.g., prospective longitudinal cohort studies)

- *Experimental*
  - Randomized clinical trial
    - Prospective
    - Optimum for evaluating the efficacy of a treatment
    - However, unable to determine causality

Observational studies may further be categorized as retrospective or prospective, depending on the line of inquiry (Figure 11.5).

- *Retrospective study*—The direction of inquiry begins with the outcome of interest and attempts to elucidate a risk factor or exposure that may contribute. The classic example of a retrospective study design is the case-control design, which is most efficient when dealing with rare events or outcomes.
- *Prospective study*—The direction of inquiry begins with defining an exposure or risk factor and waiting to observe the outcome of interest to occur. Large prospective cohort studies (e.g., Framingham Heart Study or LEAP study) are more efficient with a predictable rate of outcome or event to more quickly determine associated risk factors with the incidence of an outcome as it occurs.

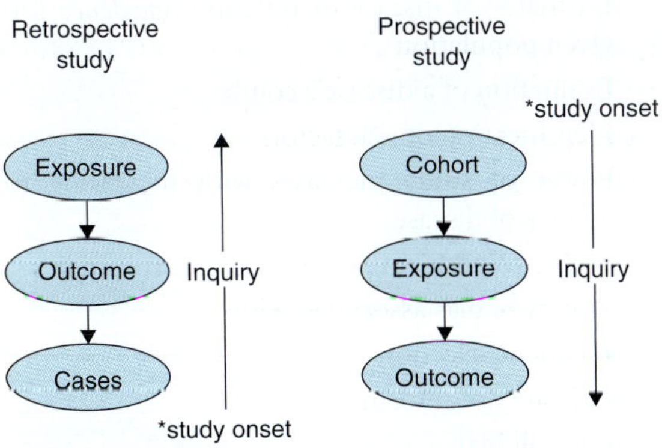

FIGURE 11.5 **Direction of inquiry in observational studies may be either retrospective or prospective.**

Description of Study Types

Case Series. Retrospective, descriptive account of a group of patients with an interesting or unique set of characteristics or who have undergone a similar treatment. The usefulness of this type of data lies in describing potential complications or success or generating background information for more sophisticated studies.

- *Example*—John Charnley's description of the successful use of methyl methacrylate in securing components used in total hip arthroplasty informed the orthopaedic community of the safety and potential success of its use.
- *Strengths*
  - Inexpensive
  - Avenue to describe results with novel treatments
  - Background data for future studies
  - May describe complication rate for a narrow population
- *Weaknesses*
  - Subject to bias, confounding, chance
  - No hypothesis

- *Type*—Observational-descriptive
- *Level IV evidence*

Cross-Sectional Study. "Snapshot" of a population at a given time. One may ascertain the epidemiology of an outcome or of a risk factor. Alternatively, population-based normative data are derived from such surveys (e.g., median household income, body mass index, intelligence quotient).

- *Strengths*
  - Quick
  - Obtain data that may be extrapolated (generalizable) to a larger population
  - May observe associations
  - Good baseline data on disease or exposure prevalence for designing future study or directing future inquiry
  - Useful for obtaining normative values of a population
  - Define the demography of a population
  - Useful for determining the prevalence of a condition at that given time
  - $\text{Prevalence} = \dfrac{\text{total \# of cases at a given time}}{\text{total \# of persons observed at risk}}$
- *Weaknesses*
  - Sampling error may limit ability to apply to general population
  - Will not provide *incidence*, which requires a time of observation typically only provided through longitudinal cohort studies or comprehensive administrative databases (e.g., government death registry).
  - $\text{Incidence} = \dfrac{\text{\# of new cases over a time interval}}{\text{total number of persons observed (in time period)}}$
- *Type*—Observational-descriptive
- *Level IV evidence*, or evidence for sampling estimates of normative values, demography, epidemiology, and deriving estimates used for power calculations

Case-Control Study. Patients with a given outcome (cases) are compared to patients without the outcome of interest (controls), and risk factors are statistically assessed for association. This method allows one to draw inferences regarding the causality of *rare* or uncommon occurrences. Typically, results are reported as an *odds ratio* or the odds of a case being exposed to a factor of interest compared to the odds of a control being exposed to the same factor.

- *Example*—Study assessing the association between fluoroquinolone antibiotics and Achilles tendon rupture. Cases: patients with Achilles tendon rupture; controls: a cohort of individuals similar to cases without Achilles tendon rupture. Both groups are then retrospectively examined for exposure to quinolones prior to tendon rupture.
- *Strengths*
  - Efficient, particularly for rare conditions
  - Inexpensive
- *Weaknesses*
  - Difficult to find appropriate control group
  - Need access to complete, thorough medical records
  - Subject to confounding, which can be addressed by:
    - Matching of cases and controls on similar attributes not directly related to the exposure of interest
    - Multivariate analysis
  - Subject to bias
    - Recall
    - Reporting
    - Sampling
- *Type*—Observational-analytical
  - Study effect presented as odds ratio (OR)
- *Level III to IV evidence*, depending on sophistication of study

Prospective Cohort. A population of interest is identified and followed prospectively to determine outcomes and statistical associations with known (and potentially unknown) risk factors.

- *Example*—Framingham Heart Study prospectively collecting information on risk factors and examining cardiovascular disease in light of these risk factors as cardiovascular events are detected.
- *Strengths*—A prospective cohort study provides:
  - Estimates of disease or outcome *incidence* for a given population
  - Evaluation of a disease's course
  - Identification of risk factors
  - Power of study increases with increasing frequency of disease
  - Ability to perform nested case-control studies
  - Minimize bias associated with:
    - Patient selection
    - Quality of information
    - Recall bias
- *Weaknesses*
  - Expensive
    - Need sustainable multiyear funding
  - Labor-intensive

- Mechanism for comprehensive prospective data collection
- Long-term (10 + years) cohorts most useful
  - Need stable population
  - Inefficient at assessing rare outcomes
  - Susceptible to bias, confounding, and error
- *Type*—Observational-analytical
  - Study effect presented as a relative risk (RR)
- *Level II to III evidence,* depending on rate of follow-up (more than 90%), data collection, and sophistication

Randomized Clinical Trial (RCT). Involves the use of concurrent (RCT), sequential (cross-over trials), or historical controls. The gold standard is the double-blind, placebo-controlled, randomized clinical trial. Randomized controlled trial requires a protocol that establishes:

- Eligibility
- Sample size
  - Ensures adequate power to detect a difference in treatments if one truly exists
- Informed consent
- Randomization
  - Minimizes selection bias and confounders (both known and unknown)
- Blinding
  - Minimizes performance, detection, interviewer, and acceptability bias
- Rules for study cessation
- Monitoring of compliance
- Safety assessment
- Data Analysis
  - Intention to treat analysis
    - Minimizes nonresponder bias

Experimental Study. These studies are expensive, timely, and logistically difficult because of patient accrual and physician acceptance. Ethically, they require equipoise (no known advantage to one arm over the other with respect to safety and benefit).

Efficacy vs. Effectiveness. Excellent internal validity (result x occurs under experimental circumstances). But this does not mean that results will be similar given different settings, patient populations, and so on.

- *Example*—AIDS patients in Africa at risk for TB given a vaccine compared to AIDS patients in Europe or the United States.
- *External validity* (is study generalizable)
  - Is studied group a representative sample of entire population or populations of interest?
  - Is the standard of care applied available?

- Weaknesses
  - Expensive
  - Timely
  - Logistically difficult
    - Patient accrual, physician acceptance
  - Ethically require equipoise (no known advantage to one arm over the other with respect to safety and benefit)
  - Not useful for determining cause and effect for rare conditions
- *Strengths*
  - Minimizes chance, bias, and confounding
  - Ideal for determining the efficacy of one treatment over another
- *Level I to II evidence,* depending on sample size, randomization technique, blinding, appropriate nontreatment (placebo) control, and percentage of retained subjects (more than 90%)

Reviews. There are several levels of review studies.

- *Level V*—An expert's assimilation of his or her knowledge of the current diagnosis or treatment of a disorder without *systematically* selecting quality studies from all available literature or statistically assessing the published literature.
- *Systematic Reviews (Levels IIa and IIIa)*—Evidenced-based summary of the medical literature that uses explicit methods to perform a complete literature search and critical appraisal of the studies. If the studies included in the systematic review are level III evidence, then the systematic review's level of evidence will also be level III.
- *Meta-Analysis (Levels Ia and IIa)*—An evidenced-based systematic review that uses quantitative methods to combine the results of several independent studies to produce summary statistics; most commonly, this refers to the systematic review of similar randomized clinical trials.
  1. Establish a summary estimate
     a. A forest plot may be created as a representation of the summary effect of a treatment (Fig. 11.6). Also known as a stem and leaf plot, a forest plot shows the summary effect of data collected from multiple studies. This graph summarizes findings from a systematic review of recurrent patellofemoral instability after lateral retinacular release alone compared to lateral release and medial reefing.
  2. Assess study homogeneity (Q-test) with respect to:
     a. Clinical treatment
     b. Methodology
     c. Measured effect (outcome)

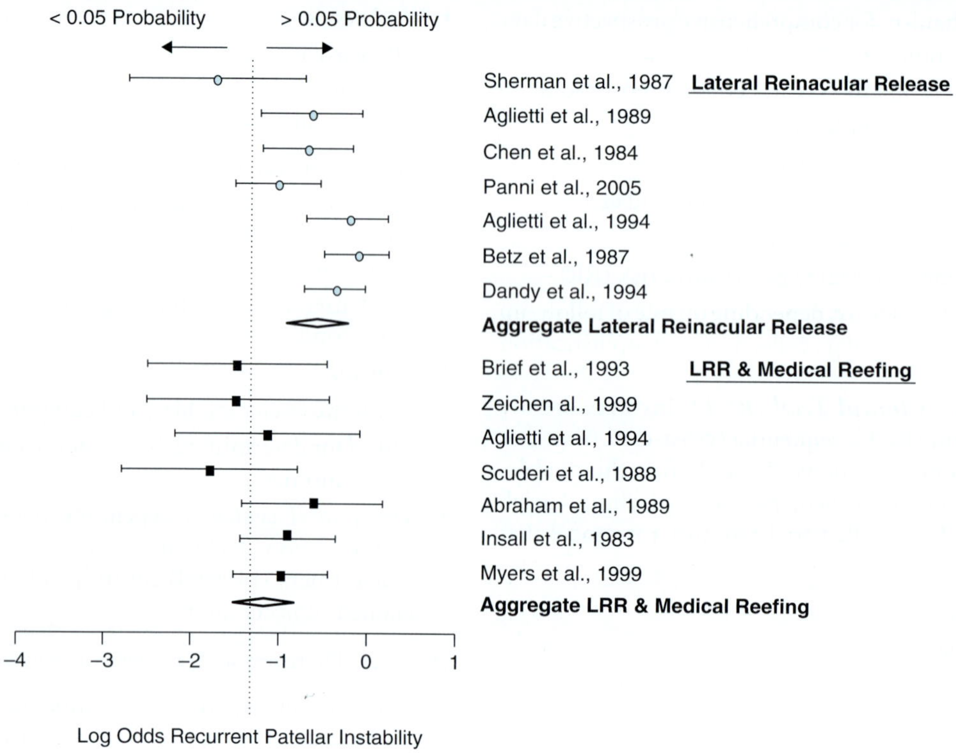

FIGURE 11.6 **Forest (or stem and leaf) plot.** ***Adapted from*** **Richetti E, Huffman GR, et al. 2006 AANA Meeting, Hollywood, FL.**

3. Assess publication bias
   a. See Funnel plot example (see Fig. 11.3)
   b. Both parametric (Egger linear regression model) and nonparametric (Begg tests) can be used to assess for publication bias

V. HYPOTHESIS TESTING

Statistical Significance. The classical approach to assessing the statistical significance involves comparing observed sample findings with theoretically expected findings (the hypothesis). This comparison allows one to compute the probability that the observed outcome could have been due to chance alone. The comparison also determines if a null hypothesis (there is no difference between treatments or there is no association between a risk factor and a given outcome) is correct or may be rejected (Figs. 11.7 and 11.8).

Statistical Significance Versus Clinical Significance. Classic methods of hypothesis testing will not help one determine statistical significance versus clinical (practical) significance. In other words, say that an investigator wants to determine whether one ACL reconstruction is superior to another. The null hypothesis is that the two are the same. Clinically,

Study Conclusion	Reality (Truth): Treatments are not different	Reality (Truth): Treatments are different
Treatments are not different	Correct Decision	Type II error (Probability = β)
Treatments are different	Type I error (Probability = α)	Correct Decision (Probability = $1 - \beta$)

FIGURE 11.7 **Hypothesis testing.**

	Disease +	Disease –
test +	A (true +)	B (false +)
test –	C (false –)	D (true –)

Sensitivity = a / (a+c)
Specificity = d / (b+d)

False-negative rate = (1 – sensitivity)
False-positive rate = (1 – specificity)

FIGURE 11.8 **Sensitivity and specificity.**

a failure is defined as 5 mm of side-to-side (ACL reconstructed to contralateral normal knee) anterior tibial displacement with KT 1000 arthrometer testing. Patients are randomized to group A and group B with significance set at 0.05 and adequate power to detect a real difference with 90% certainty given at least a 1-mm side-to-side difference. Group A patients and Group B patients do equally well clinically. However, a 1.2-mm side-to-side difference favors Group A with a p-value of 0.02. Is this result significant? Statistically, yes; however, the clinical or practical significance may be less clear.

- *p-value*
  - The probability of an event occurring by chance alone
  - Calculated with a statistical test
  - Measure of the *strength of evidence* in favor of the null hypothesis
  - If $p < \alpha$, then the evidence against the null hypothesis is strong enough for us to reject it
  - No units
  - No strength of association
  - Little precision
- *Confidence intervals*
  - Do not overlap if statistically significant
  - Provide clinical significance (magnitude of values)
  - Are precise (give range of values within a CI)

$$\alpha(\text{alpha}) = \text{probability of making a type I error}$$

α is the probability of concluding treatments differ, when in reality they do not. The lower α, the more rigorous the standard for rejecting the null hypothesis and the less likely an association may occur by chance alone.

At $\alpha = 0.05$, probability of making a type I error (concluding true association when there is none) by chance alone is 1 in 20.

At $\alpha = 0.01$, probability of association by chance alone is 1 in 100.

$$\beta(\text{beta}) = \text{probability of making a type II error}$$

or the probability of concluding the treatments do not differ when in reality they do differ.

$$\text{Power} = 1 - \text{probability of making a type II error}$$
$$= 1 - b$$

or the probability of detecting a difference between the treatments if the treatments do in fact differ.

When a study demonstrates significant association, then potential error is type I (α). However, when a study demonstrates no significant association, then potential error is type II (β), and it may be that with increased subjects or less variation, a significant association would become apparent. When no statistically significant association is detected, then the power of a study should be reported.

Elements of a Power Calculation. α, β, variance (standard deviation about the mean), the sample size, and estimated values or effect size in each group will help determine the ability of a study to detect a "significant" difference if one truly exists. Each component of the power calculation may be determined from the other elements. Statistical tests are mathematical means of determining the probability of type I error (Table 11.3).

TABLE 11.3 Types of statistical tests

Type of Data	*No. Groups*	*Independent*	*Paired*
Continuous			
Normal	2	Student t test	Paired t test
Nonnormal	2	Mann-Whitney U test	Wilcoxon signed rank test
Normal	> 2	ANOVA	Repeated-measures ANOVA
Nonnormal	> 2	Kruskal-Wallis test	Friedman test
Proportions	2 (large number of observations)	Chi square	
	2 (small number of observations)	Fischer exact	
Ordinal	2	Mann-Whitney U test	Wilcoxon signed rank test
	> 2	Kruskal-Wallis	Friedman test
Nominal	2	Fisher exact	McNemar test
	> 2	Pearson Chi square	Cochran Q test
Survival	2/> 2	Log-rank	Conditional logistic regression

Common Statistical Tests Used in Medical Research. The following tests are used to determine the statistical significance of a difference:

- *Chi square* (X^2)—Compares proportions, observed and expected
- *Fisher's exact*—Compares proportions for a small number of observations
- *Mann-Whitney U*—Compares median values
- *Student t*—Compares mean values
- *F test/analysis of variance (ANOVA)*—Compares two or more means

The following tests are used to describe or measure agreement

- *Regression coefficient*—Association between an independent variable and a dependent (outcome) variable
- *Pearson's r*—Association between two variables
- *Kappa*—A measure of agreement (interobserver) beyond the agreement that is expected due to chance. Values range from 0 (amount of agreement observed by chance alone) to 1 (perfect agreement).

Measures of Effect

- *Probability*—A value between 0 and 1, indicating how likely an event is to occur on the basis of number of events occurring per number of trials (e.g., in a coin toss, for heads, p = 0.5)
- *Odds*—Ratio of the probability of an event occurring to an event not occurring (e.g., in a coin toss, for heads, 0.5/0.5 = 1)
- *Odds ratio (OR)*—Odds of exposure to a risk factor among cases compared to the odds of exposure to a risk factor in the control group
- *Relative risk (RR)*—Incidence of disease in exposed cohort divided by the incidence of disease in the nonexposed cohort
- *Hazard function*—Probability of the event occurring at a given time point
- *Positive predictive value (PPV)*—Probability of patient having a disease when a test result is positive

$$\text{PPV} = [(\text{prevalence})(\text{sensitivity})] / [(\text{prevalence})(\text{sensitivity})] + [(1 - \text{prevalence})(1 - \text{specificity})]$$

- *Negative predictive value (NPV)*—Probability of patient not having a disease when a test result is negative

$$\text{NPV} = (1 - \text{prevalence})(\text{specificity}) / [(1 - \text{prevalence})(\text{specificity})] + [(\text{prevalence})(1 - \text{sensitivity})]$$

- *Logarithmic Regression*
  - $Px = 1/\{1 + \exp[bo + bx]\}$
  - Other nonlinear mathematical models
- *Survival Analysis*
  - Probability as function of time
  - Univariate
    - Log rank test
    - Kaplan Meier survival curve (Fig. 11.9); this is a type of time-to-event analysis in which the denominator of exposed persons (in this case, patients undergoing arthroscopic elbow capsular release) changes at each time interval. Time intervals are defined at the point at which a failure or event occurs. Patients leaving the study (for failure or lack of clinical follow-up)

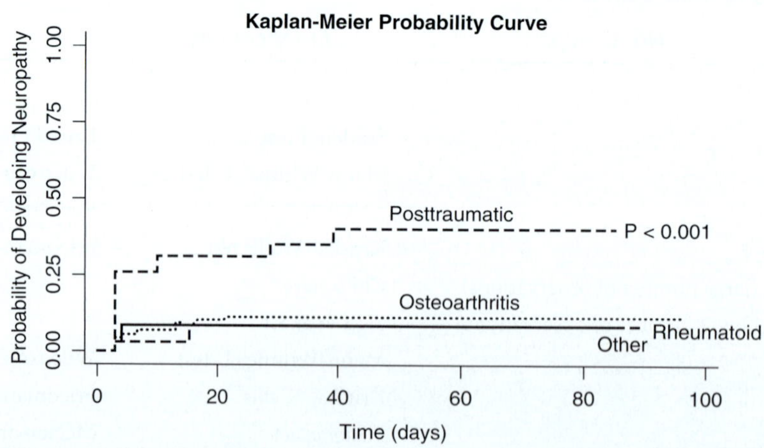

FIGURE 11.9 **Kaplan-Meier probability curve showing the probability of developing a delayed-onset ulnar neuropathy after arthroscopic elbow capsular release by preoperative diagnosis.** ***Adapted from*** **Huffman GR, O'Driscoll S. 2006 AAOS Annual Meeting, Chicago, IL.**

are removed as each event occurs. As with other statistical assessments, one assumption is that the rate of censorship (leaving a study for lack of follow-up) is the same for each group.

- Multivariate
  - Cox proportional hazard function

Model the Effects of Multiple Variables

Linear Regression. Linear regression assesses associations between risk factors and a continuous outcome. For each incremental increase in a risk factor, there is a linear increase in the outcome of interest (Fig. 11.10) according to the mathematical expression $Y = a + bX$, where X is the explanatory variable (exposure or risk factor) and Y is the dependent variable (outcome of interest). The slope of the line is b, and a is the intercept (the value of y when $x = 0$).

Logistic Regression. Logistic regression assesses associations between risk factors and a dichotomous (binary) outcome.

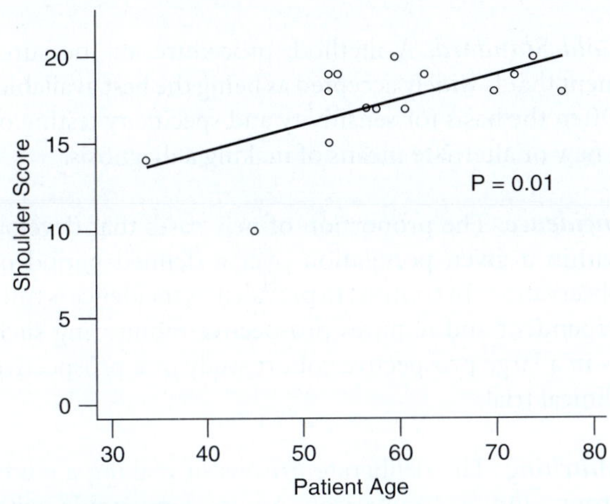

FIGURE 11.10 **Example of linear regression analysis demonstrating a significant association between increasing patient age and increasing shoulder score. Y = a + bX, where Y is the shoulder score, a is the y-intercept, b is the slope (change in shoulder score per increase in age by year), and X is the patient age. *Adapted from* Huffman GR, Wolf E. Functional results and cosmesis after arthroscopic tenotomy of the long head of the biceps brachii. *University of Pennsylvania Orthopaedic Journal* 2005; 17:15.**

Cox Proportional Hazards. Cox proportional hazards assesses associations between risk factors and a time-to-event outcome.

VI. HEALTH OUTCOMES RESEARCH

Musculoskeletal Outcomes Instruments. The AAOS and other organizations have developed measurement instruments designed to collect standardized patient-respondent data for use in clinical practice settings to assess the effectiveness of treatment regimens and in musculoskeletal research to study the clinical outcomes of treatment. These instruments have been validated (they measure what they are intended to measure) and are reliable (similar results are obtained for a given respondent at a given time when the outcomes assessment is repeated). Examples include:

- Hip Society Score
- Knee Society Score (KSS)
- DASH
- Pediatric Outcomes Data Collection Instrument
- (IKDC) International Knee Documentation Committee Subjective Knee
- ASES subjective shoulder scale

General Health Outcomes Instruments. There are two general health outcomes instruments: the Short Form 36 (SF36) and the Womac.

Visual Analog Scale. This tool is a scale 10 cm in length representing a range from worst to best for a given outcome. The respondent places a mark on the line at the point that most represents his or her experience at that particular time. To minimize bias, the scale should be free from numbers or markings (except at either extreme). It is then scored from 0 to 100 and has been shown to be valid and reliable as a simple measure of pain, satisfaction, and general outcome.

VII. GLOSSARY OF TERMS

Accuracy. The proportion of all test results, both positive and negative, that are correct.

Analysis of Variance (ANOVA). Statistical test of significance developed by Sir Ronald Fisher. It is also called the F-ratio or ANOVA (analysis of variance). The test is designed to establish whether or not a significant (nonchance/nonrandom) difference exists among several sample means. Statistically, it is the ratio of the variance occurring between the sample means to the variance occurring within the sample groups. A large F-ratio—that is, when the variance between is larger than the variance within—usually indicates a nonchance/nonrandom significant difference—that is, a difference created by the introduction of the independent variable.

Bias. Systematic error inherent in a study design. A process at any stage of inference that produces results that systematically depart from truth. Bias may occur during the collection, analysis, interpretation, publication, or review of data.

Cause and Effect. Inference of causation requires the following:

- Supporting data from nonobservational studies (RCT)
- Biologic plausibility
- Large effect size
- Reproducibility
- Temporal relationship between cause and effect
- Dose–response relationship

Cohort. A group of patients with a unifying characteristic. An example of an orthopaedic cohort is a set of patients all undergoing total knee replacement with the same implant. This group may then be followed prospectively for an outcome of interest (e.g., implant longevity, loosening, maximum achieved range of flexion) and characteristics assessed with respect to the outcome of interest (surgeon, side of surgery, year of surgery, type of bearing surface).

Confidence Interval. A measure of the precision of an estimated value. The interval represents the range of values, consistent with the data, that is believed to encompass the true value with high probability ($1 - \alpha$, where typically $\alpha = 0.05$). The confidence interval is expressed in the same units as the estimate. Wider intervals indicate lower precision; narrow intervals indicate greater precision. For a 95% CI, the distribution encompasses $+/-$ 1.96 standard error (i.e., there is a 95 percent probability that the true value of a measurement or calculated value lies within the specified range).

Confounder. A variable associated with both the outcome of interest and potential risk factors. The effect of one variable (the true risk factor associated with an outcome) is closely associated with the effect of another variable (the confounding variable) on the outcome of interest. The effect of one is distorted by the effect of the other. Confounders may be detected through the use of a demographic table to assess for statistically significant associations (the p-value or threshold for a potential confounder should be less stringent: $p \sim 0.10$). One may statistically control for confounders through the use of (1) stratified analysis or (2) multivariate analysis.

Correlation Coefficient. Allows for the measurement of relation between two variables. Correlation analysis is useful in screening known risk factors for association. For example, one studies the risk of infection after total knee replacement and in the given population, smoking, diabetes, and level of education are associated with the outcome of interest (postoperative infection). However, smoking and level of education are inversely correlated (those with higher degrees of education are less likely to smoke); therefore, the final statistical analysis must account for both factors simultaneously (a multivariate analysis).

For assessment of inter- or intraobserver agreement, the correlation coefficient fails to account for agreement that may occur by chance alone. In determining agreement, the kappa statistic is preferred for this reason.

Gold Standard. A method, procedure, or measurement that is widely accepted as being the best available. Often the basis for sensitivity and specificity testing of a new or alternate means of making a diagnosis.

Incidence. The proportion of new cases that develop within a given population over a defined period of observation. In contrast to prevalence, incidence is time dependent and requires prospective monitoring such as in a large prospective cohort study or a prospective clinical trial.

Matching. The deliberate process of making a study group and a comparison group comparable with respect to factors that are felt to be extraneous to the purpose of the investigation but that might interfere (through confounding) with the interpretation of the study's findings (for example, in case-control studies, individual cases might be matched or paired with a specific control on the basis of comparable age, gender, clinical features, or a combination of these in order to detect differences in true risk factors between cases and controls).

Mean. The average is also called sample mean—the expected value of a random variable, which is also called the population mean. The arithmetic mean is calculated as $\Sigma\ (n)/n$, where n represents the number of individual values in the sample.

Multivariate Analysis. Techniques that involve mathematical modeling to adjust or control for the effects of several variables in determining the independent effects of one variable on the outcome of interest. It is also used to determine variables that independently contribute to the overall variation in outcome. Examples include Cox proportional hazard model (time-to-event in survival analysis), logistic regression (dichotomous outcomes in case-control studies), and linear regression (continuous outcome in longitudinal cohort studies).

Negative Predictive Value. The probability of not having a disease when the test result is negative.

Normal Distribution. The frequency of a data distribution simulating a bell-shaped curve that is symmetrical around the mean and exhibits an equal chance of a data point being above or below the mean (syn.: Gaussian distribution). In this distribution, the mean and median are the same value; 68.26% of the scores lie within one standard deviation either side of the mean, 95.44% of the scores lie within 2 standard deviations either side of the mean, and 99.75% fall within 3 standard deviations.

Nonparametric. Used when data is ordinal or nominal in scale so that means testing may not be routinely applied. These tests are less sensitive than parametric tests to trends in the data (e.g., differences between conditions) but can be used with a wider range of measures.

Normative Data. Information obtained from a sample that is interpreted to represent the expected or normal value for a given measurement for the population. For example, values obtained from a random sample of 20,000 households who responded to the Knee Society Score would represent normative values for the KSS for the population from which the sample group was obtained. This data may serve as a normal control value in subsequent studies.

Null Hypothesis. The supposition that there is no true difference between 2 treatment groups or no association between risk indicator and outcome variables. The prediction that an observed difference is due to chance alone and not due to a systematic cause. In order to disprove this, we typically set the level at which we will conclude an association does not, in fact, occur by chance at less than 1 in 20 ($\alpha < 0.05$) or less than 1 in 100 ($\alpha < 0.01$).

Odds. Likelihood of an event occurring compared to it not occurring, mathematically represented by odds $= (p/1 - p)$ where p is the probability of an event occurring.

Odds Ratio. A measure of the strength or degree of association between having the risk factor if the disease or outcome is present compared to when it is absent in which a value of 1.0 means that there is no relationship between variables. An odds ratio less than 1.0 indicates an inverse or negative association. An odds ratio greater than 1.0 indicates a positive relation. The odds ratio may approximate the relative risk if (1) the cases studied are representative, with respect to exposure, of all people with the outcome; (2) the controls studied are representative, with respect to history of exposure, of all people without the outcome; and (3) the outcome of interest is uncommon.

Parametric. Parametric inferential statistical methods are mathematical procedures for statistical hypothesis testing that assume that the distributions of the variables being assessed belong to known parametrized families of probability distributions. Analysis of variance assumes that the underlying distributions are normally distributed and that the variances of the distributions being compared are similar. The Pearson product-moment correlation coefficient assumes normality.

Positive Predictive Value. The probability of disease in a patient with a positive test result. PPD $=$ Sensitivity $\times$ Prevalence/(Sensitivity $\times$ Prevalence) $+ (1 -$ specificity$) \times (1 -$ Prevalence).

Post Hoc Power Calculation. A post hoc power calculation may be performed at the end of an observational study to determine the number of observations needed in a subsequent study to determine the true effect of a risk factor (or intervention) given the observed association between a variable and an outcome of interest.

Power Calculation. The probability one will detect a meaningful difference, or effect, if that effect truly exists using a specific statistical test. In other words, a test's power is the probability that the test will reject a false null hypothesis, or in other words, that it will not make a type II error. As power increases, the chances of a type II error decrease, and vice versa. The probability of a type II error is referred to as β. Therefore power is equal to $1 - \beta$.

Prevalence. The proportion of persons in a given or defined population having the condition or disease at a given time of measurement. This may be discerned through cross-sectional or retrospective studies and may also be obtained through administrative data.

Relative Risk. The ratio of the incidence rate of a disease among individuals exposed to a specific risk factor to the incidence rate among individuals not exposed to the risk factor of interest. May only be calculated from data obtained prospectively because it is time dependent. A value of 1.0 indicates that there is no increase in the outcome of interest for the exposed population compared to the nonexposed population. Values with a 95% confidence interval greater than 1.0 indicate a statistically significant association between the risk factor and the incidence of new cases with a certainty of 95%. In case-control or retrospective studies, the relative risk cannot be calculated directly, but rather, an odds ratio (relative odds) is calculated.

Reliability. The extent to which repeated measurements by different observers and instruments obtain similar results. Qualitatively, it is the reproducibility of a test or study. This may be quantified using regression methods, a correlation coefficient, or the kappa statistic to measure agreement between observers or between different trials for the same individual observer.

Risk. The probability that an event will occur (e.g., that an individual will become sick or die) within a stated period of time or given a particular set of factors (age, gender, comorbidities, etc.). The combination of the frequency, or probability, of occurrence and the consequence of a specified hazardous event. The concept of risk always has 2 elements: the frequency or probability with which a hazardous event occurs and the consequences of the hazardous event.

Sensitivity. The proportion of people with a disease who have a positive test for the disease or true-positives plus false-negatives divided by true-negatives and false-positives as detected with a gold standard.

Specificity. The proportion of people without a disease who have a negative test, or the number of true-negatives and false-positives divided by the number of false negatives and true positives.

Standard Deviation (SD). The statistical measure of variance from the mean representing the dispersion of data (distance) from the mean and calculated as the positive square root of the variance. When scores are normally distributed (when they are part of a bell-shaped, normal curve), about two-thirds of the scores are within 1 standard deviation above and below the average (mean) score, and about 95% of scores are within 2 standard deviations of the mean. In almost any shaped distribution, all values will be within 5 standard deviations of the mean score.

Standard Error. Calculated by dividing the standard deviation of the sample by the square root of the number of subjects in the sample. A measure of an estimate's variability. The greater the standard error in relation to the size of the estimate, the less reliable the estimate.

Stratification. Analysis of data into subgroups of patients having similar characteristics (e.g., patients undergoing total hip arthroplasty with one type of implant compared to another).

Survival Analysis. Quantitative assessment of time-to-event for dichotomous outcomes and that occur only once during follow-up (e.g., time to death, time to failure of an implant or procedure).

T Test. The t test is a statistical test that computes the probability (p) that two groups of a single parameter are members of the same population. Assumptions for use of the t test in means testing are that (1) the populations should follow a normal distribution, and (2) the variances of the two populations are also assumed to be equal. However, a t test is robust enough to allow considerable deviation from normality.

Type I Error. Concluding a true association exists between variables or risk factors and outcome when in reality there is none. Typically, $\alpha < 0.05$ or < 0.01. P-values close to this level but not below may indicate a nonsignificant association that would become significant with increased study power (i.e., increasing the number of subjects observed).

Type II Error. Probability of failing to find a true association when one in fact does exist. This is represented by β, which typically is 0.2 or 0.1. The power of a study, or the study's ability to detect a true association if one exists at a given α is $1 - \beta$ and is typically 0.8 or 0.9 depending on the stringency of the study.

Univariate Analysis. Mathematical assessment of an individual risk factor and a given outcome using any appropriate statistical test. May also be used to assess the relationship of risk factors to one another in determining potential interactions or confounding.

Validity. The degree to which data measure what they are intended to measure, or the extent to which a measurement corresponds to the true value or state of that which is being measured. Qualitatively, it is the accuracy or truthfulness of a test or of data. Does a study interpretation actually draw a correct inference about a set of data? If so, then the study (or test) is valid.

- *Internal validity* is the appropriateness of a study's conclusions given the data collected after accounting for bias, confounding, and chance.

- *External validity* is the applicability of a study's conclusions to be applied to patients or populations other than at the site of initial study. If the sample of patients from which the data is obtained poorly represents the entire population or poorly represents another population, then the data may not be applicable in settings outside that in which the study was performed.

Variance. A measure of the spread or dispersion of a variable about its mean or arithmetic mean value. The variance is calculated by taking the sum of the squares of the deviations—that is, the sum of the difference between the observed value and the series mean value—and dividing by the sample size (number of observations).

References

1. Abel U, Koch A. The role of randomization in clinical studies: Myths and beliefs. *J Clin Epidemiol* 1999;52:487–497.
2. Benson K, Hartz AJ. A comparison of observational studies and randomized, controlled trials. *N Engl J Med* 2000;342:1878–1886.
3. Bernstein J, McGuire K, Freedman KB. Statistical sampling and hypothesis testing in orthopaedic research. *Clin Orthop Relat Res* 2003 Aug;(413):55–62.
4. Bradford Hill A. The environment and disease: Association and causation. *Proc R Soc Med* 1965;58:295–300.
5. Fletcher RW, Fletcher SW. *Clinical Epidemiology: The Essentials*, 4th ed. Philadelphia: Lippincott Williams & Wilkins, 2005.
6. Freedman KB, Back S, Bernstein J. Sample size and statistical power of randomized, controlled trials in orthopaedics. *J Bone Joint Surg Br* 2001 Apr;83(3):397–402.
7. Goodman SN. Toward evidenced-based medical statistics: I. The P value fallacy. *Ann Intern Med* 1999;130:995–1004.
8. Goodman SN. Toward evidenced-based medical statistics: II. The Bayes factor. *Ann Intern Med* 1999;130:1005–1013.
9. Gordis L. *Epidemiology*. Philadelphia: WB Saunders, 1996.
10. Hunsacker FG, Cioffi DA, Amadio PC, Wright JG, Caughlin B. The American Academy of Orthopaedic Surgeons Outcomes Instruments: Normative values from the general population. *J Bone Joint Surg Am* 2002;84(2):208–215.
11. Kaska SC, Weinstein JN. Historical perspective: Ernest Amory Codman (1869-1940): A pioneer of evidenced-based medicine: The end-result idea. *Spine* 1998;23:629–633.
12. Szabo RM. Principles of epidemiology for the orthopaedic surgeon. *J Bone Joint Surg Am* 1998;80:111–120.
13. The Cochrane database of systematic reviews. Available at: http://www.cochrane.org.

Key References

Bernstein J. Evidence-based medicine. *J Am Acad Orthop Surg* 2004 Mar-Apr;12(2):80–88.

The author reviewed the concept of evidenced-based medicine and commented that evidence-based medicine requires its users to embrace uncertainty in medical decision making because information that is simultaneously true and complete cannot be attained. Recognizing medicine's inherent uncertainty, proponents of evidence-based medicine advocate using a 5-step process for sound decision making: formulate answerable questions, gather evidence, appraise the evidence, implement the valid evidence, and evaluate the process.

Kocher MS, Zurakowski D. Clinical epidemiology and biostatistics: A primer for orthopaedic surgeons. *J Bone Joint Surg Am* 2004 Mar;86-A(3):607–620.

An informative review of clinical epidemiology and biostatics.

Refresher Questions

1. A prospective experimental study is being conducted to compare the relative efficacy of drug X and drug Y in treating patients with rheumatoid arthritis. Patients are randomly allocated to 1 of 2 treatment groups for 6 months, and then after 2 weeks of no treatment, the patients are switched to the other drug treatment for 6 months. This specific design is susceptible to bias if
   a) the clinical outcomes are determined in a double-blind fashion
   b) information is lacking on timing of exposure and outcome
   c) there are carryover effects from the first drug treatment
   d) there is a differential loss to follow-up in the 2 treatment groups
   e) the symmetry of unknown cofounders cannot be maintained

2. The Mangled Extremity Severity Score (MESS) predicts well for amputation when the score is greater than or equal to 7. However, when the score is less than 7, limb salvage is not well predicted. Based on this information, what is the specificity and sensitivity for the MESS score in predicting amputation?
   a) high specificity, low sensitivity
   b) high specificity, high sensitivity
   c) low specificity, low sensitivity
   d) low specificity, high sensitivity
   e) cannot determine from the information given

3. The relative risk of malignancy in a prospective cohort study looking at cancer in patients with metal-on-metal total hip arthroplasty (study group) compared to patients with metal-on-polyethylene total hip arthroplasty (control group) is defined as the
   a) incidence of cancer in patients with metal-on-polyethylene total hip arthroplasty (THA) divided by the incidence of lymphoma in patients with metal-on-metal THA
   b) incidence of cancer in patients with metal-on-metal THA divided by the incidence of cancer in patients with metal-on-polyethylene THA
   c) prevalence of cancer in patients with metal-on-polyethylene THA divided by the incidence of cancer in patients with metal-on-metal THA
   d) prevalence of cancer in patients with metal-on-metal THA divided by the incidence of cancer in patients with metal-on-polyethylene THA
   e) probability of developing cancer in patients with metal-on-metal THA divided by the probability of developing cancer in patients with metal-on-polyethylene THA

4. A researcher is interested in testing the load effects of placing osteochondral plugs at 2 different elevations with respect to the adjacent cartilaginous tissue. What is the correct statistical method for data analysis, assuming a normal distribution?
   a) analysis of variance
   b) paired student t-test
   c) Wilcoxon rank-sum test
   d) Kaplan-Meier survival curve
   e) Spearman rank correlation

5. A randomized clinical trial study design is considered appropriate for which of the following situations?
   a) identifying which of several different clinical outcomes distinguishes one treatment group from another
   b) developing a clinical text to screen for a disease
   c) demonstrating statistically that individuals with a certain disease are more likely to have a specific risk factor than are those without the disease
   d) demonstrating statistically that a clinical outcome in one treatment group is different from that in another treatment group
   e) Demonstrating statistically that individuals exposed to a risk factor are more likely to be at risk for development of a disease than those not exposed

6. In which of the following types of studies can an incidence rate be determined?
   a) cross-sectional
   b) prospective cohort
   c) case control
   d) randomized trial
   e) retrospective review

7. A father and son have aortic root widening and superior lens dislocation. The father also has scoliosis and acetabular protrusio. No other family members have significant medical problems. What is the genetic transmission of this syndrome?
   a) autosomal-recessive
   b) autosomal-dominant
   c) X-linked recessive
   d) X-linked dominant
   e) multifactorial

8. What type of study is used to determine the prevalence rates and risk factors for homologous transfusions after total knee arthroplasty in a consecutive series of patients treated at one institution for the past 10 years?
   a) experimental
   b) observational
   c) interventional
   d) descriptive
   e) case-controlled

9. A new scoring system to predict the need for amputation following high-energy lower extremity trauma is being developed. When this system is applied, a score above a threshold level will result in the decision to perform an amputation. To avoid unnecessary amputations, it is most important this scoring system have
   a) high sensitivity
   b) low sensitivity
   c) high specificity
   d) low specificity
   e) low negative predictive value

10. A study is performed on patients with total knee arthroplasty where the investigator believes that patients will have better outcomes with immediate physical therapy as opposed to delayed therapy or no therapy at all. The investigator randomly divides 60 students into 3 groups of 20. All patients undergo total knee arthroplasty. The best statistical test to determine a difference between the 3 groups is a:
    a) student t-test
    b) Chi-square
    c) analysis of variance
    d) multiple regression
    e) factor analysis

Chapter 12

Business and Practice Principles

SHARAT KUMAR KUSUMA, SELENE G. PAREKH, AND PRICE CHIPLEY FRENCH

I. HEALTH CARE COSTS

Overview. Health care spending grew nearly 4 times faster than the U.S. economy in 2002. Total health care spending per privately insured person increased 9.6% in 2002. Employers continue to see double-digit increases in premiums for employees. Increases in premiums are blamed on underlying increases in health care costs. While growth in prescription drug costs was a major component of cost growth in the 1990s, spending increases on hospital care accounted for the largest portion of cost growth recently, approximately 51% of the increase. The health share of GDP is projected to increase from 14.1% in 2001 to 17.7% in 2012. Despite such increases in health care costs, 45 million Americans are still uninsured. A recent poll indicated that more Americans are worried about health care costs than about losing their job, paying their rent or mortgage, or being a victim of a terrorist attack. Hospitals and society desire new technology and thus contribute to increased health care costs.

Role of Hospitals in Increasing Health Care Costs. Hospitals desire new technology to lure physicians and patients. Hospitals price inflate for several reasons: to pay for new technology, to pay competitive wages to employees, and simply to survive. Price inflation by hospitals contributes to increased hospital care spending. Hospital inpatient spending increased 6.8% per privately insured person in 2002. Hospitals now have stronger negotiating leverage over health plans than they had in the 1990s. Hospitals are cost shifting to insured patients to cover the underinsured and uninsured; with greater powers, hospitals now negotiate with manufacturers and are rationing care.

Role of Society in Increasing Health Care Costs. Society desires new technologies in health care. More technology availability results in greater utilization and increased health care costs, and increased health care costs produce an increased budget deficit. Premiums for active employees increased 15% on average in 2003, 13% in 2002, and 12% in 2001. Premium increases were larger than the underlying cost. Employers responded by shifting more costs to employees. Employees paid 19.3% of the cost of single coverage and 22.2% of family coverage in 2003 and saw higher deductibles. Because patients are paying more for insurance, they tend to economize on health care but demand more for their insurance dollars.

II. INSURANCE

Disability Income Insurance

Basic Principles. Most individuals have insurance coverage on homes, autos, and other tangible goods. However, the future value of their earnings from their occupation may far exceed the value of such tangible assets. If future earnings cease because of an accident or illness, the loss of income could pose a serious financial threat. Disability insurance is designed for such scenarios. Disability income insurance policies can help replace a portion of the loss of income due to disability during a person's working years. The following is a list of features that disability insurance policies can include. The items are considered essential components of a disability policy. Disability policies may be purchased by an individual or a company.

Noncancellable, Guaranteed Renewable Provisions. This is considered to be a critical provision of a disability. Such policies contain provisions that prevent the insurance company from altering or amending any of the language of the contract or the premiums due.

Cost of Living Indexing. Protection against inflation for future benefits paid. Such stipulations in a policy are referred to as cost of living adjustments (COLAs.) With such policies, benefits increase each year to offset the effects of inflation.

Elimination Periods. Policies can also have "elimination periods" before benefits commence. Generally, such periods are 30, 60, or 90 days; 6 months; or 1 year in duration. Premiums are lower when elimination periods are longer. When considering the length of elimination period to choose, individuals must consider their current level of income, cash and liquid reserves, and the length of time these reserves can sustain living expenses.

Own Occupation Definition of Disability. Some policies provide "own occupation" coverage and will pay benefits if the insured party is unable to work in his or her specific field. Such policies are designed such that if the insured is unable to practice his or her given medical specialty, then he or she is considered disabled and is eligible for benefits. These benefits are payable even if the insured chooses to work in another occupation or specialty.

Benefit Period. Policies also offer varying benefit periods. Some policies offer a lifetime benefit if the disability was caused by an accident and offer benefit to age 65 if the disability was caused by illness. Generally, the longer the benefit period, the greater the premium.

Guaranteed Insurability Option. This feature is vital to physicians who are in residency training or fellowship and to any other trainees who have yet to reach their maximum income potential. In the current medical environment, obtaining a quality disability insurance contract is difficult, and current underwriting terms are very stringent. A guaranteed insurability option (GIO) allows physicians to obtain a disability policy and secure a satisfactory health record at the commencement of the initial policy. With a GIO, the policy then allows the physician to increase coverage on the basis of increasing income at any point without the need for further health screening. As an example, imagine a scenario in which an orthopaedic surgery resident obtains a disability policy in the third year of his residency that also contains a GIO. In the fifth and final year of his residency, he sustains a severe injury to his dominant, right hand. However, the injury is not so severe that he is completely unable to practice orthopaedic surgery. After completion of his residency, he becomes a private practitioner with a salary of $250,000. However, he is concerned about how long he will be able to work as an orthopaedic surgeon given the severity of his hand injury, and he wishes to increase his coverage. Because of the GIO, he is able to do so, despite that his hand injury makes it more likely that at some point he will exercise the disability policy. If his injury had occurred prior to his policy application, he would have great difficulty obtaining a policy, or the policy would exclude his dominant hand.

Other Types of Disability Insurance. Other types of disability income insurance policies include the following:

- *Key employee disability insurance*—This type of policy is useful when owned by an employer. When an employer loses an employee secondary to disability, this type of policy can provide funds to help cover expenses of loss of services of a disabled employee, such as hiring and training a replacement.
- *Disability buy-out*—Such a policy provides funds to help effect the buy-out of a disabled business owner or professional under the terms of a buy-sell agreement.
- *Business overhead expense*—Such a policy provides funds when a business owner or professional becomes disabled. These funds are used to help cover ongoing expenses such as rent and employee salaries to keep the business open during the period of disability.
- *Disability payments*—Some disability insurance policies begin to pay benefits only when earnings drop by a certain percentage because of a disability. Other policies require a physician's certification to pay or continue benefits. Some policies provide for partial or residual disability benefits when the insured party is able to perform some, but not all, of his or her duties. It is important that purchasers of disability insurance carefully review policy language and provisions.

Life Insurance

Basic Principles. Life insurance is a type of insurance that guarantees a specific monetary benefit to a designated beneficiary at the time of demise of the insured party. Additionally, life insurance policies may allow for the insured party to receive a monetary benefit if he or she lives to a certain age. Life insurance policies involve 4 critical parties: the insurer, the insured, the policy owner, and the beneficiary. Frequently, the policy owner and the insured are one and the same. The beneficiary is the party that will receive the monetary benefit when the insured party expires. Some policies allow the insured party to change the beneficiary; others do not. Most life insurance policies contain stipulations that invalidate the policy if the insured commits suicide within a specified time period. Guaranteed renewability is another important policy feature for any prospective owner or insured to consider because it allows the insured to acquire life insurance even if he or she becomes uninsurable.

Face Amount. The face amount of the policy is monetary benefit that is disbursed when the insured party expires or lives to a certain age. Life insurance policies are most often purchased to safeguard the financial interests of the insured party. When the insured party expires, the policy will provide funds that can be used for funeral and other expenses and can also provide funds to substitute for the lost income of the expired, insured party. The benefits from the policy may be received by the beneficiary in the form of a single payment or in interval payments at regular time increments.

Premiums. Insurance companies charge premiums to the policy owner. Premiums are computed to allow the insurance company to pay for administrative costs, for the insurance company to make a profit, and also to provide a set of funds that may be used to pay out benefits when other insured parties expire. The premiums are invested by the insurance company in various financial instruments.

Term Life Insurance. This is perhaps the simplest form of life insurance in the sense that the premiums paid for the policy provide only for a monetary benefit when the insured expires. Term insurance does not offer any further benefits. Additionally, term insurance is structured such that coverage is in place for a specific number of years, or a term, for a specific premium. Term policies do not have the ability to accumulate cash value. Term insurance is considered to be more affordable than other types of life insurance. Additionally, many term policies allow physicians to convert the policy to a more permanent type of policy at any time. There are 3 important characteristics of term insurance the potential buyers should bear in mind:

1. The face amount of the policy
2. The premium
3. The length of coverage.

The face amount of the policy is simply the monetary death benefit paid when the insured expires. The length of coverage is the term. Insurance providers offer term policies with varying combinations of term, face amount, and premiums. Generally, face amounts can be constant or declining. Various insurance companies sell term insurance with many different combinations of these three parameters. The face amount can remain constant or decline. The term can be for 1 or more years. The premium can remain level or increase. There are several types of life insurance based on the term.

- *Decreasing term*—Such policies offer level premiums and a decreasing death benefit. Such policies do not allow for cash accumulation. They are often used by individuals when they wish to insure against short-term, decreasing financial liabilities such as loans.
- *Annual renewable term*—This type of insurance provides for increasing premiums with level death benefits. Annual renewable term does not allow for cash accumulation. The main advantage of this type of insurance is the low initial cost for death benefits, which can be useful for young families with limited resources and the need for maximum protection. As such young families accrue wealth and become older, they pay increasing premiums for a stable death benefit.
- *Level term*—Such policies allow for premiums that are level for a stated period of time, usually 5, 10, 15, or 20 years. Death benefits are also level. Such policies also do not allow for cash accumulation. They are frequently used to cover short or intermediate term obligations.

Permanent Life Insurance. This type differs from term insurance in that such policies remain in force until they mature. The only scenario under which permanent insurance policies can be cancelled is if premiums are not paid. Permanent policies allow cancellation by the insurer only when the insured has provided erroneous information. Permanent insurance is unique in that it accumulates a cash value; the insured party may use this cash value of the policy to borrow funds, or he or she can "surrender" the policy, in which case he or she "cashes out" the policy for a "surrender value." Therefore, permanent life insurance functions somewhat like a "forced" savings account in that individuals must pay regular premiums to maintain the policy, while at the same time, the policy builds cash value, like a savings account. There are 3 types of permanent life insurance; they include whole life, universal life, variable life, and endowment insurance. Policies such as universal life, variable life, and universal-variable life allow an individual to purchase a single financial instrument that provides for both life insurance and long-term accumulation goals. Such policies may serve as a form of "forced investment" for those who find it difficult to put funds aside on a regular basis but who routinely pay their bills.

- *Whole life insurance*—This is a very clearly defined life insurance instrument with low risk and variability. Whole insurance provides a fixed face value and a stable premium that does not change with time. Additionally, whole insurance offers the purchaser cash benefits that are detailed in a cash table. The cash values provided in these tables are guaranteed by the insurer. Therefore, the primary advantages of whole life insurance are that they provide guaranteed death benefits, guaranteed cash values, and stable premiums. The disadvantages of whole life insurance lie in the financial inflexibility of these instruments, as they have fixed rates of return that may be less than returns that can be earned in the market, fixed death benefits, and fixed premiums. Whole life insurance products are primarily used for death benefit protection and also for long-term accumulation goals. Available cash values may also serve as an "emergency reserve," if needed, or a source of loans, since life policies frequently include features permitting borrowing against these cash values. However, such policy loans or withdrawals will reduce cash values and death benefits. Such policies do provide for cash accumulation and for long-term needs, such as income for survivors. Other uses could include paying off debt and providing liquidity for estate taxes. Policies have required premiums that, if paid when billed by the insurer, provide guarantees of coverage and other benefits. Participating policies may provide dividends that can be taken in cash or used to enhance the policy. Nonparticipating policies typically provide "current" interest credits and "current" cost of insurance charges that are more favorable than the underlying guarantees.
- *Universal life insurance*—This is another form of permanent insurance, which differs primarily from whole insurance in that universal policies allow for flexible premiums and variable rates of return that are not predetermined in cash value tables. Universal policies contain a cash account that increases when premiums are paid. A portion of premiums are used to pay administrative expenses of the policy, while remaining funds are credited to the cash account. The cash account pays interest at a rate that is guaranteed by the insurer to not decline below a certain predetermined level. Generally, the interest paid on the cash account is higher than this minimum. The surrender value of the policy is the value of the cash account at the time of maturity. Universal policies have advantages over whole policies in that they allow for rates of return

that move with the levels of financial markets, while they also offer flexible premiums and variable death benefits.

- *Variable universal life insurance*—Life insurance is a modification of universal life in that the return on the cash account is directly affected by the performance of separate accounts elected by the policy owner, who allocates cash values among various types of financial instruments such as stocks funds, bond funds, or money market funds.

III. MALPRACTICE

Basic Principles. Malpractice is defined specifically as a failure to provide a professional service in a manner that is expected of skillful and conscientious practitioners of that profession. This failure results in injury, loss, or damage to the recipient of the services. In medicine, the most common reason for malpractice litigation is a charge of negligence on the part of the treating physician. *Mala praxis* is a Latin expression, meaning bad or unskillful practice in a physician whereby the health or welfare of the patient is injured. Three kinds of malpractice exist:

- *Willful malpractice*—Willful malpractice takes place when the physician purposely administers medicines or performs an operation that he or knows and expects will result in danger or death to the individual under his or her care, as in the case of criminal abortion.
- *Negligent malpractice*—This term refers to cases in which there is no criminal or dishonest object but gross negligence of that attention which the situation of the patient requires, such as if a physician administered medicines while in a state of intoxication, from which injury would arise to his patient.
- *Ignorant malpractice*—The administration of medicines, calculated to do injury, which do harm, and which a well-educated and scientific medical man would know were not proper in the case.

Existence of Malpractice. In order to prove malpractice, there must be a physician duty followed by a breach of this duty. The breach of this duty must be proven to have caused harm to the patient. The physician duties are set by standards of care.

Standard of Care/Duty of Physician. A physician, performing professional services for a patient, owes that patient the following duties of care:

- The duty to have that degree of learning and skill ordinarily possessed by reputable physicians practicing in the same or a similar locality and under similar circumstances.
- The duty to use the care and skill ordinarily exercised in like cases by reputable members of the profession practicing in the same or a similar locality under similar circumstances.
- The duty to use reasonable diligence and his or her best judgment in the exercise of skill and the application of learning.

A failure to perform any one of these duties is negligence.

Causation. The plaintiff must also prove that the alleged breach of the standard of care caused the injury, damage, or loss that resulted in this lawsuit. A physician cannot be liable for any malpractice if the malpractice did not cause the injury. The law defines cause in its own particular way. A cause of injury, damage, loss, or harm is an action or inaction that is a substantial factor in bringing about an injury, damage, loss, or harm.

Informed Consent. It is the duty of a physician to obtain the consent of a patient before treating or operating on the patient. Such consent may be express or may be implied from the circumstances. It is the duty of the physician to disclose to the patient all information to enable the patient to make an informed decision regarding the proposed operation or treatment. Material information is information that the physician knows or should know would be regarded as significant by a reasonable person in the patient's position when deciding to accept or reject a recommended medical procedure. The physician or surgeon must also disclose such additional information as a skilled practitioner of good standing would provide under the same or similar circumstances.

Malpractice Insurance

Basic Principles of Malpractice Insurance. In recent years, there has been an increase nationwide of medical malpractice suits, which has caused significant increases in rates for malpractice insurance. Some also argue that malpractice suits have caused practitioners to perform defensive medicine in which they refrain from performing highly risky procedures and in which they order excessive numbers of diagnostic tests. On the converse of these arguments are trial lawyers, who argue that the ability of patients to bring suit to their treating physicians is a force that has maintained and improved the quality of health care in the United States. They argue that the increased health care expenses generated by malpractice suits and defensive medicine are well worth the improvements in the quality of care delivered. In general, lawyers are in opposition of malpractice reform, while insurance companies and physicians are in favor of reform. Several different solutions have been proposed to reduce the growth rate of malpractice suits. These include measures such as peer review of malpractice cases by a board of medical professionals prior to cases going to trial. Also, caps on noneconomic damage awards and plaintiff liability for lost cases are other proposed solutions.

There are several different forms of malpractice insurance. The 4 most common are:

1. Claims-made coverage
2. Occurrence coverage
3. Prior acts coverage
4. Tail coverage.

Claims-Made Coverage. This type of malpractice insurance protects practitioners from suits and from incidents that take place during the time period that the insurance policy is effective. Such policies are typically renewed on an annual basis. Therefore, if they are continually renewed, the insured will have protection on a continuous basis for incidents and claims as they occur. With claims-made coverage, if a suit is filed after the policy expires, then the insured will not be protected for this suit, even if the incident that is the basis of the suit occurred at a time while the policy was in force. Once terminated, future claims arising from incidents that occurred during the policy period are not covered.

Occurrence Coverage. Occurrence policies differ from claims-made policies in that occurrence insurance provides protection for a claim that occurred during the period that the policy is in force, regardless of when such a claim is actually filed. Therefore, even if a suit is filed against a practitioner after the policy has expired, the practitioner will be protected for this suit, as long as the incident related to the suit occurred during a time period when the policy was in force. For example, if the alleged error or omission happened anytime during the residency training, it would be covered by the teaching facility's professional liability insurance even if the claim is filed after the policy has expired. Occurrence policies are no longer commonly offered but may be available through select insurance carriers or if the program self-insures its residents.

Prior Acts Coverage. Such policies are usually supplemental to claims-made policies. Prior acts coverage, which is sometimes referred to as nose coverage, protects the insured for incidents that occurred prior to the inception of the prior acts policy but which have not yet been filed against the insured. Such policies are usually purchased from a new insurance carrier when the insured changes insurance policies. Because the physician is seeking up-front coverage before securing a relationship with the insurance carrier, it is referred to as nose coverage and is usually comparable in price to tail coverage.

Tail Coverage. Tail policies are also supplemental to claims-made policies in that they provide protection for any incidents that occurred during a specified time period that the claims-made policy was in effect, even though the claim was filed after the insurer–policyholder relationship was terminated. Tail coverage is generally purchased from an existing or former insurance carrier at the expiration of a claims-made policy. Sometimes referred to as an extended reporting endorsement, tail coverage is necessary whenever a physician insured under a claims-made policy changes carriers, becomes disabled, retires, or dies.

Other Types of Liability Policies.

- *Claims-paid*—A variant of claims-made insurance, claims-paid is a professional liability insurance that provides coverage for claims arising from incidents that occur while the policy is in force. However, claims must be reported and paid before the policy is terminated.
- *Locum tenens coverage*—Covers physicians who are performing locum tenens work.
- *Slot policies*—Offer protection when services are provided at a location by several rotating providers who work at different times.
- *Self-insurance*—Many academic medical centers self-insure their staff. Instead of purchasing professional liability insurance, the resources of the training program (or its related institutions) pay any losses associated with medical malpractice claims or suits against the institution, supervising physicians, and/or physicians-in-training.
- *Liability of residents and fellows*—The Latin *respondeat superior* means "let the master answer." The educational institution conducting the residency program is responsible for the medical care provided by its residents during the training exercises. Therefore, the institution is liable for the defense costs, settlements, and awards for malpractice attributed to physicians-in-training.

IV. INVESTMENTS

Estate Planning

Basic Principles. Estate planning refers to an individual's preparation of a plan for the management of his or her tangible and intangible assets prior to or after his or her death. Important aspects of estate planning include management of estate taxes and probate fees. Legal and financial instruments that are critical in the estate planning include wills, trusts, and powers of attorney.

Probate. Probate is the legal court process by which an expired individual's estate, legal, and financial matters are concluded. The probate process can often be very expensive and time consuming. Some estimates report that the costs of probate-related processes can require between 6% and 10% of an individual's estate. However, with the use of trusts and other estate planning instruments, the probate process may be avoided altogether.

Wills and Trusts. Wills and trusts are common estate planning instruments, and they both afford individuals the ability to designate how their estate will be disbursed. Technically, a will is a legal pronouncement of an individual's designation for the distribution of his or her estate at death. Wills are usually written, legal documents. Wills also allow individuals to assign executors and guardians for remaining children. However, estates that are distributed through a will must proceed through the probate process. A trust is different from a will in that a trust is a legal entity that consists of a person or group of persons. The trust maintains control of an individual's estate. When an individual expires, the trust has control and ownership of the estate and therefore obviates the need for the probate process.

Durable Power of Attorney. Another important estate planning instrument, the durable power of attorney is a legal arrangement that allows an individual to designate another person or group of persons to make legal, financial, and even health care decisions if that individual becomes infirm or incapacitated. Individuals can maintain durable powers of attorney for various matters, including health care and finances. A durable power of attorney for health care is a kind of advance directive. It identifies an individual chosen by a patient to make health care decisions for the patient. It becomes active any time a patient is unconscious or unable to make medical decisions. Similarly, a durable power of attorney for finances makes financial decisions when an individual becomes incapacitated.

Advance Directive. An advance directive tells the physician what kind of care a patient would like to have if he or she is unable to make medical decisions. A good advance directive describes the kind of treatment the patient would want depending on how sick he or she is.

Living Will. A living will is a type of advance directive. It comes into effect only when a patient is terminally ill (less than 6 months to live). A patient can describe the kind of treatment desired in certain situations. A living will does not allow the patient to assign someone to make decisions for him or her. A living will specifies what type of life-prolonging treatments an individual desires and whether or not an individual desires to be on life support.

Do Not Resuscitate (DNR) Order. A DNR order is another kind of advance directive. A DNR is a request not to have cardiopulmonary resuscitation (CPR).

Financial Planning: Basic Investment Tools

Stocks. The terms "stock" and "share" both refer to a fractional ownership interest in a corporation. As "owners," stockholders vote for the company's board of directors and receive information on the firm's activities and business results. Stockholders may share in current profits through "dividends" declared by the firm's board. When a corporate business is first organized, investors contribute money to fund the enterprise, and in return they receive shares of stock representing their ownership in the company. If the business becomes successful, it will grow and have increasing profits, and the shares generally become more valuable. If the business is not successful, the value of the shares usually declines. Investors typically buy and hold stocks for their long-term growth potential. Stocks with a history of regular dividend payments are often held for both income and growth. The unpredictability of their performance makes stocks a risky investment, as the long-term growth of a company cannot be predicted. The short-term market value of the company's stock also can fluctuate up and down. If need or fear causes an investor to sell when the market is down, a capital loss will result. If the market is up, the investor will realize a capital gain.

Bonds. While stocks represent ownership in a business, bonds are debt. Issued by institutions such as the federal government, corporations, and state and local governments, a bond is evidence of money borrowed by the bond issuer. In return, bondholders receive interest and, at "maturity," the principal amount of the bond. When first issued, a bond will have a specified rate of return, or a "yield." For example, a 6.0% bond will pay $60.00 per year for each $1,000 invested. If a bond is traded on a public exchange, the market price will fluctuate, generally with changes in interest rates. Later investors will receive a yield that may be more or less than 6.0%, depending on price paid for the bond in the open market. Bonds are typically bought by investors seeking current, sustained, predictable income. The interest rate that bonds pay usually provides a fixed payment at regular time intervals. In some instances, bonds are also used for capital growth. Bonds also have risks. Like stocks, the market price of bonds will fluctuate up and down. If an investor sells a bond before it matures, a capital gain or loss may result. Unless the insurer defaults, bonds held to maturity will recover the principal amount. Since a bond pays a fixed return, inflation risk can be a problem; over time, the dollars received will buy less and less. Also, the interest income received may be subject to current income taxation.

Mutual Funds. A mutual fund is an organization designed to pool the assets of many investors, to achieve a common purpose. The money raised is then invested in accordance with predefined goals. This mutual effort of a number of investors provides benefits that an individual, working alone, might not be able to receive. One benefit of a mutual fund is that the funds are usually professionally managed and invested by trained, experienced investment professionals. These individuals usually perform extensive research and carefully select and monitor the assets in the common investment portfolio. Mutual funds also allow for great asset diversification. Because of the large number of investors and considerable amounts of funds available, mutual funds have the ability to purchase a large variety of assets and asset classes. Mutual funds also have the benefit of convenience. Investment programs can be started with relatively small amounts of money. Additionally, greater degrees of diversification can be achieved with smaller amounts of money than would otherwise be possible with other investment instruments. Dividends from mutual funds can be easily reinvested into the fund. Many funds offer features to automate both contributions and withdrawals. Regular fund statements ease bookkeeping by tracking an investor's purchases, withdrawals, and reinvestments, as well as providing tax information. Mutual funds are classified according to their structure and investment objectives.

- *Open-end mutual funds*—Mutual funds that issue as many shares as the public wishes to buy are called open-end mutual funds. When the public wants to sell, open-end funds redeem all shares tendered.
- *Closed-end mutual funds*—Closed-end mutual funds are those that have a fixed number of shares. Unlike shares in an open-end fund, where the fund itself sells and redeems all shares, the shares in a closed-end fund are traded on public exchanges.
- *Money market funds*—Money market funds invest in a variety of short-term, money market debt, such as Treasury bills or commercial paper.
- *Growth funds*—Growth funds have an emphasis on long-term capital growth, usually through investment in common stock.
- *Income funds*—Income funds focus on providing high, current income, using bonds and other income producing securities.
- *Balanced funds*—Balanced funds attempt to provide both income and long-term capital gain by using a combination of stocks and bonds.
- *Sector funds*—Sector funds generally invest in stocks and bonds of companies focusing on a particular sector of the economy. Typical areas of focus include technology, health, energy, and utilities. These funds usually appeal to investors with a concern or interest in a particular area of the economy.
- *Municipal bond funds*—Municipal bond funds primarily invest in municipal bonds or other short-term municipal debt. The advantages of these funds are that dividends are not charged federal taxes. Some dividends may also be exempt of state taxes. Because of their tax-free status, these funds are advantageous to high tax-bracket individuals who are seeking tax shelters.
- *Aggressive growth funds*—Typically, aggressive growth funds invest in stocks of companies with high potential earnings growth. These funds have a high risk/reward potential because their market value can be quite volatile.

It is important to understand key concepts regarding mutual funds.

- *Prospectus*—The Securities and Exchange Commission (SEC) requires that every prospective investor in an open-end mutual fund be provided a document called a prospectus. The prospectus contains valuable information concerning how the fund works, the fund's goals and risks, its history, and any expenses or charges involved. The prospectus is intended to provide the facts necessary for an investor to make an informed decision and should be reviewed carefully. For closed-end mutual funds, a prospectus is issued only when shares are first offered to the public.
- *Net asset value*—At the end of each business day, the managers of a fund add up the market value of all securities held by the fund. The total market value is then divided by the number of outstanding shares in the fund. The result is the net asset value (NAV) per share. For open-end funds, NAV is used to calculate the price per share for both purchases and sales. For closed-end funds, NAV measures only the value of the securities in the fund; the market price of shares in the fund can be higher or lower than NAV.
- *Load versus no-load*—The term *load* traditionally refers to a commission paid to purchase shares in

an open-end mutual fund. No load funds do not charge a commission to purchase their shares. Even though a fund is no-load, other fees and expenses may apply.

- *Offering price*—This is the price charged to purchase shares in an open-end fund. For a load fund, it is the NAV plus the commission charged. For a no-load fund, offering price and NAV are the same.

The rule of 72 and 115. These two simple rules are extremely useful for determining roughly how long investments will take to double or triple on the basis of a given rate of return.

- *The rule of 72*—If the number 72 is divided by the interest rate, the result is the approximate number of years required to double the investment. Therefore, for an investment that has a 1% rate of return will double in 72 years, while an investment that returns 10% will double its value in only 7.2 years
- *The rule of 115*—If the number 115 is divided by the interest, the result is the approximate number of years required to triple the investment.

Retirement Plans and Instruments

401(k) Plans. A 401(k) plan is an effective financial instrument that is useful for accumulating funds for retirement. A 401(k) is a type of retirement plan that allows employees to save and invest for their own retirement. Through a 401(k), an individual can have his or her employer deduct a predetermined amount of funds from his or her paycheck, before taxes, to be placed into an investment account. The amount of funds deducted and the financial instruments into which these funds are invested are the choice of the individual. The Internal Revenue Service (IRS) sets annual limits on the amount of money that individuals may place in their 401(k) plans. In the year 2005, this limit is $14,000 annually. A 401(k) plan offers the advantage of portability. Therefore, individuals who change employers may take their existing 401(k) plan with them. A 401(k) plan also allows the investment accounts to accumulate value on a tax-deferred basis. Another advantage is that many employers who offer 401(k) plans will match the contributions of the employee to the investment account. For example, an employer may contribute 25 cents to the investment account of an individual for every dollar that he or she contributes to the account. Finally, 401(k) plans offer the advantage of great flexibility in investment choices: individuals can choose to invest in stocks, bonds, money markets, or other types of investment funds. The federal government created 401(k) plans in 1981 to encourage individuals to save money during their working years to finance their retirement years.

403(b) Plans. A 403(b) plan is very similar to a 401(k) plan. Like a 401(k) plan, contributions are tax deductible. The main difference is that 403(b) plans are specifically available to individuals who are employed by universities, government, and nonprofit organizations. 403(b) plans also differ from 401(k) plans in that 403(b) users are not allowed to invest in individual stocks. Rather, they may invest only in annuities with insurance companies or mutual funds.

Individual Retirement Accounts (IRAs). An IRA is an investment account that allows an individual to accumulate earnings over time on a federally tax-free or tax-deferred basis. It is this tax-adjusted characteristic of IRA accounts that allows them to increase in value more quickly than other types of investment accounts, which are subject to taxes. The two most common types of IRAs are traditional IRAs and Roth IRAs.

- *Traditional IRA*—A traditional IRA allows qualified individuals to make tax-deductible contributions to their retirement investment accounts. The IRS set limits of $3,000 annual contributions in 2004, $4,000 per year for 2005 to 2007, and $5,000 per year in 2008. The assets in a traditional IRA increase in value in a tax-deferred manner. At the time of withdrawal, contributions and earnings in traditional IRAs are taxed by the federal government as regular income. If withdrawals are made prior to age 59.5, a 10% penalty must be paid to the federal government. Traditional IRAs do not have any income limits.
- *Roth IRA*—A Roth IRA differs from a traditional IRA in several ways. Like a traditional IRA, a Roth possesses certain tax shelters. A Roth IRA differs primarily from a traditional IRA in that it allows tax-free accumulation of assets and tax-free withdrawals if certain conditions are met. A Roth IRA also differs from a traditional in that the contributions to the Roth are not tax deductible. However, once the contributions are part of the retirement account, they increase in value in a tax-free manner. Additionally, when funds are withdrawn, they are not subject to federal income taxes. However, in order to qualify for a Roth IRA, a single, working individual may have a gross income of up to $95,000, or if married, a gross combined income of $150,000. Therefore, for current orthopaedic residents, the opportunity to open a Roth IRA generally exists only during residency, as most practicing orthopaedic surgeons will earn an income of higher than $95,000 during their first few years in practice, which will disqualify them from opening such a tax-sheltered retirement account.

V. HEALTH POLICY

Political Action Committees (PAC). A political action committee, or PAC, is a U.S. organization formed by a corporation, labor union, or association to raise money for political activity. A PAC can collect voluntary contributions from members of the PAC, employees of the PAC, or shareholders of the PAC. A PAC allows members of professional organizations, corporations, and other groups to combine their political contributions to give support to candidates who may advance the legislative goals of the group. PACs were initially established in the 1940s and have grown in size and popularity since the 1970s, when election reform laws set limits on levels of political contributions allowed by individuals. Many PACs were created to represent special-interest groups such as the National Rifle Association (NRA) and the American Association of Retired Persons. In general, there are 2 types of contributions that can be made to PACs: personal contributions (or hard dollars) and corporate contributions (or soft dollars). Hard dollars are contributions made by individuals from their personal accounts to the PAC and can be used to fund a particular federal political campaign. Soft dollars, which come from corporate accounts, are not allowed to be used for federal election candidates and are therefore used by PACs for administrative and operational expenses.

VI. PATIENT SAFETY AND RISK MANAGEMENT

Overview. Patient safety is defined as the prevention of errors of action in judgment, making errors visible, and mitigating the effects of these errors. Clinical data from the Advisory Board Company in Washington, D.C., reported adverse drug events as the largest group of adverse incidents, accounting for over 25% of all hospital adverse incidents. Of these, 56% could be attributed to the physician, 34% to nurses, 6% to the unit secretary, and 4% to the pharmacy staff. Types of problems with physician orders were 78% illegible signature, 58% missing order time, 24% incomplete, and 20% illegible. For nurses, the causes include math errors, calculating doses, administering wrong dose or medicine, or missing doses. Unit secretaries had mainly transcription errors. It is thought that workflow automation and process improvement can help reduce adverse drug events. Information from the National Center for Vital and Health Statistics noted that 1 in 25 hospital admissions resulted in an injured patient, and 3% resulted in permanent disabling injury. Of these, one in seven led to patient death.

The Harvard Medical Practice Study. This study involved review of over 30,000 charts from the state of Massachusetts:

- Adverse events statewide were said to occur in 3.7 % of all hospital admissions.
- Sixty-nine percent of these events were the result of a medical error and negligence was noted in 28%.
- Of the patients who experienced a medical error, total disability occurred in 27% and death in 14%.
- Four percent of the patients who experienced a medical error had been hospitalized for orthopaedic problems.

It was clear from this chart review that many of the medical errors were preventable.

The Institute of Medicine's Report, "To Err is Human." This report concluded that yearly deaths due to medical error ranged from 44,000 to 98,000 patients. Based on year 2000 mortality numbers, this made medical error the third to ninth leading cause of death. The economic impact is estimated to be over $8 billion annually.

Federal Initiative to Reduce Errors. Following the Institute of Medicine's report, President Clinton announced several government steps. A major federal initiative has been launched to reduce medical errors and improve patient safety in federally funded health care programs, and by example and partnership, in the private sector. The Leapfrog Group is an initiative driven by organizations that buy health care who are working to initiate breakthrough improvements in the safety, quality, and affordability of health care for Americans. Leapfrog and its members work together to:

- Reduce preventable medical mistakes and improve the quality and affordability of health care.
- Reward doctors and hospitals for improving the quality, safety, and affordability of health care.
- Encourage public reporting of health care quality and outcomes so that consumers and purchasing organizations can make more informed health care choices.

The National Quality Forum. The National Quality Forum published "Safe Practices for Better Healthcare: A Consensus Report" in May 2003. The report endorsed 30 practices that should be universally used in applicable clinical care settings to reduce the risk of harm to patients. Included in the 30 practices are the computer physician order entry, ICU physician staffing, and evidence-based hospital referral for certain high-risk procedures.

Wrong-Site Surgery. At a recent Joint Commission on Accreditation of Healthcare Organizations (JCAHO)

"Wrong-Site Surgery Summit," which the American Academy of Orthopaedic Surgeons (AAOS) cosponsored, participants discussed a universal protocol for preventing wrong site surgery. In addition to requiring the marking of all surgical sites in cases involving laterality, multiple structures (e.g., toes, fingers) or multiple levels (spine), the "Universal Protocol for Eliminating Wrong-Site, Wrong-Procedure, Wrong-Patient Surgery" includes a "time-out" immediately before starting the procedure. The time-out process involves the entire surgical team who, in addition to completing a final verification of the correct site, procedure, and patient, must agree on the position of the patient and, importantly, the availability of the correct implants and special equipment needed. This practice was recommended last year at a symposium for health care executives cosponsored by the Agency for Healthcare Research and Quality (AHRQ) and JCAHO.

VII. PATIENT PRIVACY

Health Insurance Portability and Accountability Act (HIPAA). HIPAA was signed into law in 1996. Its primary purpose is to provide continuous insurance coverage for workers who change jobs. It requires the adoption of standards for security, privacy, and electronic health care transactions. All health plans, clearinghouses, and providers who choose to exchange data electronically must implement HIPAA requirements. Failure to implement HIPAA will result in significant monetary penalties. The consequences of knowingly disclosing individually identifiable patient information are criminal penalties. HIPAA will affect how independent providers deal with managing both electronic transactions (claims, referrals, remittance) and medical records. HIPAA's requirements are meant to encourage health care organizations to move patient information–handling activities from manual to electronic systems in order to improve security, lower costs, and lower the error rate.

Health and Human Services (HHS). Taking effect on April 14, 2003, these new standards, developed by the Department of Health and Human Services, provide patients with access to their medical records and more control over how their personal health information is used and disclosed. They represent a uniform, federal floor of privacy protections for consumers across the country. State laws providing additional protections to consumers are not affected by this new rule.

Patient Protections. The new privacy regulations ensure a national floor of privacy protections for patients by limiting the ways that health plans, pharmacies, hospitals, and other covered entities can use patients' personal medical information. The regulations protect medical records and other individually identifiable health information. Key provisions of these new standards include:

- *Access to medical records*—Patients generally should be able to see and obtain copies of their medical records and request corrections if they identify errors and mistakes.
- *Notice of privacy practices*—Covered health plans, doctors, and other health care providers must provide a notice to their patients regarding the use of personal medical information and their rights under the new privacy regulation.
- *Limits on use of personal medical information*—The privacy rule sets limits on how health plans and covered providers may use individually identifiable health information.
- *Prohibition on marketing*—The final privacy rule sets new restrictions and limits on the use of patient information for marketing purposes.
- *Standards*—The privacy rule will set a national floor of privacy standards that protect all Americans. All state laws providing additional protections would continue to apply.
- *Confidential communications*—Under the privacy rule, patients can request that their doctors, health plans, and other covered entities take reasonable steps to ensure that their communications with the patient are confidential.
- *Complaints*—Consumers may file a formal complaint regarding the privacy practices of a covered health plan or provider. Such complaints can be made directly to the covered provider or health plan or to HHS Office for Civil Rights (OCR), which is charged with investigating complaints and enforcing the privacy regulation.

Privacy Procedures for Health Plans and Providers. The privacy rule requires health plans, pharmacies, doctors, and other covered entities to establish policies and procedures to protect the confidentiality of protected health information about their patients. Covered entities must take some additional steps to protect patient privacy:

- *Written privacy procedures*—The rule requires covered entities to have written privacy procedures, including a description of staff that has access to protected information, how it will be used, and when it may be disclosed.
- *Employee training and privacy officer*—Covered entities must train their employees in their privacy procedures and must designate an individual to be

responsible for ensuring that the procedures are followed.

- *Public responsibilities*—In limited circumstances, the final rule permits, but does not require, covered entities to continue certain existing disclosures of health information for specific public responsibilities.
- *Equivalent requirements for government*—The provisions of the final rule generally apply equally to private sector and public sector covered entities.

Outreach and Enforcement. HHS OCR oversees and enforces the new federal privacy regulations. Key elements of OCR's outreach and enforcement efforts include civil and criminal penalties.

Civil and Criminal Penalties. Congress provided civil and criminal penalties for covered entities that misuse personal health information. For civil violations of the standards, the OCR may impose monetary penalties of up to $100 per violation and up to $25,000 per year for each requirement or prohibition violated. Criminal penalties apply for certain actions such as knowingly obtaining protected health information in violation of the law. Criminal penalties can range up to $50,000 and 1 year in prison for certain offenses; up to $100,000 and up to 5 years in prison if the offenses are committed under false pretenses; and up to $250,000 and up to 10 years in prison if the offenses are committed with the intent to sell, transfer, or use protected health information for commercial advantage, personal gain, or malicious harm.

VIII. ETHICS

Advamed/PhRMA Code. Industry-driven codes of ethics, adopted by pharmaceutical (PhRMA Code) and device companies (Advamed), which regulate the interaction between the member companies and physicians, were derived to minimize the financial and personal conflicts of interest that may arise.

Principles of Medical Ethics and Professionalism in Orthopaedic Surgery. The following have been adopted by the Board of Directors of the American Academy of Orthopaedic Surgeons. They are not laws but rather standards of conduct that define the essentials of honorable behavior for the orthopaedic surgeon.

- *Physician–Patient Relationship*—The orthopaedic profession exists for the primary purpose of caring for the patient. The physician–patient relationship is the central focus of all ethical concerns. The orthopaedic surgeon should be dedicated to providing competent medical service with compassion and respect.
- *Integrity*—The orthopaedic surgeon should maintain a reputation for truth and honesty with patients and colleagues and should strive to expose through the appropriate review process those physicians who are deficient in character or competence or who engage in fraud or deception.
- *Legalities and Honor*—The orthopaedic surgeon must obey the law, uphold the dignity and honor of the profession, and accept the profession's self-imposed discipline.
- *Conflicts of Interest*—The practice of medicine inherently presents potential conflicts of interest. Wherever a conflict of interest arises, it must be resolved in the best interest of the patient.

Gifts and the Orthopaedic Surgeon's Relationship with Industry. Generally, the AAOS believes that it is acceptable for industry to provide financial and other support to orthopaedic surgeons if such support has significant educational value and has the purpose of improving patient care. All dealings between orthopaedic surgeons and industry should benefit the patient and be able to withstand public scrutiny. To avoid acceptance of inappropriate gifts or other financial support, the AAOS recommends that orthopaedic surgeons observe the following guidelines:

- *Benefit to patients*—The patient's best interest is paramount. Therefore, it is of utmost importance that any gift or other financial support accepted by an orthopaedic surgeon should primarily entail a benefit to his or her patient. A gift of any kind from industry should in no way influence the orthopaedic surgeon in determining the most appropriate treatment for his or her patient.
- *Gifts with conditions attached*—Orthopaedic surgeons should not accept gifts or other financial support with conditions attached. No gifts should be accepted with the explicit or implicit requirement that the orthopaedic surgeon use the products or services provided by that particular industry.
- *Social functions*—Social functions supported by industry in combination with significant continuing medical education events are acceptable. However, social functions supported by industry where there is no educational element should not be offered to nor accepted by orthopaedic surgeons.
- *Cash gifts*—Cash gifts from industry to orthopaedic surgeons must not be offered nor accepted.

Continuing Medical Education (CME) Events. All practitioners must accumulate a certain number of CME hours to maintain their licenses.

- *Subsidies*—Subsidies by industry to underwrite the costs of educational events where CME credits are provided can contribute to the improvement of patient care and are acceptable. A corporate subsidy received by the conference's sponsor is appropriate and acceptable so long as such support is publicly acknowledged and the location, curriculum, faculty, and educational methods of the conference or meeting are determined solely by the organization sponsoring the educational course, not by industry. Industry reimbursement, whether direct or indirect, for an orthopaedic surgeon to attend an educational event is not appropriate.
- *Faculty expenses and honoraria for CME activities*—It is appropriate for faculty at educational events where CME credits are provided to accept reasonable honoraria and to accept reimbursement for reasonable travel, lodging, and meal expenses from the conference's sponsor.
- *Consultant expenses and honoraria*—It is appropriate for consultants to industry that provide genuine services to receive reasonable compensation and to accept reimbursement for reasonable travel, lodging, and meal expenses. Token consulting or advisory arrangements cannot be used to justify compensating orthopaedic surgeons for their time, travel, lodging, or other out-of-pocket expenses.
- *Scholarships for orthopaedic surgeons-in-training*—Scholarships or other special funds from industry to permit orthopaedic surgeons-in-training to attend CME conferences are appropriate as long as the selection of students, residents, or fellows who will receive the funds is made by the orthopaedist-in-training's program director.

Evidence-Based Medicine. Evidence-based medicine is the idea that all interventions in the practice of orthopedics and medicine are based on scientifically sound and proven studies.

IX. HEALTH CARE MANAGEMENT

A summary of care-delivery systems is provided in Table 12.1.

Health Maintenance Organizations (HMOs). HMOs are the least expensive but also the least flexible of all the health insurance plans.

- *Advantages*—Low copayments, minimal paperwork, and coverage for some preventive-care and health-improvement programs.
- *Disadvantages*—The insured must choose a primary care physician (PCP) and can see only network doctors. The insured must get a referral from his or her PCP to see a specialist.

Point-of-Service Plans (POS). POS plans are more flexible than HMOs, but they also require the insured to select a PCP.

- *Advantages*—The insured may visit a doctor outside the network and still receive coverage, but at

TABLE 12.1 Types of care delivery systems

Care Delivery Systems	Advantages	Disadvantages
HMO	• Low copayments • Minimal paperwork • Coverage for some preventive-care and health-improvement programs	• Must choose a PCP • Only see network doctors • Need a referral to see a specialist
PPO	• Receive coverage for out-of-network physician visits • Offers more preventive-care and well being services	• Must choose a PCP
POS	• Nominal copayment for routine office visit • May see specialist without referral	• If physician is out-of-network, insured may be liable for the entire bill
FFS	• May choose own doctors and hospitals • May visit any specialist without referral	• A deductible must be met before the insurance company pays claims • Plans pay only for "reasonable and customary" medical expenses.

a substantially higher cost than if he or she stayed within the network. This plan offers more preventive-care and well-being services.

- *Disadvantages*—The insured must choose a PCP.

Preferred Provider Organizations (PPOs). PPOs give policyholders a financial incentive (reasonable copayments) to stay within the group's network of practitioners.

- *Advantages*—The standard copayment is $10 for a routine office visit during regular hours. The insured may go to any specialist without permission, as long as the doctor participates in the network.
- *Disadvantages*—A policyholder who sees an out-of-network doctor may have to pay the entire bill out-of-pocket and then submit it for reimbursement.

Fee-For-Service Plans (FFS), Also Called Traditional Indemnity Plans. FFS plans offer flexibility in exchange for higher out-of-pocket expenses, more paperwork, and higher premiums.

- *Advantages*—Policyholders may choose their own doctors and hospitals and may visit any specialist without getting permission from a PCP.
- *Disadvantages*—A deductible (from $500 to $1,500) is required before the insurance company starts paying claims, and then doctors are reimbursed about 80% of the bill while the insured pays the remaining 20%. Policyholders may have to pay up front for medical services and then submit the bill for reimbursement. Plans pay only for "reasonable and customary" medical expenses.

X. INSURANCE TERMINOLOGY

Children's Health Insurance Program (CHIP). The CHIP program was enacted as a partial response to census data showing that about 10 million children under age 18, or 13.8% of children, were uninsured in 1995. The two major sources of coverage for children are employer-sponsored coverage through a parent and Medicaid. In 1995, private coverage, almost all of which is employer-sponsored, reached 66.1% of children and Medicaid covered 23.2%. Medicaid plays a particularly large role for low-income children, covering almost half of all children with family incomes below 200% of the federal poverty level (FPL). (The FPL was $13,330 for a family of three in 1997.)

Deductible. A deductible is amount of a loss that an insurance policyholder has to pay out-of-pocket before reimbursement begins in accordance with the coinsurance rate.

HEDIS (Health Plan Employer Data and Information Set). HEDIS is NCQA's tool used by health plans to collect data about the quality of care and service they provide. HEDIS consists of a set of performance measures that tell how well health plans perform in key areas: quality of care, access to care, and member satisfaction with the health plan and doctors. HEDIS requires health plans to collect data in a standardized way so that comparisons are fair and valid. Health plans can arrange to have their HEDIS results verified by an independent auditor.

Product Lines. Refers to the population that the health plan covers.

- *Commercial*—Health care coverage paid for by employers or individual consumers.
- *Medicare*—A federal program that pays for certain health care expenses for people aged 65 or older and the disabled. It was established in 1965 with passage of the Social Security Amendments and is now run by the Centers for Medicare and Medicaid Services (CMMS). Enrolled individuals must pay deductibles and copayments, but much of their medical costs are covered by the program. Medicare is less comprehensive than some other health care programs, but it is an important source of postretirement health care. Medicare is divided into three parts. Part A covers hospital bills, Part B covers doctor bills, and Part C provides the option to choose from a package of health care plans. Medicare is funded by a tax on the earnings of employees that is matched by the employer and by premiums paid by enrollees. Legislation passed in 2003 provides for a drug benefit program (beginning in 2006), higher premiums for enrollees earning more than $80,000, and subsidies over 10 years to encourage private insurers to compete with Medicare.

"Opting Out" of Medicare. Since January 1, 1998, physicians have been permitted to opt out of Medicare and enter into private contracts with Medicare beneficiaries that allow them to set their own fees. A physician who opts out of Medicare agrees not to see any Medicare patients (barring emergencies or urgent services), except for those with whom he has entered into private contracts, for a period of 2 years. In order to opt out the physician must file an opt-out affidavit with the Medicare Carrier (or Carriers if the physician works in more than one Carrier jurisdiction), as well as a private contracting template. These contracts must be kept on file in the physician's office, available to be sent to the Carrier or to the Health Care Financing Administration (HCFA), which oversees the Carriers, should they be requested. New affidavits and private contracts must be completed every 2 years.

Medicaid. Medicaid is a national health insurance program in the United States for persons of low income. Established in 1965 with the passage of the Social Security Amendments and now run by the CMMS, the federal role in Medicaid is limited to setting standards, issuing regulations and guidelines, and overseeing operation of the program by the states. Of the various services covered under Medicaid, about half of the funds are used to purchase inpatient hospital services and nursing home services. The remainder covers physician services, drugs, laboratory services, x-rays, and other services.

XI. WHAT YOU SHOULD KNOW WHEN SEEKING A JOB

Before Seeking a Job. There are many things to consider before even looking for a position.

- *Accountant and Lawyer*—Before you begin your search for a practice to join, it is essential to have a trusted accountant and lawyer available to review the particulars of an offer. The accountant can help you dissect and understand the financial situation of a practice. Meanwhile, the lawyer can help you with contract issues, legal rights, and bargaining power.
- *Contract Issues*—Someone has offered you a contract. You will need legal advice about whether to sign it, whether the terms are reasonable, and whether anything needs to be changed or added.
- *Legal Consultation*—Upon the completion of residencies, many residents underestimate their value to a practice. A lawyer can determine the strength of your legal rights and the extent of your bargaining power.
- *Bargaining Power*—A lawyer can help determine how best to make use of whatever legal strengths or bargaining power you might have.
- *Residents and Fellows*—Physicians who have completed their residency or fellowship training usually arrive on the job scene armed with enthusiasm, volumes of clinical information, and all of the benefits of a modern medical education. For the most part, they have had little or no instruction on or experience in what is likely to be one of the most important decisions of their first year in practice: selecting and negotiating an employment agreement for their first job in private practice. It is important to remember that this is a 2-step process: first, decide whether the group whose contract you are reviewing offers the city or geographic area, practice type, lifestyle, and so on, that you want to pursue; second, determine if the terms of the employment agreement are reasonable in light of your goals.
- *The Employment Decision*—Physicians seeking new employment should also talk to colleagues, friends, parents, and other advisors in evaluating whether a position is right for them, both personally and professionally. Time spent carefully selecting a job in private practice will help minimize the risk of an unpleasant employment relationship.

Initial Practice Evaluation.

- *Personalities*—After meeting as many of the current members of the practice as possible, are these the type of people with whom you want to work? Do you like and respect them? Do they seem enthusiastic, or at least content, with their professional lives?
- *Geography*—Do you want to live in this town, this part of the country?
- *Quality of Life*—Based on what you are told and what you observe about the members of the practice, is their work ethic consistent with yours? Will you be able to balance your professional life with your personal life in a way that satisfies you?
- *Money*—What are the group's prospects, and what are your prospects if you join the group? Do not hesitate to inquire about the group's financial situation and projections; it is hard to succeed in a failing practice. Remember that the typical physician spends all but a few years of his or her practice as a partner or shareholder; therefore, a practice that offers relatively less during the first few years with greater opportunities thereafter will be a much better deal in the long run.
- *Partnership Terms*—When, and on what terms, will you be offered a buy-in? Employers do not want to commit to make you an owner unless you have demonstrated that you are the type of person they want to have as a partner. Therefore, few practices will commit to specific buy-in terms up front. However, it is still worthwhile to find out what the current buy-in arrangement is at the time you begin your employment. Keep in mind that the terms could change.
- *Turnover*—What is the rate of departure, and why have doctors left this practice in the past? Have the departing physicians been shareholders or nonshareholders of the practice? Having a high turnover rate among nonshareholder employees is troubling. Having a high turnover rate among shareholders may be a sign of impending disaster. Ask some of the former employers why they left. If they state that they are not at liberty to discuss the issue for legal reasons, they have told you a lot. Ask the practice for its side of the story.
- *Reputation of the Practice*—What do former physician and nonphysician employees have to say about

the practice? What do competitors say? What does the medical board say?

The Employment Agreement: Factors to Consider. If your due diligence leads you to conclude that you would be interested in practicing with the group, the next step is the negotiation of an employment agreement. The following is a list of provisions that typically need to be addressed in a written agreement:

- *Term and Termination Provisions*—Most initial employment agreements are for 1- or 2-year terms; however, termination provisions may effectively render that term meaningless.
- *Termination without Cause*—If the agreement is terminable by either party without cause, a party can terminate the physician's employment for no reason at all. Some employees request and receive agreements that do not permit termination without cause during the first year of employment.
- *Termination for Cause*—Most employment agreements include a list of events or conditions that constitute cause for termination, such as loss of license or DEA number, loss of medical staff privileges, exclusion from participation in Medicare, and failure to comply with the applicable standard of care.
- *Noncompete and Nonsolicitation Provisions*—Noncompete provisions are under scrutiny and prohibited in many states.
- *Professional Liability Insurance*—In most cases, an employer pays for professional liability insurance coverage for services provided by its physician employee during the term of employment. The employee typically is responsible for obtaining coverage for liability arising out of acts and omissions occurring after the employment relationship is terminated. Given the prevalence of claims-made insurance coverage, however, the parties typically need to agree on who will provide coverage for claims made after the termination of employment based on services provided by the physician prior to termination. Typically, the employee will be responsible for maintaining continuous coverage or purchasing tail coverage for protection against these claims.
- *Perks*—What benefits (ranging from paid time off and carryover if the time is unused, to sick time and carryover, to CME time and allowances, to health insurance, to bonuses) will the physician employee receive? If bonuses are available, the employee should look at whether bonuses are discretionary or are based on a percentage of collections. If the bonus is based on a percentage of collections, it is critical to understand exactly how the bonus will be calculated.
- *Duties*—What will the employee's job requirements consist of? At what hospitals will the physician be required to get privileges? What will the physician's call coverage obligations be? Will the physician's duties be comparable to the duties of other physician employees?
- *Alternative Dispute Resolution*—In case of a conflict between the employer and the physician employee, will the physician be required to engage in some form of alternative dispute resolution, such as forced mediation and arbitration? As a general proposition, mediation is a formalized settlement process. While mediation may be helpful where the parties are committed to finding a resolution, forced mediation can be a waste of time if one party or both parties have no interest in compromise. Arbitration is a process similar to the judicial process, although it is usually somewhat cheaper and quicker. Arbitrator's decisions usually are, and should be, binding.
- *Other Employment Opportunities*—Will the physician be permitted to engage in other work activities while working for this employer? If so, who gets the money from these extracurricular activities?

Employment Contract Negotiations

Contract Negotiation Concepts. Keep the following items in mind when negotiating your contract.

- *Abandon win-lose negotiations*—They interfere with your getting the most out of any negotiation. Instead, make a legitimate attempt to care about the other person and to meet his or her needs as well.
- *Power in negotiation*—Don't be afraid to negotiate, and don't be afraid to walk away.
- *Be humble*—Don't look so smart that you put the other party on the defense. Act professional and human.
- *The opening offer*—When you are negotiating a new employment contract, one of the most critical moments of the negotiation is when you present your initial offer. You should follow these 6 steps:
    - *Know your walk-away point*—Before you start a negotiation, you should write down all of the benefits that you would like to get from the transaction. For example, write down the salary you want, the hours per week you expect to work, the benefits you expect to receive, your anticipated on-call duties, and any other item that is relevant to you. This is your wish list; you need not share it with anyone except your spouse and your lawyer. Your wish list will enable you to focus on what

is important to you during the course of your negotiations. Once you decide on your walk-away point, do not let the other party know what it is.

- *Avoid being the first to present an offer*—You should not make 2 offers without an intervening offer from the other party. Making 2 consecutive offers is often referred to as "bidding against yourself," which is a sign of overeagerness. If the other party's initial offer is absurd, don't counter with anything concrete.
- *Never take the first offer*—Even if the first offer is reasonable, don't take it, for 2 reasons. First, it makes you look overly eager, which gives the other side a greater sense of control. Second, it makes the other side feel as though they've lost that part of the negotiation (they'll probably want to beat you on the next issue).
- *Don't use your walk-away point as your first offer*—Instead, present the other side with an initial offer that is more advantageous to you. For example, let's assume you're looking for an office-based practice and your walk-away point is $120,000. If the practice were to make an initial offer of $100,000, you might want to counter with $150,000. Your counter offer is well above your walk-away point, leaving you plenty of room to negotiate.
- *Narrowing the gap*—By now, the negotiation has begun, you and the other side have made your initial offers, and they couldn't be further apart. How do you keep the negotiation moving forward? Sweeten the deal.
- *Sweeten the deal*—To bring the other party closer to your offer, throw in something you know they want.

- *Throw-away concessions*—At some point in the negotiations, you are going to have to concede something to the other side. This may mean giving up things you really want or, if you plan it right, giving up things you don't care about but the other side does.
- *Decelerate your concessions*—Don't start out with small concessions and then concede more and more. Instead, make your concessions progressively smaller. This is perhaps the most important negotiating tip because it sets the psychological mood for the negotiation. If you make small concessions first, followed by larger ones, the other party will begin to think that if they just hang in there, you'll keep going. But by decelerating your concessions, you establish a pattern that does not look optimistic for the other party.
- *Uncover hidden agendas*—A common reason that talks stall is something called position negotiation. Don't assume you know what the other person wants. In relationship negotiating, the point is not to "beat" the other side but to get to a mutually agreeable postdeal working relationship.
- *Fait accompli*—Faced with the choice between a done deal or more negotiations with the chance of losing the deal, most people will go for the done deal.
- *Always insist on a written contract*—Although oral contracts are generally enforceable, problems often arise with regard to proof. Always insist on a written contract.
- *Merger clause*—The merger clause merges all of the oral and written communications between the parties prior to the signing of the written contract and states that the contract replaces all prior agreements or discussions.

Avoiding Physician–Employment Contract Pitfalls. There are many potential problems that can be avoided with preparation.

- *Request a "letter of intent" before receiving the contract*—A letter from the hiring organization that outlines the basics of the offer (salary, job obligations, and termination provisions) can save you time and money in attorney's fees. It helps ensure that what was agreed upon verbally ends up in the final contract.
- *Don't hesitate to negotiate*—Fearing they will lose the offer if they don't sign the contract as is, many young physicians are reluctant to negotiate.
- *Beware of one-size-fits-all contracts*—A boilerplate contract might work well for one physician but not for another. Make sure the contract reflects the actual position and scope of work and that it doesn't contain unreasonable provisions.
- *Make sure the guaranteed compensation is adequate*—Production- or collections-based compensation formulas might be detrimental for physicians new to practice because it takes time to build a patient base and start collecting receivables.
- *Consider the total compensation package*—Don't compare contracts based solely on salary. Factors such as benefits, malpractice coverage, and the time frame for and conditions of a partnership can profoundly affect earnings over several years.
- *Never accept a verbal offer or move based solely on a letter of intent*—Do not make a physical move before seeing, and signing, an actual contract. The contract may be unacceptable or, worse, may not materialize at all.

The Realities of the First Year in Practice. It may be nearly impossible to fully prepare for this transition, but residents can help ease their adjustment into practice life by assuming incrementally more duties during residency, tapping the expertise of advisors in their midst, and becoming adept at obtaining clinical information electronically. Tips for easing the transition from residency to practice are as follows:

- Physicians who are moving to a new locale should obtain a grasp of the cultural profile of their prospective or actual patient base.
- Take classes on Medicare evaluation and management coding. Learn how to code down to the fifth digit.
- Start with a slower patient volume while learning the intricacies of billing and coding and insurer contracting. Take advantage of the myriad clinical decision-support tools.
- The extent to which payer contract issues will affect physicians starting out in practice depends on the practice setting. Take practice management courses and read the medical-business journals and local publications to get a sense of both the big picture and regional market forces. Medical professional organizations (the AMA and other specialty groups) also offer excellent resources for young physicians.
- Networking can be invaluable to the newly practicing physician. There are effective and ineffective ways to go about letting other physicians know you are in town. Physicians should make the effort to arrange social encounters in the local hospital's doctors' lounge to introduce themselves and get to know other local physicians.
- Don't underestimate or "underprepare" for the credentialing process. These days, health plans and insurers face so many regulatory and reporting issues that they must ensure all providers on their panels possess the appropriate credentials. Becoming properly credentialed can take several months. Physicians should ensure that they have all license and training documentation close at hand.
- Strive for work–personal life balance, even in the difficult first years, and seek support among peers and community physicians. Residents who think they'll be "home free" when they get into practice are often dismayed to discover the stresses of their medical career. They may face productivity pressures, interrelationship issues with new colleagues, or difficulties adjusting to a new cultural environment. It is important to ensure that you have time for yourself and your family. State and local medical societies can be a valuable resource and also a source of support for newly practicing physicians and their significant others.
- Ensure an adequate financial plan is in place. In tandem with the excitement of starting the first "real" practice position and receiving a good income comes another reality: the start of education loan repayment. Loan payments are likely to account for a large portion of the household budget. It is imperative to ensure your personal finances are in order and ideally that a formal financial plan is in place to help manage the early transition years.

XII. TYPES OF PRACTICE SETTINGS

The following are descriptions of the most common types of practice settings and their lifestyle characteristics, as well as some of the perceived positives and negatives associated with each. A summary is provided in Table 12.2.

Private Practice. Also called solo practice, this setting is self-descriptive. The physician practices alone, without partners or other affiliations, usually with minimal administrative or clinical staff. Today, only about 1 in 5 residents chooses solo practice. He or she handles all aspects of the practice, from patient care to paperwork, regulatory compliance, and financial management.

- *Advantages*—The practitioner is in complete control and makes all the decisions.
- *Disadvantages*—Making all the decisions is a lot of work. In addition, solo practice generally entails more financial risk than other types of practice. Overhead is usually higher than in group practices, and because their patient base is relatively small, solo practitioners may be more acutely affected by economic and market factors. Solo practice may entail long work weeks and little time off. Some solo practitioners join independent practice associations (IPAs) to access advantages of a large physician network, or they develop relationships with other local solo physicians to lighten on-call duty and arrange weekend and vacation coverage.

Group Practice. Group practices, single-specialty and multispecialty, make up the majority of physician practice settings. As the name implies, the environment is characterized by sharing of patient care duties and physical space.

- *Advantages*—Group practice is generally viewed as less volatile than solo practice and more likely to afford a controlled lifestyle. The practitioner usually has increased financial security and the ability to have more control over lifestyle. There are added benefits of access to colleagues and mentors for help with tough diagnoses.

TABLE 12.2 Summary of types of practice settings

Practice Settings	Advantages	Disadvantages
Private practice	• Complete control • Full decision maker	• Work load • Financial risk • Higher overhead
Group practice	• Less volatility • Afford a controlled lifestyle • Increased financial security • Access colleagues and mentors for help	• Autonomy usually decreases
Staff-model HMOs	• Least risky practice model financially • Most predictable lifestyle • Guaranteed income • Work fairly regular hours	• Physicians receive a salary and some type of incentive bonus
Integrated delivery systems	• Income guarantee • Academic appointment • Good benefits package	• Policies and politics that can spark controversies
Hospital-based practice	• Predictable income • Steady patient base • Built-in referral network	• Heavy committee work • Limited autonomy • Hospital's overall financial condition could affect the practice
Locum tenens	• Practice flexibility • Schedule flexibility • Geographic flexibility	• Minimal stability

- *Disadvantages*—Autonomy usually decreases as the size of the group gets larger. Compensation methods vary widely, but in general, compensation is higher in single-specialty practices than in multispecialty practices, and most group practices employ a compensation method that includes a salary and some type of productivity bonus or incentive.

Staff-Model HMOs. Similar in structure to a large group practice, this setting is based on the traditional employment model. Physicians serve as salaried employees of an HMO and provide care only to a defined group of the HMO's members or beneficiaries, often referred to as a panel of patients. In general, clinical care delivery is dictated by the HMO, and physicians follow clearly defined practice protocols.

- *Advantages*—This model is the least risky practice model financially and the most predictable from a lifestyle standpoint. Physicians earn a guaranteed income, work fairly regular hours, and are largely relieved of paperwork and regulatory burdens.
- *Disadvantages*—Compensation is fairly standard. Physicians receive a salary and some type of incentive bonus based on productivity, patient satisfaction, or both.

Other HMO Models. One variation on the staff-model HMO is the reduced-fee-for-service or group-model HMO, in which physicians serve as contractors rather than employees. Typically, the HMO contracts with a group of physicians on either a capitated (per-member-per-month payment) or defined fee-schedule basis. Physicians are salaried and may receive a bonus for providing cost-effective care.

- *Advantages*—Patient flow is guaranteed by the HMO. In network-model HMOs, the health plan contracts with 2 or more physician groups, which often also have a patient base separate from their HMO panel.

Integrated Delivery Systems. In an integrated delivery system (IDS), the hospital and its affiliated clinics serve as the hub for care delivery. IDSs are typically formed around either a teaching hospital or a community hospital system, and the physicians are usually IDS employees.

- *Advantage*—There is an income guarantee, an academic appointment, and a good benefits package. The direct access the IDS affords to management services and support personnel can be advantageous for physicians just out of residency.

- *Disadvantages*—For physicians seeking autonomy, IDS employment is full of policies and politics that can spark controversies.

Hospital-Based Practice. In these settings, physicians work in practices or departments that are managed and owned either outright or partly by the hospital. Physicians serve as employees and are compensated by the hospital.

- *Advantage*—This model affords a predictable income, a steady patient base, and the built-in referral network via the other hospital-based practices. The setting provides camaraderie and proximity to the action.
- *Disadvantages*—There is heavy committee work, limited autonomy, and the possibility that a decline in the hospital's overall financial condition could affect the practice.

Locum Tenens. For the physician who desires practice and schedule flexibility, or who wants to try out the market before making a decision, locum tenens may be ideal. Physicians are employed by an agency to work for a short period of time, from a few weeks to several months. Locum tenens physicians have the ability to choose not only the practice setting and where they practice geographically but also how much they practice. Compensation is competitive with permanent employment, and the agency typically picks up the costs for malpractice insurance and licensure.

XIII. PHYSICIAN COMPENSATION SCHEMES

Physician Compensation Models

Overview. Today, compensation models are moving back to a focus on productivity, efficiency, and the amount of dollars a physician brings in. Most compensation models are primarily based on either a salary or a net- or gross-revenue basis, with some type of bonus or incentive component. Most income packages offered to new physicians are determined primarily by regional market factors and compensation surveys conducted by organizations such as the Medical Group Management Association (MGMA), the American Medical Group Association (AMGA), and the AMA, among others. The way an incentive plan is structured is more important than the fact that it is available. Physicians who are offered incentive plans should request details about how the plan works in practice. Even if there is little room for negotiating a compensation model or amount, it is important, nonetheless, to gain a basic understanding of the different prevailing models. Physicians should understand not only how these models are structured but also how the compensation plan may affect practice dynamics, group-member relations, and long-term earning prospects. Young physicians should calculate their living expenses and monthly personal budgets based on the compensation amount that is guaranteed. It is not advisable to count on a year-end bonus, even if it looks likely, because unforeseen factors could affect whether the bonus actually materializes. The following are common compensation models physicians are most likely to encounter during their job search.

Straight Salary/Minimum-Income Guarantee or Salary Plus Bonus/Incentive. Most often seen in large HMOs, academic settings, and large corporate- or physician-owned practices, these closely related models are perhaps the most straightforward, because the income level is set and physicians know how much they will earn. When a bonus or incentive is added in, physicians should inquire about how, when, and under what conditions the sum is paid. The minimum-income guarantee, with or without bonus, is the most prevalent model today for new physicians starting out.

- *Advantages*—These salary models are essentially worry-free for young physicians, so they offer a sense of security.
- *Disadvantages*—Without the bonus component, which is usually based on the group's total earnings, they offer little long-term financial incentive if there is no ownership track, and may ultimately either discourage entrepreneurship or support minimum-effort work standards.

Equality/Equal Shares. This model, considered the easiest from an administrative standpoint, is based purely on economics: after expenses, the remaining revenues are allocated equally among the group's physicians.

- *Advantages*—This structure discourages overutilization and doesn't require complex mathematical formulas.
- *Disadvantages*—The model presumes all physicians are equally skilled, equally productive, and most importantly perhaps, equally motivated to work in the group's best financial interest. Therefore, high producers have little long-term incentive, and low producers may be allowed to ride on the financial coattails of the more productive physicians. Nonetheless, many single-specialty groups adopt this model on the premise that all services, even those for which reimbursements are lower, are

valuable and necessary to a group seeking to operate a full service practice.

Production- or Productivity-Based Compensation. This model, with its myriad variations, can be fairly complicated. Essentially, physicians are paid a percentage of either billings or collections, or they are paid according to the resource-based relative value scale (RBRVS) units assigned to procedures or patient-visit types. The overhead costs of the practice, both fixed and variable, are allocated among the physicians.

- *Advantages*—The model both encourages and rewards extra effort by individual physicians.
- *Disadvantages*—The model can create a competitive intragroup environment that some physicians might not find appealing. The productivity model and relative overhead allocation can also be difficult to manage administratively and politically. Physicians should also determine whether their earnings in a productivity-based scheme will be based on their billings or on collections. If earnings are collections based, it behooves the physician to determine what percentage of billings the group typically collects, as well as how quickly, or slowly, reimbursement is received. Patient mix also comes into the picture in productivity-based compensation, so it is advisable to inquire about relative percentages of commercially insured, Medicare/Medicaid insured, and uninsured patients seen in the practice, as well as how new patients are assigned.

Capitation or Productivity Plus Capitation. The concept of capitation (prepaid health care premiums allocated to contracted provider groups for all coverage or specialty-services coverage of a defined enrollee population) became prevalent in the late 1980s and early 1990s. Capitation is still present in certain HMO-intensive markets, such as California, Minnesota, and the Northeast. Translated into a compensation model, capitation involves distribution of health plan payments among physicians in a nearly equal manner or based on some type of formula.

- *Advantages*—Capitation rewards groups, and in turn, those groups' individual physicians, who deliver cost-efficient, effective care.
- *Disadvantages*—From an economic standpoint, capitation-based income is dependent on marketplace factors and a group's negotiating prowess, which means that overall income levels may wax or wane from one year to the next. In addition, because global capitation contracts may entail providing all services to a group of patients, a high percentage of catastrophic diagnoses may negatively affect the group's bottom line and therefore individual physicians' income levels.

XIV. BUSINESS ORGANIZATION TYPES

The Organization of Partnerships

General Partnership. Each partner is equal in stature and risk. While different partners may have invested different amounts, each has accepted equal risk. Rewards and profits are distributed equally among the partners.

Limited Partnership. Each partner has assumed a different element of control, investment, and risk. The same is true for reward. Every partnership draws up a contract that dictates elements of control and reward. Typically, a partner who assumes greater financial risk corresponding with greater investment demands greater control. Usually in this type of partnership, there is someone called the *managing partner.* This is the partner who has assumed managerial control.

Silent Partnerships. A silent partner may exist in either a general or limited partnership. Essentially, the silent partner is an investor who is putting up money but who wishes no control over operations.

Corporations

Why Incorporate? There are many reasons to incorporate your practice:

- Protect yourself from business liabilities.
- Establish perpetual existence and transfer of ownership.
- Gain tax advantages.
- Enhance the company's image.
- Improve the ability to manage.

Types of Corporations. There are two basic types of corporations: private and public.

- *Private corporations*—Corporations that are owned by an individual or group of individuals that do not offer ownership shares for purchase by the general public.
- *Public corporations*—Corporations that are owned by large numbers of investors. Ownership shares, known as stock, are offered for sale to the general public. These shares can be purchased through a licensed broker or trader at a stock exchange. There are two different types of stock offered for sale:
    - *Common stock*—Most shares are common stock. Common stockholders are entitled to a voting share in the company and a portion of the dividend (a percentage of profits) if the company pays dividends to stockholders.

- *Preferred stock*—Limited stock issues that have no voting share. These stockholders, however, are paid a dividend, if one is offered, before common stockholders. In some cases, a dividend is paid to preferred stockholders and not common stockholders. In the event a company must divest (break apart), preferred stockholders are paid off before common stock holders.

Corporate Structure

C Corporation. A C corporation is the traditional and most common type of corporation. Forming a C corporation allows the company to have an unlimited number of shareholders. This is beneficial to companies that require many investors, as well as to companies that envision offering stock publicly.

- *Advantages*—An inherent benefit of all corporations and limited liability corporations (LLCs) is that they shield their shareholders from personal liability arising from business debts and business lawsuits.
- *Disadvantages*—The primary disadvantage of the C corporation is that it is subject to double taxation. This means that the company's profits are initially taxed at the corporate level, and then taxed again at the individual level when distributions are made to the shareholders.

S Corporation. Since its creation, the S corporation has increasingly become the preferred form for many small businesses. The S corporation is similar in structure to a C corporation but must meet a few further requirements. The C corporation can then become an S corporation when an extra step is taken by filing with the IRS.

- *Advantages*—The primary benefit of an S corporation is that it allows the shareholders to receive profits free of taxation at the corporate level. The profits will only be taxed at the individual level, thereby avoiding the double tax that C corporation shareholders are subject to. A corporation is only eligible for the S corporation election if it meets the following list of ownership requirements:
  - The company must have no more than 75 shareholders.
  - All shareholders in the company must be individuals and not other corporations or LLCs.
  - No shareholders can be nonresident aliens.
  - There can be only one class of stock in the company.
  - The company making the election cannot be a bank or thrift institution, an insurance company, or a domestic international sales corporation.
  - Each shareholder must consent to the S corporation tax status.
  - No more than 25% the company's gross corporate income may be derived from passive income.

Limited Liability Company. Many businesses are forming as an LLC and are finding that an LLC offers the best of both worlds of corporate forms. An LLC allows for pass-through taxation, thereby avoiding the double tax of a C corporation, yet also affords its owners the personal liability protection of a corporation.

- *Advantages*—The popularity of the LLC is primarily based on the tax advantage. An LLC operates in most ways as a corporation, yet the distributions to its "members" (shareholders) are not subject to taxation at the corporate level. Instead, the distributions are passed through the corporate level and are taxed only at the individual level. Therefore, the LLC avoids "double taxation."

Personal Liability Protection. Corporations and LLCs are separate entities from their owners. Since the two are separate, the personal assets of the owners (such as their personal residences and personal bank accounts) are not reachable by business creditors.

XV. PRACTICE MANAGEMENT

Governance

Effective Monthly Meeting Management. There are several proven techniques for effectively managing monthly meetings.

- Schedule meetings far in advance, with varying days so that no one doctor is inconvenienced (or unable to attend) month after month due to office, surgery, or call schedules.
- Poll all physicians before a meeting to develop an agenda. The agenda should be sent to everyone by e-mail beforehand.
- An agreed-upon individual should serve as chair of the meeting, adhering to the agenda rigorously unless an emergency arises. Votes should be taken on every issue of importance. Have a written protocol detailing the number of people who must vote to approve different levels of expenditures.
- Do not review every element of financial statements at every meeting. Instead, identify key numbers and ratios and focus on them. Wherever possible, don't look just at year-to-date (YTD) numbers but also at rolling 6- and 12-month averages.
- Allocate time for discussion.

- A secretary *and* an administrator should take minutes and compare them before they are finalized and distributed.

Finances

An understanding of financial statements, accounting, and costing will allow you to understand the health of your practice and to ask the right questions to meet your end goals.

Generally Accepted Accounting Principles (GAAP). The common set of accounting principles, standards, and procedures, GAAP is a combination of authoritative standards (set by policy boards) and the accepted ways of doing accounting.

Accrual-Based Accounting. Revenues are recognized and recorded in the books when the service is rendered, not when the payments are received. Expenses are recorded when they are realized, not when they are actually paid out.

XVI. ACCOUNTING BASICS

Assets and Liabilities. Assets equal liabilities plus equity.

- *Assets*—Anything of value that the practice owns or controls, that has a measurable cost.
- *Tangible assets*—Assets that can be touched.
- *Intangible assets*—Assets that cannot be touched, such as cash, accounts receivable, and securities.
- *Liabilities*—Sources of funding from creditors who expect to be repaid.

Financial Statements. The elements of financial statements are described here.

- *Balance sheet*—Represents the financial position of a practice at a specific time. It does not provide a "true value" of the practice.
- *Current assets*—All assets used in the operation of the practice. Includes cash and its equivalents, accounts receivable, securities, inventories, and prepaid expenses.
- *Non-current assets*—Items not expected to be used in 1 year of the practice operations. Includes properties, equipment, investment, and goodwill.
- *Current liabilities*—Financial obligations due within 1 year. Includes accounts payable, accrued expenses, and settlements with third parties.
- *Non-current liabilities*—Obligations due outside of 1 year. Includes mortgages, long-term debts, capital leases, and bonds.
- *Equity*—Funds obtained from investors or retained profits and earnings.
- *Operating cash balance*—A measure of liquidity of the practice.
- *Income statement*—A statement of the practice operations and changes in net assets over 1 year. It reports the profitability of operations.

Revenues and Expenses. Net income equals revenue minus expenses.

- *Revenue*—Includes charges, surgeries, casts, E&M, depositions, charity care, contractual allowances, ancillary services, and wages from other entities.
- *Expenses*—Includes salaries, benefits, billing and institutional fees, rent, malpractice, research, depreciation, and so on.
- *Statement of cash flows*—Details the amount of cash flow that has changed over the accounting period. Reports inflows and outflows of cash in the practice. Cash flows are affected by operating, investing, and financing activities.
- *Detailed report of expenses*—Provides the specific information for the general categories in other statements, which is useful for planning budgets.

XVII. PRACTICE MANAGEMENT METRICS

Practice management metrics are used to follow and track aspects of the practice from physician productivity to billing to collections, accounts receivable, and denials.

Billing and Coding. Billing and coding is a methodology developed to describe procedures and services.

- *Current procedure terminology (CPT)*—Created and maintained by the AMA. These are 5-digit codes with 2-digit modifiers.
- *International classification of diseases (ICD)*—Used to report diagnoses, ICD is used by all third-party payors in the United States and can be 3-, 4-, or 5-digit codes.
- *Resource-based relative value scale (RBRVS)*—Each CPT code is assigned a relative value. The RBRVS for an ICD code is then multiplied by a geographic practice multiplier (GPCI) in order to generate a physician's payment.
- *Collections*—Monies collected for services rendered.
  - Gross collection percentage = (total payments)/(total unadjusted charges).

Useful to internally track the performance of one physician from year to year.

- Net collection percentage = (total payments)/(total adjusted charges).
  Demonstrates the amount of the collectable charge being collected.

- *Payor mix analysis*—Proportion of total charges from all payors during a specific period.
- *Accounts receivable*—Charges that have been dispensed but not received into the office.
- *Days in accounts receivables*—How long it takes for a payment to be received.
- *Aged trial balance*—Accounts receivable divided into aging categories, usually in 30-day increments.

XVIII. MARKETING AND PATIENT RELATIONS

Overview. Marketing is not advertising. It is the strategy behind advertising. Try to understand who your patients/customers are and how you would like your practice to be perceived. Patients make their first impression about a practice and physician in about 15 to 45 seconds. Develop a concise, uniform message that communicates the image you want to portray. Marketing may include the creation of a logo, a selection of colors, and so on. All items in the office and communications with patients should then support this message.

The "4 Ps of Marketing" are as follows:

1. Place
2. Price
3. Promotion
4. Product and Perception

The "5 As of Product and Perception" are as follows:

1. Available
2. Affable
3. Amenable
4. Adaptable
5. Accommodating

Advertising. Advertising can be found in print, over the Internet, through brochures, the media, and community outreach programs.

Branding. A unique set of associations within the mind of the patient, branding represents a reputation for quality and a promise of values, and it creates trust and relevance.

Appointment Scheduling and Evening Hours. Stay open late at least 1 evening per week.

Internet Access. Install computers for use by patients. While waiting, patients can compose letters, use the Internet to pay bills online, and so forth.

Apologizing. In business, the customer is always right. In medicine, this applies to the patient. At the end of the day, you and your office exist to treat patients. Try to accommodate their needs and requirements and take ownership of any mistake that your office may have made.

Patient Information Materials. Communications materials, including a Web site, brochure, appointment cards, and script pads should all portray the same brand image. Hire a graphic design consultant to create a "look" for the practice. The logo should match and promote the name, color scheme, and a common appearance to everything that patients or referring doctors see.

XIX. MEDICAL RECORDS

How Long Should Records Be Retained? Per the AMA, medical considerations are the primary basis for deciding how long to retain medical records. If a particular record no longer needs to be kept for medical reasons, the physician should check state laws to see if there is a requirement that records be kept for a minimum length of time. Medical records should be kept for at least as long as the length of the statute of limitations for medical malpractice claims. The statute of limitations may be 3 or more years, depending on the state law. State medical associations and insurance carriers are the best resources for this information. Physicians should measure time from the last professional contact with the patient. If a patient is a minor, the statute of limitations for medical malpractice claims may not apply until the patient reaches the age of majority.

XX. TECHNIQUES TO INCREASE PRACTICE REVENUES

- Increase surgical and clinical volume
- Increase collections
- Other clinical services
- Radiology
- Physical therapy
- Rehabilitation
- Pharmacy
- Orthotics/prosthetics

- Ambulatory surgical center
- Distributorship
- Addition of a physiatrist to screen patients in the office, which may free you to do more surgery

XXI. DEPOSITIONS

Overview. A deposition is a legal proceeding conducted in accordance with certain court rules for the purpose of preserving the testimony of a witness for use in court. Because a physician's deposition is taken by counsel for plaintiff, the deposition is usually held in the plaintiff attorney's office, although the physician's attorney's office or a court reporter's office can sometimes be used. Physicians should not to have their deposition taken in their own offices, primarily because physicians should not allow opposing counsel the opportunity to look around the physician's office. Those present at the deposition will be the physician, a lawyer representing the physician, the plaintiff's attorney who will question the physician, and a court reporter who will swear the physician in and record the testimony. Physicians are often paid for their time by the party that their testimony will support, but the report should be as factual as possible.

The following are the goals of the attorney asking questions in a deposition:

- Discover what the physician knows concerning the matters involved in the case.
- Look for evidence favorable to the plaintiff's case.
- Commit the physician to statements under oath.
- Look for ways to discredit or impeach the physician's testimony.
- Discover the physician's defenses in the lawsuit.

XXII. STARK LAWS

Stark I Amendment. The Stark I amendment is a federal law that prohibits physicians from referring a Medicare patient to an entity for the furnishing of laboratory services if the physician or an immediate family member of the physician has a direct or indirect financial interest in the entity providing such services.

Stark II Amendment. The Stark II amendment extends this prohibition by prohibiting physicians from referring Medicare and Medicaid patients for certain types of services known as "designated health services." A financial interest includes an ownership interest or a compensation arrangement (the latter includes both the giving and receiving of compensation).

References

1. "2001 First Year Physician Starting Salary Survey." National Association of Physician Recruiters. Available at: www.napr.org. 2001.
2. Baker L, Birnbaum H, Geppert J, et al. "The Relationship Between Technology Availability and Health Care Spending." Health Affairs Nov 2003.
3. Berren M. Round-Up, Maricopa Medical Society. "Contracts: What you need to know" and "Annotated model physician employment agreement," both published by the American Medical Association. Available at: www.ama-assn.org. May 2002.
4. Brealey RA, Myers SC, Allen F. *Principles of Corporate Finance*, 8th ed. Boston: Irwin/McGraw-Hill, 2005;15–120.
5. Heffler S, Smith S, Keehan S, et al. Health Spending Projections For 2002–2012, Feb 2003.
6. Kaiser Health Poll Report, March/April 2003. Available at: http://www.kaiseredu.org
7. Kapoor JR, Dlabay LR, Hughes RJ. *Personal Finance*, 7th ed. Boston: Irwin/McGraw-Hill, 2003;416–556.
8. Kieso DE, Weygandt JJ, Warfield TD. *Intermediate Accounting*, 11th ed. Danvers, MA: Wiley 2003;33–269.
9. Standard & Poor's.
10. Towers Perrin Employer Survey.

Key References

Groeneveld PW, Laufer SB, Garber AM. Technology diffusion, hospital variation, and racial disparities among elderly Medicare beneficiaries 1989–2000. *Med Care* 2005 Apr;43(4):320–329.

Researchers conducted a study of 2,348,952 elderly Medicare beneficiaries potentially eligible for 1 of 5 emerging technologies within 90 days after admission (1989–2000). Hospitals with more than 20% black inpatients were less likely to utilize technologies on both white and black patients than were hospitals with less than 9% black inpatients.

WEB RESOURCES

Ethics

www.advamed.org/publicdocs/coe.html

www.phrma.org/publications/policy/2004-01-19.391.pdf

www.aaos.org/wordhtml/papers/ethics/prin.htm

www.aaos.org

Practice Management

www.nejmjobs.org/resource_center/First_Year_Practice.asp

Medical Records

www.ama.org

Refresher Questions

1. Which of the following characteristics of disability insurance policies is FALSE?
   a) cost of living indexing: a stipulation in a policy that provides for increasing benefits on an annual basis to keep pace with inflation
   b) own occupation definition of disability: a stipulation in a policy that provides an individual with benefits if he or she is unable to practice medicine within his or her given medical or surgical specialty
   c) guaranteed insurability option: a stipulation in a policy that allows the insured to complete one health examination at the commencement of the policy; after this examination is completed, the insured may increase his or her disability benefits without any further health screening
   d) cash-out option: a stipulation that the disabled policyholder can at any time acquire the total cash value of the disability policy
2. Which characteristic of term life insurance is FALSE?
   a) *decreasing term:* offers level insurance premiums with a decreasing death benefit
   b) *annual renewable term:* provides for increasing premiums and a level death benefit
   c) *level term:* allows for premiums that are level for a stated period of time, usually 5, 10, 15, or 20 years; death benefits are also stable with such a policy
   d) *variable term:* starts at a low fixed value for 3 years, then allow for variable premium rates that are tied to interest rates
3. Which type of malpractice insurance policy is FALSE?
   a) *claims-made coverage:* protects practitioners from suits and incidents that take place during the time period that the insurance policy is effective
   b) *occurrence coverage:* provides protection for any claims/suits that are filed during the period that the policy is actually in force, regardless of when such a claim is actually filed
   c) *prior acts coverage:* protects the insured for incidents that occurred prior to the inception of the prior acts policy but which have not yet been filed against the insured
   d) *tail coverage:* provides protection for any incidents that occurred during a specified time period that the claims-made policy was in effect, even though the claim was filed after the insurer–policyholder relationship was terminated
   e) none of the above
4. Based on the rule of 72, how much will an investment initially valued at $100,000 be worth in 12 years if the yield on the investment is 6% annually? At this yield rate, how long will this investment require to triple in value?
   a) the investment will be worth $200,000 in 12 years and will require 19.2 years to triple in value
   b) the investment will be worth $300,000 in 12 years and will require 9 years to triple in value
   c) the investment will be worth $400,000 in 12 years and will require 12 years to triple in value
5. Which of the following is not one of the 5 Ps of marketing?
   a) place
   b) price
   c) promotion
   d) power
   e) product
6. Which of the following represents the financial position of a practice at a specific time?
   a) balance sheet
   b) income statement
   c) statement of cash flows
   d) operating cash balance
   e) net profits
7. Which of the following corporate structures allows owners and partners to avoid the double tax?
   a) P corporation
   b) S corporation
   c) C corporation
   d) LLC corporation
8. Which of the following is a recommended negotiation technique?
   a) always think of situations in a win-lose framework
   b) never negotiate; just take what they give you
   c) be overly confident, to the point of offending the other party
   d) let the other party make the opening offer
   e) accept verbal contracts

9. Which of the following is not a benefit of HMOs?
   a) Low copayments
   b) minimal paperwork
   c) coverage for some preventive-care and health-improvement programs
   d) all the above are benefits of an HMO

10. Which of the following federal programs pays for certain health care expenses the disabled?
    a) Medicaid
    b) CHIP
    c) Medicare
    d) HEDIS

11. According to the National Center for Vital and Health Statistics, what ratio of hospital admissions resulted in an injured patient?
    a) 1:25
    b) 1:50
    c) 1:75
    d) 1:100

12. The estimated annual health care cost is:
    a) 10 billion
    b) 8 billion
    c) 6 billion
    d) 4 billion

Chapter 13

Tips for the OITE, Written and Oral Boards, and Recertifying Examinations

SAMEER NAGDA, SAMIR MEHTA, KINGSLEY R. CHIN, and WARREN D. YU

I. TIPS FOR THE ORTHOPAEDIC-IN-TRAINING EXAMINATION (OITE)

While some orthopaedic training programs may view the orthopaedic-in-training examination (OITE) as a nuisance and others as a rite of passage, the examination is an annual event in the residency education and training process. The examination is administered to all orthopaedic residents PGY-2 and higher (PGY-1s can take the examination at the discretion of their program) on the same day across the country. The examination is scored on the basis of the test-takers' percentile rank within their own postgraduate year (for example, a PGY-3 is scored relative to other PGY-3s across the country). Because of the large variability in knowledge base during the more junior years, the bell curve of score distributions is quite broad. As residents mature in their educational process, the bell curve becomes narrower. Therefore, one or two questions correct or incorrect can result in large swings in an individual's percentile score. However, the OITE does provide residents with objective feedback that can be applied as they prepare for Part I of the American Board of Orthopaedic Surgery (ABOS) examination. There is some data and a significant amount of anecdotal experience that correlates performance on the OITE with passing of Part I of the ABOS.

Preparation Overview

Preparing for the OITE is a dynamic, fluid process. In reality, the goal is to gather and store as much orthopaedic information as possible during your residency so that you can pass Part I (and Part II) of the ABOS examination.

Residents cannot expect to cram all the necessary information they need to know for the OITE in four weeks prior to the examination. Focused preparation for the OITE should begin 12 to 16 weeks prior to the examination (Fig. 13.1). However, constant and consistent review and reading provide the best foundation upon which to take the OITE and the ABOS examinations.

In the weeks and months prior to the OITE, residents should not only focus on reading for their cases and conferences but also begin preparing for the examination via the multitude of resources available. The most basic is a comprehensive orthopaedic review text that summarizes all of the high-yield, testable, and salient points of various orthopaedic diseases and conditions. This review text should be annotated, highlighted, and show the wears of having been used over and over again. By having one review source in which to keep notes or add information, the resident will have a primary resource to turn to at a time when rapid review is needed. Along with reading a comprehensive review text, residents should also try to do as many questions as possible. Every year, the American Academy of Orthopaedic Surgeons (AAOS) offers a CD-ROM containing questions that cover 3 subspecialty areas within orthopaedic surgery. Each subspecialty test contains 100 questions with annotated explanations. The topics recycle every three years. In addition, reviewing previous OITEs is critical because many topics are often repeated or restructured. The AAOS allows residents to keep a copy of the examination. Furthermore, in the late winter or early spring months, the AAOS publishes the correct answers with at least 2 references for each question (the source material for the correct answer). Reviewing previous examinations, by obtaining copies from more senior residents, provides a feel for the style and level of difficulty for each question.

After the OITE is over, residents should continue to read for their services. Subspecialty review books, fracture textbooks, and review articles (such as those from the *Journal of the American Academy of Orthopaedic Surgeons*) are critical in establishing a foundation in orthopaedic surgery. As residents become more senior, reading can shift from general orthopaedic surgery to

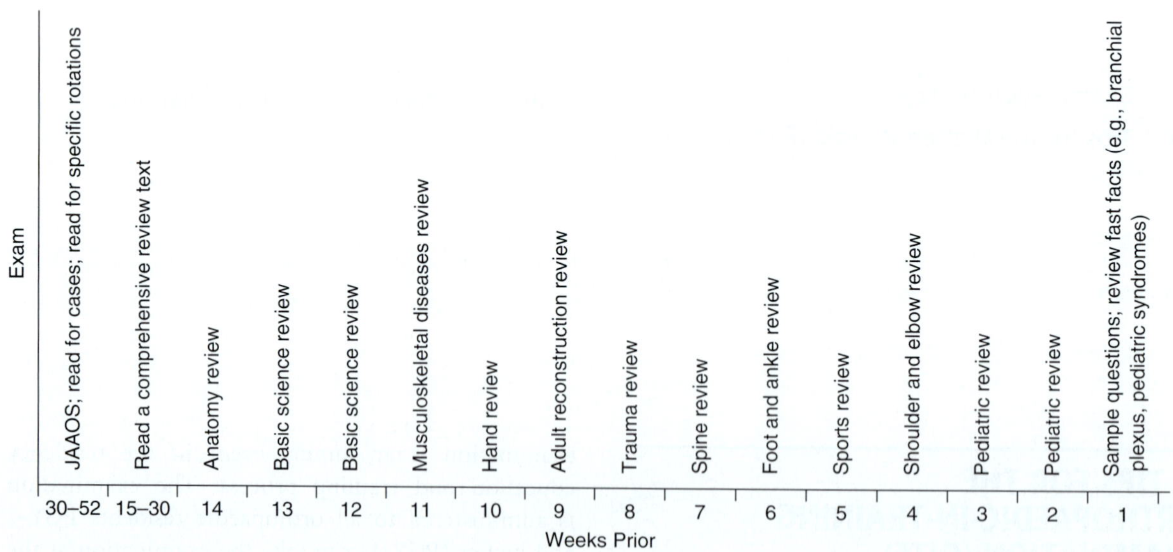

FIGURE 13.1 **Timeline for Board Preparation.**

more specialty-based reading in specialty textbooks or journals. Also, resources like the *Journal of Bone & Joint Surgery* serve as an excellent well of information to keep current with orthopaedic literature.

During the time after the OITE, residents should further familiarize themselves with the comprehensive review text they have been using. Notations and references from outside reading should be made directly in the review text to provide for the most comprehensive resource that addresses individual strengths and weaknesses immediately prior to an examination (like the OITE or ABOS).

PGY-1

If your department allows you to take the OITE during your internship, take advantage of this opportunity. Most orthopaedic departments do not make their interns take the examination because their training has barely reached the 5-month mark. However, by taking the examination during your internship, you can better focus your reading and preparation for the examination in the future.

Aside from learning how to manage patients in critical and noncritical situations, the goal of the intern year should be to establish a foundation in orthopaedic surgery upon which to build future years of learning. Reading should focus on a comprehensive text book or review book that can be completed in 1 year. Given the new work hour regulations, interns may also consider reading the *Journal of the American Academy of Orthopaedic Surgeons*, which provides review articles on select topics on a monthly basis.

PGY-2

Preparation for the OITE should have already started during internship through reading a comprehensive review book or textbook. In the months preceding the OITE, PGY-2s should obtain copies of the previous 3 years of examinations from more senior residents. Examinations beyond 3 years serve little value as the orthopaedic knowledge base expands. Furthermore, PGY-2s should purchase the AAOS Orthopaedic Special Interest Assessment Examinations for the past 3 years (which amounts to 900 questions). Finally, reading during the months prior to the examination should focus on topics that will provide a large return over the course of the residency (e.g., trauma).

PGY-3

Having had at least 1 year of the examination under your belt, you will have a better idea of what to expect on the day of the OITE. Studying should focus on reviewing previous years' examinations (including thoroughly reviewing your own examination from the previous year with particular attention paid to those questions that were incorrect) and also obtaining the Special Interest Examination for that given year. By the time of the examination, you should plan to complete a comprehensive review text from cover to cover. As you read for specific conferences, cases, or rotations, notations should be made in one resource so as to provide a rapid review prior to the examination.

PGY-4

Preparedness and performance on the OITE at this level are often indicative of maintaining diligent reading habits over the course of the PGY-3 and PGY-4 years. Reading should be expanding beyond review books and texts and should now include journals and other current resources. Practical information from these resources should be amassed in the comprehensive review text you have used over the past few years. Continuing to review this text will also benefit you by reinforcing important concepts as you gain current information. Reviewing previous OITEs and doing sample questions through the AAOS also provide a valuable learning experience. It is important to establish fellow residents you can study and prepare with because doing so will help during your PGY-5 and board-studying years. Furthermore, you should identify areas that you are not strong in and focus your preparation and note-taking in those areas.

PGY-5

The PGY-5 is the last check prior to the ABOS Part I Examination. Your performance on the OITE may serve as a platform from which you can create a specific Part I studying schedule. The culmination of your efforts over the previous years (in terms of diligence with reading, maintaining a review text, attending educational conferences, etc.) can correlate with your performance on the OITE. Using your previous OITEs along with all of the AAOS questions you have amassed provides one way of reviewing the existing material. The comprehensive review text that you have been annotating over the last 3 years is your most valuable resource. Since many senior residents are now focusing on the ABOS Part I, the bell curve for score distributions is extremely narrow at this level. Therefore, a few questions right or wrong could amount to a 15 or 20 percentile swing.

Morning of the Examination

Arrive promptly at your designated test site at the time indicated by your department proctor. You should have one or two #2 pencils. Make sure that you have had an adequate breakfast, but do not hesitate to bring snacks and drinks with you into the examination.

The Examination

The OITE is usually administered nationwide on the second Saturday in November. It is not a computerized examination. The exam consists of 275 multiple-choice questions, with no matching or K-type questions. Residents are typically given 6 hours to complete the examination. All residents receive the same examination, which is written and scored by the AAOS. The examination writers are board-certified orthopaedic surgeons who volunteer their time and effort through the AAOS. While the examination has an emphasis on orthopaedic basic science, traumatology, and pediatrics, it covers all of the subspecialties within orthopaedic surgery, including hand and spine. The material covered on the examination is not dated, but some questions may have controversial answers. The examination is reviewed and pretested by question writers, members of the AAOS, and specialists within a specific field of orthopaedics.

After the Examination

You are done for the day. Relax, enjoy, and spend the next few weeks unwinding from a busy fall season of studying. Your score will be sent to your department in December.

Summary

Ultimately, performance on the OITE is related to the amount of effort put into preparing for it and the amount of time spent utilizing existing resources, like this one, in an effort to comprehend the vast amount of knowledge that exists in our ever-changing specialty.

Good luck!

II. TIPS FOR THE WRITTEN BOARDS (PART I)

Organization of Part I

30% basic science and pathology
17% pediatric orthopaedics
20% orthopaedic trauma
33% orthopaedic specialties

The ABOS Part I Written Examination is the first of 2 examinations required to become board certified in orthopaedic surgery. The examination is administered in mid-July each year at the Hyatt Regency Hotel in downtown Chicago, Illinois. Theoretically, all candidates may pass because there is no curve, but in reality the passage rate is usually around 77% to 88% (Table 13.1). This examination represents the last written hurdle in your quest to become a board-certified orthopaedic surgeon. This chapter is meant to provide a timeline for preparing for this examination as well as some tips that will increase your chances of passing the examination on your first attempt.

Eligibility

Completion of an accredited orthopaedic surgery residency is required to be eligible to sit for the examination. Senior orthopaedic residents must apply to sit for the examination in January or February of the year they will graduate. Apply early for the examination because the late fee is hundreds of dollars. Information on eligibility requirements and fees can be found on the ABOS Web site: www.abos.org.

PGY 2 to 4 Preparation

Preparation for the Part 1 examination really should begin early in your orthopaedic residency. The OITE is meant to serve as a gauge of how well you are acquiring the knowledge base necessary for passing the Part 1

TABLE 13.1 Pass/fail rates for the Part I Written Boards

PART I	*2001*		*2002*		*2003*		*2004*		*2005*	
	Candidates	%	Candidates	%	Candidates	%	Candidates	%	Candidates	%
Passes	607	77%	637	79%	628	83%	645	88%	703	84%
Fails	182	23%	168	21%	132	17%	92	12%	113	16%
Total Candidates	789		805		760		737		703	

Source: Adapted from the ABOS report, February 2006.

examination. Preparing for this practice examination on a yearly basis will inevitably pay off as you prepare for the Part 1 examination. In addition to reading for your cases and specific rotations, reading through a review book such as this one or others is an important aspect of preparation. While these texts do not cover everything in detail, they do highlight the pertinent key facts that test-makers like to ask about. Picking one review text and reading through it every year from your PGY-2 year on will leave you far ahead of the pack when spring of your PGY-5 year comes along. In particular, highlighting and taking notes on what you have read in the margins of the review book will allow you to jog your memory faster each time you read the book. As you progress from your PGY-2 through your PGY-4 years, you will find yourself picking up points each year that you will have glanced over the year before. Also, some topics that you have not had a rotation in will seem like a foreign language early on but will make much more sense as you go through your different rotations.

In the month or two before the OITE, your residency may have special review sessions run by staff members who have gone through this process and who may have even written questions for the examination. These sessions may vary widely in how useful they are. However, if you use each weekly review session as a schedule for reviewing the different topics, you will cover all the topics before the exam.

If you have gotten this far in your training, you know that one of the most effective ways of test preparation is going through old questions. Your senior residents will have their old OITE tests from the last few years, which you should copy. Inevitably, there are repeat questions. Even more common are repeat concepts that are tested in a slightly different manner each year. Going through old tests will give you the most bang for your buck in achieving a good OITE score. However, this practice will leave you with some deficiencies in your knowledge base that will become apparent when you prepare for the board examination in your PGY-5 year. Therefore, it is essential that you continue to read every year.

In addition, the AAOS publishes a CD-ROM every year with 300 questions meant for OITE and board preparation. These questions are very helpful and are divided into 9 categories. Every 3 years, the AAOS publishes 100 questions on a topic. Each CD-ROM contains 100 questions on 3 different topics. You can purchase the current and past CD-ROMs from the AAOS Web site. You should try to go through at least 100 questions from each topic as well as 2 to 3 old OITE examinations in the month preceding the OITE. Doing so will get you into the mode of focusing on taking a test and answering questions for a few hours. In my experience, I started doing 50 questions on a topic every night about 4 weeks prior to the OITE. In the last 2 weeks before the test, I increased this to 100 questions per night. And in the last week, I would go over the old OITEs and try to do 200 to 300 questions per night. This helped me to build my test-taking stamina. If you are not ready to sit down and answer 300 questions in one day, you will find yourself making really dumb mistakes for the last half of the test.

The AAOS also publishes a series of review books called *Orthopaedic Knowledge Update* (OKU). There is the general OKU, numbered 1 to 8, with a new one published every 3 years. Also, there are subspecialty OKU books as well. I found these subspecialty books to be helpful for different rotations but found them to be not as helpful for OITE preparation. If you are preparing as previously discussed, you will likely not have time to also review the different OKU books or the larger OKU that averages 800 pages. A review of the larger, general OKU may also be difficult early in your residency because it assumes a level of knowledge that you may not yet have achieved. For this reason, I recommend leaving the OKU for your PGY-5 year. Other subspecialty review books are available, and some are very good. I recommend reading these along with your rotations.

Also, as you near the completion of your PGY-4 year, talk to the current chiefs about their studying and what they thought of the courses they may have gone to. Ask them if they would have done anything differently. And most importantly, ask them if they have any review course material that they do not want after they take their board examination. You may be able to use their old course material in preparing for your OITE.

Overall, reading and acquiring knowledge during your PGY-2-4 years not only will provide you with the foundation for your orthopaedic career but also will make your board preparation during your PGY-5 year much easier.

PGY-5 Preparation

July–November

If you have been a good resident and have diligently read for your cases and rotations, and prepared for your OITE during your PGY-2 through PGY-4 years, you will reap the benefits during your PGY-5 year. You should by now have covered all the tested topics in at least one rotation. You should also have your review book you bought in your PGY-2 year covered with highlights and notes from the last few years. If so, then going through your review book should not take long at all. This is the time to add the OKU to your library. Purchase it during the summer and start to read through it for the first few months of your year. At this point, you will have a good knowledge base on which you can add the information found in the OKU. You should also try to spend the first half of this year focusing on your weak topics. Go through your scores from prior OITEs and discern your weaknesses. As you prepare for your OITE, you will find that reading through your review book, going through the AAOS questions, and reviewing old OITEs will not take you very long. Take the extra time to perform an in-depth review of your weak areas. While preparing for my final OITE, I spent 75% of my study time on basic science, hand, and spine (my 3 weak areas). It paid off because I improved my score even though I barely covered some topics that I knew well.

December–January

This is your time to relax. Your only goal during this time is to sign up for your Part I examination and plan your next 6 months. This examination is not cheap, so sign up before the deadline to avoid even higher fees. Also, look through your OITE score from November to see how you did on your weak areas. Use your OITE score from your PGY-5 year to plan the next 6 months in terms of when and what to study. If you did very well on your OITE, the thought may cross your mind that you may not need to study much for the Part I examination. Erase that thought. No matter how well you did, you must study for this test to pass it. However, you can use your score to determine whether you may or may not need to attend a course. Also, look at your finances and your personal situation. Can you find the time and money to take a course? My wife and I were expecting our first child at the time of one of the courses, so I did not go. The curve for this examination will be much higher than for OITEs. Everyone is studying harder than they have for any OITE. Most senior residents attend a course and are therefore exposed to an intense curriculum that will jump-start their studying. If you do not attend a course, you should plan a week to study 8 to 10 hours a day as if you were at a course. Also, does your residency allow time at the end of June for graduating residents to study for the board examination? In my residency, I operated all the way until June 30 at 5 p.m. When in July is the examination? During my residency, the date of the examination varied by as much as 14 days. You may find that you will be relieved of your clinical duties by June 15 and have until July 18 to study. Conversely, you may have to work till June 30, and the examination may be July 7. This is very important to factor into planning your studying schedule.

February–April

February through April are the months to start planning your studying in detail. You should have all your relevant material and organize your notes. Sign up for any course you may want to attend.

And, if you have not done so already, read up on the topics that you consider your weakest. At this point, you may also want to review your stronger topics, those you are more interested in. Doing so will ease you into the studying mode. If you know your rotations at the end of the year will be more time consuming, you may want to study harder during these months. There are some residents in my program who read through current *JBJS* and *JAAOS* articles to prepare for the examination. Consider doing so during these months. However, you should remember that the test you will take was created at least 1 to 2 years ago, so reading the most current *JBJS* will not help you directly for the examination. It will, however, keep your knowledge current. If you did poorly on the OITE, you should be studying more during these months to improve on your weak areas. You may find your last 2 months of residency will be filled with social events, alumni dinners, graduation dinners and so on. Also, you will most likely be in the process of moving to a new location. All of these activities require time. Plan for them by taking care of as much as you can now. Or know that you will have to do it later and study more now.

May–June

May and June are the months to kick your studying into high gear. You should try to find a partner to study with. Create a schedule that you will stick to. Having a partner will keep you honest in this regard. Try your hardest not to pick you favorite drinking buddy for this endeavor. You should plan to study at least a few hours a day and for a significant portion of the weekends. This is not to say that you cannot go out and enjoy some of your chief year of residency. If you have planned this into your studying schedule, then by all means go enjoy your time off. Read through your review book one last time, and do as many questions as you can. Also, if you go to a review course, be sure to use the material they give you. They often have lists of key facts and different questions that you may not have seen before.

There are two main courses most residents attend: the Maine Review Course and the Colorado Review Course. They both last for 6 to 9 days and cost about $1,500 dollars to attend. Many residencies will pay for their residents to attend one or the other. Take advantage of this opportunity. If you do not attend a course, plan to study for a week as if you were at one. This means studying 8 to 10 hours per day to improve your concentration and stamina. Most residents I have spoken with were pleased with the course they attended. Strengths of the Colorado course include the lectures, handouts, and DVD version of the course that you can purchase if you attend the course. These materials are key because you will invariably lose your focus on some of the lectures and will need to revisit them in the few weeks before the examination. The Maine course provides you access to an extremely large test-question bank. However, both courses give attendees many practice questions. If you can afford a course and you can find the time, it will be to your benefit to attend one. The AAOS also holds a 1-day review course at the AAOS annual meeting in February or March. Residents who have attended that course did not feel that they could substitute that 1-day course for one of the other two later courses.

Early July

You should be studying 8 to 10 hours a day and going through 100 to 200 questions a day as part of this routine. At this time, you should be focusing on test-taking skills and stamina. Also, make lists of key testable items. For example, one list might include all the pediatric syndromes, the inheritance pattern, the genetic defect, and the chromosome. Start to make these lists to have for your trip to Chicago. Plan to look these lists over the night before the examination. Your studying partner and you should take 15 to 20 minutes a day when you are tired of reading and quiz each other from the different lists. The more lists you make, the less you will panic the night before the examination when you cannot recall the one key fact that you know will be on the test. Take some time to make sure everything is in order for your test. Make sure your examination ticket is correct, your flight and hotel arrangements are set, and you know what you want to take with you.

Making Arrangements to Travel

Book your flight preferably to arrive early the day before the examination. You should not book the last flight leaving your city or the last connecting flight to Chicago from an interim city. This advice is intuitive, but considering the magnitude of this examination you should be ultra-conservative. Book your room at the Hyatt Regency Chicago (on Wacker Drive) early to avoid having to travel from an outside hotel. Also, book your own room unless you know for sure that your friend who offers to split a room does not snore.

Arriving at the Hotel

Check into your room and make sure everything is functional. Also, make sure it is not too noisy. One of my classmates got a room next to the elevator. He could hear the elevator open and shut every 5 minutes. They switched his room immediately. Also, call and order room service for breakfast and lunch the next day. My morning room service also served as one of my wakeup calls. Also, I did not have to wait in any line for lunch. I just went to my room and waited 15 minutes for my lunch to arrive. For dinner, talk to your classmates and decide where you want to go after the examination. Make dinner reservations for the next night so you are not stuck calling around after the examination.

Morning of the Examination

The ABOS provides a continental breakfast the morning of the examination, but you may prefer a more hearty breakfast from room service. Go through your usual test day routine. Make sure to drink your coffee early because you do not want to waste test time going to the bathroom. Pencils are provided. Do not forget your test ticket. Make sure to update your address on it if you know your new address. You are allowed to take a candy or protein bar with you to the examination. A snack may save you in case your brain burns too much glucose thinking about the gene for achondroplasia. Remember, you have to focus for 210 minutes straight. Use earplugs if you need to, and leave your cell phone in your room. Also, digital watches are not permitted. Make sure you have a watch that will not be taken away, because there are no clocks in the room, and even if there is one, chances are you will not be able to see it. The hotel gift shop sells regular watches if you do not bring one.

The Examination

The examination is split into 2 sessions of about 160 questions each. You will have $3\frac{1}{2}$ hours to take each section. That amounts to 160 questions in 210 minutes, or about 75 seconds per question. That is a pretty swift pace to maintain for 7 hours, which is why you should have built your stamina by doing hundreds of questions a day. I paced myself to do 50 questions per hour, which left me with 10 questions and some time to go over a few other questions in the last 30 minutes. The ABOS states that a passing score usually equates to getting about 67% of the questions correct. Keep this in mind when you do your practice examination and when you take the test. If you hit a question that you have no idea how to answer, do not fret or panic; make your best guess and move on. In my experience, I found about 33% of the questions to be easy, 33% of the questions to be somewhat challenging and for which I was able to narrow the answer choices to two, and 33% to be very challenging and for which I was not really sure of the answer. Invariably, I got many of the ones I did not know correct. Go with your gut on questions. You may not know why something looks right, but chances are, it probably is and your mind is leading you to the right answer. You will find that one of the two sections is black and white, and the other has color slides. The color one will have the majority of the pathology in it. If you find that you have that section in the afternoon, you may want to prime your eyes by looking at some pathology pictures at lunch time. Or you may want to be normal and just eat your lunch during the lunch break.

After the Examination

You are done. Go relax and enjoy. Your score will take a few months to get. Start looking in the mail in late September.

Summary

Overall, this review is meant as a guide from one person's perspective on taking the ABOS Part I examination. Since you have made it this far, you clearly know how to prepare for and score well on an examination such as this. You will likely have your own methods for studying and preparing for your examination. Do what works best for you. If this chapter does nothing else for you, hopefully it will take some of the anxiety out of the test. Many other residents have graduated and have passed this examination. You too will pass. The keys to passing this test are to not blow off your annual OITE and to read throughout your residency. No one should be able to learn the salient aspects of orthopaedics in 1, 3, or even 6 months. If you have read throughout your residency, preparing for and passing this examination will be even easier than your previous USMLE exams. Remember, no one will remember how you did on the ABOS Part I; they will just remember whether you passed or failed. Hopefully, some of my comments will help you. Good luck!

III. TIPS FOR THE ORAL BOARDS (PART II)

The ABOS Part II oral examination is the final examination required to become board certified in orthopaedic surgery. The examination is administered in late July each year at the Palmer House Hilton Hotel in Chicago. Theoretically, all candidates may pass, since there is no curve, but in reality the passage rate ranges from 85% to 93% (Table 13.2). This chapter provides some tips to increase your awareness before taking the examination and possibly improve your chances of passing on your first attempt.

Eligibility

Completion of an accredited orthopaedic surgery residency and successful completion of the ABOS Part I written examination are required to be eligible. Eligible candidates must hold a full and unrestricted license to practice medicine in the United States or Canada, or be in full-time practice in the U.S. federal government. They must be continuously and actively engaged in the practice of orthopaedic surgery in the United States, its territories, Canada, or a U.S. service installation for 22 months immediately prior to the examination. Of the 22 months, 12 consecutive months must be in one location. Time spent in fellowships cannot be counted. The candidate must have started the job before September 1 of the year prior to collecting cases for the examination. This is important to know because you may be inclined to take a long vacation immediately after your fellowship. Make sure that it does not extend past September 1. The 6-month case collection period starts July 1 of the year prior to the

TABLE 13.2 Pass/fail rates for the Part II Oral Boards

PART II	*2001*		*2002*		*2003*		*2004*		*2005*	
	Candidates	%	Candidates	%	Candidates	%	Candidates	%	Candidates	%
Passes	621	86%	631	89%	563	92%	594	85%	645	93%
Fails	104	14%	76	11%	52	8%	104	15%	52	7%
Total Candidates	725		707		615		698		697	

Source: Adapted from the ABOS report, February 2006.

examination. All cases done during that period are eligible for testing. Registration is usually open online at abos.org by June before your collection period, and the deadline is October 31 with a late deadline of November 30. All relevant information is on this Web site.

Case Collection

Be proactive in choosing your cases carefully during this period to ensure that you have sound indications and are doing cases appropriate in difficulty to your level. Avoid the macho instinct to do cases that are difficult or cutting edge even if you are comfortable doing such cases. You should set the bar for determining suitable cases at a level that most surgeons would think is appropriate for your level and not on the basis of your confidence in your abilities. Doing so may be difficult if you are in an academic setting or the only surgeon trained to treat relatively rare and difficult cases in your practice area. In such unusual cases, focus on appropriate documentation of your diagnostic evaluation and indications, including outside consultation from your fellowship director or other colleagues. Ensure that all your patients exhaust appropriate nonoperative intervention for at least 4 months for nonemergent cases, and document these interventions. You should dictate your own notes in a standard format in anticipation that these notes may be read by an examiner. Your physical examination, interpretation of the radiologic studies, and treatment plan will be scrutinized by one examiner while you are talking to the other examiner. Do not cut corners in your diagnostic work-up and documentation. List pertinent negative findings on physical examination. You are graded on data collection, so include any supportive documentation, including the patient intake sheet. Especially ensure that you get all appropriate radiologic studies because the examiners will anticipate that you would have ordered a study during the diagnostic evaluation of the patient even if the diagnosis seemed apparent from the clinical examination or one radiologic study. Every patient should have a plain radiograph of the involved anatomy. Keep all radiologic studies until after your examination. Ensure that your secretary does not return films to patients. For patients who insist on having their films, you should insist in return that they get new copies made for themselves. Follow the postoperative course carefully of each patient at appropriate intervals to show that you are still involved in their care. Even if the patients are doing very well at their first postoperative follow-up, they should return at least once before the examination. If not, you may find that some of your chosen cases will have inadequate follow-up 2 months before the examination and you will be chasing after these patients. Document all complications, such as medical complications, whether they are yours or peripheral to your care. There seems to be a tendency for the ABOS to choose cases with complications. The important tip is that they are more interested in how you handle the complications than the complications themselves. However, you should try to minimize your surgical complications more diligently, especially if you are working with residents. It is highly recommended that you list your case online the same day that you completed the surgery and diligently keep your records; otherwise, it becomes a major undertaking to add information later in the year, and you risk losing critical information, if not entire cases, if your records are not accurate. If you fall behind, as is likely the case for most of us who take the examination, ensure that you have a case log on your personal computer or in a written form describing the details of the cases. Patient follow-ups can be found in the clinic records, but it is more tedious to review before the deadline, so be proactive during clinic. The deadline for your cases is January 31, 6 months before your examination.

Selecting Cases for the Examination

You are allowed to select 10 of 12 cases chosen by the ABOS for your examination. Use Table 13.1 to guide your selection. Avoid selecting "cool" cases that you think show off your superior technical skills. Rather, choose cases that are managed appropriately that can be defended by data published in the literature. Also, choose cases for which you have all the images and sound documentation, but err on choosing cases that had the best outcome and not unusual complications. If you were selecting appropriate operative cases with sound indications during your collection period, choosing your 10 should be an easy endeavor. Obviously, trauma cases do not fall into this category. The caveat on trauma cases is that during your collections period, you may have been able to avoid complex trauma cases by asking your partners to cover such cases. Your partners would have already been through this examination, and I would be surprised if they were not willing to cover these cases. However, you MUST take enough trauma calls to demonstrate that you are not above taking trauma, and I believe the trauma cases are the easiest to defend. This is more true if you are presenting to a nontrauma examiner—for instance, if you listed yourself as a spine specialist. You MUST prepare for all 12 cases and not select your 10 cases too early. I heard of one experience in which the examinee prepared for the wrong case and did not realize until the night before. Had he not had an 11th case, it would have been a disaster. The mistake was made on the sheet sent to him from the board, so check the case number and not just the case description when you receive the sheet listing the 12 cases. First, select 10 of the 12 cases that you think are the easiest to defend. Next, check to see if you have complete records on all 12 cases, including radiologic studies. If you are missing significant information, such as important radiologic studies, then you will be able to choose an alternate case from the remaining 2 cases with complete records. However, if you are missing only 1 radiologic study but you have all other preoperative and postoperative radiologic studies that can provide enough information on the case as well as convincing documentation that shows appropriate selection, technique, and outcome, then you may include that case, especially if it is an easy case to defend. In this case, you must have the radiology report of the study and an explanation for not having the study. I suggest that you contact all 12 patients for a final follow-up before the examination to obtain all missing information.

Organizing Cases for the Examination

You are required to have 3 copies of each patient record: 1 for you and 1 for each of the two examiners. Remember the KISS principle: keep it simple stupid. Use plenty of labels and color to make it easy to present each patient. Dedicate 1 folder per patient or 1 binder with 10 different major compartments, 1 for each patient, and multiple subcompartments. I found that 1 chart per patient was easy for me and the examiners to manage during the examination. The patient name and case number (1 to 12) should be clearly marked on the front of the chart. It is critically important that you add a summary sheet on the cover of the chart for you to use to present the case and also to allow the examiner to get the entire picture of the case, and then seek specific information from the inside of the chart. If you use a binder with all the patients, this is much harder to manage. The examiners choose each case according to their number on the list of 12 cases, since there are no names on this list. The radiologic studies should be separated by type and dates. Plain radiographs should be in a holder for radiographs; MRI should be in a holder for MRI; CT scans should be in a holder for CT scans. Go to your radiologic department and get extra folders of these types. Next, separate each study so that you present 1 or 2 films at a time. For instance, separate T1 sagittal MRI from T2 sagittal MRI and bone window CT scans from soft tissue windows, and label them accordingly. Use a red marker to highlight the pathology so that the examiners do not have to search for the pathology. Label the axial images, especially spinal levels; otherwise, you will be asked to show the levels. Only select studies that you feel are necessary to your case, but it is better to have more than less. Make sure that your records, including radiologic studies, can be carried on to the plane to avoid having to check them as luggage. That could be a disaster waiting to happen.

Studying for the Examination

Tables 13.3 and 13.4 list the areas that you will be tested on. Use this information to guide your preparation. However, it is helpful, but not mandatory, to take a board review course. You should at least run your cases by a colleague who can give you a mock examination to get you thinking about your answers and the types of questions the examiners may be interested in asking about each case. You should speak to colleagues about their experiences to get a sense of what to expect. You should know the differential diagnosis of the disease; the algorithm that led you to your diagnosis, including an understanding of the radiologic studies; the treatment options and why you would choose one over the other; and the techniques, including the tips and pitfalls, how would you manage the pitfalls, the salient anatomy, the postoperative management, and the expected outcomes. You should read the appropriate literature on all aspects of the case, and you MUST plan to cite selected studies to support your treatment plan. A good place to start is with this text and the OKU series published by the AAOS for your specialty.

TABLE 13.3 Case list rating definitions

Definitions	*Excellent Rating*
Surgical indications	Surgical procedures are performed for conditions with well-established indications; procedures listed treat clearly recognizable pathology
Surgical complications	Complications are infrequent and typical for the patient group treated
Ethics and professionalism	Candidate provides compassionate, beneficent, confidential care in the best interests of his or her patients and demonstrates professional attributes

Source: Adapted from the ABOS Examination Package Instructions, July 2006.

TABLE 13.4 Definitions for rating for skills

Skills	Excellent Rating
Data gathering and interpretive skills (history, physical examination, imaging, etc.)	Presents and appropriately interprets all data pertinent to the case
Diagnosis	Examiner considers the diagnosis presented correct
Treatment plan	Examiner considers the plan satisfactory for the condition
Technical skill	Examiner considers the candidate performed the procedures correctly
Outcomes	Patient outcomes as expected for the condition when treated by a competent physician
Applied knowledge	No apparent gaps in knowledge of disease or treatment protocols, superb citing of published medical information to support treatment plan

Source: Adapted from the ABOS examination package instructions, July 2006.

Making Arrangements to Travel

Book your flight to arrive at least the day before the examination. You should not book the last flight leaving your city or the last connecting flight to Chicago from an interim city. This advice is intuitive, but considering the magnitude of this examination, you should be ultra-conservative. For example, many flights were diverted from Chicago to Indianapolis the day before the examination because of severe thunderstorms. We all made it in, but not until late that evening. Experiences like this could heighten your anxiety level and give you less time for some last-minute preparation. Book your room at the Palmer House early to avoid having to travel from an outside hotel. Try not to check in any of your examination materials as luggage on your flight.

Arrival at the Hotel

Avoid mingling with your colleagues who have already taken the examination. Everyone seems to have different experiences, and you may be unlucky to talk to someone who will make you very anxious. I suggest in-room dining. It helps to go down to the examination room to sit in your booth to calm the nerves and to be aware of the surroundings the night before (Fig. 13.2). There is a well-equipped gym on the eighth floor.

Morning of the Examination

You are required to be there 45 minutes before the examination for a briefing and to register. There is no breakfast, so give yourself time to get breakfast before registering. Avoid too much conversation during this period, and stay focused but calm. You are given a list of your examiners and given the last opportunity to remove an examiner whom you might know.

The Examination

Keep a light mood, but stay focused and businesslike. Avoid being dogmatic or defensive on any issue. Try to lead the discussion by jumping in to continue your formal presentation at any sign of a break in the questioning. It is assumed that your case summary lists exactly what you would like the examiners to see and hear, so try to stick to it rather than allow the examiners to go off in directions that you may not be prepared to handle on the fly. Keep a deliberate pace. You have 35 minutes for each session with 2 examiners, so do not try to rush from case to case because you will appear disorganized and will be likely to be fumbling with multiple radiologic studies and charts on the

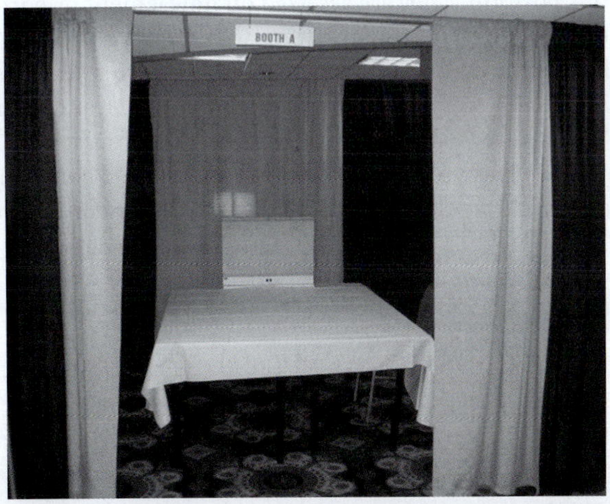

FIGURE 13.2 A testing booth at the ABOS Part II oral examination.

table. Begin each case by first placing the preoperative plain radiographs on the light box. Collect yourself and make sure that the table is cleared before narrating the history. Continue your presentation directly from the summary sheet until either you are finished or the examiners interrupt with a question. At the end, you can then discuss the films. I found that by the end of my presentation, the examiners just wanted to see the postoperative films. They have a clear picture of the case and what happened. Stay humble, and avoid any signals that you are being defensive or hiding something. If you do not have an answer, try admitting to not knowing, but if you are comfortable to guess, preface it with a statement such as "if I were to guess."

After the Examination

There is a debriefing session for the group of examinees. Nothing you do may matter here, but still try to maintain a calm persona and avoid being controversial and critical of the examination. Seek out a colleague to share a cab to the airport, but avoid discussing your examination if possible. If you have less than 1.5 hours to spare to get to the airport, you MUST take the blue line (subway) directly to the airport to avoid being stuck in traffic. The train station is 2 blocks from the hotel, and the train goes directly to the airport as the last stop. The fare is only $2. The bellman will accompany you to the station and onto the platform, carrying your bags for a nominal tip. I would have missed my flight back home had I not taken this advice from one of the examiners. You may have done as well as you could have hoped and still fail the examination because it is a subjective test, and since your cases are different from those of your colleagues, it is difficult to have true parity. Bear in mind that the examiners take an entire week out of their practice to volunteer for this position. They are assessed on how lenient or hard they grade; it is human nature that they are probably keeping a mental tab on their grading scheme. This means not everyone will pass (see Table 13.2), and your "stellar" record will not be known by the examiners. You are just a number. Therefore, you should consider approaching this examination with the assumption that the examiners are there to fail you—be prepared from the day of your collections the year before, and avoid being overconfident. This means that when you return to your practice, you should continue to treat all patients as if they could be your cases for next year's examination if you failed. The results will be mailed in early September. Candidates who do not pass Part II within 5 years (as measured in Section IV) of passing Part I must retake and repass Part I before applying to take Part II. Recertification is required after 10 years.

IV. THE RECERTIFICATION EXAMINATIONS

The Recertification Examinations are for practicing, board-certified orthopaedic surgeons in practice who periodically and voluntarily want to recertify. Surgeons must have received 120 credits of Category I–relevant CME during the 3-year period immediately prior to the date of filing an application for the examination. For surgeons with certificates expiring in or prior to 2009, this is done through CME, credentialing, and examination. Surgeons with certificates expiring in 2010 and thereafter will have some additional components as part of the new MOC process. Surgeons are given the choice to take a computerized practice profile or an oral-based examination. The written examinations are taken on an IBM-compatible computer at Prometric Technology Centers. The examination can be taken anytime during the months of March and April that the sites are operational and available. A successful candidate on the examination will receive a 10-year certificate (Table 13.5). If unsuccessful, the application is valid for 4 years.

Computer-Administered Clinical Examination

This method consists of approximately 200 multiple-choice questions over 4 hours. The questions cover general orthopaedics.

TABLE 13.5 Annual recertification pass/fail rates

Recertification	*2001*		*2002*		*2003*		*2004*		*2005*	
	Candidates	%	Candidates	%	Candidates	%	Candidates	%	Candidates	%
Passes	558	98%	666	98%	684	99%	728	98%	1041	97%
Fails	13	2%	17	98%	9	1%	12	2%	29	3%
Total Candidates	571		683		693		740		1070	

Source: Adapted from the ABOS report, February 2006.

Practice Profile Examinations

The Practice Profile Recertification examinations are offered in the subspecialty areas of adult reconstruction, sports medicine, and surgery of the spine. Each examination is broken down into approximately 50% general clinical questions and 50% clinical questions in the chosen subspecialty area.

Practice-Based Oral Examination

This test is based on the surgeon's practice and is similar to the Part II examination. The surgeon submits a list to the board of all operative cases for a 6-month period within the 2 years prior to the examination. The Board will choose 12 cases, and the surgeon gets to select 10 of the cases to present at the examination. The surgeon is responsible for bringing all pertinent materials for the chosen cases. The examination is approximately 2 hours, divided into three 35 minute periods with 2 examiners in each period. Specific skills that are evaluated are data gathering and interpretive skills, diagnosis, treatment, technical skill, outcomes, and applied knowledge. The oral examination is given at the Palmer House in Chicago around July 10.

Combined Hand Examination

This pathway is available only to candidates who currently hold a CAQ in surgery of the hand. It is a computer-based examination consisting of approximately 160 CAQ-hand surgery questions and 80 general orthopaedic surgery questions over a 6-hour period. The examination focuses on questions designed to evaluate cognitive knowledge of clinical surgery and basic science relevant to surgery of the hand.

The recertification examination application is usually available online on January 1 of the year before. The deadline is usually May 1, with an absolute deadline June 1. A $250 late fee is charged. More detailed information is available online at www.abos.org.

Answers

CHAPTER 1

1. A
2. B
3. C
4. C
5. C
6. A
7. B
8. A
9. A
10. C
11. D
12. A
13. C
14. B
15. C

CHAPTER 2

1. E
2. A
3. E
4. A
5. D
6. C
7. B
8. D
9. C
10. C

CHAPTER 3

1. D
2. D
3. A
4. B
5. D
6. C
7. E
8. D
9. C
10. B
11. D
12. E

CHAPTER 4

1. C
2. A
3. B
4. D
5. A
6. D
7. B
8. B
9. A
10. D

CHAPTER 5

1. D
2. B
3. C
4. D
5. A
6. C
7. E
8. E
9. E
10. B
11. C
12. E
13. D
14. B
15. C

CHAPTER 6

1. A
2. D
3. D
4. E
5. E
6. B
7. D
8. D
9. C
10. A

CHAPTER 7

1. D
2. D
3. C
4. C
5. D
6. C
7. C
8. B
9. C
10. D

CHAPTER 8

1. B
2. C
3. D
4. A
5. A
6. E
7. C
8. C
9. D
10. C

CHAPTER 9

1. B
2. D
3. D
4. C
5. C
6. B
7. A
8. A
9. B
10. D

CHAPTER 10

1. A
2. C
3. A
4. A
5. E
6. C
7. D
8. D
9. D
10. B

CHAPTER 11

1. C
2. A
3. B
4. B
5. D
6. B
7. B
8. B
9. C
10. C

CHAPTER 12

1. D
2. D
3. E
4. A
5. D
6. B
7. B
8. D
9. D
10. C
11. A
12. B

Index

Note: Page numbers followed by *f* indicate figures; those followed by *t* indicate tables.

G

H

J

K

L

T

U

V

W

Y